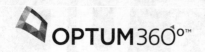 **OPTUM**360°™

RENEW TODAY

SAVE UP TO 25%

when you renew your coding essentials.

Buy 1–2 items, save 15%
Buy 3–5 items, save 20%
Buy 6+ items, save 25%

ITEM #	TITLE INDICATE THE ITEMS YOU WISH TO PURCHASE	QUANTITY	PRICE PER PRODUCT	TOTAL
			Subtotal	
	(AK, DE, HI, MT, NH & OR are exempt)		Sales Tax	
	1 item $10.95 • 2–4 items $12.95 • 5+ CALL		Shipping & Handling	
			TOTAL AMOUNT ENCLOSED	

Save up to 25% when you renew.

 Visit **optumcoding.com** and enter your promo code.

 Call **1-800-464-3649, option 1,** and mention the promo code.

 Fax this order form with purchase order to **801-982-4033.** *Optum360 no longer accepts credit cards by fax.*

Mail this order form with payment and/or purchase order to:
Optum360, PO Box 88050, Chicago, IL 60680-9920.
Optum360 no longer accepts credit cards by mail.

Name

Address

Customer Number   Contact Number

○ CHECK ENCLOSED (PAYABLE TO OPTUM360)

○ BILL ME ○ P.O.#

(   )
Telephone
(   )
Fax

E-mail

Optum360 respects your right to privacy. We will not sell or rent your email address or fax number to anyone outside Optum360 and its business partners. If you would like to remove your name from Optum360 promotions, please call 1-800-464-3649, option 1.

PROMO CODE
FOBA15A

Coders' Desk
Reference *for* HCPCS

2015

Publisher's Notice

Coders' Desk Reference for HCPCS was conceived to be an authoritative source of information about coding and reimbursement issues. Every effort has been made to verify accuracy, and information is believed reliable at the time of publication. Absolute accuracy cannot be guaranteed, however. This publication is made available with the understanding that the publisher is not engaged in rendering legal or other services requiring a professional license. Please address questions regarding this product to the Optum customer service department at 1.800.464.3649, option 1 or e-mail us at customerservice@optum.com.

Our Commitment to Accuracy

Optum is committed to producing accurate and reliable materials. To report corrections, please visit www.optumcoding.com/accuracy or email accuracy@optum.com. You can also reach customer service by calling 1.800.464.3649, option 1.

Copyright

Acknowledgments

Julie Orton Van, CPC, CPC-P, *Product Manager*
Karen Schmidt, BSN, *Technical Director*
Stacy Perry, *Manager, Desktop Publishing*
Lisa Singley, *Project Manager*
Elizabeth Leibold, RHIT, *Clinical/Technical Editor*
Regina Magnani, RHIT, *Clinical/Technical Editor*
Jacqueline Petersen, RHIT, CPC, *Clinical/Technical Editor*
Tracy Betzler, *Senior Desktop Publishing Specialist*
Hope M. Dunn, *Senior Desktop Publishing Specialist*
Katie Russell, *Desktop Publishing Specialist*
Kimberli Turner, *Editor*

Clinical/Technical Editors

Elizabeth Leibold, RHIT

Ms. Leibold has expertise in hospital outpatient coding and compliance. Her experience includes conducting coding audits and providing staff education to both tenured and new coding staff. She has a background in professional component coding, with CPT expertise in interventional procedures. Most recently Ms. Leibold was responsible for outpatient coding audits and compliance for a health information management services company. She is an active member of the American Health Information Management Association (AHIMA).

Regina Magnani, RHIT

Ms. Magnani has more than 30 years of experience in the health care industry in both health information management and patient financial services. Her areas of expertise include facility revenue cycle management, patient financial services, CPT/HCPCS and ICD-9-CM coding, the outpatient prospective payment system (OPPS), and chargemaster development and maintenance. She is an active member of the Healthcare Financial Management Association (HFMA), the American Health Information Management Association (AHIMA), and the American Association of Healthcare Administrative Management (AAHAM).

Jacqueline Petersen, RHIT, CPC

Ms. Petersen is a clinical/technical editor with Optum. She recently served as Senior Clinical Product Research Analyst with Optum developing business requirements for edits to support correct coding for claims processing applications. Her experience includes development of data-driven and system rules for professional and facility claims and in-depth analysis of claims data inclusive of ICD-9-CM, CPT, HCPCS, and modifiers. Ms. Petersen is a member of the American Academy of Professional Coders (AAPC) and the American Health Information Management Association (AHIMA).

Contents

Introduction to HCPCS

Coding is a complicated business. It is not enough to have current copies of the International Classification of Diseases, 9th Revision, Clinical Modification (ICD-9-CM), Physicians Current Procedural Terminology, Fourth Edition (CPT®), and Healthcare Common Procedure Coding System (HCPCS Level II) books. Medical coders also need dictionaries and specialty texts if they are to accurately translate physicians' operative reports or patient charts into reimbursement codes.

That's why Optum has developed the *Coders' Desk Reference* series—to provide a one-stop resource with answers to a wide variety of coding questions. We polled the medical reimbursement community and our technical staff to determine the issues causing bottlenecks in a coder's workload.

We found that experienced coders are frustrated by limited definitions accompanying many CPT, ICD-9-CM, and HCPCS Level II codes. Beginning coders need guidelines on the use of ICD-9-CM, ICD-10-CM, CPT, and HCPCS Level II codes and basic information about medical and reimbursement issues. Everyone requires up-to-date information about the anticipated changes to these coding systems.

Coders' Desk Reference for HCPCS answers the questions of both experienced and novice medical coders concerning medical supplies and equipment, as well as select services provided on an outpatient basis. It is a compendium of answers to a wide variety of coding questions and an introduction to new systems in coding structures. In order to code accurately, you must first have an understanding of the coding systems.

Coding Systems

Coding is the means by which providers and suppliers communicate their services with Medicare, Medicaid, third-party payers, and managed care organizations (MCOs). The correct use and reporting of modifiers and codes have become the defining elements in the reimbursement process for medical and surgical services, including services and items of durable medical equipment, prosthetics, orthotics, and supplies (DMEPOS). Assignment of the appropriate codes and adequate medical record documentation are necessary to avoid or minimize risk of fraud and abuse charges.

Diagnosis Coding

Diagnostic statements contained within medical records and other medical documentation are assigned codes from the ICD-9-CM and soon ICD-10-CM. The correct use and reporting of ICD-9-CM and ICD-10-CM codes is an important facet of the reimbursement process.

Diagnosis codes establish the necessity for which medical and surgical services, procedures, and DMEPOS items are furnished. Coding with ICD-9-CM, and effective October 1, 2015, ICD-10-CM, is mandatory for all Medicare claims, Medicaid claims, third-party payer claims, and most MCO claims. In rare instances, claims for services or procedures submitted to self-funded insurance pools and workers' compensation carriers do not require ICD-9-CM or ICD-10-CM codes, but do require a clearly descriptive diagnostic statement.

When reporting the appropriate diagnosis codes on claims for services, procedures, and DMEPOS items furnished to patients, ICD-9-CM or ICD-10-CM (as appropriate) diagnosis codes, CPT codes, and HCPCS Level II codes must be linked to identify the reason each service or procedure is rendered.

Providers and suppliers nationwide have discovered that many payers, including Medicare and Medicaid programs, will deny or delay claims because of incorrect or inappropriate ICD-9-CM or ICD-10-CM code assignments. Many providers and suppliers have experienced these costly denials and delays. Following are some of the problem areas identified by payers in the use of ICD-9-CM codes:

- Invalid ICD-9-CM codes used
- ICD-9-CM codes not reported to the highest level of specificity (e.g., four-digit and five-digit codes must be reported if appropriate)
- Additional digits, particularly zeroes, added to valid three-digit or four-digit ICD-9-CM codes to make them five-digit codes. This invalidates the ICD-9-CM codes
- No medical record or supplier documentation given to support the use of a particular ICD-9-CM code
- ICD-9-CM code reported does not match the sex of the patient
- ICD-9-CM code reported does not adequately support the service billed, or is not a diagnosis code recognized under medical necessity policy for the service reported

On October 1, 2015, the health care community will begin using the International Classification of

Diseases, 10th Revision, Clinical Modification (ICD-10-CM) coding system. Overall, the 10th revision goes into greater clinical detail than does ICD-9-CM and addresses information about previously classified diseases, as well as those diseases discovered since the last revision. Conditions are grouped with general epidemiological purposes and the evaluation of health care in mind. New features have been added and conditions have been reorganized, although the format and conventions of the classification remain unchanged for the most part. Please see the entry on *Code Sets* under the chapter "The Health Insurance Portability and Accountability Act (HIPAA) of 1996" for additional information.

CPT Codes (HCPCS Level I)

CPT is a standardized system of five-digit codes and descriptive terms developed, maintained, and copyrighted by the American Medical Association (AMA). Updated quarterly, CPT codes communicate to payers, and in some instances other providers and even patients, the procedures and services performed during a medical encounter.

CPT codes are the most widely accepted procedure codes for reporting medical services performed by physicians and facilities for many outpatient services. Considered HCPCS Level I codes, Medicare and Medicaid carriers are required to use CPT codes on health care claims, as designated in The Health Insurance Portability and Accountability Act of 1996 (HIPAA). An example of a CPT code follows:

30115. Excision, nasal polyp(s), extensive

Codes are grouped by body system, site, and/or type of procedure or service. They compose a nationally recognized system of codes that describe various services and procedures, including the following:

- Evaluation and management
- Anesthesia
- Surgery
- Radiology
- Laboratory and pathology
- Medicine
- Supplemental tracking or Category II codes
- Emerging technology services or Category III codes

HCPCS Level II Codes

HCPCS is an acronym (pronounced "hick-picks") for the Healthcare Common Procedure Coding System. This coding system presents national codes used to report supplies and equipment, as well as select services provided on an outpatient basis. HCPCS codes are published by CMS and updated quarterly. These codes can be obtained through the federal government and through publishers such as Optum,

which produce a complete annual and updateable edition of the HCPCS Level II codes.

HCPCS Level II codes may be used throughout the United States in all Medicare regions. They consist of one alpha character (A through V) followed by four digits. For example:

J7308   Aminolevulinic acid HCL for topical administration, 20%, single unit dosage form (354 mg)

L4350   Ankle control orthotic, stirrup style, rigid, includes any type interface, prefabricated, includes fitting and adjustment

HCPCS Level II codes describe:

- DME equipment, devices, accessories, supplies, and repairs; prosthetics; orthotics; medical and surgical supplies
- Medications
- Provider services
- Temporary Medicare codes (most commonly found in the G codes)
- Other disparate items and services, such as ambulance services
- Temporary national codes (non-Medicare) (S codes)

The majority of services and procedures performed are reported with CPT codes. However, because the CPT coding system does not describe specific drugs, durable medical equipment (DME), prosthetics, orthotics, supplies, and certain other services, the HCPCS Level II coding system must be used.

CPT and HCPCS Level II codes are designated code sets for use in electronic HIPAA complaint transactions. CPT codes are widely accepted by third-party payers with minimal problems. HIPAA covered entities are by law required to accept HCPCS Level II codes. However, providers may encounter problems with some HCPCS Level II codes. For example, Medicare does not accept HCPCS Level II codes that begin with an S and many third-party payers do not accept codes that begin with a G.

Payers who accept HCPCS Level II codes require the code that most accurately describes the item provided. For example, a Medicare patient is given a physician's order for a gastrostomy tube. Durable medical equipment Medicare administrative contractors (DME MAC) instructs providers to report HCPCS code B4087 Gastrostomy/jejunostomy tube, standard, any material, any type, each. If this patient had been a non-Medicare beneficiary covered by a plan that did not accept HCPCS Level II codes, the CPT code 99070 Supplies and materials (except spectacles), provided over and above those usually included with the office visit or other services rendered (list drugs, trays, supplies, or materials provided), would be reported with a description of the gastrostomy tube.

Keeping Current in Coding

The various coding systems change quarterly. To correctly report and be reimbursed for DMEPOS services and items, providers and suppliers must keep up-to-date with respect to these changes. Additionally, to maintain compliance in reporting services and items furnished to patients—especially Medicare and state Medicaid patients—providers and suppliers are required to report the most current codes and be knowledgeable about appropriate code reporting.

Some of the changes these coding systems undergo include:

- Code and modifier additions
- Code and modifier deletions
- Revisions of code and modifier descriptions
- Changes in grammar
- Parenthetical and instructional note changes
- Guideline changes
- Index entry changes

Providers and suppliers can choose from a variety of coding resources and educational seminars to keep up-to-date on quarterly changes. Providers and suppliers of DMEPOS should attend, at a minimum, an annual Medicare update for correct coding and billing procedures. This will help ensure compliance with federal standards.

HCPCS Level II Lay Descriptions

HCPCS Level II lay descriptions are written by Optum technical staff for people with medical training. They may not offer the details office personnel need to choose a code based on the contents of an operative report or patient's chart. Ordered numerically, each HCPCS Level II code is followed by a detailed description of the procedure that code represents.

Coders' Desk Reference for HCPCS was developed to help providers comply with the emerging standards by which DMEPOS supplies, medications, provider services, temporary Medicare codes, and other disparate items and services are coded, reported, and paid. Remember that *Coders' Desk Reference for HCPCS* is a medical reference and, as such, it is inappropriate to use this manual to select medical treatment.

The dental (D) codes are not included in the official 2015 HCPCS Level II code set. The American Dental Association (ADA) holds the copyright on those codes and instructed CMS to remove them. As a result, Optum has removed them from this product; however, Optum has additional resources available for customers requiring the dental codes. Please go to www.optumcoding.com or call 1.800.464.3649.

Using Modifiers

The HCPCS Level II codes are alphanumeric codes developed by CMS as a complementary coding system to the AMA's CPT codes. HCPCS Level II codes describe procedures, services, and supplies not found in the CPT® manual.

Similar to the CPT coding system, HCPCS Level II codes contain modifiers that serve to further define services and items without changing the basic meaning of the HCPCS Level II code with which they are reported.

It is important to note that HCPCS Level II modifiers may be used in conjunction with CPT codes, such as 69436 LT Tympanostomy (requiring insertion of ventilating tube), general anesthesia, left ear. Likewise, CPT modifiers can be used when reporting HCPCS Level II codes, such as L4396 50 Ankle contracture splint, bilateral (this scenario can also be reported with modifiers RT and LT, depending on the third-party payer's protocol). In some cases, a report may be required to accompany the claim to support the need for a particular modifier's use, especially in cases when the presence of a modifier causes suspension of the claim for manual review and pricing.

Ambulance Modifiers

For ambulance services modifiers, there are single alpha characters with distinct definitions that are paired together to form a two-character modifier. The first character indicates the origination of the patient (e.g., private residence, physician office, etc.) and the second character indicates the destination of the patient (e.g., hospital, skilled nursing facility, etc.). When reporting ambulance services, the name of the hospital or facility should be included on the claim. If reporting the scene of an accident or acute event (character S) as the origin of the patient, a written description of the actual location of the scene or event must be included with the claim.

Ambulance modifiers must be reported as two characters. For example, an ambulance transport from an accident scene to an acute care hospital would have modifier SH appended to the ambulance HCPCS code.

Ambulance Modifier Listing

D   Diagnostic or therapeutic site other than "P" or "H" when these are used as origin codes

E   Residential domiciliary, custodial facility (other than 1819 facility)

G   Hospital-based ESRD facility

H   Hospital

I   Site of transfer (for example, airport or helicopter pad) between modes of ambulance transport

J   Freestanding ESRD facility

N   Skilled nursing facility

P   Physician's office

R   Residence

S   Scene of accident or acute event

X   Intermediate stop at physician's office on way to hospital (destination code only). Note: Modifier X can only be used as a designation code in the second position of a modifier

HCPCS Level II Modifiers

Alphabetical Listing

A1   Dressing for one wound

A2   Dressing for two wounds

A3   Dressing for three wounds

A4   Dressing for four wounds

A5   Dressing for five wounds

A6   Dressing for six wounds

A7   Dressing for seven wounds

A8   Dressing for eight wounds

A9   Dressing for nine or more wounds

AA   Anesthesia performed personally by anesthesiologist

- CPT codes approved for use with modifier AA are 00100–01999.
- If an anesthetist assists the physician in the care of a single patient, the service is considered personally performed by the physician. The anesthesiologist should report this service with modifier AA and the appropriate CPT code from series 00100–01999.
- Modifier AA affects Medicare payment.

AD   Medical supervision by a physician; more than four concurrent anesthesia procedures

- Modifier AD affects Medicare payment as a distinct fee schedule amount exists.

AE   Registered dietitian

AF   Specialty physician

AG   Primary physician

AH   Clinical psychologist

AI   Principal physician of record

AJ   Clinical social worker

- Medicare limits allowable to 75 percent of the physician fee schedule.

AK Nonparticipating physician

AM Physician, team member service

- The physician member of a team is required to perform one out of every three visits made by a team member.
- Modifier AM should be used to indicate a team member visit was performed by the physician.
- Team member visits will be denied if only one person rendering services is billing for team services, as this is inappropriate billing practice.
- Modifier AM has no effect on payment.

AO Alternate payment method declined by provider of service

AP Determination of refractive state was not performed in the course of diagnostic ophthalmological examination

- Modifier AP has no effect on payment.

AQ Physician providing a service in an unlisted health professional shortage area (HPSA)

AR Physician scarcity area

AS PA, nurse practitioner, or clinical nurse specialist services for assistant-at-surgery

AT Acute treatment

- This modifier should be used when reporting services 98940, 98941, or 98942.
- Modifier AT has no effect on payment for Medicare and many third-party carrier claims.

AU Item furnished in conjunction with a urological, ostomy, or tracheostomy supply

AV Item furnished in conjunction with a prosthetic device, prosthetic, or orthotic

AW Item furnished in conjunction with a surgical dressing

AX Item furnished in conjunction with dialysis services

AY Item or service furnished to an ESRD patient that is not for the treatment of ESRD

AZ Physician providing a service in a dental health professional shortage area for the purpose of an electronic health record incentive payment

BA Item furnished in conjunction with parenteral enteral nutrition (PEN) services

BL Special acquisition of blood and blood products

BO Orally administered nutrition, not by feeding tube

BP The beneficiary has been informed of the purchase and rental options and has elected to purchase the item

BR The beneficiary has been informed of the purchase and rental options and has elected to rent the item

BU The beneficiary has been informed of the purchase and rental options and after 30 days has not informed the supplier of his/her decision

CA Procedure payable only in the inpatient setting when performed emergently on an outpatient who expires prior to admission

CB Service ordered by a renal dialysis facility (RDF) physician as part of the ESRD beneficiary's dialysis benefit, is not part of the composite rate, and is separately reimbursable

CC Procedure code change

- Modifier CC is used by the carrier when the procedure code submitted had to be changed for administrative reasons or because an incorrect code was filed.
- Payment rule: Payment determination will be based on the new code used by the contractor carrier/fiscal intermediary.
- Modifier CC has no effect on payment.

CD AMCC test has been ordered by an ESRD facility or MCP physician that is part of the composite rate and is not separately billable

CE AMCC test has been ordered by an ESRD facility or MCP physician that is separately reimbursable based on medical necessity

CF AMCC test has been ordered by an ESRD facility or MCP physician that is not part of the composite rate and is separately billable

- Effective for claims with dates of service on or after January 1, 2011, all ESRD-related laboratory services are included in the ESRD PPS base rate and must be reported by the ESRD facility and are not separately paid. The 50/50 rule no longer applies to independent laboratory claims for AMCC tests furnished to ESRD beneficiaries and modifiers CD, CE, and CF are no longer used. However, modifiers CD, CE, and CF are still required for use by ESRD facilities that are receiving the transitional blended payment amount (the transition ends in CY 2014).

CG Policy criteria applied

CH 0 percent impaired, limited or restricted

CI At least 1 percent but less than 20 percent impaired, limited or restricted

CJ At least 20 percent but less than 40 percent impaired, limited or restricted

CK At least 40 percent but less than 60 percent impaired, limited or restricted

CL At least 60 percent but less than 80 percent impaired, limited or restricted

CM At least 80 percent but less than 100 percent impaired, limited or restricted

CN   100 percent impaired, limited or restricted

- These modifiers are to be used with the functional limitation HCPCS codes reported by therapists.

CR   Catastrophe/disaster related

CS   Item or service related, in whole or in part, to an illness, injury, or condition that was caused by or exacerbated by the effects, direct or indirect, of the 2010 oil spill in the gulf of Mexico, including but not limited to subsequent clean up activities

DA   Oral health assessment by a licensed health professional other than a dentist

E1   Upper left, eyelid

E2   Lower left, eyelid

E3   Upper right, eyelid

E4   Lower right, eyelid

EA   Erythropoetic stimulating agent (ESA) administered to treat anemia due to anticancer chemotherapy

EB   Erythropoetic stimulating agent (ESA) administered to treat anemia due to anticancer radiotherapy

EC   Erythropoetic stimulating agent (ESA) administered to treat anemia not due to anticancer radiotherapy or anticancer chemotherapy

- Report modifiers EA, EB, and EC when ESA is administered to a patient who is not ESRD or who is not on maintenance dialysis. Report these modifiers with HCPCS Level II codes J0881 and J0885 only.

ED   Hematocrit level has exceeded 39% (or hemoglobin level has exceeded 13.0 g/dl) for three or more consecutive billing cycles immediately prior to and including the current cycle

EE   Hematocrit level has not exceeded 39% (or hemoglobin level has not exceeded 13.0 g/dl) for three or more consecutive billing cycles immediately prior to and including the current cycle

- Report modifier ED or EE on claims for EPO for ESRD patients receiving dialysis in renal dialysis facilities. Claims reporting no modifier or both modifiers will be returned to the provider for correction.

EJ   Subsequent claims for a defined course of therapy (e.g., EPO, sodium hyaluronate)

EM   Emergency reserve supply (for ESRD benefit only)

EP   Service provided as part of Medicaid Early Periodic Screening Diagnosis and Treatment (EPSDT) program

ET   Emergency services

- This modifier should be applied to report dental procedures performed in emergency situations.

EY   No physician or other licensed health care provider order for this item or service

F1   Left hand, second digit

F2   Left hand, third digit

F3   Left hand, fourth digit

F4   Left hand, fifth digit

F5   Right hand, thumb

F6   Right hand, second digit

F7   Right hand, third digit

F8   Right hand, fourth digit

F9   Right hand, fifth digit

FA   Left hand, thumb

FB   Item provided without cost to provider, supplier or practitioner, or full credit received for replaced device (examples, but not limited to, covered under warranty, replaced due to defect, free samples)

- Modifier FB is used to indicate a device used in a procedure was provided without cost.
- Report modifier FB with the procedure.

FC   Partial credit received for replaced device

- Report modifier FC when a credit greater than or equal to 50 percent and less than 100 percent has been given for a replaced device.
- Report modifier FC with the procedure.

FP   Service provided as part of family planning program

G1   Most recent URR reading of less than 60

G2   Most recent URR reading of 60 to 64.9

G3   Most recent URR reading of 65 to 69.9

G4   Most recent URR reading of 70 to 74.9

G5   Most recent URR reading of 75 or greater

G6   ESRD patient for whom less than six dialysis sessions have been provided in a month

- URR is the urea reduction ratio, a calculation that demonstrates the effectiveness of renal dialysis.
- ESRD facilities must use modifiers to reflect the most recent urea reduction ratio (URR), along with CPT code 90999 *Unlisted dialysis procedure inpatient or outpatient*, on all claims filed to Medicare for hemodialysis. Consequently, it will be necessary for ESRD facilities to also report a HCPCS code with the dialysis revenue code (0820, 0821, and 0829). ESRD facilities (both hospital-based and free-standing) should report CPT code 90999 and one of the G modifiers as appropriate, on all claims filed for hemodialysis services. This information will provide data to CMS regarding the adequacy

of hemodialysis for quality improvement initiatives. ESRD facilities must monitor hemodialysis adequacy monthly for all facility patients. Home hemodialysis patients may be monitored less frequently, but not less often than quarterly.

G7   Pregnancy resulted from rape or incest, or pregnancy certified by physician as life threatening

- This modifier is appended to the CPT procedure code for abortion services and indicates that the pregnancy resulted from rape or incest, or that the physician considers the pregnancy to be life threatening to the mother.

- Reporting this modifier on a claim communicates to the contractor that the physician certifies that the abortion meets Medicare's coverage policy. Medicare will cover an abortion when:

  - the pregnancy is the result of an act of rape or incest

  - the woman suffers from a physical disorder, physical injury, or physical illness, including a life-endangering physical condition caused by or arising from the pregnancy itself, that would, as certified by a physician, place the woman in danger of death unless an abortion is performed

- Claims submitted with modifier G7 for abortion services may be subject to postpayment review by the contractor.

- Third-party payers, other than Medicare, may not accept this modifier. Individual payers should be queried for claim submission requirements.

G8   Monitored anesthesia care (MAC) for deep complex, complicated or markedly invasive surgical procedure

G9   Monitored anesthesia care for patient who has a history of severe cardio-pulmonary condition

GA   Waiver of liability statement issued as required by payer policy, individual case

- This modifier indicates that the provider or supplier has a required signed advance beneficiary notice (ABN) retained in the patient's chart.

- The purpose of the waiver of liability is to ensure that the provider will be paid for the services performed, and to protect the beneficiary from receiving unnecessary services. Providers who acquire a waiver of liability for a covered service should use modifier GA directly following a procedure code to indicate that a beneficiary has signed a waiver of liability form. The provider should keep the form on file. No

other statement regarding the waiver of liability is required when modifier GA is used. Modifier GA at the end of a procedure code is sufficient evidence that the beneficiary has signed an advance notice. If the beneficiary subsequently requests a review of the denial, Medicare will request the provider or supplier to forward a copy of the notice for their files.

- An advanced notice may be applied to an extended course of treatment provided the notice identifies each service for which Medicare is likely to deny payment. A separate notice is required, however, if additional services for which Medicare is likely to deny payment are furnished later in the course of treatment.

- Medicare will deny payment for services reported with modifier GA. The beneficiary can appeal the denial.

GB   Claim being resubmitted for payment because it is no longer covered under a global payment demonstration

GC   This service has been performed in part by a resident under the direction of a teaching physician

- When a teaching physician's services are billed using this modifier, the teaching physician is certifying that he or she was present during the key portion of the service and was immediately available during the other portions of the service.

- When an anesthesiologist uses modifier QK for two to four medically directed procedures, he or she would not also append modifier GC to the anesthesia code. Only modifier QK is used.

- When there is a one-on-one situation with a resident and a teaching anesthesiologist (teaching setting), the anesthesiologist would append modifier GC only.

- Modifiers QK and GC are never used together.

- Modifier GC has no effect on payment.

GD   Units of service exceeds medically unlikely edit value and represents reasonable and necessary services

GE   This service has been performed by a resident without the presence of a teaching physician under the primary care exemption

- This modifier identifies services being billed under the primary care exception to the guideline for governing presence during the key portion of a service by the teaching physician.

- Modifier GE has no effect on payment.

GF   Nonphysician (e.g., nurse practitioner (NP), certified registered nurse anesthetist (CRNA), certified registered nurse (CRN), clinical nurse specialist (CNS), physician assistant (PA)) services in a critical access hospital

GG   Performance and payment of a screening mammogram and diagnostic mammogram on the same patient, same day

- Report modifier GG when the radiologist who interprets a screening mammography orders and interprets additional films based on the results of the screening mammogram while the beneficiary is still at the facility for the screening exam. When this occurs, Medicare will pay for both the screening and diagnostic mammograms.

GH   Diagnostic mammogram converted from screening mammogram on same day

- Report modifier GH when the radiologist's interpretation results in additional films and no additional payment is requested. When this modifier is reported, Medicare pays only for the diagnostic mammogram.

- The radiologist is considered the ordering physician in this situation and must furnish his or her national provider identifier (NPI) for Medicare claims. Diagnostic mammography claims submitted to Medicare without the ordering physician's NPI will be denied and returned as unprocessable.

GJ   Opt out physician or practitioner emergency or urgent service

- Use this modifier for claims submitted to Medicare for services rendered by an opt out provider who has not signed a private contract with the Medicare patient requiring emergent or urgent medical care.

- The provider may not charge the Medicare beneficiary more than what a nonparticipating provider would be permitted to charge, and must submit the claim to Medicare on the beneficiary's behalf.

- If modifier GJ is not reported on the claim for emergency or urgent care rendered to a Medicare beneficiary by the opt out provider, the claim will be denied and returned as unprocessable.

GK   Reasonable and necessary item/service associated with GA or GZ modifier

GL   Medically unnecessary upgrade provided instead of nonupgraded item. No charge. No advance beneficiary notice (ABN).

GM   Multiple patients on one ambulance trip

GN   Service delivered under an outpatient speech-language pathology plan of care

GO   Service delivered under an outpatient occupational therapy plan of care

GP   Service delivered under an outpatient physical therapy plan of care

GQ   Via asynchronous telecommunications system

GR   This service was performed in whole or in part by a resident in a department of veteran's affairs medical center or clinic, supervised in accordance with VA policy

GS   Dosage of erythropoietin stimulating agent has been reduced and maintained in response to hematocrit or hemoglobin level

GT   Via interactive audio and video telecommunication systems

GU   Waiver of liability statement issued as required by payer policy, routine notice

GV   Attending physician not employed or paid under arrangement by the patient's hospice provider

GW   Service not related to hospice patient's terminal condition

GX   Notice of liability issued, voluntary under payer policy

- Use this modifier when the provider has a signed voluntary advance beneficiary notice (ABN) in the patient's chart.

- This should be used if the provider wants a patient's statement of liability for services that are excluded by statute.

- Services with modifier GX will be denied.

GY   Item or service statutorily excluded, does not meet the definition of any Medicare benefit or for non-Medicare insurers, is not a contract benefit

GZ   Item or service expected to be denied as not reasonable and necessary

H9   Court-ordered

HA   Child/adolescent program

HB   Adult program, non-geriatric

HC   Adult program, geriatric

HD   Pregnant/parenting women's program

HE   Mental health program

HF   Substance abuse program

HG   Opioid addiction treatment program

HH   Integrated mental health substance abuse program

HI   Integrated mental health and mental retardation/developmental disabilities program

HJ   Employee assistance program

HK   Specialized mental health programs for high-risk populations

HL   Intern

HM   Less than bachelor degree level

HN   Bachelors degree level

HO   Masters degree level

HP   Doctoral level

HQ Group setting

HR Family/couple with client present

HS Family/couple without client present

HT Multi-disciplinary team

HU Funded by child welfare agency

HV Funded state addictions agency

HW Funded by state mental health agency

HX Funded by county/local agency

HY Funded by juvenile justice agency

HZ Funded by criminal justice agency

J1 Competitive acquisition program (CAP) no-pay submission for a prescription number

J2 Competitive acquisition program (CAP), restocking of emergency drugs after emergency administration

J3 Competitive acquisition program (CAP), drug not available through CAP as written, reimbursed under average sales price methodology

J4 DMEPOS item subject to DMEPOS competitive bidding program that is furnished by a hospital upon discharge

JA Administered intravenously

JB Administered subcutaneously

- Report modifier JA or JB to indicate the route of administration when erythropoiesis-stimulating agents (ESA), such as epoetin alfa and darbepoetin alfa, are reported. When both methods of administration are used, such as in a renal dialysis facility, report separate lines to identify the number of administrations provided using each method.

JC Skin substitute used as a graft

JD Skin substitute not used as a graft

JE Administered via dialysate

JW Drug amount discarded/not administered to any patient

K0 Lower extremity prosthesis functional level- 0; does not have the ability or potential to ambulate or transfer safely with or without assistance and a prosthesis does not enhance their quality of life or mobility

K1 Lower extremity prosthesis functional level-1: has the ability or potential to use a prosthesis for transfers or ambulation on level surfaces at fixed cadence. Typical of the limited and unlimited household ambulator

K2 Lower extremity prosthesis functional level-2: has the ability or potential for ambulation with the ability to traverse low level environmental barriers such as curbs, stairs or uneven surfaces. Typical of limited community ambulator

K3 Lower extremity prosthesis functional level-3: has the ability or potential for ambulation with

variable cadence. Typical of community ambulator who has the ability to traverse most environmental barriers and may have vocational, therapeutic or exercise activity that demands prosthetic utilization beyond simple locomotion

K4 Lower extremity prosthesis functional level-4: has the ability or potential for prosthetic ambulation that exceeds the basic ambulation skills, exhibiting high impact, stress or energy levels, typical of the prosthetic demands of the child, active adult, or athlete

KA Add-on option/accessory for wheelchair

KB Beneficiary requested upgrade for ABN, more than 4 modifiers identified on claim

KC Replacement of special power wheelchair interface

KD Drug or biological infused through DME

KE Bid under round one of the DMEPOS competitive bidding program for use with noncompetitive bid base equipment

KF Item designated by FDA as Class III device

KG DMEPOS item subject to DMEPOS competitive bidding program number 1

KH DMEPOS item, initial claim, purchase or first month rental

- DMEPOS is the acronym for durable medical equipment, prosthetics, orthotics, and supplies.
- Report with modifier RR for rented DME.

KI DMEPOS item, second or third month rental

- Report with modifier RR for rented DME.

KJ DMEPOS item, parenteral enteral nutrition (PEN) pump or capped rental, months four to 15

KK DMEPOS item subject to DMEPOS competitive bidding program number 2

KL DMEPOS item delivered via mail

KM Replacement of facial prosthesis including new impression/moulage

KN Replacement of facial prosthesis using previous master model

KO Single drug unit dose formulation

KP First drug of a multiple drug unit dose formulation

KQ Second or subsequent drug of a multiple drug unit formulation

KR Rental item–billing for partial month

KS Glucose monitor supply for diabetic beneficiary not treated with insulin using previous master model

KT Beneficiary resides in a competitive bidding area and travels outside that competitive bidding area and receives a competitive bid item

KU DMEPOS item subject to DMEPOS competitive bidding program number 3

KV DMEPOS item subject to DMEPOS competitive bidding program that is furnished as part of a professional service

KW DMEPOS item subject to DMEPOS competitive bidding program number 4

KX Requirements specified in the medical policy have been met

KY DMEPOS item subject to DMEPOS competitive bidding program number 5

KZ New coverage not implemented by managed care

L1 Provider attestation that the hospital laboratory test(s) is not packaged under the hospital OPPS

LC Left circumflex coronary artery;

LD Left anterior descending coronary artery

LL Lease/rental (use the LL modifier when DME equipment rental is to be applied against the purchase price)

LM Left main coronary artery

- Report modifiers LC, LD, LM, RC, and RI to indicate which coronary artery was involved in the percutaneous coronary intervention (PCI). PCI codes are in the range of 92920–92944. (*Medicare One-time Notification*, Pub. 100-20 [trans. 1136, November 1, 2012])

LR Laboratory round trip

LS FDA-monitored intraocular lens implant

LT Left side

- This modifier indicates the side of the body on which a procedure is performed. It does not indicate a bilateral procedure.

- Modifiers LT and RT have no effect on payment; however, failure to use when appropriate could result in delay or denial (or partial denial) of the claim.

M2 Medicare secondary payer (MSP)

MS Six-month maintenance and servicing fee for reasonable and necessary parts and labor, which are not covered under any manufacturer or supplier warranty

NB Nebulizer system, any type, FDA-cleared for use with specific drug

NR New when rented (use the NR modifier when DME which was new at the time of rental is subsequently purchased)

NU New equipment

P1 Anesthesia physical status—Normal, healthy patient

P2 Anesthesia physical status—Patient with mild, systemic disease

P3 Anesthesia physical status—Patient with severe, systemic disease

P4 Anesthesia physical status—Patient with severe, systemic disease that is a constant threat to life

P5 Anesthesia physical status—Moribund patient who is not expected to survive without the operation

P6 Anesthesia physical status—Declared brain-dead patient whose organs are being removed for donor purposes

PA Surgical or other invasive procedure on wrong body part

- Medicare will not pay for surgery performed on the wrong patient or wrong body part, or an incorrect procedure performed on a patient. All payments for these mistakenly performed procedures and any related services will be denied.

- For outpatient services, one of the three modifiers (PA, PB, or PC) should be appended to line items related to the surgical error.

PB Surgical or other invasive procedure on wrong patient

- Medicare will not pay for surgery performed on the wrong patient or wrong body part, or an incorrect procedure performed on a patient. All payments for these mistakenly performed procedures and any related services will be denied.

- For outpatient services, one of the three modifiers (PA, PB, or PC) should be appended to line items related to the surgical error.

PC Wrong surgery or other invasive procedure on patient

- Medicare will not pay for surgery performed on the wrong patient or wrong body part, or an incorrect procedure performed on a patient. All payments for these mistakenly performed procedures and any related services will be denied.

- For outpatient services, one of the three modifiers (PA, PB, or PC) should be appended to line items related to the surgical error.

PD Diagnostic or related non diagnostic item or service provided in a wholly owned or operated entity to a patient who is admitted as an inpatient within 3 days

- Modifier PD must be appended to physician preadmission diagnostic and admission-related non-diagnostic services, reported with HCPCS/CPT codes, that are subject to the three-day inpatient payment window policy. When modifier PD is present, Medicare pays only the professional component for CPT/HCPCS codes with a technical component (TC)/professional component (PC) split that are provided in the three-day (one-day in the case of non-IPPS hospitals) payment window, or the facility rate for codes without a TC/PC split.

PI   Positron Emission Tomography (PET) or PET/Computed Tomography (CT) to inform the initial treatment strategy of tumors that are biopsy proven or strongly suspected of being cancerous based on other diagnostic testing, once per cancer diagnosis

PL   Progressive additional lenses

PM   Post-mortem visits

PO   Services, procedures and/or surgeries provided at off-campus provider-based outpatient departments

PS   Positron Emission Tomography (PET) or PET/Computed Tomography (CT) to inform the subsequent treatment strategy of cancerous tumor when the beneficiary's treating physician determines that the PET study is needed to inform subsequent anti-tumor strategy

PT   Colorectal cancer screening test; converted to diagnostic test or other procedure

•   Append HCPCS Level II modifier PT to the diagnostic procedure code reported instead of the colorectal cancer screening. When reported with modifier PT, the deductible will be waived for all surgical services on the same date as the planned screening colonoscopy, planned flexible sigmoidoscopy, or barium enema.

Q0   Investigational clinical service provided in a clinical research study that is in an approved clinical research study

Q1   Routine clinical service provided in a clinical research study that is in an approved clinical research study

Q2   HCFA/ORD demonstration project procedure/service

Q3   Live kidney donor surgery and related services

•   Use modifier Q3 to identify postoperative live kidney donor services that are reimbursed at 100 percent of the Medicare fee schedule amount.

Q4   Service for ordering/referring physician qualifies as a service exemption

•   Use this modifier when the ordering or referring provider has a financial relationship with the entity performing the service, and for which the service qualifies as one of the service-related exemptions.

Q5   Service performed by a substitute physician under a reciprocal billing arrangement

•   Modifier Q5 is to be applied to the end of a procedure code to indicate that the service was provided by a substitute physician. The regular physician should keep a record on file of each service provided by the

substitute physician, associated with the substitute physician's UPIN, and make this record available to Medicare upon request.

•   This modifier has no effect on payment.

Q6   Service furnished by a locum tenens physician

•   Locum tenens physicians generally have no practice of their own; they usually move from area to area as needed. The patient's regular physician may submit a claim and receive Medicare Part B payment for a covered and medically necessary visit of a locum tenens physician who is not an employee of the regular physician and whose services for patients of the regular physician are not restricted to the regular physician's office. The locum tenens physician should not provide the visit services to Medicare patients for a continuous period of longer than 60 days.

•   This modifier has no effect on payment.

Q7, Q8, and Q9—Foot care

•   Documentation of the systemic conditions and class findings must be in the patient's record. The record must be maintained in the physician's office and available for medical review by the carrier. Documentation should indicate the course of treatment and length of treatment for infectious conditions. Documentation should include the affected toe, including the clinical evidence of mycosis, the manner in which and to what extent the nail was debrided, and the antifungal agent used in the office note/progress note.

•   A description of the qualifying symptoms should be documented

•   Ambulatory patients must exhibit a marked limitation in ambulation, pain, or secondary infection resulting from the thickening and dystrophy.

•   Non-ambulatory patients must suffer from pain or secondary infection resulting from the thickening and dystrophy of the infected nail plate.

•   Routine foot care is excluded from Medicare coverage.

•   General diagnosis such as ASHD, circulatory problems, vascular disease, and venous insufficiency are not sufficient to permit payment for routine foot care.

Q7   One Class A finding

•   Class A findings: Nontraumatic amputation of foot or integral skeletal portions thereof.

•   This modifier was established to allow the provider to report class findings without having to write a narrative description on the claim form or submit additional documentation with the claim. This modifier should be used in conjunction with foot care procedures (e.g., 11720, 11721) to indicate the severity of the patient's systemic condition and justify the medical necessity of a procedure that is usually denied as routine.

Q8   Two Class B findings

- Class B findings:
  - absent posterior tibial pulse
  - absent dorsalis pedis pulse
  - advance trophic changes such as (three required):
    - hair growth (decrease or absence)
    - nail changes (thickening)
    - pigmentary changes (discoloration)
    - skin texture (thin, shiny)
    - skin color (rubor or redness)
- This modifier was established to allow the provider to report class findings without having to write a narrative description on the claim form or submit additional documentation with the claim. This modifier should be used with foot care procedures (e.g., 11720, 11721) to indicate the severity of the patient's systemic condition and to justify the medical necessity of a procedure that is usually denied as routine.

Q9   One Class B and two Class C findings

- Class C findings:
  - claudication
  - temperature changes (e.g., cold feet)
  - edema
  - paresthesia
  - burning
- This modifier was established to allow the provider to report class findings without having to write a narrative description on the claim form or submit additional documentation with the claim. This modifier should be used in conjunction with foot care procedures (e.g., 11720, 11721) to indicate the severity of the patient's systemic condition and to justify the medical necessity of a procedure that is usually denied as routine.

QC   Single channel monitoring

QD   Recording and storage in solid state memory by a digital recorder

- This modifier has no effect on payment.

QE   Prescribed amount of oxygen is less than one liter per minute (LPM)

QF   Prescribed amount of oxygen exceeds four liters per minute (LPM) and portable oxygen is prescribed

QG   Prescribed amount of oxygen is greater than four liters per minute (LPM)

QH   Oxygen conserving device is being used with an oxygen delivery system

QJ   Services/items provided to a prisoner or patient in state or local custody, however the state or local government, as applicable, meets the requirements in 42 CFR 411.4 (B)

QL   Patient pronounced dead after ambulance called

QM   Ambulance service provided under arrangement by a provider of services

- Modifiers QM and QN should be used when a patient has an inpatient status at one hospital and is transferred to another hospital or facility for tests or treatment and then is returned to the first hospital.
- This modifier is valid for Medicare; however, the service would be denied under Medicare Part B since it is considered a Medicare Part A expense.

QN   Ambulance service furnished directly by a provider of services

- Modifiers QM and QN should be used when a patient has an inpatient status at one hospital and is transferred to another hospital or facility for tests or treatment, and then is returned to the first hospital.
- This modifier is valid for Medicare; however, the service would be denied under Medicare Part B since it is considered a Medicare Part A expense.

QP   Documentation is on file showing that the laboratory test(s) was ordered individually or ordered as a CPT-recognized panel other than automated profile codes 80002-80019, G0058, G0059, and G0060

- Sufficient documentation would be the requisition form showing that the physician had individually ordered tests either by code or the corresponding code definition.
- The individual tests that constitute an organ or disease related CPT panel do not need to be ordered individually in order for the laboratory to use modifier QP. The laboratory may bill using the CPT code for organ or disease oriented panel with modifier QP when the physician orders the components of the panel.
- CMS does not require laboratories to use this modifier, but some contractors (fiscal intermediary or carrier) strongly advise its use.

QS   Monitored anesthesia care services

- Monitored anesthesia care (MAC) services will be closely watched to ensure medical necessity is documented. ICD-9-CM codes should accurately describe the condition requiring MAC anesthesia. CMS collects data for MAC, even though it is paid the same as general anesthesia. The anesthesiologist or CRNA monitors the patient's vital signs, furnishes the preanesthesia exam, prescribes the necessary anesthesia care, administers medications, and furnishes required postoperative anesthesia care.

QT Recording and storage on tape by an analog tape recorder

- This modifier has no effect on payment.

QW CLIA waived test

QX CRNA service: with medical direction by a physician

- Payment rule: Limits payment to 55 percent of the amount that would have been allowed if personally performed by a physician or nonsupervised CRNA.

QY Medical direction of one certified registered nurse anesthetist (CRNA) by an anesthesiologist

QZ CRNA service: without medical direction by a physician

- Payment rule: No effect on payment. Payment would be equal to the amount that would have been allowed if personally performed by a physician.

RA Replacement of a DME, orthotic or prosthetic item

RB Replacement of a part of DME, orthotic or prosthetic item furnished as part of a repair

RC Right coronary artery

RD Drug provided to beneficiary, but not administered "incident-to"

RE Furnished in full compliance with FDA-mandated risk evaluation and mitigation strategy (REMS)

RI Ramus intermedius coronary artery

- Report modifiers LC, LD, LM, RC, and RI to indicate which coronary artery was involved in the percutaneous coronary intervention (PCI). PCI codes are in the range of 92920–92944. (*Medicare One-time Notification,* Pub. 100-20 [trans. 1136, November 1, 2012])

RR Rental (use the RR modifier when DME is to be rented)

- Use this modifier in conjunction with the appropriate "rental" modifiers KH, KI, and KJ.
- Modifier RR is placed directly after the HCPCS Level II code for the DME followed by the appropriate rental modifier as above.

RT Right side (used to identify procedures performed on the right side of the body)

- There are many procedure codes that require a physician to indicate the side of the

body on which a procedure was performed by using modifiers RT and LT.

- When billing for a separately identifiable/unrelated surgical procedure performed during the postoperative period of another surgical procedure, procedure code modifiers RT (right) and LT (left) must be indicated on the claim as appropriate. In addition, modifier 79 (unrelated procedure or service by the same physician during the postoperative period) must be submitted on the subsequent claim.

- This modifier indicates the side of the body on which a procedure is performed. It does not indicate a bilateral procedure.

- Modifiers LT and RT have no effect on payment; however, failure to use when appropriate could result in delay or denial (or partial denial) of the claim.

SA Nurse practitioner rendering service in collaboration with a physician

SB Nurse midwife

SC Medically necessary service or supply

SD Services provided by registered nurse with specialized, highly technical home infusion training

SE State and/or federally-funded programs/services.

SF Second opinion ordered by a professional review organization (PRO) per section 9401, p.l. 99-272 (100% reimbursement—no Medicare deductible or coinsurance)

- Use this modifier when the second opinion is ordered or requested by QIO.
- For Medicare beneficiaries, when this modifier is reported the service is eligible for 100 percent reimbursement. The usual deductible and/or coinsurance amounts are not applied.

SG Ambulatory surgery center (ASC) facility service

- This modifier is no longer required on Medicare claims. Physician and nonphysician practitioner fees must be billed on a separate claim form from the ASC facility fees.

SH Second concurrently administered infusion therapy

SJ Third or more concurrently administered infusion therapy

SK Member of high risk population (use only with codes for immunization)

SL State supplied vaccine

SM Second surgical opinion

SN Third surgical opinion

SQ Item ordered by home health

SS	Home infusion services provided in the infusion suite of the IV therapy provider

ST	Related to trauma or injury

SU	Procedure performed in physician's office (to denote use of facility and equipment)

SV	Pharmaceuticals delivered to patient's home but not utilized

SW	Services provided by a certified diabetic educator

SY	Persons who are in close contact with member of high-risk population (use only with codes for immunization)

SZ	Habilitative services

T1	Left foot, second digit

T2	Left foot, third digit

T3	Left foot, fourth digit

T4	Left foot, fifth digit

T5	Right foot, great toe

T6	Right foot, second digit

T7	Right foot, third digit

T8	Right foot, fourth digit

T9	Right foot, fifth digit

TA	Left foot, great toe

TC	Technical component. Under certain circumstances, a charge may be made for the technical component alone. Under these circumstances, the technical component charge is identified by adding modifier TC to the usual procedure number. Technical component charges are institutional charges and not billed separately by physicians. However, portable x-ray suppliers only bill for technical component and should utilize modifier TC. The charge data from portable x-ray suppliers will then be used to build customary and prevailing profiles.

- There are stand-alone procedure codes that describe technical component only codes (e.g., staff and equipment costs) of diagnostic tests. They also identify procedures that are covered only as diagnostic tests and, therefore, do not have a related professional component. Do not use modifier TC on these codes. Technical component services only are institutional and should not be billed separately by the physicians. However, portable x-ray suppliers only bill for the technical component and should use modifier TC.

TD	RN

TE	LPN/IVN

TF	Intermediate level of care

TG	Complex/high tech level of care

TH	Obstetrical treatment/services, prenatal or postpartum

TJ	Program group, child and/or adolescent

TK	Extra patient or passenger, non-ambulance

TL	Early intervention/individualized family service plan (IFSP)

TM	Individualized education program (IEP)

TN	Rural/outside providers' customary service area

TP	Medical transport, unloaded vehicle

TQ	Basic life support by volunteer ambulance provider

TR	School-based individualized education program (IEP) services provided outside the public school district responsible for the student

TS	Follow-up service

TT	Individualized service provided to more than one patient in same setting

TU	Special payment rate, overtime

TV	Special payment rates, holidays/weekends

TW	Back-up equipment

U1	Medicaid level of care 1, as defined by each state

U2	Medicaid level of care 2, as defined by each state

U3	Medicaid level of care 3, as defined by each state

U4	Medicaid level of care 4, as defined by each state

U5	Medicaid level of care 5, as defined by each state

U6	Medicaid level of care 6, as defined by each state

U7	Medicaid level of care 7, as defined by each state

U8	Medicaid level of care 8, as defined by each state

U9	Medicaid level of care 9, as defined by each state

UA	Medicaid level of care 10, as defined by each state

UB	Medicaid level of care 11, as defined by each state

UC	Medicaid level of care 12, as defined by each state

UD	Medicaid level of care 13, as defined by each state

UE	Used durable medical equipment

- Use this modifier when the used equipment is purchased by a beneficiary.

UF	Services provided in the morning

UG	Services provided in the afternoon

UH	Services provided in the evening

UJ	Services provided at night

UK	Services provided on behalf of the client to someone other than the client (collateral relationship)

UN	Two patients served

UP	Three patients served

UQ	Four patients served

UR	Five patients served

US	Six or more patients served

V5	Vascular catheter (alone or with any other vascular access)

V6   Arteriovenous graft (or other vascular access not including a vascular catheter)

V7   Arteriovenous fistula only (in use with 2 needles)

•   ESRD facilities are required to report V5, V6, or V7 for the type of vascular access used for the delivery of hemodialysis at the last hemodialysis session of the month. The modifier must be reported on the latest line-item date of service billing for revenue code 0821.

VP   Aphakic patient

XE   Separate encounter, a service that is distinct because it occurred during a separate encounter

XP   Separate practitioner, a service that is distinct because it was performed by a different practitioner

XS   Separate structure, a service that is distinct because it was performed on a separate organ/structure

XU   Unusual non-overlapping service, the use of a service that is distinct because it does not overlap usual components of the main service

Documentation Standards

Medical Records Documentation for Providers

Documentation in the medical record must contain information justifying hospitalization, an observation stay, an encounter or visit, or services provided for a patient. It must indicate that services are provided using current medical knowledge and treatment for the condition or injury, and that the services are medically necessary. In addition, the documentation must stand up to the scrutiny of others.

To meet the requirements of medical necessity for all health care services reported to the Medicare program, the patient's medical record must reflect the nature and extent of the diagnosis or injury, with clear documentation of the following patient-specific facts:

- Physical examination findings
- Diagnostic tests/analyses results
- Relation of diagnosis to the DMEPOS item
- Complicating comorbidities
- Physical functional abilities and/or limitations (ability to ambulate or transfer, amount of time needed to be spent in a bed, extent of use of a wheelchair, types/frequencies of activities recommended for outside the home, etc.)
- Duration of the diagnosis (acute, acute but refractory to treatment, chronic)
- Overall expected course/prognosis
- Rehabilitation potentials

In most instances, an evaluation and management (E/M) service is rendered before or during the same session that an order for DMEPOS is given. Requirements for the correct reporting of E/M services are beyond the scope of this publication; however, in addition to the criteria listed above for medical record documentation, an appropriate patient history must be obtained.

In general, the following three criteria (known as key elements of E/M documentation) should appear in the patient's medical record to correctly report an E/M service:

- Patient history
- Physical examination
- Level of medical decision-making

This is a requirement under both the American Medical Association's (AMA) and the Centers of Medicare and Medicaid Services' (CMS) guidelines.

Providers who dispense DMEPOS should take note that during audits of E/M services, a prevalent finding is the lack of review of systems information. This is an integral part of the patient's history. The absence or inadequate documentation of this part of the patient's history will cause an auditor to downgrade the original level of E/M, resulting in an overpayment situation in which the provider will have to refund the reimbursement difference to the payer or the patient.

Providers may receive requests from DMEPOS suppliers for copies of patient medical records that support the medical necessity of the provider's order. This is generally in response to a direct demand made upon the supplier from the Medicare contractor to substantiate the need for DMEPOS items. Providers should respond promptly to any requests made by the DMEPOS supplier for additional information. Suppliers do report certain difficulties in obtaining copies of medical records from provider offices.

General DME Documentation Standards

The following documentation is necessary for DMEPOS items regardless of the payer:

- The provider should sign and date an order for the DMEPOS item.
- If the treating provider is also supplying the item, the clinical notes should substantiate the need for the item.
- The diagnosis establishing the medical necessity for the item must be documented in the medical record.
- If the medical necessity for the item, as determined by the payer, cannot be established due to the nature of the patient's condition, injury, or illness, then the patient must sign a waiver before receiving the item. For Medicare patients, this waiver is called the advance beneficiary notice (ABN). This document must be kept on file in case the Medicare contractor, Medicaid agency, third-party payer, or managed care plan requests proof of the advance notice.
- It is recommended that the provider keep a copy of the Certificate of Medical Necessity (CMN) in the patient's medical record. An order or CMN on its own will not justify medical necessity even if the physician signs it.
- If a DME Information Form (DIF) is used instead or in conjunction with the CME, a copy of the DIF should be kept in the patient's medical record. In some cases, the DIF replaces the CMN for certain

DME supplies. The DIF must be signed by the supplier. The DIF contains much of the same information and does not require a narrative description of the equipment, cost, or a physician signature. *See the section below for more information on DIFs.*

- Provider records must substantiate the information and answers contained in the CMN.

Documentation for DMEPOS Suppliers

Suppliers are required to have the following information on file before submitting a claim to the durable medical equipment Medicare administrative contractor (DME MAC):

- Dispensing order
- Certificate of medical necessity (CMN) if applicable
- DME MAC information form (DIF) if applicable
- Patient's diagnosis from the provider
- Information for the use of specific modifiers required in certain DME program safeguard contractors' (PSC) policies
- Attestation statements required in certain DME PSC policies

Suppliers must keep documentation on file for seven years.

Suppliers are required to maintain proof of delivery in their files and it must be available to the DME PSC on request. If this information is not provided, claims will be denied and the supplier will have to refund the payment amount. Suppliers who consistently do not provide documentation to support services may be referred to the Office of Inspector General (OIG) for imposition of sanctions.

The three methods of delivery are:

- Delivering directly to the beneficiary or authorized representative
- Utilizing a delivery/shipping service to deliver items
- Delivery of items to a nursing facility on behalf of the beneficiary

Suppliers have the responsibility to ensure that coverage criteria are met before providing an item, or they risk having payment for the claim rejected. The supplier is liable for the dollar amount involved unless an appropriate ABN has been obtained. This is a CMS directive to all DMEPOS suppliers, one that is routinely scrutinized during supplier audits.

Provider Orders for DMEPOS

Provider orders for DMEPOS usually take the form of clinical record or progress note annotations, or they can take the form of separate, individual orders. These separate orders can be written on:

- Prescription forms
- Internally generated practice DMEPOS order forms
- Forms supplied by the third-party payer for DMEPOS authorization and reimbursement

In any case, a copy of the order may have to accompany the claim to the payer (if a paper claim) or must be retained on file (if an electronic claim).

For DMEPOS items billed to third-party payers, the provider must have documentation that adequately demonstrates the medical necessity of the item. This is true for any medical service. This information must be a permanent part of the patient's medical record, as should the original order for the DMEPOS item. An order or CMN on its own will not justify medical necessity even if the physician signs it.

In many instances, an entry made directly into the clinical record notes or progress notes can aptly serve as the provider order for the DMEPOS item, especially in situations where the DMEPOS supplier and the health care provider are one and the same. In these cases, the medical record entry must be complete and disclose all of the same information necessary for separate provider order documents.

Face-to-Face Encounter

42 CFR 410.38(g) currently states that "as a requirement for payment, CMS may determine through carrier instructions, or carriers may determine that an item of durable medical equipment requires a written physician order before delivery of the item." For covered items as defined in 42 CFR 410.38(g), a physician must document that the physician, physician assistant (PA), nurse practitioner (NP), or clinical nurse specialist (CNS) had a face-to-face encounter with the beneficiary within six months prior to completing the detailed written order. On claims selected for review if there is no face-to-face encounter, contractors shall deny the claim.

The contractor will ensure that the physician saw the beneficiary (including through the appropriate use of telehealth) and conducted a face-to-face assessment. Face-to-face documentation includes information supporting that the beneficiary was evaluated or treated for a condition that supports the item(s) of DME ordered. If this information is not included, the contractor shall deny the claim. If the physician completed the detailed written order before the face-to-face encounter, the contractor shall deny the claim.

If the DMEPOS item was ordered by a PA, NP, or CNS, the physician must sign or cosign and date the portion of the medical record that indicates that the face-to-face assessment occurred. If this information is not included, the contractor shall deny the claim. (*Medicare Program Integrity Manual*, Pub. 100-08, chap. 05, sec. 5.2.3.2-5.2.3.2.3)

Detailed Written Order

Any detailed written order must contain:

- Patient's name; insured's name
- Other patient identifying information (third-party payer ID number, patient's Social Security number, date of birth, patient's address and telephone number)
- DMEPOS item ordered with full description
- DMEPOS options or features that will be billed separately or that may require an upgraded HCPCS Level II code—if these codes are recognized by the payer—for the item
- Expected duration of use of the DMEPOS item; prognosis as it is known at the time of the DMEPOS order
- Patient's diagnosis, including ICD-9-CM code and narrative description
- State date of DMEPOS order
- Prescribing practitioner's NPI number
- Signature of the ordering practitioner (physician, PA, NP, or CNS)

Medicare requires that the detailed written order be completed after the face-to-face encounter. If the date of the detailed written order is prior to the date of the face-to-face encounter, the claim will be denied. (*Medicare Program Integrity Manual*, Pub. 100-08, chap. 05, sec. 5.2.3.2.3)

Orders for supplies to be used on a continuing or periodic basis must contain information about the quantities of the supplies needed, frequency of change (for dressings, pads, and so on), and expected duration of use.

If the DMEPOS item is a drug, the order must specify the name of the drug, concentration (if applicable), dosage, frequency of administration, and duration of infusion (if applicable).

Someone other than the physician may complete the detailed description of the item. However, the treating physician must review the detailed description and personally sign and date the order to indicate agreement.

The *Medicare Program Integrity Manual*, Pub. 100-08, chapter 5, section 5.2.2, advises that except as noted below, suppliers may dispense most items of DMEPOS based on a verbal order. This verbal dispensing order must include:

- A description of the item

- The patient's name
- The physician's name
- The start date of the order

Suppliers must maintain written documentation of the verbal order and this documentation must be available to Medicare upon request. For items that are dispensed based on a verbal order, the supplier must obtain a written order that meets the requirements of this section.

Verbal orders are unacceptable for certain DME billable to Medicare. A written order prior to delivery is required for:

- Pressure reducing pads
- Mattress overlays, mattresses, and beds
- Seat lift mechanisms
- TENS units
- Power operated vehicles and power wheelchairs
- Other items as denoted by contractor local or regional coverage decisions

For these items, the supplier must have received a written order that has been both signed and dated by the treating physician before dispensing the item.

If replacement supplies are needed for the use of purchased DMEPOS, the provider must specify on the prescription, or on the CMN, the type of supplies needed and the frequency with which they must be replaced, used, or consumed. "As needed" or "PRN" statements are not acceptable.

A new order is required when:

- There is a change in the order for the accessory, supply, drug, or item
- An item is replaced
- There is a change in the supplier
- The documentation section of a particular medical policy may require a new order on a regular basis (even if there is no change in the order)

For items that require a CMN, and for accessories, supplies, and drugs related to an item requiring a CMN, the CMN may serve as the written order IF the narrative description of the item is detailed enough. This applies to both hard copy and electronic orders and CMNs.

For DMEPOS products that are supplied as refills to the original order, suppliers must not automatically ship the refills, even if authorized by the patient. Suppliers must contact the patient prior to dispensing the refill. This will be done to ensure that the refilled item remains reasonable and necessary, existing supplies are approaching exhaustion, and to confirm any changes or modifications to the order. Contact with the patient or designee regarding refills must take place no sooner than 14 calendar days prior to the delivery or shipping date. The supplier must deliver the refill no sooner than 10 calendar days prior to the end of usage for the current product, regardless of which delivery method is utilized.

Separate Physician and Provider Orders

Suppliers of DMEPOS must conform to the demands of their participating contracts with the various third-party payers. DMEPOS items require an official order signed and dated by the ordering provider. The order must detail the patient's identifying information, including but not limited to a description of the DMEPOS item and the reason the patient requires the DMEPOS prescription. The provider's signature may or may not be a stamp facsimile or other substitute; some payers require an original signature. A faxed copy of the original order is usually sufficient for suppliers to fill the DMEPOS order and submit their claim for the item furnished.

However, in the case of illegible or faded faxed copies of DMEPOS orders, suppliers should insist on the original order being mailed or delivered by courier in prompt fashion. When the payer requires special forms (supplied by the payer) to be completed before the authorization, dispensation, and reimbursement of the DMEPOS item, these forms are generally viewed as a substitution for the provider order. The forms are usually supplied in duplicate or triplicate so the physician or provider has an immediate copy; the copy must become a permanent part of the patient's medical record.

Maintenance of Ordering and Certifying Documentation

The physician who writes the orders, as well as the provider or supplier that furnishes covered ordered items of durable medical equipment, prosthetics, orthotics and supplies (DMEPOS), clinical laboratory, imaging services, or covered ordered or certified home health services, is required to maintain documentation for seven years from the date of service. The parties must provide access to that documentation upon the request of CMS or a Medicare contractor.

The maintained documentation must include written and electronic documents related to written orders, certifications, and requests for payment; the National Provider Identifier (NPI) of the physician who ordered/certified the home health services; and the NPI of the physician or other eligible professional (when permitted) who ordered items of DMEPOS or clinical laboratory or imaging services.

Medicare billing privileges may be revoked if the provider, supplier, physician, or eligible professional (as applicable) fails to maintain this documentation or to furnish this documentation upon request.

Documentation cannot be requested for written orders and certifications dated prior to July 6, 2010.

A contractor may request documentation if it has reason to believe that the provider, supplier, physician, or eligible professional is not maintaining the documentation. A request may also be appropriate when:

- The contractor has detected an unusually high number of denied claims, or the Fraud Prevention System has generated an alert with respect to the provider

- The provider has been the subject of a recent Zone Program Integrity Contractor referral

- The provider maintains an elevated surety bond amount

The contractor will prepare and send a request letter to the provider via mail when it believes that a request for documentation is warranted. The provider has 30 calendar days from the date of the contractor's request to respond. If the provider fails to respond within the time limit, the contractor can revoke the provider's Medicare billing privileges and bar reenrollment for one year. (*Medicare Program Integrity Manual*, pub. 100-08, chap. 15, sec. 15.18)

Durable Medical Equipment, Prosthetics, Orthotics, and Supplies (DMEPOS)

The DMEPOS Industry

Wheelchairs, artificial limbs, braces, surgical dressings, and medications are all examples of durable medical equipment, prosthetics, orthotics, and supplies, known by the acronyms DME and POS, or simply DMEPOS.

The DMEPOS industry includes manufacturers, pharmaceutical companies, medical equipment and supply companies (suppliers and vendors), and providers. Entities peripheral to the DMEPOS industry, but having direct impact on its operations, include the Food and Drug Administration (FDA), which approves the use of medical devices and pharmaceuticals in the United States, and federal and state health care programs such as Medicare and Medicaid, which provide DMEPOS coverage and/or reimbursement for millions of beneficiaries. Other third-party payers, various preferred provider organizations (PPOs), workers' compensation carriers, and managed care organizations (MCOs) also influence the DMEPOS industry.

Health insurance benefits for DMEPOS, in general, are entangled in a mesh of rules and regulations governing coverage and reimbursement. The Centers for Medicare and Medicaid Services (CMS) is the federal agency that runs the Medicare program and oversees the Medicaid program. CMS has strict criteria that must be met by both suppliers and providers of DMEPOS, as well as numerous rules and regulations covering every aspect of the DMEPOS reimbursement process. These include coding, claims preparation, provider and supplier certifications, options for equipment rental and purchase, and a host of other billing directives. CMS's model of DMEPOS reimbursement, viewed as generally effective even if somewhat cumbersome, has inspired a number of third-party payers to pattern their own reimbursement protocol after it to some degree. While a state Medicaid program has some degree of flexibility, many will follow the Medicare program guidelines.

Special Federal and Third-Party Payer Definitions

For federally funded health care programs, such as Medicare and the Children's Health Insurance Program (CHIP), and for programs that are partially funded by the federal government, such as state Medicaid programs, there are strict definitions of what constitutes DMEPOS. A number of commercial insurance plans also follow this same framework, or a similar one, constructed around the prescription, dispensation, reporting, and reimbursement of DMEPOS.

Defining DME

According to CMS, DME must meet specific criteria to be eligible for coverage. These criteria are shown here in the form of questions. The provider or supplier must be able to answer yes to all of these questions for the equipment or device to be recognized as eligible for reimbursement under the Medicare program:

- **Can the medical equipment withstand repeated use?** Medicare Fact: Many items, though durable in nature, such as braces (orthoses) and prostheses, are not considered DME. These items fall into different categories of DMEPOS classifications. Medical supplies such as incontinent pads, catheters, bandages, stockings, irrigating kits, sheets, and bags are expendable in nature and do not qualify as DME.

- **Is the medical equipment primarily and customarily used for medical purposes?** Medicare Fact: Certain types of medical equipment are considered "presumptively medical," meaning the sole purpose of the equipment is to provide medical benefits to the patient. A variety of devices and equipment fall into this category, including hospital beds, respirators, nebulizers, commodes, traction devices, and oxygen tents. Other types of medical equipment are considered "presumptively nonmedical," meaning that the devices and equipment are not only used for medical benefits, but also for purposes of personal comfort, ambient control, environmental enhancement, or convenience. For example, an

DMEPOS

air conditioner might yield certain medical benefits to a patient recuperating from a cardiac event. The air conditioner will lower the room temperature, which may in turn assist the patient with fluid retention by minimizing fluid loss. However, because the primary and customary use of the air conditioner is not for the purpose of body fluid maintenance, it is not considered DME and payment will not be made for this equipment under the Medicare program.

- **Is the medical equipment not of use to a person without illness or injury or in need of improvement of a malformed body part?** Medicare Fact: An order or CMN on its own will not justify medical necessity even if the physician signs it. There must be documentation in the patient's medical record to substantiate the medical necessity for the item.

- **Is the medical equipment appropriate for home use?** Medicare Fact: For a patient's DME rental or purchase to be eligible for coverage under this criterion, the patient's home must be a personal dwelling or apartment, a relative's home, a home for the aged, or some other type of institution fulfilling the domiciliary needs of the patient. However, it cannot be a skilled nursing facility or a hospital.

An answer of no to any of the preceding questions could render the DME as ineligible for Medicare coverage.

The *Medicare Program Integrity Manual*, Pub. 100-08, chapter 5, section 5.1, further clarifies that a rental start date may coincide with the patient's discharge date from a facility that is not the patient's home.

Orthotic and prosthetic devices are not subject to the home use requirement for coverage and payment purposes.

Special exceptions can be made by the Medicare program, some state Medicaid programs, and other third-party payers even when the DME equipment or device does not meet the accepted definition of DME by specifically contradicting two of the criteria: (1) the equipment or devices are not primarily and customarily used for medical purposes, and/or (2) the equipment or devices can be used in the absence of illness, injury, or deformity. A DMEPOS item, described by one or both of these contradicting criteria, may be eligible for Medicare coverage if the therapeutic purpose is clearly distinguished, such as in the use of a heat lamp where the medical need for heat therapy has been established. The fact that the patient's course of treatment is under the supervision of the physician must also be in evidence.

Defining Prostheses

Prosthetic devices, as recognized by CMS and many third-party payers, are those devices that replace all or part of an internal body organ, or replace all or part of the function of a permanently inoperative or malfunctioning internal body organ. This category of devices includes:

- Artificial limbs
- Breast and eye prostheses
- Maxillofacial devices
- Joint implants
- Devices that replace all or part of the ear or nose
- Ostomy and colostomy bags
- Irrigation and flushing equipment directly related to ostomy/colostomy care

An example of a prosthesis is a urinary collection and retention system that replaces the function of the bladder in cases of permanent urinary incontinence. Replacement of a prosthetic device may be covered, but only when the replacement is required because of a change in the beneficiary's physical condition. Adjustments to an artificial limb or other prosthetic device required by wear or by a change in the beneficiary's physical condition may be likewise covered when ordered by a physician.

While parenteral and enteral nutrition (PEN) is covered by the Medicare program in many instances, there is a disparity between information in the Code of Federal Regulations (CFR) and information provided by the durable medical equipment Medicare administrative contractors (DME MAC) in the classification of PEN as a prosthetic. The CFR, in chapter 42, section 414.202, states that PEN and related accouterments are not considered to be prosthetic, while the DMERC supplier manuals list these items as general prosthetics. The *Publications 100* likewise details PEN as covered under the prosthetic device benefit. The conditions for coverage are not affected by this classification disparity. PEN is covered for patients who, due to chronic illness or injury, cannot take in sustenance through oral feeding and/or who have a permanently inoperative internal body organ or function and must receive life-sustaining nutrients via parenteral or enteral means.

Defining Orthoses

An orthosis or orthotic device is used for the correction or prevention of skeletal deformities. This includes braces for the neck, shoulder and arm, forearm, wrist and hand, hip, leg, ankle, and foot, as well as spinal or back devices. If there is a change in the beneficiary's physical condition that requires replacements and adjustments, those may also be covered. However, according to CMS, to be classified as an orthotic, the brace must be a rigid or semi-rigid device used for supporting a weak or deformed body member, or for restricting or eliminating motion in a diseased or injured part of the body.

DMEPOS

Orthoses can be classified as prefabricated or custom fabricated. A prefabricated orthosis is typically manufactured and sold without specific patient data, or in other words, without the patient's personal measurements and orthotic requirements. These devices and appliances can usually be bent, trimmed, and molded many times (with or without heat) to meet specific patient physical and therapeutic needs. An orthosis that is assembled at the point of service from prefabricated component parts is still considered to be a prefabricated orthosis.

A custom fabricated orthosis is one that has been made by following a specific patient's physical measurements and therapeutic requirements. These devices and appliances require more than bending, trimming, or simple molding to properly fit the specific patient. The creation of custom fabricated orthoses involves a significant amount of detailed work, such as building each orthotic device from component materials of plastic, metal, and fabrics. A molded-to-patient, custom, fabricated orthosis is one in which an impression of the patient's body part is taken and the resultant impression cast is used to construct the orthosis.

Defining Supplies

Within the DMEPOS industry, a supply is an item or accessory needed for the effective use of a DME, prosthetic or orthotic device, or appliance. Such supplies include those drugs and biologicals that must be placed directly into equipment to achieve the therapeutic benefit of the DME or to ensure the proper functioning of the equipment. An example of this is the use of heparin within a home dialysis system. To be eligible for coverage by Medicare, Medicaid, and third-party payers, supplies must be medically necessary and must be prescribed by the treating provider. Supplies eligible for reimbursement by these programs and payers are typically not those bought off the shelf or over the counter at local drug stores and grocery stores, with the exception of recent additions to the list of covered supplies for a patient's home use, such as supplies needed with a glucometer for the monitoring of diabetes mellitus.

Medical supplies are considered to be part of a provider's practice expense, and payment for many supplies by the Medicare program and most state Medicaid programs is included in the practice expense portion of the payment or fee schedule amount reimbursed to the provider for the primary medical or surgical service. The supplies are considered incidental to the primary medical or surgical service. Other third-party payers follow the definition of billable medical and surgical supplies found in the CPT book, which is stated in CPT guidelines as "supplies and materials provided by the physician (e.g., sterile trays/drugs), over and above those usually included with the office visit or other services rendered." Many payers require the use of the only CPT code used to report medical and surgical supplies, which is 99070 Supplies and materials (except spectacles) provided by the physician over and above those usually included with the office visit or other services rendered (list drugs, trays, supplies, or materials provided). Because this CPT code is general in its description, additional documentation or a special notation in the appropriate field for electronic claims is needed to describe the specific supply being reported.

Health care facilities must follow federal guidelines for each type of facility (hospital inpatient, hospital outpatient, ASC, skilled nursing facility, etc.) when reporting supplies to Medicare for separate payment.

Defining Customized DME

Implemented July 19, 2013, but retroactively effective January 1, 1992, CMS is clarifying the definition of customized durable medical equipment. The agency believes that customized items are rarely necessary and are rarely furnished.

In accordance with a longstanding definition in 42 CFR, Section 414.224, the criteria listed in 42 CFR, Section 414.224(a) state, "To be considered a customized item for payment purposes under paragraph (b) of this section, a covered item (including a wheelchair) must be uniquely constructed or substantially modified for a specific beneficiary according to the description and orders of a physician and be so different from another item used for the same purpose that the two items cannot be grouped together for pricing purposes. (b) Payment is made on a lump sum basis for the purchase of a customized item based on the carrier's individual consideration and judgment of a reasonable payment amount for each customized item. The carrier's individual consideration takes into account written documentation on the costs of the item including at least the cost of labor and materials used in customizing an item."

The Omnibus Budget Reconciliation Act (OBRA) of November 1990 amended the criteria for treatment of wheelchair as a customized item. This alternative definition of customized wheelchairs was never adopted for Medicare payment purposes and should not be confused with the definition of customized items referenced above. (*Medicare Claims Processing Manual*, Pub. 100-04, chap. 20, sec. 30.3 [trans.2687, April 19, 2013]; *Medicare Program Integrity Manual* Pub. 100-08, chap. 5, sec. 5.15 [trans. 460, April 19,2013]; *Medicare One-time Notification*, Pub. 100-20 [trans.1239, May 21, 2013])

Accreditation

The Medicare Modernization Act of 2003 (MMA) mandates that the Secretary of Health and Human Services establish and implement quality standards for suppliers of DMEPOS. All suppliers that furnish items or services listed below must comply with the quality standards in order to receive Medicare Part B payments and to retain a supplier billing number. Suppliers of the following items or services must be accredited:

- DME
- Medical supplies
- Home dialysis supplies and equipment
- Therapeutic shoes
- Parenteral and enteral nutrient, equipment, and supplies
- Transfusion medicine
- Prosthetic devices, prosthetics, and orthotics

Suppliers of the following items are not included:

- Medical supplies furnished by home health agencies
- Drugs used in DME, such as inhalation drugs and drugs infused with a DME pump
- Other Part B drugs, such as immunosuppressive drugs and antiemetic drugs

The Medicare Improvements for Patients and Providers Act of 2008 (MIPPA) requires all DMEPOS suppliers to meet quality standards for Medicare accreditation by September 30, 2009. Certain professionals and persons do not have to meet this deadline unless quality standards are developed specifically for these professionals and persons. CMS will work in collaboration with the medical and professional groups to develop specific quality standards. Providers and suppliers exempt from the September 30, 2009 deadline are:

- Physicians (as defined in Section 1861(r) of the Act)
- Physician assistants
- Nurse practitioners
- Physical therapists
- Occupational therapists
- Speech-language pathologists
- Clinical nurse specialists
- Certified registered nurse anesthetists
- Certified nurse-midwives
- Clinical social workers
- Clinical psychologists
- Registered dietitians
- Nutritional professionals

The Patient Protection and Affordable Care Act, Public Law 111-148, exempts a pharmacy from accreditation if it meets all of the following criteria:

- Total billings by the pharmacy for DMEPOS are less than 5 percent of total pharmacy sales.
- The pharmacy has been enrolled as a supplier of durable medical equipment, prosthetics, orthotics, and supplies, and has been issued a provider number for at least five years.
- No final adverse action has been imposed on the pharmacy in the past five years.
- The pharmacy submits an attestation, as determined by CMS, that the pharmacy meets the first three criteria.
- The pharmacy agrees to submit materials as requested during the course of an audit conducted on a random sample of pharmacies selected annually.

Existing DMEPOS suppliers, except identified exempt professionals, that are enrolled in the Medicare program must obtain and submit proof of accreditation to the National Supplier Clearinghouse (NSC).

New suppliers, except those currently exempt, submitting an enrollment application to the NSC must be accredited prior to submitting the application.

All DME suppliers must comply with the quality standards in order to retain their Medicare supplier number and to receive Medicare payment. The quality standards are comprised of two parts. The first part is supplier business services and covers the following areas:

- Administration
- Financial management
- Human resource management
- Consumer services
- Performance management
- Information management
- Product safety

The second part of the quality standards includes general product services, such as preparation, delivery and setup, training, and follow-up. Detailed standards are included for respiratory equipment, supplies, and services; manual wheelchairs, power mobility devices, including complex rehabilitative wheelchairs, and assistive technology; custom-fabricated and custom-fitted orthoses, external breast prostheses, therapeutic shoes and inserts, and their accessories and supplies; and custom-made somatic, ocular, and facial prostheses. A list of accrediting organizations and detailed quality standards are available at https://www.cms.gov/Medicare/Provider-Enrollment-and-Certification/MedicareProviderSupEnroll/DMEPOSAccreditation.html.

DME Competitive Bidding Program

Section 302 of the Medicare Prescription Drug, Improvement, and Modernization Act of 2003 (MMA) (Pub. L. 108-173) required Medicare to replace the current durable medical equipment (DME) payment methodology for certain items with a competitive acquisition process to improve the effectiveness of its methodology for setting DME payment amounts. The bidding process establishes payment amounts for certain durable medical equipment, enteral nutrition, and off-the-shelf orthotics. Competitive bidding provides a way to harness marketplace dynamics to create incentives for suppliers to provide high-quality items and services efficiently and at reasonable cost. The Medicare DME competitive bidding program has five objectives:

- To use competitive bidding for DME and to use this to determine appropriate prices for categories of DME covered by Medicare Part B

- To protect beneficiary access to high-quality DME throughout the program

- To reduce the amount Medicare pays for DMEPOS and bring the reimbursement amount more in line with that of a competitive market

- To limit the burden on beneficiaries by reducing their out-of-pocket expenses

- To mitigate proliferation of use of certain items of DMEPOS by contracting with suppliers who engage in a business model that is beneficial for the program and for Medicare beneficiaries

CMS has awarded a contract to the durable medical equipment, prosthetics, orthotics, and supplies (DMEPOS) competitive bidding implementation contractor (CBIC), Palmetto GBA, LLC, of Columbia, S.C.

Palmetto GBA will conduct certain functions related to the Medicare DMEPOS competitive bidding program, such as preparing the request for bids (RFB), performing bid evaluations, selecting qualified suppliers, and setting payments for all competitive bidding areas. In addition, Palmetto will be responsible for overseeing an education program for beneficiaries, suppliers, and referral agents. Palmetto will also help CMS and its contractors monitor program effectiveness, access, and quality.

DME in a designated competitive bidding area must be supplied by a Medicare-contracted supplier in order to bill Medicare for specifically identified DME. Restrictions will be based upon ZIP codes where beneficiaries receiving these items maintain their permanent residence. All suppliers of competitively bid DME must bill the DME MAC for these specified items.

The competitive bidding items are identified by HCPCS codes. General categories of items include:

- Oxygen supplies and equipment
- Standard power wheelchairs, scooters, and related accessories
- Complex rehabilitative power wheelchairs and related accessories (Group 2)
- Mail-order replacement diabetic supplies
- Enteral nutrients, equipment and supplies
- CPAP, RADs, and related supplies and accessories
- Hospital beds and related accessories
- Walkers and related accessories
- Support surfaces (Group 2 mattresses and overlays) in Miami

MIPPA designated the metropolitan statistical areas (MSA) for the round 1 rebid of the competitive bidding program.

The round 1 affects the following MSAs:

- Cincinnati – Middletown (Ohio, Kentucky, and Indiana)
- Cleveland – Elyria – Mentor (Ohio)
- Charlotte – Gastonia – Concord (North Carolina and South Carolina)
- Dallas – Fort Worth – Arlington (Texas)
- Kansas City (Missouri and Kansas)
- Miami – Fort Lauderdale – Pompano Beach (Florida)
- Orlando – Kissimmee (Florida)
- Pittsburgh (Pennsylvania)
- Riverside – San Bernardino – Ontario (California)

After many delays, the DME competitive bidding program began January 1, 2011.

Round 2 and national mail-order contracts and prices are scheduled to become effective on July 1, 2013.

Round 2 product categories are:

- Oxygen equipment and supplies
- Standard (power and manual) wheelchairs, scooters, and related accessories
- Enteral nutrients, equipment, and supplies
- Continuous positive airway pressure (CPAP) devices and respiratory assist devices (RAD) and related supplies and accessories
- Hospital beds and related accessories
- Walkers and related accessories
- Negative pressure wound therapy pumps and related supplies and accessories
- Mail-order diabetic testing supplies

A list of the specific items in each product category is available on the Competitive Bidding Implementation Contractor (CBIC) website,

DMEPOS

http://www.dmecompetitivebid.com/palmetto/cbic.nsf/DocsCat/Home. Specific ZIP codes in each round 2 competitive bidding area are also available on this website. The mail-order competition includes all parts of the United States, including the 50 states, the District of Columbia, Puerto Rico, the U.S. Virgin Islands, Guam, and American Samoa.

When bidding for a product category in a competitive bidding area (CBA), the supplier must have all required state licenses for that product category on file with the NSC. Every location must be licensed in each state in which it provides services. If a supplier has only one location and is bidding in a CBA that includes more than one state, the supplier must have all required licenses for every state in that CBA. Similarly, if a supplier has more than one location and is bidding in a CBA that includes more than one state, the supplier must have all required licenses for the product category for every state in that CBA. Suppliers bidding in the national mail-order competition must have the applicable licenses for all 50 states, the District of Columbia, Puerto Rico, the U.S. Virgin Islands, Guam, and American Samoa.

Suppliers must be accredited for all items in a product category in order to submit a bid for that product category. Your accreditation organization will need to report any accreditation updates to the NSC. CMS cannot contract with suppliers that are not accredited by a CMS-approved accreditation organization. Further information on the DMEPOS accreditation requirements along with a list of the accreditation organizations and those professionals and other persons exempted from accreditation may be found at the CMS website: www.cms.hhs.gov/MedicareProviderSupEnroll/01_Overview.asp.

In a report dated April 2012, CMS reports that an analysis of claims from 2010 to 2011 shows that the competitive bidding program has reduced DMEPOS spending by $202.1 million in the nine Round 1 areas. This represents an overall percentage reduction of 42 percent from lower prices and reduced inappropriate utilization. Three product categories resulted in the bulk of the savings: oxygen and oxygen supplies, mail-order diabetic supplies, and standard power wheelchairs.

Real-time claims monitoring and subsequent follow-up has indicated that beneficiaries' access to necessary and appropriate items and supplies has been preserved. Utilization rates of hospital services, emergency room visits, physician visits, and skilled nursing facility care have remained consistent with the patterns and trends seen throughout the rest of the country.

CMS is required by law to recompete contracts under the DMEPOS Competitive Bidding Program at least once every three years.The round 1 recompete of the

DMEPOS Competitive Bidding Program included the following categories of items and services:

- Respiratory equipment and related supplies and accessories—includes oxygen, oxygen equipment, and supplies; continuous positive airway pressure (CPAP) devices and respiratory assist devices (RAD) and related supplies and accessories; and standard nebulizers

- Standard mobility equipment and related accessories—includes walkers, standard power and manual wheelchairs, scooters, and related accessories

- General home equipment and related supplies and accessories—includes hospital beds and related accessories, group 1 and 2 support surfaces, transcutaneous electrical nerve stimulation (TENS) devices, commode chairs, patient lifts, and seat lifts

- Enteral nutrients, equipment, and supplies

- Negative pressure wound therapy pumps and related supplies and accessories

- External infusion pumps and supplies

The round 2 and national mail-order program contract periods expire on June 30, 2016. CMS is conducting the round 2 recompete for seven product categories in the same geographic areas that were included in round 2. Most round 2 recompete metropolitan statistical areas (MSA) have one competitive bidding area (CBA). But the three largest MSAs (Chicago, Los Angeles, and New York) are subdivided into multiple CBAs. CBAs in multistate MSAs have been defined so that there are no multistate CBAs. This results in 117 CBAs in the round 2 recompete.

The national mail-order recompete for diabetic testing supplies is occurring at the same time as the round 2 recompete. The national mail-order recompete includes all 50 states of the United States, the District of Columbia, Puerto Rico, the U.S. Virgin Islands, Guam, and American Samoa.

The round 2 recompete includes the following categories of items and services:

- Respiratory equipment and related supplies and accessories—includes oxygen, oxygen equipment, and supplies; continuous positive airway pressure (CPAP) devices and respiratory assist devices (RADs) and related supplies and accessories

- Standard mobility equipment and related accessories—includes walkers, standard power and manual wheelchairs, scooters, and related accessories

- General home equipment and related supplies and accessories—includes hospital beds and related accessories, group 1 and 2 support surfaces, transcutaneous electrical nerve stimulation (TENS) devices, commode chairs, patient lifts, and seat lifts

- Enteral nutrients, equipment, and supplies
- Negative pressure wound therapy pumps and related supplies and accessories
- Nebulizers and related supplies

The 2015 OIG Workplan notes that the OIG is going to look at the process CMS used to conduct competitive bidding and to make subsequent pricing determinations for certain medical equipment items and services in selected competitive bidding areas under rounds 1 and 2 of the competitive bidding program. Federal law requires the OIG to conduct post-award audits to assess this process. Additionally, as required by Federal law, the OIG will determine the market share of different types of diabetic testing strip types immediately following implementation of round 2. The law requires that in rounds subsequent to the round 1 rebid, contracts for mail order diabetic testing strips be awarded to suppliers that provide at least 50 percent, by volume, of all types of diabetic testing strips.

For additional information, see https://www.cms.gov/Medicare/Medicare-Fee-for-Service-Payment/DMEPOSCompetitiveBid/index.html.

DMEPOS

Durable Medical Equipment, Prosthetics, Orthotics, and Supplies and the Office of Inspector General

The Office of Inspector General (OIG) Work Plan published October 2013 explains ongoing assignments from years past and the planned assignments for 2014 with respect to the programs and operations of the Department of Health and Human Services (HHS). The entire Work Plan for FY 2014 is available for viewing at http://oig.hhs.gov/reports-and-publications/workplan/index.asp#current or you may obtain a copy by calling the OIG's Office of External Affairs at 202.619.1343. To report possible instances of waste, fraud, or abuse, you may file a report with the OIG Hotline at 800.447.8477 or go to http://oig.hhs.gov/fraud/report-fraud/report-fraud-form.asp.

For fiscal year 2014, the OIG expected recoveries of more than $4.9 billion consisting of nearly $834.7 million in audit receivables and about $4.1 billion in investigative receivables, which include about $1.1 billion in non-HHS investigative receivables resulting from work in areas such as the states' shares of Medicaid restitution. The agency also identified about $15.7 billion in savings estimated for fiscal 2014 on the basis of prior-period legislative, regulatory, or administrative actions that were supported by OIG recommendations.

Fiscal year 2014 saw exclusions of 4,017 individuals and entities from participation in federal health care programs; 971 criminal actions against individuals or entities that engaged in crimes against HHS programs; and 533 civil actions, which include false claims and unjust-enrichment lawsuits filed in federal district court, civil monetary penalties (CMP) settlements, and administrative recoveries related to provider self-disclosure matters.

Medicare Part B and Medicaid Payments for Home Blood-Glucose-Testing Supplies

The OIG continues to review Medicare Part B payments made for home blood glucose test strips and lancet supplies.

The agency will also review the effectiveness of DME MACs' claims processing edits (special system controls) designed to prevent payments to multiple suppliers of home blood-glucose test strips and lancets. All four DME MACs have LCDs that preclude the DME supplier from dispensing test strips and lancets until a beneficiary has nearly exhausted the previously dispensed supplies. The patient or a caregiver must specifically request the refill of test strips and lancets before the DME supplier dispenses them. Prior OIG reports noted inappropriate payments to multiple DME suppliers for test strips and lancets dispensed to the same patient with overlapping service dates.

Prior OIG reviews determined that suppliers of diabetic related supplies did not always comply with federal requirements. Local coverage determinations (LCD) issued by the Medicare contractors that process medical equipment and supply claims require that physicians' orders for items billed to Medicare must include certain elements and be retained by the suppliers to support billing for the services. Suppliers of diabetes testing supplies are required to add a modifier code on claims to identify when a patient is treated with insulin or not treated with insulin. The amount of supplies allowable for Medicare reimbursement differs depending on the applicable service code modifier.

As required by federal law, the OIG determines the market share of different types of diabetic testing strip types immediately following implementation of round 2. The law requires that in rounds subsequent to the round 1 rebid, contracts for mail order diabetic testing strips be awarded to suppliers that provide at least 50 percent, by volume, of all types of diabetic testing strips.

Continuing its scrutiny of diabetic testing supplies, the OIG will review Medicare's claims processing edits designed to prevent payments to multiple suppliers of home blood-glucose test strips and lancets and determine whether they are effective in preventing inappropriate payments. Prior OIG work found that inappropriate payments were made to multiple medical equipment suppliers for test strips and lancets dispensed to the same beneficiaries with overlapping service dates. The LCDs issued by the pertinent claims processing contractors state that medical equipment suppliers may not dispense test strips and lancets until patients have nearly exhausted the previously dispensed supplies. The LCDs also require that patients or their caregivers specifically request the refills before the suppliers dispense them.

The OIG continues to look for opportunities to lower Medicaid payments for home blood-glucose test strips through rebates, competitive bidding, or other means. The agency will also review the rebates that some states collected on test strips to determine whether the states properly reimbursed the federal share of the rebates.

DME Competitive Bidding Program

The 2015 OIG Workplan notes that the OIG is going to look at the process CMS used to conduct competitive bidding and to make subsequent pricing determinations for certain medical equipment items and services in selected competitive bidding areas under rounds 1 and 2 of the competitive bidding program. Federal law requires the OIG to conduct post-award audits to assess this process.

Medicare Part B Payments for Drugs

The OIG periodically reviews widely available market prices (WAMP) for selected prescription drugs covered by Part B and compares them to ASPs for those drugs to identify a designated payment-related threshold. In 2005, Medicare began paying for most Part B drugs using a new methodology based on the ASP. Federal law requires OIG to conduct studies that compare ASPs to WAMPs for Part B-covered drugs. If OIG finds that the ASP of a drug exceeds the WAMP by a certain threshold (now 5 percent), Medicare may disregard the ASP for the drug when setting reimbursement amounts (e.g., apply a price substitution policy).

The OIG continues to review Medicare payments for drugs and biologicals used on an off-label basis in cancer chemotherapeutic regimens. Medicare covers FDA-approved drugs used for off-label indications in anticancer chemotherapeutic regimens when such uses are supported in specified authoritative compendia.

The OIG will review states' claims for the federal share of Medicaid payments for the drug Herceptin, which is used to treat breast cancer, to determine whether providers properly billed the states for the drug. The agency will review providers' claims for completion and accuracy and to determine if the claim was billed in accordance with the regulations of the selected states. Prior OIG audits have shown provider noncompliance with Medicare billing requirements. The agency feels that similar issues may occur in Medicaid.

The OIG is going to determine how much Medicare Part B spending could be reduced if Medicare were able to share in the savings for 340B-purchased drugs. The agency will calculate the amount by which ASP-based payments exceed 340B prices and estimate potential savings on the basis of various shared-benefit methodologies. The 340B program requires drug manufacturers to provide discounted outpatient drugs to approximately 10,000 covered entities. Medicare Part B reimburses for almost all covered outpatient drugs (including those purchased by 340B entities) on the basis of the average sales price (ASP), without regard to the amount paid for the drug. Medicare Part B providers that purchase drugs under the 340B program can keep the full difference between the ASP-based payment amount and the 340B purchase price.

The OIG is going to examine Medicare administrative contractors' policies and procedures for reviewing and processing Part B claims for compounded drugs and assess the appropriateness of such claims. Pharmacy compounding is a practice in which pharmacists combine, mix, or alter ingredients to create unique medications that meet specific needs of individual patients. Compounded drugs may be eligible for coverage under Medicare Part B if they are produced in accordance with the federal Food, Drug, and Cosmetic Act.

The OIG will determine whether Medicare Part B payments for immunosuppressive drugs billed with modifier KX met Medicare documentation requirements. Medicare covers FDA-approved immunosuppressive drugs when a beneficiary receives an organ transplant for which immunosuppressive therapy is appropriate. Suppliers that furnish an immunosuppressive drug are supposed to append modifier KX to signify that the supplier retains documentation of the beneficiary's transplant date and that such transplant date preceded the date of service for furnishing the drug.

Lower Limb Prostheses

Prior OIG work found that suppliers frequently submitted claims that did not meet certain Medicare requirements, were for beneficiaries with no claims from their referring physicians, and had other questionable billing characteristics, such as billing lower limb prostheses for beneficiaries with no history of an amputation or missing limb. A national review of suppliers of lower limb prosthetics identified 267 suppliers that had questionable billings.

This review will look at Medicare Part B payments for claims submitted by medical equipment suppliers for lower limb prosthetics to determine whether the requirements of the *Medicare Benefits Policy Manual*, Pub. 100-02, chapter 15, section 120, were met. Providers must have and furnish upon request the information necessary to determine the payment

DMEPOS and OIG

amount due and that the items or services are reasonable and necessary.

Power Mobility Devices

Medicare requires that the treating physician conduct a face-to-face examination to determine the medical necessity of a power mobility device (PMD) and write a prescription for the PMD. The OIG will review Medicare Part B payments for PMD to determine whether the Medicare requirements for a face-to-face examination were met. Compensation for conducting the face-to-face examination is available when the prescribing physician bills for an evaluation and management (E/M) service and has the option of billing Medicare for an add-on payment for the sole purpose of documenting the need for the PMD. Prior OIG work found that when the prescribing physician did not bill the code for the add-on payment in addition to the E/M code, the resulting PMD claim was likely to be unallowable.

The OIG will further review Medicare Part B payments for suppliers of PMD to determine whether such payments were in accordance with Medicare requirements. Focus will be on whether Medicare payments for PMD claims submitted by medical equipment suppliers are medically necessary and are supported in accordance with requirements at 42 CFR § 410.38.

In another review, the OIG will determine if potential savings can be achieved by Medicare when certain PMD are rented over a 13-month period rather than acquired through a lump-sum purchase.

DMEPOS and OIG

General Billing, Claims, and Coverage Issues

ASC X12N 837 Claim Formats

Physicians and suppliers must submit all electronic Medicare Claims data to Medicare using the ASC X12N 837 claim format. The current version of the standards is 005010X0223A2 for institutional claims, 005010X0222A for professional claims, 005010X224A2 for dental claims, and the National Council for Prescription Drug Programs [NCPDP] version D.0. for pharmacy transactions.

Providers can keep up to date with the version 5010 schedule by accessing the CMS website links at http://www.cms.gov/Regulations-and-Guidance/HIPAA-Administrative-Simplification/Versions5010andD0/index.html?redirect=/Versions5010andD0/.

DMEPOS for Hospital Inpatients

Medicare does not allow separate payment for durable medical equipment, prosthetics, orthotics, and supplies (DMEPOS) when a patient is in a covered inpatient stay. These claims were related to DME dates of service greater than two days prior to Part A discharge date or Part A discharge status was not to home. Effective July 1, 2013, the DME claim will be rejected or, if paid, the contractor will institute payment recovery when all of the following conditions are met:

- There is a covered Medicare Part A inpatient claim with a TOB of 0111

- The DME and the inpatient claims are for the same beneficiary HICN

- The DME claim has a line item within the HCPCS Level II category 03 for orthotics and/or prosthesis

- The from date of service (DOS) of the durable medical equipment item is within the Part A admit and discharge dates

- The from DOS of the durable medical equipment line items is greater than two days prior to the beneficiary's Part A inpatient discharge date

- If the from DOS of the DME line items is within the beneficiary's Part A inpatient admission and discharge date and the patient discharge status (FL 17) is NOT equal to 01 Discharged to home or self-care (routine discharge)

(*Medicare Claims Processing Manual*, Pub. 100-4, Chap. 20, Sec. 01, 10, 30, 30.6, 110.2, 110.3.3, 130.5, 160.1, 160.2, 170, 210)

The CMS Recovery Audit Contractor (RAC) Program, which is responsible for identifying and correcting improper payments in the Medicare fee-for-service payment process, identified this issue. The contractor identified DMEPOS claims for patients who received DMEPOS items while in an inpatient stay in a hospital. Since Medicare does not allow separate payments for DMEPOS for the patient during a covered inpatient hospital stay, these payments associated with these claims are considered overpayments.

Medicare will cover DME that falls within an inpatient stay when the claim is for maintenance and servicing of capped rental items and when the claim contains modifier MS. (*Medicare Claims Processing Manual*, Pub. 100-4, Chap. 20, Sec. 210)

Provider Taxonomy Codes

Provider taxonomy codes are 10-character, alphanumeric codes that identify the specialty of the provider. HIPAA regulations require the use of these taxonomy codes. The taxonomy code must be used to identify the provider or supplier's specialty when the taxonomy code affects claim adjudication.

The current list of provider taxonomy codes is available from http://www.wpc-edi.com. Regional DME MACs may be able to provide a current list.

Medical Necessity and DMEPOS

For DMEPOS items or services to be billed to a Medicare contractor, the physician or provider must have documentation demonstrating the medical necessity of the item. This information must be a part of the patient's medical record. For suppliers of DMEPOS items, an official order signed and dated by the ordering provider must be obtained. The order must detail the following:

- The patient's identifying information

- A description of the DMEPOS item

- The reason for the DMEPOS prescription, which can take the form of the ICD-9-CM and ICD-10-CM code and/or diagnosis narrative information

General Billing

- The start date of the order must be clearly specified

- If the order is for supplies that will be provided on a periodic basis, the order should include information on the quantity used, frequency of change, and duration of need (e.g., an order for surgical dressings might specify one 4x4 hydrocolloid dressing that is changed one to two times per week for one month or until the ulcer heals)

- The order must be sufficiently detailed, including all options or additional features that will be separately billed or that will require an upgraded code. The description can be a narrative description (e.g., lightweight wheelchair base) or a brand name/model number

- If the order is for a rented item or if the coverage criteria in a policy specify length of need, the order must include the length of need

- If the supply is a drug, the order must specify the name of the drug, concentration (if applicable), dosage, frequency of administration, and duration of infusion (if applicable)

The provider's signature must be an original signature. A faxed copy of the original order temporarily satisfies the requirement for most Medicare contractors, and allows the supplier to begin to fulfill the DMEPOS order so the patient can begin using the DMEPOS item as soon as possible. At some point, however, the supplier must obtain the original document from the provider. The supplier must then keep the original DMEPOS order on file. A copy of the order must be sent to the Medicare contractor when requested. If the item requires a Certificate of Medical Necessity (CMN), a separate provider written order is not necessary; the CMN acts as the original provider order. A copy of the CMN faxed to the supplier is considered sufficient documentation by federal auditors as long as the supplier retains the faxed copy and the provider retains the original.

The following are certain DMEPOS items for which the supplier must obtain the signed original detailed order before fulfilling the order:

- Seat-lift mechanisms

- Transcutaneous electrical nerve stimulator (TENS) units (purchase only)

- Power-operated vehicles

- Pressure reducing pads

- Mattress overlays, mattresses, and beds

- Other items as denoted by contractor local or regional coverage decisions

The first item requires only a written physician order; the remainder of the items requires CMNs to be completed by the provider and supplier.

(*Medicare Program Integrity Manual,* Pub. 100-8, Chap. 5, Sec. 5.2.2-5.2.3.1)

Certificates of Medical Necessity

The Medicare program requires the completion of specific forms to establish the medical necessity of certain durable medical equipment, supplies, and services. Six of these particular forms, called Certificates of Medical Necessity (CMN), have been developed by the DME MAC. These forms have been given official form numbers by CMS and are generally referred to by these numbers. The form numbers are primarily used to identify each CMN submitted with electronic claims to the DME MAC.

Once a supplier receives a verbal or written order for a DMEPOS item that requires a CMN, the supplier generates a DMEPOS-specific CMN form and completes portions of the form. The supplier then sends it to the ordering provider for completion of patient-specific clinical information and final certification, which requires the provider to sign and date the order. The supplier must send the provider both sides of the CMN, as the reverse side of the form contains instructions for appropriate completion. The CMN forms cannot be modified in any way. Within the CMN forms there are specific sections for the DMEPOS supplier to fill out, and certain sections the provider must complete; in fact, the supplier is forbidden to assist the provider by completing these sections (see below).

The CMN forms generally follow a four-section format:

Section A	Patient and physician identifying information; HCPCS codes
	May be completed by the supplier
Section B	DMEPOS-specific information
.	Completed by the physician, staff, or other clinician involved in the care of the patient; cannot be completed by the supplier
Section C	Narrative description of equipment and cost
.	Completed by the supplier
Section D	Physician attestation, signature, and date
.	Completed by the physician

CMNs are currently required for:

- Oxygen

- Pneumatic compression devices

- Osteogenesis stimulators

- Transcutaneous electrical nerve stimulators (TENS) (purchase only)

- Seat lift mechanisms

CMN Form Specifics

CMS issued guidance for certain aspects of the CMN. Previously faxed copies of the CMN from the provider were not considered valid documentation under CMS rules for the supplier to fulfill the DMEPOS order. In many cases, this resulted in both a delay of medical equipment being delivered to the patient and a delay in supplier reimbursement. As of CMS allowed the use of faxed copies of provider-completed CMNs to

alleviate these situations. The faxed copy is all that is required to be kept on file by the supplier, as long as the ordering provider retains the original CMN. Note that if an audit were to be undertaken by Medicare contractors, the supplier would need to obtain the original CMN documents from the providers, or risk postpayment denial of the claims or assessment of overpayments, fines, or penalties.

| DEPARTMENT OF HEALTH AND HUMAN SERVICES
CENTERS FOR MEDICARE & MEDICAID SERVICES | Form Approved
OMB No. 0938-0679 |

CERTIFICATE OF MEDICAL NECESSITY
DME 06.03B
CMS-848 — TRANSCUTANEOUS ELECTRICAL NERVE STIMULATOR (TENS)

SECTION A Certification Type/Date: INITIAL ___/___/___ REVISED ___/___/___ RECERTIFICATION ___/___/___

PATIENT NAME, ADDRESS, TELEPHONE and HIC NUMBER	SUPPLIER NAME, ADDRESS, TELEPHONE and NSC or applicable NPI NUMBER/LEGACY NUMBER
(___ ___ ___) ___ ___ ___ - ___ ___ ___ ___ HICN _____	(___ ___ ___) ___ ___ ___ - ___ ___ ___ ___ NSC or NPI #_____

PLACE OF SERVICE_____	HCPCS CODE	PT DOB ___/___/___ Sex ___ (M/F) Ht. ___(in) Wt ___(lbs.)
NAME and ADDRESS of FACILITY *if applicable (see reverse)*		PHYSICIAN NAME, ADDRESS, TELEPHONE and applicable NPI NUMBER or UPIN
		(___ ___ ___) ___ ___ ___ - ___ ___ ___ ___ UPIN or NPI #_____

SECTION B Information in this Section May Not Be Completed by the Supplier of the Items/Supplies.

EST. LENGTH OF NEED (# OF MONTHS): _____ 1-99 *(99=LIFETIME)* DIAGNOSIS CODES (ICD-9): _____ _____ _____ _____

ANSWERS	ANSWER QUESTIONS 1-6 for purchase of TENS (Circle Y for Yes, N for No,)
Y N	1. Does the patient have chronic, intractable pain?
_____ Months	2. How long has the patient had intractable pain? (Enter number of months, 1 - 99.)
1 2 3 4 5	3. Is the TENS unit being prescribed for any of the following conditions? (Circle appropriate number) 1 - Headache 2 - Visceral abdominal pain 3 - Pelvic pain 4 - Temporomandibular joint (TMJ) pain 5 - None of the above
Y N	4. Is there documentation in the medical record of multiple medications and/or other therapies that have been tried and failed?
Y N	5. Has the patient received a TENS trial of at least 30 days?
___/___/___	6. What is the date that you reevaluated the patient at the end of the trial period?

NAME OF PERSON ANSWERING SECTION B QUESTIONS, IF OTHER THAN PHYSICIAN (Please Print):
NAME: _____TITLE: _____EMPLOYER:_____

SECTION C **Narrative Description of Equipment and Cost**

(1) Narrative description of all items, accessories and options ordered; (2) Supplier's charge; and (3) Medicare Fee Schedule Allowance for each item, accessory, and option. (see instructions on back)

SECTION D **PHYSICIAN Attestation and Signature/Date**

I certify that I am the treating physician identified in Section A of this form. I have received Sections A, B and C of the Certificate of Medical Necessity (including charges for items ordered). Any statement on my letterhead attached hereto, has been reviewed and signed by me. I certify that the medical necessity information in Section B is true, accurate and complete, to the best of my knowledge, and I understand that any falsification, omission, or concealment of material fact in that section may subject me to civil or criminal liability.

PHYSICIAN'S SIGNATURE_____ DATE ____/____/____

Form CMS-848 (09/05) EF 08/2006

General Billing

For Section B of the CMN form, all information entered in support of the DMEPOS must be present in the patient's medical record; the CMN and the medical record documentation should match in essential information. A standing directive by CMS is that Section B of the CMN may not be completed by the supplier of the DMEPOS, even under the guidance or at the request of the ordering provider. The supplier can complete section C, Narrative Description of Equipment and Cost. If the supplier-entered information in Section C does not accurately reflect the information provided by the ordering provider, CMS will return the CMN unsigned to the supplier for correction.

Providers and suppliers should note that CMS, in its quest to halt fraud and abuse, has issued a directive related to correcting errors on the CMN forms. Similar to the long standing malpractice protocol involving the patient's medical record, CMS requires the incorrect information on the CMN to be struck through with a single line, the correct information entered just above the strike-through entry, and the provider's or supplier's initials annotated adjacent to the new entry. The correction must be dated as well. If the DMEPOS supplier feels that the corrected CMN may cause confusion, the supplier may request that a new CMN be completed with the accurate information.

Camera-ready copies of these forms are available on the websites of the DME MAC or at CMS website http://www.cms.hhs.gov/CMSForms/CMSForms/list.asp#TopOfPage. If more space is needed when completing Section C of these forms (Narrative Description of Equipment and Cost) then a special CMN—CMS Form 854, Section C Continuation Form—may be used to convey the remainder of the essential information. CMS Form 854 can only be used as an addendum to CMS forms 843 and 844, not with any other CMN form. If CMS Form 854 is used, it must be signed and dated (certified) by the ordering provider. The supplier must also keep it on file. For paper claim submitters, the form must accompany the primary form; for electronic submitters, the supplier need not transmit Form 854, but must retain it in case the form is requested by the DME MAC for review.

The CMN form for oxygen—CMS Form 484—includes the addition of Section C, the listing of the supplier's charge and Medicare fee schedule allowance for the equipment requested, as required by federal law. Section C also contains an area for a brief narrative description of the oxygen delivery system requested, whether it is compressed gas, liquid or concentrated, and stationary or portable. Other pertinent information should be listed in Section C (and confirmed by the ordering provider) such as the need for a cannula or mask, the prescribed oxygen flow rates, and so on.

Also contained within the CMS Form 484 is a revised question regarding the blood gas or oximetry test result that qualifies the oxygen for Medicare coverage. This question helps establish the medical necessity for the oxygen by asking if the test was performed "either with the patient in a chronic stable state as an outpatient, or within two days before discharge from an inpatient facility to [the patient's] home." If multiple tests have been performed, CMS views the most recent test as the qualifying results for home oxygen coverage. If the patient is one with a chronic cardiopulmonary condition requiring the use of oxygen, a test result reported for determining home oxygen coverage cannot be one that was obtained during an acute cardiopulmonary episode or acute exacerbation of the patient's disease process.

The physician currently responsible for the patient's pulmonary condition must complete the oxygen CMN. Suppliers must maintain their records so they can identify the new treating physicians and obtain new CMNs when necessary.

Providers and suppliers must be aware of a defined timeline when ordering and fulfilling orders for DMEPOS. If more than three months elapse from the time a CMN is completed by the ordering provider to the time the DMEPOS item is delivered, a new CMN must be completed. This directive ensures the continued medical necessity of the DMEPOS item, as a patient may no longer require the ordered item. The timeline is more prohibitive for an initial order for oxygen, which involves certain blood gases analysis. The order must be filled in 30 days for the supplier to be reimbursed. If this timeline is not met, a new CMN must be completed. The provider cannot complete the initial CMN for oxygen dispensation more than 30 days before the expected fulfillment of the order.

A copy of the initial CMN should accompany the following:

- All initial claims for the reported DMEPOS items or services
- Changes in the original
- Initial provision of nutrients and supplies

CMNs can be submitted both by electronic means and by paper submission. If the CMN is submitted in hard copy, the supplier need only include a copy of the front of the form. If the CMN is transmitted electronically in the NSF format, only information from Sections A, B, and D (not C) is required. The HIPAA 837 professional claim format can accommodate all CMN fields.

CMN Cover Letters

A supplier must generate a cover letter for each CMN-required DMEPOS order to be sent to the provider for completion. These letters are seen as written confirmation of provider orders and are used

General Billing

as basic forums for communication between the ordering provider and the supplier. Traditionally the supplier has been limited in what to write in the letter in that it cannot influence the provider regarding the medical necessity of the DMEPOS item. However, CMS issued a statement about the use of cover letters for CMNs, in effect stating that it had no jurisprudence or regulatory control over CMN cover letters, and cannot restrict the information contained in them. It states that the burden of proof in terms of medical necessity for the DMEPOS remains with the ordering provider and the supplier.

The cover letters may include the following elements:

• An explanation of the section of the CMN to be completed by the ordering provider

• Instructions or guidance on where to send the completed CMN, and the expected time frame in which the CMN is to be returned to the supplier

• A request for a copy of any pertinent laboratory or other test results necessary for the order of the DMEPOS item

• Information related to CMS policy regarding coverage limitations or requirements for the DMEPOS being ordered of which the physician or provider should be aware

Modifier KX

Modifier KX is used on the CMS-1500 claim form to indicate that the DMEPOS supplier is maintaining medical necessity documentation in the supplier's files. This documentation only needs to be submitted to the DME MAC entity upon request. The DMEPOS supplier should create internal mechanisms to ensure the proper use of modifier KX. Improper use of the modifier may result in the submission of false claims. The OIG recommends that the DMEPOS supplier's written policies and procedures address the supplier's protocol for using this modifier.

Death of the Physician Who Completed the CMN

Suppliers are required to obtain new orders and new CMNs for customers whose originating physician has died. To avoid interruptions of payments for rentals, oxygen, or transfers of care, a grace period of 15 months from the date of death will be allowed for DME claims. At the end of the grace period, the supplier should have obtained new orders and CMNs. The supplier will then bill with the replacement physician's NPI and CMN. This applies even to lifetime orders of oxygen.

Claims requiring CMNs that are signed by a deceased physician may be medical necessity denials. The supplier will have the opportunity to appeal any claims denied due to this reason. Claims denied due to the use of a deceased physician's NPI would be

denied using the message that the NPI is invalid. These claims may also be appealed.

It is imperative that suppliers take note of this issue. Carriers' files have been updated and cross-matched against the AMA's deceased physician database and the Social Security Administration's database. Claims with a deceased physician's NPI or CMN, whose date of service is after the physician's date of death, will be rejected.

Providers Prohibited from Charging for CMN Preparation

If a patient requires an item of DMEPOS, the completion of the CMN is considered a service to the patient rather than to the supplier. Providers cannot charge the patient or the supplier for the completion of the CMN. Section 4152 of the Omnibus Reconciliation Act of 1990 requires a provider to complete the CMN or DMEPOS order. The language in the statute does not authorize providers to separately charge the patient or the supplier for completing the CMN forms. Allegations of providers charging for completion of the CMN forms will be investigated as one or more of the following:

• Potential kickback situations under Section 1128B(b) of the Social Security Act

• A false representation with respect to the provider's actual charge for professional services furnished on or near the date of the DMEPOS order for the patient

• A potential assignment violation on claims for professional services on or near the date the provider orders the DMEPOS item for the patient

• A potential charge limit violation on unassigned claims for professional services on or near the date the provider ordered the DMEPOS item for the patient

The federal government has become aggressive in its efforts against fraud, waste, and abuse, and in doing so has actively included the patient in its campaigns.

DME Information Form

A DME Information Form (DIF) replaces the CMN for certain DME supplies. A DIF is completed and signed by the supplier. The DIF contains many of the same elements as the CMN, but does not require a narrative description of equipment and cost or a physician signature. DIFs are subject to the same requirements and restrictions as CMNs.

DIFs need to be completed to provide information for enteral and parenteral nutrition (PEN) and external infusion pumps.

Contractors may ask for supporting documentation beyond a CMN or DIF. Copies of CMNs and DIFs can be downloaded at

General Billing

http://www.cms.hhs.gov/CMSForms/CMSForms/list.asp#TopOfPage.

DMEPOS Prior Authorizations/Advance Determination of Medicare Coverage

For reimbursement for some DMEPOS items, typically those requiring CMN forms, the items must have prior authorization or an advance determination of Medicare coverage (ADMC) from the DME MAC. For certain items of DMEPOS, an ADMC process must be undertaken before the delivery of the item to the patient (the DMERC entities will advise the providers and suppliers of these particular DMEPOS items). In these cases, the supplier must submit the CMN in advance of the claim for the purchase of the DMEPOS and specifically request an ADMC. The irony inherent in this process is that the prior authorization does not guarantee Medicare reimbursement for the item in question, and only indicates that the medical necessity criteria for the DMEPOS item have been met. A supplier or patient may request an ADMC before delivery of an item to determine whether payment for the item may be denied if:

- The item is a customized item
- The patient to whom the item is to be furnished, or the supplier, requests that such advance determination be made
- The item is not an inexpensive item

Customized DME is defined as items of DME that have been uniquely constructed or substantially modified for a specific patient according to the description and orders of the beneficiary's treating physician.

ADMCs are not initial determinations as no request for payment is being made and they cannot be appealed.

ADMCs must be made in writing. For submitters who usually transmit the CMN electronically with the claim, items subject to prior authorization require that both the CMN and the ADMC request be made by paper submission only. This documentation should be submitted to the DME MAC.

The Medicare contractor must render a written decision on an ADMC within 30 calendar days. An affirmative ADMC decision will provide the supplier and the patient assurance that, based on the information submitted with the request, Medicare medical necessity requirements have been met as established for the item.

An affirmative ADMC decision does not provide assurance that the patient meets Medicare eligibility requirements nor does it assure that any other Medicare requirements (MSP, etc.) have been met. Only upon submission of a complete claim can the Medicare contractor make a full and complete determination. An affirmative ADMC decision does not extend to the price that Medicare will pay for the item. An affirmative ADMC decision is valid for a period of six months from the date the decision is rendered. Medicare contractors reserve the right to review claims on a pre- or post-payment basis and may deny claims and take appropriate remedy if they determine that an affirmative ADMC decision was made based on incorrect information.

A negative ADMC decision communicates to the supplier and the patient that, based on the information submitted with the request, the patient does not meet the medical necessity requirements Medicare has established for the item. The negative ADMC decision should indicate why the request was denied. A patient or a supplier can resubmit an ADMC request if additional medical documentation is obtained that could affect the prior negative ADMC decision. However, requests may only be submitted once during a six-month period.

DME MACs publish examples of the types of items for which ADMCs are available. These are published annually in the DME MAC's Supplier Manual or Bulletin. Examples will be published in the form of HCPCS codes eligible for this program. This list is not a list of specific items, but rather a general list of the categories of types of items eligible for this program.

In 2014, the four DME MACs listed the following manual and power wheelchairs and accessories as eligible for an ADMC:

E1161	Manual adult size wheelchair, includes tilt-in-space
E1231	Wheelchair, pediatric size, tilt-in-space, rigid, adjustable, with seating system
E1232	Wheelchair, pediatric size, tilt-in-space, folding, adjustable, with seating system
E1233	Wheelchair, pediatric size, tilt-in-space, rigid, adjustable, without seating system
E1234	Wheelchair, pediatric size, tilt-in-space, folding, adjustable, without seating system
K0005	Ultralightweight manual wheelchair
K0008	Custom manual wheelchair/base
K0009	Not otherwise classified manual wheelchair base
K0835–K0843	Power Group 2
K0848–K0855	Power Group 3 provided with an alternative drive control interface (E2321–E2322, E2325, E2327–E2330)
K0856–K0864	Power Group 3
K0868–K0871	Power Group 4 provided with an alternative drive control interface (E2321–E2322, E2325, E2327–E2330)
K0877–K0886	Power Group 4
K0890–K0891	Power Group 5

General Billing

Not all DME MACs provide ADMCs for all types of wheelchairs and accessories listed above. Check the website for each DME MAC for the specific ADMCs offered.

Local Coverage Determination (LCD)

Local coverage determinations (LCD) are contractor decisions developed to specify when clinical circumstances for a service are reasonable and necessary. They serve as an administrative and educational tool to assist providers in submitting claims correctly for payment. LCDs may apply to specific state regions, all submitters, or to a specific contractor. Each LCD lists the jurisdiction for which it applies. LCDs may be accessed at the contractor's website or through the CMS coverage database at http://www.cms.gov/medicare-coverage-database/overview-and-quick-search.asP&

Medicare Program Requirements

Provider/Supplier Identifiers

Federal laws mandate the use of specific codes to identify the provider or supplier of services on the claim. These national identifiers include:

- National Provider Number (NPI)
- National Supplier Identification Number (NSIN)

The National Provider Identifier Number

The National Provider Identifier (NPI) number is part of the National Provider System developed by CMS and by various federal government and Medicaid state agencies. It was developed to standardize and simplify the provider and supplier enumeration process. Under this system, every provider and supplier is assigned an individual national identification number. This 10-digit number consists of a seven-digit base number, a one-digit mathematical algorithm, and a two-digit alphanumeric suffix to identify the provider setting or location. This number must be used on all claims filed to the DME MAC. Health care providers may apply for an NPI at http://nppes.cms.hhs.gov/NPPES/Welcome.do.

Keep NSC Files Updated

DMEPOS supplier standard number 2 requires that all suppliers notify the National Supplier Clearinghouse (NSC) with any change that is made to the Medicare enrollment application or Form CMS-855S within 30 days of the change. DMEPOS suppliers should use the March 2009 version of Form CMS-855S and should update the following information:

- List of products and services found in section 2.D

- Authorized official information in sections 6A and 15
- Correspondence address in section 2A2

This is important for suppliers who are involved in the Medicare DMEPOS Competitive Bidding Program. All suppliers must be sure that all information on their application form is current and up to date. For guidance on how to submit a change of information, please access the NSC website at http://www.palmettogba.com/nsc.

Accreditation

In November 2006, CMS approved 10 national accreditation organizations that accredit suppliers of durable medical equipment, prosthetics, orthotics, and supplies (DMEPOS) as meeting new quality standards under Medicare Part B. In order to enroll or maintain Medicare billing privileges, all DMEPOS suppliers must comply with the Medicare program's supplier standards (found at 42 CFR §424.57 (c)) and quality standards. The accreditation requirement applies to suppliers of durable medical equipment, medical supplies, home dialysis supplies and equipment, therapeutic shoes, parenteral/enteral nutrition, transfusion medicine and prosthetic devices, and prosthetics and orthotics. The Medicare Improvement for Patients and Providers Act of 2008 (MIPPA) specified professionals and other persons exempt from accreditation requirements. The Patient Protection and Affordable Care Act, Public Law 111-148, further exempted a pharmacy from accreditation if it meets all of the following criteria:

- Total billings by the pharmacy for DMEPOS are less than 5 percent of total pharmacy sales.
- The pharmacy has been enrolled as a supplier of durable medical equipment, prosthetics, orthotics, and supplies, and has been issued a provider number for at least five years.
- No final adverse action has been imposed on the pharmacy in the past five years.
- The pharmacy submits an attestation, as determined by CMS, that the pharmacy meets the first three criteria.
- The pharmacy agrees to submit materials, as requested, during the course of an audit conducted on a random sample of pharmacies selected annually.

Further information on the DMEPOS accreditation requirements, including a list of the accreditation organizations for DMEPOS suppliers, can be found at http://www.cms.gov/MedicareProviderSupEnroll/07_DMEPOSAccreditation.asp#TopOfPage.

General Billing

Mandatory Provider and Supplier Claim Submission

The Omnibus Budget Reconciliation Act of 1989 (OBRA '89) mandates that the provider or supplier, within a one-year filing limit, must submit all patient claims for reimbursement when furnishing covered items on Medicare claims. This is true whether or not the provider is participating with the Medicare program. The provider or supplier is relieved of this obligation when furnishing noncovered items, unless the patient requests a Medicare payment determination (usually to receive a written denial from the Medicare program for secondary insurance purposes).

Claims to Medicare contractors are usually transmitted by CMS-1500 form, or by electronic means (called electronic data interchange [EDI] or electronic media claims [EMC]). Medicare carriers, DME MACs, and most major third-party payers do not accept practice superbills or encounter forms as appropriate formats for claim submissions.

In certain situations, a provider who has not entered into a private contract with the Medicare beneficiary (called an opt out agreement) does not have to submit a claim for a covered service for a Medicare patient. In these cases, typically the Medicare patient or the patient's legal representative decides not to authorize the provider to submit a claim, or the patient wishes not to divulge the confidential medical information that is on a claim to the Medicare program. A common example is when the patient does not want information about mental illness or a sexually transmitted disease (STD) to be disclosed to any person or entity. The Medicare patient has the latitude to change this order and later authorize the submission of the claim for the service. In this case, the provider is obligated to prepare and submit the claim.

Electronic DMEPOS Claims

Medicare requires providers to submit electronic media claims (EMC) using the professional 837 V5010 transmission format updated as appropriate with addendum information. An electronic claim is submitted via a central processing unit (CPU) to CPU transmission, tape, direct data entry, direct wire, or personal computer upload or download. A claim that is submitted via digital fax/OCR, diskette, or touch-tone telephone is not considered as an electronic claim.

A paper claim is submitted and received on paper, including fax print-outs. This also includes a claim that the contractor receives on paper and then reads electronically with OCR technology.

For the last 10 years, Medicare has been prohibited by regulation from paying clean electronic claims earlier than the 14th day after the receipt of the claim. This holding period is commonly referred to as the payment floor. The payment floor is 29 days effective January 1, 2006, for paper and non-HIPAA compliant electronic claims. Providers can avoid this added delay in payment by submitting HIPAA compliant clean electronic claims. CMS states that only claims using ANSI V005010X0222A will be considered HIPAA-compliant (*Medicare Claims Processing Manual*, Pub. 100-04, chap. 1, sec. 80.2).

Clean claims do not require the MAC to investigate or develop them external to Medicare claims operations on a prepayment basis. These claims pass all edits, both contractor or MAC-specific and common working file (CWF), and are processed electronically.

For claims not considered clean, the Medicare contractor may need to do the following:

- Request additional information from the provider or supplier or other external source; this includes routine data not submitted with the claim, additional medical information, or information to resolve discrepancies detected within the claim and other documentation submitted for consideration

- Request information or assistance from another Medicare contractor; this includes development data obtained through the carrier-intermediary data exchange or requests for charge data from other contractors

- Develop or investigate Medicare Secondary Payer program information

- Request information from the provider or supplier necessary for a judicial coverage determination

- Perform sequential processing when an earlier claim is currently in development

- Perform outside claim development as a result of a common working file edit

The payment floor for paper claims is 29 calendar days. Clean electronic claims not paid by Medicare after 30 days will accrue interest, payable to the provider or supplier, beginning on the 31st day. The provider or supplier can also obtain automatic electronic funds transfer (EFT) and receive electronic remittance notices. In fact, a provider or supplier need not submit claims electronically to take advantage of EFT, as paper submitters can also receive EFT.

Funds deposited electronically are available in the provider's or supplier's bank account the day after the DME MAC transmits the EFT to the bank. Every EFT transaction has a tracking number in case a payment must be traced. Errors in EFT deposits usually occur when the provider or supplier has changed banks or closed the existing account currently being used for EFT by the DME MAC. All necessary information should be sent to the DME MAC as quickly as possible when the provider or supplier changes banks or bank accounts.

Many Medicare contractor supply the necessary EDI or EMC software programs free of charge; others charge a nominal fee or an inconsequential annual software maintenance fee. Certificates of Medical Necessity (CMNs) can be filed electronically as well, allowing the providers and suppliers of DMEPOS to forward all necessary documentation electronically. Physician orders, other than CMNs, currently do not have an electronic format for submission unless the note area within the electronic claim record is used for brief annotations.

Electronic Submission of Medical Documentation

At the request of providers and Medicare review contractors, CMS developed an electronic method for the submission of medical documentation. Electronic Submission of Medical Documentation (esMD) is a system that allows providers or health information handlers (HIH) to submit medical documentation over secure electronic means.

CMS uses "gateways" to securely exchange electronic private health information. The gateways are built on the sender and receiver ends. Gateways built for the esMD project follow the set of health information exchange standards, services, and policies that the Office of the National Coordinator for Health IT (ONC) has adopted. CMS esMD Gateway is built using the open source CONNECT software. This solution enables secure exchange of electronic health information adhering to various Health Information Technology (HIT) interoperability standards. Currently the gateway securely receives the electronic medical documents submitted by various HIHs on behalf of providers.

Any provider that wants to electronically submit medical documentation to a CMS review contractor must build a gateway themselves or procure gateway services from the HIH of their choice. A list of HIHs may be found at http://www.cms.gov/Research-Statistics-Data-and-Systems/Computer-Data-and-Systems/ESMD/index.html. Click on the link to the left called "Which HIHs Offer esMD Gateway Services to Providers?"

CMS encourages all Medicare administrative contractors (MAC), comprehensive error rate testing (CERT) contractors, and recovery auditors to post a statement to their websites indicating whether they do or do not accept esMD transactions along with a link to an instructional website about how a provider HIH can submit medical documentation via the esMD. MACs and CERT contractors that accept esMD are encouraged to state in their additional documentation request (ADR) how providers can get

more information about using this system. Information about the esMD system can be found at http://www.cms.gov/esMD.

Phase 1 of esMD, which went live in September 2011, allows providers to receive medical documentation requests on paper, but to have the option to electronically send medical documentation to the requesting review contractor. Phase 2, which is in process, will allow providers to receive electronic documentation requests.

In addition to medical documentation requests/responses, the esMD system supports the power mobility devices (PMD) prior authorization request process. As of June 2013, all DME MACs accept these requests through the esMD. The DME MACs, all Recovery Audit Contractors (RACs), Comprehensive Error Rate Testing (CERT) Contractor, Program Error Rate Measurement (PERM) Contractor, Supplemental Medical Review Contractor (SMRC) (Strategic Health Solutions), and ZPIICs for Zones 1, 2, and 7 accept responses to medical documentation requests through esMD systems.

Signature on File (SOF) Requirements

The patient's authorization for the release of confidential medical information is a necessary legal requirement to process medical claims. It is also a requirement by the Medicare program, state Medicaid programs, and all third-party payers, including managed care organizations. Providers and suppliers can retain in their files a blanket signature-on-file authorization form for each patient. In some cases, the patient's legal representative can complete the form. The signature-on-file authorization applies to any current and future services or items the provider or supplier may furnish to the patient. The signature-on-file form is valid for covered services only; it should not be confused with an advance beneficiary notice (ABN) for noncovered services or services deemed not medically necessary. It should be updated when the patient changes insurers, when benefits change, or when the patient's health status changes and a legal representative is assigned to care for the patient's legal matters. The signature-on-file document retained by the provider or supplier can be revoked by the patient or the patient's representative at any time.

Providers and suppliers using electronic claims processing with Medicare and other carriers must obtain the signature-on-file document. To implement this procedure, the supplier must incorporate the following language in addition to the patient's name and ID or policy number into the signature-on-file document to be acknowledged and signed by the patient or their legal representative:

General Billing

"I request that payment of authorized [Medicare or other carrier] benefits be made either to me or on my behalf for any services furnished me by [Name of provider/supplier], including physician services. I authorize any holder of medical or other information about me to release to the [Centers for Medicare and Medicaid Services or other insurance company] and its agents any information needed to determine these benefits or benefits for related services."

Many patient scenarios involve the use of a signature-on-file document, including the following:

- The patient signs the document
- The provider or supplier uses an SOF entry
- An illiterate or handicapped person acknowledges the signature-on-file authority given to the provider or supplier
- A legal representative for the patient provides the signature-on-file authorization

Beneficiary Right to Itemized Statements

Section 4311(b) of the Balanced Budget Act of 1997 provides Medicare patients the right to submit a written request to the provider or supplier for an itemized statement detailing the DMEPOS services or items furnished. Providers and suppliers must comply with the beneficiary's request within 30 days, or risk civil monetary penalties of $100 for each unfulfilled request. Once the patient receives the provider's or supplier's itemized statement, the patient can request the Medicare contractor to conduct a review for specific issues. These can be a range of issues including the following:

- The patient doesn't think these services or items were provided
- There are irregularities in the provider's or supplier's billing that seem suspicious to the patient
- The provider or supplier received overpayment

Medicare contractors routinely advise Medicare patients of their right to an itemized statement. The Explanation of Medicare Benefits (EOMB) and Medicare Summary Notice (MSN) contain the following statement:

. "You have a right to request an itemized statement that details each Medicare item or service you have received from your physician, hospital, or any other health supplier or health professional. Please contact them directly if you would like an itemized statement."

Providers and suppliers cannot charge for furnishing the Medicare patient the itemized statement.

Itemization may mean providing the following information:

- Name of the patient
- Date of service
- Description of the service or item furnished
- Number of services or items furnished
- Provider or supplier charges
- Any internal tracking number used by the provider or supplier
- Amount paid by Medicare
- Patient's coinsurance liability
- Medicare claim number

The provider or supplier should also include the name and telephone number of the contact person at the provider/supplier's office if the patient has questions about the statement.

Medicare Secondary Payer Policies and DMEPOS

Under current federal regulations, it is possible for Medicare to make a secondary payment (e.g., act as the secondary insurer under the Medicare secondary payment (MSP) program), even if the primary insurer reimburses the provider or supplier more than the Medicare-allowed amount. In MSP cases, the patient has other insurance that is considered primary, and Medicare is considered the secondary insurer. A Medicare patient can expect to receive coverage through another primary insurer, such as the following:

- Employer group health plan coverage
- Automobile medical or no-fault insurance
- Liability insurance
- Disability insurance
- Workers compensation
- Federal Black Lung program
- Veteran's Administration claims

When the Medicare contractor receives a claim as the secondary payer, the determination for amount of benefits will be the lower of two calculations:

- The amount Medicare would pay if there was no primary insurer
- The primary insurer's payment minus the higher of the Medicare allowance or primary insurer's allowance

Medicare's final MSP liability is the lower of the two calculations, which is then considered for payment at 100 percent.

For paper claims to be considered for Medicare secondary benefits, a copy of the primary insurer's explanation of benefits (EOB) or remittance notice must accompany the claim form for proper adjudication. If the primary insurance EOB is not submitted, Medicare will deny the claim.

Of particular interest to providers and suppliers of DMEPOS is that for all assigned claims, the secondary insurance claim must be prepared and submitted by the provider or supplier. This is true even in cases when the claim is unassigned (assignment was not accepted by the provider or supplier), but the patient furnishes a copy of the primary insurer's EOB and requests the provider or supplier to submit the claim to Medicare for secondary insurance determination.

Particular rules and regulations must be followed when submitting DMEPOS claims under the MSP for Medicare patients. Details of these rules and regulations fall outside of the scope of this publication; contact the Medicare contractor and the DME MAC for specific guidance.

The MSP can be confusing; the following checklist helps decipher the reason a claim has been denied by Medicare for secondary insurance payment:

- An EOB or denial from the primary insurer was not attached to the claim, or, for an electronic claim, the appropriate field was not completed

- The explanation of the denial code on the primary insurance EOB is missing. The reverse side of the EOB may have to be copied as it is common for this information to appear on the back of the EOB

- The date of service billed to Medicare does not match the date indicated on the primary insurer's EOB

- Charges submitted to Medicare do not match the charges submitted to the primary insurer as seen on the primary insurer's EOB

- Charges sent to Medicare on the secondary insurance claim are for the coinsurance amount only, instead of the full fees for the service

- The EOB attached to the Medicare claim is not from the primary insurance company on file with the Medicare contractor. A statement must be attached to the claim to alert the Medicare contractor in the event the primary insurance company has changed

- The CPT and HCPCS Level II codes on the claim do not match those submitted to the primary insurer

There is one designated contractor who will handle all coordination of benefit (COB) functions for the entire Medicare program. Group Health Incorporated (GHI) has been designated as the COB contractor. The payment safeguard functions have been assigned to one of 12 Program Safeguard Coordinators (PSCs).

These PSCs have been assigned specific tasks and specific geographic areas. Your DME MAC should advise you of the PSC assigned to your area. In some cases, the PSC may be communicating directly with you on certain claims.

The DMEPOS Patient Waiver of Liability

Advance notice to a patient of the likelihood of denial means the patient was sufficiently apprised of the situation before having the item or service furnished. The patient must sign a waiver of liability that absolves the provider or supplier from liability for the item or service, and confirms the patient's financial obligation for the item or service should the payer, in fact, deny it. The waiver of liability should include the following:

- Date of service or date the item was furnished

- Identification of the service or DMEPOS item name; narrative description

- A summarized statement explaining that the payer is likely to deny payment due to its own medical necessity determination

- The patient's agreement to pay, signed and dated before the item is delivered

Obtaining the signed waiver of liability also ensures smoother claims processing and patient billing, as all aspects of the process are known. If the claim is submitted to the carrier for a noncovered or not medically necessary item or service, a denial will ensue. In this situation, patients who signed the liability waiver notice in advance are well aware of their financial obligation and can be billed in person, either on the date-of-service or after the carrier's denial is received.

Providers and suppliers should explain to patients who sign a waiver of liability that it is the payer's own determination that has caused the patient to incur the financial liability for the DMEPOS service or item. In the view of the provider, the item is medically necessary. This medical necessity of the DMEPOS service or item may have to be explained to the patient in basic terms by a clinically trained staff member, if not the practitioner. Providers should always ensure the patient is fully aware of the financial liability before obtaining the patient's signature on the waiver form.

Medicare Coverage for Beneficiaries in State or Local Custody Under a Penal Authority

The OIG conducted a study in 2002 that determined that Medicare was incorrectly paying for services or items for beneficiaries that were in the custody of a state or local penal authority. Regulations in the Social Security Act prohibit Medicare payment for services that are paid directly or indirectly by any governmental entity. Medicare payment may be made only if the state or local law requires individuals to repay the cost of their medical services while in custody. The state or local government entity must also equally enforce these laws by billing all individuals, regardless of payer source, and must pursue the collection of this debt with the same vigor that it pursues other collection of debts.

CMS is attempting to enforce this regulation by adding fields to the CWF that contain the dates that a beneficiary is in state or local custody. All claims submitted will be checked against these date spans.

If a state or local government meets the requirements for payment as noted in the first paragraph, then the provider or supplier must append modifier QJ to claims. This is a line item modifier and it must be added to every service or item billed during the date span of the beneficiary's custody. Claims billed without a modifier for beneficiaries who are in custody will be denied.

If the state or local government does not require all individuals to repay the cost of their care and/or does not attempt to collect this payment from the individual, you will need to bill the appropriate governmental agency. State and local laws vary widely. If you are uncertain as to the details of your area, consult with an attorney or source at the government agency.

Medicaid is a federal program administered by each individual state. Medicaid may not follow the same regulations as Medicare does for this situation. Check with your state Medicaid agency for specific regulations pertaining to covered individuals who are in state or local custody.

Other payers including managed care organizations may or may not specifically address this situation. Coverage for individuals in state or local custody will most likely be addressed in the policy exclusion section of each insurance contract. If the policy does not specifically exclude coverage for this situation, you may bill the insurance carrier.

DMEPOS Claims Jurisdictions

In section 911 of the Medicare Prescription Drug, Improvement, and Modernization Act (MMA), Congress mandated that the Secretary of Health and Human Services replace the current Medicare contracting system. The Centers for Medicare and Medicaid Services (CMS) must use competitive procedures to replace its current fiscal intermediaries (FI) and carriers with a uniform type of administrative entity, Medicare administrative contractors (MAC). These administrative contractors will process both institutional and professional claims in specified geographic jurisdictions of the country. MACs are to

be phased in over the next few years with all jurisdictions to be operational by October 2011.

Home health and hospice will continue to have a specialty MAC separate from the other contractors.

As of August 2008, the SADMERC was replaced by the pricing, data analysis, and coding (PDAC) contractor. The PDAC is located in Fargo, North Dakota and is administered by Noridian Administrative Services, LLC (NAS): https://www.dmepdac.com/.

Palmetto GBA continues to provide the NSC services: http://www.palmettogba.com/palmetto/providers. nsf/DocsCatHome/National%20Supplier%20 Clearinghouse.

For further information, please go to the CMS website at http://www.cms.gov/Medicare/Medicare-Contracting/Medicare-Administrative-Contractors/ MACContractStatus.html.

Each of the DME MACs processes a multitude of individual states' DMEPOS claims within established jurisdictions. DMEPOS claims must be filed to the local Medicare carrier or the DME MAC, depending on the services or DMEPOS furnished. Providers and suppliers must be sure to check with the Medicare carrier bulletins and DME MAC bulletins for accurate claims point submissions, as there may be differences between carriers' guidelines.

The DME MACs adjudicate claims are based on the residence of the patient, not the place of service where the DMEPOS items were furnished (unless the claim in question is a foreign claim, in which case the site of service serves as the DME MAC jurisdiction marker). Suppliers must obtain the patient's permanent address, defined as the place of residence where the patient intends to spend more than six months of the calendar year. Using that information, the provider or supplier must submit the DMEPOS claim to the appropriate DME MAC entity.

DMEPOS Jurisdiction Tables

Each DME MAC entity issues a DMEPOS jurisdiction table on an annual basis (otherwise, this information is available from the DME MAC entity upon request). The tables indicate where the claims should be submitted and provide the HCPCS Level II codes (and code ranges) with general descriptions that must be reported for the DMEPOS items. (Items or services not listed can be referenced in the *Medicare Carriers Manual* or the *DME MAC Supplier Manual*.) The presence of a code in these tables does not guarantee that the Medicare contractor will accept the code, or that it represents a covered service.

Jurisdiction tables are generally issued in the spring. They are effective for July 1 of that year through June 30 of the following year. DMEPOS suppliers should

General Billing

review this table annually to note any changes and ensure that they are billing the correct contractor.

Medicare and DME MAC Claims Denials

Technical Denials

Coverage and exclusion determinations are defined in the Social Security Act, which are implemented through the following:

- Federal regulations and policies in the *Medicare Claims Processing Manual*
- Instructions from CMS
- Decisions made by the individual DME MAC entities that administer the Medicare program for specific items of DMEPOS

Many claim denials fall under the technical category of exclusions. The following are a few of these exclusions that preclude claim reimbursement:

- Disposable items and supplies used by patients at home, other than surgical dressings or supplies required for the effective use of covered DME, prosthetics, or orthotics
- Equipment that does not serve exclusive medical therapeutic functions
- Most oral or self-administered parenteral medications

Other services and items may be denied as not reasonable and necessary for the diagnosis and treatment of illness or injury or to improve the functioning of a malformed body member. These are generally national guidelines issued by CMS and are binding in all DME MAC jurisdictions. The DME MAC entities do have the authority to make medical necessity determinations on aspects of DMEPOS claims not defined by national CMS policy. There is a forced trend, however, for the national coalescence of CMS policy, which is expected to be in full effect in the next several years.

Experimental or investigational services, goods, and supplies are typically denied. Though the Medicare program has authorized coverage for several preventive medicine services and procedures, usually these services are excluded under the technical category as well.

Fragmented coding will lead to claims denials. This situation arises when an individual HCPCS code, one that includes several component items, is billed in addition to the codes for the component items. These are considered not separately payable items. Additionally, the National Correct Coding Initiative (CCI) edits contain many code combinations that, when reported together on a claim, will be denied due to one or more of the following reasons:

- Unbundling
- Using mutually exclusive codes
- Reporting sequential procedures/services
- Reporting separate procedures/services
- Reporting most extensive procedures
- Practicing certain standards of medical and surgical practice
- Including anesthesia in surgical procedures
- Reporting supplemental or add-on services

Truncated diagnosis coding is another coding error that frequently leads to claims denials. Codes having fourth or fifth digits but submitted with fewer digits are termed truncated. All ICD-9-CM diagnostic codes must be submitted at their highest level of specificity; codes should be expanded to the fourth or fifth digits, where applicable. Some codes only have three digits, however, and should not be appended with .0 or .00 to expand them to the fourth and fifth places.

The Advance Beneficiary Notice (ABN) of Noncoverage

The Medicare program puts forth great efforts to educate providers and suppliers. Updates, changes, and new policies are regularly published in bulletins, program memoranda, the *Federal Register,* and various program Internet web sites. Given this level of mass education, most physicians and health care professionals, including suppliers, are anticipating when a denial of reimbursement will occur for certain DMEPOS services or items.

For nonassigned claims, if Medicare adjudicates the claim as not medically necessary, the beneficiary is liable for payment to the provider or supplier. For assigned claims, the provider or supplier is usually held responsible for the item or service. The provider or supplier may not bill the patient for reimbursement. However, there are two major exceptions to this guideline:

- If it is clear and obvious that the patient did know, prior to receiving a service or item, that Medicare payment for that service or item would be denied, liability can shift to the patient. For example, if the patient admits that he or she had prior knowledge that payment for a service or item would be denied, no further evidence is required. No written notice is required.

- If the supplier provided advance notice to the patient in writing before providing the item or service, and if the patient agreed to pay for the item or service if it was denied by Medicare, then the patient would be liable for payment to the provider or supplier.

Advance notice to the patient of the likelihood of denial by Medicare means the patient was sufficiently

General Billing

apprised of the situation before the item or service was furnished to them. Patients must sign an ABN, waiving the provider's responsibility and attesting to their ultimate financial obligation for the item or service should Medicare deny the item or service. The ABN must include the following:

- Date of delivery of the service or item
- Service or item name; narrative description
- A statement that Medicare is likely to deny payment
- An accurate reason why the provider or supplier believes that Medicare is likely to deny payment
- The patient's agreement to pay, signed and dated before the item is delivered

To communicate to the local Medicare contractor or the DME MAC entity that advance notice was furnished and is on file, the HCPCS code for the service or item furnished must be appended with modifier GA. This notifies Medicare that the appropriate guidelines were followed, and allows the patient to obtain a denial from Medicare. The claim in question can then be forwarded to the patient's secondary insurer for possible coverage of the service or item.

For services not covered by Medicare, modifier GZ should be used on claims to indicate that a service or item is expected to be denied, but must still be billed to Medicare to engage the patient's secondary insurance. This modifier is not reported for DMEPOS services or items expected to be denied due to medical necessity issues. Modifier GA must be reported instead.

Equipment and Service Upgrades

The upgrading of equipment and services usually refers to features or enhanced DMEPOS equipment or services that are over and above the covered DMEPOS item. For example: a service may be performed daily when it is covered only as a three times a week service; or a wheelchair may be provided with enhanced or additional equipment that is more than would be medically necessary. An upgrade is an item with features that go beyond what the physician ordered. The extent of, number of, duration of, or expense for an item, feature, or service may be more extensive and/or more expensive than the item or service that is considered reasonable and necessary under the payer's coverage requirements.

Upgraded equipment or services are usually offered in place of the covered equipment or service for one of three reasons:

- The patient may request features or enhancements beyond the usual
- The physician may order a specific item with the enhancements

- The supplier may offer the enhanced equipment or service at no charge.

The last reason may occur when a supplier prefers to carry only higher-level equipment in order to reduce inventory and repair costs. Many payers have specific guidelines for each scenario.

Most payers will generally pay only for the DMEPOS that is necessary for the patient's medical conditions. Specific restrictions and coverage is available from the payer. Many payers may treat upgrades in the same manner as Medicare, which has the most restrictive criteria.

Medicare Requirements for Upgrades

CMS has released several notices about the upgrades of equipment and services for Medicare beneficiaries. This service or equipment is normally not medically necessary. CMS states that guidelines for equipment upgrades apply to both assigned and unassigned claims.

If a supplier provides upgraded equipment at no charge, a modifier is required. Use the HCPCS code for the non-upgraded item and modifier GL. Modifier GL is defined as a medically unnecessary upgrade provided instead of standard item at no charge with no ABN issued. Additionally, the claim should contain only the charge for the non-upgraded item. Item 19 of the claim (or the attachment) must contain the make and model of the upgraded equipment. The supplier further needs to explain why this model is an upgrade. Payment is based on Medicare's payment for the non-upgraded equipment.

CMS will include a message on the Medicare Summary Notice (MSN) and on the remittance that tells the beneficiary that he/she is not liable for any additional charge as the result of receiving an upgraded item or service.

If a beneficiary requests an upgrade, the supplier should have the beneficiary sign an ABN. The ABN should be signed for both assigned and unassigned claims. The ABN should be used when the supplier expects Medicare to reduce the payment and issue a medical necessity partial denial of coverage for the expenses attributable to the upgrade. If an ABN is not signed, the supplier cannot collect from the beneficiary regardless of whether or not the claim was assigned.

The upgrade must be billed as two line items on the same claim. The first line of the claim would contain the HCPCS code for the upgraded DMEPOS item or service with modifier GA or modifier GZ appended. Use modifier GA if an ABN was signed or modifier GZ if no ABN was signed. The second line on the claim must include the appropriate HCPCS code for the DMEPOS that was ordered by the physician. Suppliers must append modifier GK to this line. Modifier GK has the definition of "Actual item or service ordered by physician." Modifier GK cannot be billed alone. It must be used in conjunction with modifier GA or modifier GZ.

The charges submitted on the claim should be the supplier's full charge for the upgraded item or service and the full charge for the physician ordered item or service. Do not bill the expected Medicare allowable as the charge. Both of the DMEPOS items or services must appear in sequential order on the same claim. If the upgrade is within the same HCPCS code, suppliers must submit the two line items on the claim. The first line item for the upgraded DMEPOS should reflect the higher price.

The MSN and remittance will reflect the message that applies to ABNs. If an ABN was signed, the message will state that the beneficiary is liable for payment of the full charge or a portion of the full charge. If an ABN was not signed, the message will tell the beneficiary that they should not pay the supplier and that they are not liable for any charge.

If the physician orders an upgrade, the supplier should bill the HCPCS code for the upgraded item or service. There is no change from prior billing instructions on this issue. The carrier will review the claim and use its discretion to determine if the item or service will be covered. If the supplier believes that the ordered upgrade will not be covered, an ABN should be obtained. The ABN should explain that the physician ordered this upgrade, but Medicare may decide that it is not medically necessary.

In summary:

- An upgrade may be from one item to another within a single HCPCS code description. This would apply if one description is appropriate to either the non-upgraded item or service and the more expensive, enhanced item or service. An upgrade may also be a change from one HCPCS code to another similar HCPCS code

- An upgrade must be within the range of items or services ordered by the attending physician. The item or service must be medically appropriate for the beneficiary's medical condition. ABNs should not be used for substitutions of a different item or service that is not medically appropriate for the beneficiary's medical condition when the original item ordered was medically appropriate

- Having an ABN signed by the beneficiary does not release the supplier from any payment restrictions, coverage provisions, rules, or instructions that apply to the non-upgraded item or service. These issues still apply as if the standard item or service were being provided rather than the upgrade

- If the standard item or service is covered on a rental basis, the upgraded item or service must be provided on a rental basis

- If a supplier has an ABN signed, the claim must indicate the upgraded item or service on the claim. The item or service must be billed with modifier GA when an ABN is signed or with modifier GZ if an ABN was not signed. The upgraded item or service must be listed in Item 19 or as an attachment to the claim whether it is billed on a CMS-1500 form or as an electronic claim

- Any denials should be medical necessity denials

Other Payers

For payers other than Medicare, the supplier should check coverage criteria for upgrades. Medicaid and managed care companies may require prior approval for an upgrade. Some payers may not make any provision for upgrades and may bar the supplier from billing the customer or insured. A supplier should issue a notice of non-coverage, similar to an ABN, if the payer will not cover more than the standard fee schedule amount.

Duplicate Claim Denials

Medicare Duplicate Claims Edits

A duplicate claim is defined as a claim for the same beneficiary, from the same provider or supplier, for the same date of service, for the same HCPCS code. In most circumstances this edit is a valid one.

There are, however, instances where the claim is legitimate and not a duplicate. For example, per CMS, if a pharmacy dispenses several drugs on one date of service, the pharmacy is entitled to a dispensing fee for each drug. Medicare will allow patients to have more than one disposable nebulizer, mastectomy bra, platform for walkers, and similar DME items as identified in the regulations and manuals. For these cases, the DME MAC can override the duplicate claim rejection and pay for all items.

If a duplicate claim rejection is received for a legitimate item, contact your DME MAC and request that they review the denial. If the item can legitimately be dispensed in quantities greater than one per day (or in the case of pharmacy dispensing fees, charged more than once per day), all items may be reimbursed.

Billing Medicare for Non-Covered Items or Services

There may be circumstances when a provider or supplier will submit a bill for a non-covered item or service to Medicare. These circumstances may include claim submission at the beneficiary's insistence or submission to obtain a denial for secondary-payer coverage.

Providers and suppliers may submit the claim with the appropriate modifier attached to the corresponding HCPCS code. Modifiers GA, GY, and GZ apply. If there is no specific HCPCS code to describe the item or supply, use A9270 Non-covered item or service. Code A9270 should be used when the item is statutorily non-covered and does not meet the definition of a Medicare benefit.

If you are billing A9270, describe the item or supply on the claim form or as a claim attachment.

The Purchase and Rental of DMEPOS Items

In many instances, Medicare patients have the option of purchasing or renting (leasing) certain items of DME. Expenses incurred for this are reimbursable if the following requirements are met:

1. **The equipment meets the definition of DME under Medicare guidelines.**

2. **The equipment is necessary and reasonable for the treatment of the patient's illness or injury, or to improve the functioning of the patient's malformed body member.**

Although an item may be classified as DME, it may not be covered for every patient presentation. The previous considerations will bar payment for equipment that cannot reasonably be expected to perform a therapeutic function, or will permit only partial payment when the type of equipment furnished substantially exceeds that required for the treatment of the illness or injury. Sufficient evidence of medical necessity is of particular importance in Medicare coverage determinations for items of DME.

DME is considered medically necessary (eligible for coverage) under the Medicare program when it can be expected to make a meaningful contribution to the treatment of the patient's illness or injury or to the improvement of the patient's malformed body member. In most cases, the provider's prescription for the equipment and other medical information available will be sufficient to establish that the equipment fully serves this purpose and meets this requirement for coverage.

Even though an item of DME may serve a useful medical purpose, the Medicare carrier or DME MAC entity must also consider to what extent, if any, it would be reasonable for the Medicare program to pay for the item prescribed. The following considerations should be made:

- Is the expense of the DME item clearly disproportionate to the therapeutic benefits ordinarily derived from use of the equipment?

- Is the DME item substantially more costly than a medically appropriate and realistically feasible alternative pattern or regimen of care?

- Does the DME item essentially serve the same purpose as other equipment already available to the patient?

Claims for payment of equipment found to be not reasonable will be denied except in cases where it is determined that there exists a medically appropriate and realistically feasible alternative pattern or regimen of care for which payment could be made. In these exceptional cases, Medicare payment will be based on the reasonable charge for this alternative.

3. **The equipment is used in the patient's home.**

For purposes of purchase or rental of DME, a patient's home may be the patient's own dwelling, an apartment, a relative's home, a home for the aged, or some other type of institution. However, an institution may not be considered a patient's home under the following circumstances:

- It meets at least the basic requirement in the definition of a hospital (i.e., it is primarily engaged in providing diagnostic and therapeutic services or rehabilitation services to patients)

- It meets at least the basic requirement in the definition of a skilled nursing facility (i.e., it is primarily engaged in providing skilled nursing care and related services to inpatients, or rehabilitation services for injured, disabled, or sick persons)

If a patient is in an institution or distinct part of an institution that provides the services described above, then the patient is not entitled to have payment made for the purchase or rental of DME since such an institution may not be considered the patient's home.

Renting or Buying DME

The Medicare program provides the option of renting (leasing) certain items of DME, specifically costly items, rather than burdening the beneficiary with the need to purchase the item, alleviating the beneficiary's 20 percent coinsurance amount. The decision to rent or to purchase an item of DME resides strictly with the patient or the patient's legal representative. A rule of thumb in making the decision is to compare the rental charges for the anticipated number of months the DME will be medically necessary to the total purchase price of the item. Note that strict regulations exist under the

Medicare program, as well as state agency Medicaid programs, for the renting of DME such as oxygen, walkers, hospital beds, TENS units, wheelchairs, and other items.

Renting DME and Capped Rental Parameters

A capped rental DME item is one in which the Medicare program will only reimburse the supplier for the rental of the item for a specified period of time. Suppliers must offer patients the option of converting capped rental DME to a purchased status during the DME's 10th continuous rental month (including power-driven wheelchairs not purchased when initially furnished). Patients have one month from the date the supplier makes the offer to accept the purchase option. If the patient does not accept the purchase option, payment continues on a rental basis not to exceed a period of continuous use of longer than 13 months.

After 13 months of rental payments made by Medicare, the supplier must continue to provide the item without charge—other than a charge for maintenance and servicing fees—until medical necessity ends or Medicare coverage ceases. If the patient accepts the purchase option, payment continues on a rental basis not to exceed a period of continuous use of longer than 13 months. On the first day after 13 continuous rental months during which Medicare payment is made, the supplier must transfer the title of the equipment to the patient.

Medicare payment is made on a monthly rental basis not to exceed a period of continuous use of the DME for 13 months or on a purchase option basis, or on a purchase basis for electric wheelchairs. For the first three rental months, the rental fee schedule is calculated to limit the monthly rental to 10 percent of the average allowed purchase price for new equipment during a base period, updated as necessary to account for inflation. For each of the remaining months, the monthly rental is limited to 7.5 percent of the average allowed purchase price.

All claims submitted to the DME MAC entity for consideration for reimbursement must show if the DME is rented or purchased. For a purchased DME, the claim must show whether the equipment is new or used. If the supplier does not indicate whether the equipment is new or used, the carrier will assume that the DME is used. Suppliers must also indicate on claims the amount of the rental or purchase charge. If this information is missing, or the purchase price appears to be out-of-line with charges of other suppliers for the same item, the carrier will make the buy or rent decision based on the prevailing charge for the item.

If interest or carrying charges are imposed on the patient because the supplier has made arrangements for the patient to pay deductible or coinsurance amounts in installments, these charges should be shown on the submitted documentation as well. DME suppliers must notify all patients of the purchase vs. rental options at the time the DME is obtained.

Special Parameters

When DME is available only for purchase, such as when the DME item must be custom made, then the claim is processed by the DME MAC as a DME purchase. When DME is available only as rented DME, then it will be reimbursed as a rented DME item. However, if a similar item of DME is available for purchase in the locality, the supplier must inform the patient that a similar item is available and that the DME MAC will make a rental vs. purchase determination for reimbursement. A similar item is a DME that meets the provider's prescription for the DME. DME is considered available for purchase in a locality if it is available by catalogue purchase in that locality.

There are also special parameters of DME purchase and rental when the DME is $120 or less (in which the DME MAC will generally not authorize a rental option and will cover the equipment outright, provided all other requirements are met or exceeded), and when the Medicare patient alleges financial hardship.

Oxygen Equipment

The Medicare Improvements for Patients and Providers Act of 2008 (MIPPA) repeals the transfer of ownership to the beneficiary for oxygen equipment after 36 months of rental. The supplier will retain ownership of the equipment and be required to provide necessary service to the equipment at no cost to the beneficiary.

DMEPOS Repairs and Maintenance

Payment for DME repairs and maintenance can be made under the Medicare program to both suppliers of DME and patients who have purchased (or are in the process of purchasing) the DME. This extends to payment for expendable and non-reusable items that are essential to the effective use of the DME.

Suppliers or renters of DME equipment usually recover the expenses incurred in maintaining the DME from the rental charges. Because of this, separately itemized charges billed to the Medicare program for repair, maintenance, and replacement of rented equipment are not covered, with a special exception for dialysis equipment. Payment is also not generally made for repair, maintenance, and replacement of patient-purchased equipment requiring frequent and substantial servicing, as well as capped rental equipment and oxygen equipment.

General Billing

DME Repairs

The Medicare program covers repairs to DME that a patient has purchased or is in the process of purchasing when necessary to make the DME serviceable. If the expense for repairs exceeds the estimated expense of purchasing or renting another item of equipment for the remaining period of medical need, no payment will be made for the amount in excess.

DME Maintenance

The Medicare program does not cover the routine or periodic servicing of DME, such as testing, cleaning, regulating, and checking of the patient's equipment. The owner of the DME rather than by a retailer or some other person who may charge the patient generally performs routine maintenance. Normally, purchasers of DME are given operating manuals that describe the type of servicing an owner may perform to properly maintain the equipment. Thus, hiring a third-party contractor to do such work is viewed by the Medicare program as something done for the convenience of the supplier or patient, and is not covered. However, based on the manufacturer's recommendations, the Medicare program covers a more extensive maintenance or repair of the DME that must be performed by authorized technicians. This repair might include, for example, breaking down sealed components or performing tests that require specialized testing equipment not available to the supplier or patient.

Medicare covers the replacement of patient-owned DME in cases of loss or irreparable damage or wear, and in cases when replacement is required due to a change in the patient's condition. Expenses for replacement due to loss or irreparable damage may be reimbursed without a provider's order when Medicare determines the DME still meets the patient's medical needs. However, claims involving replacement equipment necessitated because of wear or a change in the patient's condition must be supported by a new provider's order.

Cases suggesting malicious damage, culpable neglect, or wrongful disposition of equipment will be investigated and denied if the Medicare carrier or DME MAC determines that it is unreasonable to make program payment under the circumstances.

Reasonable charges for delivery of DME, whether rented or purchased, are covered if the supplier customarily makes separate charges for delivery and it is a common practice among other local suppliers.

Renal Dialysis Equipment

Effective January 1, 2011, ESRD services are reimbursed on a bundled prospective payment system (PPS). The ESRD PPS replaces the basic case-mix adjusted composite payment system and the methodologies for the reimbursement of separately billable outpatient ESRD-related items and services. The ESRD PPS provides a single payment to ESRD facilities that covers all the resources used in providing an outpatient dialysis treatment, including supplies and equipment used to administer dialysis in the ESRD facility or at a patient's home, drugs, biologicals, laboratory tests, training, and support services. Since all ESRD PPS payments will be made to the dialysis facility only, the method II home dialysis election was terminated effective December 31, 2010. All method II home dialysis patients became method I patients.

Please see the chapter on *Reimbursement Guidelines* in this book for a list of items subject to ESRD consolidated billing.

DMAC Billing Guidelines

The *Medicare Claims Processing Manual*, Pub. 100-4, chapter 20 details the billing rules for providers and suppliers who bill for DMEPOS. Several items are highlighted in the following list:

Once-a-Month Billing is the Maximum. DMEPOS claims should not be submitted to the DME MAC more than once a month. CMS advises the DME MAC entities to initiate review processes for claims to determine whether or not providers and suppliers are billing too frequently.

Submit DMEPOS Claims in Sequence. Claims must be submitted in sequence for each Medicare patient for continuous periods of service. For example, if certain capped rental equipment is being furnished to a patient from May through August, the supplier should submit the claim for May before submitting the claim for June, and so on.

DMEPOS is by Order Only. CMS warns that suppliers and manufacturers are not permitted to provide DMEPOS to patients unless the patient (or patient's legal representative) or the patient's provider has requested the DMEPOS. CMS says this "is to ensure that the DMEPOS are actually needed." This directive extends to prescription refills for medications and similar supplies as well. The patient "must specifically request refills of repetitive services or supplies before they are dispensed.

"A supplier may not initiate a refill of an order. The supplier must not automatically dispense a quantity of supplies on a predetermined basis." This is consistent with the DME MAC Supplier Manual, which states, "The description of the item (on an order) may be completed by someone other than the physician (usually the supplier). However, the physician must review the order and sign and date it to indicate agreement." But the supplier is prohibited from automatically mailing or delivering DMEPOS to a patient until it is requested.

Requests for Prescriptions. Considering the preceding official instructions to suppliers and manufacturers, CMS states that a request for a refill is different than a request for a renewal of a prescription. "The beneficiary or his/her representative will rarely keep track of when a prescription will run out. The physician is very unlikely to keep track of this either.

The supplier is the one who will need to have the order on file and will know when the prescription will run out and a new order is needed." In these cases, the supplier is expected to take an active role in continuing the patient's prescription by contacting the physician to ask if the order should be renewed.

General Billing

Appeals, Grievances, and Sanctions

Medicare Appeals

Providers and suppliers of DMEPOS have the right to request an adjustment or review of a claim felt to be inaccurately or unfairly adjudicated by the Medicare or DME Medicare administrative contractor (DME MAC) entity. In most cases, it behooves the provider or supplier to have specific internal protocol established for these claim re-evaluation options. There are important steps to follow when pursuing a re-evaluation of a claim determination.

If a supplier requests a review or other type of appeal on a nonassigned claim, the request must be made in writing and a patient authorization must accompany the request. Without the appropriate patient authorization, the request will be denied. Acceptable review requests must also include the following pieces of information:

- Beneficiary name
- Beneficiary date of birth
- Medicare health insurance claim (HIC) number
- Name and address of provider/supplier of item/ervice
- Date of initial determination
- Date of service for which the initial determination was issued (dates must be reported in a manner that comports with the Medicare claims filing instructions; ranges of dates are acceptable only if a range of dates is properly reportable on the Medicare claim form)
- Item and/or service, if any, at issue in the appeal

If the Medicare contractor or DME MAC entity return an initial claim for DMEPOS services or items to the supplier or provider, calling it unprocessable, then there are no immediate appeal rights. The claim must be refiled as a new claim.

CMS has determined that appeal rights should be granted only to the initial claim determination. Some providers and suppliers had been submitting another claim to extend the appeal time frame. Additional claims that duplicate the originally denied claim will be rejected as duplicates. DME MAC remittance remarks and beneficiary notices will be changed to state that the claim was a duplicate of a previously processed claim and that there are no appeal rights for a duplicate claim.

DMEPOS Claims Adjustments

When a claim is processed incorrectly due to an error made by the DME MAC, the provider or supplier can request an adjustment to the claim. In most cases this can be done over the telephone with a DME MAC representative. Examples of DME MAC errors necessitating claims adjustments include the following:

- Incorrect date of death
- Incorrect number of DMEPOS units or services
- Incorrect date of service

DMEPOS Claims Reviews

If a patient, provider, or supplier is dissatisfied with a claim determination for DMEPOS, the dissatisfied party has the right to request an appeal of the claim adjudication. A request for a claims appeal is now more commonly called a request for a review. DMEPOS claims denied due to medical necessity may only be appealed through the review process; claim adjustments cannot be made to these claims.

Parties who hold the right to request a review of a claim include the following:

- The patient
- The patient's choice of a representative
- A provider or supplier who has accepted assignment
- A supplier responsible for indemnification
- Medicaid state agency or the party authorized to act on behalf of the Medicaid state agency

Medicare has a five-level appeals process and each level must be completed before an appeal can proceed to the next level. The five levels are (1) redetermination, (2) reconsideration, (3) administrative law judge, (4) Departmental Appeals Board (DAB) review Appeals Council, and (5) federal court review. The first two levels of appeal are the quickest and least costly for both the contractor and the provider. The majority of claims are resolved at one of these two levels.

Level One—Redeterminations

An initial review can be requested up to 120 days following the initial date of the claim determination, as indicated on the EOMB or electronic remittance notice. In most cases the review is considered an "independent, critical re-examination of the entire claim, by staff that did not participate in the initial decision, along with all medical necessity documentation submitted with the request." Reviews generally include the existing claim information—as originally submitted—along with any pertinent additional documentation, claim modifications, or other material evidence.

A request for redetermination must be filed with the proper contractor based on the Medicare claims processing jurisdiction rules. The jurisdiction for Part B DME claims is the state where the beneficiary resides.

To help ensure that a request for a claim review is processed as swiftly and accurately as possible by the DME MAC entity, the following steps should be taken whenever appropriate:

- Be specific in the request, citing exactly what is to be reviewed by the DME MAC and why it is felt the review of the claim is necessary

- Clearly identify the patient and the claim in question by providing:
  - health insurance claim (HIC) number;
  - date of service;
  - internal control number assigned to the claim;
  - provider's or supplier's NSC number; and
  - provider's UPIN.

- Provide any other specific information that further identifies the claim, including:
  - surgery date;
  - equipment pick up or delivery date;
  - DMEPOS-specific model number, make of the DMEPOS; and
  - purpose or use of the DMEPOS.

- When requesting a review of a claim that involves the review of the CMN as well, be sure all required fields (questions) are completed; be certain the CMN has been certified (signed and dated by the physician or provider)

- Provide additional information that may support the need for the DMEPOS

- Highlight appropriate areas of EOMBs that are included with the request for review

- Ensure handwritten requests for review are completely legible

Requests for reviews do not have to be submitted on the CMS-20027 form, but can be made in writing, and must specifically cite the reason for the request for review. A telephone review can be requested if the claim correction will result in additional payment to the provider or supplier, and the review does not require a formal medical review of the case (many telephone reviews are considered claim adjustments and not true reviews). A request for review may be written on the EOMB if space allows, with any additional information annotated neatly on the EOMB or attached to it.

However, if writing directly on the EOMB will cause the information to appear messy and possibly confuse or mislead the DME MAC officials, it is probably best not to use the EOMB as the format to request the review.

Decisions in answer to the requests for reviews are typically provided within 45 days and must be completed within 60 days of receipt of the request.

If a provider or supplier is still dissatisfied with the outcome once a decision has been rendered by the DME MAC, the provider or supplier has a right to pursue the matter further. This is done by requesting a reconsideration.

The Qualified Independent Contractors (QIC) may be handling medical review appeals for your DME MAC.

Level Two—DMEPOS Reconsiderations

A reconsideration is defined as the second level of appeal following the review process. The reconsideration process essentially gives dissatisfied providers or beneficiaries the opportunity to present the reasons for their dissatisfaction with the way their claims were processed. A QIC adjudicator or clinical health panel conducts a new impartial review and an independent decision is rendered based on the information contained in the hearing file and medical documentation. The provider or beneficiary may request a hearing, in writing, within 180 days after the date of the first formal review determination.

A request for reconsideration must be filed with the proper contractor based on the Medicare claims processing jurisdiction rules. The jurisdiction for Part B DME claims is the state where the beneficiary resides.

The request for a reconsideration must include:

- The beneficiary's name
- The beneficiary's Medicare health insurance claim number
- The specific service and item for which the reconsideration is requested, and the specific date of service
- The name and signature of the party or representative of the party
- The name of the contractor that made the redetermination

As soon as practical, but no later than 30 days after the review, the QIC will issue a decision based on the record developed at the review.

Claimants still dissatisfied with the decision generated by the QIC can request an administrative law judge (ALJ) hearing, so long as the amount in question is $130.00 (singly or in aggregate) for 2012 and $140.00 for 2013. The request for an ALJ must be made within 60 days of the QIC review.

Signatures can be mailed, faxed, or submitted via a CMS approved portal application. A signature stamp or indication that a signature is on file is not acceptable by hard copy or fax.

Level Three—Administrative Law Judge Hearings

Although less than 1 percent of all claims processed ever go beyond the contractor (fiscal intermediary or carrier) level, there are three remaining appeal levels. It would be prudent to request a copy of the appeals file at this time. It will contain all of the information used thus far in the process.

A written request must be filed with the contractor or Health and Human Services Office of Medicare Hearing and Appeals (OMHA) field office within 60 days of the date of the QIC's decision. This is requesting an in-person hearing before a federal administrative law judge (ALJ) from the Office of Hearings and Appeals of the Social Security Administration. Following a QIC Review, and pending a requested ALJ hearing, the provider may submit additional information that might affect the appeal outcome.

Level Four—Departmental Appeals Board Review

If dissatisfied with the ALJ decision, the provider may request an Departmental Appeals Board (DAB) review Appeals Council. This appeal must also be in writing. The request must be received within 60 days of the ALJ decision. It may be submitted to the DAB or ALJ hearing office.

The DAB may review an ALJ's decision/dismissal if:

- There was an error of law
- The ALJ's decision/dismissal was not supported by substantial evidence
- The ALJ abused their discretion
- There is a broad policy or procedural issue that may affect the general public

The ALJs are required to follow all national coverage decisions published in a CMS manual or the *Federal Register*.

Level Five—Federal Court Review

If dissatisfied with the appeals council review, and if the amount in controversy exceeds $1,350.00 for 2012 and $1,400.00 for 2013, the provider may request a hearing before the federal court. This is an extremely expensive proposition and it rarely occurs. Considering the staggering legal fees it would cost to undertake this type of review, it is not often attempted. This final appeal requires the provider to have an attorney file the court papers and have legal representation.

LCD (Local Coverage Determination) Appeals (Reconsiderations)

The LCD reconsideration process is a mechanism by which interested parties can request a revision to an LCD. The whole LCD or any part of the LCD may be reconsidered. Reconsiderations are only accepted for LCDs published in final form. Requests are not accepted for other documents including:

- National Coverage Determinations (NCD)
- Coverage provisions in interpretive manuals
- Draft LCDs
- Template LCDs, unless or until they are adopted by the contractor
- Retired LCDs
- Individual claim determinations
- Bulletins, articles, training materials
- Any instance in which no LCD exists (i.e., requests for development of an LMRP)

LCD Reconsideration Requests

Requests should be submitted in writing. The request must identify the specific language the provider wants changed or deleted. The provider must also submit justification and published evidence to support the request. The level of evidence is the same as that needed to validate the need for a new LCD.

The contractor will determine whether the request is valid or invalid within 30 days. If the request is invalid, the contractor will respond, in writing, to the requestor explaining why the request was invalid.

If the request is determined valid, the contractor will make a final LCD reconsideration decision and notify the requestor of the decision with a rationale within 90 days.

If the contractor decides to not make any changes or to retire the LCD, the provider is notified within 90 days of the day of the request of the decision.

Third-Party Payer Appeals

Most private third-party payers grant the privilege to rebut or appeal a claim determination that is thought by the provider or supplier to have been inaccurately or unfairly adjudicated by the payer.

With the automated provider response systems in use by most major payers, some of the claims that require a reconsideration of benefits can be handled directly over the telephone. These cases frequently involve inaccurate coding and the omission of essential information. In these situations, all of the necessary information for correction or modification of the initial claim submission should be at hand during the telephone appeal. Not all requests for claim reconsideration can be handled in such a convenient fashion. Often a formal or written request for a claim appeal must be submitted to the payer.

A formal request for reconsideration of a claim determination must be made in writing and should be addressed to the payer's provider services unit or department. Many times the payer will provide special forms (such as a Provider Inquiry Form) that must be completed in lieu of a written request by letter. In cases where provider or supplier appeal correspondence to these units has resulted in procrastinated responses or have even been ignored by the payer (e.g., "We haven't received it. Can you send it again?" is a typical response reported by many practices), the payer's area representative can be a good resource in tracking down an appeal and in getting the matter expedited for a second determination. Generally, third-party payers have area representatives who are specifically assigned to geographical areas within the payer's purview.

The written request for an appeal must disclose the reasons the initial claim determination is felt to be inaccurate or unfair. Additional information and other supporting documentation for the service or item should be sent to the payer with the appeal request, including a copy of the original EOB form. The request for the appeal should always outline the reasons for the DMEPOS service or item in relation to the patient's clinical condition, and should detail the medical benefits the provider or supplier expects the patient to derive from the service or item. If a claim for a specialized item of DMEPOS is in question, the unique characteristics of the item, as well as the medical benefits anticipated from its use, should always be clearly discussed in the appeal request.

A claim that has been denied by the payer (not adjudicated or processed) does not usually require an appeal for reprocessing. A claim, once denied, is typically not recorded in the claim processing system, and does not need to undergo appeal procedures, but should simply be amended (in whatever way necessary to have it properly adjudicated) and resent to the payer.

The appeal process can vary among payers. Providers and suppliers should always ascertain the preferred appeal process for each payer. Much of this information can be gathered from the provider's or supplier's participating manual, or from the area payer representative. Some payers provide for an expedited appeal process in cases where delays in a claim reconsideration may be detrimental to the patient's health or long-term recovery potential. The time limit for filing an appeal should be noted and disclosed to all billing staff involved in appeals processes.

Additional Claims Determinations and Grievances

When the provider or supplier remains dissatisfied with the outcome of a claim appeal, most payers provide for yet another claim reconsideration request. These requests are almost uniformly required in writing, and like the written appeal request, they must outline why the physician, provider, or supplier feels the initial and appealed claim determinations were unsatisfactory.

Sometimes these secondary appeal requests are termed a medical director's review, as the plan medical director, or his/her staff will assess the situation and formulate a new claim determination. For some third-party payers, this step is considered the filing of a provider or supplier grievance and is handled by an independent grievance committee. The committee is usually composed of claims adjudication officials, clinical personnel, and the payer's medical director.

Often the outcome of an additional claim appeal, or a grievance filed in connection with a claim determination, is considered final. Participating providers and suppliers cannot bill the patient for the amount in dispute; however, another resource is available that might be of invaluable assistance: the state insurance commissioner.

Insurance Commissioner

Another avenue for providers and suppliers who feel a claim adjudication process has been unfairly undertaken by the third-party payer is to alert the state's insurance commissioner. While the state insurance commissioner's office does not enter into general payment amount disputes, since this is seen as a function of the participating contract that the provider or supplier enters into with the payer, it can assist in the following:

- Unfair reimbursement decisions
- General reimbursement determinations
- A payer's protracted reimbursement time
- A payer's denial to pay a claim for a DMEPOS service or item timely and correctly filed

The billing manager of the provider or supplier should become acquainted with the state's insurance commissioner's role in third-party payer disputes. The insurance commissioner's office can also supply the provider or supplier with essential information, such as:

- State requirements in force for payment floors for claim reimbursement
- A payer's rights when claim data submitted by the health care professional is incorrect or not specific

- Provider or supplier appeal rights, grievance rights, and rights to rebut sanctions established by the state

Any correspondence to the insurance commissioner's office should detail all of the necessary information to address the matter with the payer. Send a copy of the letter to the payer and the patient. The letter should also include copies of EOBs, appeal denial notices, or other third-party payer correspondence related to the claim in question. Copies of pertinent clauses of the provider's or supplier's participating contract should also be included.

Third-Party Payer Sanctions

The imposition of provider and supplier sanctions is a right reserved by the third-party payer, as specified in the participating contract. Sanctions can take the form of a written warning, or can be quite severe, resulting in termination from the plan and notification of the action by the payer to the National Practitioner Data Bank. Termination from the plan can result in isolation of the provider or supplier within the professional community, as this information must be disclosed upon application for privileges to hospitals and participation with other third-party payers and MCOs.severe sanction or termination from the plan occurs when the provider or supplier has rendered substandard care to a plan member. Substandard care, in most cases, means the care has resulted or can result in imminent harm to the patient, whether acute or long-term. Sanctions can also occur when the provider or supplier has breached the participating contract and has ignored fair warnings of such breach.

If a decision is made to terminate the provider or supplier from the plan due to perceived medical negligence, the payer will report the matter to the National Practitioner Data Bank. Termination from a participating contract with a third-party payer, for whatever reason, is generally performed in the following manner:

- The provider* is notified in writing of the termination

- The facts or basis of the termination are fully disclosed to the provider

- The provider's rights to appeal the termination are also fully disclosed

- The provider is apprised of the process to file an appeal of the payer's termination decision

*Provider = physician, other health care provider, or supplier.

The steps for notifying and educating the physician, provider, or supplier about sanctions to be imposed (other than termination from the plan) usually follow the same course as described above.

When the provider or supplier is terminated from the plan, the provider or supplier is typically held to the termination decision until the appeal has been filed and processed. If a reversal is concluded, then the provider or supplier will be reinstated to the plan and all records of the incident will be kept confidential within the plan's files. No record of the proceeding is sent to the National Practitioner Data Bank.

Fraud, Abuse, and Compliance

Introduction

The DMEPOS industry has been under intense scrutiny by the federal government. Suppliers of DME, including providers who dispense DME and providers who certify the DME as medically necessary, have repeatedly surfaced as prominent targets for the Office of the Inspector General's (OIG's) annual work plan. This work plan focuses on almost every segment of the health care industry to expose areas of fraud, waste, and abuse. Physician practices, physician billing companies, DMEPOS suppliers, home health agencies, skilled nursing facilities, laboratories, and hospitals are all currently under the OIG's microscope. Given the fact that the OIG and other federal government agencies claim they have recouped inappropriate payments, overpayments, penalties, and fines of up to several billion dollars, it is unlikely that current aggressive fraud and abuse identification activities will subside.

The best and most powerful method of preventing or defending the provider and supplier's operations against fraud and abuse accusations is to prepare for such events. Preparation includes the following:

- Being fully aware of what composes fraud, abuse, and compliance
- Having a compliance plan that is reasonable and able to be practiced on a daily basis
- Performing internal self-audits

Questions that must be asked with each and every encounter or recertification include those that could incur an audit liability, such as:

- Is a copy of the original Certificate of Medical Necessity (CMN) on file for Medicare patients?
- Is the copy of the provider's order on file (that specifies the patient's exact clinical condition) in support of both the type of hospital bed ordered as well as hospital bed accessories?
- Is the need for the item and for specific accessories, including diagnosis, documented in the patient's clinical notes?

Definitions of Fraud and Abuse

CMS states that fraud occurs when a provider or supplier knowingly and willfully deceives the Medicare program, or misrepresents information, to obtain the benefit of monetary value, resulting in unauthorized Medicare payment to themselves or to another party.

The violator may act individually or in agreement with others, and may include a participating or nonparticipating provider, a supplier of DMEPOS, a Medicare patient, or even an individual or business entity unrelated to a patient.

Defrauding the Medicare program of federal monies includes but is not limited to the following practices:

- Billing for services or supplies that were not provided. This includes billing the Medicare program for no-show patients or DMEPOS clients
- Altering claim forms to obtain higher payment amounts
- Deliberately submitting claims for duplicate payment
- Soliciting, offering, or receiving a kickback, bribe, or rebate. Common examples of these practices are (1) paying an individual or business entity for the referral of a patient and (2) routinely waiving a patient's deductible or coinsurance
- Providing falsified CMN forms for patients not professionally known by the provider or supplier, or a supplier completing a CMN for the provider (in effect, ordering DMEPOS not originating from the provider's orders)
- Falsely representing the nature, level, or number of services rendered or the identity of the patient, dates of service, and so forth. This includes billing a telephone call as if it was an actual patient visit
- Being involved in collusion, whether between a provider and a patient or a provider and a supplier, resulting in higher costs or unnecessary charges to the Medicare program
- Using another person's Medicare card to authorize services for a different patient or non-Medicare patient
- Altering claims history records to generate fraudulent payment
- Repeatedly violating the assignment agreement or limiting charge amounts
- Falsely representing provider ownership in a clinical laboratory
- Using the Medicare program's name or logo without authorization. A person or entity may

use neither the Medicare program's name nor logo in marketing or other efforts, and cannot use the Social Security emblem in advertising for items or services as Medicare approved

Most state Medicaid programs and many third-party payers follow the same basic outline for the definition of abuse.

CMS defines abuse of the federal Medicare program as "incidents or practices of providers, physicians, or suppliers of services and equipment which are inconsistent with accepted sound practices." Although often these incidents or practices cannot be considered flagrantly fraudulent, in some cases they may directly or indirectly result in unnecessary costs to the federal Medicare program. One of the most prevalent kinds of abuse is overutilization of medical and health care services.

Abuse of federal monies supporting the Medicare program includes but is not limited to the following practices:

- Excessive charges for services, procedures, or supplies

- Claims for services not medically necessary, or for services not medically necessary to the extent rendered. For instance, a panel of tests is ordered when, based upon the patient's working diagnosis, only a few of the tests within the panel were actually necessary

- Breaches of assignment agreements resulting in patients being billed for disallowed amounts

- Improper billing practices, such as when the provider exceeds the Medicare imposed limiting charge (115 percent of the Medicare—allowed amount for nonparticipating providers and for all providers of certain other services)

- The submission of claims to Medicare when another third-party payer, managed care organization (MCO), or workers compensation carrier is the primary payer

- Higher fee charges for Medicare patients than for non-Medicare patients

Again, many state Medicaid programs and third-party payers follow a similar definition when identifying abusive provider and supplier activities. Under the auspices of HIPAA, private payers have also been empowered to conduct fraud and abuse detection and prevention activities.

Definition of Compliance

Compliance is a broad term that has been applied to certain administrative aspects of health care in recent times. Compliance specifically encompasses the appropriate coding, billing (reporting), and documentation of medical services. In particular, being in compliance suggests the correct reporting of

health care services to federal programs such as Medicare or the Children's Health Insurance Program (CHIP). This also applies to other federally funded programs, such as state Medicaid or medical assistance. Likewise, being in compliance is often germane to correctly documenting and billing health care services under participating contracts with third-party payers, such as Blue Cross/Blue Shield and Aetna/U.S. Healthcare. Compliance edicts may also be imposed by other payers, such as many of the common private or commercial third-party payers; MCOs, including preferred provider organizations (PPOs) and health maintenance organizations (HMOs); workers compensation carriers; and self-funded plans.

Noncompliance can lead to expulsion from private payers, hefty penalties, and possible criminal charges. Expulsion from a major health care plan such as Blue Cross/Blue Shield can permanently harm a provider's or supplier's DMEPOS business. Numerous payers consistently publish the names of sanctioned providers and suppliers. This can potentially lead to an irreparably damaged professional reputation for the exposed provider or supplier.

Criminal and Civil Statutes

Fraud and abuse against the Medicare program may be prosecuted under a variety of provisions of the United States code. A number of criminal and civil statutes are used to prosecute fraud and abuse cases involving the Medicare and Medicaid programs.

The laws used most commonly to prosecute for Medicare fraud and abuse include the Medicare-Medicaid Anti-Fraud and Abuse Amendments to the Social Security Act, the federal False Claims Act, Civil Monetary Penalties, and Assessments and Exclusion from Program Participation. It is a felony to steal from the Medicare program under these laws and depending on the validity of the case, penalties may result in criminal prosecution, civil proceedings, or administrative sanctions that may result in restitution, fines, imprisonment, and exclusion from the Medicare program.

In cases of suspected Medicare fraud and abuse, the United States attorney's office decides whether to file a civil suit or settle a case. Convicted individuals are required to pay back what was stolen plus additional fines, and they are barred from doing business with Medicare in the future. The amount stolen plus additional money is paid to the government in the form of penalties and fines as further defined below. Administrative sanctions include taking action to exclude the provider from the Medicare program, referral to state licensing boards of medical or professional societies, or withdrawal of favorable waiver presumption.

CMS and the OIG have the authority to suspend, exclude, or terminate payment to providers, practitioners, and suppliers of Medicare services. The laws used to support this authority are described below.

Fraud Alerts

To keep providers and payers informed of fraud and abuse issues, OIG and CMS periodically issue national fraud alerts. The alerts are usually issued when there is a need to advise Medicare carriers, fiscal intermediaries (FIs), the quality improvement organizations (QIOs), providers, and beneficiaries about an activity that involves false claims. Not all of the alerts pertain to all providers, however, it is important for providers to keep abreast of the issues currently under investigation.

The alerts are for educational and informational purposes so that providers and suppliers can become more aware of fraudulent situations. Claims that are denied based on these fraud alerts will be denied based on facts obtained independent of the alerts.

OIG Fraud Alerts

The OIG issues special fraud alerts to address problems it is identifying in the health care industry. The alerts put the health care industry on notice that the OIG is pursuing certain abusive practices. They are the initial tools used to get providers to review their practices and comply with Medicare regulations. The OIG distributes the alerts directly to Medicare providers and publishes new fraud alerts in the Federal Register.

CMS National Fraud Alerts

CMS fraud alerts represent examples of fraudulent and abusive billing practices that are currently being investigated and hope to be prevented in the future. CMS issues national alerts when the fraud or abuse is perceived or has the potential to be widespread (i.e., crossing contractor [fiscal intermediary or carrier] jurisdictions).

Federal Fraud and Abuse Investigative Programs

The federal government's war on fraud and abuse has been aggressive over the past several years, and only continues to intensify. Spearheaded by the OIG of the Department of Health and Human Services (DHHS), the FBI, the Department of Justice (DOJ), and CMS, the federal government has been successful in consistently uncovering what it deems "fraudulent activities aimed at the Medicare and Medicaid programs." Whether or not the providers or suppliers actually intended to commit fraud is another matter; these successful efforts have fueled and increased the intensity and number of federal (and state)

investigations, and there have been more indictments and convictions as a result.

A number of disparate programs and initiatives have evolved out of the DHHS. They include the following:

Annual OIG Workplan. In conjunction with CMS, the Public Health Service (PHS), and the Administrations for Children, Families, and Aging (all DHHS entities), the OIG Annual Workplan mission statement reads, in part, "We improve HHS programs and operations, and protect them against fraud, waste and abuse. By conducting independent and objective audits, evaluations and investigations, we provide timely, useful and reliable information and advice to Department officials, the Administration, the Congress, and the public." The OIG Workplan assists the DHHS in pursuing criminal convictions by recovering maximum dollar amounts through judicial and administrative methods, and recycling recouped program monies back into the federal programs.

Medicare Fraud Strike Force. The strike force investigates and tracks down individuals and entities defrauding Medicare and other government health care programs. The Medicare Fraud Strike Force operations are part of the Health Care Fraud Prevention and Enforcement Action Team (HEAT), a joint initiative announced in May 2009 between the DOJ and HHS. HEAT aims to focus their efforts on the prevention and deterrence of fraud and on the enforcement of antifraud laws around the country. Since its inception through February 2011, Strike Force operations in nine districts have charged over 1,000 individuals who have falsely billed Medicare for more than $2.3 billion.

OIG's Most Wanted Fugitives List. February 2011 marked the beginning of the OIG's Most Wanted Fugitives List. The list seeks to focus public attention on the individuals most sought by authorities on charges of health care fraud and abuse. CMS is working to promote this list to beneficiaries, providers, and other stakeholders, and engage proactive participation in efforts to track down these fugitives.

Blow the Whistle on Medicaid Fraud Initiative. CMS is trying to educate the public and to encourage reporting of suspected abuses to government entities. To this end, the agency is hosting outreach conferences to educate the states, contractors, and others about provider fraud and abuse.

Regional Summits on Prevention. HHS, which includes CMS and the OIG, and the DOJ have co-hosted a series of regional summits on health care fraud prevention. These summits bring together federal and state officials, law enforcement experts, private insurers, health care providers, and beneficiaries for a comprehensive discussion on the scope of fraud, weaknesses in the current health care system, and opportunities for collaborative solutions.

Fraud and Abuse Hotline. HHS has expanded the 1-800-HHS-TIPS hotline for reporting fraud in the Medicare and Medicaid programs. Since 1995, more than 32,000 tips and complaints called into the program have warranted specific follow-up action.

Medicare Integrity Program

The Health Insurance Portability and Accountability Act (HIPAA) includes a provision formally establishing the Medicare Integrity Program (MIP). CMS has had a MIP in place for several years. This provision gives CMS the authority to enter into contracts with entities to promote the integrity of the Medicare program. MIP was established, in part, to strengthen CMS's ability to deter fraud and abuse in the Medicare program. There are basically two overall areas of concern. One area deals with the Coordination of Benefits (COB) functions that ensure that Medicare is appropriately paying for services when any other type of insurance covers the beneficiary.

The second area of concern is the safeguard or monitoring and integrity of the data and payment of Medicare services.

CMS has issued a pamphlet aimed at physicians, providers, and suppliers to provide information on the MIP. The information explains how the program works, answers questions, and promotes the goal of program integrity to pay it right the first time and to pay the right amount to the right provider, for the right service, to the right beneficiary.

Medicare has two prepayment review programs intended to assist in the identification of billing and reporting errors. These are the National Correct Coding Initiative (NCCI) Edits and the Medically Unlikely Edits (MUE).

CMS developed the NCCI to promote national correct coding methodologies and to control improper coding that leads to inappropriate payment in Medicare Part B claims. NCCI policies are based on coding conventions defined in the American Medical Association's (AMA's) Current Procedural Terminology (CPT) manual, Healthcare Common Procedure Coding System (HCPCS) manual, national and local Medicare policies and edits, coding guidelines developed by national societies, standard medical and surgical practice, or current coding practice. NCCI edits are updated quarterly. NCCI edits are available to the public on the NCCI website: http://www.cms.hhs.gov/NationalCorrectCodInitEd/.

CMS established units of service edits for Medicare Part B benefit claims, referred to as MUEs. An MUE for a CPT or HCPCS Level II code is the maximum units of service under most circumstances that a provider would report for a code for a single patient on a single date of service. Not all codes have an MUE, and not all MUEs are published.

MUEs are based on anatomic considerations, code descriptions, CPT coding instructions, established CMS policies, the nature of service or procedure, the nature of equipment, and clinical judgment. There are quarterly updates to MUEs on the same schedule as the quarterly updates to NCCI. CMS continues to add MUEs for additional HCPCS/CPT codes in these updates.

Providers and suppliers reporting DMEPOS items most likely will not be affected by the NCCI edits, but may find claims returned due to MUEs. Claim lines that pass the MUE edits continue to be processed. On facility claims, the claim is returned to the provider for correction when a line item fails the MUE. When a line item fails the MUE on physician and supplier claims, the line item is denied. Claim line denials can be appealed.

Program Safeguard Coordinators (PSCs)/Zone Program Integrity Contractor (ZPIC)

CMS has awarded Indefinite Delivery, Indefinite Quantity (IDIQ) contracts to PSCs or ZPICs to perform program integrity and data analysis activities as defined in specific task orders. A PSC or ZPIC can perform one, some, all, or any sub-set of the work associated with the following payment safeguard functions:

- Medical review

- Cost report audit

- Data analysis

- Provider education

- Fraud detection and prevention

- Medical utilization and fraud review including the review of claims, medical records, and medical necessity documentation and the analysis of utilization patterns for inappropriate use of services

- Identification of MSP situations

Among other activities, the PSCs or ZPICs will review claims on both a post- and prepayment basis. They will be able to deny claims for several reasons including services that are not covered, services that are not reasonable and necessary, and services that are not billed in compliance with local and national billing requirements. PSCs or ZPICs will do targeted claims reviews of services that are at high risk of being noncovered, misrepresented, or fraudulent. They will also do random reviews of all types of claims as well as task orders issued by CMS.

These organizations may be responsible also for conducting Coordinated Comprehensive Provider Reviews when they suspect fraud or abuse or that an overpayment has occurred. These reviews will involve a thorough analysis of a provider's processed claims and claims data, including medical records, beneficiary payment history, and other documentation.

Many companies submitted proposals to perform any or all of these functions. Contracts were awarded to one or more companies depending on the scope of each task order.

Program Integrity

The *Medicare Program Integrity Manual* (PIM), CMS Pub. 100-08, is one of the completely online manuals, available on the Internet at http://www.cms.hhs.gov/Manuals/IOM/list.asp. The PIM details benefit integrity action taking place all across CMS and its contractors. The chapters in this manual are as follows:

Chapter 1.   Overview of Medical Review (MR) and Benefit Integrity (BI) Programs

Chapter 2.   Data Analysis

Chapter 3.   Verifying Potential Errors and Taking Corrective Actions

Chapter 4.   Benefit Integrity

Chapter 5.   Items and Services Having Special DME Review Considerations

Chapter 6.   Intermediary MR Guidelines for Specific Services

Chapter 7.   MR Reports

Chapter 8.   Administrative Actions and Statistical Sampling for Overpayment Estimates

Chapter 9.   Reserved for Future Use

Chapter 10. Medicare Provider/Supplier Enrollment

Chapter 11. Fiscal Administration

Chapter 12. Comprehensive Error Rate Testing Program

Chapter 13. Local Coverage Determinations

Chapter 14. National Provider Identifier

Chapter 15. Medicare Enrollment

Exhibits

This manual details the actions taken by medical review departments, gives information about the progressive corrective action program, discusses particular risk areas, and talks to contractors about dealing with the new program safeguard contractors.

Recovery Audit Contractors

The Medicare Prescription Drug, Improvement, and Modernization Act (MMA) of 2003 required CMS to conduct a demonstration project to identify Medicare underpayments and overpayments and to recoup overpayments for Part A and Part B services. This was entitled "Demonstration Project for Use of Recovery Audit Contractors." Recovery audit contractors (RAC) were any non-Medicare secondary payer (MSP) recovery audit contractors tasked with identifying and correcting improper Medicare payments through the efficient detection and collection of overpayments made on claims of health care services provided to Medicare beneficiaries, and the identification of underpayments to providers. The demonstration project ran between 2005 and 2008 and resulted in more than $900 million in overpayments being returned to the Medicare Trust Fund and nearly $38 million in underpayments returned to health care providers. Congress then required the Secretary of the Department of Health and Human Services to institute a permanent and national recovery audit program.

The mission of the current RAC program is to identify and correct Medicare and Medicaid improper payments through the efficient detection and collection of overpayments made on claims for health care services provided to Medicare and Medicaid beneficiaries, and the identification of underpayments to providers so that the Centers for Medicare and Medicaid Services (CMS) and states can implement actions that will prevent future improper payments. In addition, recovery auditors are responsible for highlighting common billing errors, trends, and other Medicare payment issues to CMS.

The CMS oversees several different RAC programs, such as those for fee-for-service (FFS) Medicare and Parts C and D. States oversee their own Medicaid recovery audit programs in accordance with federal guidelines set by CMS.

Each recovery auditor is responsible for identifying overpayments and underpayments in their area with the country being divided into four areas. The RAC jurisdictions match the DME MAC jurisdictions. The RAC in each region is as follows:

- Region A (CT, DC, DE, MA, MD, ME, NH, NJ, NY, PA, RI, and VT): Performant Recovery

- Region B (IL, IN, KY, MI, MN, OH, and WI): CGI Federal, Inc

- Region C (AL, AR, CO, FL, GA, LA, MS, NC, NM, OK, SC, TN, TX, VA, WV, Porto Rico, and U.S.Virgin Islands): Connolly, Inc.

- Region D (AK, AZ, CA, HI, IA, ID, KS, MO, MT, ND, NE, NV, OR, SD, UT, WA, WY, Guam, American Samoa, and Northern Marianas): HealthDataInsights, Inc.

RACs are paid on a contingency basis. The RAC receives a percentage of under- and overpayments that it identifies. The Medicare fee for service (FFS) RAC program consists of a number of payment systems. It has a network of contractors that process more than one billion claims each year, submitted by more than one million health care providers, including hospitals, physicians, skilled nursing facilities (SNF), labs, ambulance companies, and durable medical equipment, prosthetics, orthotics, and supplies (DMEPOS) suppliers. These Medicare Administrative Contractors (MAC) process claims, make payments to providers in accordance with Medicare regulations, and educate providers on how to submit accurately coded claims that meet Medicare guidelines.

In fiscal 2013, RACs collectively identified and corrected 1,532,249 claims for improper payments, which resulted in $3.75 billion dollars in improper payments being corrected. The total corrections identified include $3.65 billion in overpayments collected and $102.4 million in underpayments repaid to providers and suppliers. After taking into consideration all fees, costs, and first-level appeals, the Medicare FFS RAC program returned more than $3 billion to the Medicare Trust Funds. These savings do not take into account program costs and administrative expenses incurred at the third and fourth levels of appeal (Office of Medicare Hearings and Appeals [OMHA] and Medicare Appeals Council within the Departmental Appeals Board [DAB], respectively), which are funded through a different avenue.

In late fiscal 2012, CMS implemented a demonstration to use recovery auditors for the purpose of reviewing claims before they are paid. Fiscal 2013 was the first full year of the RAC prepayment review demonstration. The demonstration started on September 1, 2012 and is scheduled for three years in the following 11 states: Florida, California, Michigan, Texas, New York, Louisiana, Illinois, Pennsylvania, Ohio, North Carolina, and Missouri. The goal of the demonstration is to lower the number of improper payments for those claims, which are shown through Comprehensive Error Rate Testing (CERT) reports and other data analysis to have high rates of improper payments. This demonstration has shown that RACs have prevented $22.3 million in improper payments by reviewing claims before they were paid. (CMS website: http://www.cms.gov/Research-Statistics-Data-and-Systems/Monitoring-Programs/Medicare-FFS-Compliance-Programs/Recovery-Audit-Program/.)

Physician Order Fraud

The OIG's office published a special fraud alert in the *Federal Register* concerning physician liability for certifications in the provision of DMEPOS. The OIG's special fraud alerts typically address national trends in health care fraud, including potential violations of the Medicare anti-kickback statute. The special fraud alert related to DMEPOS specifically highlighted providers' responsibilities in making certifications for DMEPOS and the legal significance of these certifications.

The fraud alert addressed the following aspects of a provider's involvement in the DMEPOS certification process:

- The importance of physician and provider certification for Medicare patients

- How improper physician and provider certifications can foster fraud

- The potential consequences for knowingly signing a false or misleading certification, or signing such certification with reckless disregard for the truth

While the OIG believes that the actual incidence of providers who intentionally submit false or misleading CMN forms for durable medical equipment is relatively infrequent, provider laxity in reviewing and completing these certifications contributes to fraudulent and abusive practices by unscrupulous DMEPOS suppliers and home health agencies.

All providers should be aware that they are subject to criminal, civil, and/or administrative penalties if they sign a CMN form or physician order for DMEPOS knowing that the information relating to medical necessity is false, or if they sign a certification with reckless disregard for the truth of the information being submitted. While a provider can mistakenly sign a false or misleading certification (by simple, unintended negligence or by inadvertently agreeing to or omitting critical details), the provider may unwittingly facilitate the perpetration of supplier fraud. It is important that all providers and their coding or billing staff be aware of this information.

The OIG has found numerous examples of providers who have ordered DMEPOS—or more commonly have signed CMN forms—without reviewing the medical necessity for the item, or who have signed the CMN without even knowing the patient.

Certificate of Medical Necessity and DME MAC Information Form

Medicare requires claims for certain kinds of DME to be accompanied by a CMN form, signed and dated by the treating provider (unless the DME is prescribed as part of a plan of care for home health services). When a CMN is required, the provider or supplier must keep on file the CMN. The Medicare contractor may request these documents at any time.

A DME MAC Information Form (DIF) is completed and signed by the supplier. Narrative descriptions of the equipment, cost, and physician signatures are not required on a DIF. The supplier must keep a copy of the DIF.

Forms can be found at http://www.cms.gov/CMSForms/CMSForms/list.asp#TopOfPage.

Generally, a CMN form has four sections that must be completed:

- Section A contains general information on the patient, supplier, and provider. The supplier may complete section A.

- Section B contains the medical necessity justification for the DME. The supplier cannot complete this area. The provider, a nonphysician clinician involved in the care of the patient, or a physician employee must complete section B. If the provider did not personally complete section B, the name of the person who did complete section B and the person's title and employer must be specified.

- Section C contains a description of the equipment and its cost. The supplier completes section C.

- Section D is the treating provider's attestation and signature, which certifies that the provider has reviewed sections A, B, and C of the CMN, and that the information in section B is true, accurate, and complete. Signature stamps and date stamps are acceptable.

By signing the CMN, the ordering provider attests to the following:

- He/she is the patient's treating provider and the information regarding the provider's address and unique physician identification number (UPIN) or National Provider Identifier (NPI) is correct

- The entire CMN, including the sections filled out by the supplier, was completed before the provider's signature

- The information in section B relating to medical necessity is true, accurate, and complete to the best of the ordering provider's knowledge

Improper or Unauthorized CMN Forms

Unscrupulous suppliers and providers may steer other providers into signing or authorizing improper CMN forms. In some instances, the certification forms or statements are completed by DMEPOS suppliers and presented to the provider, who then signs the forms without verifying the actual need for the items or services. In many cases, the provider may obtain no personal benefit when signing these unverified orders, and is only accommodating the supplier or other provider. When the provider knows the information is false or acts with reckless disregard for the truth of the statement, the provider risks incurring criminal, civil, or administrative penalties.

Providers may receive compensation in exchange for their signatures. Compensation can take the form of cash payments, free goods, free or reduced rent, patient referrals, supplies, equipment, or free labor. Even if the provider does not receive any financial or other benefits, they can be held liable for making false

or misleading certifications. Such cases may trigger additional criminal and civil penalties under the anti-kickback statute.

The following are examples of inappropriate certifications uncovered by the OIG in the provision of DMEPOS items:

- At the prompting of a DMEPOS supplier, a provider signs a stack of blank CMN forms for transcutaneous electrical nerve stimulator (TENS) units. The CMNs are later completed with false information in support of fraudulent claims for the equipment. The false information purports to show that the provider ordered and certified the medical necessity for the TENS units for which the supplier has submitted claims.

- A provider accepts fees from a DMEPOS supplier for each prescription the provider signs for oxygen concentrators and nebulizers.

- A provider submits a claim with a UPIN/NPI that is different than the UPIN/NPI of the physician who signed the CMN. CMS recently reported that a study of DME claims revealed that a high volume were ordered or referred using UPINs/NPIs of deceased physicians. In these instances, the physician who signed the CMN was alive, but the UPIN/NPI of a different deceased physician was submitted.

Fraud Related to CMN Forms and DMEPOS Orders

A provider is generally not personally liable for erroneous claims due to mistakes, inadvertence, or simple negligence. However, knowingly signing a false or misleading CMN form or DMEPOS order, or signing these documents with reckless disregard for the truth, can lead to serious criminal, civil, and administrative penalties, including the following:

- Criminal prosecution

- Fines as high as $10,000 per false claim, plus triple damages

- Administrative sanctions, including exclusion from participation in federal health care programs, withholding or recovery of payments, and disciplinary actions by state regulatory agencies or loss of license

Realigning Internal Operations

The internal operations of the provider's practice or supplier's medical equipment company should always be geared to securing patient understanding and acknowledgment of services rendered. This is a simple but effective tactic in avoiding frivolous malpractice accusations or suspicions of fraud and abuse under Medicare and state Medicaid programs. Most malpractice carriers would agree that the number of malpractice claims drops when there is effective

Fraud, Abuse, Compliance

communication between patients and providers. Patients must understand all of the billing processes and requirements related to securing their own medical care benefits for DMEPOS, so they do not misinterpret information and report it as possible fraud. Given that many Medicare patients are elderly, the likelihood of confusion about DMEPOS items and services is probably greater than if most were younger patients. If a legal guardian handles the patient's business affairs, the guardian should be aware of medical services provided to the patient.

This educational approach takes a combined effort by all staff members and may require a realignment of internal operations. Providers and clinical staff should always explain specific services before they are rendered, and why these services are needed. For medical providers, checkout staff should review the superbill or encounter form with each patient as the patient is departing, and explain the coinsurance and deductible rules. The supplier's technical and billing staff should review the needed DMEPOS item with the patient. Provider and supplier billing personnel should further reinforce this sometimes fragile bridge of understanding between the patient and the provider or supplier by (1) being clinically informed so they are able to answer questions about clinical services, and (2) being able to answer all billing questions with confidence.

The OIG's Compliance Program Guidance for the DMEPOS Industry

Released by the OIG in June 1999, the Compliance Program Guidance for the DMEPOS Industry is designed to assist in the elimination of fraud, waste, and abuse. The compliance program guidance is completely voluntary, and follows the basic outlines used in the OIG's program guidance for other areas of the health care community (hospitals, laboratories, home health agencies, etc.). It contains the seven major elements the OIG has determined as fundamental to an effective compliance program:

- Implementing written policies, procedures, and standards of conduct

- Designating a compliance officer and/or a compliance committee

- Conducting effective training and education programs for pertinent employees

- Developing effective lines of communication

- Enforcing standards through well-publicized disciplinary guidelines

- Conducting internal monitoring and auditing

- Responding promptly to detected offenses and developing corrective actions

Recognizing the size differentials of the organizations that make up the DMEPOS industry, the OIG crafted the compliance program guidance to be applicable in numerous DMEPOS settings regardless of company size, number of locations, type of DMEPOS items or services provided, or corporate structure. The actual applicability of the recommendations and guidelines provided in the compliance program depends on the circumstances of each individual DMEPOS provider or supplier.

The *Federal Register* dated October 5, 2000, contained an important notification for providers, particularly for the solo practitioner and for small group providers. Entitled "OIG Compliance Program for Individual and Small Group Physician Practices," this notice attempts to assist physician practices in the development of a useful compliance plan. It also forewarns providers about the importance of internal detection, prevention, and continual monitoring of health care fraud and abuse. The seven major elements listed above remain the same. The official appendices to this notification address reasonable and necessary services (including advice about the completion and certification of CMNs), physician relationships with hospitals, physician billing services, and other risk areas including kickbacks and unlawful advertising.

Lines of Communication

The OIG suggests that the DMEPOS supplier establish protocols to increase the communication among treating providers, the patients, and the DMEPOS supplier. It recommends that such protocols be included in the DMEPOS supplier's written policies and procedures. These protocols may include:

- The DMEPOS supplier periodically calling the patient to ensure the equipment is still being used and is operating properly

- The DMEPOS supplier periodically calling the treating provider to ensure the provided items continue to be medically necessary for a patient

In addition, it is recommended the DMEPOS supplier create mechanisms to ensure communication between different departments within its own company (such as sales and billing) to prevent the filing of incorrect claims.

Anti-Kickback and Self-Referral Concerns

The DMEPOS supplier must have established policies and procedures for compliance with federal and state laws, including the anti-kickback statute and the Stark physician self-referral law. These policies and procedures should address the following issues:

- The DMEPOS supplier's contracts and arrangements with actual or potential referral sources (such as providers) are reviewed by counsel (if appropriate) and comply with all applicable statutes and regulations, including the anti-kickback statute and the Stark physician self-referral law.

- The DMEPOS supplier will not submit or cause to be submitted to health care programs claims for patients who were referred to the DMEPOS supplier pursuant to contracts or financial arrangements that were designed to induce such referrals in violation of the anti-kickback statute or similar federal/state statute or regulation, or that otherwise violate the Stark physician self-referral law.

- The DMEPOS supplier does not offer a provider or other referral source more than fair market value for space rented to store items or supplies (e.g., consignment closet).

- The DMEPOS supplier does not offer or provide gifts, free services, or other incentives or things of value to patients, relatives of patients, physicians, home health agencies, nursing homes, hospitals, contractors, assisted living facilities, or other potential referral sources for the purpose of inducing referrals that violate any anti-kickback statute or federal or state statute or regulation.

Further, the OIG recommends that the written policies and procedures should specifically reference and take into account the OIG's safe harbor regulations, which describe those payment practices that are immune from criminal and administrative prosecution under the anti-kickback statute.

Auditing and Monitoring

Auditing and monitoring—two of the most important elements of a compliance program—must work in harmony toward a common goal.

Audits, according to the OIG's compliance program guidance, determine whether a provider is complying with laws governing medical coding and billing, marketing, and other high-risk areas. Audits can be done internally or externally.

Monitoring is the job of the compliance officer or a regulatory affairs or legal department worker. Monitoring includes identifying variations from an established baseline and then measuring improvement. Establish baselines when providing a new service or compliance program. Auditors can provide a basic listing of operations to use as the baseline to manage potential areas of vulnerability. Determine the root cause of any significant adverse variation from the baseline. Then, correct the problem and monitor it for a reasonable period to make sure the issue does not resurface.

Use on-site visits, interviews, questionnaires, forms and written materials reviews, and trend analyses to monitor compliance. Consider the following tips when monitoring:

- Stay independent of line management
- Maintain access to all personnel and documentation
- Present written evaluation reports to governing bodies
- Identify areas where corrective actions are needed

An ongoing internal evaluation or auditing process is critical to a successful compliance program. The extent and frequency of the evaluation or audit may vary depending on:

- The size of the provider's practice or the DMEPOS supplier's company
- The resources available
- The provider or supplier's prior history of noncompliance
- The risk factors that might be inherent in a particular DMEPOS supplier

Although many monitoring techniques are available, one effective tool to promote and ensure compliance is the performance of regular, periodic compliance audits by internal or external auditors who have expertise in federal and state health care statutes, regulations, and other requirements. The audits should focus on the different aspects or departments of the provider or supplier, including external relationships with third-party contractors. At a minimum, these audits should address the DMEPOS provider and supplier's compliance with laws governing:

- Anti-kickback arrangements
- The physician self-referral prohibition
- Pricing
- Contracts
- Claim development and submission
- Reimbursement
- Sales (if appropriate)
- Marketing (if appropriate)

Whistleblowers

The OIG has stated that whistleblowers should be protected against employer and other retaliation, a concept embodied in the provisions of the False Claims Act. (See 31 U.S.C. ¤ 3730(h).) In many cases, employees become whistleblowers and report, incriminate, or sue their employers under the False Claims Act's "qui tam" provisions. They usually do this out of frustration because of the provider's or supplier's failure to take action when a questionable,

Fraud, Abuse, Compliance

fraudulent, or abusive situation is brought to the attention of the practice or company principal.

Billing Companies: OIG Guidelines

In 1998, the OIG released the Compliance Program Guidance for Third-Party Medical Billing Companies. In doing so, the OIG issued a statement that said, "This guidance, designed to assist companies that process bills for the nation's health care providers in preventing fraud, waste and abuse, affects virtually every segment of the health care industry."

According to the OIG, billing companies are becoming a vital segment of the national health care industry. Increasingly, health care providers and suppliers are relying on billing companies to assist them in processing claims in accordance with applicable statutes and regulations. Some health care providers are also consulting with billing companies to provide timely and accurate advice regarding reimbursement matters.

Billing companies are in a unique position to discover various types of fraud, waste, abuse, and billing errors on the part of the provider or supplier for whom they work. This unique access to information may place the billing company in a precarious position. On the one hand, the billing company's allegiance is to its client, the provider or supplier. On the other hand, the billing company should maintain a commitment to comply with the applicable federal and state laws, and the program requirements of federal, state, and private health care plans.

The OIG recognizes the importance of maintaining a positive and interactive communication between billing companies and the providers or suppliers they service. It is with this understanding that the OIG has addressed certain obligations for third-party medical billing companies with regard to provider and supplier misconduct. If the billing company finds evidence of misconduct on the part of the provider or supplier, it should refrain from the submission of questionable claims and notify the provider or supplier in writing within 30 days of such a determination. This notification should include all claim-specific information and the rationale for such a determination.

If the billing company discovers credible evidence of the provider's or supplier's continued misconduct, or flagrant fraudulent or abusive conduct, the company should (1) refrain from submitting any false or inappropriate claims, (2) terminate the contract, or (3) report the misconduct to the appropriate federal and state authorities within a reasonable time frame (i.e., no more than 60 days after determining that there is credible evidence of a violation).

When reporting misconduct to federal or state government officials, a billing company should provide all evidence relevant to the alleged violation of applicable federal or state law and the potential cost impact. Providers and suppliers should be aware that the compliance officer of the billing company, with guidance from governmental authorities, could be requested to continue to investigate the reported violation. Once the investigation is completed, the compliance officer may be required to notify the appropriate governmental authority of the outcome of the investigation, including a description of the impact of the alleged violation on the operation of the applicable health care programs or their patients. If the investigation ultimately reveals that criminal, civil, or administrative violations have occurred, the appropriate federal and state officials must be notified immediately.

Risk Assessment

The OIG has identified the following areas of risk as being particularly problematic for billing companies (but providers and suppliers who perform their own billing operations should also take note of this information):

- Billing for items or services not actually documented
- Unbundling of procedure codes
- Upcoding of procedure codes
- Failing to properly use modifiers
- Doing inappropriate balance billing
- Inadequately resolving overpayments
- Using computer software programs that encourage billing personnel to enter data in fields indicating services were rendered, although they were not actually performed or documented
- Failing to maintain the confidentiality of information or records
- Willfully misusing provider or supplier identification numbers, which may result in improper billing
- Rendering outpatient services in connection with inpatient stays
- Doing duplicate billing in an attempt to gain duplicate payments
- Billing for discharge in lieu of transfer
- Providing billing company incentives that violate the anti-kickback statute or other similar federal or state statutes or regulations
- Participating in joint ventures
- Routinely waving copayments and billing third-party insurance only
- Providing discounts and professional courtesies

Billing Companies and DMEPOS Coding Services

Any billing company used by providers and suppliers of DMEPOS should have written policies and procedures concerning proper coding, and should reflect the current reimbursement principles set forth in applicable federal, state, or private-payer health care program requirements. The company's written policies and procedures should ensure that coding and billing are based on medical record documentation. Particular attention should be paid to issues of appropriate diagnosis codes, individual Medicare Part B claims (including documentation guidelines for evaluation and management services) and the use of patient discharge codes. The billing company should also institute a policy to require the coder or the coding department to review all rejected claims that pertain to diagnosis and procedure codes. Among the risk areas that billing companies should address while providing coding services are the following:

- Internal coding practices
- Assumption coding
- Alteration of the documentation
- Coding without proper documentation of all physician and other professional services
- Billing for services provided by unqualified or unlicensed clinical personnel
- Availability of all necessary documentation at the time of coding
- Employment of sanctioned individuals

Billing companies that provide coding services should maintain an up-to-date, user-friendly index for coding policies and procedures to ensure that specific information can be readily located. The billing company should ensure that essential coding materials, including quarterly updates, are readily accessible to all coding staff. These recommendations also apply to providers and suppliers who perform their own coding.

Billing companies that do not code bills for their clients should notify the provider or supplier to follow compliance safeguards with respect to the documentation of services rendered. The OIG recommends that billing companies that do not code for their clients incorporate in their contracts an agreement from each provider or supplier to address all coding compliance concerns.

Credit Balances

Credit balances occur when payments, allowances, or charge reversals posted to an account exceed the charges to the account. The matter of overpayments is of prime concern by the OIG and other federal officials. Providers and suppliers must establish or be aware of the billing company's policies and procedures for timely identification and resolution of these overpayments.

A billing company's information system should produce copies of individual patient accounts that reflect a credit balance, which simplifies tracking of these balances. Likewise, a credit balance report should be generated, typically on a monthly basis, for the timely reconciliation of these accounts. The billing company should always maintain a complete audit trail of all credit balances, and document the steps taken to reconcile the accounts.

Failure to notify authorities about an overpayment within a reasonable period of time could be interpreted as an attempt to conceal the overpayment from the government. That, in turn, could establish a basis for a criminal violation with respect to the billing company, as well as any individual who may be involved. For this reason, billing company compliance programs should ensure that overpayments are identified quickly, and encourage their provider and supplier clients to promptly return overpayments obtained from Medicare or other federal health care programs.

Fraud and Abuse and Medicare Patients

CMS continues to actively engage beneficiaries and their caregivers to reduce fraud, waste, and abuse in Medicare and Medicaid.

The Administration on Aging (AoA) heads the Senior Medicare Patrol (SMP) program. The program aims to empower seniors to identify and fight fraud though education and community outreach. Since its inception, the program has educated more than 4.2 million beneficiaries and reached more than 25 million people through community education outreach events. Medicare is partnering with AoA to expand the size of the SMP program and to engage more people in the community in the fight against fraud.

Medicare maintains a secure website, www.mymedicare.gov, where beneficiaries can check their claims within 24 hours of the processing date. This information is also available through the 1.800.MEDICARE automated system. CMS encourages beneficiaries to review their Medicare claims summaries thoroughly. The agency is working with beneficiaries to redesign Medicare Summary Notices (MSN) to make it easier to understand and easier to spot potential fraud or irregularities on claims submitted for their care.

Medicare patients are being instructed to watch for and report the following activities related to provider and supplier services:

- Duplicate billing of services

- Charges for services not performed or items not dispensed

- Inappropriate or unnecessary services

- Charges billed for a more expensive procedure than the one received

- Low-cost new or used medical equipment, which is charged to the Medicare program as higher-cost or new equipment

- Services provided free to the patient but billed to Medicare

- CMN forms completed by the supplier or medial equipment vendor instead of the provider

Medicare reinforces to Medicare beneficiaries that they should:

- Guard their Medicare number and treat it as they would a credit card.

- Look for suspicious activities and be wary of salespeople who knock on the door or call uninvited and try to sell products or services.

- Use a calendar or personal journal to record all doctor appointments, tests, and services. Then compare quarterly claims statement to the record. Call the doctor's office or health care provider and ask about any discrepancies. If they can't resolve questions or concerns, call 1.800.MEDICARE.

- Report suspected misuse of the patient's Medicare number, call 1.800.MEDICARE. If identity theft is suspected, or if someone incorrectly possesses personal information, call the Federal Trade Commission's ID Theft Hotline at 1.877.438.4338.

Fraud and abuse may be reported to the OIG hotline 1.800.HHS.TIPS [800.477.8477] or online at http://oig.hhs.gov/fraud/report-fraud/index.asp. More information about CMS fraud prevention efforts is available at http://www.cms.gov/Outreach-and-Education/Outreach/Partnerships/DMEPOS_Toolkit.html or http://www.cms.gov/Outreach-and-Education/Outreach/Partnerships/FraudPrevention Toolkit.html.

In early 2014, the Departments of Justice and Health and Human Services announced recoveries of $4.3 billion in fiscal 2013 and $19.2 billion over the last five years resulting from joint efforts to combat health care fraud. These recoveries were made from individuals and companies who attempted to defraud federal health programs serving seniors or who sought payments from taxpayers to which they were not entitled.

Since the inception of the program in1997, the Health Care Fraud and Abuse Control (HCFAC) program has returned more than $25.9 billion to the Medicare Trust Funds and treasury. The success of this joint Department of Justice and HHS effort was made possible in part by the Health Care Fraud Prevention and Enforcement Action Team (HEAT), created in 2009 to prevent fraud, waste, and abuse in Medicare and Medicaid and to crack down on individuals and entities that are abusing the system and costing American taxpayers billions of dollars. The Justice Department and HHS are currently operating Medicare Fraud Strike Force teams in nine areas across the country. The strike force teams use advanced data analysis techniques to identify high-billing levels in health care fraud hot spots so that interagency teams can target emerging or migrating schemes as well as chronic fraud by criminals masquerading as health care providers or suppliers. The Justice Department's enforcement of the civil False Claims Act and the Federal Food, Drug and Cosmetic Act has produced similar record-breaking results. These combined efforts coordinated under HEAT have expanded local partnerships and helped educate Medicare beneficiaries about how to protect themselves against fraud.

For additional information, visit websites https://oig.hhs.gov/reports-and-publications/hcfac/index.asp and http://www.stopmedicarefraud.gov/newsroom/index.html.

The Health Insurance Portability and Accountability Act (HIPAA) of 1996

The HIPAA that has taken shape in Washington evolved from a straightforward effort to guarantee employees the right to transfer the security of their group health insurance coverage from one job to another—the "portability" of HIPAA's name. However, the biggest effect of HIPAA on those that provide health care services comes from the Administrative Simplification Provisions of HIPAA.

HIPAA Administrative Simplification

The Administrative Simplification provisions of HIPAA, Title II require the Department of Health and Human Services (HHS) to establish national standards for electronic health care transactions and national identifiers for providers, health plans, and employers. It also addresses the security and privacy of health data. HHS believes that by adopting these standards, the efficiency and effectiveness of the nation's health care system will increase by encouraging the widespread use of electronic data interchange in health care. This includes the transmission and processing of claims containing health care data. *Any and all* parties that submit or process health care claims are subject to regulations in HIPAA. DMEPOS suppliers must comply with HIPAA requirements.

Essentially, Administrative Simplification is several sets of regulations that deal with protecting the confidentiality of certain medical information and that contain standards for the safe and accurate exchange of that information

Privacy Standards

On December 28, 2000, the initial publication of the Standards for Privacy of Individually Identifiable Health Information Final Rule, was published. The purpose of these privacy requirements is five fold:

1. To limit the use and release of identifiable health information.

2. To give patients new rights to access their medical records and to know who else has accessed them.

3. To restrict most disclosures of personal health information to the minimum amount necessary to complete a given task.

4. To establish comprehensive federal criminal and civil sanctions for improper use and disclosure.

5. To establish new requirements for access of personal health information (PHI) by researchers and others.

Although these goals seem fairly simple and straightforward, HIPAA has established a complex set of requirements to meet them. Prior to beginning the steps for implementation of these complex requirements, determine if your organization is considered a "covered entity" under the HIPAA privacy regulations. Covered entities include all health plans, health care clearinghouses, and health care providers that transmit health information in electronic transactions covered under another part of the Administrative Simplification, the Standards for Electronic Transactions. Health care providers are defined as "any person or organization that furnishes, bills, or is paid for health care in the normal course of doing business." Most any provider of health care services that does billing in an electronic fashion will be a covered entity under HIPAA.

Transaction Standards and Code Sets

Transaction Standards

HIPAA required that the secretary of HHS adopt standards for the electronic transfer of medical, billing, and administrative information within the health care systems. In addition, standardized code sets are vital under HIPAA for accurate and efficient electronic data interchange for diagnoses, procedures, and drugs. Overall, these standards were expected to reduce the administrative burdens on health care plans and providers by eliminating the estimated 400 different claim formats that were in use.

The final rule concerning transaction standards and code sets was implemented in October 2000.

Compliance was required by October 2002, although small health care plans had until October 2003 to comply. However, passage of H.R. 3323, Public Law 107-105 (also known as the Administrative Simplification Compliance Act) on January 3, 2002, delayed the implementation date for a year. The final deadline for compliance with the transaction standards was October 16, 2003.

These standards were required to be adopted by all government health care plans, including Medicare, Medicaid, the Military Health System for active duty and civilian personnel, and the health information programs of the Indian Health Service and the Veterans Administration. In addition, all private sector health plans (except certain small, self-administered plans) must use these standards, including managed care organization and ERISA plans, health care clearinghouses, and all health care providers who elect to submit or receive electronic transactions. The standards apply to electronic data interchange (EDI) only. They are not applicable to data that is stored, which can be in any format as long as it can be translated into the standard transaction format when necessary.

Although health care clearinghouses are required to comply with the standards, they may accept transactions that are not standardized in order to translate them into standard transactions for customers to send, or they may receive standard transactions and translate them into nonstandard formats for customers.

Use of these standards does not mean that a health plan has to change its payment policies. Although health plans have to accept and process bills submitted in the standard format, they do not have to provide benefits for any service or item that would not be paid prior to implementation of the standards, such as noncovered cosmetic procedures.

These standards are applicable to the following types of transactions:

- Health care claims and equivalent encounter information
- Enrollment and disenrollment in a health care plan
- Health insurance plan eligibility
- Health care payment and remittance advice
- Health insurance plan premium payments
- Health care claim status
- Certification and authorization of referrals
- Coordination of benefits

Although HIPAA also requires electronic submission standards for the first report of injury, these will be adopted at a future date. In addition, a standard for the electronic transmission of health care claims attachments will also be adopted.

All of the transaction standards were created by standards development organizations in the private sector. With the exception of the retail pharmacy standards, all are from the Accredited Standards Committee. For purposes of electronic transactions, version 4010 of ANSI ASC X12N was selected.

The standards for retail pharmacy transactions are from the National Council for Prescription Drug Programs (NCPDP) since these standards are currently in widespread use. A February 20, 2003 final rule authorized the National Council for Prescription Drug Program's Telecommunication Standard Implementation Guide, version 5, release 1 (version 5.1), September 1999, and equivalent NCPDP Batch Standard Batch Implementation Guide, version 1, release 1 (version 1.1), January 2000, as the standards for transactions for the retail pharmacy sector.

A physician, practitioner, facility, or supplier with fewer than 10 FTEs is considered a small employer. Providers and suppliers that qualify as a small employer automatically qualify for waiver of the requirement that their claims be submitted to Medicare electronically. CMS encourages these providers to submit their claims electronically, but they are not required to do so under the law. The small provider exception does not apply to health care claim clearinghouses that are agents for electronic claim submission for small providers. HIPAA required that clearinghouses submit claims electronically effective October 16, 2003, without exception.

Code Sets

The standard medical code sets, which are already in use by most health plans, health care clearinghouses, and health care providers, include:

- **ICD-9-CM, Volumes 1 and 2 (including the official ICD-9-CM guidelines for coding and reporting):** required for diseases, injuries, impairments, other health problems and manifestations, and causes of injuries, diseases, impairments, and other health problems

- **ICD-9-CM, Volume 3 (including the official ICD-9-CM guidelines for coding and reporting):** required for reporting diagnostic, preventive, therapeutic, or management procedures or actions taken by hospitals on inpatients

- **CPT:** required for reporting physician and other health care services

- **HCPCS Level II:** required for reporting physician and other health care services, equipment, supplies, substances, and other items used for health care services

- **CDT-4 (Current Dental Terminology):** required for reporting dental services

- **National Drug Codes (NDC):** required for reporting drugs and biologics by retail pharmacies

On January 16, 2009, HHS published two final rules to adopt updated HIPAA standards. In the first rule, HHS adopted X12 version 5010 and NCPDP version D.0 for HIPAA transactions. For versions 5010 and D.0, the compliance date for all covered entities is January 1, 2012, giving the health care industry enough time to test standards internally and externally before the compliance date. Active testing with electronic trading partners has been going on through 2011.

In the second final rule published in January 2009, HHS modified the standard medical data code sets for coding diagnoses and inpatient hospital procedures by adopting the International Classification of Diseases, Tenth Revision, Clinical Modification (ICD-10-CM) for diagnosis coding, including the Official ICD-10-CM Guidelines for Coding and Reporting, and the International Classification of Diseases, Tenth Revision, Procedural Coding System (ICD-10-PCS) for inpatient hospital procedure coding, effective October 1, 2014. The most current 2012 draft update release is available for public viewing, and additional updates are expected before implementation. At this time, ICD-10 codes are not valid for any purpose or use other than for reporting mortality data for death certificates.

On April 17, 2012, a proposed rule was released that would delay implementation of the ICD-10-CM and ICD-10-PCS data sets until October 1, 2014, a one-year delay. CMS believes this change gives covered entities the additional time needed to synchronize system and business process preparation and to make the necessary changes for the updated medical data code sets. The final rule on the delayed implementation was published in the *Federal Register* on September 5, 2012.

Patient Protection and Affordable Care Act of 2010

The Patient Protection and Affordable Care Act of 2010 (PPACA, Public Law 111-148), section 1104, Administrative Simplification adds new and expanded provisions to the HIPAA regulations. Among the provisions are:

- A standard for electronic funds transfer.

- Operating rules for each of the HIPAA covered transactions must be adopted. This is intended to reduce current variations in transaction standard implementation and usage by individual health plans and clearinghouses. The intent is for a non-profit entity to develop these rules that will then be reviewed by the National Committee for Vital and Health Statistics (NCVHS) and HHS. Top priority is to be given to operating rules for eligibility verification, claim status, claim remittance or payment, and electronic funds transfer.

- Transaction set standards not yet implemented must be complete (e.g., the unique plan identifier). Additional plans must be adopted with accompanying operating rules to expand transaction standardization.

- The requirement that health plans certify their compliance with the standards and operating rules. Established deadlines range from 2013 to 2015 with increased penalties for noncompliance.

- HHS is to seek input on activities and items relating to the following areas no later than January 1, 2012:

  - the electronic standardization of the application process, including the use of a uniform application form, for enrollment of health care providers by health plans

  - whether electronic exchange and transaction standards (section 1173 of the Social Security Act) should apply to the health care transactions of automobile insurance, workers' compensation, and other programs or persons not currently covered

  - whether standardized forms could apply to financial audits required by health plans, federal and state agencies, including state auditors, the OIG, and CMS

  - whether there could be greater transparency and consistency of methodologies and processes used to establish claim edits used by health plans

  - whether health plans should be required to publish their timeliness of payment rules

Administrative Simplification is further amended to require that NCVHS establish a review committee to coordinate HIPAA administrative standards with those of the health information technology activities for electronic health records. HHS is directed to conduct a review every three years to determine if additional areas could be made more uniform to improve the operations of the health care system and reduce administrative costs.

Health Plan Identifier

The idea of a standardized identification number to be used by all parties to represent a specific health plan was first discussed in the Health Insurance Portability and Accountability Act (HIPAA) that was passed by Congress and enacted into law in August of 1996. Further pushed along by the Affordable Care Act, a health plan identification number or HPID was touted as a "cut in red tape" that would "save up to $6 billion over 10 years."

HIPAA

The Department of Health and Human Services purports that a health plan may use a wide range of different identifiers that do not have a standard format. As a result, it is claimed that health care providers run into time-consuming problems, such as misrouting or rejection of transactions due to insurance identification errors. The HPID and its associated other entity identifier (OEID) is intended to address this issue. The final rule for the NPID was published on September 5, 2012.

Title 45, section 160.103 of the Code of Federal Regulations defines a health plan as "an individual or group plan that provides, or pays the cost of, medical care (as defined in section 2791(a)(2) of the PHS Act, 42 U.S.C. 300gg-91(a)(2))." The term health plan includes, but is not limited to the following:

- A group health plan
- A health insurance issuer
- An HMO
- Part A, Part B, Part C (Medicare Advantage), and Part D (Prescription Drug Benefit) of the Medicare (title XVIII) program
- Medicaid (title XIX) program
- Medicare supplemental policy
- The health care program for uniformed services under title 10
- The veterans' health care program under 38 U.S.C. chapter 17
- Indian Health Service program under the Indian Health Care Improvement Act
- Federal Employees Health Benefits Program
- Any other individual or group plan, or combination of individual or group plans, that provides or pays for the cost of medical care

Title 42, section 300gg-91(a)(2) of the Code of Federal Regulations defines medical care as:

- (A) The diagnosis, cure, mitigation, treatment, or prevention of disease, or amounts paid for the

purpose of affecting any structure or function of the body
- (B) Amounts paid for transportation primarily for and essential to medical care referred to in subparagraph (A)
- (C) Amounts paid for insurance covering medical care referred to in subparagraphs (A) and (B)

Health plans are further divided into a controlling health plan (CHP) and a subhealth plan (SHP).

CHPs must obtain an HPID for itself. A CHP may obtain an HPID for its subhealth plans or may direct them to obtain their own HPID. A SHP is not required to obtain a HPID, but may do so.

Health plans, except for small health plans, have until November 5, 2014 to obtain their HPID.

Small health plans should obtain their HPID by November 7, 2015. Health plans, covered health care providers, and health care clearinghouses must fully implement the use of the HPID by November 7, 2016.

On September 23, 2014, the National Committee on Vital and Health Statistics (NCVHS), as an advisory body to HHS, recommended that HHS rectify in rulemaking that all covered entities (health plans, health care providers and clearinghouses, and their business associates) not use the HPID in the HIPAA transactions (see http://ncvhs.us/wp-content/uploads/2014/10/140923lt5.pdf). This enforcement discretion will allow HHS to review the NCVHS's recommendation and consider any appropriate next steps.

HPIDs and OEIDs can be obtained through the Health Plan and Other Entity Enumeration System (HPOES). HPOES is housed within the CMS Health Insurance Oversight System (HIOS) (https://portal.cms.gov/wps/portal/unauthportal/home/).

Reimbursement Guidelines

Many providers attempt to furnish items of DMEPOS as a convenience to their patients. Providers also furnish DMEPOS items to ensure that the proper application or fit of those items is achieved for maximum medical benefit to their patients. Very few providers actually proceed into DMEPOS dispensing with the idea that this activity will result in big profits. In this environment of stiff provider competition, however, the practice with an expansive service base will likely attract a larger and steadier patient base than a similar practice with a more limited scope of service. The one-stop shopping approach for medical services is a powerful tool in creating high patient volume and maintaining the fiscal health of the practice. This business principle is also true of DMEPOS supplier facilities.

DMEPOS Utilization and Authorization

Utilization, one of the most significant factors in the cost of medical care, is the primary focus of managed care and DMEPOS industry interface. To help control member utilization, the typical managed care policy requires the MCO member to obtain a provider order for any DMEPOS item. Under some MCO stipulations, this order can be generated by the treating specialist, who in turn must notify the MCO and receive authorization to either (1) dispense the item directly to the patient, or (2) allow the patient to obtain the item from a supplier. Under other MCO rules, the order for the DMEPOS must be routed from the specialist to the provider for approval, and then the MCO must be notified by the provider for final approval.

Prior authorizations, preauthorizations, and precertifications are mandatory (and many times burdensome) communications with the MCO generally required for performing special services (such as surgical procedures), making referrals, treating a patient in the emergency department (ED) admitting a patient to a skilled nursing facility, and ordering DMEPOS. This policy mandate affects all participating provider offices and involved suppliers as well.

Once approval is obtained from the MCO for the DMEPOS item, an authorization number or form is given to the provider. Providers should insist on receiving the MCO's permission in writing to obtain the DMEPOS item. The provider, whether a PCP or a specialist, must then contact the approved supplier and furnish the information necessary for DMEPOS dispensation. The supplier will need the patient's personal data (name, date of birth, address, etc.) and

insurance information. In many cases, the supplier may also need information such as the following:

- Type of DMEPOS item with specific characteristics, if appropriate
- Patient's diagnosis
- Patient's prognosis
- Length of time the DMEPOS is needed (for items such as oxygen)
- Written physician order, personally signed and dated

These special reimbursement provisions clarify three basic facts:

- Which services and items are covered when pre-authorization is obtained from the plan
- Which services and items are specifically excluded
- Who is responsible for payment for excluded or noncovered items or services, and for covered items or services denied as not medically necessary when the patient has been given advance written notice of the probable denial

By signing the advance notice (similar to the Medicare program's ABN), the patient waives the provider's or supplier's liability and acknowledges financial responsibility for the item or service furnished. Obtaining the signed advance notice form ahead of time also ensures smoother claims processing and patient billing, as all facets of the process are known. If the claim is submitted to the carrier for a noncovered or not medically necessary item or service, a denial will ensue. Patients who signed the liability waiver notice in advance are aware of their financial obligation and can be billed on the date of service (for noncovered items) or after the carrier's denial is received (for items deemed not medically necessary).

PPS and Consolidated Billing

In an effort to contain costs, CMS has been instituting prospective payment systems (PPS) for each of its covered types of services. Acute care hospital stays are reimbursed by diagnosis-related groups (DRGs). The payment is based on the patient's diagnoses, age, and procedures performed. The majority of the services provided to the hospital inpatient are covered in that one payment to the hospital.

CMS has expanded its cost containment efforts. A prospective payment system based on resource utilization was put into place for Skilled Nursing

Reimbursement

Facilities (SNFs) in 1999. A prospective payment system based on resource utilization for Home Health Agencies (HHAs) was instituted in 2000. The End-Stage Renal Disease (ESRD) PPS began implementation January 1, 2011. Other PPS reimbursement plans have been instituted for hospital outpatients, long term acute care hospitals, and rehabilitation hospitals.

Customized prosthetic devices are excluded from these requirements for all PPS payments. A number of other items and services that are considered DMEPOS are included. Among the included items are ostomy supplies, surgical dressings, drugs, and some equipment.

Suppliers need to know the mechanics of the programs if they are going to enter into agreements with the SNF or HHA to provide DMEPOS. They also need to know what to do if their routine customer is now receiving SNF level services or HHA services.

Hospital Inpatients

Medicare does not allow separate payment for durable medical equipment, prosthetics, orthotics, and supplies (DMEPOS) when a patient is in a covered inpatient stay. These claims were related to DME dates of service greater than two days prior to Part A discharge date or Part A discharge status was not to home. Effective July 1, 2013, the DME claim will be rejected or, if paid, the contractor will institute payment recovery when all of the following conditions are met:

- There is a covered Medicare Part A inpatient claim with a TOB of 111

- The DME and the inpatient claims are for the same beneficiary HICN

- The DME claim has a line item within the HCPCS Level II category 03 for orthotics and/or prosthesis

- The from date of service (DOS) of the durable medical equipment item is within the Part A admit and discharge dates

- The from DOS of the durable medical equipment line items is greater than two days prior to the beneficiary's Part A inpatient discharge date

- If the from DOS of the DME line items is within the beneficiary's Part A inpatient admission and discharge date and the patient discharge status (FL 17) is NOT equal to 01 Discharged to home or self-care (routine discharge)

(*Medicare One-time Notification*, Pub. 100-20 [trans. 1183, February 8, 2013])

The CMS Recovery Audit Contractor (RAC) Program, which is responsible for identifying and correcting improper payments in the Medicare fee-for-service payment process, identified this issue. The contractor

identified DMEPOS claims for patients who received DMEPOS items while in an inpatient stay in a hospital. Since Medicare does not allow separate payments for DMEPOS for the patient during a covered inpatient hospital stay, these payments associated with these claims are considered overpayments.

Skilled Nursing Facilities

The consolidated billing requirement confers on the SNF the billing responsibility for the entire package of care that residents receive during a covered Part A SNF stay and physical, occupational, and speech therapy services received during a non-covered stay.

Exception: there are a limited number of services specifically excluded from consolidated billing and therefore separately payable.

For Medicare beneficiaries in a covered Part A stay, these separately payable services are:

- Physician's professional services

- Certain dialysis-related services, including covered ambulance transportation to obtain the dialysis services

- All ambulance services except when a medically necessary transport from one SNF to another SNF occurs, when the beneficiary is discharged from the first SNF and admitted to the second, and covered ambulance transportation to obtain dialysis

- Erythropoietin for certain dialysis patients

- Chemotherapy

- Chemotherapy administration services

- Radioisotope services

- Customized prosthetic devices

- Hospital's "facility charge" in connection with clinic services of a physician

- Certain cardiac catheterizations

- Certain computerized axial tomography (CT) scans

- Certain magnetic resonance imaging (MRIs)

- Certain radiation therapies

- Certain angiographies and lymphatic and venous procedures

- Emergency services

- Certain ambulatory surgeries involving the use of a hospital operating room

- Hospice care related to a beneficiary's terminal illness

- Screening services

A Part A covered stay means that the resident or patient meets Medicare coverage guidelines that deem they are receiving a skilled level of care. The patient's medical condition, potential for improvement, the intensity of the services provided, and their ability to perform daily functions are among the issues that are taken into account when determining if a patient is receiving skilled levels of care. Many long-term residents in SNFs or nursing homes are not receiving Medicare skilled levels of care. However, even a long-term resident may have a status change that can change their level of care. A resident may have a cerebral vascular accident or may fall and break a bone. The resident would most likely be transferred to an acute care hospital. Upon the resident's return, they would probably qualify for skilled levels of care.

The SNF receives an all-inclusive payment for Part A covered stays. This payment depends on the resource utilization group (RUGs) to which their situation falls. The payment is intended to cover all services except those listed above. The payment does not change based upon the cost of the items or services.

Many DMEPOS supplies and some devices or equipment may not be billed separately by the SNF or by any other provider or supplier. These certain DMEPOS items are considered a part of the nursing home's PPS reimbursement. The supplier should bill the nursing home for these items and should have a formal agreement with the home for payment of these items.

If a patient in a nursing home is not receiving a skilled level of care and is not being reimbursed under Part A, then the supplier has a choice. Billing may be submitted directly by the supplier or may be submitted by the nursing home. Suppliers should have an agreement with the nursing home specifying which party will bill in these situations. Such an agreement will eliminate duplicate billing and concerns related to fraud and abuse. Only one party should submit the bill for the service. Do not bill the nursing home and then bill the DME MAC if the nursing home is taking too long to pay.

Home Health Agencies

CMS has a PPS program in place for Home Health Agencies (HHAs). Resource utilization groups take into account the patient's medical condition and the intensity of the services performed among other things to group HHA patients. If the patient is under a plan of care, many of the DMEPOS items should be billed to the Home Health Agency (HHA). The supplies are considered a part of the HHA's PPS reimbursement. The supplier should bill the HHA for these items and should have a formal agreement with the home for payment of these items.

The HHA must have its own physician order for the DMEPOS item. This is true even if the supplier has a long-standing order to supply an item, such as ostomy supplies to a patient or customer. Many DMEPOS items must be provided under an arrangement. If the

supplier was unaware of the HHA services and there is no agreement with the HHA about the provision of the ostomy supplies, the supplies will not be reimbursed by any party. The patient has a freedom of choice that allows them to accept the HHA services. At that point, the HHA becomes responsible for all related care including the provision of many DMEPOS items.

If the patient is not on a plan of care or is not receiving Part A reimbursable services, the supplier may still be required to bill the HHA. Many DMEPOS items are subject to consolidated billing regulations. This means that the HHA must submit all charges for these services. The HHA will receive additional payment for these items. The supplier should bill the HHA for these items and should probably have an agreement with the home for payment of these items.

Applicable Consolidated Billing

The types of services, supplies, and equipment subject to consolidated billing regulations vary for SNFs and for HHAs. SNF regulations also vary depending upon whether the patient is receiving a skilled level of care and is covered under PPS. These items are usually listed by HCPCS code.

A provider or supplier may not be aware of changes in the customer's medical condition or types of care unless the supplier actively tracks all of their patients or customers. Even then, it may be difficult to make a determination. The supplier may only become aware of the issue upon receipt of a denial from the DME MAC. If the supplier routinely supplies nursing home or SNF patients, the supplier should work out an agreement with the SNF that would alert them prior to billing when billing should be sent to the SNF instead of the DMERC.

ESRD Prospective Payment System

Effective January 1, 2011, ESRD services are reimbursed on a bundled prospective payment system (PPS). The ESRD PPS replaces the basic case-mix adjusted composite payment system and the methodologies for the reimbursement of separately billable outpatient ESRD-related items and services. The ESRD PPS provides a single payment to ESRD facilities that covers all the resources used in providing an outpatient dialysis treatment, including supplies and equipment used to administer dialysis in the ESRD facility or at a patient's home, drugs, biologicals, laboratory tests, training, and support services.

Since all ESRD PPS payments will be made to the dialysis facility only, the method II home dialysis election terminated effective December 31, 2010. All method II home dialysis patients became method I patients.

Reimbursement

A per-dialysis treatment base rate for adult patients is adjusted to reflect differences in wage levels among the areas in which ESRD facilities are located, by patient-level adjustments for case-mix, an outlier adjustment (if applicable), facility-level adjustments, a training add-on (if applicable), adjustments specific to pediatric patients (dialysis patients that are under the age of 18), and a budget neutrality adjustment during the transition period.

Effective January 1, 2011, all drugs reported on the renal dialysis facility claim are considered included in the ESRD PPS. The list of drugs and biologicals for consolidated billing are designated as always ESRD-related and no separate payment is to be made to ESRD facilities.

The Medicare Improvements for Patients and Providers Act (MIPPA) eliminated method II home dialysis claims effective with dates of service January 1, 2011, and later. All home dialysis claims must be billed by a renal dialysis facility and paid under the ESRD PPS. ESRD patients are no longer required to file CMS-382 form with the Medicare contractor. Report modifier AY to indicate that an item, drug, or biological is unrelated to the ESRD treatment and payment may be made separately.

Financial Management Guidelines

This section of the *Coders' Desk Reference for HCPCS* reviews important areas of DMEPOS dispensing that every provider's practice and supplier's office should be intimately familiar with. Applying these formulas, tips, and guidelines will help to monitor profit and loss, and ultimately help the DMEPOS provider and supplier remain profitable.

DMEPOS dispensers should have knowledge of or develop the following:

- Financial formulas related to medical care used to regularly monitor the charges and reimbursements for DMEPOS items and services furnished
- Business formulas to monitor overhead and associated expenses
- Tips on how to perform a cost study and a reimbursement analysis
- Guidelines for doing a managed-care viability analysis to determine a managed-care plan's contribution or detriment to the business's bottom line; this should be done for both regular capitation or fee-for-service scenarios and for managed-care contracts that include DMEPOS as a carve-out service
- A checklist of simple office controls for tighter financial management

Financial Formulas

Financial management for DMEPOS providers and suppliers has become quite complicated over the past several years. A great deal of financial management concern has been placed on the numerous managed-care plans with which the DMEPOS provider and supplier must participate.

The DMEPOS provider and supplier must regularly monitor the financial trends of each health insurance plan they contract with by conducting a basic financial analysis of collections and accounts receivable (A/R). The fundamental structure of collections and A/R analysis begins with three key financial elements:

- Charges
- Adjustments
- Payments

Every provider and supplier's office should generate monthly financial information in these areas, either by a computerized billing system or by manual bookkeeping reports. These key elements, when used in the basic formulas provided in this section, will provide a snapshot of the provider and supplier's financial strength or weakness in terms of collections and A/R status.

Conducting Cost and Reimbursement Analyses

Becoming or remaining profitable when furnishing patients with DMEPOS items involves monitoring all aspects of the financial investment made to furnish those items. Patient charges, mandatory health insurance adjustments, and other types of adjustments and insurance and patient payments (reimbursements) must be meticulously followed and studied. Becoming or remaining profitable also involves tracking all associated costs for dispensing DMEPOS items. These costs are easy to track, and include a range of considerations from the actual purchase price of the DMEPOS item to the costs of any supplies used in furnishing the item. The payer must track reimbursement for the DMEPOS items because the profit margin for a single item of DMEPOS can vary greatly between one payer and another.

A cost and reimbursement analysis should be performed at least every six months, and no less than once every year.

DMEPOS Cost Study

The costs of furnishing DMEPOS items must be closely monitored, as many times escalating costs can out-rise reimbursement for those items, thereby nullifying any potential profits. If all of the costs are not tracked alongside the reimbursements, a deceptively healthy financial picture surrounding

DMEPOS dispensing activities can emerge, fooling providers and suppliers into thinking the DMEPOS profit center is fiscally sound.

Typical costs associated with furnishing DMEPOS to patients, for both providers and suppliers, include the following:

- Actual item purchase price
- Shipping and freight charges
- Taxes
- Physician or provider time involved in the dispensation process
- Staff time involved in the dispensation process
- Office or medical supplies expended when ordering, receiving, and furnishing the items

Most of the information needed to perform the cost study is taken directly from the invoices for the DMEPOS items. Using a computerized spreadsheet gives the provider or supplier the ability to assign formulas to each cell for automatic calculations, resulting in a re-calculation of each DMEPOS item. This makes it convenient to keep all information current and to perform the study on a semi-annual basis. Many DMEPOS suppliers have software programs that can pull specific data fields, collate the data into a requested format, and dump the information into a report. In these cases, cost reports should be done more frequently than semi-annually simply because the convenience of obtaining this information makes it easier to monitor the cost data.

The final cost information for each DMEPOS item furnished, when considered in aggregate (the total number of each item dispensed on an annual basis), is the cost data that should be used in the final profit or loss determinations. Manufacturer and vendor discounts, such as that given for paying the amount due earlier than specified or those given when purchasing DMEPOS items in bulk, become important when considered on an annual basis. For example, a $2 early-pay discount received for each of 10 items paid early in one month (a total of $20 in savings) can add up to a considerable amount of savings over the space of a year.

The final calculated cost of each DMEPOS item should be organized by CPT or HCPCS Level II code and associated code description (instead of patient name, account number, etc.) for easy interface with reimbursement data. This will facilitate the next step in the financial analysis process—conducting a reimbursement analysis.

DMEPOS Reimbursement Analysis

The reimbursement analysis is the final portion of the financial management analysis needed to determine a particular DMEPOS item's profit or loss margin. Simply stated, the cost data are compared against the reimbursement information and a determination is made.

Reimbursement data for DMEPOS can come from a variety of sources, including the following:

- Health insurance payments (third-party payers, Medicare, Medicaid, managed-care plans, workers compensation carriers, private or self-funded plans)
- Patient copayments
- Patient coinsurance amounts (secondary insurance payments)
- Other patient payments (in the cases of insurance denials, noncovered items, self-pay patients, etc.)

The reimbursement analysis must also contain pertinent adjustment information, such as mandatory participating provider or supplier adjustments, courtesy and professional adjustments, and bad debt and charity write-offs.

Reimbursement information is obtained from the health insurance explanations of benefit forms (EOBs) or the explanations of Medicare benefit forms (EOMBs) that accompany each payment. These forms can vary widely in the type of payment information provided, but most will supply the following:

- The patient's name
- Plan identification number
- Provider's or supplier's name
- Provider's or supplier's plan identification number
- Date of service
- CPT or HCPCS Level II code for the DMEPOS item
- Modifier, if reported
- Diagnosis code linked to the CPT or HCPCS Level II code
- The provider's or supplier's charge
- The amount to be adjusted
- Patient copayment/coinsurance amounts
- Amount reimbursed

Some EOBs may only contain the patient and provider's or supplier's names, date of service, a description of the DMEPOS item and the amounts charged, adjusted, and reimbursed. In addition, most EOBs/EOMBs will note any amount applicable to the patient's annual deductible.

Reimbursement data is also obtained from the patient accounts for copayment and coinsurance amounts paid, deductibles collected, and retrieval of self-pay patient information. Self-pay patient information also includes patients with health insurance who, because the insurance did not cover the DMEPOS item, have paid for the item out of pocket when appropriate.

Reimbursement

Like the cost study, the reimbursement analysis is set up in a spreadsheet format. The easiest method of setting up the spreadsheet is to arrange the CPT or HCPCS Level II codes and item descriptions horizontally (in the spreadsheet bars), from left to right, with the payer, charge, adjustment, and reimbursement information running vertically in the columns. Reimbursement for the items, whether received from the patient or from insurance carriers, must be tracked (entered onto the spreadsheet) by payer and CPT or HCPCS Level II code to dovetail with the previously collected cost data. DMEPOS volume data must be entered onto the spreadsheet as well to account for the number of specific items purchased and dispensed during the time period being studied.

Additional spreadsheets can be added when space does not allow for all of the information to be entered onto one spreadsheet.

Costs and Reimbursements

All of the information is to be considered individually and in aggregate when assessing the value of dispensing items of DMEPOS. In making the final determination, providers and suppliers should weigh the necessity of dispensing items against not dispensing items, especially if the items carry a significant margin of loss. This financial data must be assessed for each item of DMEPOS against such factors as:

- The item's necessity to other related DMEPOS items that carry a significant profit margin (supplies needed when using a certain DME apparatus)

- The possible loss of business because the patient prefers to obtain the related DME elsewhere, where all of the necessary DMEPOS items are available

- The impact of striking various unprofitable DMEPOS items from the service menu, thereby restricting provider options, forcing them to refer their patients to other suppliers

Medicare Guidelines for Selected Topics

ESRD Equipment, Supplies, and Drugs and Biologicals

Effective January 1, 2011, ESRD services are reimbursed on a bundled prospective payment system (PPS). The ESRD PPS replaces the basic case-mix adjusted composite payment system and the methodologies for the reimbursement of separately billable outpatient ESRD-related items and services. The ESRD PPS provides a single payment to ESRD facilities that covers all the resources used in providing an outpatient dialysis treatment, including supplies and equipment used to administer dialysis in the ESRD facility or at a patient's home, drugs, biologicals, laboratory tests, training, and support services.

Since all ESRD PPS payments will be made to the dialysis facility only, the method II home dialysis election terminated effective December 31, 2010. All method II home dialysis patients became method I patients.

A per-dialysis treatment base rate for adult patients is adjusted to reflect differences in wage levels among the areas in which ESRD facilities are located, by patient-level adjustments for case-mix, an outlier adjustment (if applicable), facility-level adjustments, a training add-on (if applicable), adjustments specific to pediatric patients (dialysis patients that are under the age of 18), and a budget neutrality adjustment during the transition period.

Outpatient Drugs and Biologicals Subject to Consolidated Billing

Effective January 1, 2011, all drugs reported on the renal dialysis facility claim are considered included in the ESRD PPS. The list of drugs and biologicals for consolidated billing are designated as always ESRD-related and no separate payment is to be made to ESRD facilities. The following ESRD-related drugs and biologicals must be billed by the renal dialysis facility. Other drugs and biologicals may be considered separately payable to the dialysis facility if the drug was not for the treatment of ESRD. The facility must append modifier AY to indicate it was not for the treatment of ESRD.

Effective January 1, 2015, ESRD facilities must report the composite rate drugs identified on the consolidated billing list on the claim. No other composite rate drugs, items, or services are to be

reported on the claim. (*Medicare Claims Processing Manual,* Pub. 100-4, Chap. 8, Sec. 5.3 [trans. 3125, November 14, 2015])

Access Management

C9121	J1642	J1644
J1945	J2993	J2997
J3364–J3365		

Anemia management

J0882	J0886	J0890
J1750	J1756	J2916
J3420	Q0139*–Q2047	Q4081
Q9970*	Q9972*	

Cellular Management

J1955

Anti-infectives

J0878	J3370

When reporting vancomycin, J3370, or daptomycin, J0878, the ESRD facility must also report the diagnosis code for which the drug is indicated. The diagnosis code reported should be in accordance with ICD-9-CM guidelines.

Bone and Mineral Metabolism

J0610	J0630	J0635
J0636	J0895	J1270
J1740	J2430	J2501
J2487	J3487*	S0169

Composite Rate Drugs and Biologicals*

A4802	J0670	J1200
J1205	J1240	J1940
J2001	J2150	J2720
J2795	J3410	J3480*
Q0163		

*Consolidate billing requirements effective January 1, 2015.

Medicare Guidelines

Method II ESRD Services Billed to the DME MAC

The Medicare Improvements for Patients and Providers Act (MIPPA) eliminated method II home dialysis claims effective with dates of service January 1, 2011, and later. All home dialysis claims must be billed by a renal dialysis facility and paid under the ESRD PPS. ESRD patients are no longer required to file CMS-382 form with the Medicare contractor.

The following method II home dialysis service HCPCS codes will be denied when billed separately by a DME supplier. Report modifier AY to indicate that an item is unrelated to the ESRD treatment and payment may be made separately.

Method II supplies and equipment subject to consolidated billing

A4216–A4218	A4450	A4452
A6215–A6216	A6402	E0210

The following method II home dialysis service HCPCS codes will be denied when billed separately by a DME supplier. Modifier AY cannot be used to indicate that an item is unrelated to the ESRD treatment. All claims for the following items and services must be billed by a renal dialysis facility and paid under the ESRD PPS.

Method II supplies and equipment payable only to the ESRD facility

A4215	A4244–A4248	A4651–A4653
A4657	A4660	A4663
A4670–A4674	A4680	A4690
A4706–A4709	A4714	A4719–A4726
A4728	A4730	A4736–A4737
A4740	A4750	A4755
A4760	A4765–A4766	A4770–A4774
A4802	A4860	A4870
A4890	A4911	A4913
A4918	A4927–A4731	A6204
A6250	A6260	E1500
E1510	E1520	E1530
E1540	E1550	E1560
E1570	E1575	E1580
E1590	E1592	E1594
E1600	E1610	E1615
E1620	E1625	E1630
E1632	E1634–E1637	E1639

Diabetic Supplies and Services

CMS generally defines diabetes mellitus as a condition of abnormal glucose metabolism diagnosed using the following criteria: a fasting blood sugar greater than or equal to 126 mg/dL on two different occasions; a two-hour post-glucose challenge greater than or equal to 200 mg/dL on two different occasions; or a random glucose test greater than 200 mg/dL for a person with symptoms of uncontrolled diabetes.

Medicare

Insulin and Syringes

When insulin is furnished to inpatients in a covered hospital stay it is covered and payment is included in the reimbursement for the inpatient stay. For outpatient services, insulin is a self-administrable drug that is not covered unless administered in an emergency situation, such as to a patient in a diabetic coma.

Insulin syringes are covered only when they are furnished incident to a physician's professional services. To be covered under this provision an insulin syringe must have been used by the physician or under his or her direct personal supervision, and the insulin injection must have been given in an emergency situation (e.g., diabetic coma). Home use of an insulin syringe by a diabetic is not covered.

Blood Glucose Monitors and Related Supplies

Blood glucose monitors are meter devices that read color changes produced on specially treated reagent strips by glucose concentrations in the patient's blood. There are several different types of blood glucose monitors. Medicare coverage of these devices varies depending on both the type of device and the medical condition of the patient for whom the device is prescribed.

Reflectance colorimeter devices used for measuring blood glucose levels in clinical settings are not covered as durable medical equipment for use in the home because the need for frequent professional re-calibration makes them unsuitable for home use.

Some types of blood glucose monitors that use a reflectance meter specifically designed for home use by diabetic patients may be covered as durable medical equipment, subject to the conditions and limitations described below.

Lancets, reagent strips, and other supplies necessary for the proper functioning of the device are also covered for patients for whom the device is indicated. Coverage of home blood glucose monitors and related supplies is limited to patients meeting the following conditions:

- The patient has diabetes (ICD-9-CM codes 250.00–250.93) that is being treated by a physician.

- The patient's physician states that the patient is capable of being trained to use the particular device prescribed in an appropriate manner. In some cases, the patient may not be able to perform this function, but a responsible individual can be trained to use the equipment and monitor the patient to assure that the intended effect is achieved. This is permissible if the patient's physician properly documents it in the medical record.

- The glucose monitor and related accessories and supplies have been ordered by the physician who is treating the patient's diabetes and the treating physician maintains records reflecting the care provided including, but not limited to, evidence of medical necessity for the prescribed frequency of testing.

- The device is designed for home use rather than clinical.

There is a blood glucose monitoring system designed especially for use by those with visual impairments. The monitors used in such systems are identical in terms of reliability and sensitivity to the standard blood glucose monitors described above. They differ by having such features as voice synthesizers, automatic timers, and specially designed arrangements of supplies and materials to enable the visually impaired to use the equipment without assistance. These blood glucose monitoring systems are covered under Medicare if the following conditions are met:

- The patient and device meet the conditions listed above for coverage of standard home blood glucose monitors.

- The patient's physician certifies that a visual impairment is severe enough to require use of this special monitoring system.

The additional features and equipment for use with these monitors justifies a higher reimbursement amount than allowed for standard blood glucose monitors.

Supplies used in home glucose monitoring are covered when the monitor is covered. The supplier must have an order that is signed and dated by the treating physician. The order for home blood glucose monitors and/or diabetic testing supplies must include all of the following elements:

- Item to be dispensed

- Quantity of items to be dispensed

- Specific frequency of testing

- Whether the patient has insulin-treated or non-insulin-treated diabetes

- Treating physician's signature

- Date of the treating physician's signature

- Start date of the order (only required if the start date is different from the signature date)

An order that states "as needed" will result in those items being denied as not medically necessary. The supplier is required to have a renewal order from the treating physician every 12 months. This renewal order must also contain the information specified above.

An order for supplies must also meet the following criteria:

- The patient has nearly exhausted the supply of test strips and lancets or useful life of one lens shield cartridge previously dispensed.

- When the treating physician has ordered a frequency of testing that exceeds utilization guidelines, there must be documentation in the patient's medical record stating the specific reason.

- The treating physician has seen the patient and has evaluated his or her diabetes control within six months prior to ordering strips and lancets or lens shield cartridges that exceed utilization guidelines.

- If refills of supplies that exceed utilization guidelines are dispensed, there must be documentation in the physician's records (e.g., a specific narrative statement that adequately documents the frequency at which the patient is actually testing or a copy of the beneficiary's log) or in the supplier's records (e.g., a copy of the beneficiary's log) stating the patient is testing at a frequency that corroborates the quantity of supplies that have been dispensed. If the patient is regularly using quantities of supplies that exceed utilization guidelines, new documentation must be present at least every six months.

The quantity of test strips, lancets, and replacement lens shield cartridges that are covered depends on the usual medical needs of the diabetic patient.

Suppliers must not dispense a quantity of supplies exceeding a beneficiary's expected utilization. Suppliers should stay attuned to atypical utilization patterns on behalf of their clients and verify with the ordering physician that the atypical utilization is, in fact, warranted. Regardless of utilization, a supplier must not dispense more than a three-month quantity of glucose testing supplies at a time.

Suppliers may contact the treating physician to renew an order; however, the request for renewal may only be made with the patient's continued monthly use of

Medicare Guidelines

testing supplies and only with the patient's request to the supplier for order renewal.

Laser skin piercing devices are not medically necessary. If a laser skin piercing device is ordered for use with a covered home blood glucose monitor, payment will be based on the allowance for the least costly medically appropriate alternative. Since the laser skin-piercing device is not medically necessary, replacement lens shield cartridges are also not medically necessary. If replacement lens shields are ordered, payment will be based on the allowance for the least costly medically appropriate alternative (A4259).

Alcohol or peroxide and Betadine or pHisoHex are not covered since these items are not required for the proper functioning of the device.

Urine test reagent strips or tablets are not covered since they are not used with a glucose monitor.

The ICD-9-CM or ICD-10-CM diagnosis code describing the condition that necessitates glucose testing must be included on each claim for the monitor, accessories, and supplies.

If the patient is being treated with insulin injections, modifier KX must be appended to the code for the monitor and each related supply on every claim submitted. Modifier KX must not be used for a patient who is not receiving insulin injections. If the patient is not being treated with insulin injections, modifier KS must be appended to the code for the monitor and each related supply on every claim submitted.

All diabetic testing supplies dispensed via mail-order are subject to the DME competitive billing program. This includes all parts of the United States, including the 50 states, the District of Columbia, Puerto Rico, the U.S. Virgin Islands, Guam, and American Samoa.

Glucose Monitor Modifiers

All DME MACs have LCDs that require the supplier to append an appropriate modifier to claims for glucose monitors. One of the following modifiers should be appended:

EY   No physician or other licensed health care provider order for this item or service
KS   Glucose monitor supply for diabetic beneficiary not treated by insulin
KX   Requirements specified in the medical policy have been met

Hospital Use of Glucometers

Glucometers are simple devices that determine blood glucose. Most are FDA-approved for home use by the patient. All home use of these devices automatically qualifies under the CLIA waiver. Some of these devices are also reimbursable when used by health care professionals in a facility under the CLIA waiver.

Professional use of these devices is reviewed on a case-by-case basis.

Diabetes Self-Management Training

Medicare covers outpatient diabetes self-management training (DSMT) services when furnished by a certified provider who meets certain quality standards. DSMT is intended to educate beneficiaries in the successful self-management of diabetes. The program includes instructions in self-monitoring of blood glucose, education about diet and exercise, an insulin treatment plan developed specifically for the patient who is insulin-dependent, and motivation for patients to use the skills for self-management.

Medicare covers the initial training for a patient who has one or more of the following medical conditions present prior to the physician's or nonphysician practitioner's order:

- New onset diabetes or a patient with diabetes who is newly eligible for Medicare
- Inadequate glycemic control as evidenced by a glycosylated hemoglobin (HbA1C) level of 8.5 percent or more on two consecutive HbA1C determinations three or more months apart in the year before the patient begins receiving training
- Change in treatment regimen from diet control to oral diabetes medication, or from oral diabetes medication to insulin
- High risk for complications based on inadequate glycemic control (documented acute episodes of severe hyperglycemia occurring in the past year during which the beneficiary needed emergency room visits or hospitalization)
- High risk based on at least one of the following documented complications:
  - Lack of feeling in the foot or other foot complications such as foot ulcers, deformities, or amputation
  - Pre-proliferative or proliferative retinopathy or prior laser treatment of the eye
  - Kidney complications related to diabetes, when manifested by albuminuria, without other cause, or elevated creatinine

The physician or qualified nonphysician practitioner treating the condition must order the training. The order must include a statement signed by the physician indicating the service is needed, the number of initial or follow-up hours ordered, the topics to be covered in training, and a determination as to whether individual or group training is appropriate.

The condition requiring training must be documented in the medical record maintained by the referring physician or qualified nonphysician practitioner. Patients are eligible to receive follow-up training each calendar year following the year in which they have been certified as requiring initial training. When training under the order is changed, the physician or qualified nonphysician practitioner treating the patient must sign the training order or referral. A copy must be maintained in the patient's file in the DSMT program's records.

Providers billing these codes must provide a copy of the American Diabetes Association's or the Indian Health Service's Education Recognition Program certificate prior to submitting the first claim.

CMS will not reimburse services rendered to a patient in the hospital or SNF, hospice care, nursing home, or in an RHC/FQHC.

Initial DSMT cannot exceed 10 hours. It must be furnished within a continuous 12-month period. Except for one hour, training must be furnished in a group setting, unless there are no group sessions available within two months of when the training is ordered, the beneficiary has documented special needs, or the physician orders additional insulin training.

Follow-up training can consist of no more than two hours of individual or group training per year. Group training consists of two to 20 individuals. Follow-up training must follow the year during which initial training occurred. The physician must document the specific medical condition the training must address.

Medical Nutrition Therapy Services

Medicare covers medical nutrition therapy (MNT) services when furnished by a registered dietitian or nutrition professional meeting certain requirements. The benefit is available for beneficiaries with diabetes or renal disease when a physician makes the referral.

Medicare will cover an initial three-hour visit for an assessment, follow-up visits for interventions not to exceed two hours, and reassessments as necessary during the 12-month period beginning with the initial assessment ("episode of care") to assure compliance with the dietary plan.

For Medicare purposes, MNT is a separate benefit from DSMT. A patient may receive the full amount of both benefits in the same period, which is 10 hours of initial DSMT and three hours of MNT. However, providers are not allowed to bill DSMT and MNT on the same date of service for the same patient.

Medicare will cover MNT if the following conditions are met:

- The treating physician makes a referral and indicates a diagnosis of diabetes or renal disease.

- The number of hours covered in an episode of care are not exceeded unless a second referral is received from the treating physician.

MNT services may be provided on an individual or group basis without restrictions. MNT services are not covered for beneficiaries receiving maintenance dialysis.

The referring physician must maintain documentation in the patient's medical record. Referrals must be made for each episode of care and reassessments prescribed as a result of a change in medical condition or diagnosis.

Additional hours of MNT services may be covered when the treating physician determines there is a change of diagnosis or medical condition that necessitates diet modification.

A qualified registered dietitian or nutrition professional must provide MNT services. In order to file Medicare claims for MNT, a registered dietitian/nutrition professional must be enrolled as a provider in the Medicare program and meet the qualification requirements. Registered dietitians and nutrition professionals must accept assignment. These services can be billed to the FI when performed in a hospital outpatient setting if the nutritionist or registered dietitian reassigns the patient's benefits to the hospital. There is no facility fee payment for these services.

MNT may be billed with CPT codes 97802, 97803, or 97804. HCPCS Level II codes G0270 and G0271 are reported for reassessment and subsequent intervention following a second referral in the same year for a change in diagnosis, medical condition, or treatment regimen.

Dressings

Medicare

Coverage of surgical dressings are limited to primary and secondary dressings required for the treatment of a wound caused by or treated by a surgical procedure that has been performed by a physician or other health care professional. Surgical dressings required after debridement of a wound are also covered, irrespective of the type of debridement, as long as the debridement was reasonable and necessary and was performed by a health care professional acting within the scope of his or her legal authority when performing this function. Surgical dressings are covered for as long as they are medically necessary.

Primary dressings are therapeutic or protective coverings applied directly to wounds or lesions on the skin or caused by an opening to the skin. Secondary dressing materials that serve a therapeutic or protective function and that are needed to secure a primary dressing are also covered. Items such as adhesive tape, roll gauze, bandages, and disposable compression material are examples of secondary dressings. Some items, such as transparent film, may be used as a primary or secondary dressing.

Elastic stockings, support hose, foot coverings, leotards, knee supports, surgical leggings, gauntlets, and pressure garments for the arms and hands are examples of items that are not ordinarily covered as surgical dressings.

Porcine skin dressings are covered if reasonable and necessary for the individual patient as a dressing for burns, donor sites of a homograft, and decubiti and other ulcers. Gradient pressure dressings are Jobst elasticized heavy-duty dressings and are covered when used to reduce hypertrophic scarring and joint contractures following burn injury.

Surgical dressings furnished to an inpatient in a hospital or skilled nursing facility are considered therapeutic items covered under the inpatient stay. Supplies including surgical dressings furnished to an inpatient for use only outside the hospital are not usually covered as inpatient hospital services. However, a temporary supply that is medically necessary to permit or facilitate the patient's discharge from the hospital and is required until the patient can obtain a continuing supply is covered as an inpatient hospital service.

Surgical dressings applied on an outpatient basis in a hospital or skilled nursing facility are covered when provided in connection with a clinic visit or a practitioner's treatment of the outpatient.

If a physician or nonphysician practitioner applies surgical dressings as part of a professional service that is billed to Medicare, the surgical dressings are considered incident to the professional services of the health care practitioner.

Surgical dressings used by a home health agency in its visits are generally considered routine supplies that are included in the cost per visit of home health care services. Routine supplies would not include those supplies that are specifically ordered by the physician or are essential to HHA personnel in order to effectuate the plan of care.

When surgical dressings are not covered incident to the services of a health care practitioner and are obtained by the patient from a supplier (e.g., drugstore, physician, or other health care practitioner that qualifies as a supplier) on an order from a physician or other health care professional, the surgical dressings are covered separately under Part B. These dressings would be billed by the supplier to the DME MAC.

Consolidated Billing

All surgical dressings and related supplies dispensed to a nursing home patient/resident or home health services recipient are included in the consolidated billing requirements and each provider's prospective payment system (PPS).

For home health services recipients, all billing related to these items must be performed by the home health agency. For nursing home patients/residents receiving skilled care reimbursed under Part A, these items are considered to be a component of the inpatient stay. If a source other than the skilled nursing facility dispenses these items, the source must look to the nursing home for payment and cannot bill Medicare directly for these items. If the nursing home patient/resident is not receiving a skilled level of care and is not being reimbursed under Part A, then suppliers have a choice. The first option is for the supplier to bill these items directly to the DME MAC. The second option is for the supplier to bill the nursing home directly and the home would bill Medicare.

Drugs, Biologicals, and Radiopharmaceuticals

Medicare

Drugs, biologicals, and radiopharmaceuticals for use in a hospital or skilled nursing facility that are ordinarily furnished by the hospital for the care and treatment of inpatients are covered. Payment is included in the reimbursement for the inpatient Part A covered stay.

Drugs and biologicals furnished by a hospital to an inpatient for use outside the hospital are, in general, not covered as inpatient hospital services. When a drug or biological is deemed medically necessary to permit or facilitate the patient's departure from the hospital, and a limited supply is required until the patient can obtain a continuing supply, the limited supply is covered as an inpatient hospital service.

Medicare Part B provides limited benefits for outpatient drugs. The program covers drugs that are furnished "incident to" a physician's service provided that the drugs are not usually self-administered by the patients who take them.

When reporting concurrent administration for drugs and biologicals that are mixed together, hospitals should report the HCPCS code and quantity of each product. If the hospital is compounding drugs that have no assigned HCPCS code, the hospital should report the unlisted HCPCS Level II drug code J9999 or J3490.

Generally, drugs, biologicals, and radiopharmaceuticals are covered only if all of the following requirements are met:

- They meet the definition of drugs or biologicals
- They are of the type that is not usually self-administered
- They meet all the general requirements for coverage of items as incident to a physician's services
- They are reasonable and necessary for the diagnosis or treatment of the illness or injury for which they are administered according to accepted standards of medical practice
- They are not excluded as noncovered immunizations
- They have not been determined by the Food and Drug Administration (FDA) to be less than effective

The drug must be approved for marketing by the FDA and must be used for indications specified on the labeling.

In order to meet all the general requirements for coverage under the incident-to provision, an FDA approved drug or biological must:

- Be of a form that is not usually self-administered
- Must be furnished by a physician
- Must be administered by the physician or by auxiliary personnel employed by the physician and under the physician's personal supervision

The charge, if any, for the drug, biological, or radiopharmaceutical must be included in the physician's bill, and the cost must represent an expense to the physician. Drugs, biologicals, and radiopharmaceuticals furnished by other health care professionals must also meet these requirements.

Self-administrable Drugs

Medicare Part B does generally not cover drugs that can be self-administered, such as those in pill form or those self-injected. Certain self-administered drugs are covered. Examples of self-administered drugs that are covered include blood-clotting factors, drugs used in immunosuppressive therapy, erythropoietin for dialysis patients, osteoporosis drugs for certain homebound patients, certain oral cancer drugs, and drugs that are necessary for the effective use of durable medical equipment (DME) or prosthetic devices. It is up to the Medicare contractor to determine is a self-administrable drug is covered. Contractors have proscribed instructions to follow when determining if a self-administrable drug is covered. Generally if the drug and route of administration will be covered. If a drug is available in both oral and injectable forms, the injectable form of the drug must be medically reasonable and necessary as compared to using the oral form. Self-administrable

drugs that are integral to a procedure (e.g., eye drops used prior to or in cataract surgery) are covered.

Antineoplastic Drugs

Antineoplastic drugs, biologicals, or radiopharmaceuticals are covered on an inpatient or outpatient basis for FDA-approved uses. Coverage of off-label uses of antineoplastic drugs, biologicals, or radiopharmaceuticals is dependent upon the Medicare contractor. Check local coverage determinations that may be specific to the contractor.

CMS will cover off-label use of oxaliplatin, irinotecan, cetuximab, or bevacizumab when used in one of nine clinical trials identified by CMS and sponsored by the National Cancer Institute. A list of clinical trials is available at http://cms.hhs.gov/coverage/download/id90b.pdf. When billing for oxaliplatin, irinotecan, cetuximab, or bevacizumab used in one of the nine clinical trials identified by CMS and sponsored by the National Cancer Institute, modifier QR must be appended to the HCPCS Level II code. ICD-9-CM diagnosis code V70.7 must be reported as a secondary diagnosis.

Oral Antineoplastic Drugs

Oral antineoplastic drugs are covered if it has the same active ingredient as the injectable drug. It may have a different chemical composition than the injectable drug but body metabolizing of the drug must result in the same chemical composition in the body. A cancer diagnosis code must be reported when billing for these HCPCS Level II codes. If there is no cancer diagnosis the claim will be denied.

Oral Antiemetic Drugs

Medicare covers oral antiemetic drugs when used as full therapeutic replacement for intravenous dosage forms as part of a cancer chemotherapeutic regimen when the drug is administered or prescribed by a physician for use immediately before, at, or within 48 hours after the time of administration of the chemotherapeutic agent. A cancer diagnosis code must be reported when billing for these HCPCS codes.

The allowable period of covered therapy includes day one, the date of service of the chemotherapy drug (beginning of the time of treatment), plus a period not to exceed two additional calendar days, or a maximum period up to 48 hours. Some drugs are limited to 24 hours; some to 48 hours. The hour limit is included in the narrative description of the HCPCS Level II code.

The oral antiemetic drug should be prescribed only on a per chemotherapy treatment basis. For example, only enough of the oral antiemetic for one 24- or 48-hour dosage regimen (depending upon the drug) should be prescribed/supplied for each incidence of chemotherapy treatment. These drugs may be supplied by the physician in the office, by an inpatient or outpatient provider (e.g., hospital, CAH, SNF, etc.), or through a supplier (e.g., a pharmacy).

The physician must indicate on the prescription that the beneficiary is receiving the oral antiemetic drug as full therapeutic replacement for an intravenous antiemetic drug as part of a cancer chemotherapeutic regimen. When the drug is provided by a facility, the patient's medical record maintained by the facility must be documented to reflect that the patient is receiving the oral antiemetic drug as full therapeutic replacement for an intravenous antiemetic drug as part of a cancer chemotherapeutic regimen.

Take-home Supplies of Oral Antiemetic and Antineoplastic Drugs

Hospitals, including CAHs, cannot bill the contractor for take-home supplies of oral anti-cancer drugs, oral antiemetic drugs, or inhalation drugs, in addition to the previous prohibition on immunosuppressive drugs. Hospitals can bill the contractor and be paid for only a single day's dose administered or dispensed during a defined encounter in a hospital outpatient department. Medicare has specifically defined this encounter as "an encounter with a physician or mid-level professional (e.g., a physician assistant or nurse practitioner) during which one or more specimens are collected for laboratory work, treatment is monitored (including anticancer drugs, either oral or infused), and a drug is administered."

A problem arises only when more than a single day's supply of a drug is dispensed to the patient for take-home use. The hospital has three choices:

1. The hospital may dispense the drugs and not charge for them. They cannot bill the patient for covered drugs and these drugs are covered under Part B in most circumstances.

2. The hospital may issue a prescription for the drugs.

3. The hospital can enroll as a pharmacy supplier with the DME MAC and bill the dispensed drugs and a dispensing fee to the DME MAC via the National Council for Prescription Drug Programs (NCPDP) electronic transaction.

Claims for SNF patients in a non-covered stay, or for hospital or SNF inpatients that have exhausted Part A benefits (TOB 12X or 22X) are not affected. TOBs 12X and 22X would be billed to the contractor as usual. Payment is dependent on the applicable reimbursement methodology for the type of hospital (e.g., OPPS for OPPS hospitals or reasonable cost for CAHs and non-OPPS hospitals).

Drugs Used in DME

Drugs and biologicals that are necessary for the effective use of durable medical equipment are covered if they are reasonable and necessary for treatment of the illness or injury or to improve the functioning of a malformed body member. These drugs and biologicals include those which must be put directly into the equipment in order to achieve the therapeutic benefit of the durable medical equipment or to assure the proper functioning of the equipment (e.g., tumor chemotherapy agents used with an infusion pump or heparin used with a home dialysis system).

Drugs and biologicals dispensed for use in DME must be billed to the DME MAC by a supplier who possesses a current license to dispense prescription drugs in the state in which the drug is dispensed. A supplier that is not the entity that dispenses the drugs or biologicals cannot purchase the item used in conjunction with DME for resale to the beneficiary.

Immunosuppressive Drugs

Immunosuppressive drugs are covered following discharge from a hospital for a Medicare covered organ transplant. Covered drugs include those immunosuppressive drugs that have been specifically labeled as such and approved for marketing by the FDA. (This is an exception to the standing drug policy that permits coverage of FDA-approved drugs for non-labeled uses, where such uses are found to be reasonable and necessary in an individual case.)

Covered drugs also include those prescription drugs, such as prednisone, that are used in conjunction with immunosuppressive drugs as part of a therapeutic regimen reflected in FDA-approved labeling for immunosuppressive drugs. Antibiotics, hypertensives, and other drugs that are not directly related to organ rejection are not covered

Prescriptions for immunosuppressive drugs generally should be non-refillable and limited to a 30-day supply. The 30-day guideline is necessary because dosage frequently diminishes over a period of time, and further, it is not uncommon for the physician to change the prescription from one drug to another. Unless there are special circumstances, contractors will not consider a supply of drugs in excess of 30 days to be reasonable and necessary and will deny payment. OPPS hospitals cannot dispense and bill for 30-day supplies of immunosuppressive drugs unless they are enrolled DME suppliers.

Hemophilia Clotting Factors

Medicare covers blood-clotting factors for hemophilia patients competent to use such factors to control bleeding without medical supervision, and items related to the administration of such factors. For purposes of Medicare Part B coverage, hemophilia encompasses the following conditions:

- Factor VIII deficiency (classic hemophilia)
- Factor IX deficiency (also termed plasma thromboplastin component (PTC) or Christmas factor deficiency)
- von Willebrand's disease

The amount of clotting factors determined to be necessary to have on hand and thus covered under this provision is based on the historical utilization pattern or profile developed by the contractor for each patient. It is expected that the treating source (e.g., a family physician or comprehensive hemophilia diagnostic and treatment center) have such information.

Unanticipated occurrences involving extraordinary events, such as automobile accidents or inpatient hospital stays, will change this base line data and should be appropriately considered. In addition, changes in a patient's medical needs over a period of time require adjustments in the profile.

Medicare will cover anti-inhibitor coagulant complex (AICC) for patients with hemophilia A and inhibitor antibodies to factor VIII who have major bleeding episodes and who fail to respond to other, less expensive therapies.

Reimbursement is based upon the least expensive medically necessary blood clotting factors. Blood clotting factors are available both in virally inactivated forms and a recombinant form. The FDA has determined that both varieties are safe and effective. Therefore, unless the prescription specifically calls for the recombinant form, payment is based on the less expensive, non-recombinant forms.

Consolidated Billing

For nursing home patients/residents receiving skilled care reimbursed under Part A, these items are considered to be a component of the inpatient stay. If a source other than the skilled nursing facility dispenses these items, the source must look to the nursing home for payment and cannot bill Medicare directly for these items. If the nursing home patient/resident is not receiving a skilled level of care and is not being reimbursed under Part A, then suppliers must bill these items directly to the DME MAC. Drugs and biologicals dispensed to home health services recipients must be billed directly by the supplier.

Medicare pays for drugs in one of three ways: some drugs are paid on a cost basis; some under its prospective payment system (PPS) plans; but for most drugs outside of a facility setting, Medicare pays the lower of billed charges or the payment limit based on the Average Sales Price (ASP).

The items paid for under this last method include but are not limited to drugs furnished incident to a

physician's service, immunosuppressive drugs furnished by pharmacies, drugs furnished by pharmacies under the durable medical equipment benefit, covered oral anticancer drugs, and blood clotting factors. The table below indicates the payment methodology for drugs and biologicals by type and setting.

Enteral Nutrition

Medicare

These nutrient solutions, devices, and accessories are billed to the DME MAC and not to facility or professional contractors. In place of a CMN, a DME information form (DIF) needs to be completed to provide information for enteral and parenteral nutrition (PEN). For PEN, this form is CMS-10126. A DIF is completed and signed by the supplier. It does not require a narrative description of equipment and cost or a physician signature. DIFs are subject to the same requirements and restrictions as CMNs. This form must be submitted with the CMS-1500 claim form. Electronic filers can use the electronic CMN format.

Typical examples of conditions that would qualify for coverage are anatomic in nature, such as head and neck cancer with reconstructive surgery; and disorders impairing motility, such as a central nervous system disease leading to interference with the neuromuscular mechanisms of ingestion, of such severity that the patient cannot be maintained with oral feeding. However, claims for Part B coverage of enteral nutrition therapy for these and any other conditions must be approved on a case-by-case basis. Enteral therapy is not covered for clinical reasons like anorexia, nausea associated with mood disorders, or end stage renal disease.

The patient must have permanent impairment. However, this judgment does not preclude the possibility that the patient will improve. If, in the judgment of the provider, the condition is of long and/or indefinite duration (at least three months), then the test of permanence is considered to be met.

Baby food and other regular grocery products that can be blended and used with the enteral system will be denied as non-covered. Of special note: Ensure will only be covered if the criteria for parenteral and enteral nutrition (PEN) therapy are met; Medicare does not reimburse for Ensure if it is taken orally.

A total daily calorie intake of 20-35 cal/kg/day is considered sufficient to achieve or maintain appropriate body weight in most patients. The ordering provider must document the medical necessity for a caloric intake outside this range in an individual patient. This information must be available to the DME contractor on request.

Medicare Guidelines

Consolidated Billing

For nursing home patients/residents receiving skilled care reimbursed under Part A, these items are considered to be a component of the inpatient stay. If a source other than the skilled nursing facility dispenses these items, the source must look to the nursing home for payment and cannot bill Medicare directly for these items. If the nursing home patient/resident is not receiving a skilled level of care and is not being reimbursed under Part A, then suppliers must bill these items directly to the DME MAC. Enteral solutions, supplies, and accessories dispensed to home health services recipients should be billed directly by the supplier.

Documentation Standards

Additional documentation must be included with the first claim for enteral nutrition if the nutrient solutions are to be delivered via a pump, or if special nutrient solutions are needed. Refer to the DME MAC Supplier Manual for specific instructions.

Each claim must contain a physician's written order or prescription and sufficient medical documentation (e.g., hospital records, clinical findings from the attending physician, etc.) to permit an independent conclusion that the patient's condition meets the requirements of the prosthetic device benefit, and that enteral nutrition therapy is medically necessary. Allowed claims are to be reviewed at periodic intervals of no more than three months by the contractor's medical consultant or specially trained staff, and additional medical documentation considered necessary should be obtained as part of this review. (Note: DME MACs may have differing recertification requirements, e.g., every six months instead of every three months.)

An interval recertification for continued coverage of the PEN therapy, usually three to six months (depending on the DME contractor policy), must include a provider's statement describing the continued need for parenteral nutrition. Some recertifications must include specific test results; refer to the DME MAC Supplier Manual for these rules.

If there are changes in the patient's condition causing the reporting of different codes other than those initially certified with the original CMN, or if the patient has an interval of two or more months since the previous enteral nutrition administration, or if the method of administration changes from syringe or gravity to that of a pump, a new CMN and/or recertification must be filed.

The ordering physician is expected to see the patient within 30 days before the initial certification or required recertification (but not revised certifications). If the physician does not see the patient within this timeframe, he/she must document the reason why and describe what other monitoring methods were used to evaluate the patient's enteral nutrition needs.

Hospital Beds

Medicare

Hospital beds used in facilities are considered part of the routine equipment. Their cost should be included in the room and board charges. Specialty beds are generally considered to be included with the definition of routine equipment. Facilities are advised to check with their contractor if there are questions about the appropriateness of additional charges for rented specialty beds

A fixed height hospital bed for use in the patient's home is covered when:

- The patient's condition requires positioning of the body, for example, to alleviate pain, promote good body alignment, prevent contractures, and avoid respiratory infections, in ways not feasible in an ordinary bed. Elevation of the head/upper body less than 30 degrees does not usually require the use of a hospital bed. When the patient requires the head of the bed to be elevated more than 30 degrees due to congestive heart failure, chronic pulmonary disease, or problems with aspiration, pillows or wedges must have been considered and ruled out.

- The patient's condition requires special attachments, such as traction equipment, that cannot be fixed and used on an ordinary bed.

A physician's prescription and additional documentation must establish the medical necessity for a hospital bed for home use. The physician's prescription and supplementing documentation when required must accompany the initial claim. If the stated reason for the need for a hospital bed is the patient's condition requires positioning, the prescription or other documentation must describe the medical condition (e.g., cardiac disease, chronic obstructive pulmonary disease, quadriplegia or paraplegia) and also the severity and frequency of the symptoms of the condition. If the stated reason for requiring a hospital bed is the patient's condition requires special attachments, the prescription must describe the patient's condition and specify the attachments that require a hospital bed.

It is up to the Medicare contractor to determine if a variable height feature of a hospital bed is approved for coverage and is considered medically necessary for one of the following conditions:

- Severe arthritis and other injuries to lower extremities (e.g., fractured hip). The condition requires the variable height feature to assist the patient to ambulate by enabling the patient to

- place his or her feet on the floor while sitting on the edge of the bed
- Severe cardiac conditions where the patient is able to leave the bed, but must avoid the strain of "jumping" up or down
- Spinal cord injuries, including quadriplegic and paraplegic patients, multiple limb amputee, and stroke patients. Those patients who are able to transfer from bed to a wheelchair, with or without help
- Other severely debilitating diseases and conditions, if the variable height feature is required to assist the patient to ambulate.

A heavy duty extra wide hospital bed is covered if the patient meets criteria for hospital bed and weighs more than 350 pounds, but less than 600 pounds. An extra heavy-duty hospital bed is covered if the patient meets criteria for a hospital bed and the patient's weight exceeds 600 pounds.

Electric powered adjustments to lower and raise head and foot may be covered when the provider's medical staff determines that the patient's condition requires frequent change in body position and/or there may be an immediate need for a change in body position (i.e., no delay can be tolerated) and the patient can operate the controls and cause the adjustments. Exceptions may be made in cases of spinal cord injury and brain damaged patients. A total electric hospital bed is not covered, as the height adjustment feature is a convenience feature.

An air-fluidized bed uses warm air under pressure to set small ceramic beads in motion that simulate the movement of fluid. The patient's body weight is evenly distributed over a large surface area, which creates a sensation of floating. Medicare payment for home use of the air-fluidized bed for treatment of pressure sores can be made if such use is reasonable and necessary for the individual patient.

An air-fluidized bed may be considered reasonable and necessary when:

- The patient has a stage three full thickness tissue loss or stage four deep tissue destruction pressure sore
- The patient is bedridden or chair bound as a result of severely limited mobility
- In the absence of an air-fluidized bed, the patient would require institutionalization
- The air-fluidized bed is ordered in writing by the patient's attending physician based upon a comprehensive assessment and evaluation of the patient after completion of a course of conservative treatment designed to optimize conditions that promote wound healing. This course of treatment must have been at least one month in duration without progression toward

wound healing. This month of prerequisite conservative treatment may include some period in an institution as long as there is documentation available to verify that the necessary conservative treatment has been rendered

- Use of wet-to-dry dressings for wound debridement, begun during the period of conservative treatment and which continue beyond 30 days, will not preclude coverage of air-fluidized bed. Should additional debridement again become necessary, while a patient is using an air-fluidized bed (after the first 30-day course of conservative treatment), it will not cause the air-fluidized bed to become not covered. In all instances documentation verifying the continued need for the bed must be available.
- A trained adult caregiver is available to assist the patient with activities of daily living, fluid balance, dry skin care, repositioning, recognition and management of altered mental status, dietary needs, prescribed treatments, and management and support of the air-fluidized bed system and its problems such as leakage
- A physician directs the home treatment regimen and reevaluates and recertifies the need for the air-fluidized bed on a monthly basis
- All other alternative equipment has been considered and ruled out

Conservative treatment must include:

- Frequent repositioning of the patient with particular attention to relief of pressure over bony prominences, usually every two hours
- Use of a specialized support surface (Group II) designed to reduce pressure and shear forces on healing ulcers and to prevent new ulcer formation
- Necessary treatment to resolve any wound infection
- Optimization of nutrition status to promote wound healing
- Debridement by any means (including wet to dry dressings that do not require an occlusive covering) to remove devitalized tissue from the wound bed
- Maintenance of a clean, moist bed of granulation tissue with appropriate moist dressings protected by an occlusive covering, while the wound heals

Home use of the air-fluidized bed is not covered under any of the following circumstances:

- The patient has coexisting pulmonary disease (the lack of firm back support makes coughing ineffective and dry air inhalation thickens pulmonary secretions)

- The patient requires treatment with wet soaks or moist wound dressings that are not protected with an impervious covering such as plastic wrap or other occlusive material

- The caregiver is unwilling or unable to provide the type of care required by the patient on an air-fluidized bed

- Structural support is inadequate to support the weight of the air-fluidized bed system (it generally weighs 1,600 pounds or more)

- Electrical system is insufficient for the anticipated increase in energy consumption

- Other known contraindications exist

Coverage of an air-fluidized bed is limited to the equipment itself. Payment for this covered item may only be made if the written order from the attending physician is furnished to the supplier prior to the delivery of the equipment. Payment is not included for the caregiver or for architectural adjustments such as electrical or structural improvement.

For hospital beds used in the home, an order for each item billed must be signed and dated by the treating physician, kept on file by the supplier, and made available to the DME contractor upon request. Items billed to the DME contractor before a signed and dated order has been received by the supplier must be submitted with modifier EY added to each affected HCPCS Level II code.

If the patient does not meet any of the coverage criteria for any type of hospital bed it will be denied as not medically necessary. If documentation does not support the medical necessity of the type of bed billed, payment will be based on the allowance for the least costly medically appropriate alternative.

If the patient's condition requires bedside rails, they can be covered as an integral part of, or an accessory to, a hospital bed. Trapeze equipment is covered if the patient needs this device to sit up because of a respiratory condition, to change body position for other medical reasons, or to get in or out of bed. A bed cradle is covered when it is necessary to prevent contact with the bed coverings. If a patient's condition requires a replacement innerspring mattress or foam rubber mattress it will be covered for a patient owned hospital bed.

A bed board or an over bed table is not covered since it is not primarily medical in nature.

Infusion Pumps, External; Equipment and Supplies

Medicare
Injectable drugs administered in a physician's office, with or without a pump, must be billed to the local carrier and not the DME MAC.

Payment is made if all of the requirements for Medicare reimbursement are met and the applicable DME MAC entity's medical necessity policies for the external infusion pump have been followed.

An external infusion pump is covered for the indications as detailed below:

I. Administration of deferoxamine for the treatment of chronic iron overload

II. Administration of chemotherapy for the treatment of primary hepatocellular carcinoma or colorectal cancer when this disease manifestation cannot be resected or when the patient refuses surgical excision of the tumor

III. Administration of morphine when used in the treatment of intractable pain caused by cancer

IV. Administration of continuous subcutaneous insulin for the treatment of diabetes mellitus, type-I, which has been documented by a serum C-peptide level < 0.5 mcg/L, if either of the following criteria (a) or (b) are met:

a. The patient has completed a comprehensive diabetes education program; has been on a program of multiple daily injections of insulin (i.e., at least three injections per day), with frequent self-adjustments of insulin dose for at least six months prior to initiation of the insulin pump; and has documented frequency of glucose self-testing an average of at least four times per day during the two months prior to initiation of the insulin pump, and meets one or more of the following criteria (1-5) while on the multiple injection regimen:

1. Glycosylated hemoglobin level (HbA1C) greater than 7 percent

2. History of recurring hypoglycemia

3. Wide fluctuations in blood glucose before mealtime

4. Dawn phenomenon with fasting blood sugars frequently exceeding 200 mg/dL

5. History of severe glycemic excursions

b. The patient with type-I diabetes has been on an external insulin infusion pump prior to enrollment in Medicare and has documented frequency of glucose self-testing an average of at least four times per day during the month prior to Medicare enrollment.

In addition to meeting Criterion A or B above, the following general requirements must be met:

The patient with diabetes must be insulinopenic per the updated fasting C-peptide testing requirement, or, as an alternative, must be beta cell autoantibody positive. The updated fasting C-peptide testing requirement is:

– Insulinopenia is defined as a fasting C-peptide level that is less than or equal to 110 percent of the lower limit of normal of the laboratory's measurement method.

– For patients with renal insufficiency and creatinine clearance (actual or calculated from age, gender, weight, and serum creatinine) 50 ml/minute, insulinopenia is defined as a fasting C-peptide level that is less than or equal to 200 percent of the lower limit of normal of the laboratory's measurement method.

– Fasting C-peptide levels will only be considered valid with a concurrently obtained fasting glucose 225 mg/dL.

– Levels only need to be documented once in the medical records.

For patients who have purchased an external insulin infusion pump prior to April 1, 2000, insulin and supplies used with the pump are covered during the period of covered use of the pump as long as the patient is a type-I diabetic as evidenced by a serum C-peptide level less than 0.5 mcg/L.

Continued coverage of an external insulin pump requires that the patient be seen and evaluated by the treating physician at least every three months. In addition, the external insulin infusion pump must be ordered and follow-up care rendered by a physician who manages multiple patients on continuous subcutaneous insulin infusion therapy, and who works closely with a team, including nurses, diabetic educators, and dietitians who are knowledgeable in the use of continuous subcutaneous insulin infusion therapy.

V. Administration of other drugs is covered if either of the following sets of criteria (1) or (2) is met:

Criteria set 1:

- Parenteral administration of the drug in the home is reasonable and necessary

- An infusion pump is necessary to safely administer the drug

- The drug is administered by a prolonged infusion of at least eight hours because of proven improved clinical efficacy

- The therapeutic regimen is proven or generally accepted to have significant advantages over intermittent bolus administration regimens or infusions lasting less than eight hours

Criteria set 2:

- Parenteral administration of the drug in the home is reasonable and necessary

- An infusion pump is necessary to safely administer the drug

- The drug is administered by intermittent infusion (each episode of infusion lasting less than eight hours), which does not require the patient to return to the physician's office prior to the beginning of each infusion

- Systemic toxicity or adverse effects of the drug is unavoidable without infusing it at a strictly controlled rate as indicated in the *Physicians Desk Reference,* American Medical Association's drug evaluations, or the U.S. pharmacopeia drug information

Coverage for the administration of other drugs, based on criteria set (1) or (2), using an external infusion pump, is limited to the following situations (a) to (e):

1. Administration of the anticancer chemotherapy drugs cladribine, fluorouracil, cytarabine, bleomycin, floxuridine, doxorubicin (non-liposomal), vincristine, or vinblastine by continuous infusion over at least eight hours when the regimen is proven or generally accepted to have significant advantages over intermittent administration regimens

2. Administration of narcotic analgesics (except meperidine) in place of morphine to a patient with intractable pain caused by cancer, who has not responded to an adequate oral/transdermal therapeutic regimen and/or cannot tolerate oral/transdermal narcotic analgesics

3. Administration of the following antifungal or antiviral drugs: acyclovir, foscarnet, amphotericin B, and ganciclovir. Liposomal amphotericin B is covered for patients who meet one of the following criteria:

   - The patient has suffered some significant toxicity that would preclude the use of standard amphotericin B and is unable to complete the course of therapy without the liposomal form

Medicare Guidelines

- The patient has significantly impaired renal function

- Payment for the liposomal form will be based on the allowance for the least-costly medically appropriate alternative, standard amphotericin B, unless accompanied by a statement from the provider substantiating the medical need for the liposomal form of amphotericin B for a particular patient

4. Administration of parenteral inotropic therapy, using the drugs dobutamine, milrinone, and/or dopamine, for patients with congestive heart failure and depressed cardiac function if a patient meets all of the following criteria:

  - Dyspnea at rest is present despite treatment with maximum or near maximum tolerated doses of digoxin, a loop diuretic, and an angiotensin converting enzyme inhibitor or another vasodilator (e.g., hydralazine or isosorbide dinitrate), used simultaneously (unless allergic or intolerant). Doses are within the following ranges (lower doses will be covered only if part of a weaning or tapering protocol from higher dose levels):

    - Dobutamine 2.5-10 mcg/kg/min
    - Milrinone 0.375-0.750 mcg/kg/min
    - Dopamine < 2 mcg/kg/min

  - Invasive hemodynamic studies performed within six months prior to the initiation of home inotropic therapy show (a) cardiac index (CI) is less than or equal to 2.2 liters/min/meter squared and/or pulmonary capillary wedge pressure (PCWP) is greater than or equal to 20 mm Hg before inotrope infusion on maximum medical management and (b) at least a 20 percent increase in CI and/or at least a 20 percent decrease in PCWP during inotrope infusion at the dose initially prescribed for home infusion

  - There has been an improvement in patient well being (less dyspnea, improved diuresis, improved renal function, and/or reduction in weight), with the absence of dyspnea at rest at the time of discharge and the capability of outpatient evaluation by the prescribing provider at least monthly

  - In the case of continuous infusion, there is documented deterioration in clinical status when the drug is tapered or discontinued under observation in the hospital, or, in the case of intermittent infusions, there is documentation of repeated hospitalizations for congestive heart failure despite maximum medical management

  - Any life threatening arrhythmia is controlled prior to hospital discharge and there is no need for routine electrocardiographic monitoring at home

  - The patient is maintained on the lowest practical dose, and efforts to decrease the dose of the drug or the frequency/duration of infusion are documented during the first three months of therapy

  - The patient's cardiac symptoms, vital signs, weight, lab values, and response to therapy are routinely assessed and documented in the patient's medical record

5. Administration of parenteral epoprostenol for patients with pulmonary hypertension if they meet the following disease criteria:

  - The pulmonary hypertension is not secondary to pulmonary venous hypertension (e.g., left-sided atrial or ventricular disease, left-sided valvular heart disease, etc.) or disorders of the respiratory system (e.g., chronic obstructive pulmonary disease, interstitial lung disease, obstructive sleep apnea or other sleep disordered breathing, alveolar hypoventilation disorders, etc.)

  - The patient has primary pulmonary hypertension or pulmonary hypertension that is secondary to one of the following conditions:

    - connective tissue disease
    - thromboembolic disease of the pulmonary arteries
    - human immunodeficiency virus (HIV) infection
    - cirrhosis
    - diet drugs
    - congenital left-to-right shunts

  - If these conditions are present, the following criteria must be met:

    - the pulmonary hypertension has progressed despite maximal medical and/or surgical treatment of the identified condition
    - the mean pulmonary artery pressure is greater than 25 mm Hg at rest or greater than 30 mm Hg with exertion

- the patient has significant symptoms from the pulmonary hypertension (i.e., severe dyspnea on exertion, and either fatigability, angina, or syncope)

- treatment with oral calcium channel blocking agents has been tried and failed, or has been considered and ruled out

6. Administration of gallium nitrate for the treatment of symptomatic cancer-related hypercalcemia (ICD-9-CM diagnosis code 275.42). Generally, patients should have serum calcium (corrected for albumin) equal to or greater than 12 mg/dl.

   The recommended usage for gallium nitrate is daily for five consecutive days. Use for more than five days will be denied as not medically necessary. More than one course of treatment for the same episode of hypercalcemia will be denied as not medically necessary.

Other Supplies

External infusion pumps and related drugs and supplies will be denied as not medically necessary when the criteria described by the above indications are not met. When an infusion pump is covered, the drug necessitating the use of the pump and necessary supplies are also covered. When a pump has been purchased by the Medicare program, other insurer, or the patient, or the rental cap has been reached, the drug necessitating the use of the pump and supplies are covered as long as the coverage criteria for the pump are met.

An IV pole is covered only when a stationary infusion pump is covered. It is considered not medically necessary if it is billed with an ambulatory infusion pump.

Supplies used with an external infusion pump (excluding external insulin infusion pumps) are covered during the period of covered use of an infusion pump. Allowance is based on the number of cassettes or bags prepared. For intermittent infusions, no more than one cassette or bag is covered for each dose of drug. For continuous infusion, the concentration of the drug and the size of the cassette or bag should be maximized to result in the fewest cassettes or bags in keeping with good pharmacologic and medical practice. Drugs and supplies that are dispensed, but not used for unforeseen circumstances (e.g., emergency admission to hospital, drug toxicity, etc.) are covered. Suppliers are expected to anticipate changing needs for drugs (e.g., planned hospital admissions, drug level testing with possible dosage change, etc.) in their drug and supply preparation and delivery schedule.

Charges for drugs administered via a DME infusion pump may only be billed by the entity that actually dispenses the drug to the Medicare patient, and that entity must be permitted under all applicable federal, state, and local laws and regulations to dispense drugs. Drugs and related supplies and equipment billed by a supplier who does not meet these criteria will be denied as not medically necessary.

The DME MAC does not process claims for implantable infusion pumps or drugs and supplies used in conjunction with an implantable infusion pump. Hospitals submit claims for these items to their intermediary. Claims for implantable pumps, drugs, and supplies from other providers are billed to the local carrier.

Drugs used in a DME infusion pump should be coded using the appropriate HCPCS codes or NDC number. If the drug does not have a distinct code, then use the unclassified drug code J7799. Do not use J9999; this code is not valid for claims billed to the DME MAC.

Any entity billing drugs to a DME MAC must use the NDC number.

Medicare Noncovered Items/Services

External insulin infusion pumps for type-II diabetics, including insulin-treated type-II diabetics, will be denied as not medically necessary.

An external infusion pump and related drugs and supplies will be denied as not medically necessary in the home setting for the treatment of thromboembolic disease and/or pulmonary embolism by heparin infusion.

An infusion controller device has been considered by the Medicare program as not medically necessary.

Documentation Standards

For an item to be considered for coverage and payment by Medicare, the information submitted by the supplier must be corroborated by documentation in the physician's medical records that Medicare coverage criteria have been met. The patient's medical records include the provider's office records, hospital records, nursing home records, home health agency records, or records from other health care professionals. This documentation must be available to the DME MAC upon request.

An order for the item that has been signed and dated by the treating provider and a DIF (CMS form 10125) that has been filled out, signed, and dated by the treating provider must be kept on file by the supplier. For external infusion pumps, an ICD-9-CM diagnosis code (specific to the fifth digit) describing the condition that necessitates the pump must be included on each order and DIF for the pump, drug/insulin, and/or supplies.

If a patient begins using an infusion for one drug and subsequently the drug is changed or if another drug is added, a revised DIF must be submitted for use of the pump with the new or additional drug. In the case of an additional drug, all drugs for which the pump is used should be included on the revised DIF.

If an inotropic drug is ordered, the initial claim must include a copy of the order (prescription and documentation from the treating physician), which includes information relating to each of the criteria defined in the aforementioned guidelines. This must include the before and after inotropic drug infusion values.

Medical necessity related to specific clinical data may not be completed by the supplier or by anyone in a financial relationship with the supplier. If coverage criteria as stated in the Medicare policy are not met, the claim should be accompanied by a letter from the physician detailing the patient's history (e.g., dates of past hospitalization for heart failure, prior use of parenteral inotropics and the results, etc.). If invasive hemodynamic studies were not performed, a letter and any supporting documentation should accompany the claim explaining the rationale for not performing the tests.

Intravenous Immune Globulin

The Medicare Intravenous Immune Globulin (IVIG) demonstration is being implemented to evaluate the benefits of providing payment and items for services needed for the in-home administration of intravenous immune globulin for the treatment of primary immune deficiency disease (PIDD). This is a three-year demonstration that began with services on October 1, 2014. It will continue for three years, as long as funding remains available. This demonstration will pay a bundled payment for items and services needed for the in-home administration of intravenous immune globulin for the treatment of PIDD.

Suppliers do not need to apply for this demonstration. However, they must meet all Medicare, national, state, and local standards and regulations applicable to the provision of demonstration covered services. The demonstration is limited to no more than 4,000 Medicare patients and $45 million, which includes benefit costs and administrative expenses. Participation is voluntary and may be terminated by the patient at any time.

Under this demonstration, Medicare will issue under Part B a bundled payment for all items and services that are necessary to administer IVIG in the home to enrolled beneficiaries who are not otherwise homebound and receiving home health care benefits. In processing all services and supplies needed for the administration of IVIG, CMS is not making any changes to existing coverage determinations to receive the IVIG drug in the home or for services and supplies that are otherwise not covered under the traditional fee-for-service (FFS) Medicare Part B

benefit. The demonstration covered services will be paid as a bundle and will be subject to coinsurance and deductible in the same manner as other Part B services.

Providers and suppliers billing for the services and supplies covered under the demonstration must meet all Medicare as well as other national, state, and local standards and regulations applicable to the provision of services related to home infusion of IVIG.

The demonstration only applies to situations where the patient requires IVIG for the treatment of PIDD or is currently receiving subcutaneous immune globulin to treat PIDD and wishes to switch to IVIG. This demonstration does not apply if the immune globulin is intended to be administered subcutaneously. Only those beneficiaries with PIDD who are eligible to receive IVIG under the current Medicare benefit (have Part B, and have traditional FFS Medicare) will be eligible to enroll in the demonstration and have the services paid under the new demonstration.

The demonstration will not change how subcutaneous administration of immune globulin is covered and paid for under traditional Medicare FFS programs. Also, nothing in this demonstration impacts how IVIG is paid by Medicare for patients covered under a home health episode of care.

Payment for this demonstration will be made only if the following requirements are met:

The patient must:

1. Be enrolled in the demonstration (on the eligibility file provided by NHIC, Corp., the implementation support contractor).

2. Be eligible to have the IVIG drug paid for at home (has a diagnosis of PIDD) under the traditional Medicare benefit.

3. Be enrolled in Medicare Part B and not be enrolled in a Medicare Advantage plan (i.e. have traditional FFS Medicare coverage).

4. Not be covered on the date of service in a home health episode (which covers the services under the home health episode payment).

5. Receive services in their home or a setting that is "home like" (the place of service).

Patient enrollment is currently closed.

The following Q code is to be reported for services, supplies, and accessories used in the home under the Medicare IVIG demonstration:

Q2052 Services, supplies, and accessories used in the home under Medicare Intravenous immune globulin (IVIG) demonstration

The code is for use with the IVIG demo only and the jurisdiction for this code is the DME MAC.

Code Q2052 must be billed as a separate claim line on the same claim for the IVIG drug.

Claims billed without an associated J code for the IVIG drug will not be payable. For 2014, the nationwide Medicare allowable for Q2052 will be $300 each time the IVIG is administered. While this is expected to be approximately monthly, it can be more or less frequent depending upon a patient's medical need.

The following J codes represent immune globulin drugs that are administered intravenously and payable in 2014 under Medicare Part B for services rendered in the home (or home-like setting) for beneficiaries with PIDD: Privigen, (J1459), Bivigam (J1556), Gammaplex (J1557), Gamunex (J1561), Immune Globulin Not Otherwise Specified (J1566 and J1599), Octagam (J1568), Gammagard liquid (J1569), and Flebogamma (J1572). The claim for Q2052 must have the same place of service code on the claim line as the IVIG (J code) for which it is applicable. In cases where the drug is mailed or delivered to the patient prior to administration, the date of service for the administration of the drug may be no more than 30 calendar days after the date of service on the drug claim line.

(*MLN Matters* article, SE1424, August 28, 2014)

Lens

Medicare
Refractive lenses are covered when they are medically necessary to restore the vision normally provided by the natural lens of the eye of an individual lacking the organic lens because of surgical removal or congenital absence. Covered diagnoses are limited to Pseudophakia (ICD-9-CM code V43.1), Aphakia (ICD-9-CM code 379.31), and congenital Aphakia (ICD-9-CM code 743.35). Lenses provided for other diagnoses will be denied as noncovered.

Aphakia is the absence of the lens of the eye. Pseudophakia is an eye in which the natural lens has been replaced with an artificial intraocular lens (IOL).

After each cataract surgery with insertion of an intraocular lens (ICD-9-CM code V43.1), coverage is limited to one pair of eyeglasses or contact lenses. Replacement glasses and lenses are noncovered. If a patient has a cataract extraction with IOL insertion in one eye, subsequently has a cataract extraction with IOL insertion in the other eye, and does not receive spectacles or cataract lenses between the two surgical procedures, Medicare covers only one pair of eyeglasses or contact lenses after the second surgery. If a patient has a pair of eyeglasses, has a cataract extraction with IOL insertion, and receives only new lenses, but not new frames after the surgery, the benefit would not cover new frames at a later date (unless it follows subsequent cataract extraction in the other eye).

Refractive lenses are covered even though the surgical removal of the natural lens occurred before Medicare entitlement.

For patients who are aphakic who do not have an IOL (ICD-9-CM codes 379.31 and 743.35), the following lenses or combinations of lenses are covered when determined to be medically necessary:

• Lenses in frames for far vision and lenses in frames for near vision

• Contact lenses for far vision (including for cases of binocular and monocular aphakia); payment will be made for the contact lenses, as well as lenses in frames for near vision to be worn at the same time as the contact lens, and lenses in frames to be worn when the contacts have been removed

When billing claims for a progressive lens, use the appropriate code for the standard bifocal (V2200-V2299) or trifocal (V2300-V2399) lens, and a second line item using V2781 for the difference between the charge for the progressive lens and the standard lens.

If aphakia is the result of the removal of a previously implanted lens, the date of the surgical removal of the lens must accompany the claim.

Medicare Noncovered Items/Services
Lenses used as sunglasses (pseudophakic patient) in addition to regular prosthetic lenses are not covered.

Ostomy Devices and Supplies

Medicare
Ostomy bags supplies and necessary accessories required for attachment are covered as prosthetic devices. This coverage also includes irrigation and flushing equipment and other items and supplies directly related to ostomy care, whether the attachment of a bag is required.

Ostomy supplies are exempt DME in a hospital setting under certain restrictions. When the ostomy supply is associated with the surgery that created the opening or a revision to the opening, it is an exempt DME item. In that situation, hospitals bill their intermediary. If the ostomy supply is used in other circumstances it does not qualify as an exempt DME. Freestanding ambulatory surgery centers are also allowed the same exemptions as hospitals.

They may bill the items listed as exempt DME to their carrier.

Ostomy supplies used in the home for routine care must be dispensed and billed by a DME supplier.

Consolidated Billing

All ostomy devices, supplies, and accessories dispensed to a nursing home patient/resident or home health services recipient are included in the consolidated billing requirements and each provider's prospective payment system (PPS).

For home health services recipients, all billing related to these items must be performed by the home health agency. For nursing home patients/residents receiving skilled care reimbursed under Part A, these items are considered to be a component of the inpatient stay. If a source other than the skilled nursing facility dispenses these items, the source must look to the nursing home for payment and cannot bill Medicare directly for these items. If the nursing home patient/resident is not receiving a skilled level of care and is not being reimbursed under Part A, then suppliers have a choice. The first option is for the supplier to bill these items directly to the DME MAC. The second option is for the supplier to bill the nursing home directly and the home would bill Medicare.

Oxygen (O_2) and O_2 Equipment

Medicare

Oxygen furnished to hospital inpatients is covered as a part of the inpatient stay as a supply. Oxygen furnished to hospital outpatients is covered as a part of the outpatient visit or surgery. Routine supplies furnished by the physician in the course of performing his or her services (e.g., gauze, ointments, bandages, and oxygen) are covered. Charges for such services and supplies must be included in the physician's bill.

Home oxygen and oxygen equipment is covered by Medicare as reasonable and necessary only for patients with significant hypoxemia who meet the medical documentation, laboratory evidence, and health conditions as specified below.

Coverage is available for patients with significant hypoxemia in the chronic stable state (e.g., not during a period of acute illness or an exacerbation of their underlying disease) when the patient has:

- A severe lung disease, such as chronic obstructive pulmonary disease, diffuse interstitial lung disease, cystic fibrosis, bronchiectasis, widespread pulmonary neoplasm

- Hypoxia-related symptoms or findings that might be expected to improve with oxygen therapy (e.g., pulmonary hypertension, recurring congestive heart failure due to chronic cor pulmonale, erythrocytosis, impairment of the cognitive process, nocturnal restlessness, and morning headache)

If the patient has one of these conditions the following further requirements apply:

- Group I—Patients with significant hypoxemia evidenced by any of the following:

  - An arterial PO_2 at or below 55 mm Hg or an arterial oxygen saturation at or below 88 percent, taken at rest, breathing room air

  - An arterial PO_2 at or below 55 mm Hg or an arterial oxygen saturation at or below 88 percent, taken during sleep for a patient who demonstrates an arterial PO_2 at or above 56 mm Hg or an arterial oxygen saturation at or above 89 percent, while awake; or a greater than normal fall in oxygen level during sleep (a decrease in arterial PO_2 more than 10 mm Hg or decrease in arterial oxygen saturation more than 5 percent) associated with symptoms or signs reasonably attributable to hypoxemia (e.g., impairment of cognitive processes and nocturnal restlessness or insomnia). In either of these cases, coverage is provided only for use of oxygen during sleep, and then only one type of unit will be covered. Portable oxygen would not be covered in this situation

  - An arterial PO_2 at or below 55 mm Hg or an arterial oxygen saturation at or below 88 percent, taken during exercise for a patient who demonstrates an arterial PO_2 at or above 56 mm Hg, or an arterial oxygen saturation at or above 89 percent, during the day while at rest. In this case, supplemental oxygen is provided during exercise if there is evidence the use of oxygen improves the hypoxemia that was demonstrated during exercise when the patient was breathing room air

- Group II—Patients whose arterial PO_2 is 56 to 59 mm Hg or whose arterial blood oxygen saturation is 89 percent, if there is evidence of:

  - Dependent edema suggesting congestive heart failure

  - Pulmonary hypertension or cor pulmonale, determined by measurement of pulmonary artery pressure, gated blood pool scan, echocardiogram, or "P" pulmonale on EKG (P wave greater than 3 mm in standard leads II, III, or AVF)

- Erythrocythemia with a hematocrit greater than 56 percent

- Group III—The Medicare contractor's reviewing physician will review on a case-by-case basis instances where oxygen is ordered for patients arterial PO$_2$ levels at or above 60 mm Hg or arterial blood oxygen saturation at or above 90 percent.

Initial claims for oxygen services must include a completed CMN (CMS form 484) to establish whether coverage criteria are met and to ensure that the oxygen services provided are consistent with the physician's prescription or other medical documentation. The documentation must indicate the other forms of treatment that have been tried (e.g., medical and physical therapy directed at secretions, bronchospasm, and infection) and that these treatments have not been sufficiently successful.

The medical and prescription information in section B of the CMN can be completed only by the treating physician, the physician's employee, or another clinician (e.g., nurse, respiratory therapist, etc.) as long as that person is not the DME supplier. Although hospital discharge coordinators and medical social workers may assist in arranging for physician-prescribed home oxygen, they do not have the authority to prescribe the services. Suppliers may not enter this information. While this section may be completed by a nonphysician clinician or a physician employee, it must be reviewed and the CMN must be signed by the attending physician.

Claims for oxygen must also be supported by medical documentation in the patient's record. Separate documentation is used with electronic billing. This documentation may be in the form of a prescription written by the patient's attending physician who has recently examined the patient, usually within a month of the start of therapy, and must specify:

- A diagnosis of the disease requiring home use of oxygen
- The oxygen flow rate
- An estimate of the frequency, duration of use (e.g., 2 liters per minute, 10 minutes per hour, 12 hours per day), and duration of need (e.g., six months or lifetime) Note that a prescription for "Oxygen PRN" or "Oxygen as needed" does not meet this requirement

The attending physician should specify the type of oxygen delivery system to be used (e.g., gas, liquid, or concentrator).

New medical documentation written by the patient's attending physician must be submitted in support of revised oxygen requirements when there has been a change in the patient's condition and need for oxygen therapy. Repeat arterial blood gas studies are appropriate when evidence indicates that an oxygen recipient has undergone a major change in his or her condition relevant to home use of oxygen.

A physician's certification of medical necessity for oxygen equipment must include the results of specific testing before coverage can be determined. Initial claims for oxygen therapy must include the results of a blood gas study that has been ordered and evaluated by the attending physician. This is usually in the form of a measurement of the partial pressure of oxygen (PO$_2$) in arterial blood. A measurement of arterial oxygen saturation obtained by ear or pulse oximetry is also acceptable when ordered and evaluated by the attending and performed under his or her supervision or when performed by a qualified provider or supplier of laboratory services.

When the arterial blood gas and the oximetry studies are both used to document the need for home oxygen therapy and the results are conflicting, the arterial blood gas study is the preferred source of documenting medical need. Blood gas tests can be conducted by a hospital certified to do such tests. The conditions under which the laboratory tests are performed must be specified in writing and submitted with the initial claim (i.e., at rest, during exercise, or during sleep).

It is expected that virtually all patients who qualify for home oxygen coverage for the first time have recently been discharged from a hospital where they have had arterial blood gas tests; these hospital tests can be submitted in support of initial claims for home oxygen. If more than one arterial blood gas test is performed during the patient's hospital stay, the test result obtained closest to, but no earlier than two days prior to the hospital discharge date, is required as evidence of the need for home oxygen therapy. For those patients whose initial oxygen prescription did not originate during a hospital stay, blood gas studies should be done while the patient is in the chronic stable state (i.e., not during a period of an acute illness or an exacerbation of the underlying disease).

Medicare Noncovered Items/Services
Conditions for which oxygen therapy is not covered include:

- Angina pectoris in the absence of hypoxemia. This condition is generally not the result of a low oxygen level in the blood, and there are other preferred treatments.

- Breathlessness without cor pulmonale or evidence of hypoxemia. Although intermittent oxygen use is sometimes prescribed to relieve this condition, it is potentially harmful and psychologically addicting.

- Severe peripheral vascular disease that results in clinically evident desaturation in one or more extremities. There is no evidence that increased

PO_2 improves the oxygenation of tissues with impaired circulation.

- Terminal illnesses that do not affect the lungs.

The Medicare program assumes any delivery charges for home O_2 equipment are included in the price charged for the equipment. Separate reimbursement for delivery is not typically paid and separate charges are prohibited from being charged.

Medicare does not reimburse for O_2 when the Medicare beneficiary is traveling on an airplane.

Oxygen equipment that is purchased is not eligible for Medicare coverage.

Claims for supplies and accessories, including drugs, will be denied if submitted in advance of claims for the base equipment. If the DME MAC cannot determine that the patient either owns or rents the O_2 base equipment, the supplies and accessories will be denied payment. A denial may also occur if the DME MAC cannot establish whether or not the patient meets the medical necessity requirements for the base O_2 equipment.

Consolidated Billing

If oxygen and related equipment are dispensed to a nursing home patient/resident receiving skilled care reimbursed under Part A, these items are considered to be a component of the inpatient stay. If a source other than the skilled nursing facility dispenses these items, the source must look to the nursing home for payment and cannot bill Medicare directly for these items. If the nursing home patient/resident is not receiving a skilled level of care and is not being reimbursed under Part A, then suppliers should bill these items directly to the DME MAC. For home health services recipients, suppliers should bill these items to the HHA as they are included in consolidated billing requirements.

Parenteral Nutrition

Medicare

For parenteral nutrition therapy to be covered under Part B, the claim must be accompanied by the physician's or provider's certified DIF, and there must be evidence of written medical documentation to permit an independent conclusion that the requirements of a prosthetic device benefit are met, and that parenteral nutrition therapy is medically necessary. An example of a condition that would typically qualify for coverage is a massive small bowel resection resulting in severe nutritional deficiency in spite of adequate oral intake. However, coverage of parenteral nutrition therapy for this and any other condition must be approved (certified) on a case-by-case basis initially and at periodic intervals of no more than three months by the carrier's medical

consultant or specially trained staff, relying on medical and other documentation as the carrier may require.

Nutrient solutions for parenteral therapy are routinely covered. However, Medicare will not pay for more than one month's supply of nutrients at any one time. Claims submitted retroactively (vs. prospectively, for qualified providers) may include multiple months.

Reimbursement for nutrient solutions is based on the reasonable charge for the solution components (vs. a pre-mixed solution). However, if the patient's medical record establishes that the patient, due to physical or mental state, is unable to safely or effectively mix the solution, and there is no family member or other person who can assist the patient, payment can be made on the basis of the reasonable charge for the more expensive premixed solutions. The medical record must include a signed statement from the attending physician that attests that the premixed solutions are required.

The patient must have (a) a condition involving the small intestine and/or its exocrine glands that significantly impairs the absorption of nutrients, or (b) a disease of the stomach and/or intestine that is a motility disorder and impairs the ability of nutrients to be transported through the gastrointestinal (GI) system. There must be objective evidence supporting the clinical diagnosis.

Parenteral nutrition is noncovered for the patient with a functioning gastrointestinal tract whose need for parenteral nutrition is only due to the following:

- A swallowing disorder
- A temporary defect in gastric emptying, such as a metabolic or electrolyte disorder
- A psychological disorder impairing food intake, such as depression
- A metabolic disorder inducing anorexia, such as cancer
- A physical disorder impairing food intake, such as the dyspnea of severe pulmonary or cardiac disease
- A side effect of a medication
- Renal failure and/or dialysis

Parenteral nutrition is covered in any of the following situations:

A. The patient has undergone recent (within the past three months) massive small bowel resection leaving less than five feet of small bowel beyond the ligament of Treitz.

B. The patient has a short bowel syndrome that is severe enough that the patient has net gastrointestinal fluid and electrolyte malabsorption, such that on an oral intake of 2.5

to 3.0 liters/day, the enteral losses exceed 50 percent of the oral/enteral intake and the urine output is less than 1 liter/day.

C. The patient requires bowel rest for at least three months and is receiving intravenously 20-35 cal/kg/day for treatment of symptomatic pancreatitis with/without pancreatic pseudocyst, severe exacerbation of regional enteritis, or a proximal enterocutaneous fistula where tube feeding distal to the fistula is not possible.

D. The patient has complete mechanical small bowel obstruction where surgery is not an option.

E. The patient is significantly malnourished (10 percent weight loss over three months or less and serum albumin less than 3.4 gm/DL) and has severe fat malabsorption (fecal fat exceeds 50 percent of oral/enteral intake on a diet of at least 50 gm of fat/day as measured by a standard 72 hour fecal fat test).

F. The patient is significantly malnourished (10 percent weight loss over three months or less and serum albumin less than 3.4 gm/Dl) and has a severe motility disturbance of the small intestine and/or stomach that is unresponsive to prokinetic medication, and is demonstrated either (1) scintigraphically (solid meal gastric emptying study demonstrates that the isotope fails to reach the right colon by six hours following ingestion), or (2) radiographically (barium or radiopaque pellets fail to reach the right colon by six hours following administration). These studies must be performed when the patient is not acutely ill and is not on any medication that would decrease bowel motility. Unresponsiveness to prokinetic medication is defined as the presence of daily symptoms of nausea and vomiting while taking maximal doses.

For criteria A through F above, the conditions are deemed to be severe enough that the patient would not be able to maintain weight and strength on only oral intake or tube enteral nutrition. Patients who do not meet criteria A through F above must meet criteria 1 and 2, which is modification of diet and pharmacologic intervention, plus criteria G and H below:

G. The patient is malnourished (10 percent weight loss over three months or less and serum albumin less than 3.4 gm/Dl).

H. A disease or clinical condition has been documented as being present and it has not responded to altering the manner of delivery of appropriate nutrients (e.g., enteral therapy — slow infusion of nutrients through a tube with the tip located in the stomach or jejunum).

The following are some examples of moderate abnormalities that would require a failed trial of tube enteral nutrition before parenteral nutrition would be covered:

• Moderate fecal fat malabsorption that exceeds 25 percent of oral/enteral intake on a diet of at least 50 gm of fat/day as measured by a standard 72 hour fecal fat test

• Diagnosis of malabsorption with objective confirmation by methods other than 72-hour fecal fat test (e.g., Sudan stain of stool, d-xylose test, etc.)

• Gastroparesis that has been demonstrated (a) radiographically or scintigraphically as described in F above with the isotope or pellets failing to reach the jejunum in three to six hours, or (b) by manometric motility studies with results consistent with an abnormal gastric emptying, and which is unresponsive to prokinetic medication

• A small bowel motility disturbance that is unresponsive to prokinetic medication, demonstrated with a gastric to right colon transit time between three to six hours

• A small bowel resection leaving greater than five feet of small bowel beyond the ligament of Treitz

• A short bowel syndrome that is not severe (as defined in B)

• A mild to moderate exacerbation of regional enteritis, or an enterocutaneous fistula

• A partial mechanical small bowel obstruction where surgery is not an option as long as the following criteria are met: 1a) a permanent condition of the alimentary tract is present that has been deemed to require parenteral therapy because of its severity (criteria A-F); or 1b) a permanent condition of the alimentary tract is present that is unresponsive to standard medical management (criterion H); and 2) the person is unable to maintain weight and strength (criterion G)

If the coverage requirements for parenteral nutrition are met, medically necessary nutrients, administration supplies, and equipment are covered.

There are specific guidelines that contain stipulations for patients who require intradialytic parenteral nutrition (IDPN), as well as parameters of coverage for total caloric daily intake; nutrition solutions containing little or no amino acids and/or carbohydrates; solutions with proteins outside of the range of 0.8-1.5 gm/kg/day; dextrose concentration less than 10 percent, or lipid use; and guidelines for patients with the ability to obtain partial nutrition from oral intake or a combination of oral/enteral (or even oral/enteral/parenteral) intake.

Medicare Guidelines

Consolidated Billing

For nursing home patients/residents receiving skilled care reimbursed under Part A, these items are considered to be a component of the inpatient stay. If a source other than the skilled nursing facility dispenses these items, the source must look to the nursing home for payment and cannot bill Medicare directly for these items. If the nursing home patient/resident is not receiving a skilled level of care and is not being reimbursed under Part A, then suppliers must bill these items directly to the DME MAC. Parenteral solutions, supplies, and accessories dispensed to home health services recipients should be billed directly by the supplier.

Documentation Standards

Additional documentation must be included with the first claim for parenteral nutrition, depending on the type of solution that is medically necessary.

An interval recertification for continued coverage of the PEN therapy, usually three to six months (depending on the DME MAC policy), must include a physician's statement describing the continued need for parenteral nutrition. Some recertifications must include specific test results; refer to the DME MAC Supplier Manual for these rules.

The ordering physician is expected to see the patient within 30 days before the initial certification or required recertification (but not revised certifications). If the physician does not see the patient within this timeframe, the provider must document the reason why and describe what other monitoring methods were used to evaluate the patient's nutrition needs.

If there are changes in the patient's condition that cause the reporting of different codes other than those initially certified with the original DIF, a new DIF and/or recertification must be filed.

Pressure Reducing Support Surfaces: Groups I, II, and III

Medicare

General Coverage: Codes E0185 and E0197-E0199 identified as "pressure pad for mattress" describe nonpowered pressure reducing mattress overlays. These devices are designed to be placed on top of a standard hospital or home mattress. A gel/gel-like mattress overlay (E0185) is characterized by a gel or gel-like layer with a height of 2 inches or greater. An air mattress overlay (E0197) is characterized by interconnected air cells having a cell height of 3 inches or greater that are inflated with an air pump. A water mattress overlay (E0198) is characterized by a filled height of 3 inches or greater. A foam mattress overlay (E0199) is characterized by all of the following:

- Base thickness of 2 inches or greater and peak height of 3 inches or greater if it is a convoluted overlay (e.g., egg crate-type), or an overall height of at least 3 inches if it is a non-convoluted overlay
- Foam with a density and other qualities that provide adequate pressure reduction
- Durable, waterproof cover

Codes E0186, E0187, and E0196 describe nonpowered pressure-reducing mattresses. A foam mattress (E0184) is characterized by all of the following:

- Foam height of 5 inches or greater
- Foam with a density and other qualities that provide adequate pressure reduction
- Durable, waterproof cover
- Can be placed directly on a hospital bed frame

An air, water, or gel mattress (E0186, E0187, E0196) is characterized by all of the following:

- Height of 5 inches or greater of the air, water, or gel layer (respectively)
- Durable, waterproof cover
- Can be placed directly on a hospital bed frame

Codes E0180, E0181, E0182, and A4640 describe powered pressure-reducing mattress overlay systems (alternating pressure or low air loss). They are characterized by all of the following:

- An air pump or blower that provides either sequential inflation and deflation of air cells or a low interface pressure throughout the overlay
- Inflated cell height of the air cells through which air is being circulated 2.5 inches or greater
- Height of the air chambers, proximity of the air chambers to one another, frequency of air cycling (for alternating pressure overlays), and air pressure provide adequate patient lift, reduce pressure, and prevent bottoming out

The staging (grading) of pressure ulcers used in Medicare's policy follows:

- Stage I—nonblanchable erythema of intact skin
- Stage II—partial thickness skin loss involving epidermis and/or dermis
- Stage III—full thickness skin loss involving damage or necrosis of subcutaneous tissue that may extend down to, but not through, underlying fascia
- Stage IV—full thickness skin loss with extensive destruction, tissue necrosis, or damage to muscle, bone, or supporting structures

"Bottoming out" is the finding that an outstretched hand, placed palm up between the undersurface of the overlay or mattress and the patient's bony prominence (coccyx or lateral trochanter), can readily palpate the bony prominence. This bottoming out criterion should be tested with the patient in the supine position with their head flat, in the supine position with their head slightly elevated (no more than 30 degrees), and in the side-lying position.

A group I mattress overlay or mattress (A4640, E0181-E0187, E0196-E0199) is covered if the patient meets criterion 1 or criteria 2 or 3 and at least one of criteria 4 through 7:

Criteria:

1. Completely immobile (i.e., patient cannot make changes in body position without assistance)

2. Limited mobility (i.e., patient cannot independently make changes in body position significant enough to alleviate pressure)

3. Any stage pressure ulcer on the trunk or pelvis

4. Impaired nutritional status

5. Fecal or urinary incontinence

6. Altered sensory perception

7. Compromised circulatory status

When the coverage criteria for a group I overlay or mattress are not met, a claim will be denied as not medically necessary unless there is clear documentation that justifies the medical necessity for the item in the individual case. A group I support surface billed without modifier KX (see later in this section) will usually be denied as not medically necessary.

A foam overlay or mattress that does not have a waterproof cover is not considered durable (i.e., DME) and will be denied as noncovered by the Medicare program.

The support surface provided for the patient should be one in which the patient does not bottom out.

Clinical information for Group I support surfaces: Patients needing pressure-reducing support surfaces should have a care plan that has been established by the patient's physician or home care nurse, which is documented in the patient's medical records, and which generally should include the following:

- Education of the patient and caregiver on the prevention and/or management of pressure ulcers

- Regular assessment by a nurse, physician, or other licensed health care practitioner

- Appropriate turning and positioning

- Appropriate wound care (for a stage II, III, or IV ulcer)

- Appropriate management of moisture/incontinence

- Nutritional assessment and intervention consistent with the overall plan of care

Note: Products containing multiple components are categorized according to the clinically predominant component (usually the topmost layer of a multi-layer product). For example, a product with 3 inch powered air cells on top of a 3 inch foam base would be coded as a powered overlay (E0181), not as a powered mattress (E0277).

Group II support surfaces: E0277 describes a powered pressure-reducing mattress (alternating pressure, low air loss, or powered flotation without low air loss) that is characterized by all of the following:

- An air pump or blower that provides either sequential inflation and deflation of the air cells or a low interface pressure throughout the mattress

- Inflated cell height of the air cells through which air is being circulated is 5 inches or greater

- Height of the air chambers, proximity of the air chambers to one another, frequency of air cycling (for alternating pressure mattresses), and air pressure provide adequate patient lift, reduce pressure, and prevent bottoming out

- A surface designed to reduce friction and shear

- Can be placed directly on a hospital bed frame

Code E0193 describes a semielectric or total electric hospital bed with a fully integrated powered pressure-reducing mattress that has all of the characteristics defined previously under code E0277 characteristics.

Code E0371 describes an advanced nonpowered pressure-reducing mattress overlay that is characterized by all of the following:

- Height and design of individual cells that provide significantly more pressure reduction than a group I overlay, and prevent bottoming out

- Total height of 3 inches or greater

- A surface designed to reduce friction and shear

Documented evidence to substantiate that the product is effective for the treatment of conditions described by the coverage criteria for group II support surfaces

Code E0372 describes a powered pressure reducing mattress overlay (low air loss, powered flotation without low air loss, or alternating pressure) that is characterized by all of the following:

- An air pump or blower that provides either sequential inflation and deflation of the air cells or a low interface pressure throughout the overlay
- Inflated cell height of the air cells through which air is being circulated is 3.5 inches or greater
- Height of the air chambers, proximity of the air chambers to one another, frequency of air cycling (for alternating pressure overlays), and air pressure to provide adequate patient lift, reduce pressure, and prevent bottoming out
- A surface designed to reduce friction and shear

Code E0373 describes an advanced nonpowered pressure-reducing mattress that is characterized by all of the following:

- Height and design of individual cells that provide significantly more pressure reduction than a group I mattress, and prevent bottoming out
- Total height of 5 inches or greater
- A surface designed to reduce friction and shear
- Can be placed directly on a hospital bed frame

The staging of pressure ulcers for group II support surfaces is the same as that for group I support surfaces.

A group II support surface is covered if the patient meets criterion 1, 2, and 3; criterion 4; or criterion 5 and 6.

Criteria:

1. Multiple stage II pressure ulcers located on the trunk or pelvis

2. Patient on a comprehensive ulcer treatment program for at least the past month, which includes the use of an appropriate group 1 support surface

3. The ulcers have worsened or remained the same over the past month

4. Large or multiple stage III or IV pressure ulcer on the trunk or pelvis

5. Recent myocutaneous flap or skin graft for a pressure ulcer on the trunk or pelvis (surgery within the past 60 days)

6. The patient on a group II or III support surface immediately prior to a recent discharge from a hospital or nursing facility (discharge within the past 30 days)

The comprehensive ulcer treatment described in criterion two above should generally include:

- Education of the patient and caregiver on the prevention and/or management of pressure ulcers

- Regular assessment by a nurse, physician, or other licensed health care practitioner (usually at least weekly for a patient with a stage III or IV ulcer)
- Appropriate turning and positioning
- Appropriate wound care (for a stage II, III, or IV ulcer)
- Appropriate management of moisture/incontinence
- Nutritional assessment and intervention consistent with the overall plan of care

If the patient is on a group II surface, a care plan should be established by the physician or home care nurse that includes the above elements. The support surface provided for the patient should be one in which the patient does not bottom out.

When a group II surface is covered following a myocutaneous flap or skin graft, coverage generally is limited to 60 days from the date of surgery.

When the stated coverage criteria for a group II mattress or bed are not met, a claim will be denied as not medically necessary unless there is clear documentation that justifies the medical necessity for the item in the individual case. A Group II support surface billed without modifier KX will usually be denied as not medically necessary.

Clinical Information for Group II Support Surfaces: Continued use of a group II support surface is covered until the ulcer is healed, or if healing does not continue, there is documentation in the medical record to show that: (1) other aspects of the care plan are being modified to promote healing, or (2) the use of the group II support surface is medically necessary for wound management.

Appropriate use of modifier KX is the responsibility of the supplier billing the DME MAC. The supplier should maintain adequate communication on an ongoing basis with the clinician providing the wound care, in order to accurately determine that use of modifier KX still reflects the clinical conditions that meet the criteria for coverage of a group II support surface, and that adequate documentation exists in the medical record reflecting these conditions. Such documentation should not be submitted with a claim, but should be available for review if requested by the DME MAC.

In cases where a group II product is inappropriate, a group I or III support surface could be covered if coverage criteria for that group are met.

Group III support surfaces: Code E0194 for an air-fluidized bed is a device employing the circulation of filtered air through silicone-coated ceramic beads creating the characteristics of fluid. The staging of pressure ulcers for group III support surfaces is the same as that for groups I and II.

An air-fluidized bed is covered only if all of the following criteria are met:

- The patient has a stage III (full thickness tissue loss) or stage IV (deep tissue destruction) pressure sore
- The patient is bedridden or chair bound as a result of severely limited mobility
- In the absence of an air-fluidized bed, the patient would require institutionalization
- The air-fluidized bed is ordered in writing by the patient's attending physician based upon a comprehensive assessment and evaluation of the patient after conservative treatment has been tried without success

Treatment should generally include the following:

- Education of the patient and caregiver on the prevention and/or management of pressure ulcers
- Assessment by a physician, nurse, or other licensed health care practitioner at least weekly
- Appropriate turning and positioning
- Use of a group II support surface, if appropriate
- Appropriate wound care
- Appropriate management of moisture/incontinence
- Nutritional assessment and intervention consistent with the overall plan of care

The patient must generally have been on the conservative treatment program for at least one-month prior to use of the air-fluidized bed, with worsening or no improvement of the ulcer. Generally, the evaluation must be performed within a week prior to initiation of therapy with the air-fluidized bed. An air-fluidized bed will be covered under the following circumstances:

- A trained adult caregiver is available to assist the patient with activities of daily living, fluid balance, dry skin care, repositioning, recognition and management of altered mental status, dietary needs, prescribed treatments, and management and support of the air-fluidized bed system and its problems, such as leakage
- A physician directs the home treatment regimen, and reevaluates and recertifies the need for the air-fluidized bed on a monthly basis
- All other alternative equipment has been considered and ruled out

An air-fluidized bed will be denied as not medically necessary under any of the following circumstances:

- The patient has coexisting pulmonary disease (the lack of firm back support makes coughing ineffective and dry air inhalation thickens pulmonary secretions)
- The patient requires treatment with wet soaks or moist wound dressings that are not protected with an impervious covering, such as plastic wrap or other occlusive material
- The caregiver is unwilling or unable to provide the type of care required by the patient on an air-fluidized bed
- Structural support is inadequate to support the weight of the air-fluidized bed system (it generally weighs 1,600 pounds or more)
- The electrical system is insufficient for the anticipated increase in energy consumption
- Other known contraindications exist

Payment is not included for the caregiver or for architectural adjustments, such as electrical or structural improvement.

If the stated coverage criteria for an air-fluidized bed are not met, the claim will be denied as not medically necessary unless there is clear documentation that justifies the medical necessity for the item in the individual case.

Clinical Information for Group III Support Surfaces: The continued medical necessity of an air-fluidized bed must be documented by the treating physician every month. Continued use of an air-fluidized bed is covered until the ulcer is healed, or, if healing does not continue, there is documentation to show the following:

- Other aspects of the care plan are being modified to promote healing
- The use of the bed is medically necessary for wound management

Documentation Standards

Group I Support Surfaces

An order for the overlay or mattress, which is signed and dated by the treating physician, must be kept on file by the supplier. The written order must be obtained prior to the delivery of the item.

For Medicare beneficiaries, the supplier should obtain all necessary information prior to dispensing the pressure-reducing support surface. A DME MAC data collecting form, Statement of Ordering Physician Group I Support Surfaces, should be provided to the treating physician for completion. Questions pertaining to medical necessity on any form used to collect this information may not be completed by the supplier or anyone in a financial relationship with the supplier. This statement must be supported by information in the patient's medical record, which would be available to the DME MAC on request. Do not send this form to the DME MAC unless specifically requested.

Group II Support Surfaces

An order for the mattress or bed, which is signed and dated by the treating provider, must be kept on file by the supplier. The written order must be obtained prior to the delivery of the item.

For Medicare beneficiaries, the supplier should obtain all necessary information prior to dispensing the pressure-reducing support surface. A DME MAC data collecting form, Statement of Ordering Physician Group II Support Surfaces, should be provided to the treating physician for completion. Questions pertaining to medical necessity on any form used to collect this information may not be completed by the supplier or anyone in a financial relationship with the supplier. This statement must be supported by information in the patient's medical record, which would be available to the DMERC on request. Do not send this form to the DMERC unless specifically requested.

Group III Support Surfaces

An order for the bed, which has been signed and dated by the attending physician who is caring for the patient's wounds, must be kept on file by the supplier. The written order must be obtained prior to the delivery of the air-fluidized bed.

Prosthetic and Orthotic Devices

Medicare

Prosthetic devices (other than dental) are covered under Part B when the device replaces all or part of an internal body organ or replaces all or part of the function of a permanently inoperative or malfunctioning internal body organ. Orthotics, which include leg, arm, back, and neck braces; trusses; and artificial limbs and eyes are covered under Part B when furnished incident to physician services or on a physician's order.

A brace includes rigid and semi-rigid devices that are used for the purpose of supporting a weak or deformed body member or restricting or eliminating motion in a diseased or injured part of the body. Back braces include, but are not limited to, special corsets (e.g., sacroiliac, sacrolumbar, dorsolumbar corsets) and belts. A terminal device (e.g., hand or hook) is covered under this provision whether the patient requires an artificial limb. Stump stockings and harnesses (including replacements) are also covered when these appliances are essential to the effective use of the artificial limb. Elastic stockings, garter belts, and similar devices do not come within the scope of the definition of a brace.

Replacements or repairs of such devices are covered when furnished incident to physician services or on a physician's orders. Adjustments to an artificial limb or other appliance required by wear or by a change in the patient's condition are covered when ordered by a physician. Adjustments, repairs, and replacements are covered even when the item has been in use before the user enrolled in Part B of the program so long as the device continues to be medically required.

Prefabricated prosthetics and orthotics, other than ostomy supplies, are exempt DME that may be billed by the nursing home or hospital to the FI. When furnished to inpatients in a Part A covered stay, the prefabricated prosthetics and orthotics is included in the inpatient reimbursement. When the patient is not in a covered Part A inpatient stay or is an outpatient, separate payment will be made under the DMEPOS fee schedule. Customized prosthetics and orthotics should be billed directly by the supplier to the DME MAC.

Please note that there are nine states that currently require an orthotist or prosthetist furnish orthotics and prosthetics. As of October 2005, the nine states include Alabama, Florida, Illinois, New Jersey, Ohio, Oklahoma, Rhode Island, Texas, and Washington. When a supplier from one of these states bills customized fabricated orthotics and prosthetics to the DME MAC, the supplier must have a specialty code that includes orthotists or prosthetists or Medicare will deny the claim.

Off-the-Shelf Orthotics

The Social Security Act, section 1847(a)(2), defines Off-The-Shelf (OTS) orthotics as those orthotics described in section 1861(s)(9) of the Act for which payment would otherwise be made and which require minimal self-adjustment for appropriate use and do not require expertise in trimming, bending, molding, assembling, or customizing to fit to the individual. Orthotics that are currently paid are described as leg, arm, back, and neck braces. The *Medicare Benefit Policy Manual*, publication 100-02, chapter 15, section 130 provides the longstanding Medicare definition of braces. Braces are defined in this section as "rigid or semi-rigid devices which are used for the purpose of supporting a weak or deformed body member or restricting or eliminating motion in a diseased or injured part of the body."

CMS regulations also define the term "minimal self-adjustment" to mean an adjustment that the patient, caretaker, or supplier of the device can perform and that does not require the services of a certified orthotist or an individual who has specialized training.

The list below contains the final 2014 list that identifies HCPCS Level II codes considered OTS orthotics. Items classified under these codes require minimal self-adjustment for appropriate use and do not require expertise in trimming, bending, molding, assembling, or customizing to fit the beneficiary. Subsequent coding updates to the OTS list will be included in program instructions.

Suppliers of any orthotic other than an OTS orthotic must be in compliance with Appendix C of the DMEPOS quality standards, which specifies that suppliers must possess specialized education, training, and experience in fitting and certification and/or licensing.

Note that in some cases there are two HCPCS Level II codes that describe a particular prefabricated orthotic product: one code for when the device is furnished OTS and a second code for when the device is furnished with custom fitting. In these cases, and in the case of any code for a prefabricated orthotic that requires more than minimal self-adjustment and requires expertise in fitting or customizing, the code that describes a custom fitted orthotic cannot be used unless the custom fitting services have been performed and the supplier is in compliance with Appendix C of the DMEPOS quality standards.

OTS orthotics is one of the categories of items subject to competitive bidding. CMS has not determined the schedule for bidding OTS orthotics, but will identify the specific OTS orthotic codes.

L0120	L0160	L0172
L0174	L0450	L0455
L0457	L0467	L0469
L0621	L0623	L0625
L0628	L0641	L0642
L0643	L0648	L0469
L0650	L0651	L0980
L0982	L0984	L1812
L1830	L1833	L1836
L1848	L1850	L1902
L1906	L3100	L3170
L3650	L3660	L3670
L3675	L3678	L3710
L3762	L3908	L3912
L3916	L3918	L3924
L3925	L3927	L3930
L4350	L4361	L4370
L4387	L4397	L4398

Consolidated Billing

For nursing home patients/residents receiving skilled care reimbursed under Part A, non-customized

prosthetics and orthotics are considered to be a component of the inpatient stay. If a source other than the skilled nursing facility dispenses these items, the source must look to the nursing home for payment and cannot bill Medicare directly for these items. If the nursing home patient/resident is not receiving a skilled level of care and is not being reimbursed under Part A, then suppliers may bill these items to the facility or directly to the DME MAC. Prosthetics and orthotics dispensed to home health services recipients are exempt from consolidated billing requirements and may be billed directly by the supplier.

Ankle-Foot Orthosis (AFO) and Knee-Ankle-Foot Orthosis (KAFO); Related Additions and Replacements; Repairs

Medicare

For an item to be considered for Medicare coverage under the orthotic benefit category, it must be a rigid or semirigid device used for the purpose of supporting a weak or deformed body member or restricting or eliminating motion in a diseased or injured part of the body.

A nonambulatory AFO may be either an ankle contracture splint or a foot drop splint.

AFOs and KAFOs that are molded-to-patient-model (custom fabricated) are covered for ambulatory patients when the basic coverage criteria listed previously are met and one of the following criteria are met:

- The patient could not be fit with a prefabricated AFO

- The condition necessitating the orthosis is expected to be permanent or of longstanding duration (more than six months)

- There is a need to control the knee, ankle, or foot in more than one plane

- The patient has a documented neurological, circulatory, or orthopedic status that requires custom fabricating over a patient model to prevent tissue injury

- The patient has a healing fracture that lacks normal anatomical integrity or anthropometric proportions

If the specific criteria for a molded-to-patient-model orthosis are not met, but the criteria for a prefabricated, custom fitted orthosis are met, payment will be based on the allowance for the least costly medically appropriate alternative.

The allowance for the labor involved in replacing an orthotic component that is coded with the

Medicare Guidelines

miscellaneous code L4210 is separately payable in addition to the allowance for that component.

Claims for prefabricated or custom fabricated devices that contain a concentric adjustable torsion style mechanism in the knee or ankle joint and that are being used to treat a joint contracture should be coded as E1810 *Dynamic adjustable knee extension/flexion device* or E1815 *Dynamic adjustable ankle extension/flexion device* for the device itself and the interface material (represented by code E1820). If a concentric adjustable torsion style mechanism in the knee or ankle joint is used in a custom-fabricated orthosis to provide and assist function to joint motion during ambulation, it should be coded as L2999.

Medicare Noncovered Items/Services

Evaluation of the patient, measurement and/or casting, and fitting of the orthosis are included in the allowance for the orthosis. There is no separate payment for these services.

If the expense for repairs exceeds the estimated expense of providing another entire orthosis, no payment will be made for the amount in excess.

The allowance for the labor involved in replacing an orthotic component is included in the allowance for that component.

Modifiers

If an AFO or KAFO is used solely for the treatment of edema and/or for the prevention or treatment of a heel pressure ulcer, modifier GY should be added to the base code and any related addition code. A short narrative statement should be documented in the medical record explaining why modifier GY is reported, such as "Used to prevent pressure ulcer," "Used to treat pressure ulcer," or "Used to treat edema." This statement should be entered in the HAO record of an electronic claim or attached to a hard copy claim.

Facial Prosthesis

Medicare

Modifications may be billed to Medicare when they occur more than 90 days after delivery of the prosthesis and they are required because of a change in the patient's condition.

Repairs are covered when there has been accidental damage or extensive wear to the prosthesis that can be repaired. The expense for the repairs cannot exceed the estimated expense for a replacement prosthesis.

Replacement of a facial prosthesis is covered in cases of loss or irreparable damage or wear or when required because of a change in the patient's condition that cannot be accommodated by

modification of the existing prosthesis. When replacement involves a new impression/moulage rather than use of a previous master model, the reason for the new impression/moulage must be clearly documented in the supplier's records and be available to the DME MAC on request.

Claims for facial prostheses from nonphysicians provided in an office or nursing home setting are submitted to the DME MAC. Claims for facial prostheses from physicians in these settings are submitted to the local carrier. Claims for facial prostheses provided in an outpatient hospital setting are submitted to the local intermediary. Facial prostheses provided in an inpatient hospital setting are included in the payment made to the hospital and should not be submitted to the DME MAC. Implanted prosthesis anchoring components should not be billed to the DME MAC.

If an ocular prosthesis is dispensed to the patient as an integral part of a facial prosthesis, the supplier of the facial prosthesis must bill the ocular prosthesis component.

When a new ocular prosthesis component is provided as an integral part of an orbital, upper facial, or hemi-facial prosthesis, it should be billed using code V2623 or V2629 on a separate claim line. When a replacement facial prosthesis utilizes an ocular component from the prior prosthesis, the ocular prosthesis code should not be billed.

If a facial prosthesis has a component that is used to attach it to a bone-anchored implant or to an internal prosthesis (e.g., maxillary obturator), that component should be billed separately using code L8048. This code should not be used for implanted prosthesis anchoring components.

When a prosthesis is needed for adjacent facial regions, a single code must be used to bill for the item whenever possible. For example, if a defect involves the nose and orbit, this should be billed using the hemi-facial prosthesis code and not separate codes for the orbit and nose. This would apply even if the prosthesis is fabricated in two separate parts.

Medicare Noncovered Items/Services

Follow-up visits that occur more than 90 days after delivery and that do not involve modification or repair of the prosthesis are not covered.

Modifiers

When a replacement prosthesis is fabricated from a new impression/moulage, modifier KM should be added to the code. When a replacement prosthesis is fabricated using a previous master model, modifier KN should be added to the code.

The right (RT) and left (LT) modifiers should be used with facial prosthesis codes when applicable. If bilateral prostheses using the same code are billed on the same date of service, the code should be entered on a single claims line using modifiers LT and RT and billed with 2 units of service.

Lower Limb Prostheses; Related Additions and Replacements; Miscellaneous Prostheses and Services

Medicare

Prostheses are covered when furnished incident to physician's services or on a physician's order.

Accessories (e.g., stump stockings for the residual limb, harness [including replacements]) are covered when these appliances aid in or are essential to the effective use of the artificial limb. A lower limb prosthesis is covered when the patient:

- Will reach or maintain a defined functional state within a reasonable period of time
- Is motivated to ambulate

This information must be documented in the medical record.

A functional status level is a determination of the medical necessity for certain components/additions to the prosthesis. Potential functional ability is based on the reasonable expectations of the prosthetist and ordering physician, considering factors including, but not limited to:

- The patient's past history (including prior prosthetic use if applicable)
- The patient's current condition, including the status of the residual limb and the nature of other medical problems
- The patient's desire to ambulate

Clinical assessments of patient rehabilitation potential should be based on the following classification levels:

- Level 0: The patient does not have the ability or potential to ambulate or transfer safely with or without assistance and a prosthesis does not enhance their quality of life or mobility.
- Level 1: The patient has the ability or potential to use a prosthesis for transfers or ambulation on level surfaces at fixed cadence. This is typical of the limited and unlimited household ambulator.
- Level 2: The patient has the ability or potential for ambulation with the ability to traverse low-level environmental barriers such as curbs, stairs, or uneven surfaces. This is typical of the limited community ambulator.
- Level 3: The patient has the ability or potential for ambulation with variable cadence. This is typical of the community ambulator who has the ability to traverse most environmental barriers, and may

have vocational, therapeutic, or exercise activity that demands prosthetic utilization beyond simple locomotion.

- Level 4: The patient has the ability or potential for prosthetic ambulation that exceeds basic ambulation skills, exhibiting high impact, stress, or energy levels. This is typical of the prosthetic demands of the child, active adult, or athlete.

Basic lower extremity prostheses include a single axis, constant friction knee. Coverage is extended only if there is sufficient clinical documentation of functional need for the technologic design feature of a given type of knee prosthesis. This information must be retained in the physician or prosthetist's files.

Any prosthesis or prosthetic component provided in an inpatient hospital setting should not be submitted to the DME MAC.

The submitted charge for replacements reflects both the cost of the component and the labor associated with the removal, replacement, and finishing of that component. Labor associated with replacement should not be reported using L7520.

Adjustments to a prosthesis due to wear or by change in the patient's condition are covered under the initial provider's order for the prosthesis for the life of the prosthesis.

Repairs to a prosthesis are covered when necessary to make the prosthesis functional.

If the expense for repairs exceeds the estimated expense of purchasing another entire prosthesis, no payments can be made for the amount of the excess. Maintenance, which may be necessitated by manufacturer's recommendations or the construction of the prosthesis (and must be performed by the prosthetist), is covered as a repair.

Replacement of a prosthesis or prosthetic component is covered in cases of loss or irreparable damage or wear, or when required because of a change in the patient's condition. Expenses for replacement of a prosthesis or prosthetic components required because of loss or irreparable damage may be reimbursed without a provider's order when it is determined that the prosthesis, as originally ordered, still fulfills the patient's medical needs. However, claims involving replacement of a prosthesis or major component (foot, ankle, knee, socket) necessitated by wear or a change in the patient's condition must be supported by a new provider's order. When the DMERC determines that malicious damage, culpable neglect, or wrongful disposition of the prosthesis has occurred, an investigation will be undertaken to determine whether it is unreasonable to make program payment under the circumstances.

Medicare Guidelines

Medicare Non-Covered Items/Services

A prosthesis will be denied as not medically necessary if the patient's potential functional level is 0. The above functional levels are reflected in modifiers K0 through K4.

The following items are included in the reimbursement for a prosthesis and are not separately billable to Medicare:

- Evaluation of the residual limb and gait
- Fitting of the prosthesis
- Cost of base component parts and labor contained in HCPCS base codes
- Repairs due to normal wear or tear within 90 days of delivery
- Adjustments of the prosthesis or the prosthetic component made when fitting the prosthesis or component, and for 90 days from the date of delivery when the adjustments are not necessitated by changes in the residual limb or the patient's functional abilities
- Routine periodic servicing, such as testing, cleaning, and checking of the prosthesis, is noncovered

Speech Generating Devices and Speech Aids

Medicare

Electronic speech aids are covered as prosthetic devices when the patient has had a laryngectomy or his or her larynx is permanently inoperative. There are two types of speech aids. One operates by placing a vibrating head against the throat and the other amplifies sound waves through a tube that is inserted into the user's mouth.

A tracheostomy-speaking valve is covered as an element of the trachea tube, which makes the tube more effective. The trachea tube and valve are covered prosthetic devices.

Augmentative and alternative communication devices or communicators, which are generally referred to as speech generating devices, are covered prosthetic devices if the contractor's medical staff determines that the patient suffers from a severe speech impairment and that the medical condition warrants the use of a device.

Speech generating devices are defined as speech aids that provide an individual who has severe speech impairment with the ability to meet his or her functional speaking needs. Speech generating devices include the following characteristics:

- Dedicated speech device, used solely by the individual who has a severe speech impairment

- Digitized speech output, using prerecorded messages, less than or equal to eight minutes recording time
- Digitized speech output, using prerecorded messages, greater than eight minutes recording time
- Synthesized speech output that requires message formulation by spelling and device access by physical contact with the device-direct selection techniques
- Synthesized speech output that permits multiple methods of message formulation and multiple methods of device access
- Software that allows a laptop computer, desktop computer, or personal digital assistant (PDA) to function as a speech generating device

Devices that would not meet the definition of speech generating devices and are not covered are characterized by:

- Devices that are not dedicated speech devices, but are devices that are capable of running software for purposes other than for speech generation (e.g., devices that can also run a word processing package, an accounting program, or perform other than non-medical function).
- Laptop computers, desktop computers, or PDAs that may be programmed to perform the same function as a speech generating device, are not covered since they are not primarily medical in nature and do not meet the definition of DME. For this reason, they cannot be considered speech-generating devices for Medicare coverage purposes.
- A device that is useful to someone without severe speech impairment is not considered a speech-generating device for Medicare coverage purposes.

A tracheostomy-speaking valve and electronic speech aids are devices that may be billed by any facility just as any other exempt prosthetic and orthotic. Speech generating devices must be supplied and billed by an enrolled DME supplier.

Transcutaneous Electrical Nerve Stimulation

Medicare

Transcutaneous electrical nerve stimulation (TENS) is an accepted modality as a rehabilitation therapy. TENS may be used for the relief of acute postoperative pain and its use is covered under Medicare. TENS may be covered whether used as an adjunct to the use of drugs or as an alternative to drugs in the treatment of acute pain resulting from surgery. TENS, when used for acute postoperative pain, is expected to be necessary for relatively short periods of time, usually 30 days or less. TENS devices, whether durable or disposable, may be used in furnishing this service. TENS devices are considered supplies when used for the purpose of treating acute postoperative pain. As such they may be hospital supplies furnished to inpatients covered under Part A, or supplies incident to a physician's service when furnished in connection with surgery done on an outpatient basis, and covered under Part B.

When TENS is used for chronic pain, the TENS device may be covered as DME. An assessment of the effectiveness of the TENS to treat chronic pain should be made before the device is prescribed. This assessment usually involves attachment of a transcutaneous nerve stimulator to the surface of the skin over the peripheral nerve to be stimulated. The patient uses it on a trial basis and its effectiveness in modulating pain is monitored by the physician or physical therapist.

When used for the treatment of chronic, intractable pain, the TENS unit must be used by the patient on a trial basis for a minimum of one month (30 days), but not to exceed two months. Document the medical necessity for such services that are furnished beyond the first month. The trial period must be monitored by the physician to determine the effectiveness of the TENS unit in modulating the pain. For coverage of a purchase, the physician must determine whether the patient is likely to derive a significant therapeutic benefit from continuous use of a TENS. The medical records must document a reevaluation of the patient at the end of the trial period, must indicate how often the patient used the TENS unit, the typical duration of use each time, and the results.

If TENS significantly alleviates pain, it may be considered as primary treatment. If it produces no relief or greater discomfort than the original pain, then the TENS therapy cannot be covered.

The physician or physical therapist providing the services usually furnishes the equipment necessary for assessment. Where the physician or physical therapist advises the patient to rent the TENS from a supplier during the trial period rather than supplying it himself or herself, Medicare payment may be made for rental of the TENS, as well as for the services of the physician or physical therapist who is evaluating its use.

A four lead TENS unit may be used with two leads or four leads, depending on the characteristics of the patient's pain. If it is ordered for use with four leads, the medical record must document why two leads are insufficient to meet the patient's needs.

During the rental of a TENS unit from a DME supplier, supplies for the unit are included in the rental allowance. There is no additional allowance for

electrodes, lead wires, batteries, etc. If a TENS unit (E0720 or E0730) is purchased, the allowance includes lead wires and one month's supply of electrodes, conductive paste or gel (if needed), and batteries.

When supplied by a DME supplier, separate payment may be made for DME replacement supplies when they are medically necessary and are used with a TENS unit that has been purchased. If two TENS leads are medically necessary, then a maximum of one unit of HCPCS Level II code A4595 would be allowed per month. If four leads were necessary, a maximum of two units per month would be allowed. If the use of the TENS unit is less than daily, the frequency of billing for the TENS supply code should be reduced proportionally.

There should be no billing and there will be no separate allowance for replacement electrodes, conductive paste or gel, replacement batteries, or a battery charger used with a TENS unit.

When supplied by a DME supplier, replacement of lead wires will be covered when they are inoperative due to damage and the TENS unit is still medically necessary. Replacement more often than every 12 months would rarely be medically necessary. Other supplies, including but not limited to the following, will not be separately allowed: adapters (e.g., snap, banana, alligator, tab, button, clip), belt clips, adhesive remover, additional connecting cable for lead wires, carrying pouches, or covers.

TENS can ordinarily be delivered to patients through the use of conventional electrodes, adhesive tapes, and lead wires. There may be times where it might be medically necessary for certain patients receiving TENS treatment to use, as an alternative to conventional electrodes, adhesive tapes and lead wires, a form-fitting conductive garment (i.e., a garment with conductive fibers that are separated from the patient's skin by layers of fabric).

A form-fitting conductive garment (and medically necessary related supplies) may be covered under the program only when it has been approved by the FDA and it has been prescribed by a physician for use in delivering covered TENS treatment. Additionally one of the medical indications below must be met:

- The patient cannot manage without the conductive garment because there is such a large area or so many sites to be stimulated and the stimulation would have to be delivered so frequently that it is not feasible to use conventional electrodes, adhesive tapes, and lead wires.

- The patient cannot manage without the conductive garment for the treatment of chronic intractable pain because the areas or sites to be stimulated are inaccessible with the use of conventional electrodes, adhesive tapes, and lead wires.

- The patient has a documented medical condition such as skin problems that preclude the application of conventional electrodes, adhesive tapes, and lead wires.

- The patient requires electrical stimulation beneath a cast to treat disuse atrophy, where the nerve supply to the muscle is intact, or to treat chronic intractable pain.

- The patient has a medical need for rehabilitation strengthening (pursuant to a written plan of rehabilitation) following an injury where the nerve supply to the muscle is intact.

TENS treatments performed in a facility or professional office are billed as a rehabilitation therapy modality. TENS devices when used by the patient in the home for covered therapy would be billed by the DME supplier to the DME MAC.

When the TENS is rented or purchased from a DME supplier, an order for each item billed must be signed and dated by the treating physician, kept on file by the supplier, and made available to the DME MAC upon request. Items delivered before the supplier has received a signed written order must be submitted with modifier EY added to each affected HCPCS Level II code.

When the TENS purchased from a DME supplier, a CMN (CMS form 848) must be completed, signed, and dated by the treating physician. The CMN must be kept on file by the supplier and made available to the DME MAC on request. The CMN may act as a substitute for a written order if it contains all the required elements of an order. The initial claim must include a copy of the CMN. A TENS CMN is not necessary for rentals.

Urological Supplies

Medicare

Permanent urinary retention is defined as retention that is not expected to be medically or surgically corrected in that patient within three months.

Most use in hospitals is on a temporary basis, which means that these items do not meet the definition of DME. When used on a temporary basis, these supplies should be billed without a HCPCS Level II code using revenue codes 0270, 0271, or 0272 as routine supplies. If the patient is permanently impaired and the supplies qualify as DME, then they should be reported with a HCPCS Level II code under revenue code 0274 as orthotics and prosthetics.

If the catheter or the external urinary collection device meets the coverage criteria, then the related supplies

that are necessary for their effective use are also covered.

The patient must have a permanent impairment of urination. This does not require a determination that there is no possibility that the patient's condition may improve sometime in the future. If the medical record, including the judgment of the attending physician, indicates the condition is of long and indefinite duration (ordinarily at least three months), the test of permanence is considered met.

When urological supplies are furnished in a physician's office, they may be billed to the DME MAC only if the patient's condition meets the definition of permanence. The use of a urological supply for the treatment of chronic urinary tract infection or other bladder condition in the absence of permanent urinary incontinence or retention is not covered by Medicare. Since the patient's urinary system is functioning, the criteria for coverage under the prosthetic benefit provision are not met.

Nonroutine catheter changes are covered when documentation substantiates medical necessity, such as for the following indications:

- The catheter is accidentally removed (e.g., pulled out by the patient)

- A malfunction of catheter has occurred (e.g., the balloon does not stay inflated, a hole has developed in the catheter)

- The catheter is obstructed by encrustation, mucous plug, blood clot, etc.

- There is a history of recurrent obstruction or urinary tract infection for which it has been established that an acute event is prevented by a scheduled change at intervals of less than once per month

A urinary drainage collection system will be covered for routine changes of the urinary drainage collection system, as noted in the following table.

Additional charges will be allowed for medically necessary nonroutine changes when the documentation substantiates the medical necessity (e.g., obstruction, clotting of blood, or chronic, recurrent urinary tract infection).

If there is a catheter change and an additional drainage bag change within a month, the combined utilization for the items should be considered when determining if additional documentation should be submitted with the claim for appropriate adjudication.

Intermittent irrigation of an indwelling catheter requires the use of certain supplies. These supplies are covered when they are used on an as-needed (nonroutine) basis in the presence of acute obstruction of the catheter. Supplies for the routine intermittent irrigation of a catheter will be denied as not medically necessary. Routine irrigation is defined as being performed at predetermined intervals. In some cases, the DMERC may request a copy of the order for irrigation and documentation in the patient's medical record of the presence of acute catheter obstruction when irrigation supplies are billed.

Covered supplies for medically necessary nonroutine irrigation of a catheter include either an irrigation tray or an irrigation syringe, and sterile saline or sterile water. When syringes, trays, sterile saline, or water are used for routine irrigation, they will be denied as not medically necessary. Irrigation solutions containing antibiotics and chemotherapeutic agents will be denied as noncovered. Irrigating solutions such as acetic acid or hydrogen peroxide used for the treatment or prevention of urinary obstruction will be denied as not medically necessary. Irrigation supplies that are used for care of the skin or perineum of incontinent patients are noncovered.

Supplies for the continuous irrigation of an indwelling catheter are covered if there is a history of obstruction of the catheter and the patency of the catheter cannot be maintained by intermittent irrigation in conjunction with medically necessary catheter changes. Continuous irrigation as a primary preventive measure (i.e., there is no history of catheter obstruction) will be denied as not medically necessary. Documentation must substantiate the medical necessity of catheter irrigation and, in particular, continuous irrigation as opposed to intermittent irrigation. The medical records must also indicate the rate of solution administration and the duration of need. This documentation may be requested by the DME MAC.

Covered supplies for medically necessary continuous bladder irrigation include a three-way Foley catheter, irrigation tubing set, and sterile saline or sterile water. Payment for irrigating solutions such as acetic acid or hydrogen peroxide will be based on the allowance for sterile water or sterile saline.

Continuous irrigation is a temporary measure. Continuous irrigation for more than two weeks is rarely medically necessary. The patient's medical records should indicate this medical necessity; these medical records may be requested by the DME MAC.

For each episode of covered sterile catheterization, Medicare will cover the following:

- One catheter and an individual packet of lubricant
- An intermittent catheter kit

The kit code should be used for billing even if the components are packaged separately rather than together as a kit. If sterile catheterization is not medically necessary, sterile supplies will be denied as not medically necessary.

Male external catheters (condom type) or female external urinary collection devices are covered for patients who have permanent urinary incontinence when used as an alternative to an indwelling catheter. The utilization of male external catheters generally should not exceed 35 per month. Greater use of these devices must be accompanied by documentation that supports the medical necessity of the increased quantity.

Adhesive strips or tape used with a male external catheter are included in the allowance for the catheter and are not separately payable. If adhesive strips or tape are used with the male external catheter, payment will be denied as not medically necessary.

When billing for urological supplies furnished in a physician's office for a permanent impairment, use the place of service code (POS) corresponding to the patient's current place of residence (POS=12); do not use POS 11 for the physician's office.

Medicare Noncovered Items/Services

Other supplies used in the management of incontinence include, but are not limited to, the following items:

- Creams, salves, lotions, barriers (liquid, spray, wipes, powder, paste), or other skin care products
- Catheter care kits
- Adhesive remover (coverage remains for use with ostomy supplies)
- Catheter clamp or plug
- Disposable underpads, e.g., Chux pads
- Diapers, drip collectors, or incontinent garments, disposable or reusable
- Drainage bag holder or stand
- Urinary suspensory without leg bag
- Measuring container
- Urinary drainage tray
- Gauze pads and other dressings (coverage remains under other benefits, e.g., surgical dressings)
- Other incontinence products not directly related to the use of a covered urinary catheter or external urinary collection device

These items will be denied as noncovered because they are not prosthetic devices, nor are they required for the effective use of a prosthetic device.

Irrigation solutions containing antibiotics and chemotherapeutic agents should be coded A9270 Non-covered item or service. Irrigating solutions such as acetic acid or hydrogen peroxide that are used for the treatment or prevention of urinary obstruction should be coded A4321 *Therapeutic agent for urinary catheter irrigation.*

Catheter insertion trays will be denied as not medically necessary for clean, nonsterile intermittent catheterization.

Catheters and related supplies will be denied as noncovered if it is expected that the condition will be temporary.

If the patient's condition is expected to be temporary, urological supplies may not be billed to the DME MAC. In this situation, they are considered supplies provided incident to a physician's service, and payment is included in the allowance for the physician's services, which are processed by the local carrier.

Urological supplies, that are not used with, or for which use is not related to covered catheters or external urinary collection devices (i.e., drainage and/or collection of urine from the bladder), will be denied as noncovered.

The use of leg bags for bedridden patients will be denied as not medically necessary.

Irrigation solutions containing antibiotics and chemotherapeutic agents will be denied as noncovered.

Consolidated Billing

All urological supplies dispensed to a nursing home resident or home health recipient are included in the consolidated billing requirements and the prospective payment system (PPS) reimbursement. This means that the supplier will need to know the patient status when the supplies are dispensed.

For patients in a nursing home: If the patient is receiving skilled nursing level care and is covered under Part A benefits, the supplies may not be billed separately by the SNF or by any other provider or supplier. This would be duplicate billing. The supplies are considered a part of the nursing home's PPS reimbursement. The DME supplier should bill the nursing home for these items and should probably have an agreement with the home for payment of these items.

If a patient in a nursing home is not receiving a skilled nursing level of care and is not being reimbursed under Part A, then the DME supplier has a choice: billing may be submitted directly by the supplier or may be submitted by the nursing home. DME suppliers should have an agreement with the nursing home specifying which party will bill in these situations. Such an agreement will eliminate duplicate billing and concerns related to fraud and abuse. Only

one party should submit the bill for the service. Do not bill the nursing home and then bill the DME MAC if the nursing home is taking too long to pay.

For patients receiving home health services: If the patient is under a plan of care, urological supplies should be billed to the Home Health Agency (HHA). The supplies are considered a part of the HHA's PPS reimbursement. The DME supplier should bill the HHA for these items and should probably have an agreement with the home for payment of these items.

The HHA must have an order for the urological supplies and the supplies must be provided under an arrangement. If the supplier was unaware of the HHA services and there is no agreement with the HHA about the provision of the supplies, the supplies will not be reimbursed by any party. The patient has the freedom to accept the HHA services. At that point, the HHA becomes responsible for all related care, including the provision of urological supplies, but excluding any other DME.

If the patient is not on a plan of care or is not receiving Part A reimbursable services, the supplier must still bill the HHA. These urological supplies are subject to consolidated billing regulations. This means that the HHA must submit all charges for these services. The HHA will receive additional payment for these items. The supplier should bill the HHA for these items and should probably have an agreement with the home for payment of these items.

Documentation Standards

The order on file must include the type of supplies ordered and the approximate quantity to be used per unit of time. There must be a statement indicating whether the patient has permanent or temporary urinary incontinence or retention, or other indication for use of a catheter or urinary collection device. If the order indicates permanent urinary incontinence or urinary retention, and if the item is a catheter, an external urinary collection device, or a supply used with one of these items, modifier KX should be added to the code for each urological supply on each claim submitted.

When billing for quantities of supplies greater than those approved for coverage, the claim must include documentation supporting the medical necessity for the higher utilization.

The initial claim for catheters or kits used for sterile intermittent catheterization in the home must be accompanied by documentation supporting the medical necessity for sterile technique.

Medicare Guidelines

Wheelchairs and Power Mobility Devices

Physicians, physician assistants, nurse practitioners, or clinical nurse specialists may prescribe wheelchairs and power mobility devices (PMD). Wheelchairs and PMDs do not require a CMN. The treating practitioner must conduct a face-to-face examination of the beneficiary and write a written prescription for the PMD. The written prescription must be signed and dated by the treating practitioner who performed the face-to-face examination. The written prescription must include the beneficiary's name, the date of the face-to-face examination, the diagnoses and conditions that the PMD is expected to modify, a description of the item, and the length of need. This written prescription for the PMD must be received by the supplier within 45 days after the face-to-face examination. For those instances of a recently hospitalized beneficiary, the supplier must receive the written prescription within 45 days after the date of discharge from the hospital.

The face-to-face examination requirement does not apply when only accessories for PMDs are ordered, nor does it apply for the ordering of replacement PMDs. A replacement PMD would be the same device as previously ordered. For instance, if a beneficiary has a POV but would like to replace the POV with a power wheelchair, a face-to-face examination would need to be conducted.

Prior to dispensing a PMD, the DME supplier must obtain from the treating practitioner who performed the face-to-face examination the written prescription accompanied by supporting documentation of the beneficiary's need for the PMD in the home. Supporting documentation of the patient's need for the PMD in the home must accompany the prescription. This documentation must be specific to the patient's PMD evaluation and may include the history, physical examination, diagnostic tests, and summary of findings, diagnoses, and treatment plans. Submit only those parts of the medical record that clearly demonstrate medical necessity, including the history of events that led to the request for the PMD, the mobility deficits to be corrected by the PMD, documentation demonstrating that other treatments do not obviate the need for the PMD, documentation that the patient lives in an environment that supports the use of the PMD, and documentation that the patient or caregiver is capable of operating the PMD.

CMS will pay a separate add-on payment in addition to the office visit for the additional physician and treating practitioner work and resources required for submitting pertinent parts of the medical record. Report HCPCS Level II code G0372 Physician service required to establish and document the need for a power mobility device (use in addition to primary evaluation and management code), to obtain this add-on payment. Code G0372 must be reported on the same claim as the E/M code.

Prior Authorization of Power Mobility Devices Demonstration

On November 15, 2011, CMS announced a demonstration project to require prior authorization of power mobility devices (PMD) for people with Medicare who reside in seven states with high populations of fraud- and error-prone providers. These seven states are California, Florida, Illinois, Michigan, New York, North Carolina, and Texas. CMS delayed the demonstration start date so the agency could make necessary improvements based on comments received from the public. This demonstration project began for orders written on or after September 1, 2012.

This demonstration project requires that patients who reside in one of the demonstration states obtain prior authorization for the following items paid by Medicare:

- All power operated vehicles (K0800–K0802 and K0812)
- All standard power wheelchairs (K0813–K0829)
- All group 2 complex rehabilitative power wheelchairs (K0835–K0843)
- All group 3 complex rehabilitative power wheelchairs without power options (K0848–K0855)
- All pediatric and group 4 power wheelchairs (K0887–K0891)
- Miscellaneous power wheelchairs (K0898)
- Group 3 complex rehabilitative power wheelchairs with power options (K0856–K0864) are excluded. The prior authorization request is submitted by the patient's physician or treating practitioner. The supplier may submit this request on the physician's behalf.

No prior authorization decisions will be made on any code NOT on the above list. If a DME MAC receives a prior authorization request for a code not on this list, the DME MAC will not review the request and will not issue a decision letter.

For additional information, see http://www.cms.gov/Research-Statistics-Data-and-Systems/Monitoring-Programs/CERT/PADemo.html.

In an update posted April 23, 2013, CMS announced that the agency had begun collecting data to analyze and evaluate the effectiveness of the demonstration. Based on data initially collected, spending per month on power mobility devices in the seven demonstration states decreased after September 2012, as did spending per month on PMD in the non-demonstration states. Further analysis showed that as of March 12, 2013:

Medicare Guidelines

- Prior authorization requests were submitted for more than 12,000 Medicare patients.

- Approximately 50 percent of the prior authorization requests were not approved because the patient did not qualify for the benefit based on the documentation submitted. PMDs were approved for all patients who met all of the requirements.

- More than 700 prior authorization requests were submitted electronically through CMS's electronic submission of medical documentation (esMD) program.

CMS will continue to closely monitor and evaluate the effectiveness of the demonstration. CMS plans to analyze demonstration data to assist in the investigation and prosecution of fraud.

Medicare Guidelines

Medicare Noncovered Codes

The following is a list of Medicare noncovered HCPCS Level II codes (as indicated in the HCPCS code set master file):

A0021	A4570	E0242	G9052	H0036	H2032
A0080	A4575	E0243	G9053	H0037	H2033
A0090	A4580	E0244	G9054	H0038	H2034
A0100	A4590	E0245	G9055	H0039	H2035
A0110	A4611	E0270	G9056	H0040	H2036
A0120	A4612	E0273	G9057	H0041	H2037
A0130	A4613	E0274	G9058	H0042	J1055
A0140	A4627	E0315	G9059	H0043	J1680
A0160	A4670	E0446	G9060	H0044	J2271
A0170	A6000	E0457	G9061	H0045	J2275
A0180	A6413	E0459	G9062	H0046	J3487
A0190	A6530	E0481	G9147	H0047	J3488
A0200	A6533	E0571	H0001	H0048	J3520
A0210	A6534	E0625	H0002	H0049	J3535
A0225	A6535	E0637	H0003	H0050	J3570
A0380	A6536	E0638	H0004	H1000	J7184
A0382	A6537	E0641	H0005	H1001	J7300
A0384	A6538	E0642	H0006	H1002	J7301
A0390	A6539	E0936	H0007	H1003	J7302
A0392	A6540	E0970	H0008	H1004	J7303
A0394	A6541	E1085	H0009	H1005	J7304
A0396	A6544	E1086	H0010	H1010	J7306
A0398	A6549	E1089	H0011	H1011	J7307
A0420	A9152	E1090	H0012	H2000	J8499
A0422	A9153	E1130	H0013	H2001	J8515
A0424	A9180	E1140	H0014	H2010	J9001
A0888	A9270	E1250	H0015	H2011	J9002
A0998	A9272	E1260	H0016	H2012	J9010
A4210	A9273	E1285	H0017	H2013	K0740
A4232	A9274	E1290	H0018	H2014	L2861
A4250	A9275	E1300	H0019	H2015	L3215
A4252	A9276	E8000	H0020	H2016	L3216
A4261	A9277	E8001	H0021	H2017	L3217
A4264	A9278	E8002	H0022	H2018	L3219
A4266	A9279	G0122	H0023	H2019	L3221
A4267	A9280	G0219	H0024	H2020	L3222
A4268	A9281	G0235	H0025	H2021	L3891
A4269	A9282	G0252	H0026	H2022	L7600
A4466	A9283	G0255	H0027	H2023	L8680
A4490	A9300	G0282	H0028	H2024	L8685
A4495	B4100	G0295	H0029	H2025	L8686
A4500	E0172	G0428	H0030	H2026	L8687
A4510	E0203	G9013	H0031	H2027	L8688
A4520	E0231	G9014	H0032	H2028	L8692
A4554	E0232	G9016	H0033	H2029	M0075
A4555	E0240	G9050	H0034	H2030	M0076
A4566	E0241	G9051	H0035	H2031	M0100

M0300	S0169	S0506	S2112	S3708	S4022
M0301	S0170	S0508	S2115	S3711	S4023
P2031	S0171	S0510	S2117	S3713	S4025
P7001	S0172	S0512	S2118	S3721	S4026
Q0090	S0174	S0514	S2120	S3722	S4027
Q0144	S0175	S0515	S2140	S3800	S4028
Q3026	S0176	S0516	S2142	S3818	S4030
Q3028	S0177	S0518	S2150	S3819	S4031
S0012	S0178	S0580	S2152	S3820	S4035
S0014	S0179	S0581	S2202	S3822	S4037
S0017	S0181	S0590	S2205	S3823	S4040
S0020	S0182	S0592	S2206	S3828	S4042
S0021	S0183	S0595	S2207	S3829	S4981
S0023	S0187	S0596	S2208	S3830	S4989
S0028	S0189	S0601	S2209	S3831	S4990
S0030	S0190	S0610	S2225	S3833	S4991
S0032	S0191	S0612	S2230	S3834	S4993
S0034	S0194	S0613	S2235	S3835	S4995
S0039	S0195	S0618	S2260	S3837	S5000
S0040	S0197	S0620	S2265	S3840	S5001
S0073	S0199	S0621	S2266	S3841	S5010
S0074	S0201	S0622	S2267	S3842	S5011
S0077	S0207	S0625	S2270	S3843	S5012
S0078	S0208	S0630	S2300	S3844	S5013
S0080	S0209	S0800	S2325	S3845	S5014
S0081	S0215	S0810	S2340	S3846	S5035
S0088	S0220	S0812	S2341	S3847	S5036
S0090	S0221	S1001	S2342	S3848	S5100
S0091	S0250	S1002	S2344	S3849	S5101
S0092	S0255	S1015	S2348	S3850	S5102
S0093	S0257	S1016	S2350	S3851	S5105
S0104	S0260	S1030	S2351	S3852	S5108
S0106	S0265	S1031	S2360	S3853	S5109
S0108	S0270	S1034	S2361	S3854	S5110
S0109	S0271	S1035	S2400	S3855	S5111
S0117	S0272	S1036	S2401	S3860	S5115
S0119	S0273	S1037	S2402	S3861	S5116
S0122	S0274	S1040	S2403	S3862	S5120
S0126	S0280	S1090	S2404	S3865	S5121
S0128	S0281	S2053	S2405	S3866	S5125
S0132	S0302	S2054	S2409	S3870	S5126
S0136	S0310	S2055	S2411	S3890	S5130
S0137	S0315	S2060	S2900	S3900	S5131
S0138	S0316	S2061	S3000	S3902	S5135
S0139	S0317	S2065	S3005	S3904	S5136
S0140	S0320	S2066	S3600	S3905	S5140
S0142	S0340	S2067	S3601	S4005	S5141
S0144	S0341	S2068	S3620	S4011	S5145
S0145	S0342	S2070	S3625	S4013	S5146
S0148	S0353	S2079	S3626	S4014	S5150
S0155	S0354	S2080	S3628	S4015	S5151
S0156	S0390	S2083	S3630	S4016	S5160
S0157	S0395	S2095	S3645	S4017	S5161
S0160	S0400	S2102	S3650	S4018	S5162
S0164	S0500	S2103	S3652	S4020	S5165
S0166	S0504	S2107	S3655	S4021	S5170

S5175	S8421	S9211	S9443	S9992	T2022
S5180	S8422	S9212	S9444	S9994	T2023
S5181	S8423	S9213	S9445	S9996	T2024
S5185	S8424	S9214	S9446	S9999	T2025
S5190	S8425	S9325	S9447	T1000	T2026
S5199	S8426	S9326	S9449	T1001	T2027
S5497	S8427	S9327	S9451	T1002	T2028
S5498	S8428	S9328	S9452	T1003	T2029
S5501	S8429	S9329	S9453	T1004	T2030
S5502	S8430	S9330	S9454	T1005	T2031
S5517	S8431	S9331	S9455	T1006	T2032
S5518	S8450	S9335	S9460	T1007	T2033
S5520	S8451	S9336	S9465	T1009	T2034
S5521	S8452	S9338	S9470	T1010	T2035
S5522	S8460	S9339	S9472	T1012	T2036
S5523	S8490	S9340	S9473	T1013	T2037
S5550	S8930	S9341	S9474	T1014	T2038
S5551	S8940	S9342	S9475	T1015	T2039
S5552	S8948	S9343	S9476	T1016	T2040
S5553	S8950	S9345	S9480	T1017	T2041
S5560	S8990	S9346	S9482	T1018	T2042
S5561	S8999	S9347	S9484	T1019	T2043
S5565	S9001	S9348	S9485	T1020	T2044
S5566	S9007	S9349	S9490	T1021	T2045
S5570	S9015	S9351	S9494	T1022	T2046
S5571	S9024	S9353	S9497	T1023	T2048
S8030	S9025	S9355	S9500	T1024	T2049
S8032	S9034	S9357	S9501	T1025	T2101
S8035	S9055	S9359	S9502	T1026	T4521
S8037	S9056	S9361	S9503	T1027	T4522
S8040	S9061	S9363	S9504	T1028	T4523
S8042	S9075	S9364	S9529	T1029	T4524
S8049	S9083	S9365	S9537	T1030	T4525
S8055	S9088	S9366	S9538	T1031	T4526
S8080	S9090	S9367	S9542	T1502	T4527
S8085	S9097	S9368	S9558	T1503	T4528
S8092	S9098	S9370	S9559	T1505	T4529
S8096	S9109	S9372	S9560	T1999	T4530
S8097	S9110	S9373	S9562	T2001	T4531
S8100	S9117	S9374	S9590	T2002	T4532
S8101	S9122	S9375	S9810	T2003	T4533
S8110	S9123	S9376	S9900	T2004	T4534
S8120	S9124	S9377	S9901	T2005	T4535
S8121	S9125	S9379	S9960	T2007	T4536
S8130	S9126	S9381	S9961	T2010	T4537
S8131	S9127	S9401	S9970	T2011	T4538
S8185	S9128	S9430	S9975	T2012	T4539
S8186	S9129	S9433	S9976	T2013	T4540
S8189	S9131	S9434	S9977	T2014	T4541
S8210	S9140	S9435	S9981	T2015	T4542
S8262	S9141	S9436	S9982	T2016	T4543
S8265	S9145	S9437	S9986	T2017	T4544
S8270	S9150	S9438	S9988	T2018	T5001
S8301	S9152	S9439	S9989	T2019	T5999
S8415	S9208	S9441	S9990	T2020	V2025
S8420	S9209	S9442	S9991	T2021	V2702

V2787	V5095	V5230	V5253	V5267	V5286
V2788	V5100	V5240	V5254	V5268	V5287
V5008	V5110	V5241	V5255	V5269	V5288
V5010	V5120	V5242	V5256	V5270	V5289
V5011	V5130	V5243	V5257	V5271	V5290
V5014	V5140	V5244	V5258	V5272	V5298
V5020	V5150	V5245	V5259	V5273	V5336
V5030	V5160	V5246	V5260	V5274	V5362
V5040	V5170	V5247	V5261	V5275	V5363
V5050	V5180	V5248	V5262	V5281	V5364
V5060	V5190	V5249	V5263	V5282	
V5070	V5200	V5250	V5264	V5283	
V5080	V5210	V5251	V5265	V5284	
V5090	V5220	V5252	V5266	V5285	

Glossary

An increasingly complex reimbursement climate means new terminology develops every year. The following glossary includes terms not only used when coding, it includes terms used by major insurers and the federal government.

AAPA. American Academy of Physician Assistants.

AAPC. American Academy of Professional Coders. National organization for coders and billers offering certification (CPC, CPC-H, and CPC-P) based upon physician-, outpatient facility-, or payer-specific guidelines.

AAPCC. Adjusted average per capita cost. Estimated average cost of Medicare benefits for an individual, based upon criteria including age, sex, institutional status, Medicaid, disability, and end-stage renal failure.

AAPPO. American Association of Preferred Provider Organizations.

abduction. Pulling away from a central reference line, such as moving away from the midline of the body.

abduction pillow. Device that immobilizes the hips and legs of hip surgery patients postoperatively.

ABN. Advance beneficiary notice.

abstractor. Person who selects and extracts specific data from the medical record and enters the information into computer files.

accrual. Amount of money set aside to cover a health care benefit plan's expenses based upon estimates using a combination of data, including the claims system and the plan's prior history. In facility accounting, accrual accounting records the expenses as they are incurred and the revenue as it is generated. This contrasts with cash accounting where expenses are recorded only when payment is made or revenues are recorded only when payment is received.

ACLS. Advanced cardiac life support. Certification for health care professionals who have achieved proficiency in providing emergent care of cardiac and respiratory systems and medication management.

ACR. 1) American College of Radiology. **2)** Adjusted community rate, calculation of what premium the plan charges to provide Medicare-covered benefits for greater frequency of use by participants.

activities of daily living. Self-care activities often used to determine a patient's level of function such as bathing, dressing, using a toilet, transferring in and out of bed or a chair, continence, eating, and walking.

actuarial assumptions. Characteristics used in calculating the risks and costs of a plan, including age, sex, and occupation of enrollees; location; utilization rates; and service costs.

adduction. Pulling toward a central reference line, such as toward the midline of the body.

adjudication. Processing and review of a submitted claim resulting in payment, partial payment, or denial. In relationship to judicial hearings, it is the process of hearing and settling a case through an objective, judicial procedure.

admission. Formal acceptance of a patient by a health care facility.

ADS. Alternative delivery system. Any health care delivery system other than traditional fee-for-service.

advance beneficiary notice. Written communication with a Medicare beneficiary given before Part B services are rendered, informing the patient that the provider (including independent laboratories, physicians, practitioners, and/or suppliers) believes Medicare will not pay for some or all of the services to be rendered. Form CMS-R-131 (revised 03/201*1)* may be used for all situations where Medicare payment is expected to be denied.

adverse selection. In health care contracting, the risk of enrolling members who are sicker than assumed and who will utilize expensive services more frequently.

age restriction. In health care contracting, limitation of benefits when a patient reaches a certain age.

age/sex rating. In health care contracting, structuring capitation payments based on members' ages and genders.

aggregate amount. Contracted maximum for which a member is insured for any single event in a health plan.

AHA. American Hospital Association. Health care industry association that represents the concerns of institutional providers. The AHA hosts the National Uniform Billing Committee (NUBC), which has a formal consultative role under HIPAA. The AHA also publishes Coding Clinic for ICD-9-CM.

AHIMA. American Health Information Management Association. Association of health information management professionals that offers professional and educational services, providing these certifications: RHIA, RHIT, CCS, CCS-P, CCA, CHDA, and CHPS.

Al-Anon, Alateen. Alcoholic support groups.

AMA. American Medical Association. Professional organization for physicians. The AMA is the secretariat of the National Uniform Claim Committee (NUCC), which has a formal consultative role under HIPAA. The AMA also maintains the Physicians' Current Procedural Terminology (CPT) coding system.

ambulatory surgery. Surgical procedure in which the patient is admitted, treated, and released on the same day.

AMCRA. American Managed Care Review Association.

ANA. American Nursing Association.

AOA. American Osteopathic Association.

AP-DRG. All patient diagnosis-related group. 3M HIS made revisions and adjustments to the DRG system, now referred to as the All Patient DRGs. Early features of AP-DRGs included MDC 24, specifically devoted to HIV, and restructuring of the major diagnostic categories governing newborns.

APA. American Psychiatric Association.

APG. Ambulatory patient group. Reimbursement methodology developed for the Centers for Medicare and Medicaid Services.

apnea. Absence of breathing or breath.

apnea monitor. Device used to monitor breathing during sleep that sounds an alarm if breathing stops for more than the specified amount of time.

appeal. Specific request made to a payer for reconsideration of a denial or adverse coverage or payment decision and potential restriction of benefit reimbursement.

appropriateness of care. Proper setting of medical care that best meets the patient's care or diagnosis, as defined by a health care plan or other legal entity.

APR. Average payment rate. Amount of money CMS could pay an HMO for services provided to Medicare recipients under a risk contract.

ART. Accredited record technician. Former AHIMA certification describing medical records practitioners; now known as a registered health information technician (RHIT).

AS. Associate of Science.

ASN. Associate of Science, Nursing.

ASO. Administrative services only. Contractual agreement between a self-funded plan and an insurance company in which the insurance company assumes no risk and provides administrative services only.

assignment. In medical reimbursement, the arrangement in which the provider submits the claim on behalf of the patient and is reimbursed directly by the patient's plan. By doing so, the provider agrees to accept what the plan pays.

assignment of benefits. Authorization from the patient allowing the third-party payer to pay the provider directly for medical services. Under Medicare, an assignment is an agreement by the hospital or physician to accept Medicare's payment as the full payment and not to bill the patient for any amounts over the allowance amount, except for deductible and/or coinsurance amounts or noncovered services.

at risk. In medical reimbursement, a type of contract between Medicare and a payer or a payer and a provider in which the payer (in the case of Medicare) and the provider (in the case of the payer contracts) gets paid a set amount for care of a patient base. If costs exceed the amount the payer or provider were paid, the patients still receive care during the term of the contract.

attained age. In medical reimbursement, the age of the member as of the last birthday.

auditor. Professional who evaluates a provider's utilization, quality of care, or level of reimbursement.

AWP. *1)* Average wholesale price. Pharmaceutical price based on common data that is included in a pharmacy provider contract. *2)* Any willing provider. Describing statutes requiring a provider network to accept any provider who meets the network's usual selection criteria.

backlog. In medical reimbursement, the queue of claims that have not been adjudicated.

balance billing. Arrangement prohibited in Medicare regulations and some payer contracts whereby a provider bills the patient for charges not reimbursed by the payer.

basic coverage. Insurance providing coverage for hospital care.

basic health services. Defined set of benefits all federally qualified HMOs must offer enrollees.

BCBS. Blue Cross Blue Shield.

binder. Broad bandage that supports a body part.

board certification. Certification in a particular specialty based on the physician's demonstration of expertise and experience.

boarder. Individual who receives lodging, such as a parent, caregiver, or other family member, who is not a patient but may wish or need to be near the patient.

book of business. Payer's list of clients and contracts.

brace. Orthotic device that supports, in correct position, any moveable body part, and allows for limited movement. Medicare has a strict definition of a brace that includes only rigid or semirigid devices.

BSN. Bachelor of Science, Nursing.

Buck traction. Type of skin traction of the extremities maintained by using an apparatus such as a special splint, applied by dressings to the affected body part. Buck traction may be used on burn patients to hold the arm in a suspended upward position to prevent swelling, reduce skin shrinkage, and allow for greater range of motion with healing.

bundled. *1)* Gathering of several types of health insurance policies under a single payer. *2)* Inclusive grouping of codes related to a procedure when submitting a claim.

business coalition. Employers who form a cooperative to purchase health care less expensively.

cafeteria plan. Employer's offer of various services of many payers as separate elements in a health care plan.

Cap. *1)* Capitation. *2)* Contract maximum.

capitation. Contractual agreement whereby the provider is paid a fixed amount for treating enrolled patients regardless of utilization.

carve-out. Medical benefits for a specific type of care considered covered by separate guidelines or not covered by the payer.

case management. Ongoing review of cases by professionals to assure the most appropriate utilization of services

case manager. Medical professional (usually a nurse or social worker) who reviews cases every few days to determine necessity of care and to advise providers on payers' utilization restrictions. Certifies ongoing care.

casting. Material used for encasing a body part to immobilize it for injury repair; usually made from plaster or fiberglass.

casting tape. Material used for molding casts, usually made from fiberglass, but can be composed of plaster strips.

catastrophic case management. Method of reviewing ongoing cases in which the patient sustains catastrophic or extremely costly medical problems.

catchment area. Geographical area from which a health care organization draws its members.

CC. Complication or comorbid condition.

CDC. Centers for Disease Control and Prevention.

census. In medical reimbursement, number and demographics of patients or members

Certificate of Medical Necessity. Form required by Medicare to establish the medical necessity of certain DMEPOS. It is completed by both the physician and the supplier, detailing the medical diagnosis and other information specific to the device ordered.

certification. Approval by a payer's case manager to continue care for a given number of days or visits.

CFR. Code of Federal Regulations.

churning. *1)* Performance-based reimbursement system emphasizing provider productivity. *2)* When a provider sees a patient more than medically necessary with the intent of generating more revenue.

Civilian Health and Medical Program of the Uniformed Services. Federal program that covered the health benefits for families of all uniformed service employees. The program has been replaced by TRICARE.

CLA. Certified laboratory assistant.

claim. Statement of services rendered requesting payment from an insurance company or a government entity.

claim lag. Time incurred between the date of a claim and its submission for payment. c. manual Administrative guidelines used by claims processors to adjudicate claims according to company policy and procedure.

claim manual. Administrative guidelines used by claims processors to adjudicate claims according to company policy and procedure.

claims manager. Payer's manager who oversees the employee who processes routine claims.

claims reviewer. Payer employee who reviews claims like an auditor, looking at coding, prior authority, contract violations, etc.

CLIA. Clinical Laboratory Improvement Amendments. Requirements set in 1988, CLIA imposes varying levels of federal regulations on clinical procedures. Few laboratories, including those in physician offices, are exempt. Adopted by Medicare and Medicaid, CLIA regulations redefine laboratory testing in regard to laboratory certification and accreditation, proficiency testing, quality assurance, personnel standards, and program administration.

Glossary

Glossary

closed claim. Claim for which all apparent benefits have been paid.

closed panel. Arrangement in which a managed care organization contracts providers on an exclusive basis, restricting the providers from seeing patients enrolled in other payers' plans.

closed treatment. Realignment of a fracture or dislocation without surgically opening the skin to reach the site. Treatment methods employed include with or without manipulation and with or without traction.

CMA. Certified medical assistant.

CMN. Certificate of medical necessity.

CMP. Competitive medical plan. Federal designation allowing plans to obtain eligibility to receive a Medicare risk contract without having to qualify as an HMO.

CMS. Centers for Medicare and Medicaid Services. Federal agency that administers the public health programs.

CMS-1500. Universal form used to file professional claims.

COA. Certificate of authority. State license to operate as an HMO.

COB. Coordination of benefits. In health care contracting, method of integrating benefits payable when there is more than one group insurance plan so that the insured's benefits and the payment of insurance benefits from all sources do not exceed 100 percent of the allowed medical expenses.

COBRA. Consolidated Omnibus Reconciliation Act. Federal law that allows and requires past employees to be covered under company health insurance plans for a set premium, allowing individuals to remain insured when their current plan or position has been terminated.

coder. Professional who translates documented, written diagnoses and procedures into numeric and alphanumeric codes.

coding conventions. Each space, typeface, indentation, and punctuation mark determining how ICD-9-CM codes are interpreted. These conventions were developed to help match correct codes to the diagnoses documented.

coinsurance. Percentage of the allowed charges paid by a beneficiary toward the cost of care.

collagen. Protein based substance of strength and flexibility that is the major component of connective tissue, found in cartilage, bone, tendons, and skin.

collar. Device that encircles the neck to immobilize it, provide support, and/or severely limit its mobility.

commercial carriers. For-profit insurance companies issuing health coverage.

common working file. System of local databases containing total beneficiary histories developed by CMS to improve Medicare claims processing. Medicare fiscal intermediaries, and/or carriers, interact with these databases to obtain data on eligibility, utilization, Medicare secondary payer (MSP), and other detailed claims information.

community rating. Methodology of state and federal governments that require qualified HMOs to request the same amount of money for each member in a plan.

comparative performance report. Report that provides an annual comparison of a physician's services and procedures with those of another physician in the same specialty and geographic area.

complex repair. Surgical closure of a wound requiring more than layered closure of the deeper subcutaneous tissue and fascia (i.e., debridement, scar excision, placement of stents or retention sutures, and sometimes site preparation or undermining that creates the defect requiring complex closure).

complication. Condition arising after the beginning of observation and treatment that modifies the course of the patient's illness or the medical care required, or an undesired result or misadventure in medical care.

component code. In the National Correct Coding Initiative (NCCI), the column II code that cannot be charged to Medicare when the column I code is reported.

component coding. Coding a service that represents only a portion of the entire service provided, meant to standardize the reporting of interventional radiology services. Component coding allows a physician, regardless of specialty, to specifically identify and report those aspects of the service he or she provided, whether the procedural component, the radiological component, or both.

comprehensive codes. In the National Correct Coding Initiative (NCCI), the column I code that is reported to Medicare and precludes reporting column II codes.

consultation. Advice or opinion regarding diagnosis and treatment or determination to accept transfer of care of a patient rendered by a medical professional at the request of the primary care provider.

continuity of coverage. In health care contracting, transfer of benefits from one plan to another without a lapse in coverage.

continuous positive airway pressure device. Pressurized device used to maintain the patient's airway for spontaneous or mechanically aided breathing. Often used for patients with mild to moderate sleep apnea.

contractor. Entity who enters into a contractual agreement with CMS to service a component of the Medicare program administration, for example, fiscal intermediaries, carriers, program safeguard coordinators.

conversion. In health care contracting, shifting a member under a group contract to an individual contract in accordance with contract terms and occurring with a change in employer benefits or when the covered person leaves the group.

conversion factor. *1)* Dollar value for each relative value unit. When this dollar amount is multiplied by the total relative value units, it yields the reimbursement rate for the service. *2)* National multiplier that converts the geographically adjusted relative value units into Medicare fee schedule dollar amounts that applies to all services paid under the MPFS.

coordinated care. In health care contracting, system of health care delivery that influences utilization, quality of care, and cost of services. Managed care integrates financing and management with an employed or contracted organized provider network that delivers services to an enrolled population.

copayment. Cost-sharing arrangement in which a covered person pays a specified portion of allowed charges. In relation to Medicare, the copayment designates the specific dollar amount that the patient must pay and coinsurance designates the percentage of allowed charges.

Correct Coding Initiative. Official list of codes from the Centers for Medicare and Medicaid Services' (CMS) National Correct Coding Policy Manual for Medicare Services that identifies services considered an integral part of a comprehensive code or mutually exclusive of it.

corridor deductible. Fixed out-of-pocket amount the member must pay before benefits are available.

COT. Certified ophthalmic technician.

COTA. Certified occupational therapy assistant.

counseling. Discussion with a patient and/or family concerning one or more of the following areas: diagnostic results, impressions, and/or recommended diagnostic studies; prognosis; risks and benefits of management (treatment) options; instructions for management (treatment) and/or follow-up; importance of compliance with chosen management (treatment) options; risk factor reduction; and patient and family education.

Coverage Issues Manual. Revised and renamed the National Coverage Determination Manual in the CMS manual system, it contained national coverage decisions and specific medical items, services, treatment procedures, or technologies paid for under the Medicare program. This manual has been converted to the Medicare National Coverage Determinations Manual (NCD manual), Pub. 100-03.

covered charges. Charges for medical care and supplies that are medically necessary and met coverage and program guidelines.

covered person. Any person entitled to benefits under the policy, whether a member or dependent.

CPR. Cardiopulmonary resuscitation. Substitutionary action made for both the heart and lungs in sudden death cases by artificial respiration and external cardiac compression.

CPT. Current Procedural Terminology. Definitive procedural coding system developed by the American Medical Association that lists descriptive terms and identifying codes to provide a uniform language that describes medical, surgical, and diagnostic services for nationwide communication among physicians, patients, and third parties, used in outpatient reporting of services.

CPT codes. Codes maintained and copyrighted by the AMA and selected for use under HIPAA for noninstitutional and nondental professional transactions.

CPT modifier. Two-character code used to indicate that a service was altered in some way from the stated CPT or HCPCS Level II description, but not enough to change the basic definition of the service.

credentialing. *1)* Reviewing the medical degrees, licensure, malpractice, and any disciplinary record of medical providers for panel and quality assurance purposes and to grant hospital privileges. *2)* Coding certification.

CRNA. Certified registered nurse anesthetist. Nurse trained and specializing in the administration of anesthesia. Anesthesia services rendered by a CRNA must be reported with HCPCS Level II modifier QX, QY, or QZ.

crosswalk. Cross-referencing of CPT codes with ICD-9-CM, anesthesia, dental, or HCPCS Level II codes.

CRT. Certified respiratory therapist.

CSO. Clinical service organization. Health care organization developed by academic medical centers to integrate medical school, faculty practice plan, and hospital.

CST. Certified surgical technologist.

CTLSO. Cervical-thoracic-lumbar-sacral orthosis.

Glossary

custom fitted. Premanufactured orthotics that can be adjusted to fit the patient by bending, trimming, or other minimal efforts.

cutback. Reduction of the amount or type of insurance for a member who attains a specified age or condition (e.g., age 65, retirement).

daily benefit. Specified maximum benefit payable for room and board charges at a hospital.

DAW. Dispense as written. Notation from a physician to a pharmacist requesting that the brand name medication be given in lieu of a generic medication.

DC. *1)* Doctor of chiropractic medicine. *2)* Discontinue. *3)* Direct current.

decubitus ulcer. Progressively eroding skin lesion produced by inflamed necrotic tissue as it sloughs off caused by continual pressure to a localized area, especially over bony areas, where blood circulation is cut off when a patient lies still for too long without changing position.

deductible. Predetermined dollar amount of covered billed charges that the patient must pay toward the cost of care.

diagnosis. Determination or confirmation of a condition, disease, or syndrome and its implications.

diagnostic. Examination or procedure to which the patient is subjected, or which is performed on materials derived from a hospital outpatient, to obtain information to aid in the assessment of a medical condition or the identification of a disease. Among these examinations and tests are diagnostic laboratory services such as hematology and chemistry, diagnostic x-rays, isotope studies, EKGs, pulmonary function studies, thyroid function tests, psychological tests, and other tests given to determine the nature and severity of an ailment or injury.

direct contract model. Plan that contracts directly with individual private practice physicians rather than through an intermediary.

disarticulation. Removal of a limb through a joint.

discharge plan. Treatment plan by the provider for continued patient care after discharge that may include home care, the services of case managers or other health care providers, or transfer to another facility.

discharge status. Disposition of the patient at discharge (e.g., left against medical advice, discharged home, transferred to an acute care hospital, expired).

discharge transfer. Discharge of a patient from one facility to another.

disposition of patient. Description of the patient's status and destination at discharge (e.g., discharged to home) used for data and quality assurance purposes.

DME. Durable medical equipment. Medical equipment that can withstand repeated use, is not disposable, is used to serve a medical purpose, is generally not useful to a person in the absence of a sickness or injury, and is appropriate for use in the home. Examples of durable medical equipment include hospital beds, wheelchairs, and oxygen equipment.

DME MAC. Durable medical equipment Medicare administrative contractor. Entity where claims for specific DMEPOS must be submitted for processing and reimbursement.

DMEPOS. Durable medical equipment, prosthetics, orthotics, and supplies.

DO. Doctor of osteopathy.

DOS. Date of service. In health care contracting, day the encounter or procedure is performed or the day a supply is issued.

DPM. Doctor of podiatric medicine.

drug formulary. List of prescription medications preferred for use by a health plan and dispensed through participating pharmacies to covered persons.

dual option. Offering of an HMO and traditional plan by one carrier.

dual-lead device. Implantable cardiac device (pacemaker or implantable cardioverter-defibrillator [ICD]) in which pacing and sensing components are placed in only two chambers of the heart.

DUR. Drug utilization review. Review to assure prescribed medications are medically necessary and appropriate.

DVM. Doctor of Veterinary Medicine.

dynamic flexion device. Highly specialized orthotic brace that allows for a controlled range of motion of a joint or joints during postoperative or post-traumatic convalescence.

E code. ICD-9-CM diagnosis code that describes the circumstance that caused an injury, not the nature of the injury. E codes are used to classify external causes of injury, poisoning, or other adverse effects. An E code should not be used as a principal diagnosis because the intermediary will reject the claim.

e.g.. For example.

E/M. Evaluation and management services. Assessment, counseling, and other services provided to a patient and reported through CPT codes.

Glossary

E/M service components. Key components in determining the correct level of E/M codes are history, examination, and medical decision-making.

EAP. Employee assistance program. Services designed to help employees, their family members, and employers find solutions for workplace and personal problems that affect morale, productivity, or financial issues such as workplace stress, family/marital concerns, legal or financial problems, elder care, child care, substance abuse, emotional/stress issues, and other daily living concerns.

ecchymosis. Bruise.

EdD. Doctor of education.

EDI. Electronic data interchange. Transference of claims, certifications, quality assurance reviews, and utilization data via computer in X12 format. May refer to any electronic exchange of formatted data.

EHO. Emerging healthcare organizations. Hospitals and other providers that are emerging or affiliating.

electronic media claim. Automated claims processing method that uses a data storage tool to transfer claims data to the payer. EMC has been replaced by electronic data interchange (EDI).

emergency department. Organized hospital-based facility for the provision of unscheduled episodic services to patients who present for immediate medical attention. The facility must be available 24 hours a day.

emergency outpatient. Patient admitted for diagnosis and treatment of a condition requiring immediate attention but who will not stay at that facility or be transferred to another.

EMT. Emergency medical technician.

EMT-P. Paramedic.

encounter. Direct personal contact between a registered hospital outpatient (in a medical clinic or emergency department, for example) and a physician (or other person authorized by state law and hospital bylaws to order or furnish services) for the diagnosis and treatment of an illness or injury. Visits with more than one health professional that take place during the same session and at a single location within the hospital are considered a single visit.

enrollee. In medical reimbursement, person who subscribes to a specific health plan.

enrollment. Number of lives covered by the plan.

enteral nutrition. Feeding of a nutrient mixture directly into or just proximal to the upper end of the small bowel via a tube or through an existing stoma. Patients are usually able to absorb the nutrients.

EOB. Explanation of benefits. Statement mailed to the member and provider explaining claim adjudication and payment.

EOMB. Explanation of Medicare benefits. Explanation of Medicaid benefits. Explanation of member benefits. Typically sent to the provider and the patient, an explanation of how Medicare, Medicaid, or member benefits were paid, that is, the allowable amount paid, the coinsurance due to the provider or payable by the patient, or the reason why a claim may have been rejected or paid less or more than the original amount charged.

episode of care. One or more health care services received during a period of relatively continuous care by a hospital or health care provider.

EPO. *1)* Epoetin alpha. *2)* Exclusive provider organization. In health care contracting, an organization similar to an HMO, but the member must remain within the provider network to receive benefits. EPOs are regulated under insurance statutes rather than HMO legislation.

ERISA. Employee Retirement Income Security Act of 1974, Public Law 93-406. Mandates reporting, disclosure of grievance and appeals requirements, fiduciary standards for private group life and health plans, and preempts state benefit mandates and premium tax laws for self-funded group health plans.

ESRD. End stage renal disease. Progression of chronic renal failure to lasting and irreparable kidney damage that requires dialysis or renal transplant for survival.

established patient. *1)* Patient who has received professional services in a face-to-face setting within the last three years from the same physician/qualified health care professional or another physician/qualified health care professional of the exact same specialty and subspecialty who belongs to the same group practice. *2)* For OPPS hospitals, patient who has been registered as an inpatient or outpatient in a hospital's provider-based clinic or emergency department within the past three years.

exclusions. Services excluded from a plan's coverage by the employer or payer because of risk or cost.

experience rating. In medical reimbursement, designation of a group's previous claims history to help determine premium rates.

explanation of benefits. Statement mailed to the member and provider explaining claim adjudication and payment.

explanation of Medicare benefits. Medicare statement mailed to the member and provider explaining claim adjudication and payment.

extrication collar. Cervical collar with opening at the throat for patients who have a tracheotomy or tracheostomy.

fab fragment. Immunoglobulin molecule fragment that is antigen binding with a light and heavy chain.

facility. Place of patient care, including inpatient and outpatient, acute or long term.

fact-oriented V codes. Codes that do not describe a problem or a service; they simply state a fact. These generally do not serve as an outpatient primary or inpatient principal diagnosis.

FAR. Federal acquisition regulations. Regulations of the federal government's acquisition of services.

FDA. Food and Drug Administration. Federal agency responsible for protecting public health by substantiating the safety, efficacy, and security of human and veterinary drugs, biological products, medical devices, national food supply, cosmetics, and items that give off radiation.

Federal Register. Government publication listing changes in regulations and federally mandated standards, including coding standards such as HCPCS Level II and ICD-9-CM.

federally qualified HMO. HMO that meets CMS guidelines for Medicare reimbursement.

fee for service. Payment model where each service performed is individually paid. Fee-for-service arrangements may be discounted or undiscounted rates.

fee schedule. List of codes and related services with pre-established billing amounts by a provider, or payment amounts by a payer that could be percentages of billed charges, flat rates, or maximum allowable amounts established by third-party payers. Medicare fee schedules apply to clinical laboratory, radiology, and durable medical equipment services.

FEHB. Federal Employee Health Benefits Program. Provides health plans to federal workers.

FEHBAR. Federal Employee Health Benefits Acquisition Regulations. Federal regulations for acquisition of health services used by government agencies and subcontractors.

FFS. Fee for service. *1)* Payment for services, usually physician services, on a service-by-service basis rather than an alternative payment system like capitation. Fee-for-service arrangements may be discounted or undiscounted rates. *2)* Situation in which the payer pays full charges for medical services.

FO. Finger orthosis.

formulary. List of prescription medications preferred for use by the health plan and dispensed through participating pharmacies to covered persons.

fraternal insurance. Cooperative plan provided to members of an association or fraternal group.

FTE. Full time employee. Accounting equivalent of one full time employee that includes wages, benefits, and other costs.

gatekeeper. Primary care physician in a health care system in which a member's care must be provided by a primary care physician unless the physician refers the member to a specialist or approves the care provided by a specialist.

GHAA. Group Health Association of America. HMO trade organization.

global surgery package. Services included in a surgical procedure that include all of the elements needed to perform the procedure and routine follow-up care.

gm. Gram.

government mandates. Services mandated by state or federal law.

grace period. Set number of days past the due date of a premium payment during which medical coverage may not be canceled and the premium payment may be made, or after employment termination. It varies by health plan contract and state law but is generally 30 to 60 days.

group model. HMO that contracts with a group of providers.

group practice. Group of providers that shares facilities, resources, and staff, and who may represent a single unit in a managed care network.

HCl. Hydrochloric acid.

HCPCS. Healthcare Common Procedure Coding System. *HCPCS Level I:* Healthcare Common Procedure Coding System Level I. Numeric coding system used by physicians, facility outpatient departments, and ambulatory surgery centers (ASC) to code ambulatory, laboratory, radiology, and other diagnostic services for Medicare billing. This coding system contains only the American Medical Association's Physicians' Current Procedural Terminology (CPT) codes. *HCPCS Level II:* Healthcare Common Procedure Coding System Level II. National coding system, developed by CMS, that contains alphanumeric codes for physician and nonphysician services not included in the CPT coding system. HCPCS Level II codes cover such things as ambulance services, durable medical equipment, and orthotic and prosthetic devices. *HCPCS modifiers:* Two-character code (AA-ZZ) that identifies circumstances that alter or enhance the description of a service or supply. They are recognized by carriers nationally.

Hct. Hematocrit.

Health Insurance Portability and Accountability Act of 1996. Federal law that allows persons to qualify immediately for comparable health insurance coverage when they change their employment relationships. Title II, subtitle F, of HIPAA gives the Department of Health and Human Services the authority to mandate the use of standards for the electronic exchange of health care data; to specify what medical and administrative code sets should be used within those standards; to require the use of national identification systems for health care patients, providers, payers (or plans), and employers (or sponsors); and to specify the types of measures required to protect the security and privacy of personally identifiable health care information.

heel cup. Plastic or rubber cup that fits into the back portion of the patient's shoe to provide protection, support, and stabilization.

HFO. Hand-finger orthosis.

HHA. Home health agency. Health care provider, licensed under state or local law, that provides skilled nursing and other therapeutic services. HHAs include visiting nurse associations and hospital-based home care programs. To participate in Medicare, an HHA must meet health and safety standards established by the U.S. Department of Health and Human Services (HHS). Home health services usually are provided in the patient's home, although some outpatient services performed in a hospital, SNF or rehabilitation center may be covered under home health if the equipment is required and cannot be used in the patient's home.

HHS. Health and Human Services. Cabinet department that oversees the operating divisions of the federal government responsible for health and welfare. HHS oversees the Centers for Medicare and Medicaid Services, Food and Drug Administration, Public Health Service, and other such entities.

HIAA. Health Insurance Association of America. Trade organization for payers.

hierarchy. Ranking or ordering of information or people.

HIPAA. Health Insurance Portability and Accountability Act of 1996. Federal law that allows persons to qualify immediately for comparable health insurance coverage when they change their employment relationships. Title II, subtitle F, of HIPAA gives the Department of Health and Human Services the authority to mandate the use of standards for the electronic exchange of health care data; to specify what medical and administrative code sets should be

used within those standards; to require the use of national identification systems for health care patients, providers, payers (or plans), and employers (or sponsors); and to specify the types of measures required to protect the security and privacy of personally identifiable health care information.

HKAFO. Hip-knee-ankle foot orthosis.

HMO. Health maintenance organization. Medical health insurance coverage that pays claims based on a provider cost, per diem, or charge basis. Hospitals contract with an HMO to provide care at a contractually reduced price. HMO members pay a set monthly amount for coverage and are treated without additional cost, except for a copayment or deductible amount, payable by the patient. Like all managed care organizations, HMOs use a variety of mechanisms to control costs, including utilization management, discounted provider fee schedules, and financial incentives. HMOs use primary care physicians as gatekeepers and tend to emphasize preventive care.

hold harmless. Contractual clause stating that if either party is held liable for malpractice, the other party is absolved.

home health. Palliative and therapeutic care and assistance in the activities of daily life to home bound Medicare and private plan members.

horseshoe. U-shaped device that stabilizes or immobilizes the patella when used with a knee orthosis.

hospice. Organization that furnishes inpatient, outpatient, and home health care for the terminally ill. Hospices emphasize support and counseling services for terminally ill people and their families, pain relief, and symptom management. When the Medicare beneficiary chooses hospice benefits, all other Medicare benefits are discontinued, except physician services and treatment of conditions not related to the terminal illness.

hypopnea. Abnormal respiratory event lasting at least 10 seconds, with at least a 30 percent reduction in thoracoabdominal movement or airflow as compared to a baseline, and with at least a 4 percent oxygen desaturation.

IA. Intra-arterial.

IBNR. Incurred but not reported. Amount of money the payer's plan accrues to forestall unknown medical expenses.

ICD-10. International Classification of Diseases, 10th Revision. Classification of diseases by alphanumeric code, used by the World Health Organization.

ICD-10-CM. International Classification of Diseases, 10th Revision, Clinical Modification. It is a clinical modification of the alphanumeric classification of diseases used by the World Health Organization, already in use in much of the world, and used for mortality reporting in the United States. The implementation date for ICD-10-CM diagnostic coding system to replace ICD-9-CM in the United States is October 1, 2014.

ICD-9-CM. International Classification of Diseases, 9th Revision, Clinical Modification. Clinical modification of the international statistical coding system used to report, compile, and compare health care data, using numeric and alphanumeric (E codes and V codes) codes to help plan, deliver, reimburse, and quantify medical care in the United States.

ICF. Intermediate care facility. Health care facility that furnishes services to patients who do not require the degree of care provided by a hospital or skilled nursing facility or a step-down facility for patients who are leaving the hospital but who cannot be discharged to home because of continuing medical needs.

ID card. Wallet card carried by a plan member providing name, member and group numbers, effective dates, deductibles, and other information.

immobilizer. Device used to restrain a part of the body, keeping the body part from moving.

implant. Material or device inserted or placed within the body for therapeutic, reconstructive, or diagnostic purposes.

in plan. Services chosen from a network provider.

incontestable clause. Provision in a policy that prohibits the plan from disputing coverage for certain conditions after a specified period of time.

INF. 1) Inferior. 2) Infusion.

infusion pump. Device that delivers a measured amount of drug or intravenous solution through injection over a period of time.

inpatient hospitalization. Period in which a patient is housed in a single hospital usually without interruption.

insoles. Rubber or plastic orthotics that fit inside the shoes to correct a deformity or help aid in the healing of an injury.

insurance carrier. Insurer or health plan that may underwrite, administer, or sell a range of health benefit programs.

intermediate repair. 1) Surgical closure of a wound requiring closure of one or more of the deeper subcutaneous tissue and non-muscle fascia layers in addition to the skin. 2) Contaminated wounds with single layer closure that need extensive cleaning or foreign body removal.

internal skeletal fixation. Repair involving wires, pins, screws, and/or plates placed through or within the fractured area to stabilize and immobilize the injury.

IOL. Intraocular lens.

IPA. Individual practice association. Organization made up of providers who, along with the rest of a group, contract with payers at a discounted fee-for-service or capitated rate.

IPO. Individual practice organization. Organization made up of providers who, along with the rest of a group, contract with payers at a discounted fee-for-service or capitated rate.

IS. Information services. Administrators of the computer systems used by payers and providers.

IV. 1) Intravenous. 2) Cranial nerve on the brainstem responsible for motor control of the superior oblique muscle (trochlear).

JCAHO. Joint Commission on Accreditation of Healthcare Organizations. Organization that accredits health care organizations. In the future, the JCAHO may play a role in certifying these organizations' compliance with the HIPAA A/S requirements. Previously known as the Joint Commission for the Accreditation of Hospitals.

JD. Doctor of jurisprudence.

KAFO. Knee-ankle-foot orthosis. External apparatus utilized to improve motor control, gait stabilization, and reduce pain. The device is attached to the leg in order to help correct flexible deformities and to halt the progression of fixed deformities.

key components. Three components of history, examination, and medical decision making are considered the keys to selecting the correct level of E/M codes. In most cases, all three components must be addressed in the documentation. However, in established, subsequent, and follow-up categories, only two of the three must be met or exceeded for a given code.

KOH. Potassium hydroxide.

lapse. Terminated policy.

late effect. Abnormality, dysfunction, or other residual condition produced after the acute phase of an illness, injury, or disease is over. There is no time limit on when late effects can appear.

LCD. Local coverage determination. Published decision by a Medicare contractor regarding coverage guidelines for a particular service and is valid only in the contractor's jurisdiction. LCDs replaced local medical review policies for CMS as of 2006.

LCSW. Licensed clinical social worker.

limiting charge. Maximum amount a nonparticipating physician or provider can charge for services rendered to a Medicare patient.

limits. In medical reimbursement, the ceiling for benefits payable under a plan.

line of business. Different health plans offered by a larger insurer or insurance broker as a product line.

lives. Unit of measurement used by plans to determine the number of people covered. Calculated by multiplying the number of members by 2.5.

local coverage determination. Decision of coverage and related usage specific to a Medicare administrative contractor (MAC), fiscal intermediary or carrier, or in a designated geographic area.

long-term care facility. Nursing home or, more specifically, a facility offering extended, nonacute care to a resident patient whose illness does not require acute care.

loss ratio. Ratio between the cost to deliver medical care and the amount of money taken in by the plan.

LPN. Licensed practical nurse.

LSO. Lumbar sacral orthosis.

LVN. *1)* Licensed visiting nurse. *2)* Licensed vocational nurse.

MA. *1)* Master of arts degree. *2)* Medical assistant. *3)* Mental age.

MAC. Medicare administrative contractor. One of 15 jurisdictional organizations that contract with CMS to adjudicate professional claims under Part A and Part B, responsible for daily claims processing, utilization review, record maintenance, dissemination of information based on CMS regulations, and whether services are covered and payments are appropriate. Four of the jurisdictions also include home health services. There are four separate MAC jurisdictions for DME services.

malingering. Feigning of illness, as the result of intentional deceit or as the result of mental illness.

managed health care. *1)* Managing active cases to ensure care is the most appropriate, efficient, and effective. *2)* System of health care meant to manage overall cost. *3)* Method of health care whereby contracted physicians participate in managing health care costs.

mandated benefits. Services mandated by state or federal law such as child abuse or rape, not necessarily covered by insurers.

maximum allowable charge. Amount set by the insurer as the highest amount that can be charged for a particular medical service or by a pharmacy vendor.

MCE. Medical care evaluation.

mcg. Microgram.

MCO. Managed care organization. Generic term for various health benefit plans that provide coverage for health care services in conjunction with management and review of services provided to ensure that services are medically necessary and appropriate.

MD. Medical doctor.

ME. Medical examiner.

MEd. Master of education.

Medicaid. Joint federal and state program that covers medical expenses for people with low incomes and limited resources who meet the criteria. The benefits for recipients vary from state to state.

medical consultation. Advice or an opinion rendered by a physician at the request of the primary care provider.

medical loss ratio. Ratio between the cost to deliver medical care and the amount of money taken in by the plan.

medical necessity. Medically appropriate and necessary to meet basic health needs; consistent with the diagnosis or condition and national medical practice guidelines regarding type, frequency, and duration of treatment; rendered in a cost-effective manner.

Medicare. Federally funded program authorized as part of the Social Security Act that provides for health care services for people age 65 or older, people with disabilities, and people with end-stage renal disease (ESRD).

Medicare administrative contractor. Uniform type of Medicare administrative entity that processes both institutional and professional claims in specified geographic jurisdictions of the country. There are 15 A/B MACs that are scheduled to be combined into a total of 10 A/B MACS, while maintaining four DME MACs, and four home health/hospice MACs.

Medicare fee schedule. Fee schedule based upon physician work, expense, and malpractice designed to slow the rise in cost for services and standardize payment to physicians regardless of specialty or location of service with geographic adjustments.

Medicare Part A. Hospital insurance coverage that includes hospital, nursing home, hospice, home health, and other inpatient care. Claims are submitted to intermediaries for reimbursement.

Medicare Part B. Supplemental medical insurance that includes outpatient hospital care and physician and other qualified professional care. Claims from providers or suppliers other than a hospital are

Glossary

submitted to carriers for reimbursement. Hospital outpatient claims are submitted to their FI/MAC.

Medicare secondary payer. Specified circumstance when other third-party payers have the primary responsibility for payment of services and Medicare is the secondary payer. Medicare is secondary to workers' compensation, automobile, medical no-fault and liability insurance, EGHPs, LGHPs, and certain employer health plans covering aged and disabled beneficiaries. The MSP program prohibits Medicare payment for items or services if payment has been made or can reasonably be expected to be made by another payer, as described above.

Medicare supplement. Private insurance coverage that pays the Medicare deductible and copayments and may also pay the costs of services not covered by Medicare.

Medigap policy. Health insurance or other health benefit plan offered by a private company to those entitled to Medicare benefits. The policy covers charges not payable by Medicare because of deductibles, coinsurance amounts, or other Medicare-imposed limitations.

member. In medical reimbursement, subscriber of a health plan.

member months. In medical reimbursement, total of months each member was covered.

member services. In health care contracting, the payer department that works as a patient advocate to solve problems and may take claims appeals to a final committee after all other processes have been exhausted.

mental health substance abuse. Payer term for services rendered to members for emotional problems or chemical dependency.

mental or nervous. Payer term for services rendered to members for emotional problems or chemical dependency.

mEq. Milliequivalent.

MeSH. Medical staff-hospital organization.

MET. Multiple employer trust. Group of employers that join together to purchase health insurance using a self-funded approach to lower costs by the broadening membership pool to prevent an adverse selection.

MEWA. Multiple employer welfare association. Group of employers that join together to purchase health insurance using a self-funded approach to lower costs by the broadening membership pool to prevent an adverse selection.

mg. Milligram.

MHA. Master of health administration.

minor procedure. Self-limited procedure, usually with an assignment of 0 or 10 follow-up days by payers. A minor procedure may be considered by many payers to be part of the global package for a primary surgical service and cannot be billed separately from the primary procedure.

MIS. Management information system. Hardware and software facilitating claims management.

mixed model. HMO that includes both an open panel and closed panel option.

ml. Milliliter.

MLP. Midlevel practitioners. Professionals such as nurse practitioners, nurse midwives, physical therapists, physician assistants, and others who provide medical care but do so with physician input.

MLT. Medical laboratory technician.

modality. *1)* Form of imaging (e.g., x-ray, fluoroscopy, ultrasound, nuclear medicine, duplex Doppler, CT, and MRI). *2)* Any physical agent applied to produce therapeutic changes to biologic tissue including, but not limited to, thermal, acoustic, light, mechanical, or electric energy.

modifier. Two characters that can be appended to a HCPCS code as a means of identifying circumstances that alter or enhance the description of a service or supply.

morbidity rate. In health care contracting, an actuarial term describing predicted medical expense rate.

MP. Metacarpal phalangeal.

MPH. Master of public health. Advanced degree.

MSA. Medical savings account.

MSN. Master of science in nursing.

MSW. Master's in social work.

MT. *1)* Medical technologist. *2)* Medical transcriptionist.

multiple birth. Two or more infants delivered at the same time.

multiple employer group. Group of employers who contract together to subscribe to a plan, broadening the risk pool and saving money. Different from a multiple employer trust.

multiple-lead device. Implantable cardiac device (pacemaker or implantable cardioverter-defibrillator [ICD]) in which pacing and sensing components are placed in at least three chambers of the heart.

NA. Nurse assistant.

NAHMOR. National Association of HMO Regulators.

NAIC. National Association of Insurance Commissioners. Organization of state insurance regulators.

national coverage determination. National policy statement regarding the circumstances under which a service, item, or test is considered reasonable and necessary or otherwise not covered for Medicare purposes.

National Supplier Clearinghouse. Entity that approves providers and medical equipment vendors as "suppliers" under the Medicare program, issuing an identification number to approved applicants.

national supplier identification number. Number with which providers or other health care professionals who disperse DMEPOS submit their claims. This number is obtained through an application to the National Supplier Clearinghouse, a centralized agency for DMEPOS suppliers.

NBICU. Newborn intensive care unit. Special care unit for premature and seriously ill infants.

NCD. National coverage determinations. National policy statements granting, eliminating, or excluding Medicare coverage for a service, item, or test and indicate CMS policy regarding the circumstances under which the service, item, or test is considered reasonable and necessary or otherwise not covered for Medicare purposes.

NCHS. National Center for Health Statistics. Division of the Centers for Disease Control and Prevention that compiles statistical information used to guide actions and policies to improve the public health of U.S. citizens. The NCHS maintains the ICD-9-CM and ICD-10-CM coding systems.

NCQA. National Committee for Quality Assurance. Organization that accredits managed care plans, or HMOs. In the future, the NCQA may play a role in certifying these organizations' compliance with the HIPAA A/S requirements.

ND. Doctor of naturopathy.

nebulization device. Device used to vaporize liquid medication for the airborne delivery of the medication to the patient. The medication is absorbed into the body via the respiratory tract. Medications can also be administered with a nebulizer to fragment and mobilize thick, excess mucous in the respiratory tract; these medications are broadly termed mucolytics.

NEC. Not elsewhere classifiable. Condition or diagnosis that is not provided with its own specified code in ICD-9-CM, but included in a more broadly defined code for other specified conditions.

neonatal period. Period of an infant's life from birth to the age of 27 days, 23 hours, and 59 minutes.

network model. Plan that contracts with multiple groups of providers, or networks, to provide care.

new patient. Patient who is receiving face-to-face care from a provider/qualified health care professional or another physician/qualified health care professional of the exact same specialty and subspecialty who belongs to the same group practice for the first time in three years. For OPPS hospitals, a patient who has not been registered as an inpatient or outpatient, including off-campus provider based clinic or emergency department, within the past three years.

NOS. Not otherwise specified. Condition or diagnosis remains ill-defined and is unspecified without the necessary information for selecting a more specific code.

NP. *1)* Nurse practitioner. *2)* Neuropsychiatry.

NPI. National provider identifier. Standard eight-digit alphanumeric provider identifier implemented under the Health Insurance Portability and Accountability Act of 1996 (HIPAA) requirements. The first seven digits identify the provider and the eighth position is a check digit. Providers are required to report their NPI number for electronic and paper billing.

O2. Oxygen.

occupational therapy. Training, education, and assistance intended to assist a person who is recovering from a serious illness or injury perform the activities of daily life.

OIG. Office of Inspector General. Agency within the Department of Health and Human Services that is ultimately responsible for investigating instances of fraud and abuse in the Medicare and Medicaid and other government health care programs. OIG work plan Annual plan released by the Office of Inspector General (OIG) that details the areas of focus for fraud and abuse investigations.

open enrollment period. Time period during which subscribers in a health benefit program have the opportunity to re-enroll or select an alternative health plan being offered to them, usually without evidence of insurability or waiting periods.

open panel. Arrangement in which a managed care organization that contracts with providers on an exclusive basis is still seeking providers.

OPL. Other party liability. In coordination of benefits, the decision that the other plan is the primary plan.

Glossary

orthosis. Derived from a Greek word meaning "to make straight," it is an artificial appliance that supports, aligns, or corrects an anatomical deformity or improves the use of a moveable body part. Unlike a prosthesis, an orthotic device is always functional in nature.

orthotic. Associated with the making and fitting of an orthosis(es).

osteogenesis stimulator. Device used to stimulate the growth of bone by electrical impulses or ultrasound.

ostomy. Artificial (surgical) opening in the body used for drainage or for delivery of medications or nutrients.

OTR. Occupational therapist registered.

out of plan. In health care contracting, services of a provider who is not a member of the preferred provider network.

out of service area. In health care contracting, medical care received out of the geographic area that may or may not be covered, depending on the plan.

outpatient. Person who has not been admitted as an inpatient but who is registered on the hospital or CAH records as an outpatient and receives services (rather than supplies alone) directly from the hospital or CAH. (Code of Federal Regulations, section 410.2)

outpatient visit. Encounter in a recognized outpatient facility.

overutilization. Services rendered by providers more frequently than usual.

PA. *1)* Physician assistant. Medical professional who receives additional training and can assess, treat, and prescribe medications under a physician's review. *2)* Posteroanterior. *3)* Pulmonary artery. *4)* HCPCS Level II modifier used to denote a surgical or other invasive procedure that was performed on the wrong body part.

paneled. In health care contracting, provider contracted with an HMO.

par provider. Provider who is participating in a health plan or Medicare program.

parenteral nutrition. Nutrients provided subcutaneously, intravenously, intramuscularly, or intradermally for patients during the postoperative period and in other conditions, such as shock, coma, and renal failure.

partial disability. Congenital or acquired inability to perform part of one's job.

partial hospitalization. Situation in which the patient only stays part of each day over a long period.

Cardiac, rehabilitation, and chronic pain patients, for example, could use this service.

partial payment. Payment to a provider or member with the expectation that other payments will be forthcoming before the claim is closed.

PATOS. Payment (received) at the time of service.

PBM. Prescription benefit managers. HMO staff who monitor amount and use of drugs prescribed.

PCP. Primary care physician. Physician who makes an initial diagnosis and referral and retains control over the patient and utilization of services both in and outside of the plan.

pediatric patient. Patient usually younger than 14 years of age.

peer review. Evaluation of the quality of the total health care provided by medical staff with equivalent training, such as a physician-to-physician or nurse-to-nurse evaluation.

PEPM. Per employee per month.

PEPP. Payment error prevention program. Program to help reduce Medicare PPS inpatient hospital payment errors.

per diem reimbursement. In health care contracting, reimbursement to an institution based on a set rate per day rather than on a charge-by-charge basis.

percutaneous skeletal fixation. Treatment that is neither open nor closed and the injury site is not directly visualized. Fixation devices (pins, screws) are placed through the skin to stabilize the dislocation using x-ray guidance.

pessary. Device placed in the vagina to support and reposition a prolapsing or retropositioned uterus, rectum, or vagina.

PharmD. Doctor of pharmacy.

PhD. Doctor of philosophy.

PHO. Physician-hospital organization.

physician assistant. Medical professional who receives additional training and can assess, treat, and prescribe medications under a physician's review.

PIN. Physician identification number.

plan manager. Payer employee managing all of the contracts and contract negotiations for one or more specific plans.

PMPM. Per member per month.

PMPY. Per member per year.

pneumatic splint. Splint filled with air or gas to provide circumferential protection and support.

pooling. Health payers' practice of combining risk.

POS. Point of service. Health benefit plan allowing the covered person to choose to receive a service from a participating or nonparticipating provider, with different benefit levels associated with the use of participating providers.

posting date. Date a charge is posted to a patient account by the provider, frequently not the same as the actual date of service, but usually within five days of the actual date of service.

PPA. Preferred provider arrangement. Similar to a PPO.

PPO. Preferred provider organization. Program that establishes contracts with providers of medical care. Usually the benefit contract provides significantly better benefits and lower member cost for services received from preferred providers, encouraging covered persons to use these providers, who may be reimbursed on a discounted basis.

PPS. Prospective payment system. Reimbursement methodology that uses predetermined rates for each type of discharge, procedure, service, or item based on a standard type of case. For hospital inpatients, the Medicare PPS system of DRGs was implemented in 1983 to hold down the rising cost of health care. For hospital outpatients, OPPS has been based on ambulatory payment classifications effective August 1, 2000. For skilled nursing facilities, it is based on the RUG-IV system, and for home health it is based on the HHRGs.

precertification. Confirmation that a payer covers a given procedure for a given patient, including admission or continued stay.

preexisting condition. Symptom that causes a person to seek diagnosis, care, or treatment for which medical advice or treatment was recommended or received by a physician within a certain time period before the effective date of medical insurance coverage. The preexisting condition waiting period is the time the beneficiary must wait after buying health insurance before coverage begins for a condition that existed before coverage was obtained.

prehensile. Ability to grasp, seize, or hold.

presenting problem. Disease, condition, illness, injury, symptom, sign, finding, complaint, or other reason for the patient encounter

primary care. Basic or general health care, traditionally provided by family practice, pediatrics, and internal medicine practitioners.

primary diagnosis. Current, most significant reason for the services or procedures provided.

principal diagnosis. Condition established after study to be chiefly responsible for occasioning the admission of the patient to the hospital for care.

principal procedure. Procedure performed for definitive treatment rather than for diagnostic or exploratory purposes, or that was necessary to treat a complication. Usually related to the principal diagnosis.

problem-oriented V codes. ICD-9-CM codes that identify circumstances that could affect the patient in the future but are neither a current illness nor an injury. Use these codes to describe an existing circumstance or problem that may influence future medical care.

prodrug. Inactive drug that goes through a metabolic process when given resulting in a chemical conversion that changes the drug into an active pharmacological agent.

professional association plans. Plan provided by a professional association that affords self-employed professionals (e.g., physicians, CPAs, lawyers) less expensive coverage.

program safeguard coordinator. Contractor charged with maintaining the integrity of the Medicare program. Duties include data analysis, audit, review, and monitoring related to beneficiary information (such as COB data), medical review, cost reports, provider education, and fraud detection and prevention.

prosthetic. Device that replaces all or part of an internal body organ or body part, or that replaces part of the function of a permanently inoperable or malfunctioning internal body organ or body part.

provider. All-inclusive, generic term for people or institutions that provide health care. The provider may be a physician, hospital, pharmacy, other facility, or other health care provider.

PSC. Program safeguard coordinators.

PT. Physical therapy.

PTA. Physical therapy assistant.

PTMPY. Per thousand members per year.

QA. Quality assurance. Monitoring and maintenance of established standards of quality for patient care.

QM. Quality management. Monitoring and maintenance of established standards of quality.

RBRVS. Resource-based relative value scale. Fee schedule introduced by CMS to reimburse physician Medicare fees based on the amount of time and

Glossary

resources expended in treating patients with adjustments for overhead costs and geographical differences.

reasonable and customary. Fees charged for medical services that are considered normal, common, and in line with the prevailing fees in the provider's geographical area.

referral. Approval from the primary care physician to see a specialist or receive certain services. May be required for coverage purposes before a patient receives care from anyone except the primary physician.

rehabilitation. Restoration of physical and mental functions to allow the usual daily activities of life.

reimbursement. Payment of actual charges or allowable incurred as a result of accident or illness.

reinsurance. Insurance purchased by an HMO, insurance company, or self-funded employer from another insurance company to protect itself against all or part of the losses that may be incurred in the process of honoring the claims of its participating providers, policy holders, or employees and covered dependents.

residual limb. Portion of an arm or leg that remains attached to the body after an amputation.

review committee. Multidisciplinary committee that considers denied cases being appealed, catastrophic cases, or fee-for-service cases.

RHIA. Registered health information administrator. Accreditation for medical record administrators, previously known as a registered records administrator (RRA), through AHIMA.

RHIT. Registered health information technician. Accreditation for medical records practitioners, previously known as accredited records technician (ART), through AHIMA.

rib belt. Device that encircles the abdomen and provides support for injured ribs while they heal.

risk contract. Contract between Medicare and a payer or a payer and a provider in which the payer (in the case of Medicare) and the provider (in the case of the payer contracts) receive a set amount for care of a patient base. If costs exceed the amount the payer or provider was paid, the patients still receive care during the term of the contract.

risk factor reduction. Reduction of risk in the pool of health plan members.

risk manager. Person charged with keeping financial risk low, including malpractice cases.

risk pool. Pool of people who will be in the insured group, their medical and mental histories, other factors such as age, and their predicted health.

RN. Registered nurse.

RPh. Registered pharmacist.

RPT. Registered physical therapist.

RRA. Registered records administrator.

RRT. Registered respiratory therapist.

rush charge. Charge for expeditious test results.

RVS. Relative value study. Guide that shows the relationship between the time, resources, competency, experience, severity, and other factors necessary to perform procedures that is multiplied by a dollar conversion factor to determine a monetary value for the procedure.

RVU. Relative value unit. Value assigned a procedure based on difficulty and time consumed. Used for computing reimbursement under a relative value study.

SACH. Solid ankle, cushion heel.

sanction. Imposition of penalties or exclusion of a provider for fraud or infractions such as an inappropriate use of services, providing procedures that may harm the patient, or applying inferior techniques.

schedule. Listing of amounts payable for specific procedures.

second opinion. Medical opinion obtained from another health care professional, relevant to clinical evaluation, before the performance of a medical service or surgical procedure. Includes patient education regarding treatment alternatives and/or to determine medical necessity.

secondary insurer. In a COB arrangement, the insurer that reimburses for benefits pending after payment by the primary insurer.

self-funded plan. Plan where the risk is assumed by the employer rather than the insurer. The employer generally pays claims directly from a general fund account that may be managed by a third party.

self-insured. Individual or organization that assumes the financial risk of paying for health care.

self-pay patients. Patients who pay for medical care out-of-pocket.

SEO. Shoulder-elbow orthosis.

service date. Date a charge is incurred for a service.

service plan. *1)* Plan that has contracts with providers but is not a managed care plan. *2)* Another name for Blue Cross/Blue Shield plans.

service-oriented V codes. ICD-9-CM codes that identify or define examinations, aftercare, ancillary services, or therapy. Use these V codes to describe the patient who is not currently ill but seeks medical services for some specific purpose such as follow-up visits. You can also use this type of V code as a primary diagnosis for outpatient services when the patient has no symptoms that can be coded and screening services are provided.

shadow pricing. Setting rates just below a competitor's rates. Maximizes profits but raises medical costs.

simple repair. Surgical closure of a superficial wound, requiring single layer suturing of the skin (epidermis, dermis, or subcutaneous tissue).

skeletal traction. Applying direct pulling force on the long axis of bones by inserted wires or pins and using weights and pulleys to keep the bone in proper alignment.

skin traction. Application of a pulling force to a limb accomplished by a device fixed to felt dressings or strappings applied to the body surface.

small subscriber group aggregate. Aggregate of professional associations, small business, or other entities formed to be considered a single, large subscriber group.

SNF. Skilled nursing facility. Institution or a distinct part of an institution that is primarily engaged in providing skilled nursing care and related services for residents who require medical or nursing care; or rehabilitation services for the rehabilitation of injured, disabled, or sick persons.

SO. *1)* Shoulder orthosis. *2)* Sacroiliac orthosis.

SOF. Signature on file.

softgoods or soft goods. DMEPOS industry term for medical devices such as braces, splints, joint supports and protectors, cervical pillows, and other similar orthopaedic-oriented items.

specimen. Tissue cells or sample of fluid taken for analysis, pathologic examination, and diagnosis.

splint. Brace or support for an anatomical structure after surgery or injury.

split inventory technique. Keeping highly-utilized DMEPOS easily accessible to staff, while keeping surplus in a central storage area.

SSA. Social Security Act.

SSN. Social security number.

staff model. HMO that employs its own providers.

standard anesthesia formula. Reimbursement formula that consists of base units plus time units plus modifying units (e.g., physical status and qualifying circumstances) plus other allowed unit/charges that is multiplied by a conversion factor.

stat charge. Charge for expeditious test results.

state insurance commission. State group that approves insurance certificates for each state and regulates the industry based on statutes.

steering. Providing financial incentives to plan members to use the managed care provider panel.

stockinet. Material used to wrap an injured body part before applying a cast; usually of breathable material to wick moisture away from skin.

stop loss. In health care contracting, a form of reinsurance that protects health insurance above a certain limit and minimizes risks for providers.

subrogation. Recovery of monies or benefits from a third party who is liable for the payment.

subsidiary codes. Services that are not included as part of the primary procedure but that are not performed alone and may be identified as each additional, or list-in-addition-to services. Phrases that help identify subsidiary codes include, but are not limited to: each additional, list in addition to, and done at time of other major procedure

subtraction. Process of using an image to remove an overlying structure in another image to better visualize the area underneath the overlying structure.

superbill. Multipurpose sheet used for all patient encounters that typically contains a check-off list of ICD-9-CM diagnosis codes, evaluation and management codes, and procedure and HCPCS Level II codes in the outpatient setting.

supplemental health services. Optional services that a health plan may cover or provide.

support. Article that provides stabilization, but not immobilization, to an injured or disabled body part.

surgical package. Normal, uncomplicated performance of specific surgical services, with the assumption that, on average, all surgical procedures of a given type are similar with respect to skill level, duration, and length of normal follow-up care.

TCC. Transitional care center. Facility used in lieu of an extended care facility or before discharge to an extended care facility.

technical component. Portion of a health care service that identifies the provision of the equipment, supplies, technical personnel, and costs attendant to

Glossary

the performance of the procedure other than the professional services.

TEFRA. Tax Equity and Fiscal Responsibility Act. Protects the rights of full-time employees to remain on the company's health plan to age 69.

terminal device. Addition to an upper limb prosthesis that replaces the function and/or appearance of a missing hand.

tertiary care facility. Hospital providing specialty care to patients referred from other hospitals because of the severity of their injuries or illnesses.

therapeutic. Act meant to alleviate a medical or mental condition.

therapeutic procedure. Treatment of a pathological or traumatic condition through the use of activities performed to treat or heal the cause or to effect change through the application of clinical skills or services that attempt to improve function.

therapeutic services. Services performed for treatment of a specific diagnosis. These services include performance of the procedure, various incidental elements, and normal, related follow-up care.

thermoplastic. Item that can be softened by heat, but hardens upon cooling.

third-party administrator. Firm that performs administrative functions for a self-funded plan but assumes no risk.

third-party payer. Public or private organization that pays for or underwrites coverage for health care expenses for another entity, usually an employer (e.g., Blue Cross Blue Shield, Medicare, Medicaid, commercial insurers).

THKAO. Thoracic-hip-knee-ankle orthosis.

time limit. In health care contracting, a set number of days in which a claim can be filed according to the payer or state insurance commission.

TPA. Third-party administrator. Firm that performs administrative functions for a self-funded plan but assumes no risk.

TPL. Third party liability. Payer liable for the cost of an illness or injury, such as auto or homeowner insurer.

TQM. Total quality management. Concept that quality is an organic part of a plan's service and a provider's care and can be quantified and constantly improved.

traction. Drawing out or holding tension on an area by applying a direct therapeutic pulling force.

transaction standard. Set of rules, conditions, or requirements describing the classification and

components or a transaction. Transaction standards define the data elements and code sets that must be used in a transaction.

transcutaneous electrical nerve stimulator. Device that delivers a controlled amount of electricity to an area of the body to stimulate healing and/or to mitigate post-surgical or post-traumatic pain.

transfer. Situation in which the patient is transferred to another acute care hospital for related care.

treatment plan. Plan of care established by the provider outlining specific deficits and planned treatment that may be submitted to the case manager when seeking certification for a plan member.

triage. Medical screening of patients to determine priority of treatment based on severity of illness or injury and resources at hand.

triple option. Offering of an HMO, indemnity plan, and preferred provider organization by one insurance firm.

type A emergency department. Emergency department licensed and advertised to be available to provide emergent care 24 hours a day, seven days a week. Type A emergency departments must meet both the CPT book definition of an emergency department and the EMTALA definition of a dedicated emergency department.

type B emergency department. Emergency department licensed and advertised to provide emergent care less than 24 hours a day, seven days a week. Type B emergency departments must meet the EMTALA definition of a dedicated emergency department.

uCi. Microcurie.

UCR. Usual, customary, and reasonable. Fees charged for medical services that are considered normal, common, and in line with the prevailing fees in a given geographical area.

unbundling. Separately packaging costs or services that might otherwise be billed together including billing separately for health care services that should be combined according to the industry standards or commonly accepted coding practices.

underwriting. Evaluating and determining the financial risk a member or member group has on an insurer.

unlisted procedure. Procedural descriptions used when the overall procedure and outcome of the procedure are not adequately described by an existing procedure code. Such codes are used as a last resort and only when there is not a more appropriate procedure code.

unspecified. Codes for use when documentation is insufficient to assign a more specific code.

upcoding. Practice of billing a code that represents a higher reimbursement than the code for the procedure actually performed.

URAC. Utilization Review Accreditation Commission. Accrediting body of case management.

urgent admission. Admission in which the patient requires immediate attention for treatment of a physical or psychiatric problem.

USP. United States pharmacopoeia.

USPHS. United States Public Health Service.

utilization review. Formal assessment of the medical necessity, efficiency, and/or appropriateness of health care services and treatment plans on a prospective, concurrent, or retrospective basis.

utilization review nurse. Nurse who evaluates cases for appropriateness of care and length of service and can plan discharge and services needed after discharge.

volume. *1)* Number of services performed. *2)* Number of patients. *3)* Number of patients in a DRG during a specific time.

weighting. Assigning more worth to a fee based on the number of times it is charged, weighting the resource-based relative value fees for an area.

withhold. Percentage of payment to providers held by an HMO until the cost of referral or services has been determined. If the provider goes over the amount determined appropriate, the HMO keeps that amount.

workers' compensation. State-governed system designated to administer and regulate the provision and cost of medical treatment and wage losses arising from a worker's job-related injury or disease, regardless of who is at fault. In exchange, the employer is protected from being sued.

wraparound plan. Insurance or health plan coverage for copays and deductibles not covered under a member's base plan.

ZPIC. Zone Program Integrity Contractor. CMS contractor that replaced the existing Program Safeguard Contractors (PSC). Contractors are responsible for ensuring the integrity of all Medicare-related claims under Parts A and B (hospital, skilled nursing, home health, provider, and durable medical equipment claims), Part C (Medicare Advantage health plans), Part D (prescription drug plans), and coordination of Medicare-Medicaid data matches (Medi-Medi).

Glossary

HCPCS Lay Descriptions

A

A0021

A0021   Ambulance service, outside state per mile, transport (Medicaid only)

Lay Description
This code represents a per mile charge for ambulance transportation outside of the state where the ambulance provider is based. This code is used only for Medicaid claims. Consult the local Medicaid office in the state that the provider is located for further definition and usage requirements.

A0080-A0210

A0080   Nonemergency transportation, per mile - vehicle provided by volunteer (individual or organization), with no vested interest

A0090   Nonemergency transportation, per mile - vehicle provided by individual (family member, self, neighbor) with vested interest

A0100   Nonemergency transportation; taxi

A0110   Nonemergency transportation and bus, intra- or interstate carrier

A0120   Nonemergency transportation: mini-bus, mountain area transports, or other transportation systems

A0130   Nonemergency transportation: wheelchair van

A0140   Nonemergency transportation and air travel (private or commercial) intra- or interstate

A0160   Nonemergency transportation: per mile - caseworker or social worker

A0170   Transportation ancillary: parking fees, tolls, other

A0180   Nonemergency transportation: ancillary: lodging-recipient

A0190   Nonemergency transportation: ancillary: meals, recipient

A0200   Nonemergency transportation: ancillary: lodging, escort

A0210   Nonemergency transportation: ancillary: meals, escort

Lay Description
These codes provide for reporting nonemergency transportation and related ancillary services. Different types of vehicles used and/or the areas traveled, as well as additional fees are specified in these codes. This range reports nonemergency transport services such as a vehicle provided by a volunteer or family member; wheelchair van, taxi, bus, or air transport (private or commercial); mountainous area transport, or transportation outside the state. Examples of ancillary services include parking fees and tolls, lodging or meals for the recipient or for the escort, and per mile transportation of a caseworker or social worker.

A0225

A0225   Ambulance service, neonatal transport, base rate, emergency transport, one way

Lay Description
Use this code for the emergency transport of a neonate by ambulance, one way only, at base rate.

A0380

A0380   BLS mileage (per mile)

Lay Description
A basic life support (BLS) ambulance provides transportation plus the equipment and staff needed for basic life support services, such as controlling bleeding, splinting fractures, treating shock, delivering babies, and performing cardio-pulmonary resuscitation (CPR). BLS transport is reported on a per mile basis.

A0382

A0382   BLS routine disposable supplies

Lay Description
Basic life support (BLS) routine disposable supplies include such items as cervical collar, gauze, dressings, and ice packs. Report a unit of one for all routine disposable supplies that are used.

A0384

A0384   BLS specialized service disposable supplies; defibrillation (used by ALS ambulances and BLS ambulances in jurisdictions where defibrillation is permitted in BLS ambulances)

Lay Description
Specialized disposable basic life support (BLS) defibrillation supplies include such items as defibrillator electrodes (AED), pacing pads, combination pads, and gel pads. This code is used in jurisdictions where defibrillation is permitted in BLS ambulances.

A0390

A0390   ALS mileage (per mile)

Lay Description
Advanced life support (ALS) mileage is paid on a per mile basis based on the patient's condition. Some local governments may require an ALS response for all calls, but Medicare pays only for the level of service provided, and only when the service is medically necessary. This applies to ground and air transports.

A0392

A0392   ALS specialized service disposable supplies; defibrillation (to be used only in jurisdictions where defibrillation cannot be performed in BLS ambulances)

Lay Description
Specialized disposable advanced life support (ALS) defibrillation supplies include such items as defibrillator electrodes (AED), pacing pads, combination pads, and gel pads.

A0394

A0394   ALS specialized service disposable supplies; IV drug therapy

Lay Description
Specialized disposable advanced life support (ALS) IV drug therapy supplies include items such as IV start kits, IV tubing, disposable armboard, catheter, pump sets, micro drip, and Y-site tubing. Report this code once for all IV drug therapy supplies used.

A0396

A0396   ALS specialized service disposable supplies; esophageal intubation

Lay Description
Specialized disposable advanced life support (ALS) esophageal intubation supplies, which are used for airway management, include such items as esophageal obturator, esophageal gastric tube, stylette, inflation syringe, endotracheal tube, laryngoscope blade, cricotracheotomy kits, and disposable bag valve mask.

A0398

A0398   ALS routine disposable supplies

Lay Description
Advanced life support (ALS) routine disposable supplies include such items as EKG electrodes, cervical collar, gauze, and dressings. Report a unit of one for all routine disposable supplies that are used.

A0420

A0420   Ambulance waiting time (ALS or BLS), one-half (1/2) hour increments

Lay Description
This code reports ambulance waiting time for both BLS and ALS services. Time is reported in one-half hour increments. Do not report waiting time of less than one-half hour. Report one unit for each half-hour increment or portion thereof for waiting times of one-half hour or more.

A0422

A0422   Ambulance (ALS or BLS) oxygen and oxygen supplies, life sustaining situation

Lay Description
This code reports the oxygen and oxygen supplies used in a life-sustaining situation during ambulance transportation (ALS or BLS). There are two levels of ambulance service, basic medical care or basic life support (BLS) and advanced emergency medical care or advanced life support (ALS).

A0424

A0424   Extra ambulance attendant, ground (ALS or BLS) or air (fixed or rotary winged); (requires medical review)

Lay Description
This code reports charges for an additional ambulance attendant for both ground (BLS and ALS) and air (fixed wing and rotary transports). The need for an additional ambulance attendant must be substantiated by report.

A0425

A0425   Ground mileage, per statute mile

Lay Description
This code reports ground mileage. Mileage and reimbursement rates are generally defined by and under the jurisdiction of state statutes.

A0426-A0427

A0426   Ambulance service, advanced life support, nonemergency transport, level 1 (ALS 1)

A0427   Ambulance service, advanced life support, emergency transport, level 1 (ALS 1 - emergency)

Lay Description
Advanced life support, non-emergency transport, level 1 (ALS 1) is the transportation by ground ambulance vehicle and the provision of medically necessary supplies and services. Report these codes for advanced life support, emergency ambulance transport, level 1 (ALS 1-emergency), which includes the provision of an ALS assessment or at least one ALS intervention. Advanced life support intervention means a procedure that is in accordance with state and local laws, beyond the scope of authority of an emergency medical technician-basic (EMT-basic).

A0428-A0429

A0428 Ambulance service, basic life support, nonemergency transport, (BLS)

A0429 Ambulance service, basic life support, emergency transport (BLS, emergency)

Lay Description
Basic life support, non-emergency transport (BLS) is transportation by ground ambulance vehicle and the provision of medically necessary supplies and services, including BLS ambulance services as defined by state laws. The ambulance must be staffed by an individual who is qualified in accordance with state and local laws as an emergency medical technician-basic (EMT-basic). These laws may vary from state to state or within a state. For example, only in some jurisdictions is an EMT-basic permitted to operate limited equipment on board the vehicle, assist more qualified personnel in performing assessments and interventions, and establish a peripheral intravenous (IV) line.

A0430-A0431

A0430 Ambulance service, conventional air services, transport, one way (fixed wing)

A0431 Ambulance service, conventional air services, transport, one way (rotary wing)

Lay Description
Fixed wing (FW) ambulance (airplane) conventional air service is the transportation by a fixed wing aircraft that is certified by the Federal Aviation Administration (FAA) as a fixed wing air ambulance along with the provision of medically necessary services and supplies. Rotary wing (RW) ambulance (helicopter) conventional air service is the transportation by helicopter that is certified by the Federal Aviation Administration (FAA) as a rotary wing ambulance, including the provision of medically necessary supplies and services.

A0432

A0432 Paramedic intercept (PI), rural area, transport furnished by a volunteer ambulance company which is prohibited by state law from billing third-party payers

Lay Description
Paramedic intercept (PI) services are advanced life support (ALS) services provided with the ambulance transport by a volunteer ambulance company that is prohibited from doing any third-party billing by state laws. Use this code for PI services provided in a rural area.

A0433

A0433 Advanced life support, level 2 (ALS 2)

Lay Description
Advanced life support, level 2 (ALS 2) is the transportation by ground ambulance vehicle and the provision of medically necessary supplies and services including at least three separate administrations of one or more medications by intravenous push/bolus or by continuous infusion (excluding crystalloid fluids), or ground ambulance transport and the provision of at least one ALS 2 procedure, such as manual defibrillation/cardioversion, endotracheal intubation, central venous line, cardiac pacing, chest decompression, surgical airway, or intraosseous line.

A0434

A0434 Specialty care transport (SCT)

Lay Description
Specialty care transport (SCT) is hospital-to-hospital transportation of a critically injured or ill beneficiary by a ground ambulance vehicle, including the provision of medically necessary supplies and services, at a level of service beyond the scope of the EMT paramedic. SCT is necessary when a beneficiary's condition requires ongoing care that must be furnished by one or more health professionals in an appropriate specialty area (e.g., emergency or critical care nursing, emergency medicine, respiratory care, cardiovascular care, or a paramedic with additional training).

A0435-A0436

A0435 Fixed wing air mileage, per statute mile

A0436 Rotary wing air mileage, per statute mile

Lay Description
Use these codes to report each statutory mile a patient is transported in a fixed wing or a rotary wing aircraft.

A0888

A0888 Noncovered ambulance mileage, per mile (e.g., for miles traveled beyond closest appropriate facility)

Lay Description
Mileage for an ambulance trip is covered only to the nearest, appropriate facility. However, there are instances when a beneficiary requests to be transported to a facility that is not the closest appropriate facility. In these situations, there is additional mileage that is not covered. Use this code to report these additional, noncovered miles. This policy applies to both ground and air ambulance services.

A0998

A0998 Ambulance response and treatment, no transport

Lay Description
Report this code when an ambulance is dispatched and treatment is provided to the patient without the patient being transported to another site.

A

A0999

A0999 Unlisted ambulance service

Lay Description

This code is used for any ambulance service that is not described by other HCPCS Level II codes. It should be used as a last resort and only when there is not a more appropriate procedure code. When reporting an unlisted code, provide a detailed explanation of the services in remarks, billing notes, or as an attachment.

A4206-A4209

A4206 Syringe with needle, sterile, 1 cc or less, each

A4207 Syringe with needle, sterile 2 cc, each

A4208 Syringe with needle, sterile 3 cc, each

A4209 Syringe with needle, sterile 5 cc or greater, each

Lay Description

A sterile syringe with a needle is used for injecting or withdrawing liquids into or from any vessel or cavity. Each may vary in size and content capacity.

A4210

A4210 Needle-free injection device, each

Lay Description

This code reports a needle free injection instrument. These could be injectors such as hypodermic jet pressure powered devices for insulin injections.

A4211

A4211 Supplies for self-administered injections

Lay Description

Patients may administer injectable medications, such as insulin or calcitonin, themselves. Supplies for self-administered injections are rarely covered unless an emergency situation exists.

A4212

A4212 Noncoring needle or stylet with or without catheter

Lay Description

Noncoring needles or stylets are most often used to cleanly penetrate rubber self-sealing septums that are part of indwelling ports and pumps. The reservoirs on these surgically implanted devices can be refilled numerous times when noncoring needles are used.

A4213

A4213 Syringe, sterile, 20 cc or greater, each

Lay Description

This code reports supply of a sterile syringe with a capacity of 20 cc or greater. Syringes of this size may be used for injection of medications by intravenous or intraarterial push. These types of syringes may also be used for wound irrigation.

A4215

A4215 Needle, sterile, any size, each

Lay Description

This code reports any size sterile needle. This code is for a single needle and may be reported multiple times or with multiple units if more than one needle is used.

A4216-A4217

A4216 Sterile water, saline and/or dextrose, diluent/flush, 10 ml

A4217 Sterile water/saline, 500 ml

Lay Description

Use these codes to report sterile water, saline, or dextrose for injection or irrigation.

A4218

A4218 Sterile saline or water, metered dose dispenser, 10 ml

Lay Description

A metered dose dispenser of sterile saline or water may be used with a nebulizer or inhaler for dispensing inhalation medications. A metered dose dispenser delivers a precise amount of sterile saline or water for use in the device. This allows proper dilution of the medication.

A4220

A4220 Refill kit for implantable infusion pump

Lay Description

Implantable infusion pumps are typically small, biocompatible, stainless steel units that are surgically placed subcutaneously near the target drug delivery area. A refillable reservoir delivers a constant, prescribed rate of liquid drug to the target site. Drug delivery may be by spring or piston pressure against the reservoir. Routes of administration include intravenous, intra-arterial, intraperitoneal, and intraventricular. The refill kit may contain appropriate noncoring needles, filters, connectors, and other items, but not the drug itself.

A4221

A4221 Supplies for maintenance of drug infusion catheter, per week (list drug separately)

Lay Description

Drug infusion catheters embrace a range of approaches, including peripheral intravenous lines, peripherally inserted central catheters (PICC), and centrally inserted intravenous lines. Maintenance supplies for such drug infusion catheters may include flush solutions, dressings, cannulas, and needles. This code is not drug specific.

A4222-A4223

A4222 Infusion supplies for external drug infusion pump, per cassette or bag (list drugs separately)

A4223 Infusion supplies not used with external infusion pump, per cassette or bag (list drugs separately)

Lay Description

These codes report infusion supplies for external drug infusion pumps, which may be portable units worn on belts outside of the body or larger stationary units. Use these codes per cassette or bag, with drugs, such as diluting solutions, tubing, and other administration supplies, such as port caps listed separately. They also report infusion supplies not used with an external infusion pump, per cassette or bag. These codes are not drug specific.

A4230-A4231

A4230 Infusion set for external insulin pump, nonneedle cannula type

A4231 Infusion set for external insulin pump, needle type

Lay Description

These codes report infusion supplies pertaining to external insulin pumps. These are portable, battery-operated devices worn by the patient on a belt or sling. The device connects to a drug reservoir and the system is designed to deliver continuous subcutaneous insulin therapy over an extended period of time. The device usually delivers insulin into subcutaneous fat in the abdominal region and the infusion set must be changed out every few days. Cassettes or bags are included, as are diluting solutions, tubing, and other administration supplies, such as port caps. These codes are drug specific to insulin.

A4232

A4232 Syringe with needle for external insulin pump, sterile, 3 cc

Lay Description

This code is designated for a syringe with needle for external insulin pump, sterile, 3 cc, and describes the insulin reservoir for use with the external insulin infusion pump. The reservoir may be either glass or plastic and includes the needle for drawing up the insulin. This code does not include the insulin for use in the reservoir.

A4233-A4236

A4233 Replacement battery, alkaline (other than J cell), for use with medically necessary home blood glucose monitor owned by patient, each

A4234 Replacement battery, alkaline, J cell, for use with medically necessary home blood glucose monitor owned by patient, each

A4235 Replacement battery, lithium, for use with medically necessary home blood glucose monitor owned by patient, each

A4236 Replacement battery, silver oxide, for use with medically necessary home blood glucose monitor owned by patient, each

Lay Description

Glucometers with associated accessories and supplies are used for patients with all types of diabetes mellitus to monitor blood glucose, and are available in a variety of models. A replacement battery for a medically necessary, patient-owned home blood glucose monitor (glucometer) is reported based on the type of battery required.

A4244-A4248

A4244 Alcohol or peroxide, per pint

A4245 Alcohol wipes, per box

A4246 Betadine or pHisoHex solution, per pint

A4247 Betadine or iodine swabs/wipes, per box

A4248 Chlorhexidine containing antiseptic, 1 ml

Lay Description

Glucometers and associated accessories and supplies are used for patients with all types of diabetes mellitus to monitor blood glucose levels. Supplies used in monitoring blood glucose levels include a variety of antiseptics and antimicrobials to cleanse the skin prior to piercing the skin to obtain a blood sample to perform the glucose test. Betadine, pHisoHex, and iodine are other types of anti-infective solutions used on the skin and are available in both pints or individually wrapped swabs or wipes. A chlorhexidine containing antiseptic such as Hibiclens may also be used to prevent skin infections. Chlorhexidine has antiseptic activity and an antimicrobial effect against a wide range of microorganisms.

A

A4250-A4259

A4250　Urine test or reagent strips or tablets (100 tablets or strips)

A4252　Blood ketone test or reagent strip, each

A4253　Blood glucose test or reagent strips for home blood glucose monitor, per 50 strips

A4255　Platforms for home blood glucose monitor, 50 per box

A4256　Normal, low, and high calibrator solution/chips

A4257　Replacement lens shield cartridge for use with laser skin piercing device, each

A4258　Spring-powered device for lancet, each

A4259　Lancets, per box of 100

Lay Description

Glucometers and associated accessories and supplies are used for patients with all types of diabetes mellitus to monitor blood glucose levels, and are available in a variety of models. Accessories and supplies for these devices range from alcohol prep pads to lancets for piercing the skin to obtain the required blood sample to perform the test. Many of these supplies must be used each time the test is performed and are not reusable. Many diabetics require frequent, if not daily, blood glucose monitoring, whether or not the patient is on insulin. For Type I diabetes mellitus patients who require insulin (the patient's body does not manufacture insulin and therefore it must come from an external source, such as injections), blood glucose monitoring is a life-sustaining requirement. The accessories and supplies are medically necessary to properly and accurately perform the blood glucose monitoring. Blood glucose test or reagent strips are used with home glucose monitoring devices and are usually covered for insulin-dependent diabetics whose monitor has been prescribed by the physician. Platforms are used with lancing devices to prevent cross infection and to control depth of penetration of the lancing device. Calibrator solutions or chips are used with a home glucose monitoring device to check the integrity of the glucometer and the test strips. Calibrator solutions or chips are provided in normal, low, and high levels. Lancing devices use lasers or springs. Use of a laser device requires a lens shield cartridge. A lancet is a pointed surgical knife with two edges.

A4261

A4261　Cervical cap for contraceptive use

Lay Description

A cervical cap is a thimble shaped latex device that covers the cervix and is used with a spermicide as a barrier method of contraception.

A4262-A4263

A4262　Temporary, absorbable lacrimal duct implant, each

A4263　Permanent, long-term, nondissolvable lacrimal duct implant, each

Lay Description

Report A4262 for use of a temporary, absorbable tear duct implant. Report A4263 when a permanent, long-term nondissolvable lacrimal duct implant is used.

A4264

A4264　Permanent implantable contraceptive intratubal occlusion device(s) and delivery system

Lay Description

An intratubal occlusion device is a permanent, implantable, contraceptive occlusive device and system used for nonincisional sterilization. This process is performed using a hysteroscopic approach. The system is comprised of a micro-insert implantable stainless steel inner coil with polyester fibers and a super-elastic nitinol outer anchoring coil. The micro-insert, when released, expands to conform and anchor in the fallopian tube.

A4265

A4265　Paraffin, per pound

Lay Description

Paraffin is a waxy, white, tasteless, odorless mixture of solid hydrocarbon made from petroleum. It is often used as the base for an ointment or wound dressing.

A4266

A4266　Diaphragm for contraceptive use

Lay Description

A diaphragm is a rubber or plastic cup that fits over the cervix uteri and is used for contraceptive purposes.

A4267-A4268

A4267　Contraceptive supply, condom, male, each

A4268　Contraceptive supply, condom, female, each

Lay Description

A condom is a thin, flexible sheath used by a man to prevent pregnancy and/or sexually transmitted diseases. A female condom is made for sheathing the internal anatomy of the female.

A4269

A4269　Contraceptive supply, spermicide (e.g., foam, gel), each

Lay Description

Spermicides are contraceptive agents used to kill spermatozoa.

A4270

A4270 Disposable endoscope sheath, each

Lay Description
This code reports the use of a disposable sheath that covers an endoscope, a device consisting of a tube and optical system for viewing the inside of a hollow organ or cavity.

A4280

A4280 Adhesive skin support attachment for use with external breast prosthesis, each

Lay Description
This code is used to report the adhesive skin support attachment used with a breast prosthesis, a man-made substitute for a missing breast.

A4281-A4286

A4281 Tubing for breast pump, replacement

A4282 Adapter for breast pump, replacement

A4283 Cap for breast pump bottle, replacement

A4284 Breast shield and splash protector for use with breast pump, replacement

A4285 Polycarbonate bottle for use with breast pump, replacement

A4286 Locking ring for breast pump, replacement

Lay Description
A breast pump is a mechanical device used to extract milk from a lactating mother. Pumps may be manual, electronic, or battery-powered. These codes represent replacement parts for the breast pump.

A4290

A4290 Sacral nerve stimulation test lead, each

Lay Description
There are five pairs of spinal or sacral nerves. This code is used to report each test lead used in a sacral nerve stimulation examination.

A4300

A4300 Implantable access catheter, (e.g., venous, arterial, epidural subarachnoid, or peritoneal, etc.) external access

Lay Description
A catheter is a tube inserted into the body to evacuate or inject fluids into body cavities.

A4301

A4301 Implantable access total catheter, port/reservoir (e.g., venous, arterial, epidural, subarachnoid, peritoneal, etc.)

Lay Description
This code reports the supply of an integrated vascular port/reservoir and catheter designed for subdermal implantation. The system is designed for patients requiring regular or continuous intravenous or intra-arterial infusion of drugs. The system may be used to deliver any of a variety of medicines, particularly those for oncology therapy. In some instances, the implanted port and catheter delivers drugs to the spinal cord (epidural), the brain (subarachnoid), or to the abdominal (peritoneal) cavity. Implantable infusion pumps are typically small biocompatible stainless steel units that are surgically placed subcutaneously near the site of optimal drug delivery. The port and reservoir can be smaller in diameter than a nickel coin. A refillable reservoir delivers a constant, prescribed rate of liquid drug to the target site. Typically, the reservoir features a rubber diaphragm that can be penetrated by a non-coring needle to refill the drug.

A4305-A4306

A4305 Disposable drug delivery system, flow rate of 50 ml or greater per hour

A4306 Disposable drug delivery system, flow rate of less than 50 ml per hour

Lay Description
These disposable drug delivery systems comprise devices that deliver liquid drugs by the elastic pressure of the reservoir container. The term elastomeric infusion pump may be used. These codes are not drug specific.

A4310-A4316

A4310 Insertion tray without drainage bag and without catheter (accessories only)

A4311 Insertion tray without drainage bag with indwelling catheter, Foley type, 2-way latex with coating (Teflon, silicone, silicone elastomer or hydrophilic, etc.)

A4312 Insertion tray without drainage bag with indwelling catheter, Foley type, 2-way, all silicone

A4313 Insertion tray without drainage bag with indwelling catheter, Foley type, 3-way, for continuous irrigation

A4314 Insertion tray with drainage bag with indwelling catheter, Foley type, 2-way latex with coating (Teflon, silicone, silicone elastomer or hydrophilic, etc.)

A4315 Insertion tray with drainage bag with indwelling catheter, Foley type, 2-way, all silicone

A4316 Insertion tray with drainage bag with indwelling catheter, Foley type, 3-way, for continuous irrigation

Lay Description
Urinary catheters and external urinary collection devices are used to drain or collect urine from a patient who has permanent urinary incontinence or permanent urinary retention. Supplies or accessories are also used with the catheters and are part of the service provided.

A4320-A4322

A4320   Irrigation tray with bulb or piston syringe, any purpose

A4321   Therapeutic agent for urinary catheter irrigation

A4322   Irrigation syringe, bulb or piston, each

Lay Description

These codes are reported for cleaning and irrigation items for incontinence care.

A4326

A4326   Male external catheter with integral collection chamber, any type, each

Lay Description

Male external catheters (condom-type) are used by patients who have permanent urinary incontinence as an alternative to an indwelling catheter. A male external catheter is used over the external genitalia as an incontinence guard. This code reports a male external catheter with integral collection chamber, any type, each.

A4327-A4328

A4327   Female external urinary collection device; meatal cup, each

A4328   Female external urinary collection device; pouch, each

Lay Description

A female external urinary collection device is used to collect urine as it passes to the outside of the body.

A4330

A4330   Perianal fecal collection pouch with adhesive, each

Lay Description

A perianal pouch is applied to the outside of the body with adhesive to manage stool incontinence.

A4331

A4331   Extension drainage tubing, any type, any length, with connector/adaptor, for use with urinary leg bag or urostomy pouch, each

Lay Description

Extension drainage tubing is used with a urostomy pouch or latex urinary leg bag for patients who are ambulatory or are chair or wheelchair bound but not bedridden. Report this code for any type, any length of extension drainage tubing with the connector or adaptor.

A4332-A4334

A4332   Lubricant, individual sterile packet, each

A4333   Urinary catheter anchoring device, adhesive skin attachment, each

A4334   Urinary catheter anchoring device, leg strap, each

Lay Description

Urinary catheters may be held in place by means of an adhesive patch or a strap that goes around the leg. Lubricant is used for the insertion of the catheter into the bladder.

A4335

A4335   Incontinence supply; miscellaneous

Lay Description

Incontinence supplies are leak proof undergarments worn by the patient who cannot retain or control the release of urine, semen, or feces. This code reports miscellaneous incontinence supplies.

A4336

A4336   Incontinence supply, urethral insert, any type, each

Lay Description

Urethral inserts are designed for the female patient to manage and/or treat urinary incontinence. A self-inserted, single use, disposable intra-urethral device results in instant control of severe stress urinary incontinence (SUI).This insert is a small, latex free, narrow silicone tube that is totally encased in a soft, thin, mineral oil-filled sleeve. The sleeve forms a balloon at the internal tip and a soft, oval shaped external retainer at the opposite end. The device is inserted using a disposable applicator.

A4338-A4346

A4338   Indwelling catheter; Foley type, 2-way latex with coating (Teflon, silicone, silicone elastomer, or hydrophilic, etc.), each

A4340   Indwelling catheter; specialty type, (e.g., Coude, mushroom, wing, etc.), each

A4344   Indwelling catheter, Foley type, 2-way, all silicone, each

A4346   Indwelling catheter; Foley type, 3-way for continuous irrigation, each

Lay Description

Urinary catheterization involves insertion of a drainage tube up the urethra and into the bladder where it is often held in place by an inflated balloon. For these indwelling catheters, a reservoir is typically attached to contain the drained urine, which, for many patients, may be monitored for volume and tested for content. A topical anesthetic may be employed and the catheter is lubricated.

A4349

A4349   Male external catheter, with or without adhesive, disposable, each

Lay Description
Male external catheters (condom-type) are used by patients who have permanent urinary incontinence as an alternative to an indwelling catheter. A male external catheter is used over the external genitalia as an incontinence guard.

A4351-A4353

A4351   Intermittent urinary catheter; straight tip, with or without coating (Teflon, silicone, silicone elastomer, or hydrophilic, etc.), each

A4352   Intermittent urinary catheter; Coude (curved) tip, with or without coating (Teflon, silicone, silicone elastomeric, or hydrophilic, etc.), each

A4353   Intermittent urinary catheter, with insertion supplies

Lay Description
Urinary catheterization involves insertion of a drainage tube up the urethra and into the bladder where it is often held in place by an inflated balloon. For these indwelling catheters, a reservoir is typically attached to contain the drained urine, which, for many patients, may be monitored for volume and tested for content. This code range, however, reports intermittent catheterization, a treatment approach for certain urinary disorders, and patient profiles. The catheter is inserted using antiseptic technique by the patient or a caregiver four times a day, or more often as needed. A topical anesthetic may be employed and the catheter is lubricated. The bladder is completely voided into a container and the catheter withdrawn after each procedure. The catheter may be disinfected and reused or discarded.

A4354

A4354   Insertion tray with drainage bag but without catheter

Lay Description
This code reports the supply of a urinary catheterization insertion tray. This type of sterile tray typically includes a preloaded syringe, absorbent pads, drapery, gloves, and lubricants. A drainage bag or graduated container is included in the code description, but the catheter itself is specifically excluded.

A4355

A4355   Irrigation tubing set for continuous bladder irrigation through a 3-way indwelling Foley catheter, each

Lay Description
This code reports the supply of a specific continuous bladder irrigation set. Bladder catheterization is generally called for in patients unable to void urine naturally and following certain surgeries. Continuous irrigation is usually temporary and may be required in certain circumstances involving obstructions. The bladder is a sterile environment and sterile hardware and technique is ordinarily required to catheterize it. A Foley catheter features a balloon tip that is inflated upon entry into the bladder to hold the device in place (indwelling). A three-way catheter features a lumen for urine drainage, one to inflate and deflate the Foley balloon, and one for irrigation fluids and medications.

A4356

A4356   External urethral clamp or compression device (not to be used for catheter clamp), each

Lay Description
This code reports the supply of external urethral clamps, also known as penile clamps, Cunningham clamps, or Knuttsen clamps. These reusable metal devices fit over the penis. Typically, soft foam that contours to the shape of the penis is compressed, closing off the urethra. Compression on the devices must be relieved every several hours.

A4357

A4357   Bedside drainage bag, day or night, with or without antireflux device, with or without tube, each

Lay Description
Patients with urinary ostomies may use a bedside drainage bag during the day or night. The bedside drainage bag is used for the collection of urinary output from a urinary pouch. It is sometimes necessary, especially at night, for the bag to be connected to the pouch to prevent urinary overflow and excessive weight in the pouch, which could cause urinary leakage and disruption of the pouch seal. The bag is made of a high grade PVC and can hold up to 2,000 cc. The anti-reflux device prevents backflow.

A4358

A4358   Urinary drainage bag, leg or abdomen, vinyl, with or without tube, with straps, each

Lay Description
Leg or abdomen urinary drainage bags are indicated for patients who are ambulatory or are chair or wheelchair bound but not bedridden. The vinyl bag can be used with a suprapubic or Foley catheter for urine collection. It typically holds up to 1,000 cc. The bag is held in place next to the abdomen or around the leg by woven straps. This code describes a drainage bag, with or without tubing.

A

A4360

A4360   Disposable external urethral clamp or compression device, with pad and/or pouch, each

Lay Description
A disposable, external urethral clamp or compression device is designed for a male patient to manage and/or treat light to moderate urinary incontinence. It works by minimizing urinary incontinence by means of mechanical compression of the urethra, eliminating the leakage of urine and allowing the bladder to fill. If there is leakage that breaks through from the urethra, the moisture is restricted to the disposable pouch or pad.

A4361

A4361   Ostomy faceplate, each

Lay Description
An ostomy faceplate is a solid interface between the patient's skin and the pouch. It is usually made of plastic, rubber, or encased metal. It does not have an adhesive property and there is no pectin-based or karaya material that is an integral part of the faceplate. It can be taken off the skin and reattached repeatedly. It is held on by means of a separate adhesive and/or an elastic belt.

A4362, A5121-A5122

A4362   Skin barrier; solid, 4 x 4 or equivalent; each

A5121   Skin barrier; solid, 6 x 6 or equivalent, each

A5122   Skin barrier; solid, 8 x 8 or equivalent, each

Lay Description
Skin barriers are an interface between the patient's skin and the pouching system. They are used to create an adhesive seal between the skin and the pouch. Barriers can be curved with a built in convexity creating a more adhesive bond to the patient's skin and better protrusion of the stoma. These codes represent solid ostomy skin barriers that are used independently, usually with a pouch that does not have its own integral skin barrier.

A4363

A4363   Ostomy clamp, any type, replacement only, each

Lay Description
An ostomy clamp is a closure accessory used to prevent spillage from an open-ended (drainable) ostomy pouch. An ostomy clamp is provided with the purchase of an ostomy bag and is not billed separately. This code is used to report the replacement of the ostomy clamp.

A4364, A5126

A4364   Adhesive, liquid or equal, any type, per oz

A5126   Adhesive or nonadhesive; disk or foam pad

Lay Description
Adhesive liquids are applied directly to the skin or to a protective barrier, such as a disk or foam pad, providing increased bonding of ostomy devices. These adhesives are in liquid form or are equal to a liquid available in bottles or spray cans. They are rubber based or acrylic based and non-toxic. Proper application of adhesives is a thin, light coat on the desired area. Adhesives can be removed with petroleum-based solvents.

A4366

A4366   Ostomy vent, any type, each

Lay Description
A separate ostomy vent can be added to the ostomy pouch to allow the release of gas. This code must not be used for pouches in which a vent with a filter is incorporated in the pouch by the manufacturer.

A4367

A4367   Ostomy belt, each

Lay Description
An ostomy belt is used to secure and conceal ostomy appliances. They are made of lightweight cotton and Lycra/elastic. Belts are designed to be used with one or two-piece systems for left, right, or center stomas and vary in width depending on the patient's need. Some belts provide a pocket for the appliance that has a Velcro closure that allows for easy emptying.

A4368

A4368   Ostomy filter, any type, each

Lay Description
An ostomy filter prevents the buildup of gas trapped in the pouch by allowing the gas to be effectively expelled through a vent. Filters may be incorporated into a pouch, inserted into a venting ring on the pouch, or attached to the pouch exterior. They may also include deodorizing materials such as charcoal for the vented gas.

A4369-A4373

A4369 Ostomy skin barrier, liquid (spray, brush, etc.), per oz

A4371 Ostomy skin barrier, powder, per oz

A4372 Ostomy skin barrier, solid 4 x 4 or equivalent, standard wear, with built-in convexity, each

A4373 Ostomy skin barrier, with flange (solid, flexible or accordian), with built-in convexity, any size, each

Lay Description
This range of codes reports skin care and conditioning supplies for patients fitting adhesive pouches over an ostomy, a surgically created opening through the skin to divert bowel contents into an external container or pouch. Peristomal skin can become difficult to care for over time due to the irritating nature of fecal material, enzymes, and the repeated application and removal of adhesives. Barriers are an interface between the patient's skin and the pouching system and have a variety of options such as built-in convexity, locking or non-locking flanges, and use with or without faceplates. Barriers offer a level of protection to the skin while providing a surface to adhere the ostomy faceplate.

A4375-A4378

A4375 Ostomy pouch, drainable, with faceplate attached, plastic, each

A4376 Ostomy pouch, drainable, with faceplate attached, rubber, each

A4377 Ostomy pouch, drainable, for use on faceplate, plastic, each

A4378 Ostomy pouch, drainable, for use on faceplate, rubber, each

Lay Description
These codes represent drainable ostomy pouches. Ostomy pouches are used by patients who have had a surgically created opening for diversion of the urine or feces. An ostomy faceplate is a solid interface between the patient's skin and the pouch. It is usually made of plastic, rubber, or encased metal. It can be taken off the skin and reattached repeatedly. It is held on by means of a separate adhesive and/or an elastic belt.

A4379-A4384

A4379 Ostomy pouch, urinary, with faceplate attached, plastic, each

A4380 Ostomy pouch, urinary, with faceplate attached, rubber, each

A4381 Ostomy pouch, urinary, for use on faceplate, plastic, each

A4382 Ostomy pouch, urinary, for use on faceplate, heavy plastic, each

A4383 Ostomy pouch, urinary, for use on faceplate, rubber, each

A4384 Ostomy faceplate equivalent, silicone ring, each

Lay Description
These codes represent urinary ostomy pouches for use on barrier, with flange. Urinary ostomy pouches are used by patients who have had a surgically created opening for diversion of the urine. An ostomy faceplate is a solid interface between the patient's skin and the pouch. It is usually made of plastic, heavy plastic, rubber, or silicone. It can be taken off the skin and reattached repeatedly. It is held on by means of a separate adhesive and/or an elastic belt.

A4385

A4385 Ostomy skin barrier, solid 4 x 4 or equivalent, extended wear, without built-in convexity, each

Lay Description
An ostomy is a surgically created opening through the skin to divert bowel contents into an external container or pouch. Peristomal skin can become difficult to care for over time due to the irritating nature of fecal material, enzymes, and the repeated application and removal of adhesives. Barriers are an interface between the patient's skin and the pouching system and have a variety of options, such as built-in convexity, locking or non-locking flanges, and use with or without faceplates. Barriers offer a level of protection to the skin while providing a surface to adhere the ostomy faceplate.

A4387-A4390

A4387 Ostomy pouch, closed, with barrier attached, with built-in convexity (1 piece), each

A4388 Ostomy pouch, drainable, with extended wear barrier attached, (1 piece), each

A4389 Ostomy pouch, drainable, with barrier attached, with built-in convexity (1 piece), each

A4390 Ostomy pouch, drainable, with extended wear barrier attached, with built-in convexity (1 piece), each

Lay Description
An ostomy pouch is a device used for the collection of stomal or urinary output for patients who have undergone procedures causing a temporary or

permanent interference with normal excretion. The ostomy pouch with barrier attached is a one-piece system in which a solid barrier serving to create an adhesive seal is part of the ostomy pouch. The barrier may be pectin-based or karaya-based for normal wear, or pectin-based with special additives for extended wear. The pouch may contain an opening at the bottom through which the contents can be drained, or be sealed without an outlet.

A4391-A4393

A4391   Ostomy pouch, urinary, with extended wear barrier attached (1 piece), each

A4392   Ostomy pouch, urinary, with standard wear barrier attached, with built-in convexity (1 piece), each

A4393   Ostomy pouch, urinary, with extended wear barrier attached, with built-in convexity (1 piece), each

Lay Description
Urinary ostomy pouches are for use with patients who have had a surgically created opening for diversion of the urine. The ostomy pouch with barrier attached is a one-piece system in which a solid barrier serving to create an adhesive seal is part of the pouch. The barrier may be pectin-based or karaya-based for normal wear, or pectin-based with special additives for extended wear. The use of convexity is commonly indicated when a pouch seal is unable to fasten properly for an acceptable length of time or when persistent skin irritation occurs even without leakage.

A4394-A4395

A4394   Ostomy deodorant, with or without lubricant, for use in ostomy pouch, per fl oz

A4395   Ostomy deodorant for use in ostomy pouch, solid, per tablet

Lay Description
These codes report deodorants for use with ostomy pouches, devices for collecting stomal or urinary output in patients who have undergone procedures causing a temporary or permanent interference with normal excretion. Deodorants are available in liquid or solid form and eliminate urine and fecal odors.

A4396

A4396   Ostomy belt with peristomal hernia support

Lay Description
This code reports an ostomy belt with peristomal hernia support. Ostomy belts are used to secure and conceal ostomy appliances. They are made of lightweight cotton and Lycra/elastic. Belts are designed to be used with one or two-piece systems for left, right, or center stomas and vary in width depending on the patient's need. Some belts provide a pocket for the appliance that has a Velcro closure that allows for easy emptying. This ostomy belt

utilizes a rigid hernia support plate in the pouch pocket of the belt to provide necessary support for a herniated stoma.

A4397-A4400

A4397   Irrigation supply; sleeve, each

A4398   Ostomy irrigation supply; bag, each

A4399   Ostomy irrigation supply; cone/catheter, with or without brush

A4400   Ostomy irrigation set

Lay Description
Irrigation sets are used in the cleaning and maintenance of sigmoid colostomies. Full kits include all supplies necessary for proper irrigation of colostomies, such as a water bag regulator, cone, faceplate, belt, and sleeves. An irrigation bag is used for holding the warm water necessary for flushing out the ostomy. The replacement of an irrigation ostomy bag or cone/catheter, including brush, every three months would be appropriate.

A4402

A4402   Lubricant, per oz

Lay Description
The lubricants used for ostomy supplies are water soluble, greaseless, odorless gels. These gels lubricate ostomy supplies such as catheters to reduce irritation.

A4404

A4404   Ostomy ring, each

Lay Description
This code is used to report an ostomy ring. An "o" ring is a round rubber ring used as an additional security measure to hold a pouch clip closed. It can be found in any hardware store and looks like a thick, black ring.

A4405-A4406

A4405   Ostomy skin barrier, nonpectin-based, paste, per oz

A4406   Ostomy skin barrier, pectin-based, paste, per oz

Lay Description
Pastes are applied directly to the skin to act as a protective sealant beneath ostomy appliances. They may have a synthetic or natural base. Non-pectin based paste (e.g., karaya) is required for skin sensitive to synthetic barriers.

A4407-A4411

A4407 Ostomy skin barrier, with flange (solid, flexible, or accordion), extended wear, with built-in convexity, 4 x 4 in or smaller, each

A4408 Ostomy skin barrier, with flange (solid, flexible or accordion), extended wear, with built-in convexity, larger than 4 x 4 in, each

A4409 Ostomy skin barrier, with flange (solid, flexible or accordion), extended wear, without built-in convexity, 4 x 4 in or smaller, each

A4410 Ostomy skin barrier, with flange (solid, flexible or accordion), extended wear, without built-in convexity, larger than 4 x 4 in, each

A4411 Ostomy skin barrier, solid 4 x 4 or equivalent, extended wear, with built-in convexity, each

Lay Description

An ostomy skin barrier (wafer) with built-in convexity is one in which an outward curve is usually achieved with plastic embedded in the barrier, allowing better protrusion of the stoma and adherence to the skin. Skin barriers are an interface between the patient's skin and the pouching system. They are used to create an adhesive seal between the skin and the pouch.

A4412-A4413

A4412 Ostomy pouch, drainable, high output, for use on a barrier with flange (2 piece system), without filter, each

A4413 Ostomy pouch, drainable, high output, for use on a barrier with flange (2-piece system), with filter, each

Lay Description

These codes report the supply of a high-output, drainable ostomy pouch to be used with a two-piece barrier with flange system. These pouches have been specifically designed for high stomal output. A high-output ostomy pouch must have a capacity of greater than or equal to 0.75 liters, an anti-reflux valve, and a large bore solid spout with cap or plug.

A4414-A4415

A4414 Ostomy skin barrier, with flange (solid, flexible or accordion), without built-in convexity, 4 x 4 in or smaller, each

A4415 Ostomy skin barrier, with flange (solid, flexible or accordion), without built-in convexity, larger than 4 x 4 in, each

Lay Description

These codes represent ostomy skin barriers with a flange, solid, flexible, or accordion type, without built-in convexity, not specified as extended wear. Skin barriers are an interface between the patient's skin and the pouching system. They are used to create an adhesive seal between the skin and the pouch.

A4416-A4420, A4423

A4416 Ostomy pouch, closed, with barrier attached, with filter (1 piece), each

A4417 Ostomy pouch, closed, with barrier attached, with built-in convexity, with filter (1 piece), each

A4418 Ostomy pouch, closed; without barrier attached, with filter (1 piece), each

A4419 Ostomy pouch, closed; for use on barrier with nonlocking flange, with filter (2 piece), each

A4420 Ostomy pouch, closed; for use on barrier with locking flange (2 piece), each

A4423 Ostomy pouch, closed; for use on barrier with locking flange, with filter (2 piece), each

Lay Description

These codes represent ostomy pouches that are for use with patients who have had a surgically created opening for diversion of stool. Ostomy pouches collect the stomal output, in this case feces, and can be drainable or closed. Drainable pouches have an opening at the bottom through which fecal contents can be emptied. Closed pouches have a sealed bottom with no outlet for feces. There are also one-piece and two-piece systems. One-piece systems are supplied "with barrier attached" or "without barrier attached." Two-piece systems have a locking or non-locking flange that is coupled to a skin barrier with flange. Skin barriers are an interface between the patient's skin and the pouching system and have a variety of different options such as built-in convexity, filters, locking or non-locking flanges, and use with or without faceplates.

A4421

A4421 Ostomy supply; miscellaneous

Lay Description

Report this code for miscellaneous ostomy supplies for which a more specific code is not available.

A4422

A4422 Ostomy absorbent material (sheet/pad/crystal packet) for use in ostomy pouch to thicken liquid stomal output, each

Lay Description

Absorbent material such as sheets, pads, or crystals is added to the ostomy pouch to thicken the liquid output from the stoma. These materials draw liquid away from the stoma to minimize irritation, reduce splashing when emptying the pouch, and facilitate in venting of gas. Report this code for absorbent material, any type.

A

A4423

A4423 Ostomy pouch, closed; for use on barrier with locking flange, with filter (2 piece), each

Lay Description
Please refer to codes A4416–A4420 for the description, coding, and billing information.

A4424-A4427

A4424 Ostomy pouch, drainable, with barrier attached, with filter (1 piece), each

A4425 Ostomy pouch, drainable; for use on barrier with nonlocking flange, with filter (2-piece system), each

A4426 Ostomy pouch, drainable; for use on barrier with locking flange (2-piece system), each

A4427 Ostomy pouch, drainable; for use on barrier with locking flange, with filter (2-piece system), each

Lay Description
These codes represent drainable ostomy pouches. Ostomy pouches are for use with patients who have had a surgically created opening for diversion of the urine. The ostomy pouch with barrier attached is a one-piece system in which a solid barrier serving to create an adhesive seal is part of the ostomy pouch. The barrier may be pectin-based or karaya-based for normal wear or pectin-based with special additives for extended wear. Filters prevent the buildup of gas trapped in the pouch by allowing the gas to be effectively expelled through a vent. A flange or plastic ring on both the pouch and skin barrier secures the barrier and the pouch.

A4428-A4434

A4428 Ostomy pouch, urinary, with extended wear barrier attached, with faucet-type tap with valve (1 piece), each

A4429 Ostomy pouch, urinary, with barrier attached, with built-in convexity, with faucet-type tap with valve (1 piece), each

A4430 Ostomy pouch, urinary, with extended wear barrier attached, with built-in convexity, with faucet-type tap with valve (1 piece), each

A4431 Ostomy pouch, urinary; with barrier attached, with faucet-type tap with valve (1 piece), each

A4432 Ostomy pouch, urinary; for use on barrier with nonlocking flange, with faucet-type tap with valve (2 piece), each

A4433 Ostomy pouch, urinary; for use on barrier with locking flange (2 piece), each

A4434 Ostomy pouch, urinary; for use on barrier with locking flange, with faucet-type tap with valve (2 piece), each

Lay Description
These codes represent urinary ostomy pouches. Urinary ostomy pouches are for use with patients who have had a surgically created opening for diversion of the urine. The ostomy pouch with barrier attached is a one-piece system in which a solid barrier serving to create an adhesive seal is part of the ostomy pouch. The barrier may be pectin-based or karaya-based for normal wear or pectin-based with special additives for extended wear. The use of convexity is commonly indicated when a pouch seal is unable to fasten properly for an acceptable length of time or when persistent skin irritation occurs even without leakage. A flange or plastic ring on both the pouch and skin barrier secures the barrier and the pouch.

A4435

A4435 Ostomy pouch, drainable, high output, with extended wear barrier (one-piece system), with or without filter, each

Lay Description
An ostomy pouch is used for patients who have had a surgically created opening for diversion of stool. Ostomy pouches collect the stomal output, in this case feces, and can be drainable or closed. Drainable pouches have an opening at the bottom through which fecal contents can be emptied. There are also one-piece and two-piece systems. One-piece systems are supplied "with barrier attached" or "without barrier attached." Two-piece systems have a locking or nonlocking flange that is coupled to a skin barrier with flange. Skin barriers are an interface between the patient's skin and the pouching system and have a variety of different options, such as built-in convexity, filters, locking or nonlocking flanges, and use with or without faceplates.

A4450-A4452

A4450 Tape, nonwaterproof, per 18 sq in

A4452 Tape, waterproof, per 18 sq in

Lay Description

Tape is used to hold on a wound cover and can be an elastic roll gauze or non-elastic roll gauze. Additional tape is usually not required when a wound cover with an adhesive border is used. Tape change is determined by the frequency of wound cover change.

A4455-A4456

A4455 Adhesive remover or solvent (for tape, cement or other adhesive), per oz

A4456 Adhesive remover, wipes, any type, each

Lay Description

Adhesives sometimes require adhesive remover or solvent for complete removal. They are usually petroleum based. Adhesive remover or solvent for removal of tape, cement, or other adhesive is reported per ounce.

A4458

A4458 Enema bag with tubing, reusable

Lay Description

This code reports the supply of a reusable enema bag and tubing. Traditionally, these are heavy gauge rubber bags that hold about two quarts of liquid. An enema bag is designed to hang about 18 inches above the patient in the SIMM's position (lying on the side). Tubing from the bag is inserted into the rectum. Fluid from the bag is allowed to drain into the colon. The fluid is retained for a short duration and the patient voids contents of the colon/rectum.

A4461-A4463

A4461 Surgical dressing holder, nonreusable, each

A4463 Surgical dressing holder, reusable, each

Lay Description

An abdominal dressing holder is usually a slightly elastic garment that may be worn over surgical dressings where adhesives might pose problems or among patients with limited mobility. The device typically opens from side panels, allowing for easy access to the dressings.

A4465

A4465 Nonelastic binder for extremity

Lay Description

A nonelastic extremity binder is used for the treatment of lymphedema. These binders apply a gentle, gradient pressure to the affected extremity by use of a sleeve in combination with adjustable straps that provide compression. The sleeve slides over the affected extremity and then the compression bands are adjusted. Some models have gauges that assess the pressure applied over any region of the extremity.

These gauges ensure that compression applied to the patient's limb is consistently applied and in the proper range to provide optimal results.

A4466

A4466 Garment, belt, sleeve or other covering, elastic or similar stretchable material, any type, each

Lay Description

Garment, belt, sleeve or other covering made of elastic or a similar stretchable material, any type/each. This code may apply to devices, such as splints, that are not rigid or semi-rigid and/or support devices which are made up of elastic, neoprene, or a similar stretchable material. Elastic garments are considered to be elastic even if they have flexible plastic or metal stays.

A4470

A4470 Gravlee jet washer

Lay Description

The Gravlee Jet Washer is a sterile, disposable, diagnostic device for detecting endometrial cancer by obtaining a tissue sample. The use of this device is indicated where the patient exhibits clinical symptoms or signs suggestive of endometrial disease, such as irregular or heavy vaginal bleeding. The tissue obtained is preserved by the addition of an equal amount of Papanicolaou fixative to the irrigation solution from which a cell block is prepared to give a histologic specimen. The use of the Gravlee jet washer should not be confused with a diagnostic curettage.

A4480

A4480 VABRA aspirator

Lay Description

The VABRA aspirator is a vacuum operated device designed to collect endometrial samples for biopsy. The cervix may be first accessed by a sounding device to assist in dilation. A pipette tip from the VABRA device is inserted into the vaginal canal, through the cervical os, and into the endometrial lining of the uterus. Retraction of an outer sleeve of the cannula creates a gentle suction to collect the specimen. The specimen is stabilized in neutral fluid and prepared for analysis. Collection of the endometrial tissues may be timed to a particular phase of the menstrual cycle for optimal results.

A4481

A4481 Tracheostoma filter, any type, any size, each

Lay Description

This code reports the supply of a filter designed to fit the opening of a tracheostomy. Typically, this device is a soft foam filter disk to cover the air entry of a tracheal stoma. The filter may be designed to interface with a silicon button fitted to the stoma.

A

A4483

A4483 Moisture exchanger, disposable, for use with invasive mechanical ventilation

Lay Description

Patients on mechanical ventilation lose the advantage of natural moisturizing effects of air flowing over the mucous membranes of the sinuses and nasopharynx. This code reports provision of a disposable moisture exchange device fitted to the mechanical ventilation system.

A4490-A4510

A4490 Surgical stockings above knee length, each

A4495 Surgical stockings thigh length, each

A4500 Surgical stockings below knee length, each

A4510 Surgical stockings full-length, each

Lay Description

Surgical compression stockings are designed to reduce edema and enhance circulation with graduated compression. Graduated compression means that each stocking has the greatest amount of compression at the ankle and gradually decreases as the garment comes up the leg toward the heart. Graduated compression ensures that the garment will not have a constricting or strangulation affect on the leg. Surgical stockings should be properly fit to the individual patient. A surgical compression stocking will have at least 20 mmHg of compression at the ankle, which is the minimum compression considered therapeutic. Ulcerations of the legs, edema of the legs, varicose veins, and lymphedema are some of the problems aided by surgical stockings. There are many different surgical stocking lengths available, such as above the knee, thigh length, below the knee, and full length. There are also many types of surgical stockings ranging in size and custom made. These HCPCS Level II codes do not include antiembolism stocking (TED hose) as these only have a minimal gradient compression.

A4520

A4520 Incontinence garment, any type, (e.g., brief, diaper), each

Lay Description

Incontinence garments may be disposable or reusable and may be a flat diaper or a brief. Disposable garments include those commonly found at supermarkets. Flat reusable cloth diapers are generally rectangular with the same thickness throughout. Fit is accomplished by folding. Reusable briefs come in many varieties and may vary from slightly contoured to fully fitted briefs. There are also fully fitted briefs made of patented materials that are designed to be used with internal pads.

A4550

A4550 Surgical trays

Lay Description

A surgical tray comprises procedure-specific instruments, devices, and dressings within a ready-to-use sterilized package. The trays are prepared and inventoried for any of a variety of anticipated procedures (e.g., suture removal). The instruments may be sterilized and repackaged; however, a recent trend is toward the use of disposable surgical trays.

A4554

A4554 Disposable underpads, all sizes

Lay Description

Disposable underpads are designed for incontinent patients to protect bedding and furniture from leakage. Most have a soft quick-drying cover layer, an absorbent center core, and a waterproof bottom layer.

A4555

A4555 Electrode/transducer for use with electrical stimulation device used for cancer treatment, replacement only

Lay Description

Electrically-insulated surface electrodes are applied to the head of the patient for the treatment of glioblastoma multiforme (GBM). These electrodes deliver alternating electric fields that are said to slow or stop the glioblastoma cells from dividing.

A4556-A4558

A4556 Electrodes (e.g., apnea monitor), per pair

A4557 Lead wires (e.g., apnea monitor), per pair

A4558 Conductive gel or paste, for use with electrical device (e.g., TENS, NMES), per oz

Lay Description

Apnea monitors and transcutaneous electrical nerve stimulation (TENS) units consist of several components: the apnea monitor or TENS unit, lead wires, electrodes, and, for some devices, an electrode belt and conductive paste or gel. Electrodes for devices such as TENS units and apnea monitors are dispensed in pairs and may be stick-on electrodes or, in the case of an apnea monitor, contained within an electrode belt. Electrodes are placed on the proper site to deliver stimulation (in the case of a TENS unit) or to monitor breathing (in the case of an apnea monitor). Lead wires are also dispensed in pairs. They are usually color coded because each wire must be attached to the correct electrode. For example, an apnea monitoring system usually has one black and one white lead wire. The white lead wire is attached to the electrode on the right side of the chest and the black one is attached to the electrode on the left. The lead wires are then attached to the TENS unit or apnea monitor via a cable. Conductive paste or gel may be used on the skin at the site where the electrodes are placed to improve conduction of electrical impulses.

A4559

A4559   Coupling gel or paste, for use with ultrasound device, per oz

Lay Description
Coupling gels and pastes are used with ultrasonic probes and devices. The gel and/or paste acts as an agent to keep the probe from sticking to the patient's skin, probe cover, or other covers. The probes temperature can range from cool to hot and may require specific, high-heat gels or pastes. Ultrasound conductive coupling gel may be covered and separately payable if an ultrasonic osteogenesis stimulator is covered.

A4561-A4562

A4561   Pessary, rubber, any type
A4562   Pessary, nonrubber, any type

Lay Description
A pessary is a hard rubber, plastic, or silicon device that is inserted into the vagina, often to support the uterus and/or bladder from prolapse. The device may be ring-shaped, similar to the outer structure of a cervical cap or diaphragm. Other designs are also seen. The device may be prescribed for extended use or for short-term treatment. Regardless, the device should be removed regularly for hygienic considerations.

A4565

A4565   Slings

Lay Description
Typically constructed of canvas-type material or other materials such as cotton or nylon (including mesh-type products), an arm sling usually uses the shoulder/neck as the primary anchor, suspending the upper limb as needed, supporting the shoulder, upper arm, elbow, and, to a limited degree, the wrist and hand. Arm slings can be used with a cast or splint for any of these body areas, providing an added measure of support and protection. Arm slings may protect against reinjury.

A4566

A4566   Shoulder sling or vest design, abduction restrainer, with or without swathe control, prefabricated, includes fitting and adjustment

Lay Description
Abduction is a movement that draws a limb away from the median or sagittal plane of the body. An abduction restrainer is an immobilization device used to restrict movement in and around the shoulder by reducing movement and arm rotation. Most are figure eight designs that use a swathe that attaches to a sling or vest to position the arm.

A4570

A4570   Splint

Lay Description
A splint is an orthotic medical device used to immobilize a limb or the spine. A splint is usually composed of two pieces held in place by some type of cotton or nylon material. It may be used to temporarily immobilize a suspected fracture or dislocation until additional medical help can be obtained. Code A4570 is an undefined splint. Report this code only if a more appropriate HCPCS code is not available.

A4575

A4575   Topical hyperbaric oxygen chamber, disposable

Lay Description
A topical hyperbaric oxygen chamber is a device that applies oxygen at a high atmospheric pressure to a skin or surface wound. It is noninvasive and used in the home. The topical application of a limited supply of pressurized oxygen is purported to promote the healing of various acute and chronic wounds. The topical application has frequently been prescribed for decubitus ulcers and other chronic wounds of the skin and its underlying structures.

A4580-A4590

A4580   Cast supplies (e.g., plaster)
A4590   Special casting material (e.g., fiberglass)

Lay Description
Casting materials are made of plaster-imbedded strips or bandages or fiberglass wraps or strips, available in varieties pertinent to the type of fracture or post-surgical state requiring the support and protection of a cast. Some of these materials are initially dry and are water-activated, while others come pre-moistened for immediate application. Plaster varieties can be embedded with strength-adding chemical compounds such as polyurethane. Splints are used when a cast is not necessary but the injury or condition requires immobilization. Casts and casting materials support and protect fractured or strained extremities or other body areas. They hold manipulated (set) fractures in place or can assist other devices (pins, wires, screws) in doing so and protect against reinjury. These codes identify the different casting materials (e.g., fiberglass or plaster) for physicians, the type of immobilization provided (e.g., splint or cast for adult or pediatric patients), and the length or shape of casts for the different types of injuries or conditions (e.g., shoulder or body cast, long or short leg or arm cast).

A

A4595

A4595   Electrical stimulator supplies, 2 lead, per month, (e.g., TENS, NMES)

Lay Description

This code reports electrical stimulator supplies, two leads, per month (e.g., TENS, NMES). A transcutaneous electrical nerve stimulator (TENS) is a device that uses electrical current delivered through electrodes placed on the surface of the skin to decrease the patient's perception of pain by inhibiting the transmission of afferent pain nerve impulses and/or by stimulating the release of endorphins. The TENS unit can be applied in a variety of settings (in the patient's home, a physician's office, or in an outpatient clinic). A TENS unit alleviates or palliates acute postoperative pain, as well as chronic or intractable pain, depending on the etiology of the patient's condition. A four-lead TENS unit may be used with two leads or four leads, depending on the characteristics of the patient's pain. The leads direct the current from the stimulator to the electrodes to the area in which pain control is needed.

A4600

A4600   Sleeve for intermittent limb compression device, replacement only, each

Lay Description

Intermittent limb compression devices are used to inflate and deflate a compression sleeve. The sleeve is inflated to apply compressive pressure gradient against the limb which will decrease from a lower to upper portion of the limb to enhance the acceleration of the flow of blood through the limb.

A4601

A4601   Lithium ion battery, rechargeable, for nonprosthetic use, replacement

Lay Description

These battery systems fall into two major categories: primary or single-use batteries, which are cells containing lithium-metal anodes; and secondary or rechargeable batteries, which are systems utilizing lithium-ion chemistry. Primary lithium batteries have been used for implantable devices such as cardiac pacemakers, drug pumps, neurostimulators, and cardiac defibrillators. Rechargeable batteries have been used with left ventricular assist devices and total artificial hearts. All of these cells share the characteristics of high safety, reliability, energy density, and predictability of performance.

A4604

A4604   Tubing with integrated heating element for use with positive airway pressure device

Lay Description

Supply of tubing with an integrated heating element to be used with a positive airway pressure device is reported with A4604. The heating element is embedded in the outer spiral of the inspiratory limb of the tubing and has a smooth inner surface. This allows delivery of positive airway pressure with optimal humidity that does not condense in the tubing. This device is used primarily for individuals with obstructive sleep apnea who require heated humidification with positive airway pressure.

A4605

A4605   Tracheal suction catheter, closed system, each

Lay Description

A closed system tracheal suction catheter is designed to remove bronchial secretions in intubated patients. Closed suction catheters allow suctioning without requiring the patient to be disconnected from the ventilator. The advantage of a closed system is the prevention of hypoxemia during suctioning because ventilation is maintained during the suctioning process.

A4606

A4606   Oxygen probe for use with oximeter device, replacement

Lay Description

Oximetry is a noninvasive method to measure blood hemoglobin (Hb), usually to determine oxygen saturation. A probe is attached to the patient's earlobe or a fingertip. The probe emits a light source. The hemoglobin absorbs a percentage of the light, depending upon its oxygen saturation level, and the results are digitally recorded, sometimes in addition to other data, such as pulse. This code reports a replacement unit for the oxygen probe.

A4608

A4608   Transtracheal oxygen catheter, each

Lay Description

This code reports supply of a transtracheal oxygen (TTO) catheter, a small-diameter flexible tube that is fitted directly into the trachea. A stoma is surgically created to accommodate the catheter. The system is designed to directly deliver oxygen to the lungs at high efficiency. The catheter is inserted to a level several centimeters above the carinal junction. Compared to nasal cannulas, more oxygen is conserved, flow is largely uninterrupted, and arterial blood oxygen levels are better maintained. Additionally, speech is unimpeded and eating routines are unaffected. Generally, cleaning of the catheter is required several times per day. Durable catheters may require change-out about every 90 days, or earlier as needed. Other systems may feature disposable catheter components.

A4611-A4613

A4611 Battery, heavy-duty; replacement for patient-owned ventilator
A4612 Battery cables; replacement for patient-owned ventilator
A4613 Battery charger; replacement for patient-owned ventilator

Lay Description
This range of codes reports supply of batteries and related components for patient-owned ventilators. Patient-owned ventilators are likely to be conventional AC-powered devices with supplemental internal and external sealed lead acid (SLA) batteries for emergency use and portability. A 12 V or 24 V external battery and charging system with a direct current to alternating current inverter are common features of many ventilator systems. Typically, the external battery charges a 24 V internal battery, as does the AC system while in use. The internal battery always remains fully charged and is the power source of last resort. In emergencies, these systems can run on conventional 12 V car batteries. The SLA batteries are generally notable for price, reliability, charge retention, and relatively long life. Disadvantages include slow recharge time and the need to keep the charge topped off while the battery is not in use. Some patients prefer deep cycle marine batteries that stand up better to near-complete discharge and recharge. Most systems require special cables. Nickel cadmium (NiCad) batteries are usually acceptable for air travel and have other advantages, but they tend to lose charge over time while not in use.

A4614

A4614 Peak expiratory flow rate meter, hand held

Lay Description
A peak expiratory flow rate meter measures the maximum amount of air an individual can forcibly exhale. Hand held units are commonly used by asthmatics to determine a need for bronchodilation medications and to record regular readings in a daily journal. Hand held units vary in design, but many feature an air resistance cylinder that freezes a needle at the point of peak exhalation.

A4615

A4615 Cannula, nasal

Lay Description
A cannula is a hollow tube or sheath inserted into a vessel, duct, or cavity to facilitate passage of another instrument, such as a trocar or flexible tubing, fluid, or air. Use this code to report a nasal cannula, one that sits in the nostrils to facilitate the delivery of therapeutic oxygen, also called nasal prongs.

A4616

A4616 Tubing (oxygen), per foot

Lay Description
Oxygen tubing is reported by the foot but is usually supplied in lengths of 25 and 50 feet. Tubing is crush resistant to prevent interruptions in the flow of oxygen and may be supplied with tubing connectors.

A4617

A4617 Mouthpiece

Lay Description
Mouthpieces for nebulizers may be purchased separately. They are available in pediatric and adult sizes. Mouthpieces are used to deliver inhalant medications dispensed via small volume nebulizers.

A4618

A4618 Breathing circuits

Lay Description
A breathing circuit is a component array used to connect an intubated patient's airway to a gas anesthesia delivery system. The circuit creates an artificial atmosphere that the patient both draws air from as well as breathes exhaled air into. Components include: a port to deliver various anesthetic and other gases to the breathing circuit; a port to the patient's intubated airway; a reservoir bag for gas; an expiration port to release and control exhaled gas into room air; a carbon dioxide absorbing system for total rebreathing circuit; and tubes to connect the various components. A breathing circuit can be set so that no rebreathing of air is allowed (fresh gas is not mixed with exhaled gas). A partial rebreathing setting allows for a portion of exhaled gas to be mixed with fresh gas. Total rebreathing settings require that exhaled gas be purged of carbon dioxide. A variety of breathing circuit features is available, including an interface with ventilation assist and alarms.

A4619

A4619 Face tent

Lay Description
A face tent is a soft plastic face mask type of device for the delivery of oxygen or combination of gases. The device differs from a face mask in that the perimeter of the device does not come in contact with the patient's skin. Face tents are useful for individuals who have had facial surgery or who otherwise cannot tolerate the contact of a face mask or nasal cannulas. Disadvantages include difficulty in delivering therapeutic quantities of gas due to the imperfect air seal.

A4620

A4620 Variable concentration mask

Lay Description
Variable concentration masks are also known as low flow masks and deliver oxygen at variable rates

depending upon how the patient is breathing. The device is usually a simple face mask with tubing and is used in instances where a fixed concentration of oxygen is not required.

A4623

A4623 Tracheostomy, inner cannula

Lay Description
Inner cannulas are used inside of outer cannulas after a tracheostomy. A small opening is made through the stoma and a breathing tube is placed directly into the trachea (windpipe). There are three parts to the placement of a trach tube. The obturator is used to pass the trach tube into the trachea and a portion is removed leaving the outer cannula in place. The outer cannula has a plate that sits against the skin of the neck and holds the trach in place. The inner cannula fits inside the outer cannula and locks it into place.

A4624

A4624 Tracheal suction catheter, any type other than closed system, each

Lay Description
Tracheal suction catheters are used to clear the airways of excessive secretions. Catheters are made of soft rubber or hard plastic material. The diameter of each catheter is measured according to the French catheter scale, and they vary in length. Catheter tips may be a two-eye whistle tip design reducing the chance of damage to the mucosal tissue, or softer rounded style, which can be gentler on the mucosal lining. This code is for a tracheal suction catheter, any type.

A4625-A4626, A4629

A4625 Tracheostomy care kit for new tracheostomy
A4626 Tracheostomy cleaning brush, each
A4629 Tracheostomy care kit for established tracheostomy

Lay Description
A tracheostomy care kit for a new tracheostomy is used following an open surgical tracheostomy that is expected to remain open for at least three months. These kits are composed of supplies that are used to routinely clean and care for tracheostomy tubes, accessories, and the area around the tracheostomy. Tracheostomy care is necessary to reduce the chance of inflammation and infection around the tracheostomy site. Cleaning the tracheostomy tube allows air to move freely through the tube.

A4627

A4627 Spacer, bag or reservoir, with or without mask, for use with metered dose inhaler

Lay Description
A spacer, bag, or reservoir used with a metered dose inhaler increases the space between the metered dose inhaler and the mouth. It helps the patient inhale more medication into the lungs and decreases the amount of medication that is deposited at the back of the throat. Spacers, bags, and reservoirs are particularly useful for children, particularly those with asthma, due to the difficulty some children have in inhaling slowly while depressing the inhaler at the same time.

A4628

A4628 Oropharyngeal suction catheter, each

Lay Description
An oropharyngeal suction catheter is used to remove secretions from the oral cavity and pharynx.

A4629

A4629 Tracheostomy care kit for established tracheostomy

Lay Description
Please refer to codes A4625–A4626 for the description.

A4630

A4630 Replacement batteries, medically necessary, transcutaneous electrical stimulator, owned by patient

Lay Description
Transcutaneous electrical nerve stimulator (TENS) units require the use of a 9-volt, standard battery or a rechargeable cell. The initial purchase of a TENS unit generally includes a battery. When the battery for a patient-owned, medically necessary TENS unit requires replacement, report this code.

A4633-A4634

A4633 Replacement bulb/lamp for ultraviolet light therapy system, each
A4634 Replacement bulb for therapeutic light box, tabletop model

Lay Description
Light box therapy is used in the treatment of seasonal affective disorder (SAD), diurnal disorders, or sometimes to mitigate the sedating effect of medications. Although bulbs are rated for 20,000 hours of use, they generally begin to lose intensity after four to five years of use and require replacement. When long-term ultraviolet light or light box therapy is required, the bulbs must be periodically replaced.

A4635-A4637

A4635 Underarm pad, crutch, replacement, each

A4636 Replacement, handgrip, cane, crutch, or walker, each

A4637 Replacement, tip, cane, crutch, walker, each

Lay Description

Underarm pads, hand grips, and tips for patient-owned crutches, canes, and walkers periodically require replacement.

A4638

A4638 Replacement battery for patient-owned ear pulse generator, each

Lay Description

This code is used to report a replacement battery for a patient-owned ear pulse generator used in the tympanic treatment of inner ear endolymphatic fluid, also known as Ménière's disease.

A4639

A4639 Replacement pad for infrared heating pad system, each

Lay Description

An infrared heating pad system consists of a pad or pads containing mechanisms (e.g., luminous gallium aluminum arsenide diodes) that generate infrared (or near infrared) light and a power source. Use this code for each replacement pad.

A4640

A4640 Replacement pad for use with medically necessary alternating pressure pad owned by patient

Lay Description

An alternating pressure pad is designed to distribute the patient's body weight more effectively, preventing pressure points from developing. The pressure pad is attached to a pump that alternately inflates and deflates air cells in the pressure pad. Air cycling through the air cells provides patient lift and pressure reduction that assists in reducing pressure on skin and tissues and facilitates blood flow to all areas of the body that come in contact with the mattress. Alternating pressure pads are used to prevent and/or treat pressure ulcers and lesions, such as decubitus ulcers.

A4641

A4641 Radiopharmaceutical, diagnostic, not otherwise classified

Lay Description

This code is used to report the supply of radiopharmaceutical diagnostic imaging agents that do not have another specific HCPCS Level II code. Radiopharmaceuticals are radioactive isotopes, such as radioactive iodine or radioactive cobalt. They are often attached to carrier molecules and used in diagnostic nuclear medicine procedures.

A4642

A4642 Indium In-111 satumomab pendetide, diagnostic, per study dose, up to 6 millicuries

Lay Description

Satumomab pendetide is a murine monoclonal antibody that binds to a glycoprotein, a cell surface antigen produced in large amounts by colorectal and ovarian tumors. This monoclonal antibody does not generally react with normal adult tissue, but it may react with salivary gland ducts, normal post-ovulatory endometria, some benign ovarian tumors, and fetal gastrointestinal tissue. Indium 111 is a radioactive form of the metallic element indium. It has a half-life of approximately 56 hours and decays by electron capture and gamma emission. The monoclonal antibody is combined with indium 111 chloride so that it can be readily identified in images. Indium 111 satumomab pendetide is administered intravenously. It rapidly attaches itself to colorectal adenocarcinomas and common epithelial ovarian carcinomas. Optimal images are obtained 48 to 72 hours following administration. Since satumomab pendetide may attach itself to nonmalignant tissue, use of this diagnostic agent is not recommended for screening purposes. Indium 111 satumomab pendetide is indicated for patients with known colorectal or ovarian cancer to determine the extent and location of disease.

A4648

A4648 Tissue marker, implantable, any type, each

Lay Description

An implantable tissue marker is a small, non-absorbable piece of material, usually metal, that is used to mark an area of concern within soft tissue. The tissue marker is usually visible with multiple types of imaging and can be used to mark an area that needs continued follow-up. The marker can also be used to indicate an area to be removed or biopsied.

A4649

A4649 Surgical supply; miscellaneous

Lay Description

This code is used to report miscellaneous surgical supplies and should only be used if a more specific HCPCS Level II or CPT code is not available.

A4650

A4650 Implantable radiation dosimeter, each

Lay Description

An implantable radiation dosimeter is a permanent, small, non-absorbable device that is inserted into the target area that is to be irradiated with external beam ionizing radiation. The device measures the amount of

A

radiation reaching the targeted area and serves as a marker. This allows the physician to better track and calibrate the location and amount of radiation delivered.

A4651

A4651 Calibrated microcapillary tube, each

Lay Description
This code reports the supply of each calibrated microcapillary tube. These are glass laboratory tubes designed to measure and contain extremely small quantities of liquid. Some may have a coating of heparin on the inside surface to maintain blood in liquid storage. Others may be tempered to withstand extreme temperature variations. Most can be sealed for centrifuging or mechanical agitation.

A4652

A4652 Microcapillary tube sealant

Lay Description
Microcapillary tubes are glass laboratory tubes used to measure and contain small quantities of liquid. Most can be sealed for centrifuging or mechanical agitation.

A4653

A4653 Peritoneal dialysis catheter anchoring device, belt, each

Lay Description
Peritoneal dialysis is an alternative to hemodialysis. Peritoneal dialysis requires that a peritoneal catheter be inserted into the abdominal (peritoneal) cavity. The catheter consists of a 15-inch tube with two cuffs in the middle of the catheter. One section of tubing is placed into the peritoneal cavity. The cuffs in the middle section are placed just outside the peritoneal cavity in the fatty tissue and protect the catheter site from infection and leakage. The outer portion of tubing is used to connect the dialysis solution. Dialysis solution is then instilled through the catheter into the peritoneal cavity where it removes impurities, waste products, and extra fluid when this function can no longer be performed by the kidneys due to disease or injury. Patients on peritoneal dialysis sometimes require additional supplies to protect the catheter, such as an anchoring device that helps to protect the catheter from becoming dislodged.

A4657

A4657 Syringe, with or without needle, each

Lay Description
A sterile syringe is used for injecting or withdrawing fluid from any vessel or cavity. Syringes may vary in size and may be supplied with or without a needle.

A4660

A4660 Sphygmomanometer/blood pressure apparatus with cuff and stethoscope

Lay Description
This code reports the supply of a sphygmomanometer with cuff and stethoscope, a traditional blood pressure measuring device still in common use. A cuff and rubber bag are wrapped around the upper arm and secured with Velcro. Tubing connects the bag to a mercury manometer, which measures pressure within the cuff. The bag is inflated, usually by squeezing an air bulb, until pressure on the arm exceeds arterial pressure. A stethoscope over the brachial artery below the cuff confirms that no blood movement is heard. A valve slowly releases pressure on the bag. The artery first emits sound upon peak pressure from the heart, or systolic pressure. This is noted by the observer and the manometer reading is taken. As pressure on the cuff continues to drop, arterial occlusion fails even upon lowest pressure from the heart, the diastolic pressure. This characteristic sound heard through the stethoscope is also noted by the trained observer and the second manometer reading is taken. The two pressures, systolic and diastolic, are recorded as the patient's blood pressure.

A4663

A4663 Blood pressure cuff only

Lay Description
This code reports the supply of a traditional sphygmomanometer blood pressure cuff only. The cuff is the portion of the apparatus that wraps around the upper arm and is secured with Velcro. The traditional cuff contains a rubber bag that is connected to a manometer or other device to measure pressure. The bag is inflated, usually by squeezing an air bulb, placing pressure on the arteries of the arm.

A4670

A4670 Automatic blood pressure monitor

Lay Description
An automatic blood pressure monitor consists of a digital gauge and a stethoscope in one unit. Automatic blood pressure monitors are powered by batteries. The cuff may be inflated manually or automatically depending on the model. The blood pressure recording is displayed on a digital screen that will also display error messages. The error messages help ensure accurate blood pressure readings. Deflation of the cuff is automatic. Some models of automatic blood pressure monitors will also provide a paper printout of blood pressure recordings.

A4671

A4671   Disposable cycler set used with cycler dialysis machine, each

Lay Description
During automated peritoneal dialysis, also called continuous cycling peritoneal dialysis (CCPD) or nocturnal cyclical peritoneal dialysis, a sterile mixture of sugar and minerals dissolved in water (dialysis solution) flows through a catheter into the peritoneal cavity using a cycler machine. Using osmosis, the solution draws wastes, impurities, chemicals, and extra water from the tiny blood vessels in the peritoneal membrane into the solution. The cycler machine automatically infuses the dialysis solution and then drains it several times during the night. Disposable cycler kits are available that contain supplies required for CCPD.

A4672-A4673

A4672   Drainage extension line, sterile, for dialysis, each

A4673   Extension line with easy lock connectors, used with dialysis

Lay Description
Extension lines for dialysis provide added length to catheters, which can assist in patient comfort and mobility.

A4674

A4674   Chemicals/antiseptics solution used to clean/sterilize dialysis equipment, per 8 oz

Lay Description
There are two types of dialysis, hemodialysis and peritoneal dialysis. Hemodialysis removes excess fluids, wastes, impurities, and chemicals from the blood by use of a dialyzer. Hemodialysis requires the use of a dialysis machine, dialyzer, dialysis solution, treated water, and disposable supplies. Peritoneal dialysis is an alternative to hemodialysis. Peritoneal dialysis uses the thin lining in the abdomen that coats the outer surface of the intestines (peritoneal membrane) to remove waste products and balance fluids. The dialysis solution is instilled through a catheter placed through the skin into the peritoneal cavity. The dialysis solution removes waste products and excess fluid and is then drained from the abdomen and discarded. Dialysis equipment must be properly cleaned and sterilized to prevent infection.

A4680

A4680   Activated carbon filter for hemodialysis, each

Lay Description
This code represents an activated carbon filter used for hemodialysis as a component of a water purification system to remove unsafe concentrations of chloride or chloramines.

A4690

A4690   Dialyzer (artificial kidneys), all types, all sizes, for hemodialysis, each

Lay Description
This code reports the supply of a dialyzer, the portion of a hemodialysis machine that cleanses blood in patients with end-stage renal disease (ESRD). Dialysis is a physicochemical and filtration process. The dialyzer portion of a hemodialysis unit is typically a two-chambered clear plastic cylinder. The cylinder is packed with hollow fiber strands that form a membrane between the chambers. One chamber circulates blood drawn from the patient. The second circulates a solution known as dialysate in the opposite direction from movement of the blood. This semipermeable membrane between the chambers allows accumulated uremic toxins, excess ions, and water in the blood to pass into the dialysate. A similar dialyzer design, known as the parallel plate process, separates the chambers by a cellophane-type membrane. With either process, cleansed blood is returned to the patient as the dialysate is constantly refreshed. The dialyzer is generally changed out between patients, although the same patient may use a single dialyzer repeatedly.

A4706-A4707

A4706   Bicarbonate concentrate, solution, for hemodialysis, per gallon

A4707   Bicarbonate concentrate, powder, for hemodialysis, per packet

Lay Description
These codes report the supply of bicarbonate concentrate for hemodialysis. Hemodialysis is a physicochemical and filtration process. The dialyzer portion of a hemodialysis unit is typically two-chambered. One chamber circulates blood drawn from the patient. The second circulates a solution known as dialysate in the opposite direction from movement of the blood. A semipermeable membrane between the chambers allows accumulated uremic toxins, excess ions, and water in the blood to pass into the dialysate. Cleansed blood is returned to the patient as the dialysate is constantly refreshed. Bicarbonate concentrate is added to treated water and acetic acid in a fixed proportion to form the dialysate base. Low concentrations of bicarbonate in the dialysate can result in metabolic acidosis. Ordinarily, a sensor and alarm on the hemodialysis unit alert the operator of an imbalance in the dialysate solution.

A

A4708-A4709

A4708   Acetate concentrate solution, for hemodialysis, per gallon

A4709   Acid concentrate, solution, for hemodialysis, per gallon

Lay Description

These codes report the supply of acetate concentrate and acid concentrate solutions for hemodialysis. Hemodialysis is a physicochemical and filtration process. The dialyzer portion of a hemodialysis unit is typically two chambered. One chamber circulates blood drawn from the patient. The second circulates a solution know as dialysate in the opposite direction from movement of the blood. A semipermeable membrane between the chambers allows accumulated uremic toxins, excess ions, and water in the blood to pass into the dialysate. Cleansed blood is returned to the patient as the dialysate is constantly refreshed. Acetate and/or acid concentrate, as well as bicarbonate concentrate, must be mixed with dialysate in specific ratios depending on the type of dialysis equipment being used to achieve the proper chemical balance in the dialysis solution.

A4714

A4714   Treated water (deionized, distilled, or reverse osmosis) for peritoneal dialysis, per gallon

Lay Description

Peritoneal dialysis is an alternative to hemodialysis. Peritoneal dialysis uses the thin lining in the abdomen that coats the outer surface of the intestines (peritoneal membrane) to remove waste products and balance fluids. The dialysis solution is instilled through a catheter placed through the skin into the peritoneal cavity. The dialysis solution removes waste products and excess fluid and is then drained from the abdomen and discarded. Treatments are generally performed by the patient. Peritoneal dialysis requires the use of dialysis solution, treated water, and disposable supplies.

A4719

A4719   "Y set" tubing for peritoneal dialysis

Lay Description

This code reports the supply of y-set tubing for peritoneal dialysis. Peritoneal dialysis (PD) is the main alternative to hemodialysis for patients with end-stage renal disease (ESRD). In PD, used dialysate is exchanged for fresh product, usually once or twice per day. The patient will have a surgically created stoma and an indwelling peritoneal catheter. A special y-tube with clamps is connected to the PD catheter. A clamp on the y-tube is opened and used dialysate is drained from the cavity and collected. Upon completion, the drain tube is clamped and about 1.5 to 3 liters of fresh dialysate is gravity infused through the other lead of the y-tube catheter into the peritoneal cavity. The dialysate may be left in place for

one to eight hours, depending on the patient's requirements. Y-set tubing is reusable for up to several months.

A4720-A4726

A4720   Dialysate solution, any concentration of dextrose, fluid volume greater than 249 cc, but less than or equal to 999 cc, for peritoneal dialysis

A4721   Dialysate solution, any concentration of dextrose, fluid volume greater than 999 cc but less than or equal to 1999 cc, for peritoneal dialysis

A4722   Dialysate solution, any concentration of dextrose, fluid volume greater than 1999 cc but less than or equal to 2999 cc, for peritoneal dialysis

A4723   Dialysate solution, any concentration of dextrose, fluid volume greater than 2999 cc but less than or equal to 3999 cc, for peritoneal dialysis

A4724   Dialysate solution, any concentration of dextrose, fluid volume greater than 3999 cc but less than or equal to 4999 cc, for peritoneal dialysis

A4725   Dialysate solution, any concentration of dextrose, fluid volume greater than 4999 cc but less than or equal to 5999 cc, for peritoneal dialysis

A4726   Dialysate solution, any concentration of dextrose, fluid volume greater than 5999 cc, for peritoneal dialysis

Lay Description

This range of codes reports various sized supplies of dialysate solution for peritoneal dialysis. The codes are differentiated by volume of solution supplied. Peritoneal dialysis (PD) is the main alternative to hemodialysis for patients with end-stage renal disease (ESRD). In PD, used dialysate is exchanged for fresh product, usually once or twice per day. The patient will have a surgically created stoma and an indwelling peritoneal catheter. A special y-tube with clamps is connected to the PD catheter. A clamp on the y-tube is opened and used dialysate is drained from the cavity and collected. Upon completion, the drain tube is clamped and about 1.5 to 3 liters of fresh dialysate is gravity infused through the other lead of the y-tube catheter into the peritoneal cavity. The fresh solution contains dextrose (sugar) that helps to withdraw wastes and excess fluids. This range of codes is independent of dextrose concentrations in the dialysate.

A4728

A4728   Dialysate solution, nondextrose containing, 500 ml

Lay Description

There are two types of dialysis, hemodialysis and peritoneal dialysis. Both make use of a solution called dialysate to draw waste products out of the blood. Hemodialysis removes excess fluids, wastes, impurities, and chemicals from the blood by use of a dialyzer. Hemodialysis requires the use of a dialysis machine, dialyzer, dialysis solution (dialysate), treated water, and disposable supplies. Peritoneal dialysis is an alternative to hemodialysis. Peritoneal dialysis uses the thin lining in the abdomen that coats the outer surface of the intestines (peritoneal membrane) to remove waste products and balance fluids. The dialysis solution (dialysate) is instilled through a catheter placed through the skin into the peritoneal cavity. The dialysis solution removes waste products and excess fluid and is then drained from the abdomen and discarded.

A4730

A4730   Fistula cannulation set for hemodialysis, each

Lay Description
This code reports the supply of each fistula cannulation set for hemodialysis. In most cases, patients will have had a surgically created arterial-venous fistula in the wrist or elbow region, and several configurations are seen. A synthetic graft of soft plastic tubing between the artery and the vein may be chosen. The plastic graft portion of the fistula, which may lie exteriorly, can then be repeatedly accessed for hemodialysis. The cannula set is designed to interface between the fistula and the hemodialysis unit.

A4736-A4737

A4736   Topical anesthetic, for dialysis, per g
A4737   Injectable anesthetic, for dialysis, per 10 ml

Lay Description
These codes report local anesthetics used during dialysis. Local anesthetics reduce sensation or feeling in the area of the body where they are applied or injected.

A4740

A4740   Shunt accessory, for hemodialysis, any type, each

Lay Description
A hemodialysis shunt is an artificial, external blood route that provides access to the blood supply. Shunt accessories such as connectors and adapters are attached to the hemodialysis shunt to perform dialysis. Examples of items that would be reported with this code include shunt connectors, universal connectors, Teflon connectors, shunt adapters, universal adapters, and Teflon adapters.

A4750-A4755

A4750   Blood tubing, arterial or venous, for hemodialysis, each
A4755   Blood tubing, arterial and venous combined, for hemodialysis, each

Lay Description
Hemodialysis tubing consists of a plastic tube or tubes that is attached to a fistula needle or shunt connector and allows blood to flow to and from the patient and dialyzer. Blood tubing for hemodialysis may be separate arterial and venous tubing or combined arteriovenous tubing.

A4760

A4760   Dialysate solution test kit, for peritoneal dialysis, any type, each

Lay Description
Dialysate is an electrolyte solution containing elements such as potassium, sodium, chloride, etc. Dialysate that is supplied in solution or powder concentrate form must be mixed with purified water prior to use. The mixed solution requires testing to verify that electrolyte levels are correct.

A4765-A4766

A4765   Dialysate concentrate, powder, additive for peritoneal dialysis, per packet
A4766   Dialysate concentrate, solution, additive for peritoneal dialysis, per 10 ml

Lay Description
Dialysate is an electrolyte solution containing elements such as potassium, sodium, chloride, etc. Dialysate that is supplied in solution or powder concentrate form must be mixed with purified water prior to use.

A4770-A4771

A4770   Blood collection tube, vacuum, for dialysis, per 50
A4771   Serum clotting time tube, for dialysis, per 50

Lay Description
These codes report blood collection tubes for dialysis. Vacuum tubes have a precisely controlled vacuum that allows the correct amount of blood to be collected for each specimen required. Serum clotting time tubes are designed specifically to test blood samples for clotting time.

A4772-A4774

A4772 Blood glucose test strips, for dialysis, per 50

A4773 Occult blood test strips, for dialysis, per 50

A4774 Ammonia test strips, for dialysis, per 50

Lay Description
These codes report test strips used to check blood glucose, occult blood, and ammonia levels in patients undergoing dialysis.

A4802

A4802 Protamine sulfate, for hemodialysis, per 50 mg

Lay Description
Protamine sulfate is used to neutralize the effects of heparin. Protamine sulfate is a strong basic polypeptide that when administered alone has an anticoagulant effect. However, when administered with heparin, protamine sulfate complexes with the strongly acidic heparin to form an inactive stable salt and the complex has no anticoagulant activity.

A4860

A4860 Disposable catheter tips for peritoneal dialysis, per 10

Lay Description
This code is used to report a supply of 10 disposable catheter tips used during peritoneal dialysis.

A4870-A4890

A4870 Plumbing and/or electrical work for home hemodialysis equipment

A4890 Contracts, repair and maintenance, for hemodialysis equipment

Lay Description
These codes are used to report plumbing and electrical modifications required in the patient's home so that the dialysis equipment can be effectively and safely used, as well as contract work performed on hemodialysis equipment. Report A4870 for costs associated with plumbing and electrical modifications.

A4911-A4932

A4911 Drain bag/bottle, for dialysis, each

A4913 Miscellaneous dialysis supplies, not otherwise specified

A4918 Venous pressure clamp, for hemodialysis, each

A4927 Gloves, nonsterile, per 100

A4928 Surgical mask, per 20

A4929 Tourniquet for dialysis, each

A4930 Gloves, sterile, per pair

A4931 Oral thermometer, reusable, any type, each

A4932 Rectal thermometer, reusable, any type, each

Lay Description
These codes report additional supplies used during dialysis. All codes are for specific supplies except A4913, which should be used to report miscellaneous dialysis supplies when a more specific HCPCS Level II code is not available.

A5051-A5054, A5056-A5057

A5051 Ostomy pouch, closed; with barrier attached (1 piece), each

A5052 Ostomy pouch, closed; without barrier attached (1 piece), each

A5053 Ostomy pouch, closed; for use on faceplate, each

A5054 Ostomy pouch, closed; for use on barrier with flange (2 piece), each

A5056 Ostomy pouch, drainable, with extended wear barrier attached, with filter, (1 piece), each

A5057 Ostomy pouch, drainable, with extended wear barrier attached, with built in convexity, with filter, (1 piece), each

Lay Description
These codes represent ostomy pouches that are used with patients who have had a surgically created opening for diversion of stool. Ostomy pouches collect the stomal output, in this case feces, and can be drainable or closed. Drainable pouches have an opening at the bottom through which fecal contents can be emptied. Closed pouches have a sealed bottom with no outlet for feces. Drainable pouches have an opening at one end to allow the contents to be drained without removing the entire bag. There are also one-piece and two-piece systems. One-piece systems are supplied "with barrier attached" or "without barrier attached." Two-piece systems have a locking or non-locking flange that is coupled to a skin barrier with flange. Skin barriers are an interface between the patient's skin and the pouching system and have a variety of different options, such as built-in convexity, filters, locking or nonlocking flanges, and use with or without faceplates.

A5055
A5055   Stoma cap

Lay Description
Stoma caps are designed to retain discharge at the site of the stoma for patients with ostomies. A stoma is an artificial opening into a body passageway or organ. It is performed when the organ cannot function normally. Ostomies are usually permanent openings, created for drainage to the outside of the body, so that fecal or urinary materials can be eliminated. The stoma caps are extremely absorbent, flexible, waterproof covers that may also include odor control features.

A5056-A5057
A5056   Ostomy pouch, drainable, with extended wear barrier attached, with filter, (1 piece), each
A5057   Ostomy pouch, drainable, with extended wear barrier attached, with built in convexity, with filter, (1 piece), each

Lay Description
Please refer to codes A5052-A5054 for the description, coding, and billing information.

A5061-A5063
A5061   Ostomy pouch, drainable; with barrier attached, (1 piece), each
A5062   Ostomy pouch, drainable; without barrier attached (1 piece), each
A5063   Ostomy pouch, drainable; for use on barrier with flange (2-piece system), each

Lay Description
These codes represent drainable ostomy pouches. Ostomy pouches are used by patients who have had a surgically created opening for diversion of urine. The ostomy pouch with barrier attached is a one-piece system in which a solid barrier serving to create an adhesive seal is part of the ostomy pouch. The barrier may be pectin-based or karaya-based for normal wear, or pectin-based with special additives for extended wear. A flange or plastic ring on both the pouch and skin barrier secures the barrier and the pouch.

A5071-A5073
A5071   Ostomy pouch, urinary; with barrier attached (1 piece), each
A5072   Ostomy pouch, urinary; without barrier attached (1 piece), each
A5073   Ostomy pouch, urinary; for use on barrier with flange (2 piece), each

Lay Description
These codes represent urinary ostomy pouches. Urinary ostomy pouches are for use with patients who have had a surgically created opening for diversion of the urine. There are one-piece and two-piece systems. In one-piece appliances, the collection pouch and barrier cannot be separated from one another, whereas the two-piece appliance is designed so that the barrier and collection pouch are separated by a locking mechanism. An ostomy faceplate is a solid interface between the patient's skin and the pouch. It is usually made of plastic, rubber, or encased metal. It can be taken off the skin and reattached repeatedly. It is held on by means of a separate adhesive and/or an elastic belt.

A5081-A5083
A5081   Stoma plug or seal, any type
A5082   Continent device; catheter for continent stoma
A5083   Continent device, stoma absorptive cover for continent stoma

Lay Description
These codes report specific supplies for continent stomas. A continent stoma usually involves a surgically fashioned "neobladder" that allows for natural voiding capability. In some instances the pouch is created from a section of ileum, cecum, or other portions of the colon. Part of the bladder may be preserved and the intestinal graft attached to it. Nerves and blood vessels of the graft are usually preserved. The ileocecal sphincter may be preserved and used as a valve. The stoma is managed by a plug and catheter system, and these codes report the supply of these products.

A5093
A5093   Ostomy accessory; convex insert

Lay Description
A convex insert is an ostomy accessory that fits between the ostomy pouch and the ostomy pad surrounding the stoma opening. The convex insert helps to provide the ostomy pouch with a tighter fit.

A5102
A5102   Bedside drainage bottle with or without tubing, rigid or expandable, each

Lay Description
Patients with urinary ostomies may use a bedside drainage bottle. The bedside drainage bottle is reusable and collects urinary output from a pouch. It is sometimes necessary, especially at night, for the bottle to be connected to the pouch to prevent urinary overflow and excessive weight in the pouch, which could cause urinary leakage and disruption of the pouch seal. The bottle is made of a high-density polyethylene and can hold up to 2,000 cc. Report this code for rigid or expandable bedside bottle with or without tubing.

A

A5105

A5105 Urinary suspensory with leg bag, with or without tube, each

Lay Description

This code reports the supply of an external urinary suspensory garment. This garment is usually designed for males and is worn like a jock strap. A urinal sheath is attachable to a portion that fits around the penis. This in turn is attachable to a tube and leg bag to drain urine.

A5112

A5112 Urinary drainage bag, leg or abdomen, latex, with or without tube, with straps, each

Lay Description

Urinary leg bags are used with male external urinary catheters. At the top is an anti-reflux flutter valve that attaches to the urinary catheter and allows urine to drain from the bladder into the leg bag. At the bottom is a drainage valve that allows the catheter to be emptied as needed. Leg bags may be constructed of a variety of materials.

A5113-A5114

A5113 Leg strap; latex, replacement only, per set

A5114 Leg strap; foam or fabric, replacement only, per set

Lay Description

These codes are for replacement leg straps used with a urinary leg bag. These codes are not used for a leg strap for an indwelling catheter.

A5120

A5120 Skin barrier, wipes or swabs, each

Lay Description

Skin barrier wipes and swabs are used to clean and protect the stoma site. Wipes and swabs are formulated with soothing, non-sting cleanser that also provides a protective film around the stoma to prevent irritation of the stoma between pouch changes. Wipes and swabs may also be medicated to provide further protection to the stoma site.

A5121-A5122

A5121 Skin barrier; solid, 6 x 6 or equivalent, each

A5122 Skin barrier; solid, 8 x 8 or equivalent, each

Lay Description

Please refer to code A4362 for the description.

A5126

A5126 Adhesive or nonadhesive; disk or foam pad

Lay Description

Please refer to code A4364 for the description.

A5131

A5131 Appliance cleaner, incontinence and ostomy appliances, per 16 oz

Lay Description

Appliance cleaners are used to deodorize, remove crystallized deposits, and clean the inside of rubber, latex, and plastic incontinence or ostomy collection devices. Report this code for every 16 oz. of cleaner.

A5200

A5200 Percutaneous catheter/tube anchoring device, adhesive skin attachment

Lay Description

A percutaneous catheter/tube anchoring device is a dressing with adhesive that is designed to be applied directly over the cutaneous opening through which the catheter/tube passes. This dressing has a hole through which the catheter/tube passes and a mechanism for firmly anchoring the catheter/tube to the dressing.

A5500-A5501

A5500 For diabetics only, fitting (including follow-up), custom preparation and supply of off-the-shelf depth-inlay shoe manufactured to accommodate multidensity insert(s), per shoe

A5501 For diabetics only, fitting (including follow-up), custom preparation and supply of shoe molded from cast(s) of patient's foot (custom molded shoe), per shoe

Lay Description

These items include fitting with follow-up, custom preparation, and supply of off-the-shelf or custom made shoes that accommodate various shoe inserts. Shoes and shoe inserts assist the diabetic patient with ambulation, decrease pressure points that may be present in non-prescription shoes, and help prevent ulcerative conditions of the feet. They are used in patients with partial or complete amputation (opposite foot). Previous foot ulcerations and current pre-ulcerative conditions may be present. Circulation may be impaired, and deformity and/or peripheral neuropathy may be present. Report A5500 for off-the-shelf depth shoes, which are custom prepared and have multi-density (varying depths) of insert. They usually are full-length. In A5501, a molded cast of the patient's foot may be performed or may be heat-molded to fit almost any foot. They also have removable inserts that can be altered, with some form of shoe closure. Each code is reported per shoe.

A5503-A5506

A5503 For diabetics only, modification (including fitting) of off-the-shelf depth-inlay shoe or custom molded shoe with roller or rigid rocker bottom, per shoe

A5504 For diabetics only, modification (including fitting) of off-the-shelf depth-inlay shoe or custom molded shoe with wedge(s), per shoe

A5505 For diabetics only, modification (including fitting) of off-the-shelf depth-inlay shoe or custom molded shoe with metatarsal bar, per shoe

A5506 For diabetics only, modification (including fitting) of off-the-shelf depth-inlay shoe or custom molded shoe with off-set heel(s), per shoe

Lay Description
These items include fitting with follow-up, custom preparation, and supply of off-the-shelf or custom made shoes with special added features. A molded cast of the patient's foot may be performed. Shoes and shoe inserts assist the diabetic patient with ambulation, decrease pressure points that may be present in non-prescription shoes, and help prevent ulcerative conditions of the feet. They are used in patients with partial or complete amputation (opposite foot). Previous foot ulcerations and current pre-ulcerative conditions may be present. Circulation may be impaired, and deformity and/or peripheral neuropathy may be present. Rigid rocker bottoms are exterior elevations. The apex (a narrowed or pointed end) is measured from the back end of the heel, positioned behind the metatarsal heads, and tapers off sharply to the front tip of the sole. Apex height helps to eliminate pressure at the metatarsal heads. The heel tapers off in back to cause the shoe heel to strike in the middle of the heel. The steel in a patient's shoe ensures rigidity. Roller bottoms (sole or bar) are the same as rocker bottoms, but the heel is tapered from the apex to the front tip of the sole. A shoe with wedges that are either of the hind foot, fore foot, or both and may be in the middle or to the side is reported with A5504. The function is to shift or transfer weight bearing upon standing or during ambulation to the opposite side for added support, stabilization, equalized weight distribution, or balance. An exterior bar is placed behind the metatarsal heads in order to remove pressure from the metatarsal heads. The bars are of various shapes, heights, and construction depending on the purpose it serves. Report A5506 for an offset heel flanged at its base either in the middle, to the side, or a combination, that is then extended upward to the shoe in order to stabilize extreme positions of the hind foot.

A5507

A5507 For diabetics only, not otherwise specified modification (including fitting) of off-the-shelf depth-inlay shoe or custom molded shoe, per shoe

Lay Description
This code is used to report therapeutic modifications to an off-the-shelf depth-inlay or custom-made shoe for a diabetic patient not identified with a more specific HCPCS Level II code.

A5508

A5508 For diabetics only, deluxe feature of off-the-shelf depth-inlay shoe or custom molded shoe, per shoe

Lay Description
Report this code for a deluxe feature of an off-the-shelf depth-inlay or custom-made shoe that does not contribute to the therapeutic function of the diabetic shoe. It may include, but is not limited to, style, color, or type of leather.

A5510-A5513

A5510 For diabetics only, direct formed, compression molded to patient's foot without external heat source, multiple-density insert(s) prefabricated, per shoe

A5512 For diabetics only, multiple density insert, direct formed, molded to foot after external heat source of 230 degrees Fahrenheit or higher, total contact with patient's foot, including arch, base layer minimum of 1/4 inch material of shore a 35 durometer or 3/16 inch material of shore a 40 durometer (or higher), prefabricated, each

A5513 For diabetics only, multiple density insert, custom molded from model of patient's foot, total contact with patient's foot, including arch, base layer minimum of 3/16 inch material of shore a 35 durometer or higher), includes arch filler and other shaping material, custom fabricated, each

Lay Description
A diabetic shoe insert is a total contact, removable inlay that is directly molded to the patient's foot or a model of the patient's foot and that is made of a suitable material with regard to the patient's condition. There are several methods of fabrication including compression molded without the use of a heat source, direct formed with the use of a heat source, and custom molded from a model of the patient's foot. In A5510, the insert is prefabricated, multiple density, and formed using a compression mold of the patient's foot without the use of a heat

A

source. In A5512, the insert is prefabricated and direct formed to the foot using an external heat source and total contact with the patient's foot. In A5513, the insert is custom-fabricated from a model of the patient's foot. Codes A5512 and A5513 contain additional specific requirements for the insert. The inserts must provide total contact including arch support with a base layer minimum of 1/4 inch material of shore A dermometer or 3/16 inch material of shore A 40 dermometer or higher.

A6000

A6000 Noncontact wound-warming wound cover for use with the noncontact wound-warming device and warming card

Lay Description

Wound healing occurs best in a warm, moist environment that enhances subcutaneous oxygen tension and increases blood flow to the wound. A noncontact wound warming device, also referred to as noncontact normothermic wound therapy (NNWT), is a wound treatment device designed to create an optimal environment to promote wound healing. A non-contact wound warming device includes a non-contact bandage and a warming unit designed to maintain 100 percent relative humidity and to produce optimal temperatures in the wound and surrounding tissues. The bandage consists of a sterile foam collar that adheres to the skin surrounding the wound and a sterile, transparent film that covers the top of the wound without touching it. An infrared warming card or flexible heat unit is inserted into a pocket in the film covering.

A6010-A6011

A6010 Collagen based wound filler, dry form, sterile, per g of collagen

A6011 Collagen based wound filler, gel/paste, per g of collagen

Lay Description

Collagen based wound filler is a natural hydrolyzed protein available in a dry powder or a gel/paste. Collagen based wound filler may be used for chronic wounds and dermal ulcers including pressure ulcers, stasis ulcers, diabetic ulcers, first- and second-degree burns, surgical wounds, and traumatic wounds. Collagen based wound fillers provide a platform for new cell growth, supply a nutritive protein to the wound site, and protect the wound from bacteria. The powder type forms a gel when it combines with the wound exudate to provide a moist healing environment. The gel/paste type is a hydrogel that contains collagen.

A6021-A6023

A6021 Collagen dressing, sterile, size 16 sq in or less, each

A6022 Collagen dressing, sterile, size more than 16 sq in but less than or equal to 48 sq in, each

A6023 Collagen dressing, sterile, size more than 48 sq in, each

Lay Description

Surgical dressings include both primary dressings (i.e., therapeutic or protective coverings applied directly to wounds or lesions on the skin) and secondary dressings (i.e., materials needed to secure a primary dressing). Collagen dressings are sterile dressings used for moderate to heavily draining wounds to enhance healing and tissue repair. These dressings can be used on burns, pressure ulcers, scrapes, cuts, and for dermatologic conditions. They also come in wet form for burns and other wounds. In general, these products are used for direct wound care, including protecting a wound from infection, absorbing wound exudate (drainage), filtering into the wound, and/or cleansing the wound. Dressings also reduce inflammation and edema and allow for gas exchange.

A6024

A6024 Collagen dressing wound filler, sterile, per 6 in

Lay Description

Usually made from a bovine collagen, sterile collagen dressing wound filler is a hydrolysate powder that interacts with the wound site and forms a gel that provides a moist wound-healing environment when mixed with the wounds exudate. Collagen promotes new cell growth and provides protein to the wound site. The collagen wound filler is typically used for the management of chronic wounds such as pressure ulcers, diabetic ulcers, and venous insufficiency ulcers, as well as surgically or trauma induced wounds.

A6025

A6025 Gel sheet for dermal or epidermal application, (e.g., silicone, hydrogel, other), each

Lay Description

Gel sheets help create and maintain a moist environment. Increasing moisture to a wound helps keep the wound clean and assists in debridement of necrotic tissue. Gel sheets are used mainly for wounds with minimal or no exudate.

A6154

A6154 Wound pouch, each

Lay Description

A wound pouch is a waterproof collection device with a drainable port that adheres to the skin around a wound. Use this code for each wound pouch supplied.

A6196-A6199

A6196 Alginate or other fiber gelling dressing, wound cover, sterile, pad size 16 sq in or less, each dressing

A6197 Alginate or other fiber gelling dressing, wound cover, sterile, pad size more than 16 sq in but less than or equal to 48 sq in, each dressing

A6198 Alginate or other fiber gelling dressing, wound cover, sterile, pad size more than 48 sq in, each dressing

A6199 Alginate or other fiber gelling dressing, wound filler, sterile, per 6 in

Lay Description

Alginate or other fiber gelling sterile dressing covers and fillers are used for moderately to highly exudative full thickness wounds (e.g., stage III or IV ulcers). Usual dressing change is up to once per day. One wound cover sheet of the approximate size of the wound or up to two units of wound filler (one unit = 6 inches of alginate or other fiber gelling dressing rope) is usually used at each dressing change. It is usually inappropriate to use alginates or other fiber gelling dressings in combination with hydrogels.

A6203-A6205

A6203 Composite dressing, sterile, pad size 16 sq in or less, with any size adhesive border, each dressing

A6204 Composite dressing, sterile, pad size more than 16 sq in, but less than or equal to 48 sq in, with any size adhesive border, each dressing

A6205 Composite dressing, sterile, pad size more than 48 sq in, with any size adhesive border, each dressing

Lay Description

Composite dressings are products combining physically distinct components into a single dressing that provides multiple functions. These functions must include, but are not limited to (a) a bacterial barrier, (b) an absorptive layer other than an alginate or other fiber gelling dressing, foam, hydrocolloid, or hydrogel, and (c) a semi-adherent or nonadherent property over the wound site. Usual composite dressing change is up to three times per week, one wound cover per dressing change.

A6206-A6208

A6206 Contact layer, sterile, 16 sq in or less, each dressing

A6207 Contact layer, sterile, more than 16 sq in but less than or equal to 48 sq in, each dressing

A6208 Contact layer, sterile, more than 48 sq in, each dressing

Lay Description

Contact layers are thin, non-adherent sheets placed directly on an open wound bed to protect the wound tissue from direct contact with other agents or dressings applied to the wound. They are porous to allow wound fluid to pass through for absorption by an overlying dressing. Contact layer dressings are used to line the entire wound; they are not intended to be changed with each dressing change. Usual dressing change is up to once per week.

A6209-A6215

A6209 Foam dressing, wound cover, sterile, pad size 16 sq in or less, without adhesive border, each dressing

A6210 Foam dressing, wound cover, sterile, pad size more than 16 sq in but less than or equal to 48 sq in, without adhesive border, each dressing

A6211 Foam dressing, wound cover, sterile, pad size more than 48 sq in, without adhesive border, each dressing

A6212 Foam dressing, wound cover, sterile, pad size 16 sq in or less, with any size adhesive border, each dressing

A6213 Foam dressing, wound cover, sterile, pad size more than 16 sq in but less than or equal to 48 sq in, with any size adhesive border, each dressing

A6214 Foam dressing, wound cover, sterile, pad size more than 48 sq in, with any size adhesive border, each dressing

A6215 Foam dressing, wound filler, sterile, per g

Lay Description

Foam dressings are used on full thickness wounds (e.g., stage III or IV ulcers) with moderate to heavy exudate. Usual dressing change for a foam wound cover used as a primary dressing is up to three times per week. When a foam wound cover is used as a secondary dressing for wounds with heavy exudate, dressing change may also be up to three times per week. Usual dressing change for foam wound fillers is up to once per day.

A6216-A6221

A6216 Gauze, nonimpregnated, nonsterile, pad size 16 sq in or less, without adhesive border, each dressing

A6217 Gauze, nonimpregnated, nonsterile, pad size more than 16 sq in but less than or equal to 48 sq in, without adhesive border, each dressing

A6218 Gauze, nonimpregnated, nonsterile, pad size more than 48 sq in, without adhesive border, each dressing

A

A6219 Gauze, nonimpregnated, sterile, pad size 16 sq in or less, with any size adhesive border, each dressing

A6220 Gauze, nonimpregnated, sterile, pad size more than 16 sq in but less than or equal to 48 sq in, with any size adhesive border, each dressing

A6221 Gauze, nonimpregnated, sterile, pad size more than 48 sq in, with any size adhesive border, each dressing

Lay Description

Usual non-impregnated gauze dressing change is up to three times per day for a dressing without a border and once per day for a dressing with a border. It is usually not necessary to stack more than two gauze pads on top of each other in any one area.

A6222-A6233

A6222 Gauze, impregnated with other than water, normal saline, or hydrogel, sterile, pad size 16 sq in or less, without adhesive border, each dressing

A6223 Gauze, impregnated with other than water, normal saline, or hydrogel, sterile, pad size more than 16 sq in, but less than or equal to 48 sq in, without adhesive border, each dressing

A6224 Gauze, impregnated with other than water, normal saline, or hydrogel, sterile, pad size more than 48 sq in, without adhesive border, each dressing

A6228 Gauze, impregnated, water or normal saline, sterile, pad size 16 sq in or less, without adhesive border, each dressing

A6229 Gauze, impregnated, water or normal saline, sterile, pad size more than 16 sq in but less than or equal to 48 sq in, without adhesive border, each dressing

A6230 Gauze, impregnated, water or normal saline, sterile, pad size more than 48 sq in, without adhesive border, each dressing

A6231 Gauze, impregnated, hydrogel, for direct wound contact, sterile, pad size 16 sq in or less, each dressing

A6232 Gauze, impregnated, hydrogel, for direct wound contact, sterile, pad size greater than 16 sq in, but less than or equal to 48 sq in, each dressing

A6233 Gauze, impregnated, hydrogel, for direct wound contact, sterile, pad size more than 48 sq in, each dressing

Lay Description

Impregnated gauze dressings are woven or non-woven materials into which substances such as iodinated agents, petrolatum, zinc paste, crystalline sodium chloride, chlorhexidine gluconate (CHG), bismuth tribromophenate (BTP), water, aqueous saline, hydrogel, or other agents have been incorporated into the dressing material by the manufacturer.

A6234-A6241

A6234 Hydrocolloid dressing, wound cover, sterile, pad size 16 sq in or less, without adhesive border, each dressing

A6235 Hydrocolloid dressing, wound cover, sterile, pad size more than 16 sq in but less than or equal to 48 sq in, without adhesive border, each dressing

A6236 Hydrocolloid dressing, wound cover, sterile, pad size more than 48 sq in, without adhesive border, each dressing

A6237 Hydrocolloid dressing, wound cover, sterile, pad size 16 sq in or less, with any size adhesive border, each dressing

A6238 Hydrocolloid dressing, wound cover, sterile, pad size more than 16 sq in but less than or equal to 48 sq in, with any size adhesive border, each dressing

A6239 Hydrocolloid dressing, wound cover, sterile, pad size more than 48 sq in, with any size adhesive border, each dressing

A6240 Hydrocolloid dressing, wound filler, paste, sterile, per oz

A6241 Hydrocolloid dressing, wound filler, dry form, sterile, per g

Lay Description

Hydrocolloid dressings are covered for use on wounds with light to moderate exudate. Usual dressing change for hydrocolloid wound covers or hydrocolloid wound fillers is up to three times per week.

A6242-A6248

A6242 Hydrogel dressing, wound cover, sterile, pad size 16 sq in or less, without adhesive border, each dressing

A6243 Hydrogel dressing, wound cover, sterile, pad size more than 16 sq in but less than or equal to 48 sq in, without adhesive border, each dressing

A6244 Hydrogel dressing, wound cover, sterile, pad size more than 48 sq in, without adhesive border, each dressing

A6245 Hydrogel dressing, wound cover, sterile, pad size 16 sq in or less, with any size adhesive border, each dressing

A6246 Hydrogel dressing, wound cover, sterile, pad size more than 16 sq in but less than or equal to 48 sq in, with any size adhesive border, each dressing

A6247 Hydrogel dressing, wound cover, sterile, pad size more than 48 sq in, with any size adhesive border, each dressing

A6248 Hydrogel dressing, wound filler, gel, per fl oz

Lay Description

Hydrogel dressings are used on full thickness wounds with minimal or no exudate (e.g., stage III or IV ulcers). Hydrogel dressings are not usually medically necessary for stage II ulcers.

A6250

A6250 Skin sealants, protectants, moisturizers, ointments, any type, any size

Lay Description

Skin sealants and protectants are liquid barrier films made of polymers and solvents. The solvent evaporates after the sealant or protectant is applied to the skin, leaving behind a protective film. A moisturizer is a water and oil mixture. Ointments are oil in water emulsions. This code is used to report any type or size of skin sealant, protectant, moisturizer, or ointment when a more specific code is not available.

A6251-A6256

A6251 Specialty absorptive dressing, wound cover, sterile, pad size 16 sq in or less, without adhesive border, each dressing

A6252 Specialty absorptive dressing, wound cover, sterile, pad size more than 16 sq in but less than or equal to 48 sq in, without adhesive border, each dressing

A6253 Specialty absorptive dressing, wound cover, sterile, pad size more than 48 sq in, without adhesive border, each dressing

A6254 Specialty absorptive dressing, wound cover, sterile, pad size 16 sq in or less, with any size adhesive border, each dressing

A6255 Specialty absorptive dressing, wound cover, sterile, pad size more than 16 sq in but less than or equal to 48 sq in, with any size adhesive border, each dressing

A6256 Specialty absorptive dressing, wound cover, sterile, pad size more than 48 sq in, with any size adhesive border, each dressing

Lay Description

Specialty absorptive dressings are unitized multi-layer dressings that provide either a semi-adherent quality or nonadherent layer and highly absorptive layers of fibers, such as absorbent cellulose, cotton, or rayon. These may or may not have an adhesive border.

A6257-A6259

A6257 Transparent film, sterile, 16 sq in or less, each dressing

A6258 Transparent film, sterile, more than 16 sq in but less than or equal to 48 sq in, each dressing

A6259 Transparent film, sterile, more than 48 sq in, each dressing

Lay Description

Transparent film dressings are used on closed wounds or open partial thickness wounds with minimal exudate. Usual dressing change is up to three times per week.

A6260

A6260 Wound cleansers, any type, any size

Lay Description

This code reports wound cleansers of any type and any size that do not a have more specific code listed. Wound cleansers remove wound debris as the wound is cleansed and washed. Wound cleansers are often over-the-counter products that can be used as a rinse or can be sprayed on the wound.

A6261-A6262

A6261 Wound filler, gel/paste, per fl oz, not otherwise specified

A6262 Wound filler, dry form, per g, not otherwise specified

Lay Description

Wound fillers are dressing materials that are placed into open wounds to eliminate dead space and absorb exudate, or maintain a moist wound surface. Use these codes for wound fillers, gel/paste, or dry form not specifically listed elsewhere. Usual dressing change is up to once per day.

A6266

A6266 Gauze, impregnated, other than water, normal saline, or zinc paste, sterile, any width, per linear yd

Lay Description

Impregnated gauze dressings are woven or non-woven materials in which substances such as iodinated agents, petrolatum, zinc compounds, crystalline sodium chloride, chlorhexidine gluconate (CHG), bismuth tribromophenate (BTP), water, aqueous saline, or other agents have been incorporated into the dressing material by the manufacturer.

A

A6402-A6404

A6402   Gauze, nonimpregnated, sterile, pad size 16 sq in or less, without adhesive border, each dressing

A6403   Gauze, nonimpregnated, sterile, pad size more than 16 sq in, less than or equal to 48 sq in, without adhesive border, each dressing

A6404   Gauze, nonimpregnated, sterile, pad size more than 48 sq in, without adhesive border, each dressing

Lay Description

Usual non-impregnated gauze dressing change is up to three times per day for a dressing without a border and once per day for a dressing with a border. It is usually not necessary to stack more than two gauze pads on top of each other in any one area.

A6407

A6407   Packing strips, nonimpregnated, sterile, up to 2 in in width, per linear yd

Lay Description

Packing strips are placed in open wounds and are often used in wet-to-dry type of wound treatment. They are sterile supplies that are usually made of fine mesh cotton gauze. Some are impregnated with antiseptics, such as iodoform.

A6410-A6412

A6410   Eye pad, sterile, each

A6411   Eye pad, nonsterile, each

A6412   Eye patch, occlusive, each

Lay Description

Eye pads are used to protect an injured eye from further injury by keeping the eyelid closed. Eye pads are usually constructed of soft absorbent cotton covered by fine mesh gauze and contoured to fit the eye. They may be sterile or nonsterile supplies. An occlusive eye patch may be used to protect an injured eye or to treat a condition such as amblyopia. Light occlusive eye patches, in addition to providing a soft absorbent pad, contain a film on the outer surface that blocks specific wavelengths of light.

A6413

A6413   Adhesive bandage, first aid type, any size, each

Lay Description

An adhesive bandage is a sterile piece of gauze or other absorptive material affixed to a fabric or film that has been coated with a pressure-sensitive adhesive.

A6441

A6441   Padding bandage, nonelastic, nonwoven/nonknitted, width greater than or equal to 3 in and less than 5 in, per yd

Lay Description

A nonelastic, nonwoven/nonknitted padding bandage is used to pad and protect the wound surface.

A6442-A6447

A6442   Conforming bandage, nonelastic, knitted/woven, nonsterile, width less than 3 in, per yd

A6443   Conforming bandage, nonelastic, knitted/woven, nonsterile, width greater than or equal to 3 in and less than 5 in, per yd

A6444   Conforming bandage, nonelastic, knitted/woven, nonsterile, width greater than or equal to 5 in, per yd

A6445   Conforming bandage, nonelastic, knitted/woven, sterile, width less than 3 in, per yd

A6446   Conforming bandage, nonelastic, knitted/woven, sterile, width greater than or equal to 3 in and less than 5 in, per yd

A6447   Conforming bandage, nonelastic, knitted/woven, sterile, width greater than or equal to 5 in, per yd

Lay Description

Nonelastic conforming bandages are made of a knitted, crocheted, or woven material that allows them to stretch. Nonelastic conforming bandages are supplied in rolls that are then used to wrap the wound. Other dressings such as 2 X 2's or 4 X 4's may be layered under and held in place by the conforming bandage.

A6448-A6452

A6448   Light compression bandage, elastic, knitted/woven, width less than 3 in, per yd

A6449   Light compression bandage, elastic, knitted/woven, width greater than or equal to 3 in and less than 5 in, per yd

A6450   Light compression bandage, elastic, knitted/woven, width greater than or equal to 5 in, per yd

A6451   Moderate compression bandage, elastic, knitted/woven, load resistance of 1.25 to 1.34 ft lbs at 50% maximum stretch, width greater than or equal to 3 in and less than 5 in, per yd

A6452 **High compression bandage, elastic, knitted/woven, load resistance greater than or equal to 1.35 ft lbs at 50% maximum stretch, width greater than or equal to 3 in and less than 5 in, per yd**

Lay Description
Elastic, knitted/woven compression bandages are used as support wraps for conditions such as sprains, strains, and venous ulcers. They come in a variety of types, including variable stretch, limited stretch, and high stretch, that provide varying degrees of compression. The type used depends on the condition or injury being treated.

A6453-A6455

A6453 **Self-adherent bandage, elastic, nonknitted/nonwoven, width less than 3 in, per yd**

A6454 **Self-adherent bandage, elastic, nonknitted/nonwoven, width greater than or equal to 3 in and less than 5 in, per yd**

A6455 **Self-adherent bandage, elastic, nonknitted/nonwoven, width greater than or equal to 5 in, per yd**

Lay Description
Elastic, self-adherent, nonknitted/nonwoven bandages are composed of laminated nonwoven and elastic materials. The wrap is made of a material that will stick to itself, but will not adhere to other fabrics, materials, or the skin. It is supplied in rolls in a variety of widths.

A6456

A6456 **Zinc paste impregnated bandage, nonelastic, knitted/woven, width greater than or equal to 3 in and less than 5 in, per yd**

Lay Description
A nonelastic, knitted/woven zinc paste-impregnated bandage may be used as a wrap for venous insufficiency or other conditions. Zinc oxide paste-impregnated bandages stay soft and flexible and conform to the leg to promote healing. A zinc oxide paste-impregnated bandage is typically used under a compression bandage, which is reported separately.

A6457

A6457 **Tubular dressing with or without elastic, any width, per linear yd**

Lay Description
Tubular dressing is a secondary dressing used to secure the primary dressing. It is used as an alternative to a gauze wrap or adhesive tape. Tubular dressings are available in a variety of materials, including synthetic materials such as nylon or natural materials such as cotton. Some types of tubular dressings

require application using a metal cage device while others can be placed by hand.

A6501-A6513

A6501 **Compression burn garment, bodysuit (head to foot), custom fabricated**

A6502 **Compression burn garment, chin strap, custom fabricated**

A6503 **Compression burn garment, facial hood, custom fabricated**

A6504 **Compression burn garment, glove to wrist, custom fabricated**

A6505 **Compression burn garment, glove to elbow, custom fabricated**

A6506 **Compression burn garment, glove to axilla, custom fabricated**

A6507 **Compression burn garment, foot to knee length, custom fabricated**

A6508 **Compression burn garment, foot to thigh length, custom fabricated**

A6509 **Compression burn garment, upper trunk to waist including arm openings (vest), custom fabricated**

A6510 **Compression burn garment, trunk, including arms down to leg openings (leotard), custom fabricated**

A6511 **Compression burn garment, lower trunk including leg openings (panty), custom fabricated**

A6512 **Compression burn garment, not otherwise classified**

A6513 **Compression burn mask, face and/or neck, plastic or equal, custom fabricated**

Lay Description
Compression burn garments are used to reduce hypertrophic scarring and joint contractures following a burn injury.

A6530-A6535

A6530 **Gradient compression stocking, below knee, 18-30 mm Hg, each**

A6531 **Gradient compression stocking, below knee, 30-40 mm Hg, each**

A6532 **Gradient compression stocking, below knee, 40-50 mm Hg, each**

A6533 **Gradient compression stocking, thigh length, 18-30 mm Hg, each**

A6534 **Gradient compression stocking, thigh length, 30-40 mm Hg, each**

A6535 **Gradient compression stocking, thigh length, 40-50 mm Hg, each**

Lay Description
This range of codes reports the supply of below-the-knee and thigh length compression stockings. These stockings may be prescribed for a variety of conditions, such as prevention of deep vein thrombosis (DVT) or postoperative prevention of venous thromboembolisms. Gradient compression

A

refers to the difference in pressure exerted over the length of the stocking. For example, the squeezing pressure at the ankle is usually greatest, gradually diminishing proximally toward the calf area. The pressure is expressed in millimeters of mercury (mmHg). The patient's anatomical dimensions and the presence of edema can affect sizing of these stockings. Pressures less than 15 mmHg are generally considered less than therapeutic. Pressures in the 18 to 20 mmHg range are considered mildly therapeutic for minor varicosity. Pressures in the 20 to 30 mmHg range are considered firm while those above 30 mmHg are considered extra firm.

A6536-A6538

A6536   **Gradient compression stocking, full-length/chap style, 18-30 mm Hg, each**

A6537   **Gradient compression stocking, full-length/chap style, 30-40 mm Hg, each**

A6538   **Gradient compression stocking, full-length/chap style, 40-50 mm Hg, each**

Lay Description
This range of codes reports the supply of full length, chap style compression stockings. These stockings may be prescribed for a variety of conditions, such as prevention of deep vein thrombosis (DVT) or postoperative prevention of venous thromboembolisms. Gradient compression refers to the difference in pressure exerted over the length of the stocking. For example, the squeezing pressure at the ankle is usually greatest, gradually diminishing proximally toward the thigh and waist region. The pressure is expressed in millimeters of mercury (mmHg). The patient's anatomical dimensions and the presence of edema can affect sizing of these stockings. Pressures less than 15 mmHg are generally considered less than therapeutic. Pressures in the 18 to 20 mmHg range are considered mildly therapeutic for minor varicosity. Pressures in the 20 to 30 mmHg range are considered firm while those above 30 mmHg are considered extra firm.

A6539-A6544

A6539   **Gradient compression stocking, waist length, 18-30 mm Hg, each**

A6540   **Gradient compression stocking, waist length, 30-40 mm Hg, each**

A6541   **Gradient compression stocking, waist length, 40-50 mm Hg, each**

A6544   **Gradient compression stocking, garter belt**

Lay Description
This range of codes reports the supply of waist length compression stockings and related supplies for compression garments, as well as other supplies and accessories used with compression stockings. These stockings may be prescribed for a variety of conditions, such as prevention of deep vein thrombosis (DVT) or postoperative prevention of venous thromboembolisms. Gradient compression

refers to the difference in pressure exerted over the length of the stocking. For example, the squeezing pressure at the ankle is usually greatest, gradually diminishing proximally toward the thigh and waist region. The pressure is expressed in millimeters of mercury (mmHg). The patient's anatomical dimensions and the presence of edema can affect sizing of these stockings. Pressures less than 15 mmHg are generally considered less than therapeutic. Pressures in the 18 to 20 mmHg range are considered mildly therapeutic for minor varicosity. Pressures in the 20 to 30 mmHg range are considered firm, while those above 30 mmHg are considered extra firm.

A6545-A6549

A6545   **Gradient compression wrap, nonelastic, below knee, 30-50 mm Hg, each**

A6549   **Gradient compression stocking/sleeve, not otherwise specified**

Lay Description
This code reports the supply of a below knee gradient compression wrap. It uses adjustable bands to provide therapeutic compression levels. Compression wraps may be prescribed for a variety of conditions, such as lymphedema, and to treat venous disease and active venous stasis ulcers. Surgical removal of lymph nodes can cause lymphedema, a condition hallmarked by fluid retention and swelling in the affected extremity. Gradient compression refers to the difference in pressure exerted over the length of the wrap. For example, the squeezing pressure at the ankle is usually greatest, gradually diminishing proximally toward the thigh and waist region. The pressure is expressed in millimeters of mercury (mmHg). The components of the gradient wrap are a nonelastic binder that is fitted at the prescribed compression level using markers on the neoprene strip and a built in pressure system that runs posterior length of the device.

A6550

A6550   **Wound care set, for negative pressure wound therapy electrical pump, includes all supplies and accessories**

Lay Description
Negative pressure wound therapy (NPWT), also called vacuum assisted closure (VAC), uses subatmospheric pressure to assist in treatment of acute, subacute, and chronic wounds. NPWT promotes healing by increasing local vascularity and oxygenation of the wound bed, evacuating wound fluid thereby reducing edema, and removing exudates and bacteria. The subatmospheric pressure is generated using an electrical pump that is reported as a separate supply (E2402). The electrical pump conveys intermittent or continuous subatmospheric pressure through connecting tubing to a specialized wound dressing. A specialized wound dressing includes porous foam dressing that covers the entire wound surface and an airtight adhesive dressing that seals the wound and

contains the subatmospheric pressure at the wound site. Each wound care set inclusive of all supplies and accessories is reported with A6550.

A7000-A7002

A7000 Canister, disposable, used with suction pump, each

A7001 Canister, nondisposable, used with suction pump, each

A7002 Tubing, used with suction pump, each

Lay Description
Canisters to be used with suction pumps can be disposable or non-disposable. Canisters are made of a hard plastic and are used for collecting aspirated materials. Although they vary in size, they usually hold approximately 800 cc to 1200 cc and have a lid and splash guard. Tubing runs from the suction catheter to the canister to deliver the aspirated material.

A7003-A7006

A7003 Administration set, with small volume nonfiltered pneumatic nebulizer, disposable

A7004 Small volume nonfiltered pneumatic nebulizer, disposable

A7005 Administration set, with small volume nonfiltered pneumatic nebulizer, nondisposable

A7006 Administration set, with small volume filtered pneumatic nebulizer

Lay Description
Nebulizer base equipment is comprised of an air compressor for airflow nebulization or a generator for nebulization of liquid by means of ultrasonic vibrations. The actual nebulizer is the chamber in which the nebulization of the liquid medication or solution for inhalation occurs. The nebulizing chamber is attached to the aerosol compressor or an ultrasonic generator. Nebulization therapy is considered beneficial to patients with a variety of respiratory and/or pulmonary conditions and diseases, including cystic fibrosis, bronchiectasis, chronic obstructive pulmonary disease, emphysema, severe asthma (when metered dose inhalers are ineffective), as well as other conditions such as AIDS, which requires the administration of medications like pentamidine. Small volume nebulizers are designed primarily to deliver inhalation medications. Nebulization occurs when the medication and/or solution to be administered is vaporized and subsequently inspired by the patient via the lungs, through which the medication enters the patient's system, or the medication has a direct effect on mucus retained by the lungs and bronchi (known as mucolytic action). Various accessory supplies may be required for use with the nebulizer.

A7007-A7012

A7007 Large volume nebulizer, disposable, unfilled, used with aerosol compressor

A7008 Large volume nebulizer, disposable, prefilled, used with aerosol compressor

A7009 Reservoir bottle, nondisposable, used with large volume ultrasonic nebulizer

A7010 Corrugated tubing, disposable, used with large volume nebulizer, 100 ft

A7011 Corrugated tubing, nondisposable, used with large volume nebulizer, 10 ft

A7012 Water collection device, used with large volume nebulizer

Lay Description
Nebulizer base equipment is comprised of an air compressor for airflow nebulization or a generator for nebulization of liquid by means of ultrasonic vibrations. The actual nebulizer is the chamber in which the nebulization occurs. The nebulizing chamber is attached to the aerosol compressor or an ultrasonic generator. Large volume nebulizers are designed to deliver humidified gas, such as oxygen, in concentrations ranging from 28 percent to 98 percent along with medications. Large volume nebulizers are useful in the treatment of conditions such as cystic fibrosis, bronchiectasis, and tracheostomy where humidified gas assists in thinning respiratory secretions. Large volume nebulizers are also useful for administration of pentamidine in the treatment of HIV. Various accessory supplies may be required for use with the nebulizer.

A7013-A7016

A7013 Filter, disposable, used with aerosol compressor or ultrasonic generator

A7014 Filter, nondisposable, used with aerosol compressor or ultrasonic generator

A7015 Aerosol mask, used with DME nebulizer

A7016 Dome and mouthpiece, used with small volume ultrasonic nebulizer

Lay Description
Nebulizer base equipment is comprised of an air compressor for airflow nebulization or a generator for nebulization of liquid by means of ultrasonic vibrations. The actual nebulizer is the chamber in which the nebulization occurs. The nebulizing chamber is attached to the aerosol compressor or an ultrasonic generator. Various accessory supplies may be required for use with the nebulizer.

A7017

A7017 Nebulizer, durable, glass or autoclavable plastic, bottle type, not used with oxygen

Lay Description
A nebulizer is an apparatus for producing a fine spray or mist. This may be made by rapidly passing air through a liquid or by vibrating a liquid at a high frequency so that the particles produced are

A

extremely small. Use this code to report a durable, bottle-type nebulizer made of glass or plastic that can be sterilized in an autoclave and is not used with oxygen.

A7018

A7018   **Water, distilled, used with large volume nebulizer, 1000 ml**

Lay Description

Nebulizer base equipment is comprised of an air compressor for airflow nebulization or a generator for nebulization of liquid by means of ultrasonic vibrations. The actual nebulizer is the chamber in which the nebulization occurs. The nebulizing chamber is attached to the aerosol compressor or an ultrasonic generator. Large volume nebulizers are designed to deliver humidified gas, such as oxygen, in concentrations ranging from 28 percent to 98 percent along with medications. Large volume nebulizers are useful in the treatment of conditions such as cystic fibrosis, bronchiectasis, and tracheostomy where humidified gas assists in thinning respiratory secretions. Large volume nebulizers are also useful for administration of pentamidine in the treatment of HIV. Various accessory supplies may be required for use with the nebulizer.

A7020

A7020   **Interface for cough stimulating device, includes all components, replacement only**

Lay Description

Cough stimulating devices are used for people who are not able to cough to remove secretions from the lungs. Components for the cough stimulator should be replaced every two months to reduce the risk of infection and to ensure that the components are not worn out. This code represents a replacement patient interface device. Patient interface devices include a face mask, mouthpiece, or tracheal adapter.

A7025-A7026

A7025   **High frequency chest wall oscillation system vest, replacement for use with patient-owned equipment, each**

A7026   **High frequency chest wall oscillation system hose, replacement for use with patient-owned equipment, each**

Lay Description

These codes report replacement supplies that are used with a patient owned, high-frequency chest wall oscillation (HFCWO) system. The vest component consists of an inflatable vest connected by tubes to an air-pulse generator. The air-pulse generator rapidly inflates and deflates the vest, compressing and releasing the chest wall. HFCWO allows the patient to clear mucus by generating increased airflow velocities that create repetitive cough-like shear forces and decrease the viscosity of secretions.

A7027-A7039

A7027   **Combination oral/nasal mask, used with continuous positive airway pressure device, each**

A7028   **Oral cushion for combination oral/nasal mask, replacement only, each**

A7029   **Nasal pillows for combination oral/nasal mask, replacement only, pair**

A7030   **Full face mask used with positive airway pressure device, each**

A7031   **Face mask interface, replacement for full face mask, each**

A7032   **Cushion for use on nasal mask interface, replacement only, each**

A7033   **Pillow for use on nasal cannula type interface, replacement only, pair**

A7034   **Nasal interface (mask or cannula type) used with positive airway pressure device, with or without head strap**

A7035   **Headgear used with positive airway pressure device**

A7036   **Chinstrap used with positive airway pressure device**

A7037   **Tubing used with positive airway pressure device**

A7038   **Filter, disposable, used with positive airway pressure device**

A7039   **Filter, nondisposable, used with positive airway pressure device**

Lay Description

CPAP is a noninvasive method of providing air pressure through the patient's nostrils, usually through a nasal mask or flow generator system. These devices are used primarily in conservative therapy (vs. surgery) for patients with documented sleep apnea; however, not all patients benefit from this conservative approach because some cannot tolerate the CPAP device during sleep. The CPAP device assists the patient in nocturnal respiration (during sleep), particularly when the patient's oropharyngeal tissues relax, collapse, and/or otherwise obstruct the normal airflow during inspiration and expiration, causing a variety of symptoms including hypersomnolence during the day, loss of concentration, headache, agitation, depression, fatigue, and many others.

A7040-A7041

A7040   **One way chest drain valve**

A7041   **Water seal drainage container and tubing for use with implanted chest tube**

Lay Description

Chest tubes are inserted into the pleural space to drain blood, fluid, or air from the pleural cavity and to allow full expansion of the lungs. The chest tube is inserted through an incision between the ribs into the pleural space and connected to a water seal system to prevent air from being sucked into the chest cavity and to allow the continuous or intermittent removal of fluid. A water seal thoracic drainage unit for removal of fluids from the thoracic cavity of a patient can use one, two, or three containers. A single-container water seal consists of a drainage collection container that also serves as the water seal. The container is initially filled with 100 ml of sterile water to form the seal. A two-container water seal is comprised of a collection chamber for receiving fluids from the patient and a second container that provides the underwater seal. Generally, the water or other liquid for the seal is provided with the collection chamber and water seal container as a complete unit ready for use. A three-container water seal system uses a collection chamber, a water seal container, and a third container that provides suction control.

A7042

Lay Description
An implantable pleural catheter and drainage kit is used for long-term treatment of symptomatic, chronic/recurrent, malignant, pleural effusion. This type of implantable catheter allows intermittent drainage of the effusion. The small-bore catheter consists of three sections: internal, middle, and external. The internal section has a fenestrated end that is placed into the pleural space. The middle section is tunneled through the skin for several inches. The external section includes an exposed length of catheter with a one-way valve. A separate drainage kit is required that includes a lightweight, plastic, vacuum drainage bottle and tubing. Each day or as needed the patient or caregiver drains the pleural fluid by temporarily attaching the external length of catheter to the tubing, which is connected to the pre-evacuated (vacuum) drainage bottle.

A7044

A7044 Oral interface used with positive airway pressure device, each

Lay Description
This code reports the supply of each oral interface used with a positive airway pressure (PAP) device. Such devices may also be prescribed for use on a continuous basis (CPAP). The oral interface may be a removable tube-like component that the patient uses during treatment.

A7045

A7045 Exhalation port with or without swivel used with accessories for positive airway devices, replacement only

Lay Description
Some masks used with positive pressure airway devices require the use of an accessory supply called an exhalation port to function properly. An exhalation port allows predetermined amounts of exhaled air to "leak" through the exhalation port. This is necessary to properly exhaust exhaled CO_2 from the mask so the patient does not rebreathe the CO_2. Some masks have a swivel device that allows the circuit tubing to move freely.

A7046

A7046 Water chamber for humidifier, used with positive airway pressure device, replacement, each

Lay Description
Some humidifiers used with positive airway pressure devices have separate water chambers. The water chamber holds the water used in the humidifier. Removable water chambers are more easily cleaned. This code reports replacement of a removable water chamber.

A7047

A7047 Oral interface used with respiratory suction pump, each

Lay Description
Oral interface used with respiratory suction pump is a replacement piece used with a portable home model respiratory suction pump. A portable home model respiratory suction pump is a lightweight, compact, electric aspirator designed for upper respiratory oral pharyngeal and tracheal suction to be used in the home.

A7048

A7048 Vacuum drainage collection unit and tubing kit, including all supplies needed for collection unit change, for use with implanted catheter, each

Lay Description
An implantable pleural catheter and drainage kit is used for long-term treatment of symptomatic, chronic/recurrent, malignant, pleural effusion. This type of implantable catheter allows intermittent drainage of the effusion. The small-bore catheter consists of three sections: internal, middle, and external. The internal section has a fenestrated end that is placed into the pleural space. The middle section is tunneled through the skin for several inches. The external section includes an exposed length of catheter with a one-way valve. A separate drainage kit is required that includes a lightweight, plastic, vacuum drainage bottle and tubing. Each day or as needed the patient or caregiver drains the pleural fluid by temporarily attaching the external length of catheter to the tubing, which is connected to the pre-evacuated (vacuum) drainage bottle.

A

A7501-A7502

A7501 Tracheostoma valve, including diaphragm, each

A7502 Replacement diaphragm/faceplate for tracheostoma valve, each

Lay Description

This code reports the supply of a tracheostoma valve, including diaphragm. These devices are typically used by laryngectomees who retain a level of potential voice function. Designs such as the prototypical Blom-Singer provide the user a means to speak without first manually occluding the stoma with a finger. Tracheostoma valves are often two-unit devices. A faceplate inserts over the tracheostoma. A disposable diaphragm in the valve can be adjusted to control airflow through the stomal opening. When the diaphragm is closed, or near closed, speech can be accomplished. The diaphragm may be set to allow one-way airflow upon expiration.

A7503-A7506

A7503 Filter holder or filter cap, reusable, for use in a tracheostoma heat and moisture exchange system, each

A7504 Filter for use in a tracheostoma heat and moisture exchange system, each

A7505 Housing, reusable without adhesive, for use in a heat and moisture exchange system and/or with a tracheostoma valve, each

A7506 Adhesive disc for use in a heat and moisture exchange system and/or with tracheostoma valve, any type each

Lay Description

A tracheostoma heat and moisture exchange system is used by some tracheostomy patients to add warmth and water vapor to the air when they inhale. A heat and moisture exchange system can retain up to 60 percent of the humidity in the patient's airway, greatly reducing coughing and mucus production. It consists of a reusable plastic holder or cap, also referred to as a cassette, that contains a filter made of foam, paper, or other material. The holder fits into reusable plastic housing that is held in place over the tracheostoma by an adhesive disc. A heat and moisture exchanger may be used by itself or in addition to a tracheostoma valve.

A7507-A7509

A7507 Filter holder and integrated filter without adhesive, for use in a tracheostoma heat and moisture exchange system, each

A7508 Housing and integrated adhesive, for use in a tracheostoma heat and moisture exchange system and/or with a tracheostoma valve, each

A7509 Filter holder and integrated filter housing, and adhesive, for use as a tracheostoma heat and moisture exchange system, each

Lay Description

A tracheostoma heat and moisture exchange system is used by some tracheostomy patients to add warmth and water vapor to the air when they inhale. A heat and moisture exchange system can retain up to 60 percent of the humidity in the patient's airway, greatly reducing coughing and mucus production. Some heat and moisture exchange systems use integrated components.

A7520-A7522

A7520 Tracheostomy/laryngectomy tube, noncuffed, polyvinylchloride (PVC), silicone or equal, each

A7521 Tracheostomy/laryngectomy tube, cuffed, polyvinylchloride (PVC), silicone or equal, each

A7522 Tracheostomy/laryngectomy tube, stainless steel or equal (sterilizable and reusable), each

Lay Description

A tracheostomy/laryngectomy tube, also called a trach tube, is a curved tube that is inserted into a tracheostomy stoma (the surgically created hole made in the neck and windpipe). Tracheostomy tubes can be made of a variety of materials including metal, plastic, or silicone. Plastic and silicone tubes have the advantage of being lighter weight with less crusting of secretions than with metal tubes. Tracheostomy tubes come in cuffed and uncuffed models. A cuff is a soft balloon around the distal (far) end of the tube. The cuff is inflated with air, foam, or sterile water to allow for mechanical ventilation in patients with respiratory failure. Cuffs can be low or high volume. The low volume cuff is round while a high volume cuff is barrel-shaped. The high volume cuff spreads the pressure out over a larger surface area and may be better at averting complications such as stenosis than the low volume cuff that tends to push on one spot in the airway. When the balloon is deflated, the tube allows air around the tube for vocalization.

A7523

A7523 Tracheostomy shower protector, each

Lay Description

A tracheostomy shower protector is used to protect the tracheostomy stoma (the surgically created hole made in the neck and windpipe) from water, soaps, and shampoos when showering. Tracheostomy shower protectors are made of waterproof materials such as latex and fit like a bib over the stoma site to shield and deflect the water from the stoma site when showering.

A7524

A7524 Tracheostoma stent/stud/button, each

Lay Description
A tracheostoma stent, stud, or button is a rigid cannula that is placed into the tracheostoma after removal of a tracheostomy tube. These devices are used primarily for conditions such as obstructive sleep apnea where the patient requires the tracheostoma for breathing at night, but does not need it for breathing during the day. A stent, stud, or button allows the stoma to be closed and the patient to breathe through the nose and mouth instead of through the tracheostoma site during the day. These devices do not extend into the tracheal lumen so patients are able to breathe and talk normally when these types of devices are in place.

A7525

A7525 Tracheostomy mask, each

Lay Description
Tracheostomy masks are used in conjunction with nebulizers. They are composed of a flexible, mask-shaped plastic covering that fits securely over the tracheostomy tube. The outer portion has an opening that connects with the nebulizer tubing. Masks are used for ventilation and to humidify inspired air.

A7526

A7526 Tracheostomy tube collar/holder, each

Lay Description
A tracheostomy tube collar or holder attaches to each side of the tracheostomy tube and loosely wraps around the back of the neck. A tracheostomy tube holder or collar is used to secure the tracheostomy tube in place. Collars and holders are made of a variety of materials that include stainless steel metal chains, laminates of foam and nylon, plastics, and other materials.

A7527

A7527 Tracheostomy/laryngectomy tube plug/stop, each

Lay Description
This code reports the specialized plug or stopper for use with a tracheostomy, fenestration, or laryngectomy tube, which the patient has in place. The plug, also called a decannulation plug, is used to obstruct the proximal end of the tube and permit breathing through the fenestration and the upper airway. Using the plug with the tube facilitates weaning in preparation for extubation and aids in speaking.

A8000-A8004

A8000 Helmet, protective, soft, prefabricated, includes all components and accessories

A8001 Helmet, protective, hard, prefabricated, includes all components and accessories

A8002 Helmet, protective, soft, custom fabricated, includes all components and accessories

A8003 Helmet, protective, hard, custom fabricated, includes all components and accessories

A8004 Soft interface for helmet, replacement only

Lay Description
Protective helmets are head coverings used to prevent or lessen injury or damage to the head. The helmets may be composed of hard material such as hard plastic or soft material such as nylon or fabric. Protective helmets may be used to protect patients prone to falling or hitting their head. Prefabricated helmets are pre-made and are usually purchased off the shelf. Custom-fabricated helmets are constructed specifically for a patient using the patient's physical measurements and needs. Helmets may contain straps or belts to hold the helmet on the head.

A9150

A9150 Nonprescription drugs

Lay Description
This code reports drugs that do not require a prescription, also referred to as over-the-counter (OTC) drugs. Identify the specific drug provided, as well as the strength, amount, and condition being treated.

A9152-A9153

A9152 Single vitamin/mineral/trace element, oral, per dose, not otherwise specified

A9153 Multiple vitamins, with or without minerals and trace elements, oral, per dose, not otherwise specified

Lay Description
Vitamins are organic substances found in small amounts within foods. Minerals are nonorganic solid substances found in the earth's crust. Trace mineral elements occur in very small amounts. These are essential nutrients needed by the body in varying, small amounts for proper metabolic function.

A9155

A9155 Artificial saliva, 30 ml

Lay Description
Natural saliva is more than 99 percent water, with some buffering agents, enzymes, and minerals. Saliva coats, lubricates, and helps cleanse the tissues in the

A

mouth. It also begins the digestive process as we chew. When the saliva glands do not produce enough saliva, the mouth becomes dry. Artificial saliva is intended to replace natural saliva. Artificial saliva usually contains water, a mixture of buffering agents, cellulose derivatives, and flavoring agents. However, it does not contain the digestive and antibacterial enzymes, other proteins, or minerals present in real saliva. Artificial saliva is used to treat xerostomia, or dry mouth, which results from an inadequate flow of saliva. Drying irritates the soft tissues in the mouth, which can make them inflamed and more susceptible to infection.

A9180

A9180   Pediculosis (lice infestation) treatment, topical, for administration by patient/caretaker

Lay Description
A pediculicide is a topical medication applied to hair used to treat lice infestations. Pediculicides are available in both over-the-counter (OTC) formulas and by prescription. OTC formulas include pyrethrins, a natural extract from the chrysanthemum flower, sometimes in combination with piperonyl butoxide. Another OTC formula is permethrin. Treatment is the same regardless of whether an OTC or prescription medication is used. The pediculicide is applied to unwashed hair. After approximately eight to 12 hours, the hair should be checked for live lice. The hair should be combed to remove dead lice and any remaining live lice. The hair should be combed daily with a fine tooth or nit comb and checked every two to three days for the presence of live lice. The hair should be retreated seven to 10 days after the first treatment.

A9270

A9270   Noncovered item or service

Lay Description
Noncovered services are services that are billed to the patient. In many cases, the beneficiary is already aware that the services are noncovered because they are included in the information given in the Medicare handbook (e.g., oral medications, screening mammograms in less than the designated waiting period, etc.) or by their insurance provider. At other times, the services are listed as noncovered because they are considered either experimental or investigational in nature.

A9272

A9272   Wound suction, disposable, includes dressing, all accessories and components, any type, each

Lay Description
Wound suction devices are used to remove excess fluids such as blood, pus, serosanguineous fluid, and tissue secretions, from wounds. A build up of fluids

can cause infection and delay of healing. Mechanical suction uses nonelectrical powered methods, such as springs, to create suction around the wound to draw out the fluid. The fluid is collected in absorbant dressings. The device may have straps or belts to attach the device to the patient. The suction device can be left in place for several days. The system is disposable and is designed for single use. This code includes the cartridges, tubing, dressing, and any other accessories.

A9273

A9273   Hot water bottle, ice cap or collar, heat and/or cold wrap, any type

Lay Description
An ice cap or collar is a cold therapy application to deliver treatment to affected tissues, usually following a surgical procedure or trauma. Cold therapy is generally used in the immediate postoperative or post-trauma period to reduce edema and control pain. An ice cap or collar is a passive method to deliver cold therapy. A hot water bottle is a container, usually made of plastic or rubber, which may be filled with hot or cold water and applied to an injured or painful body part.

A9274

A9274   External ambulatory insulin delivery system, disposable, each, includes all supplies and accessories

Lay Description
External ambulatory insulin delivery systems, also called insulin pumps, are computerized, battery-powered delivery devices with programming capabilities. These devices are used as a treatment for people with insulin-dependent diabetes mellitus. A sterile reservoir is filled with rapid-acting insulin. The sterile reservoir is connected to the patient by a thin plastic tube that has a small catheter needle attached. The needle is usually inserted into the subcutaneous tissue of the abdomen. The device continuously delivers micro-doses of insulin at a programmed rate.

A9275

A9275   Home glucose disposable monitor, includes test strips

Lay Description
Glucometers are used for patients with all types of diabetes mellitus to monitor blood glucose and are available in a variety of models with various features, including disposable home glucose monitors. Whether or not the patient is on insulin, many diabetics require frequent, if not daily, blood glucose monitoring. For Type I diabetes mellitus patients who require insulin (the patient's body does not manufacture insulin and therefore it must come from an external source, such as injections), blood glucose monitoring is a life-sustaining requirement. Disposable types of home glucose monitors are

provided with test strips that are inserted into the monitor to provide a glucose reading. When all of the test strips have been used or upon the expiration date of the meter, whichever comes first, the patient discards the entire unit (meter and any remaining test strips).

A9276-A9278

A9276 Sensor; invasive (e.g., subcutaneous), disposable, for use with interstitial continuous glucose monitoring system, 1 unit = 1 day supply

A9277 Transmitter; external, for use with interstitial continuous glucose monitoring system

A9278 Receiver (monitor); external, for use with interstitial continuous glucose monitoring system

Lay Description
Continuous glucose monitoring systems make continuous measurements of glucose levels. Many of these devices take measurements from subcutaneous tissue rather than from blood. Most systems consist of a sensor that is attached to the back of the arm or abdomen. The sensor has a very thin wire that is inserted subcutaneously. The wire then measures the glucose level in interstitial fluid that exits between the cells. The sensor is attached to a transmitter that sends the glucose readings to a wireless receiver. The receiver is a small computerized device that records and stores the glucose readings. These HCPCS Level II codes represent replacement components for a continuous glucose monitoring system.

A9279

A9279 Monitoring feature/device, stand-alone or integrated, any type, includes all accessories, components and electronics, not otherwise classified

Lay Description
This code may be applied to numerous technologies and is a nonspecific monitoring device. It represents an entire system, whether stand-alone or integrated into a delivery system. It includes all accessories, components, and electronics. Report a more specific code if there is one available.

A9280

A9280 Alert or alarm device, not otherwise classified

Lay Description
This code reports alert or alarm devices that do not have a more specific code available. A detailed description of the device may be required when reporting this code.

A9281

A9281 Reaching/grabbing device, any type, any length, each

Lay Description
A reaching/grabbing device is used to pick up objects without twisting the wrist. It typically lifts objects that are 5 pounds. or less. It is often used by people who have difficulty lifting objects due to arthritic conditions, small hands, or who have restrictive movement.

A9282

A9282 Wig, any type, each

Lay Description
A wig is hairpiece of human or artificial hair worn as personal adornment or to conceal baldness. A wig or hairpiece is a supply for hair loss.

A9283

A9283 Foot pressure off loading/supportive device, any type, each

Lay Description
This code reflects various devices used to reduce pressure on the foot to help prevent ulcers. The device usually has an antibacterial layer and an inner layer that may contain gel, foam, small beads, or other pressure reducing material that help support and redistribute the pressure of the foot. The patient can usually adjust the device as needed.

A9284

A9284 Spirometer, nonelectronic, includes all accessories

Lay Description
A spirometer measures pulmonary function. It measures the lung output on both inspiration and expiration and is used to track and diagnose a number of respiratory and cardiac conditions. It may also be used to keep the lungs clear and functioning.

A9300

A9300 Exercise equipment

Lay Description
Report this code for exercise equipment used for rehabilitation therapy (e.g., stimulation balls, Theraputty, and Thera-Bands).

A9500

A9500 Technetium tc-99m sestamibi, diagnostic, per study dose

Lay Description
Sestamibi is a chemical complex that principally congregates in the heart, breast tissue, and parathyroid. Technetium is a radioactive metallic element that is a byproduct of uranium decay. It may also be produced by bombarding another metal, molybdenum, with specific atoms. Technetium 99m is

a widely used radionuclide with a half-life of approximately six hours, which is long enough to examine metabolic processes but short enough to minimize the radiation dose received by the patient. It decays by gamma emission, which is measured by scintillation or gamma cameras. Sestamibi is combined with technetium 99m to produce functional and physiological images of the breast, heart, or parathyroid. The radiopharmaceutical is administered by intravenous injection. Technetium Tc-99m sestamibi is used to diagnose heart disease, parathyroid diseases, and thyroid disorders. It may also be used as a second-line diagnostic tool in breast imaging after a mammography to evaluate breast lesions in patients with an abnormal mammogram or a palpable breast mass.

A9501

A9501   Technetium Tc-99m teboroxime, diagnostic, per study dose

Lay Description
Teboroxime is a chemical complex that principally congregates in the heart. Technetium is a radioactive metallic element that is a byproduct of uranium decay. It may also be produced by bombarding another metal, molybdenum, with specific atoms. Technetium 99m is a widely used radionuclide with a half-life of approximately six hours, which is long enough to examine metabolic processes, but short enough to minimize the radiation dose received by the patient. It decays by gamma emission, which is then measured by scintillation or gamma cameras. Teboroxime is combined with technetium 99m to produce functional and physiological images of the heart. Technetium Tc-99m teboroxime is used to diagnose reversible myocardial ischemia in the presence or absence of an infarction, for myocardial perfusion studies in patients with known or suspected coronary artery disease, and for the assessment of patients being evaluated for heart disease.

A9502

A9502   Technetium Tc-99m tetrofosmin, diagnostic, per study dose

Lay Description
Tetrofosmin is a chemical complex that principally congregates in the heart. Technetium is a radioactive metallic element that is a byproduct of uranium decay. It may also be produced by bombarding another metal, molybdenum, with specific atoms. Technetium 99m is a widely used radionuclide with a half-life of approximately six hours, which is long enough to examine metabolic processes but short enough to minimize the radiation dose received by the patient. It decays by gamma emission, which is then measured by scintillation or gamma cameras. Tetrofosmin is combined with technetium 99m to produce functional and physiological images of the heart. The radiopharmaceutical is administered by intravenous injection. Technetium Tc-99m

tetrofosmin is used to diagnose reversible myocardial ischemia in the presence or absence of an infarction, to study myocardial perfusion in patients with known or suspected coronary artery disease, and to assess left ventricular function (ejection fraction and wall motion) in patients being evaluated for heart disease.

A9503

A9503   Technetium Tc-99m medronate, diagnostic, per study dose, up to 30 millicuries

Lay Description
Medronate is a chemical complex that principally congregates in the bone. Technetium is a radioactive metallic element that is a byproduct of uranium decay. It may also be produced by bombarding another metal, molybdenum, with specific atoms. Technetium 99m is a widely used radionuclide with a half-life of approximately six hours, which is long enough to examine metabolic processes but short enough to minimize the radiation dose received by the patient. It decays by gamma emission, which is then measured by scintillation or gamma cameras. Medronate is combined with technetium 99m to delineate areas of altered osteogenesis. The radiopharmaceutical is administered by intravenous injection. Optimal imaging is obtained from one to four hours after administration. Technetium Tc-99m medronate is used to diagnose disorders of bone formation.

A9504

A9504   Technetium Tc-99m apcitide, diagnostic, per study dose, up to 20 millicuries

Lay Description
Apcitide is a synthetic peptide that binds to receptors on the surface of platelets. Technetium is a radioactive metallic element that is a byproduct of uranium decay. It may also be produced by bombarding another metal, molybdenum, with specific atoms. Technetium 99m is a widely used radionuclide with a half-life of approximately six hours, which is long enough to examine metabolic processes, but short enough to minimize the radiation dose received by the patient. It decays by gamma emission, which is then measured by scintillation or gamma cameras. Apcitide is combined with technetium 99m to locate areas of thrombus. The radiopharmaceutical is administered by intravenous injection. Optimal imaging is obtained from 10 to 60 minutes after administration.

A9505

A9505   Thallium Tl-201 thallous chloride, diagnostic, per millicurie

Lay Description
Thallium is a toxic heavy metal found within various rare ores. It is usually recovered from the byproducts of lead and zinc ores by dissolving the ore in

hydrochloric acid and precipitating out the thallous chloride. Thallium-201 is a radioactive isotope of thallous chloride that is used as a diagnostic imaging agent. It is administered by intravenous injection. Thallous chloride TL-201 is indicated for use in myocardial perfusion studies and localization of sites of parathyroid hyperactivity, as well as diagnosing and staging of head and neck cancer. Thallous chloride TL-201 has a half-life of 72 hours and decays by electron capture.

A9507

A9507   Indium In-111 capromab pendetide, diagnostic, per study dose, up to 10 millicuries

Lay Description
Capromab pendetide is a murine monoclonal antibody that binds to a glycoprotein, a cell surface antigen that attaches itself to the sites of prostate specific membrane antigen (PSMA). PSMA is associated with prostatic adenocarcinoma cells and is useful in diagnosing metastatic disease. Indium 111 is a radioactive form of the metallic element indium. It has a half-life of approximately 56 hours and decays by electron capture and gamma emission. The monoclonal antibody is combined with indium 111 chloride so that it can be readily identified in images. Indium In-III capromab pendetide is administered intravenously over five minutes. Optimal imaging is obtained from 72 to 120 hours after administration.

A9508

A9508   Iodine I-131 iobenguane sulfate, diagnostic, per 0.5 millicurie

Lay Description
Iobenguane sulfate is an analogue of norepinephrine that binds to receptors in the sympathetic nervous system and to related tumors. Iodine 131 is a radioactive isotope of the common element iodine. Iodine 131 has a half-life of eight days and decays by beta and gamma emissions. Iobenguane sulfate combined with Iodine 131, also known as MIBG, is a radiopharmaceutical used as a diagnostic imaging agent for neuroendocrine tumors and disorders of the adrenal medulla. It is also used for local radiation therapy in the treatment of carcinoid syndrome, pheochromocytoma, and neuroblastoma. Iodine I-131 iobenguane sulfate is injected intravenously. Multiple scans are usually performed for up to four days post administration.

A9509

A9509   Iodine I-123 sodium iodide, diagnostic, per millicurie

Lay Description
Iodine is a common nonmetallic element necessary for the proper function of the thyroid gland. Iodine 123 sodium iodide is a radioactive isotope of iodine produced in a cyclotron. It decays by electron capture

and gamma emission with a half-life of 13 hours. Iodine 123 sodium iodide is administered orally in capsule form. It is readily absorbed from the gastrointestinal tract and congregates primarily in the thyroid gland. Optimal images may be initiated six hours after administration. Sodium iodide I-123 is indicated for diagnostic use in the evaluation of thyroid function and/or morphology.

A9510

A9510   Technetium Tc-99m disofenin, diagnostic, per study dose, up to 15 millicuries

Lay Description
Disofenin is a derivative of an iminodiacetic acid that is a form of acetoacetic acid, a byproduct of metabolism that congregates in the gallbladder. Technetium is a radioactive metallic element that is a byproduct of uranium decay. It may also be produced by bombarding another metal, molybdenum, with specific atoms. Technetium 99m is a widely used radionuclide with a half-life of approximately six hours, which is long enough to examine metabolic processes but short enough to minimize the radiation dose received by the patient. It decays by gamma emission, which is then measured by scintillation or gamma cameras. Disofenin is combined with technetium 99m to provide images of the gallbladder and surrounding ducts. The radiopharmaceutical is administered by intravenous injection. Dosage is based upon the patient's body weight. Optimal imaging is obtained from one to four hours after administration. Technetium Tc-99m disofenin is used to diagnose acute cholecystitis and may be used to rule out this disease in patients with right upper quadrant pain or tenderness and jaundice.

A9512

A9512   Technetium Tc-99m pertechnetate, diagnostic, per millicurie

Lay Description
Technetium Tc-99m pertechnetate is an ionized acid of technetium. Technetium is a radioactive metallic element that is a byproduct of uranium decay. It may also be produced by bombarding another metal, molybdenum, with specific atoms. Technetium 99m is a widely used radionuclide with a half-life of approximately six hours, which is long enough to examine metabolic processes but short enough to minimize the radiation dose received by the patient. It decays by gamma emission, which is then measured by scintillation or gamma cameras. The pertechnetate form of technetium rapidly diffuses into the blood stream and localizes in the thyroid gland, gastric mucosa, salivary glands, certain areas of the brain, sweat glands, and other mucosal tissues. The radiopharmaceutical is administered primarily by intravenous injection, but it may be administered orally as an ophthalmic solution or by instillation into the urinary bladder. The dosage administered depends upon the body area being imaged.

Technetium Tc-99m pertechnetate is used to provide images of the thyroid, salivary glands, and nasolacrimal drainage system. It is also used for placental localization, brain imaging including cerebral angiography, blood pool imaging including angiography, and urinary bladder imaging for detection of vesicoureteral reflux. Technetium Tc-99m pertechnetate may also be used to prepare other technetium 99m imaging agents.

A9516

A9516   Iodine I-123 sodium iodide, diagnostic, per 100 microcuries, up to 999 microcuries

Lay Description

Iodine is a common nonmetallic element necessary for the proper function of the thyroid gland. Iodine 123 sodium iodide is a radioactive isotope of iodine produced in a cyclotron. It decays by electron capture and gamma emission with a half-life of 13 hours. Iodine 123 sodium iodide is administered orally in capsule form. It is readily absorbed from the gastrointestinal tract and congregates primarily in the thyroid gland. Optimal images may be initiated six hours after administration. Sodium iodide I-123 is indicated for diagnostic use in the evaluation of thyroid function and/or morphology.

A9517

A9517   Iodine I-131 sodium iodide capsule(s), therapeutic, per millicurie

Lay Description

Iodine is a common nonmetallic element necessary for the proper function of the thyroid gland. Iodine 131 sodium iodide is a radioactive isotope of iodine produced in a cyclotron. It decays by beta and gamma emission with a half-life of eight hours. Iodine 131 sodium iodide is administered orally in capsule or solution form. It is readily absorbed from the gastrointestinal tract and congregates primarily in thyroid tissue. Therapeutic doses of sodium iodide I-131 capsules are indicated for the treatment of hyperthyroidism and selected cases of thyroid cancer. Palliative effects may be seen in patients with papillary and/or follicular carcinoma of the thyroid. Sodium iodide I-131 is not usually used for the treatment of hyperthyroidism in patients younger than 30 years of age unless circumstances preclude other methods of treatment.

A9520

A9520   Technetium tc-99m, tilmanocept, diagnostic, up to 0.5 millicuries

Lay Description

Tilmanocept is a diagnostic macromolecule composed of DTPA, mannose (CD-206), and dextran that selectively binds with mannose receptors on the surface of macrophages and dendrite cells. It accumulates in lymphatic tissue. Technetium is a radioactive metallic element that is a byproduct of uranium decay. It may also be produced by bombarding another metal, molybdenum, with specific atoms. Technetium 99m is a widely used radionuclide with a half-life of approximately six hours, which is long enough to examine metabolic processes but short enough to minimize the radiation dose received by the patient. It decays by gamma emission, which is measured by scintillation or gamma cameras. The radiopharmaceutical is administered by intradermal, subcutaneous, or peritumoral injection. Technetium Tc-99m tilmanocept is used for lymphatic mapping using a hand-held gamma counter. It is used for sentinel node mapping, the localization of lymph nodes that drain the primary tumor site, in patients with breast cancer, melanoma, and cancers of the head and neck. The recommended dosage is 0.5 mCi and should be administered at least 15 minutes prior to imaging. Each kit contains five vials that may be used for up to four patients.

A9521

A9521   Technetium Tc-99m exametazime, diagnostic, per study dose, up to 25 millicuries

Lay Description

Exametazime, also known as hexamethylpropyleneamine oxime, is a chemical complex that is taken up by leukocytes and selectively retained in neutrophils. Technetium is a radioactive metallic element that is a byproduct of uranium decay. It may also be produced by bombarding another metal, molybdenum, with specific atoms. Technetium 99m is a widely used radionuclide with a half-life of approximately six hours, which is long enough to examine metabolic processes, but short enough to minimize the radiation dose received by the patient. It decays by gamma emission, which is then measured by scintillation or gamma cameras. Tc-99m exametazime is used to label autologous leukocytes. The labeled leukocytes are then used in imaging to localize or identify areas of intra-abdominal infection or inflammation. Optimal imaging with labeled leukocytes is two to four hours after administration. When technetium Tc-99m pertechnetate is added to the exametazime, the resulting radiopharmaceutical is taken up by lipids that can cross the blood-brain barrier. The technetium Tc-99m pertechnetate/exametazime is useful for only 30 minutes. Its useful life can be extended by the addition of methylene blue. Tc-99m pertechnetate/exametazime is used in cerebral perfusion imaging to detect regions altered by stroke. The radiopharmaceutical is administered by intravenous injection. Optimal imaging for cerebral perfusion studies may begin immediately after administration and can continue up to six hours after administration.

A9524

A9524 Iodine I-131 iodinated serum albumin, diagnostic, per 5 microcuries

Lay Description

Serum albumin is a protein component of blood. Iodine 131 is a radioactive isotope of the common element iodine. Iodine 131 has a half-life of eight days and decays by beta and gamma emissions. Serum albumin is combined with iodine 131 to provide images of the blood pool and its movement. The radiopharmaceutical is administered by intravenous injection and is dispersed within the intravascular pool within 10 minutes. Full distribution throughout the body takes from two to four days after administration. Dosage depends upon the imaging to be performed. Iodinated I-131 serum albumin is indicated for use in determinations of total blood and plasma volumes, cardiac output, cardiac and pulmonary blood volumes and circulation times, and in protein turnover studies, heart and great vessel delineation, localization of the placenta, and localization of cerebral neoplasms.

A9526

A9526 Nitrogen N-13 ammonia, diagnostic, per study dose, up to 40 millicuries

Lay Description

Nitrogen N-13 ammonia is a radioisotope composed of ammonia molecules combined with nitrogen N-13 that is widely used in cardiac imaging. Nitrogen N-13 is a radioactive isotope of nitrogen produced within a cyclotron. Nitrogen 13 has a half-life of approximately 10 minutes and decays by positron emission. The positrons are used to produce positron emission tomography (PET) images. Due to its short half-life, nitrogen N-13 ammonia must be produced shortly before use. Nitrogen N-13 ammonia is injected intravenously and is rapidly distributed to all organs of the body. Optimal imaging of the myocardium is generally obtained 15 to 20 minutes after administration. Nitrogen N-13 ammonia is currently approved only for myocardial perfusion for the diagnosis and management of patients with known or suspected coronary artery disease. The perfusion study may be performed at rest or with pharmacological stress.

A9527

A9527 Iodine I-125, sodium iodide solution, therapeutic, per millicurie

Lay Description

Iodine 125 sodium iodide is a radioactive isotope of iodine produced by the neutron irradiation of xenon-124. It decays by electron capture and gamma emission with a half-life of 60 days. Therapeutic iodine 125 sodium iodide is administered in solution form. It is used to treat hyperthyroidism and prostate and brain cancers. This code represents one millicurie of I-125 sodium iodide solution used as a therapeutic dose.

A9528-A9531

A9528 Iodine I-131 sodium iodide capsule(s), diagnostic, per millicurie

A9529 Iodine I-131 sodium iodide solution, diagnostic, per millicurie

A9530 Iodine I-131 sodium iodide solution, therapeutic, per millicurie

A9531 Iodine I-131 sodium iodide, diagnostic, per microcurie (up to 100 microcuries)

Lay Description

Iodine is a common nonmetallic element necessary for the proper function of the thyroid gland. Iodine 131 sodium iodide is a radioactive isotope of iodine produced in a cyclotron. It decays by beta and gamma emission with a half-life of eight hours. Iodine 131 sodium iodide is administered orally in capsule or solution form. It is readily absorbed from the gastrointestinal tract and congregates primarily in thyroid tissue. Therapeutic doses of sodium iodide I-131 capsules are indicated for the treatment of hyperthyroidism and selected cases of thyroid cancer. Palliative effects may be seen in patients with papillary and/or follicular carcinoma of the thyroid. Sodium iodide 1-131 is not usually used for the treatment of hyperthyroidism in patients younger than 30 years of age unless circumstances preclude other methods of treatment.

A9532

A9532 Iodine I-125 serum albumin, diagnostic, per 5 microcuries

Lay Description

Serum albumin is a protein component of blood. Iodine 125 is a radioactive isotope of the common element iodine. Iodine 125 has a half-life of 60 days and decays by beta and gamma emissions. Serum albumin is combined with iodine 125 to provide measures of the blood and plasma pool. The radiopharmaceutical is administered by intravenous injection. Dosage depends upon body weight and can vary from 5 to 50 microcuries. At five and 15 minutes after administration, blood samples are drawn from the arm that was not injected. The radioactivity of the blood samples is measured and a calculation of the patient's blood volume is determined. For plasma volume, the samples are first centrifuged and the red blood cells removed. Iodinated I-125 serum albumin is indicated for use in determinations of total blood and plasma volumes.

A

A9536

A9536 Technetium Tc-99m depreotide, diagnostic, per study dose, up to 35 millicuries

Lay Description
Depreotide is a synthetic peptide that binds to somatostatin receptors in cells. Somatostatin is a peptide that regulates the release of hormones by many different neuroendocrine cells in the brain, pancreas, and gastrointestinal tract. Technetium is a radioactive metallic element that is a byproduct of uranium decay. It may also be produced by bombarding another metal, molybdenum, with specific atoms. Technetium 99m is a widely used radionuclide with a half-life of approximately six hours, which is long enough to examine metabolic processes, but short enough to minimize the radiation dose received by the patient. It decays by gamma emission, which is then measured by scintillation or gamma cameras. Depreotide is combined with technetium 99m to determine the nature of pulmonary masses in patients who have known or suspected malignancy. The radiopharmaceutical is administered by intravenous injection. Dosage is 15 to 20 mCi. Optimal imaging is obtained from two to four hours after administration.

A9537

A9537 Technetium Tc-99m mebrofenin, diagnostic, per study dose, up to 15 millicuries

Lay Description
Mebrofenin is a derivative of an iminodiacetic acid that is a form of acetoacetic acid, a byproduct of metabolism that congregates in the gallbladder. Technetium is a radioactive metallic element that is a byproduct of uranium decay. It may also be produced by bombarding another metal, molybdenum, with specific atoms. Technetium 99m is a widely used radionuclide with a half-life of approximately six hours, which is long enough to examine metabolic processes but short enough to minimize the radiation dose received by the patient. It decays by gamma emission, which is then measured by scintillation or gamma cameras. Mebrofenin is combined with technetium 99m to provide images of the gallbladder and surrounding ducts. Technetium Tc-99m mebrofenin is rapidly cleared and has a short useful life. The radiopharmaceutical is administered by intravenous injection. Dosage is based upon patient's body weight. Optimal imaging is obtained from 10 to 60 minutes after administration.

A9538

A9538 Technetium Tc-99m pyrophosphate, diagnostic, per study dose, up to 25 millicuries

Lay Description
Pyrophosphate is a form of phosphorus formed by the breakdown of adenosine triphosphate (ATP) into adenosine monophosphate (AMP). Technetium is a radioactive metallic element that is a byproduct of uranium decay. It may also be produced by bombarding another metal, molybdenum, with specific atoms. Technetium 99m is a widely used radionuclide with a half-life of approximately six hours, which is long enough to examine metabolic processes but short enough to minimize the radiation dose received by the patient. It decays by gamma emission, which is then measured by scintillation or gamma cameras. Pyrophosphate combined with technetium 99m seems to be attracted to certain crystals found in bone and damaged heart cells. The radiopharmaceutical is administered by intravenous injection. Dosage and optimal imaging depend on the area being imaged. Technetium Tc-99m pyrophosphate is used in skeletal imaging to identify areas of altered bone, such as occurs in metastatic disease, Paget's disease, arthritis, osteomyelitis, and fractures. It is used in cardiac imaging to aid in the diagnosis of an acute myocardial infarction. Technetium Tc-99m pyrophosphate may also be used in conjunction with technetium Tc-99m pertechnetate for the labeling of red blood cells.

A9539

A9539 Technetium Tc-99m pentetate, diagnostic, per study dose, up to 25 millicuries

Lay Description
The pentetate here refers to calcium trisodium pentetate, which is a chelating agent that forms stable bounds with metals, which are then excreted in the urine. Technetium is a radioactive metallic element that is a byproduct of uranium decay. It may also be produced by bombarding another metal, molybdenum, with specific atoms. Technetium 99m is a widely used radionuclide with a half-life of approximately six hours, which is long enough to examine metabolic processes, but short enough to minimize the radiation dose received by the patient. It decays by gamma emission, which is then measured by scintillation or gamma cameras. Pentetate combined with technetium 99m is rapidly distributed throughout the body and is excreted from the body by glomerular filtration. The images of the kidneys obtained in the first few minutes after administration will show the blood pool within the kidney. Subsequent images show kidney function. Technetium Tc-99m pentetate also tends to accumulate in intracranial lesions with many new blood vessels or with an altered blood-brain barrier. The radiopharmaceutical is administered by

intravenous injection. Dosage and optimal imaging depend on the area being imaged. Technetium Tc-99m pentetate is used for kidney and brain imaging and to assess renal function and estimate the glomerular filtration rate. When in aerosol form, it is administered by inhalation. The aerosol form is used to assess airway patency, especially in conjunction with perfusion lung imaging to evaluate for a pulmonary embolism.

A9540

A9540   Technetium Tc-99m macroaggregated albumin, diagnostic, per study dose, up to 10 millicuries

Lay Description
Macroaggregated albumin, also called aggregated albumin, is an unusually large amount of albumin, a protein component of blood. Technetium is a radioactive metallic element that is a byproduct of uranium decay. It may also be produced by bombarding another metal, molybdenum, with specific atoms. Technetium 99m is a widely used radionuclide with a half-life of approximately six hours, which is long enough to examine metabolic processes, but short enough to minimize the radiation dose received by the patient. It decays by gamma emission, which is then measured by scintillation or gamma cameras. Macroaggregated albumin combined with technetium 99m pertechnetate rapidly accumulates in pulmonary alveolar capillaries. The radiopharmaceutical is administered by intravenous injection. Dosage depends upon body weight. Optimal imaging can be obtained immediately after administration. Technetium Tc-99m macroaggregated albumin is used for a lung imaging agent and may be used as an adjunct in the evaluation of pulmonary perfusion in adults and pediatric patients. It may be used in adults for evaluation of peritoneovenous (LeVeen) shunt patency.

A9541

A9541   Technetium Tc-99m sulfur colloid, diagnostic, per study dose, up to 20 millicuries

Lay Description
Sulfur colloid is suspension of very fine particles of sulfur, a nonmetallic element, in an isotonic saline liquid. Technetium is a radioactive metallic element that is a byproduct of uranium decay. It may also be produced by bombarding another metal, molybdenum, with specific atoms. Technetium 99m is a widely used radionuclide with a half-life of approximately six hours, which is long enough to examine metabolic processes but short enough to minimize the radiation dose received by the patient. It decays by gamma emission, which is then measured by scintillation or gamma cameras. Sulfur colloid combined with technetium 99m is rapidly eliminated by the reticuloendothelial system, which is a group of

cells within the immune system. The radiopharmaceutical is administered orally or by intravenous or intra-peritoneal injection. Dosage and optimal imaging depends upon body weight and intended area study. Technetium Tc-99m sulfur colloid injected intravenously is used for imaging of the liver, spleen, and bone marrow. Administered orally, it is used for the evaluation of swallowing functions, gastroesophageal reflux studies, and the detection of pulmonary aspiration of gastric contents. Technetium Tc-99m sulfur colloid injected intra-peritoneally may be used in adults for evaluation of peritoneovenous (LeVeen) shunt patency.

A9542-A9543

A9542   Indium In-111 ibritumomab tiuxetan, diagnostic, per study dose, up to 5 millicuries
A9543   Yttrium Y-90 ibritumomab tiuxetan, therapeutic, per treatment dose, up to 40 millicuries

Lay Description
Ibritumomab is a murine monoclonal antibody produced in Chinese hamster ovary cells. This antibody is specifically directed against the CD20 antigen, which is found on the surface of normal and malignant B lymphocytes. Tiuxetan is a chelating agent that allows ibritumomab to form stable bonds with metals. Indium 111 is a radioactive form of the metallic element indium. It has a half-life of approximately 56 hours and decays by electron capture and gamma emission. Indium 111 ibritumomab tiuxetan is used to determine the biodistribution pattern in preparation for the administration of yttrium 90 of ibritumomab tiuxetan. The usual dose for diagnostic purposes is 5 millicuries injected intravenously. Yttrium 90 is a radioactive form of the metallic element yttrium found in rare earth minerals. Ibritumomab tiuxetan combined with yttrium 90 is used for the treatment of relapsed or refractory low-grade, follicular, or transformed B cell non-Hodgkin's lymphoma, including rituximab-refractory follicular non-Hodgkin's lymphoma. The dosage for therapeutic yttrium 90 ibritumomab tiuxetan depends upon body weight. It is administered by intravenous injection. Both forms of ibritumomab tiuxetan are administered in conjunction with rituximab.

A9544-A9545

A9544   Iodine I-131 tositumomab, diagnostic, per study dose
A9545   Iodine I-131 tositumomab, therapeutic, per treatment dose

Lay Description
Tositumomab is a murine monoclonal antibody produced in mammalian cells. This antibody is specifically directed against the CD20 antigen, which is found on the surface of normal and malignant B lymphocytes. Iodine 131 is a radioactive isotope of the

common element iodine. It decays by beta and gamma emission with a half-life of eight hours. The diagnostic dosage of tositumomab is used to determine the biodistribution pattern in preparation for the administration of the therapeutic dosage. The usual dose for diagnostic purposes is 450 mg of tositumomab infused intravenously over one hour followed by 5 mCi of iodine 131 tositumomab infused intravenously over 20 minutes. The therapeutic dosage depends on the patient's body weight and condition. It is infused intravenously over 20 minutes. Iodine I-131 tositumomab is used for the treatment of relapsed or refractory CD20 positive follicular, non-Hodgkin's lymphoma, including rituximab-refractory follicular non-Hodgkin's lymphoma.

A9546

A9546   Cobalt Co-57/58, cyanocobalamin, diagnostic, per study dose, up to 1 microcurie

Lay Description
Cyanocobalamin Co-57/58 is a radioactive form of vitamin B12 in which portions of the molecules contain cobalt 57 or cobalt 58. The drug is administered orally and used to diagnose pernicious anemia and intestinal defects of vitamin B12 absorption.

A9547

A9547   Indium In-111 oxyquinoline, diagnostic, per 0.5 millicurie

Lay Description
Indium 111 oxyquinoline is a radioisotope used to label autologous white blood cells. These labeled cells are then administered intravenously and used to scan for abscesses and other inflammatory processes where the white cells would usually congregate. Indium 111 oxyquinoline is not the preferred technique for the initial evaluation of patients with a suspected abscess in an unknown location. It should be considered only if other methods prove unsuccessful or ambiguous. Imaging is performed approximately two hours postinjection. Indium 111 decays by electron capture with a half-life of 67.2 hours.

A9548

A9548   Indium In-111 pentetate, diagnostic, per 0.5 millicurie

Lay Description
Pentetate, also known as pentetic acid or DTPA, is a chelating agent that binds with iron. Indium 111 is a radioactive form of indium, a metallic element. Indium 111 has a half-life of 2.8 days and decays by electron capture and gamma emission. Pentetate combined with indium In-111 is used to provide images of the cerebrospinal fluid (CSF) flow. It is indicated for use in radionuclide cisternography to study the flow of CSF in the brain for identification of CSF abnormalities and sites of CSF leakage, and for evaluation of CSF shunt patency. Indium In-111 pentetate is administered by intrathecal injection into the lumbar intrathecal space. It flows up the spinal canal with the CSF to the brain. Under normal flow patterns, it does not penetrate into the ventricles. Indium In-111 pentetate is supplied as a unit dose. Each unit dose vial contains 0.7 mCi of sterile indium In-111 pentetate. The maximum recommended dose for an adult (average weight 70 kg) is 10.5 mCi. Any unused portion must be discarded.

A9550

A9550   Technetium Tc-99m sodium gluceptate, diagnostic, per study dose, up to 25 millicurie

Lay Description
Sodium gluceptate is a carbohydrate derivative. Technetium is a radioactive metallic element that is a byproduct of uranium decay. It may also be produced by bombarding another metal, molybdenum, with specific atoms. Technetium 99m is a widely used radionuclide with a half-life of approximately six hours, which is long enough to examine metabolic processes but short enough to minimize the radiation dose received by the patient. It decays by gamma emission, which is then measured by scintillation or gamma cameras. Sodium gluceptate combined with technetium 99m pertechnetate is rapidly eliminated from the body by the kidneys. It tends to accumulate in intracranial lesions with many new blood vessels or with an altered blood-brain barrier. Technetium 99m sodium gluceptate is used for kidney and brain imaging and to assess renal and brain perfusion. The radiopharmaceutical is administered by intravenous injection. The recommended adult dosage is 10 to 15 mCi for renal imaging and 15 to 20 mCi for brain imaging. Dynamic imaging may begin immediately after administration, and static images can be obtained up to several hours after administration.

A9551

A9551   Technetium Tc-99m succimer, diagnostic, per study dose, up to 10 millicuries

Lay Description
Succimer, also known as DMSA, is a chelating agent that is similar to dimercaprol and is used in the treatment of heavy metal poisoning. Technetium is a radioactive metallic element that is a byproduct of uranium decay. It may also be produced by bombarding another metal, molybdenum, with specific atoms. Technetium 99m is a widely used radionuclide with a half-life of approximately six hours, which is long enough to examine metabolic processes, but short enough to minimize the radiation dose received by the patient. It decays by gamma emission, which is then measured by scintillation or gamma cameras. Succimer combined with technetium 99m pertechnetate is rapidly eliminated

from the body by the kidneys. The radiopharmaceutical is administered by intravenous injection. Technetium 99m succimer is used in the evaluation of renal parenchymal disorders. The recommended adult dosage is 2 to 6 mCi. Optimal imaging may be obtained one to two hours after administration.

A9552

A9552   Fluorodeoxyglucose F-18 FDG, diagnostic, per study dose, up to 45 millicuries

Lay Description
Glucose is a sugar actively taken up by cells. Fludeoxyglucose F18 (FDG) is a radioisotope widely used in positron emission tomography (PET imaging). FDG is a radioactive version of glucose that is administered intravenously. Peak imaging is at 30 to 40 minutes after injection. FDG is indicated for identifying regions of abnormal glucose metabolism that can be associated with foci of epileptic seizures or evaluation of malignancy in patients who have an existing diagnosis or who have known of or suspected abnormalities identified by other methods. FDG may also be used to assess coronary artery disease and left ventricular dysfunction when used together with myocardial perfusion. It must be produced from cyclotron bombardment of fluorine F18, which is itself produced from proton bombardment of enriched water. FDG decays by positron emission and has a half-life of 109.8 minutes.

A9553

A9553   Chromium Cr-51 sodium chromate, diagnostic, per study dose, up to 250 microcuries

Lay Description
Chromium CR 51 is a radioisotope of sodium chromate, which binds to red blood cells. Chromium 51 is used to label red blood cells and the labeled cells are administered intravenously. Labeled red blood cells are used for determining red blood cell volume or mass, evaluating blood loss, and studying red blood cell survival time for conditions such as hemolytic anemia. Chromium 51 decays by electron capture and gamma emission. It has a half-life of 27.7 days.

A9554

A9554   Iodine I-125 sodium iothalamate, diagnostic, per study dose, up to 10 microcuries

Lay Description
Sodium iothalamate is a solution of iodine and sodium hydroxide that is used as a contrast agent. Iodine I-125 is a radioactive version of iodine that has a half-life of 60 days and decays by electron capture and gamma emission. Sodium iothalamate combined with iodine I-125 is used to evaluate renal glomerular filtration when diagnosing and monitoring patients with renal disease. The compound is cleared by renal glomerular filtration without tubular secretion or reabsorption. The suggested dose range employed in an adult patient (average weight 70 kg) depends on the infusion method. For continuous intravenous infusion, the dose is 20 to 100 uCi. For single intravenous injection, the dose is 10 to 30 uCi. Blood and urine samples are collected from the patient at varying intervals post administration. The concentration of iodine I-125 in each specimen is then measured using scintillation counters. These figures are used to compute clearance factors, which provide an indication of renal function.

A9555

A9555   Rubidium Rb-82, diagnostic, per study dose, up to 60 millicuries

Lay Description
Rubidium-82 is a radioisotope widely used in cardiac imaging, as it is a chemical analog to potassium. Potassium ions are metabolized by muscle tissue, including the heart. Once in the heart, the beta decay of the rubidium-82 is used to help produce a PET image. The half-life of rubidium-82 is 1.273 minutes. Due to its short half-life, rubidium-82 must be produced shortly before use by a rubidium-82 generator. Rubidium-82 is produced by the beta decay of strontium-82. Strontium-82 is an isotope that can readily be made in an accelerator and has a half-life of 25.5 days. The relatively long-lived strontium-82 in the form of a solution is loaded into the rubidium-82 generator. As the strontium-82 decays, rubidium-82 is produced. A solvent is then selectively used to remove the rubidium-82 from the solution. As the strontium-82 is continually decaying and producing rubidium-82, one can allow the rubidium to accumulate and remove the rubidium-82 as needed.

A9556

A9556   Gallium Ga-67 citrate, diagnostic, per millicurie

Lay Description
Gallium is a rare metal that is liquid at room temperature. Gallium GA 67 citrate is a radioactive version of gallium used to identify the presence and extent of Hodgkin's disease, lymphomas, and bronchogenic carcinomas. It may also be useful in detecting some inflammatory lesions. Gallium GA 67 citrate is administered intravenously and peak imaging is often 48 to 120 hours after injection. It must be produced from cyclotron proton bombardment of Zinc ZN 68 enriched metal. Gallium GA 67 decays by electron capture and gamma emission. It has a half-life of 78.3 hours.

A9557

A9557 Technetium Tc-99m bicisate, diagnostic, per study dose, up to 25 millicuries

Lay Description

Bicisate, also known as ethyl cysteinate dimer (ECD), is a lipophilic amine having the ability to cross the blood-brain barrier and localize in the brain. Technetium is a radioactive metallic element that is a byproduct of uranium decay. It may also be produced by bombarding another metal, molybdenum, with specific atoms. Technetium 99m is a widely used radionuclide with a half-life of approximately six hours, which is long enough to examine metabolic processes, but short enough to minimize the radiation dose received by the patient. It decays by gamma emission, which is then measured by scintillation or gamma cameras. Bicisate combined with technetium 99m pertechnetate is used in single photon emission computerized tomography (SPECT) imaging as an adjunct to conventional CT or MRI imaging in the localization of stroke in patients in whom stroke has already been diagnosed. The radiopharmaceutical is injected intravenously. The recommended adult dosage is 10 to 30 mCi. Optimal imaging may be obtained 30 to 60 minutes after administration.

A9558

A9558 Xenon Xe-133 gas, diagnostic, per 10 millicuries

Lay Description

Xenon is a gaseous element that is not chemically reactive. Xenon Xe133 gas is a mixture of radioactive xenon gas and carbon dioxide inhaled by the patient for use in diagnostic evaluations of pulmonary functions, pulmonary imaging, and in the assessment of cerebral blood flow. The gas is a reactor-produced by-product of uranium U235 fission. Xenon Xe133 gas decays by beta and gamma emissions with a half-life of 5.245 days.

A9559

A9559 Cobalt Co-57 cyanocobalamin, oral, diagnostic, per study dose, up to 1 microcurie

Lay Description

Cyanocobalamin Co-57 is a radioactive forms of vitamin B12 in which portions of the molecules contain cobalt 57. The drug is administered orally and used to diagnose pernicious anemia and intestinal defects of vitamin B12 absorption.

A9560

A9560 Technetium Tc-99m labeled red blood cells, diagnostic, per study dose, up to 30 millicuries

Lay Description

Technetium is a radioactive metallic element that is a byproduct of uranium decay. It may also be produced by bombarding another metal, molybdenum, with specific atoms. Technetium 99m is a widely used radionuclide with a half-life of approximately six hours, which is long enough to examine metabolic processes but short enough to minimize the radiation dose received by the patient. It decays by gamma emission, which is then measured by scintillation or gamma cameras. Technetium 99m pertechnetate is used to label autologous red blood cells, which are then injected intravenously. The recommended adult dosage is 10 to 20 mCi. Technetium Tc-99m labeled red blood cells are used for blood pool imaging, including cardiac first pass and gated equilibrium imaging, and for detection of sites of gastrointestinal bleeding.

A9561

A9561 Technetium Tc-99m oxidronate, diagnostic, per study dose, up to 30 millicuries

Lay Description

Oxidronate, also known as HDP and HMDP, is a chemical compound that is attracted to sites of bone mineralization. Technetium is a radioactive metallic element that is a byproduct of uranium decay. It may also be produced by bombarding another metal, molybdenum, with specific atoms. Technetium 99m is a widely used radionuclide with a half-life of approximately six hours, which is long enough to examine metabolic processes, but short enough to minimize the radiation dose received by the patient. It decays by gamma emission, which is then measured by scintillation or gamma cameras. Oxidronate combined with technetium 99m is used for skeletal imaging to identify areas of altered bone growth. The radiopharmaceutical is injected intravenously. The recommended adult dosage is 10 to 20 mCi. Optimal imaging is three to four hours after administration.

A9562

A9562 Technetium Tc-99m mertiatide, diagnostic, per study dose, up to 15 millicuries

Lay Description

Mertiatide is a chemical compound that binds to plasma protein. Technetium is a radioactive metallic element that is a byproduct of uranium decay. It may also be produced by bombarding another metal, molybdenum, with specific atoms. Technetium 99m is a widely used radionuclide with a half-life of approximately six hours, which is long enough to examine metabolic processes but short enough to minimize the radiation dose received by the patient. It decays by gamma emission, which is then measured by scintillation or gamma cameras. Mertiatide combined with technetium 99m pertechnetate is used for renal imaging to diagnose congenital and acquired abnormalities, renal failure, urinary tract obstruction, and calculi in adults and children. It is a diagnostic aid in providing renal function, split function, renal angiograms, and renogram curves for whole kidney and renal cortex. The radiopharmaceutical is injected intravenously. The recommended adult dosage is 5 to 10 mCi.

A9563

A9563   Sodium phosphate P-32, therapeutic, per millicurie

Lay Description
Phosphorus is a common nonmetallic element essential to the human body. It is a major component of bone, is abundant in all tissues, and is involved in some form in almost all metabolic processes. Phosphorus 32 is a radioactive form of phosphorus. It has a half-life of approximately 14.28 days and decays by beta emission. Sodium is a common metallic element, an electrolyte necessary for the proper functioning of the body. Sodium phosphate P-32 is a compound of sodium and phosphorus P-32. It concentrates largely in rapidly proliferating tissue, accumulating in the liver, spleen, and bone marrow. Sodium phosphate P-32 is used for the therapeutic treatment of polycythemia vera, chronic myelocytic leukemia, and chronic lymphocytic leukemia. It may also be used for the palliative treatment of bone pain associated with multiple areas of skeletal metastases.

A9564

A9564   Chromic phosphate P-32 suspension, therapeutic, per millicurie

Lay Description
Phosphorus is a common nonmetallic element essential to the human body. It is a major component of bone, is abundant in all tissues, and is involved in some form in almost all metabolic processes. Phosphorus 32 is a radioactive form of phosphorus. It has a half-life of approximately 14.28 days and decays by beta emission. Chromium is a metallic trace element used in glucose metabolism and is essential to the body in small amounts. Chromic phosphate P-32 is a compound of phosphorus 32 and chromium. It is administered by intraperitoneal or intrapleural instillation or interstitial injection. Chromic phosphate P-32 is used intraperitoneally or intrapleurally for the therapeutic treatment of effusions resulting from metastatic disease and interstitially in the treatment of certain ovarian and prostate carcinomas. Dosages vary from 0.1 to 20 millicuries depending on the disease being treated and method of administration.

A9566

A9566   Technetium Tc-99m fanolesomab, diagnostic, per study dose, up to 25 millicuries

Lay Description
Fanolesomab is a murine monoclonal antibody that binds to the CD15 antigen. The CD15 antigen is found on the surface of some neutrophils, eosinophils, and monocytes, which are types of leukocytes or white blood cells. Technetium is a radioactive metallic element that is a byproduct of uranium decay. It may also be produced by bombarding another metal, molybdenum, with specific atoms. Technetium 99m is a widely used radionuclide with a half-life of approximately six hours, which is long enough to examine metabolic processes, but short enough to minimize the radiation dose received by the patient. It decays by gamma emission, which is then measured by scintillation or gamma cameras. Fanolesomab combined with technetium 99m pertechnetate labels the leukocytes or white blood cells. Leukocytes gather at the site of an infection. Technetium 99m fanolesomab is used to confirm appendicitis in patients with the signs and symptoms associated with appendicitis. The radiopharmaceutical is injected intravenously. The recommended adult dosage is 10 to 200 mCi. Imaging may begin immediately after administration.

A9567

A9567   Technetium Tc-99m pentetate, diagnostic, aerosol, per study dose, up to 75 millicuries

Lay Description
The pentetate here refers to calcium trisodium pentetate, which is a chelating agent that forms stable bonds with metals, which are then excreted in the urine. Technetium is a radioactive metallic element that is a byproduct of uranium decay. It may also be produced by bombarding another metal, molybdenum, with specific atoms. Technetium 99m is a widely used radionuclide with a half-life of approximately six hours, which is long enough to examine metabolic processes but short enough to minimize the radiation dose received by the patient. It decays by gamma emission, which is then measured by scintillation or gamma cameras. Pentetate combined with technetium 99m is rapidly distributed throughout the body and is excreted from the body by glomerular filtration. The images of the kidneys obtained in the first few minutes after administration show the blood pool within the kidney. Subsequent images show kidney function. Technetium Tc-99m pentetate also tends to accumulate in intracranial lesions with many new blood vessels or with an altered blood-brain barrier. The radiopharmaceutical is administered by intravenous injection. Dosage and optimal imaging depend on the area being imaged. Technetium Tc-99m pentetate is used for kidney and brain imaging and to assess renal function and to estimate the glomerular filtration rate. When in aerosol form, it is administered by inhalation. The aerosol form is used to assess airway patency, especially in conjunction with perfusion lung imaging to evaluate for a pulmonary embolism.

A

A9568

A9568   Technetium Tc-99m arcitumomab, diagnostic, per study dose, up to 45 millicuries

Lay Description

Arcitumomab is a murine monoclonal antibody directed to the carcinoembryonic antigen (CEA), a tumor-associated antigen whose expression is increased in various carcinomas, particularly of the gastrointestinal tract, and in certain inflammatory states (e.g., Crohn's disease, inflammatory bowel disease, post-radiation therapy to the bowel). Technetium is a radioactive metallic element that is a byproduct of uranium decay. It may also be produced by bombarding another metal, molybdenum, with specific atoms. Technetium 99m is a widely used radionuclide with a half-life of approximately six hours, which is long enough to examine metabolic processes but short enough to minimize the radiation dose received by the patient. It decays by gamma emission which is then measured by scintillation or gamma cameras. Arcitumomab combined with technetium 99m pertechnetate is indicated, in conjunction with standard diagnostic evaluations, for detection of the presence, location, and extent of recurrent and/or metastatic colorectal carcinoma involving the liver, extrahepatic abdomen, and pelvis in patients with a histologically confirmed diagnosis of colorectal carcinoma. The radiopharmaceutical is administered by intravenous injection. The recommended adult dosage is 1 mg labeled with 20-30 millicuries of technetium TC 99m arcitumomab. Optimal imaging is at two to five hours after administration.

A9569

A9569   Technetium Tc-99m exametazime labeled autologous white blood cells, diagnostic, per study dose

Lay Description

Exametazime, also known as hexamethylpropyleneamine oxime, is a chemical complex that is taken up by leukocytes and selectively retained in neutrophils. Technetium is a radioactive metallic element that is a byproduct of uranium decay. It may also be produced by bombarding another metal, molybdenum, with specific atoms. Technetium 99m is a widely used radionuclide with a half-life of approximately six hours, which is long enough to examine metabolic processes but short enough to minimize the radiation dose received by the patient. It decays by gamma emission, which is then measured by scintillation or gamma cameras. Tc-99m exametazime is used to label autologous leukocytes. The labeled leukocytes are then used in imaging to localize or identify areas of intra-abdominal infection or inflammation. Optimal imaging with labeled leukocytes is two to four hours after administration. When technetium Tc-99m pertechnetate is added to the exametazime, the resulting radiopharmaceutical is taken up by lipids that can cross the blood-brain barrier. The technetium Tc-99m pertechnetate/exametazime is useful for only 30 minutes. Its useful life can be extended by the addition of methylene blue. Tc-99m pertechnetate/exametazime is used in cerebral perfusion imaging to detect regions altered by stroke. The radiopharmaceutical is administered by intravenous injection. Optimal imaging for cerebral perfusion studies may begin immediately after administration and can continue up to six hours after administration.

A9570

A9570   Indium In-111 labeled autologous white blood cells, diagnostic, per study dose

Lay Description

Indium 111 is a radioactive form of indium, a metallic element. Indium 111 has a half-life of 2.8 days and decays by electron capture and gamma emission. Indium 111 is used to label autologous white blood cells. These labeled cells are then reinfused into the patient intravenously and used to scan for abscesses and other inflammatory processes where the white cells would usually congregate. Imaging is performed approximately two hours postinjection.

A9571

A9571   Indium In-111 labeled autologous platelets, diagnostic, per study dose

Lay Description

Indium 111 is a radioactive form of indium, a metallic element. Indium 111 has a half-life of 2.8 days and decays by electron capture and gamma emission. Indium 111 is used to label autologous platelets. These labeled cells are then reinfused into the patient intravenously. Platelets tend to aggregate at areas of thrombosis or active bleeding. Indium-labeled platelets are used to scan for deep vein thrombosis, vascular integrity, and platelet survival. Imaging is performed approximately two hours postinjection.

A9572

A9572   Indium In-111 pentetreotide, diagnostic, per study dose, up to 6 millicuries

Lay Description

Pentetreotide is a mixture of pentetic acid and octreotide. Pentetic acid, also known as pentetate or DTPA, is a chelating agent that binds with iron. Octreotide is a synthetic version of somatostatin, which is a peptide that inhibits the release of growth hormone, thyrotropin, and corticotropin. Indium 111 is a radioactive form of indium, a metallic element. Indium 111 has a half-life of 2.8 days and decays by electron capture and gamma emission. Indium In-111 pentetreotide binds somatostatin receptors on cell surfaces throughout the body. After approximately an hour following intravenous injection most of the indium In-111 pentetreotide is distributed throughout the body and is seen concentrated in tumors containing a high density of somatostatin receptors. Indium In-111 pentetreotide allows imaging that identifies the presence and location of primary and metastatic neuroendocrine tumors bearing somatostatin receptors. Indium In-111 pentetreotide is administered by intravenous injection. The recommended dose for planar imaging is 3.0 mCi. The recommended dose for SPECT imaging is 6.0 mCi.

A9575

A9575   Injection, gadoterate meglumine, 0.1 ml

Lay Description
Magnetic resonance imaging (MRI) is a radiation-free, noninvasive technique used to produce high-quality sectional images of the inside of the body in multiple planes. MRI uses the natural magnetic properties of the hydrogen atoms in our bodies that emit radiofrequency signals when exposed to radio waves within a strong electromagnetic field. These signals are processed and converted by the computer into high-resolution, three-dimensional tomographic images. Gadolinium is a rare earth metal that is strongly magnetic at room temperature. Various forms of the metal are used to enhance an MRI. Gadoterate meglumine is a gadolinium-based contrast agent for use in MRI of the brain, spine, and associated tissues to detect and visualize areas with disruption of the blood brain barrier and/or abnormal vascularity. Gadoterate does not cross the intact blood-brain barrier (BBB) and, therefore, does not enhance normal brain or lesions that have a normal blood-brain barrier (eg, cysts, mature postoperative scars). However, when there is a disruption of the BBB or abnormal vascularity gadoterate meglumine allows distribution of gadoterate in brain lesions such as neoplasms, abscesses, and infarcts. Dosage depends on patient body weight with a recommended dose of 0.2 ml per kg.

A9576-A9579

A9576   Injection, gadoteridol, (ProHance multipack), per ml

A9577   Injection, gadobenate dimeglumine (MultiHance), per ml

A9578   Injection, gadobenate dimeglumine (MultiHance multipack), per ml

A9579   Injection, gadolinium-based magnetic resonance contrast agent, not otherwise specified (NOS), per ml

Lay Description
Magnetic resonance imaging (MRI) is a radiation-free, noninvasive technique used to produce high-quality sectional images of the inside of the body in multiple planes. MRI uses the natural magnetic properties of the hydrogen atoms in our bodies that emit radiofrequency signals when exposed to radio waves within a strong electromagnetic field. These signals are processed and converted by the computer into

high-resolution, three-dimensional tomographic images. Gadolinium is a rare earth metal that is strongly magnetic at room temperature. Various forms of the metal are used to enhance an MRI. The gadolinium is administered intravenously and circulates within the cardiovascular system allowing the MRI to capture greater detail. Gadolinium highlights disruptions of the blood-brain barrier and enhances areas of abnormal vascularization that is common in neoplasms, abscesses, or subacute infarcts. It is indicated for use in MRIs of the brain; spine; head and neck; thoracic, abdominal, and pelvic cavities; and retroperitoneal space. It is not indicated for use in cardiac imaging. Dosage depends on patient body weight with a recommended dose of 0.2 ml per kg.

A9580

A9580   Sodium fluoride F-18, diagnostic, per study dose, up to 30 millicuries

Lay Description
Sodium fluoride F-18 is a radiopharmaceutical used with PET scans. It is a positron emitting substance used to detect abnormal bone activity in the patient. Abnormal activity can be a result of cancer, Paget's disease, or osteomyelitis. Sodium fluoride is injected through an IV line and allowed to circulate. It accumulates in the areas of bone activity. Those areas are visible with the PET scan. The normal dose of sodium fluoride F-18 is 5 mCi to 15 mCi.

A9581

A9581   Injection, gadoxetate disodium, 1 ml

Lay Description
Gadoxetate disodium is a paramagnetic, gadolinium-based contrast agent for MRI that creates a magnetic field. It provides a brightening of blood and tissue. It is used for liver MRIs to look for lesions or liver disease. The recommended dose of gadoxetate disodium is 0.1 mL/kg based on the patient's body weight. It is administered by IV injection.

A9582

A9582   Iodine I-123 iobenguane, diagnostic, per study dose, up to 15 millicuries

Lay Description
Iobenguane sulfate is an analogue of norepinephrine that binds to receptors in the sympathetic nervous system and to related tumors. Iodine 123 is a radioactive isotope of the common element iodine produced in a cyclotron. It decays by electron capture and gamma emission with a half life of 13 hours. Iobenguane sulfate combined with Iodine 123, also known as MIBG, is a radiopharmaceutical used as a diagnostic imaging agent for neuroendocrine tumors and disorders of the adrenal medulla. Iodine I-123 iobenguane sulfate is injected intravenously. Multiple scans are usually performed for up to four days post administration.

A

A9583

A9583 Injection, gadofosveset trisodium, 1 ml

Lay Description

Gadofosveset trisodium is a contrast agent used to evaluate vascular structures with magnetic resonance angiography (MRA). The recommended dose is based on body weight and is administered intravenously.

A9584

A9584 Iodine I-123 ioflupane, diagnostic, per study dose, up to 5 millicuries

Lay Description

Iodine is a common, nonmetallic element necessary for the proper function of the thyroid gland. Iodine 123 is a radioactive isotope of iodine produced in a cyclotron. It decays by electron capture and gamma emission with a half-life of 13 hours. Ioflupane is a neuroimaging drug with an affinity for dopamine transporters in the striatal regions of the brain. Patients with Parkinson's disease have a marked reduction in dopaminergic neurons in the striatal regions of the brain. Once Iodine I-123 ioflupane has bound with the dopamine transporters, a quantitative measure and spatial distributions can be obtained. This radiopharmaceutical is used to diagnose Parkinson's disease and differentiate Parkinson's disease from other disorders that display similar symptoms.

A9585

A9585 Injection, gadobutrol, 0.1 ml

Lay Description

Gadobutrol is a paramagnetic macrocyclic contrast agent used for magnetic resonance imaging (MRI) procedures. The chemical name for gadobutrol is 10-[(1SR,2RS)-2,3-dihydroxy-l-hydroxymethylpropyl]-l, 4,7,10-tetraazacyclododecane-l,4,7-triacetic acid, gadolinium complex. Gadobutrol is used to locate defects in the blood brain barrier (BBB) and abnormalities in the vascular structure of the central nervous system. When the gadobutrol is placed in the MRI machines, it shortens the relaxation time of the spin-lattice or longitudinal (T1) and the spin-spin or transverse (T2) relaxation times. Variations based on the relaxation times and the gadobutrol concentration can be identified during the scan. The recommended dose is 0.1 mL/kg body weight for children 2 years of age or older and adults. It is administered by intravenous injections prior to the MRI imaging.

A9586

A9586 Florbetapir F18, diagnostic, per study dose, up to 10 millicuries

Lay Description

Florbetapir F-18 is a diagnostic radiopharmaceutical used with PET scans of the brain that binds with β-amyloid aggregates. This radiopharmaceutical uses fluorine (F-18) that decays by positron (β+) emission

and has a half-life of 109.77 minutes. The uptake of Florbetapir F-18 can be used to estimate β-amyloid neuritic plaques in adult patients with cognitive impairment. This radiopharmaceutical, trade name Amyvid, does not establish a diagnosis of Alzheimer's disease or other cognitive disorders or predict development of dementia or other neurologic conditions.

A9599

A9599 Radiopharmaceutical, diagnostic, for beta-amyloid positron emission tomography (PET) imaging, per study dose

Lay Description

This code represents diagnostic radiopharmaceuticals used with PET scans of the brain that bind with β-amyloid aggregates, other than florbetapir f18, which has its own assigned code of A9586. These diagnostic radiopharmaceuticals include: Florbetaben is florbetaben F18 (or AV-1, or BAY-94-9172); Flutemetamol is flutemetamol F18 (or GE-067); FDDNP is FDDNP F18; AZD4694 is AZD4694 F18 (or NAV4694); PIB is Pittsburgh Compound B C11; and other radiopharmaceuticals under development. The uptake of these radiopharmaceuticals can be used to estimate β-amyloid neuritic plaques in adult patients with cognitive impairment. The radiopharmaceuticals do not establish a diagnosis of Alzheimer's disease or other cognitive disorders or predict development of dementia or other neurologic conditions. At this time, Medicare does not cover this type of testing as it has determined that evidence is insufficient to conclude that the use of positron emission tomography (PET) amyloid-beta (Aβ) imaging is reasonable and necessary for the diagnosis or treatment of illness or injury or to improve the functioning of a malformed body member for Medicare beneficiaries with dementia or neurodegenerative disease.

A9600

A9600 Strontium Sr-89 chloride, therapeutic, per millicurie

Lay Description

Strontium is a metallic earth element that is similar to calcium, soft, and decomposes readily in water. Strontium 89 is a radioactive version of strontium. Strontium 89 has a half-life of 50.5 days and decays by beta emissions. Since strontium behaves like calcium, it is concentrated in the bone and in areas of calcium uptake. Strontium 89 is used as a source in radiation therapy. In the form of strontium 89 chloride, it is injected intravenously or delivered by catheter into a large vein. Strontium 89 chloride is indicated as a palliative treatment for debilitating bone pain in patients whose cancer has metastasized to bone. The bone metastasis should be confirmed prior to use of strontium 89. The recommended dosage is 4 mCi. Repeat treatments may be performed at 90-day intervals.

A9604

A9604   Samarium sm-153 lexidronam, therapeutic, per treatment dose, up to 150 millicuries

Lay Description
Samarium is a metallic rare earth element found in other rare earth mineral ores. Samarium 153 is a radioactive form of samarium that has a half-life of 46.7 hours and decays by beta and gamma emissions. Lexidronam, also known as ethylene diamine tetramethylene phosphonate or EDTMP, is a chemical complex that concentrates in the bone and in areas of calcium uptake. Samarium 153 lexidronam is indicated as a palliative treatment for debilitating bone pain in patients whose cancer has metastasized to bone. The bone metastasis should be confirmed prior to use of samarium 153. The recommended dosage is 1 mCi per kg of body weight. It is administered intravenously through an indwelling catheter.

A9606

A9606   Radium RA-223 dichloride, therapeutic, per microcurie

Lay Description
Radium (RA) 223 dichloride (Trade Name Xofigo) is used for the treatment of castration resistant prostate cancer, symptomatic bone metastases, and unknown visceral metastatic disease. Radium 223 dichloride is an alpha emitting radiotherapeutic drug that mimics calcium and forms a mineral compound at areas of increased bone turnover, such as bone metastases. Recommended dosage is 50 kBq/kg of body weight (1.35 microcuries/kg) administered by slow intravenous injection over one minute every four weeks for six doses. Available in single use vials containing 6 ml of solution at a concentration of 1,000 kBq/ml (27 microcuries/ml) at the reference date with a total radioactivity of 3,000 kBq/vial (162 microcuries/vial) at the reference date. Six-stage decay is by predominantly alpha emissions with some beta and gamma emissions. The high linear energy transfer of alpha emitters leads to a high frequency of DNA breaks, resulting in cell death. Since alpha particle range is less than 100 micrometers, damage to adjacent tissue is limited.

A9698

A9698   Nonradioactive contrast imaging material, not otherwise classified, per study

Lay Description
Use this code when a HCPCS code for a contrast imaging material utilized has not been issued by CMS.

A9699

A9699   Radiopharmaceutical, therapeutic, not otherwise classified

Lay Description
This code is used to report the supply of radiopharmaceutical therapeutic imaging agents that do not have another specific HCPCS Level II code. Radiopharmaceuticals are radioactive isotopes, such as radioactive iodine or radioactive cobalt. They are often attached to carrier molecules and used in therapeutic nuclear medicine procedures.

A9700

A9700   Supply of injectable contrast material for use in echocardiography, per study

Lay Description
This code is used to report the supply of injectable contrast material used in echocardiography that does not have another specific HCPCS Level II code. There are HCPCS Level II codes for perflexane lipid microspheres, octafluoropropane microspheres, and perflutren lipid microspheres.

A9900

A9900   Miscellaneous DME supply, accessory, and/or service component of another HCPCS code

Lay Description
Durable medical equipment includes any medical equipment used in the home to aid in a better quality of living. This code represents a miscellaneous DME supply, accessory, and/or service component of another HCPCS code.

A9901

A9901   DME delivery, set up, and/or dispensing service component of another HCPCS code

Lay Description
This code represents the delivery, set-up, and dispensing service component of another HCPCS code, such as hospital beds, wheelchairs, catheters, and glucose monitors.

A9999

A9999   Miscellaneous DME supply or accessory, not otherwise specified

Lay Description
This code is a catch all code for supplies, accessories, or services not covered in other DME HCPCS codes.

B

B4034-B4036

B4034 Enteral feeding supply kit; syringe fed, per day, includes but not limited to feeding/flushing syringe, administration set tubing, dressings, tape

B4035 Enteral feeding supply kit; pump fed, per day, includes but not limited to feeding/flushing syringe, administration set tubing, dressings, tape

B4036 Enteral feeding supply kit; gravity fed, per day, includes but not limited to feeding/flushing syringe, administration set tubing, dressings, tape

Lay Description
Patients with chronic illness or trauma cannot be sustained through oral feeding and must rely on enteral or parenteral therapy, depending upon the particular nature of the medical condition. Daily enteral nutrition is necessary for patients with a functioning gastrointestinal (GI) tract but nonfunctioning body structures for allowing food to reach the small bowel, or for patients with small bowel disease that impairs digestion and absorption of nutrients. Enteral nutrition is administered to a patient through a tube into the stomach or small intestine. The solutions may be administered by syringe, gravity, or infusion pump.

B4081-B4088

B4081 Nasogastric tubing with stylet
B4082 Nasogastric tubing without stylet
B4083 Stomach tube - Levine type
B4087 Gastrostomy/jejunostomy tube, standard, any material, any type, each
B4088 Gastrostomy/jejunostomy tube, low-profile, any material, any type, each

Lay Description
Patients with chronic illness or trauma cannot be sustained through oral feeding and must rely on enteral or parenteral therapy, depending upon the particular nature of the medical condition. Enteral nutrition is administered to a patient through a tube (nasogastric, jejunostomy, or gastrostomy) into the stomach or small intestine. There are several types of gastric tubes including Levin type stomach tube, gastric sump, Moss, Sengstaken Blakemore, and Miller-Abbott. Specifically, feeding tubes are generally referred to as G tubes, J tubes, NG tubes, or surgical feeding tubes. Surgical feeding tubes require intraoperative placement.

B4100

B4100 Food thickener, administered orally, per oz

Lay Description
Patients who have facial paralysis, due to a stroke, Parkinson's disease, multiple sclerosis, and other conditions, have difficulty swallowing liquids (dysphagia) and often benefit from the use of a food thickener. Thickened food has a pureed consistency necessary to help prevent choking. Commercial instant food thickener has no taste or aftertaste. It mixes with hot or cold foods and liquids and thickens in just 30 seconds. These products allow for normal hydration by releasing available fluid after consumption. The thickened food and liquid does not harden when chilled or cause constipation. Use this code per ounce of food thickener.

B4102-B4104

B4102 Enteral formula, for adults, used to replace fluids and electrolytes (e.g., clear liquids), 500 ml = 1 unit

B4103 Enteral formula, for pediatrics, used to replace fluids and electrolytes (e.g., clear liquids), 500 ml = 1 unit

B4104 Additive for enteral formula (e.g., fiber)

Lay Description
For patients who cannot be sustained through oral feedings, enteral nutrition is administered by means of a nasogastric, jejunostomy, or gastrostomy feeding tube directly into the stomach or small intestine. An enteral formula additive, such as fiber, is used to maintain normal bowel function and avoid constipation.

B4149

B4149 Enteral formula, manufactured blenderized natural foods with intact nutrients, includes proteins, fats, carbohydrates, vitamins and minerals, may include fiber, administered through an enteral feeding tube, 100 calories = 1 unit

Lay Description
For patients who cannot be sustained through oral feedings, enteral nutrition is administered by means of a nasogastric, jejunostomy, or gastrostomy feeding tube directly into the stomach or small intestine. Enteral formulas are composed of varying combinations of natural or semi-synthetic proteins, amino acids, fats, carbohydrates, vitamins, and minerals to fulfill different nutritional needs. A blenderized natural foods formula of intact nutrients includes proteins, fats, carbohydrates, vitamins and minerals, and possibly fiber per 100 cal unit. Intact nutrients are not already broken down and remain in a high molecular weight form, which require normal digestive and absorptive ability.

B4150-B4152

B4150 Enteral formula, nutritionally complete with intact nutrients, includes proteins, fats, carbohydrates, vitamins and minerals, may include fiber, administered through an enteral feeding tube, 100 calories = 1 unit

B4152 Enteral formula, nutritionally complete, calorically dense (equal to or greater than 1.5 kcal/ml) with intact nutrients, includes proteins, fats, carbohydrates, vitamins and minerals, may include fiber, administered through an enteral feeding tube, 100 calories = 1 unit

Lay Description
These codes report a nutritionally complete enteral formula or nutrient mixture administered to patients who cannot be sustained through oral feedings, given by means of a nasogastric, jejunostomy, or gastrostomy feeding tube directly into the stomach or small intestine. Tube feedings can be administered by bolus feedings, continuous drip feedings, or a combination of the two. Intact nutrients are not already broken down and remain in a high molecular weight form, which require normal digestive and absorptive ability.

B4153

B4153 Enteral formula, nutritionally complete, hydrolyzed proteins (amino acids and peptide chain), includes fats, carbohydrates, vitamins and minerals, may include fiber, administered through an enteral feeding tube, 100 calories = 1 unit

Lay Description
This code reports a nutritionally complete enteral formula or nutrient mixture administered to patients who cannot be sustained through oral feedings, given by means of a nasogastric, jejunostomy, or gastrostomy feeding tube directly into the stomach or small intestine. Tube feedings can be administered by bolus feedings, continuous drip feedings, or a combination of the two. This code reports a formula of hydrolyzed proteins of amino acids and peptide chain, including fats, carbohydrates, vitamins and minerals, and possibly fiber, per 100 cal unit. Hydrolyzed proteins have been split down into their smaller building-block forms of amino acids and peptide chains by enzymes, acids, or alkalis. They provide the same nutritive equivalent in a more easily digestible form.

B4154-B4155

B4154 Enteral formula, nutritionally complete, for special metabolic needs, excludes inherited disease of metabolism, includes altered composition of proteins, fats, carbohydrates, vitamins and/or minerals, may include fiber, administered through an enteral feeding tube, 100 calories = 1 unit

B4155 Enteral formula, nutritionally incomplete/modular nutrients, includes specific nutrients, carbohydrates (e.g., glucose polymers), proteins/amino acids (e.g., glutamine, arginine), fat (e.g., medium chain triglycerides) or combination, administered through an enteral feeding tube, 100 calories = 1 unit

Lay Description
A nutritionally complete enteral formula or nutrient mixture is administered to patients who cannot be sustained through oral feedings, given by means of a nasogastric, jejunostomy, or gastrostomy feeding tube directly into the stomach or small intestine. Tube feedings can be administered by bolus feedings, continuous drip feedings, or a combination of the two. These codes report a formula designed for special metabolic needs that are not a consequence of an inherited metabolism disorder. The formula may contain proteins, fats, and carbohydrates in altered composition, and possible fiber, per 100 cal unit. Nutritionally incomplete enteral formula of modular nutrients contains specific nutrient forms of carbohydrates, fats, or proteins to cover deficiency needs, such as glucose polymers, glutamine, arginine, and medium chain triglycerides.

B4157

B4157 Enteral formula, nutritionally complete, for special metabolic needs for inherited disease of metabolism, includes proteins, fats, carbohydrates, vitamins and minerals, may include fiber, administered through an enteral feeding tube, 100 calories = 1 unit

Lay Description
For patients who cannot be sustained through oral feedings, enteral nutrition is administered by means of a nasogastric, jejunostomy, or gastrostomy feeding tube directly into the stomach or small intestine. Enteral formulas are composed of varying combinations of natural or semisynthetic proteins, amino acids, fats, carbohydrates, vitamins, and minerals to fulfill different nutritional needs. This nutritionally complete formula is designed for the special metabolic needs of inherited metabolism disorders, per 100 cal unit.

B

B4158-B4159

B4158 Enteral formula, for pediatrics, nutritionally complete with intact nutrients, includes proteins, fats, carbohydrates, vitamins and minerals, may include fiber and/or iron, administered through an enteral feeding tube, 100 calories = 1 unit

B4159 Enteral formula, for pediatrics, nutritionally complete soy based with intact nutrients, includes proteins, fats, carbohydrates, vitamins and minerals, may include fiber and/or iron, administered through an enteral feeding tube, 100 calories = 1 unit

Lay Description

These codes report a pediatric enteral formula or nutrient mixture administered to patients who cannot be sustained through oral feedings, given by means of a nasogastric, jejunostomy, or gastrostomy feeding tube directly into the stomach or small intestine. Tube feedings can be administered by bolus feedings, continuous drip feedings, or a combination of the two in patients who require calorie and protein support. Intact nutrients are not already broken down and remain in a high molecular weight form, which require normal digestive and absorptive ability. The soy-based, pediatric enteral formula is used to avoid milk-protein sensitivity.

B4160

B4160 Enteral formula, for pediatrics, nutritionally complete calorically dense (equal to or greater than 0.7 kcal/ml) with intact nutrients, includes proteins, fats, carbohydrates, vitamins and minerals, may include fiber, administered through an enteral feeding tube, 100 calories = 1 unit

Lay Description

This code reports a pediatric enteral formula or nutrient mixture administered to patients who cannot be sustained through oral feedings, given by means of a nasogastric, jejunostomy, or gastrostomy feeding tube directly into the stomach or small intestine. Tube feedings can be administered by bolus feedings, continuous drip feedings, or a combination of the two in patients who require calorie and protein support. This code reports a calorically dense, nutritionally complete formula, with intact nutrients, greater than .7kcal/ml, and possibly including fiber, per 100 cal unit. Intact nutrients are not already broken down and remain in a high molecular weight form, which require normal digestive and absorptive ability.

B4161

B4161 Enteral formula, for pediatrics, hydrolyzed/amino acids and peptide chain proteins, includes fats, carbohydrates, vitamins and minerals, may include fiber, administered through an enteral feeding tube, 100 calories = 1 unit

Lay Description

This code reports a pediatric enteral formula or nutrient mixture administered to patients who cannot be sustained through oral feedings, given by means of a nasogastric, jejunostomy, or gastrostomy feeding tube directly into the stomach or small intestine. Tube feedings can be administered by bolus feedings, continuous drip feedings, or a combination of the two in patients who require calorie and protein support. This code reports a formula of hydrolyzed/amino acids and peptide chain proteins, including fats, carbohydrates, vitamins and minerals, and possibly fiber, per 100 cal unit. Hydrolyzed proteins have been split down into their smaller building-block forms of amino acids and peptide chains by enzymes, acids, or alkalis. They provide the same nutritive equivalent in a more easily digestible form.

B4162

B4162 Enteral formula, for pediatrics, special metabolic needs for inherited disease of metabolism, includes proteins, fats, carbohydrates, vitamins and minerals, may include fiber, administered through an enteral feeding tube, 100 calories = 1 unit

Lay Description

This code reports a pediatric enteral formula, or nutrient mixture administered to patients who cannot be sustained through oral feedings, given by means of a nasogastric, jejunostomy, or gastrostomy feeding tube directly into the stomach or small intestine. Tube feedings can be administered by bolus feedings, continuous drip feedings, or a combination of the two in patients who require calorie and protein support. This code reports a nutritionally complete pediatric formula designed for the special metabolic needs of inherited metabolism disorders, per 100 cal unit.

B4164-B4185

B4164 Parenteral nutrition solution: carbohydrates (dextrose), 50% or less (500 ml = 1 unit), home mix

B4168 Parenteral nutrition solution; amino acid, 3.5%, (500 ml = 1 unit) - home mix

B4172 Parenteral nutrition solution; amino acid, 5.5% through 7%, (500 ml = 1 unit) - home mix

B4176 Parenteral nutrition solution; amino acid, 7% through 8.5%, (500 ml = 1 unit) - home mix

B4178 Parenteral nutrition solution: amino acid, greater than 8.5% (500 ml = 1 unit), home mix

B4180 Parenteral nutrition solution: carbohydrates (dextrose), greater than 50% (500 ml = 1 unit), home mix

B4185 Parenteral nutrition solution, per 10 grams lipids

Lay Description
Parenteral nutrition is administered to the patient intravenously. Since the alimentary tract of a patient with severe pathology does not function adequately for ingesting food normally, an indwelling catheter is placed percutaneously in the subclavian vein, and then advanced into the superior vena cava for infusing nutrients intravenously. Parenteral nutrition solutions are based on the composition of ingredients or nutrient source in each product, and whether it is supplied in a home mix or a premix. These codes report home mix solutions of 1 unit equaling 500 ml.

B4189-B4216

B4189 Parenteral nutrition solution: compounded amino acid and carbohydrates with electrolytes, trace elements, and vitamins, including preparation, any strength, 10 to 51 g of protein, premix

B4193 Parenteral nutrition solution: compounded amino acid and carbohydrates with electrolytes, trace elements, and vitamins, including preparation, any strength, 52 to 73 g of protein, premix

B4197 Parenteral nutrition solution; compounded amino acid and carbohydrates with electrolytes, trace elements and vitamins, including preparation, any strength, 74 to 100 grams of protein - premix

B4199 Parenteral nutrition solution; compounded amino acid and carbohydrates with electrolytes, trace elements and vitamins, including preparation, any strength, over 100 grams of protein - premix

B4216 Parenteral nutrition; additives (vitamins, trace elements, Heparin, electrolytes), home mix, per day

Lay Description
Parenteral nutrition is administered to the patient intravenously. Since the alimentary tract of a patient with severe pathology does not function adequately for ingesting food normally, an indwelling catheter is placed percutaneously in the subclavian vein, and then advanced into the superior vena cava for infusing nutrients intravenously. Parenteral nutrition solutions are based on the composition of ingredients or nutrient source in each parenteral nutrient product, and whether it is supplied in a home mix or a premix. These codes report premix solutions, including preparation of any strength compounded amino acids and carbohydrates with electrolytes, trace elements, and vitamins.

B4220-B4224

B4220 Parenteral nutrition supply kit; premix, per day

B4222 Parenteral nutrition supply kit; home mix, per day

B4224 Parenteral nutrition administration kit, per day

Lay Description
Patients with chronic illness or trauma cannot be sustained through oral feeding and must rely on enteral or parenteral therapy, depending upon the particular nature of the medical condition. Parenteral nutrition is administered to the patient intravenously. These codes report the supply and administration kits for parenteral nutrition on a daily basis.

B5000-B5200

B5000 Parenteral nutrition solution: compounded amino acid and carbohydrates with electrolytes, trace elements, and vitamins, including preparation, any strength, renal - Amirosyn RF, NephrAmine, RenAmine - premix

B5100 Parenteral nutrition solution: compounded amino acid and carbohydrates with electrolytes, trace elements, and vitamins, including preparation, any strength, hepatic - FreAmine HBC, HepatAmine - premix

B5200 Parenteral nutrition solution: compounded amino acid and carbohydrates with electrolytes, trace elements, and vitamins, including preparation, any strength, stress - branch chain amino acids - premix

Lay Description
Parenteral nutrition is administered to the patient intravenously. Since the alimentary tract of a patient with severe pathology does not function adequately for ingesting food normally, an indwelling catheter is placed percutaneously in the subclavian vein, and then advanced into the superior vena cava for infusing nutrients intravenously. Parenteral nutrition solutions are based on the composition of ingredients or nutrient source in each parenteral nutrient product and whether it is supplied in a home mix or a premix. These codes report premix solutions, including preparation of any strength compounded amino acids

B

and carbohydrates with electrolytes, trace elements, and vitamins.

B9000-B9002

B9000 Enteral nutrition infusion pump - without alarm

B9002 Enteral nutrition infusion pump - with alarm

Lay Description
Infusion pumps are available when enteral nutrition patients experience complications associated with syringe or gravity feedings. An enteral pump is ordered when feeding problems arise such as reflux and/or aspiration, severe diarrhea, dumping syndrome, an administration rate less than 100 ml/hr, blood glucose fluctuations, or circulatory overload.

B9004-B9999

B9004 Parenteral nutrition infusion pump, portable

B9006 Parenteral nutrition infusion pump, stationary

B9998 NOC for enteral supplies

B9999 NOC for parenteral supplies

Lay Description
Permanent conditions of the alimentary tract cause the patient to be unable to maintain weight and strength through normal feeding and require parenteral therapy, the intravenous infusion of nutrients, with the use of a parenteral nutrition infusion pump.

C

C1713

C1713 Anchor/screw for opposing bone-to-bone or soft tissue-to-bone (implantable)

Lay Description
An implantable pin and/or screw is used to oppose soft tissue-to-bone, tendon-to-bone, or bone-to-bone. A screw opposes the tissue by means of drilling as follows: soft tissue-to-bone, tendon-to-bone, or bone-to-bone fixation. Pins are inserted or drilled into the bone with the intent to facilitate stabilization or oppose bone-to-bone. In many instances this may include orthopedic plates with accompanying washers and nuts.

C1714

C1714 Catheter, transluminal atherectomy, directional

Lay Description
This code represents a special type of catheter used in transluminal atherectomy procedures. Transluminal atherectomy procedures involve opening the patients blocked arteries or vein grafts by using specialized devices attached to the end of catheters, which assist

in the removal of thrombi and plaque material. Rotational atherectomy involves a high speed rotational device that grinds up the plaque material being removed from the vessel. Directional atherectomy scrapes or directs the plaque into an opening on one side of the catheter. Transluminal extraction atherectomy uses a device that cuts plaque off vessel walls and then vacuums it into a bottle.

C1715

C1715 Brachytherapy needle

Lay Description
This code pertains to needles specifically used in brachytherapy and is utilized per needle not per procedure.

C1716-C1719

C1716 Brachytherapy source, nonstranded, gold-198, per source

C1717 Brachytherapy source, nonstranded, high dose rate iridium-192, per source

C1719 Brachytherapy source, nonstranded, nonhigh dose rate iridium-192, per source

Lay Description
Brachytherapy is a form of radiotherapy in which physicians place the source of irradiation close to the tumor or within a body cavity. Brachytherapy could include placing radioactive sources inside a body cavity (intracavitary brachytherapy) or putting radioactive material directly into body tissue using hollow needles (interstitial brachytherapy). Brachytherapy may be given in addition to external beam radiation, or it may be used as the only form of radiotherapy. In some cases, the radioactive sources may be permanently left in place; in other cases, they are removed after a specified time. Placement of radioactive sources may be repeated several times. The isotope gold has a half life of 2.7 days and is used in some cancer treatments and treatments for other diseases. There are two natural isotopes of iridium, and many radioisotopes, the most stable radioisotope being Ir-192 with a half-life of 73.83 days. Ir-192 beta decays into platinum-192, while most of the other radioisotopes decay into osmium.

C1721-C1722

C1721 Cardioverter-defibrillator, dual chamber (implantable)

C1722 Cardioverter-defibrillator, single chamber (implantable)

Lay Description
Implantable cardioverter defibrillators are used in patients at risk for recurrent, sustained ventricular tachycardia or fibrillation. The defibrillators are connected to leads that are positioned inside the heart or on the heart surface. These leads deliver electrical shocks, sense the heart's rhythm, and pace the heart as necessary. Various leads are tunneled to

the pulse generator, which has been implanted in a pouch made in the skin of the abdomen or chest. When the defibrillator detects ventricular tachycardia or fibrillation, it will automatically shock the heart to restore normal rhythm.

C1724

C1724   Catheter, transluminal atherectomy, rotational

Lay Description
This code represents a special type of catheter used in transluminal atherectomy procedures. Transluminal atherectomy procedures involve opening the patient's blocked arteries or vein grafts by using specialized devices attached to the end of catheters, which assist in the removal of thrombi and plaque material. Rotational atherectomy involves a high speed rotational device that grinds up the plaque material being removed from the vessel. Directional atherectomy scrapes or directs the plaque into an opening on one side of the catheter. Transluminal extraction atherectomy uses a device that cuts plaque off vessel walls and then vacuums it into a bottle.

C1725

C1725   Catheter, transluminal angioplasty, nonlaser (may include guidance, infusion/perfusion capability)

Lay Description
A transluminal angioplasty nonlaser catheter is a small hollow tube that is inserted into the central space (or lumen) of an artery or vein .This code refers to a catheter that is not used with a laser, but is used with balloon or other device that is designed to be advanced through the blood vessels to the area of occlusion or blockage. When the catheter is in position, the device is used to compress, break up, or remove the obstruction.

C1726

C1726   Catheter, balloon dilatation, nonvascular

Lay Description
A nonvascular balloon dilatation catheter is a small hollow tube containing a deflated balloon that is inserted into body cavity, duct or other passageway. The catheter is advanced to the area of occlusion or blockage. When the catheter is in position, the balloon is inflated and used to dilate strictures or stenoses. Examples of common sites are the common bile duct, intestines, or ureter.

C1727

C1727   Catheter, balloon tissue dissector, nonvascular (insertable)

Lay Description
A balloon tissue dissector, nonvascular catheter is small hollow tube that contains a deflated balloon. The catheter is guided to the appropriate space; the balloon is inflated and sometimes elongated. It is used to create a space between soft tissues to improve operative vision and work space.

C1728

C1728   Catheter, brachytherapy seed administration

Lay Description
A brachytherapy seed administration catheter used to temporarily place encapsulated radioactive materials (seeds or sources) in or near the targeted tissue or tumor, or into a body cavity.

C1729

C1729   Catheter, drainage

Lay Description
A drainage catheter is a small hollow tube that is used to drain collected fluids from internal structures out through the skin and subcutaneous tissue. This category does not include Foley catheters or suprapubic catheters.

C1730-C1732

C1730   Catheter, electrophysiology, diagnostic, other than 3D mapping (19 or fewer electrodes)
C1731   Catheter, electrophysiology, diagnostic, other than 3D mapping (20 or more electrodes)
C1732   Catheter, electrophysiology, diagnostic/ablation, 3D or vector mapping

Lay Description
These codes describe catheters that assist in providing anatomic and physiologic information about the heart's electrical activity. Electrophysiology catheters are categorized into two main groups: (1) catheters used for mapping, pacing, and/or recording only, and (2) ablation (therapeutic) catheters that also have diagnostic capability. The electrophysiology ablation catheters are distinct from non-cardiac ablation catheters.

C1733

C1733   Catheter, electrophysiology, diagnostic/ablation, other than 3D or vector mapping, other than cool-tip

Lay Description
An electrophysiology, diagnostic/ablation catheter, other than 3D or vector mapping, other than cool-tip, is a small hollow tube that assists in providing anatomic and physiologic information about the cardiac electrical conduction system. Electrophysiology catheters are categorized into two main groups: (1) diagnostic catheters that are used for mapping, pacing, and/or recording only, and (2) ablation (therapeutic) catheters that also have diagnostic capability. The electrophysiology ablation catheters are distinct from noncardiac ablation

catheters. Electrophysiology catheters designated as "cool-tip" refer to catheters with tips cooled by infused and/or circulating saline. Catheters designated as "other than cool-tip" refer to the termister tip catheter with temperature probe that measures temperature at the tissue catheter interface.

C1749

C1749   Endoscope, retrograde imaging/illumination colonoscope device (implantable)

Lay Description
A retrograde imaging/illumination colonoscope device is a J-shaped catheter that can be inserted into endoscope working channels. The rear-facing catheter contains an imaging device that provides illumination and a continuous retrograde view of the colon. It allows the physician to look behind the folds to find lesions. The devise is intended for single patient use and is disposable.

C1750, C1752

C1750   Catheter, hemodialysis/peritoneal, long-term

C1752   Catheter, hemodialysis/peritoneal, short-term

Lay Description
These codes describe a catheter that can be a permanent or temporary placed tube with one or two cuffs. This catheter is surgically placed into the peritoneum in the abdomen via a small incision and works by permitting the exchange of fluid through the catheter, allowing dialysate in and out of the abdominal cavity.

C1751

C1751   Catheter, infusion, inserted peripherally, centrally or midline (other than hemodialysis)

Lay Description
An infusion catheter is a plastic catheter that may have multiple lumens that is inserted into a large vein and ends up in the subclavian, brachiocephalic, or iliac veins, the superior or inferior vena cava, or the right atrium. It can be inserted centrally into the jugular, subclavian, femoral vein or inferior vena cava or peripherally into the basilic or cephalic vein. It can be used to administer medication, hydration, nutrition, and for monitoring and withdrawing blood samples. There are two different types of catheters: tunnelled and non-tunnelled.

C1753

C1753   Catheter, intravascular ultrasound

Lay Description
This code describes a specially designed catheter with a very small ultrasound probe attached to the distal end of the catheter. The proximal end of the catheter

is attached to computerized ultrasound equipment. It allows the application of ultrasound technology to see from inside blood vessels out through the surrounding blood column, allowing the visualization of the inner wall of blood vessels.

C1754

C1754   Catheter, intradiscal

Lay Description
An intradiscal catheter is a small hollow tube that is inserted into a vertebral disc through which therapeutic treatments are performed. The flexible catheter is threaded percutaneously using fluoroscopic guidance. The catheter may be used to deliver electrothermal therapy.

C1755

C1755   Catheter, intraspinal

Lay Description
An intraspinal catheter is small hollow tube that is inserted into the spinal column to deliver diagnostic or therapeutic substances within the central nervous system.

C1756

C1756   Catheter, pacing, transesophageal

Lay Description
A transesophageal pacing catheter is a small hollow tube that is inserted into the esophagus and positioned near the posterior aspect of the atria. The catheter contains an electrode that delivers electrical stimulation to the heart and usually includes a device to record an electrocardiogram. The catheter may be used for therapeutic purposes, such as converting an arrhythmia during an intraoperative procedure, or for diagnostic purposes, such as in evaluations of sinus node function.

C1757

C1757   Catheter, thrombectomy/embolectomy

Lay Description
A thrombectomy or embolectomy catheter is a small hollow tube that is inserted into a blood vessel and guided to the site of the embolism or thrombus. A device that breaks up or macerates the thrombus or embolus may be inserted through the catheter. Usually, the catheter is used to aspirate the thrombus or embolus.

C1758

C1758   Catheter, ureteral

Lay Description
Ureteral catheter is a small hollow tube that is inserted into the ureter to withdraw or introduce fluid. The catheter may be inserted either through the urethra and bladder or posteriorly via the kidney.

C1759

C1759 Catheter, intracardiac echocardiography

Lay Description
An intracardiac echocardiography (ICE) catheter is a small tube inserted into a blood vessel that contains an ultrasound device. It is maneuvered into the heart to provide anatomic and physiologic real time imaging within the heart walls. A Doppler device provides imaging of blood flow and velocity and of myocardial wall motion.

C1760

C1760 Closure device, vascular (implantable/insertable)

Lay Description
A vascular closure device seals femoral artery punctures caused by invasive or interventional procedures. The closure or seal is achieved by placing the vessel ends between the device's two primary structures, which are usually an anchor and a biologic substance (e.g., collagen) or suture through the tissue tract.

C1762

C1762 Connective tissue, human (includes fascia lata)

Lay Description
Human connective tissue (includes fascia lata) is natural human cellular collagen or extracellular matrix obtained from autologous rectus fascia, decellularized cadaver fascia lata, or decellularized dermal tissue. The tissue is intended to repair or support damaged or inadequate soft tissue. They are used to treat urinary incontinence resulting from hypermobility or Intrinsic Sphincter Deficiency (ISD), pelvic floor repair, or for implantation to reinforce soft tissues where weakness exists in the urological anatomy. The category excludes those items that are used to replace skin.

C1763

C1763 Connective tissue, nonhuman (includes synthetic)

Lay Description
Nonhuman connective tissue (includes synthetic) is a natural collagen matrix typically obtained from porcine or bovine small intestinal submucosa, or pericardium. The material is acellular as all cells are removed leaving only a matrix or scaffold. This tissue is intended to promote the growth of the patient's cells within the implanted matrix. It is intended to repair or support damaged or inadequate soft tissue. Nonhuman connective tissue is used to treat urinary incontinence resulting from hypermobility or intrinsic sphincter deficiency (ISD), pelvic floor repair, or for implantation to reinforce soft tissues where weakness exists in the urological or musculoskeletal anatomy. This category excludes those items that are used to replace skin.

C1764

C1764 Event recorder, cardiac (implantable)

Lay Description
Event recorders are implanted in the left front of the chest in a pocket created in the skin. Once implanted, the patient's cardiac events are recorded. Implantable cardiac event monitors are for long-time use, enabling the recorder to capture more infrequent heart rhythms. The device can have auto activation or manual activation depending upon the needs of the patient. If the patient experiences syncopal episodes, the manual activation button can be pressed only after the patient is conscious again. If the device has auto activation, the device records rhythms automatically when the heart rate is in excess or under a preset limit.

C1765

C1765 Adhesion barrier

Lay Description
An adhesion barrier is a bioresorbable substance used on and around neural structures, minimizing the formation of scar tissue. It is mainly used in spinal surgeries, such as laminectomies and diskectomies.

C1766

C1766 Introducer/sheath, guiding, intracardiac electrophysiological, steerable, other than peel-away

Lay Description
An intracardiac electrophysiological introducer or sheath, guiding, steerable, other than peel-away, is a small hollow tube that is inserted into the heart and guided to the target area. Electrophysiological devices and catheters are then passed through the introducer to the target area.

C1767

C1767 Generator, neurostimulator (implantable), nonrechargeable

Lay Description
An implantable nonrechargeable neurostimulator generator is a device that creates small electrical impulses that are transmitted to electrodes implanted near the spinal cord or a peripheral nerve. The small electrical impulses interrupt pain signals sent to the brain. This type of generator contains a battery that cannot be recharged, but must be removed and replaced.

C1768

C1768 Graft, vascular

Lay Description
A vascular graft uses material to patch a damaged, diseased, or injured area of an artery or for replacement of whole segments of vessels. Vascular grafts may be biological or synthetic. Biological grafts are generally taken from another site in the patient,

also known as autografts. In a common autograft, the internal mammary artery is generally used in coronary artery bypass surgery. Other biological grafts can come from another member of the same species, such as the use of cadaver grafts. Synthetic grafts are usually made from Dacron or polytetrafluoroethylene (PTFE).

C1769

C1769   Guide wire

Lay Description

A guidewire is a thin piece of material that is guided into a desired blood vessel through a trocar. The trocar is then removed and the guidewire left in place. Catheters, cannulas, or other tubular devices can be inserted over the guidewire into the blood vessel and the guidewire is withdrawn.

C1770

C1770   Imaging coil, magnetic resonance (insertable)

Lay Description

An insertable magnetic resonance imaging coil is an intracavity probe that is placed in a relatively inaccessible or dense body area. The coil emits a magnetic signature that enhances images taken during the MRI.

C1771

C1771   Repair device, urinary, incontinence, with sling graft

Lay Description

A urinary incontinence repair device is used to attach or insert body tissue, synthetic material, or mesh for the purpose of strengthening the pelvic floor. The repair material is fashioned into a sling or hammock that supports the urethra. This code represents the device components used to deliver the sling graft and/or fixate (via permanent sutures or bone anchors) the sling graft. This code includes the sling graft.

C1772

C1772   Infusion pump, programmable (implantable)

Lay Description

An implantable programmable infusion pump is an electrical device that delivers drugs, nutrients, or fluids into the patient's body. It is surgically placed in a subcutaneous pocket with a catheter that is threaded into a desired position. This code represents a device that has a programmer that can be set to deliver the fluid continuously or at set intervals.

C1773

C1773   Retrieval device, insertable (used to retrieve fractured medical devices)

Lay Description

An insertable retrieval device is used to retrieve fractured medical devices that are lodged within the vascular system. This device can also be used to exchange intravascular introducers or sheaths.

C1776

C1776   Joint device (implantable)

Lay Description

A joint device is an artificial prosthetic device that is implanted in a patient as a replacement for a natural joint, such as a finger or toe. Generally a joint device is not used to oppose soft tissue-to-bone, tendon-to-bone, or bone-to-bone.

C1777

C1777   Lead, cardioverter-defibrillator, endocardial single coil (implantable)

Lay Description

An endocardial single coil cardioverter-defibrillator lead is an implanted wire with an electrode at its tip that connects a generator to the heart muscle. An electrode detects electrical changes in the heart which are recorded by the generator and transmits electrical charges created by the generator to the heart to correct and maintain a steady heart rhythm. A cardioverter-defibrillator is a device designed to detect ventricular tachycardia or fibrillation and to deliver an electrical shock to return the heart to normal rhythm. This is a lead that attaches to the heart wall of the heart muscle with the other end connected to a cardioverter-defibrillator.

C1778

C1778   Lead, neurostimulator (implantable)

Lay Description

An implantable neurostimulator lead is a wire with an electrode at its tip that connects a generator to the brain or nervous system. An electrode transmits electrical charges created by the neurostimulator. The electrical signal interrupts the brain function or nerve conduction. Neurostimulators can be used to reduce or eliminate pain, activate nerve responses, or control electrical brain discharges.

C1779

C1779   Lead, pacemaker, transvenous VDD single pass

Lay Description

A pacemaker is a device used to synchronize the beating of the heart. Single-pass VDD is a physiological stimulation mode that requires a single lead with a floating dipole to detect the atrial signal. A transvenous pacemaker lead senses and paces the ventricle and the atrium. The VDD pacemaker is used for AV nodal dysfunction with intact and appropriate sinus node behavior.

C1780

C1780   Lens, intraocular (new technology)

Lay Description
This code describes an artificial lens made of plastic, silicone, or acrylic that performs the function of the eye's natural lens, typically a quarter of an inch in diameter. The lens is usually soft enough that it can be folded and placed into the eye through a small incision. This code specifically refers to the intraocular lenses approved by CMS as "new technology IOL."

C1781

C1781   Mesh (implantable)

Lay Description
A mesh implant is a synthetic patch composed of absorbable or nonabsorbable material that is used to repair hernias, support weakened or attenuated tissue, cover tissue defects, etc.

C1782

C1782   Morcellator

Lay Description
A morcellator is a device that cuts, cores, and extracts tissue in laparoscopic procedures. The device uses suction to draw tissue into its tip where it is cut into small pieces by a rotating blade. The device removes the tissue from the field using suction.

C1783

C1783   Ocular implant, aqueous drainage assist device

Lay Description
Glaucoma is a group of ocular diseases that affect the optic nerve. High intraocular pressure frequently accompanies these diseases. This code describes a drain implanted into the anterior chamber of the eye that drains the aqueous humor to the outer eye. Drainage of the aqueous humor reduces intraocular pressure.

C1784

C1784   Ocular device, intraoperative, detached retina

Lay Description
An intraoperative ocular device for a detached retina is a carbon and fluorine (perfluorocarbon) gas that is instilled into the vitreous during a procedure to treat detached retina. The vitreous is a clear collagen gel that fills the eye that helps the retina lie smoothly and firmly against the back wall of the eyeball. The gas is injected to help return the retina to its normal position or to replace vitreous fluid removed during other retina repair procedures. The gas bubble eventually dissipates and may be replaced with body fluids.

C1785-C1786

C1785   Pacemaker, dual chamber, rate-responsive (implantable)
C1786   Pacemaker, single chamber, rate-responsive (implantable)

Lay Description
A pacemaker is a medical device that uses electrical impulses, delivered by electrodes contacting the heart muscles, to regulate the beating of the heart. The primary purpose of a pacemaker is to maintain an adequate heart rate. The dual chamber rate responsive pacemaker operates in an atrial synchronized modality when the sensed atrial rate is within a physiologic range and paces at a sensor determined rate when the atrial rate is above or below the physiologic range. The dual artificial pacemaker has two leads; one in the atrium and one in the ventricle, so electromechanical synchrony can be approximated and can deliver stimuli at a rate adjustable to some parameter independent of atrial activity. The single chamber pacemaker has only one lead in the atrium or ventricle. The pacemaker is placed beneath skin in the pectoral region.

C1787

C1787   Patient programmer, neurostimulator

Lay Description
A patient programmer is a handheld device that transmits operational commands to the neurostimulator. A patient may control the amplitude and rate of the electrical impulses delivered by the neurostimulator system

C1788

C1788   Port, indwelling (implantable)

Lay Description
An indwelling port (e.g., central venous access device) is a small medical appliance inserted subcutaneously that connects to a vein. The port contains a subcutaneous septum that allows blood to be withdrawn and drugs to be injected. The device consists of a reservoir (or portal) composed of a self-sealing silicone bubble and a catheter. The catheter runs from the port to a major vein (e.g., jugular, subclavian). Ideally it terminates in the superior vena cava near the right atrium. This position allows injected drugs to spread quickly and efficiently throughout the body.

C1789

C1789   Prosthesis, breast (implantable)

Lay Description
A breast implant is a prosthesis used to modify the size, form, and feel of a woman's breast in a post-mastectomy reconstruction; improve chest wall congenital deformities; augment the breast; or perform gender transition (male to female). Breast

implants are surgically placed in anatomical relation to the pectoralis major muscle.

C1813

C1813 Prosthesis, penile, inflatable

Lay Description
The inflatable penile prosthesis is a medical device used for men with organic or psychogenic impotence who suffer from erectile dysfunction. This prosthesis is also used in the final stages of plastic surgery phalloplasty in gender reassignment surgery, as well as in total phalloplasty in males that need genital modification. The inflatable penile prosthesis is made of three components: cylinders, pump, and reservoir. It can be inflated and deflated upon demand.

C1814

C1814 Retinal tamponade device, silicone oil

Lay Description
Silicone oil is a silicon analogue of carbon based organic compounds that can form long and complex molecules based on silicon rather than carbon. This HCPCS Level II code represents silicone oil used as a permanent or prolonged retinal tamponade for the treatment of complex retinal detachments. The vitreous is a clear collagen gel that fills the eye and helps the retina lie smoothly and firmly against the back wall of the eyeball. Silicone oil is injected to help return the retina to its normal position or to replace vitreous fluid removed during other retina repair procedures. The silicone oil eventually dissipates and may be replaced with body fluids.

C1815

C1815 Prosthesis, urinary sphincter (implantable)

Lay Description
An artificial urinary sphincter (AUS) is a medical device that closely simulates the function of a biological urinary sphincter. A donut-shaped sac that circles the urethra, an AUS offers a competent bladder outlet during urinary storage and an open, unobstructed outlet to allow voiding. When the sac is filled with fluid, it squeezes the urethra closed. When a valve implanted under the skin is pressed, the fluid is released allowing the urethra to open and urine to flow.

C1816

C1816 Receiver and/or transmitter, neurostimulator (implantable)

Lay Description
A neurostimulator, also called an implanted pulse generator, is a battery powered medical device that delivers electrical impulses through a lead to electrodes implanted near the spinal cord or an affected peripheral nerve. The device is used to stimulate the spinal cord or peripheral nerve and block the transmission of pain to the brain. The

neurostimulator system includes an integrated circuit, a radio-wave transceiver, a battery, and a connector block. There are two types of neurostimulation systems based on the location of the battery: a fully implanted system has an internal power source or one with an external power source.

C1817

C1817 Septal defect implant system, intracardiac

Lay Description
An intracardiac septal defect implant system is a an implant placed with the heart for closure of a variety of defects that may occur dividing wall that separates the left and right sides of the heart. The septal defect implant system represented by this code includes a delivery catheter.

C1818

C1818 Integrated keratoprosthesis

Lay Description
An integrated keratoprosthesis is a flexible, one-piece biocompatible polymer lens. It is used to replace diseased native corneas in conditions where traditional corneal transplantation is not indicated or possible.

C1819

C1819 Surgical tissue localization and excision device (implantable)

Lay Description
A lesion localization device is an implantable radiofrequency guide that allows for stabilization, dissection, and excision of a lesion or foreign objects. Used with stereotactic, alphanumeric grid imaging techniques and ultrasound, this device may include radiofrequency, laser, or ultrasonic components. Implantation within the body proximate to the suspect tissue or object is done prior to surgery with one or more integrated transponder tags. At the time of surgery, scanning of the body with a radiofrequency scanner or reader activates the tag or tags and provides the surgeon with signals indicative of the location.

C1820

C1820 Generator, neurostimulator (implantable), with rechargeable battery and charging system

Lay Description
An implantable rechargeable neurostimulator generator is a device that creates small electrical impulses that are transmitted to electrodes implanted near the spinal cord or a peripheral nerve. The small electrical impulses interrupt pain signals sent to the brain. This type of generator contains a battery that can be recharged. The code represents the generator, rechargeable battery and its charging system.

C1821

C1821   Interspinous process distraction device (implantable)

Lay Description

Interspinous process distraction implantable devices are implants placed between vertebral spinous processes. They aim to restrict painful motion while enabling normal motion. The implant is inserted between the spinous processes through a small incision and acts as a spacer between the spinous processes. After implantation, the device is opened or expanded to distract (open) the neural foramen and decompress the nerves. Reduction of vertebral motion may prevent pain caused by compression of blood vessels and nerves in the spine.

C1830

C1830   Powered bone marrow biopsy needle

Lay Description

A bone marrow biopsy needle is a specialized stylus used to penetrate and withdraw bone marrow. This code represents a battery-powered rotary device that is similar to a hand held drill. The device drives a single lumen needle into the medullary cavity of an adult hip. The needle contains two parts: an outer cannula and an inner bevel-tipped stylet. The device appears to deliver larger volume bone marrow specimens in a more rapid fashion. Patients report less associated pain with the powered device.

C1840

C1840   Lens, intraocular (telescopic)

Lay Description

An intraocular lens is an artificial lens made of plastic, silicone, or acrylic that performs the function of the eye's natural lens. This code represents a miniature implantable telescope lens intended to improve visual acuity in patients with age-related macular degeneration. The device magnifies images onto the healthy areas of the retina to help improve central vision. The telescopic lens is implanted into the posterior chamber of the eye's anterior segment. It is held in place with haptic loops.

C1841

C1841   Retinal prosthesis, includes all internal and external components

Lay Description

This retinal prosthesis is an implantable medical device that is intended to provide electrical stimulation of the retina to induce visual perception in patients who are profoundly blind due to retinitis pigmentosa (RP). The system employs electrical signals to bypass dead photo-receptor cells and stimulate the overlying neurons. There are three primary components: an implanted epiretinal prosthesis that is fully implanted on and in the eye (there are no percutaneous leads); external components, such as an externally worn video camera that wirelessly transmits a real-time video signal; and a "fitting" system for the clinician that is periodically used to perform diagnostic tests with the system and to custom-program the external unit. This procedure is reported with ICD-9-CM procedure code 14.81 for implantation of an epiretinal visual prosthesis, 14.82 for removal, and 14.83 for revision or replacement.

C1874

C1874   Stent, coated/covered, with delivery system

Lay Description

A stent with delivery system is a small hollow tube made of a biocompatible substance, such as phosphorylcholine, silicone, or metal, that is inserted into a natural body passage or conduit. The stent maintains the body passage or conduit allowing less restricted flow. This code represents a stent packaged with a delivery system that generally includes a stent mounted or unmounted on a balloon angioplasty catheter, introducer, and sheath.

C1875

C1875   Stent, coated/covered, without delivery system

Lay Description

A coated or covered stent without a delivery system is a small hollow tube made of a biocompatible substance, such as phosphorylcholine, silicone, or metal, that is inserted into a natural body passage or conduit. The stent maintains the body passage or conduit allowing less restricted flow. It is coated with a drug that helps prevent the conduit from becoming narrowed again. This code represents a stent packaged without a delivery system.

C1876-C1877

C1876   Stent, noncoated/noncovered, with delivery system

C1877   Stent, noncoated/noncovered, without delivery system

Lay Description

A stent is a small hollow tube made of stainless steel that is inserted into a natural body passage or conduit. The stent maintains the body passage or conduit allowing less restricted flow. These stents are not coated with any drugs or polymers. A delivery system is a method of delivering the device to its intended position in the body. Delivery systems can use balloon and guidewires or may be proprietary. These codes represent noncoated stents with and without a delivery system.

C1878

C1878 Material for vocal cord medialization, synthetic (implantable)

Lay Description

Material for vocal cord medialization is a synthetic implantable substance that is not absorbable. The substance is injected or implanted in a vocal cord to move the cord closer to midline to allow a greater strike with the opposite vocal cord.

C1880

C1880 Vena cava filter

Lay Description

A vena cava filter is a device that is inserted into the vena cava, the large vein that returns blood to the heart from the abdomen and legs (inferior vena cava). This filter is an umbrella-shaped barrier device that helps prevent blood clots that may form in the deep veins of the lower limbs from traveling to the lungs and heart where they may block blood flow. Vena cava filters are placed using a catheter inserted through a vein in the neck or groin. The device may be placed due to failure of anticoagulations, contraindications to anticoagulations, large clots in the vena cava or iliac veins, or for patients at high risk for having a pulmonary embolism.

C1881

C1881 Dialysis access system (implantable)

Lay Description

Hemodialysis requires access to the bloodstream or vascular access. The access is meant to be permanent so that it can be reused. The different types of access for hemodialysis include a fistula or a graft. A fistula is created by connecting one of the arteries to one of the veins in the lower arm. A graft uses a synthetic tube implanted under the skin of the arm to connect an artery and a vein. A temporary method using a venous catheter is usually used while permanent access develops. A catheter is placed in a vein in the neck, chest, or groin. Peritoneal dialysis access requires introduction of a catheter in the belly. Placement is usually done 10 to 14 days before dialysis starts. Because of a high risk of complications with prolonged use, these catheters are not commonly used.

C1882

C1882 Cardioverter-defibrillator, other than single or dual chamber (implantable)

Lay Description

A cardioverter-defibrillator is an electronic device that delivers an electric shock to the heart, helping re-establish normal contraction rhythms in a heart having dangerous arrhythmia or in cardiac arrest. An implantable cardioverter-defibrillator (ICD) has two components: a pulse generator and a defibrillator lead. The device is connected to leads positioned inside the heart or on its surface. These leads deliver electrical shocks, sense cardiac rhythm, and sometimes pace the heart, as needed. The various leads are connected to a pulse generator, which is implanted in a pouch beneath the skin of the chest or abdomen. The pulse generator's function is to generate energy, deliver defibrillating shocks, filter/analyze, and store electrical signals from the myocardium to distinguish normal from pathologic rhythms that require a response from the ICD. This code represents an implantable cardioverter-defibrillator, other than a single or dual chamber.

C1883

C1883 Adaptor/extension, pacing lead or neurostimulator lead (implantable)

Lay Description

A pacing or neurostimulator lead adaptor or extension is an implantable device that is placed in between an existing lead and a new generator. The end of the adaptor lead has the appropriate connector pin that enables the use of the existing lead with a new generator that has a different connecting receptacle. These are required when a generator is replaced or when two leads are connected to the same port in the connector block.

C1884

C1884 Embolization protective system

Lay Description

An embolization protective system is a system designed to trap, macerate, and remove atheromatous or thrombotic debris from the vascular system during an angioplasty, atherectomy, or stenting procedure.

C1885

C1885 Catheter, transluminal angioplasty, laser

Lay Description

A transluminal angioplasty laser catheter is a small hollow tube that is inserted into the central space (or lumen) of an artery or vein .This code refers to a catheter that has a laser at its tip. The catheter is advanced through the blood vessel to the area of occlusion or blockage. When the catheter is in position, the laser emits pulsating beams of light that break up or vaporize the obstruction.

C1886

C1886 Catheter, extravascular tissue ablation, any modality (insertable)

Lay Description

An ablation catheter is a long thin tube inside a sheath that is used to deliver destructive electrical or thermal energy to abnormal or problematic tissues. Electrodes are located in the catheter to generate the necessary energy. The catheter is inserted and maneuvered into the desired tissue Extravascular catheters are inserted into the body to treat the desired tissue. The catheter is designed to penetrate the tissue but not the vascular structure.

C1887

C1887   Catheter, guiding (may include infusion/perfusion capability)

Lay Description
A guiding catheter is a small hollow tube used to introduce interventional or diagnostic devices into the coronary or peripheral vascular system. It can be used to inject contrast material, function as a conduit through which other devices pass, and/or provide a mechanism for measuring arterial pressure, and maintain a pathway created by the guide wire during the performance of a procedure.

C1888

C1888   Catheter, ablation, noncardiac, endovascular (implantable)

Lay Description
A noncardiac endovascular ablation catheter is a small hollow tube containing a laser or radiofrequency tip that is inserted into a blood vessel. The catheter is advanced to the target area and a pulse from the laser or radiofrequency device is used to occlude or obliterate the blood vessel.

C1891

C1891   Infusion pump, nonprogrammable, permanent (implantable)

Lay Description
An implantable infusion pump is a medical device that delivers fluids, drugs, or nutrients into the patient's bloodstream in a consistent dose at a consistent rate with consistent pressure. The pump is intended to provide long-term, continuous, or intermittent drug infusion. Non-programmable pumps are used for fixed dosages of medication or fluids.

C1892

C1892   Introducer/sheath, guiding, intracardiac electrophysiological, fixed-curve, peel-away

Lay Description
A guiding, intracardiac electrophysiological, fixed-curve, peel-away introducer or sheath is a small hollow tube made of nonabsorbable material. The sheath or introducer that separates into two pieces is guided to the target area. A lead or catheter is then placed through the introducer and the sheath is removed.

C1893

C1893   Introducer/sheath, guiding, intracardiac electrophysiological, fixed-curve, other than peel-away

Lay Description
A guiding, intracardiac electrophysiological, fixed-curve, non peel-away introducer or sheath is a small hollow tube made of nonabsorbable material. The sheath or introducer, which separates into two pieces, is guided to the target area. The introducer or sheath is for cardiac use and measures the electrical activity within the heart while providing a conduit for the passage of a device. The lead or catheter is then placed through the introducer and the sheath is removed.

C1894

C1894   Introducer/sheath, other than guiding, other than intracardiac electrophysiological, nonlaser

Lay Description
An introducer or a sheath is a small hollow tube made of nonabsorbable material. The sheath or introducer, which separates into two pieces, is guided to the target area. This introducer or sheath is for anything other than cardiac electrophysiological use. The tube provides a conduit for the passage of a nonlaser device. The lead or catheter is then placed through the introducer and the sheath is removed.

C1895

C1895   Lead, cardioverter-defibrillator, endocardial dual coil (implantable)

Lay Description
A pacemaker/cardioverter-defibrillator combination is a specialized device composed of a cardiac defibrillator and a pacemaker. Pacemakers provide electrical stimulation when cardiac contractions are slow or absent. A defibrillator is designed to directly treat a cardiac tachydysrhythmia. Pacing systems consist of a pulse generator and pacing leads. A dual coil lead is a thin, flexible wire that is inserted transvenously and advanced to the right ventricle and/or atrium where it is implanted into the myocardial tissue. The pulse generator is placed subcutaneously or submuscularly in the chest wall. This code represents an endocardial dual coil that connects to a pacemaker/cardioverter-defibrillator combination (implantable).

C1896

C1896   Lead, cardioverter-defibrillator, other than endocardial single or dual coil (implantable)

Lay Description
A pacemaker/cardioverter-defibrillator combination is a specialized device composed of a cardiac defibrillator and a pacemaker. Pacemakers provide electrical stimulation when cardiac contractions are

slow or absent. A defibrillator is designed to directly treat a cardiac tachydysrhythmia. Pacing systems consist of a pulse generator and pacing leads. A coil lead is a thin, flexible wire that is inserted transvenously and advanced to the right ventricle and/or atrium where it is implanted into the myocardial tissue. The pulse generator is placed subcutaneously or submuscularly in the chest wall. Report this code for a lead other than endocardial single or dual coil that connects to a pacemaker/cardioverter-defibrillator combination (implantable).

C1897

C1897   Lead, neurostimulator test kit (implantable)

Lay Description
Neurostimulators are medical devices that transmit electrical impulses to specified nerves through an implanted wire or lead. A neurostimulator test kit (implantable) allows for the temporary use of a neurostimulator and its leads to determine if the intended usage will be beneficial to the patient.

C1898

C1898   Lead, pacemaker, other than transvenous VDD single pass

Lay Description
A pacemaker is a device used to synchronize the beating of the heart. The lead is a small wire that conducts electrical impulses from the pacemaker to the heart. The lead is passed through a vein into the heart. The pacemaker is programmed to regulate the rhythm of the heart and the electronic impulses are conducted through the leads to the heart muscle.

C1899

C1899   Lead, pacemaker/cardioverter-defibrillator combination (implantable)

Lay Description
A pacemaker/cardioverter-defibrillator combination is a specialized device composed of a cardiac defibrillator and a pacemaker. Pacemakers provide electrical stimulation when cardiac contractions are slow or absent. A defibrillator is designed to directly treat a cardiac tachydysrhythmia. Pacing systems consist of a pulse generator and pacing leads. Endocardial leads are thin, flexible wires that are inserted transvenously and advanced to the right ventricle and/or atrium where they are implanted into the myocardial tissue. The pulse generator is placed subcutaneously or submuscularly in the chest wall.

C1900

C1900   Lead, left ventricular coronary venous system

Lay Description
A left ventricular coronary venous system lead is an implanted wire with an electrode at its tip that connects a generator to the left ventricle of the heart. It is intended to treat the symptoms associated with heart failure.

C2614

C2614   Probe, percutaneous lumbar discectomy

Lay Description
A percutaneous discectomy is the removal of a herniated intravertebral disc through a small incision. The probe is a small hollow tube that is inserted in the intervertebral disc. Tiny surgical instruments are inserted through the tube to cut and/or aspirate the disc material.

C2615

C2615   Sealant, pulmonary, liquid

Lay Description
Liquid pulmonary sealant is an absorbable hydrogel formed from two components. Human serum albumin is mixed with a synthetic cross-linking component of polyethylene glycol. It is indicated to seal visceral pleural air leaks during pulmonary resection. The liquid pulmonary sealant is intended for single use. It is not recommended that more than 30 ml be used per patient.

C2616

C2616   Brachytherapy source, nonstranded, yttrium-90, per source

Lay Description
Brachytherapy is a form of radiotherapy involving implantation of radioactive sources within the tumor bed, which allows delivery of high radiation doses to the tumor site sparing adjacent normal tissue. This code uses radioactive isotope yttrium-90.

C2617

C2617   Stent, noncoronary, temporary, without delivery system

Lay Description
A noncoronary, temporary stent, without a delivery system is a small hollow tube made of a biocompatible substance, such as phosphorylcholine, silicone, or metal that is inserted into a natural body passge or conduit. The stent maintains the body passage or conduit allowing less restricted flow. This code represents a stent packaged without a delivery system. A temporary stent is designed to be removed and is placed for a period of less than one year.

C2618

C2618   Probe/needle, cryoablation

Lay Description
Cryoablation probes are hollow needles (cryoprobes) through which cooled, thermally conductive fluids are circulated. Cryoprobes are inserted into or placed adjacent to diseased tissue. Ablation occurs in tissue that has been frozen by at least three mechanisms: 1) formation of ice crystals within cells thereby disrupting membranes; 2) coagulation of blood thereby interrupting blood flow; 3) induction of apoptosis, the so-called programmed cell death cascade.

C2619-C2620

C2619   Pacemaker, dual chamber, nonrate-responsive (implantable)

C2620   Pacemaker, single chamber, nonrate-responsive (implantable)

Lay Description
A pacemaker is an electronic device that regulates contraction rhythms of the heart through electrical impulses. A pacemaker has two components: a pulse generator and lead(s). The pulse generator is connected to leads positioned inside the heart or on its surface. These leads are used to deliver electrical impulses, sense the cardiac rhythm, and pace the heart, as needed. The various leads are connected to a pulse generator, which is implanted in a pouch beneath the skin of the chest or abdomen. Dual chamber pacemakers can sense and pace in both heart chambers, atrium and ventricle. Single chamber pacemakers sense and pace in only one heart chamber, usually the ventricle. Rate responsive pacemakers sense both physiologic and nonphysiologic signals and adjust their output to meet patient needs. Nonrate-responsive pacemakers deliver a consistent fixed rate.

C2621

C2621   Pacemaker, other than single or dual chamber (implantable)

Lay Description
A pacemaker is an electronic system that monitors the electrical impulses of the heart and delivers an electrical charge when necessary to set normal heart rhythms. This code represents an implantable pacemaker that is neither a single nor dual chamber model.

C2622

C2622   Prosthesis, penile, noninflatable

Lay Description
A non-inflatable penile prosthesis consists of a pair of malleable cylinders that are surgically inserted into the penis. This prosthesis maintains the penis in a semi-rigid state. The penis must be manually positioned, up for intercourse or down for everyday activities.

C2625

C2625   Stent, noncoronary, temporary, with delivery system

Lay Description
A noncoronary, temporary stent, with a delivery system is a small hollow tube made of a biocompatible substance, such as phosphorylcholine, silicone, or metal, that is inserted into a natural body passage or conduit. The stent maintains the body passage or conduit allowing less restricted flow. A temporary stent is designed to be removed and is placed for a period of less than one year. This code represents a stent packaged with a delivery system, generally including components such as a stent mounted or unmounted on a balloon angioplasty catheter, introducer, and sheath.

C2626

C2626   Infusion pump, nonprogrammable, temporary (implantable)

Lay Description
A nonprogrammable, temporary infusion pump is a short term pain management system which is a component of a permanent implantable system used for the management of chronic pain.

C2627

C2627   Catheter, suprapubic/cystoscopic

Lay Description
A suprapubic catheter is a flexible hollow tube that is inserted through the abdomen into the urinary bladder to drain urine. It is a popular method of long-term bladder drainage in voiding dysfunction. A cystoscopic catheter is a flexible hollow tube that is used in a cystoscopy.

C2628

C2628   Catheter, occlusion

Lay Description
An occlusion catheter is a flexible hollow tube with a balloon at the tip. The device is placed into an organ or blood vessel and the balloon is inflated. This blocks or occludes the vessel stopping blood flow.

C2629

C2629   Introducer/sheath, other than guiding, other than intracardiac electrophysiological, laser

Lay Description
An intracardiac, electrophysiological introducer or sheath is a small hollow tube made of nonabsorbable material that is used in the heart. The sheath or introducer, which separates into two pieces, is guided to the target area. A laser is placed through the introducer and the sheath is removed.

C2630

C2630 Catheter, electrophysiology, diagnostic/ablation, other than 3D or vector mapping, cool-tip

Lay Description
An electrophysiology, diagnostic or ablation, other than 3D or vector mapping, cool-tip catheter is a small hollow tube containing devices that aid in providing anatomic and physiologic information about the cardiac electrical conduction system. This device has temperature sensing capability also contains a cooling mechanism which is a tip cooled by infused, circulating saline.

C2631

C2631 Repair device, urinary, incontinence, without sling graft

Lay Description
A urinary incontinence repair device is used to attach or insert body tissue, synthetic material, or mesh for the purpose of strengthening the pelvic floor. The repair material is fashioned into a sling or hammock that supports the urethra. This code represents the device components used to deliver the sling graft and/or fixate (via permanent sutures or bone anchors) the sling graft, but does not include the sling graft.

C2634-C2644

C2634 Brachytherapy source, nonstranded, high activity, iodine-125, greater than 1.01 mCi (NIST), per source

C2635 Brachytherapy source, nonstranded, high activity, palladium-103, greater than 2.2 mCi (NIST), per source

C2636 Brachytherapy linear source, nonstranded, palladium-103, per 1 mm

C2637 Brachytherapy source, nonstranded, ytterbium-169, per source

C2638 Brachytherapy source, stranded, iodine-125, per source

C2639 Brachytherapy source, nonstranded, iodine-125, per source

C2640 Brachytherapy source, stranded, palladium-103, per source

C2641 Brachytherapy source, nonstranded, palladium-103, per source

C2642 Brachytherapy source, stranded, cesium-131, per source

C2643 Brachytherapy source, nonstranded, cesium-131, per source

C2644 Brachytherapy source, cesium-131 chloride solution, per millicurie

Lay Description
Brachytherapy is a form of radiotherapy in which physicians place the source of irradiation close to the tumor or within a body cavity. Brachytherapy could include placing radioactive sources inside a body cavity (intracavitary brachytherapy) or putting radioactive material directly into body tissue using hollow needles (interstitial brachytherapy). Brachytherapy may be given in addition to external beam radiation or it may be used as the only form of radiotherapy. In some cases, the radioactive sources may be permanently left in place; in other cases, they are removed after a specified time. Placement of radioactive sources may be repeated several times. The isotope gold-198 has a half life of 2.7 days and is used in some cancer treatments and treatments for other diseases. There are two natural isotopes of iridium, and many radioisotopes, the most stable radioisotope being Ir-192 with a half-life of 73.83 days. Ir-192 beta decays into platinum-192, while most of the other radioisotopes decay into osmium.

C2698-C2699

C2698 Brachytherapy source, stranded, not otherwise specified, per source

C2699 Brachytherapy source, nonstranded, not otherwise specified, per source

Lay Description
Brachytherapy is a form of radiotherapy in which physicians place the source of irradiation close to the tumor or within a body cavity. Brachytherapy includes placing radioactive sources inside a body cavity (intracavitary brachytherapy) or putting radioactive material directly into body tissue using hollow needles (interstitial brachytherapy). Stranded sources are seeds or sources connected in a linear fashion using absorbable material.

C5271-C5278

C5271 Application of low cost skin substitute graft to trunk, arms, legs, total wound surface area up to 100 sq cm; first 25 sq cm or less wound surface area

C5272 Application of low cost skin substitute graft to trunk, arms, legs, total wound surface area up to 100 sq cm; each additional 25 sq cm wound surface area, or part thereof (list separately in addition to code for primary procedure)

C5273 Application of low cost skin substitute graft to trunk, arms, legs, total wound surface area greater than or equal to 100 sq cm; first 100 sq cm wound surface area, or 1% of body area of infants and children

C5274 Application of low cost skin substitute graft to trunk, arms, legs, total wound surface area greater than or equal to 100 sq cm; each additional 100 sq cm wound surface area, or part thereof, or each additional 1% of body area of infants and children, or part thereof (list separately in addition to code for primary procedure)

C5275 Application of low cost skin substitute graft to face, scalp, eyelids, mouth, neck, ears, orbits, genitalia, hands, feet, and/or multiple digits, total wound surface area up to 100 sq cm; first 25 sq cm or less wound surface area

C5276 Application of low cost skin substitute graft to face, scalp, eyelids, mouth, neck, ears, orbits, genitalia, hands, feet, and/or multiple digits, total wound surface area up to 100 sq cm; each additional 25 sq cm wound surface area, or part thereof (list separately in addition to code for primary procedure)

C5277 Application of low cost skin substitute graft to face, scalp, eyelids, mouth, neck, ears, orbits, genitalia, hands, feet, and/or multiple digits, total wound surface area greater than or equal to 100 sq cm; first 100 sq cm wound surface area, or 1% of body area of infants and children

C5278 Application of low cost skin substitute graft to face, scalp, eyelids, mouth, neck, ears, orbits, genitalia, hands, feet, and/or multiple digits, total wound surface area greater than or equal to 100 sq cm; each additional 100 sq cm wound surface area, or part thereof, or each additional 1% of body area of infants and children, or part thereof (list separately in addition to code for primary procedure)

Lay Description
These codes are designed to parallel the surgical procedures described by CPT codes under the heading in the 2014 CPT codebook "Skin Replacement Surgery" and the subheading "Skin Substitute Grafts." OPPS considers that skin substitute products serve as a necessary supply for these surgical repair procedures. OPPS hospitals report these C codes when the skin substitute is considered the low cost group, a cost at or below $32 in 2014. Report the appropriate code based on the area of the body and size of the wound surface. In 2014, the following are considered low cost skin substitutes: C9358, C9360, C9363, Q4100, Q4102–Q4105, Q4108, Q4111, Q4115, Q4117, Q4119–Q4121, Q4123, Q4124, Q4128–Q4129, Q4135–Q4138, Q4140–Q4143, and Q4146–Q4148. OPPS hospitals report CPT codes 15271–15278 when the skin substitute is in the high cost group (above $32 in 2014). CMS will review costs and may revise them annually. There are a few skin substitute products that are applied as liquids or powders and are employed in procedures outside of the noted CPT code range. These products will not be classified as high cost or low cost but will be packaged into the surgical procedure in which they are used.

C8900

C8900 Magnetic resonance angiography with contrast, abdomen

Lay Description
Magnetic resonance angiography (MRA) is an application of magnetic resonance imaging (MRI) that provides visualization of blood flow and images of normal and diseased blood vessels. MRA techniques typically are noninvasive because they do not require the use of contrast media. Contrast media may be used to enhance the images in MRA, but use of these agents is not necessary.

C8901

C8901 Magnetic resonance angiography without contrast, abdomen

Lay Description
Magnetic resonance angiography (MRA) is an application of magnetic resonance imaging (MRI) that provides visualization of blood flow and images of normal and diseased blood vessels. MRA techniques typically are noninvasive because they do not require the use of contrast media. Contrast media may be used to enhance the images in MRA, but use of these agents is not necessary.

C8902

C8902 Magnetic resonance angiography without contrast followed by with contrast, abdomen

Lay Description
Magnetic resonance angiography (MRA) is an application of magnetic resonance imaging (MRI) that provides visualization of blood flow and images of normal and diseased blood vessels. MRA techniques typically are noninvasive because they do not require the use of contrast media. Contrast media may be used to enhance the images in MRA, but use of these agents is not necessary.

C8903

C8903 Magnetic resonance imaging with contrast, breast; unilateral

Lay Description
Magnetic resonance imaging (MRI) is a noninvasive, painless test that assists the physician in diagnosing and treating certain medical conditions. MRI uses a powerful magnetic field, radio waves, and a computer to create detailed pictures of bone, organs, soft tissues, and other internal body structures. These detailed pictures allow the physician to better comprehend and evaluate the part of the body in question or diseased areas under scrutiny. An MRI of the breast assists in evaluating abnormalities detected via a mammography, evaluates the integrity of breast implants, differentiates between scar tissue and tumors, assesses multiple tumor locations, determines whether cancer detected by mammography or other radiological tests has spread

further into the breast or chest wall pre- or post-surgery, assesses the effect of chemotherapy, and/or provides more information on a diseased breast to make medical treatment decisions.

C8904

C8904   Magnetic resonance imaging without contrast, breast; unilateral

Lay Description
Magnetic resonance imaging (MRI) is a noninvasive, painless test that assists the physician in diagnosing and treating certain medical conditions. MRI uses a powerful magnetic field, radio waves, and a computer to create detailed pictures of bone, organs, soft tissues, and other internal body structures. These detailed pictures allow the physician to better comprehend and evaluate the part of the body in question or diseased areas under scrutiny. An MRI of the breast assists in evaluating abnormalities detected via a mammography, evaluates the integrity of breast implants, differentiates between scar tissue and tumors, assesses multiple tumor locations, determines whether cancer detected by mammography or other radiological tests has spread further into the breast or chest wall pre- or post-surgery, assesses the effect of chemotherapy, and/or provides more information on a diseased breast to make medical treatment decisions.

C8905

C8905   Magnetic resonance imaging without contrast followed by with contrast, breast; unilateral

Lay Description
Magnetic resonance imaging (MRI) is a noninvasive, painless test that assists the physician in diagnosing and treating certain medical conditions. MRI uses a powerful magnetic field, radio waves, and a computer to create detailed pictures of bone, organs, soft tissues, and other internal body structures. These detailed pictures allow the physician to better comprehend and evaluate the part of the body in question or diseased areas under scrutiny. An MRI of the breast assists in evaluating abnormalities detected via a mammography, evaluates the integrity of breast implants, differentiates between scar tissue and tumors, assesses multiple tumor locations, determines whether cancer detected by mammography or other radiological tests has spread further into the breast or chest wall pre- or post-surgery, assesses the effect of chemotherapy, and/or provides more information on a diseased breast to make medical treatment decisions.

C8906

C8906   Magnetic resonance imaging with contrast, breast; bilateral

Lay Description
Magnetic resonance imaging (MRI) is a noninvasive, painless test that assists the physician in diagnosing and treating certain medical conditions. MRI uses a powerful magnetic field, radio waves, and a computer to create detailed pictures of bone, organs, soft tissues, and other internal body structures. These detailed pictures allow the physician to better comprehend and evaluate the part of the body in question or diseased areas under scrutiny. An MRI of the breast assists in evaluating abnormalities detected via a mammography, evaluates the integrity of breast implants, differentiates between scar tissue and tumors, assesses multiple tumor locations, determines whether cancer detected by mammography or other radiological tests has spread further into the breast or chest wall pre- or post-surgery, assesses the effect of chemotherapy, and/or provides more information on a diseased breast to make medical treatment decisions.

C8907

C8907   Magnetic resonance imaging without contrast, breast; bilateral

Lay Description
Magnetic resonance imaging (MRI) is a noninvasive, painless test that assists the physician in diagnosing and treating certain medical conditions. MRI uses a powerful magnetic field, radio waves, and a computer to create detailed pictures of bone, organs, soft tissues, and other internal body structures. These detailed pictures allow the physician to better comprehend and evaluate the part of the body in question or diseased areas under scrutiny. An MRI of the breast assists in evaluating abnormalities detected via a mammography, evaluates the integrity of breast implants, differentiates between scar tissue and tumors, assesses multiple tumor locations, determines whether cancer detected by mammography or other radiological tests has spread further into the breast or chest wall pre- or post-surgery, assesses the effect of chemotherapy, and/or provides more information on a diseased breast to make medical treatment decisions.

C8908

C8908   Magnetic resonance imaging without contrast followed by with contrast, breast; bilateral

Lay Description
Magnetic resonance imaging (MRI) is a noninvasive, painless test that assists the physician in diagnosing and treating certain medical conditions. MRI uses a powerful magnetic field, radio waves, and a computer to create detailed pictures of bone, organs, soft tissues, and other internal body structures. These

detailed pictures allow the physician to better comprehend and evaluate the part of the body in question or diseased areas under scrutiny. An MRI of the breast assists in evaluating abnormalities detected via a mammography, evaluates the integrity of breast implants, differentiates between scar tissue and tumors, assesses multiple tumor locations, determines whether cancer detected by mammography or other radiological tests has spread further into the breast or chest wall pre- or post-surgery, assesses the effect of chemotherapy, and/or provides more information on a diseased breast to make medical treatment decisions.

C8909

C8909   Magnetic resonance angiography with contrast, chest (excluding myocardium)

Lay Description
Magnetic resonance angiography (MRA) is an application of magnetic resonance imaging (MRI) that provides visualization of blood flow and images of normal and diseased blood vessels. MRA techniques typically are noninvasive because they do not require the use of contrast media. This MRA procedure is designed to examine the heart and the blood vessels entering the lungs. Contrast media may be used to enhance the images in MRA, but use of these agents is not necessary.

C8910

C8910   Magnetic resonance angiography without contrast, chest (excluding myocardium)

Lay Description
Magnetic resonance angiography (MRA) is an application of magnetic resonance imaging (MRI) that provides visualization of blood flow and images of normal and diseased blood vessels. MRA techniques typically are noninvasive because they do not require the use of contrast media. This MRA procedure is designed to examine the heart and the blood vessels entering the lungs. Contrast media may be used to enhance the images in MRA, but use of these agents is not necessary.

C8911

C8911   Magnetic resonance angiography without contrast followed by with contrast, chest (excluding myocardium)

Lay Description
Magnetic resonance angiography (MRA) is an application of magnetic resonance imaging (MRI) that provides visualization of blood flow and images of normal and diseased blood vessels. MRA techniques typically are noninvasive because they do not require the use of contrast media. This MRA procedure is designed to examine the heart and the blood vessels entering the lungs. Contrast media may be used to

enhance the images in MRA, but use of these agents is not necessary.

C8912-C8914

C8912   Magnetic resonance angiography with contrast, lower extremity

C8913   Magnetic resonance angiography without contrast, lower extremity

C8914   Magnetic resonance angiography without contrast followed by with contrast, lower extremity

Lay Description
Magnetic resonance angiography (MRA) is an application of magnetic resonance imaging (MRI) that provides visualization of blood flow and images of normal and diseased blood vessels. MRA techniques typically are noninvasive because they do not require the use of contrast media. This MRA procedure is designed to examine major blood vessels in the lower extremities. Contrast media may be used to enhance the images in MRA, but use of these agents is not necessary.

C8918-C8920

C8918   Magnetic resonance angiography with contrast, pelvis

C8919   Magnetic resonance angiography without contrast, pelvis

C8920   Magnetic resonance angiography without contrast followed by with contrast, pelvis

Lay Description
Magnetic resonance angiography (MRA) is an application of magnetic resonance imaging (MRI) that provides visualization of blood flow and images of normal and diseased blood vessels. MRA techniques typically are noninvasive because they do not require the use of contrast media. This MRA procedure is designed to examine major blood vessels in the pelvis. Contrast media may be used to enhance the images in MRA, but use of these agents is not necessary.

C8921-C8922

C8921   Transthoracic echocardiography with contrast, or without contrast followed by with contrast, for congenital cardiac anomalies; complete

C8922   Transthoracic echocardiography with contrast, or without contrast followed by with contrast, for congenital cardiac anomalies; follow-up or limited study

Lay Description
Transthoracic echocardiography is performed to detect congenital cardiac anomalies. Contrast is injected into the patient's vein. Transducers are placed on the patient's chest to record an echocardiograph, which uses ultrasound to visualize the heart's function, blood flow, valves, and chambers. Report contrast material separately.

C8923-C8924

C8923 Transthoracic echocardiography with contrast, or without contrast followed by with contrast, real-time with image documentation (2D), includes M-mode recording, when performed, complete, without spectral or color doppler echocardiography

C8924 Transthoracic echocardiography with contrast, or without contrast followed by with contrast, real-time with image documentation (2D), includes M-mode recording when performed, follow-up or limited study

Lay Description

A transthoracic echocardiography is performed with real-time image documentation (2D). Contrast material is injected into the vein. An ultrasound is used to visualize the heart's function, blood flow, valves, and chambers. Two-dimensional echocardiography, also referred to as real-time imaging, is performed using multiple transducers or a rotating transducer, and these images are recorded on videotape. Computer reconstruction provides the two-dimensional image of specific planes of the heart. M-mode, when performed, provides additional detail of specific portions of the heart. A stationary ultrasound beam is directed at the area of the heart requiring additional study. Report contrast material separately.

C8925-C8926

C8925 Transesophageal echocardiography (TEE) with contrast, or without contrast followed by with contrast, real time with image documentation (2D) (with or without M-mode recording); including probe placement, image acquisition, interpretation and report

C8926 Transesophageal echocardiography (TEE) with contrast, or without contrast followed by with contrast, for congenital cardiac anomalies; including probe placement, image acquisition, interpretation and report

Lay Description

Transesophageal echocardiography (TEE) is performed. TEE is an invasive technique whereby contrast material is injected into the vein. The transducer is placed at the tip of an endoscope and introduced into the patient's esophagus to record a two-dimensional echocardiograph. The codes include probe placement, image acquisition, interpretation, and report. Report contrast material separately.

C8927

C8927 Transesophageal echocardiography (TEE) with contrast, or without contrast followed by with contrast, for monitoring purposes, including probe placement, real time 2-dimensional image acquisition and interpretation leading to ongoing (continuous) assessment of (dynamically changing) cardiac pumping function and to therapeutic measures on an immediate time basis

Lay Description

Transesophageal echocardiography (TEE) is performed to assess cardiac pumping function and for therapeutic measures on an immediate time basis. TEE is an invasive technique whereby contrast is injected into the vein. The transducer is placed at the tip of an endoscope and introduced into the patient's esophagus to record a two-dimensional echocardiograph. TEE provides high-quality, real-time images of the beating heart and mediastinal structures. This code reports ongoing hemodynamic monitoring using TEE. TEE may be used to monitor critically ill patients in the intensive care unit, as well as patients in certain operative settings. In both the intensive care unit and the operating room, it is used to monitor cardiac function including cardiac preload, contractility, and valve function in patients with acute hemodynamic decompensation. In addition, TEE may also be used to assess and monitor mediastinal, heart, lung, and aortic injury resulting from blunt chest trauma even in patients undergoing other life-saving procedures. Report contrast material separately.

C8928

C8928 Transthoracic echocardiography with contrast, or without contrast followed by with contrast, real-time with image documentation (2D), includes M-mode recording, when performed, during rest and cardiovascular stress test using treadmill, bicycle exercise and/or pharmacologically induced stress, with interpretation and report

Lay Description

Transthoracic echocardiography is performed while the patient is at rest and exercising on a treadmill or stationary bicycle with or without medication and includes M-mode recording, when performed. TEE is an invasive technique whereby contrast is injected into the vein. Transducers are placed on a patient's chest to record a two-dimensional echocardiograph, which uses ultrasound to visualize the heart's function, blood flow, valves, and chambers. Report contrast material separately.

C8929

C8929 Transthoracic echocardiography with contrast, or without contrast followed by with contrast, real-time with image documentation (2D), includes M-mode recording, when performed, complete, with spectral doppler echocardiography, and with color flow doppler echocardiography

Lay Description

Transthoracic echocardiography (TEE) is performed. TEE is an invasive technique whereby contrast is injected into the vein. Transducers are placed on a patient's chest to record a two-dimensional echocardiograph, which uses ultrasound to visualize the heart's function, blood flow, valves, and chambers. This code is for a complete evaluation that includes spectral and color flow Doppler, which provide information regarding blood flow velocity, direction, type, and hemodynamics. Report contrast material separately.

C8930

C8930 Transthoracic echocardiography, with contrast, or without contrast followed by with contrast, real-time with image documentation (2D), includes M-mode recording, when performed, during rest and cardiovascular stress test using treadmill, bicycle exercise and/or pharmacologically induced stress, with interpretation and report; including performance of continuous electrocardiographic monitoring, with physician supervision

Lay Description

Transthoracic echocardiography (TEE) is performed. TEE is an invasive technique whereby contrast is injected into the vein. Transducers are placed on the patient's chest to record a two-dimensional echocardiograph, which uses ultrasound to visualize the heart's function, blood flow, valves, and chambers. This is completed while the patient is at rest and again while exercising on a treadmill or stationary bicycle, with or without medication, and includes M-mode recording, when performed. It also includes the performance of continuous electrocardiographic monitoring with physician supervision. Supply of the contrast agent and/or the drugs used in pharmacologic stress are reported separately.

C8931-C8936

C8931 Magnetic resonance angiography with contrast, spinal canal and contents

C8932 Magnetic resonance angiography without contrast, spinal canal and contents

C8933 Magnetic resonance angiography without contrast followed by with contrast, spinal canal and contents

C8934 Magnetic resonance angiography with contrast, upper extremity

C8935 Magnetic resonance angiography without contrast, upper extremity

C8936 Magnetic resonance angiography without contrast followed by with contrast, upper extremity

Lay Description

Magnetic resonance imaging uses the natural magnetic properties of the hydrogen atoms that emit radiofrequency signals when exposed to radio waves within a strong electromagnetic field. These signals are processed and converted by the computer into high-resolution, three-dimensional tomographic images. Magnetic resonance angiography (MRA) is magnetic resonance imaging (MRI) that specifically visualizes blood vessels and blood flow to evaluate vascular disorders within the structure being studied. Unlike conventional or CT images, MRIs/MRAs do not rely on the absorption of ionizing radiation. Patients with metallic or electronic implants or foreign bodies cannot be exposed to MRI. The patient must remain still while lying on a motorized table within the large, circular MRI tunnel. A sedative may be administered, as well as contrast material for image enhancement.

C8957

C8957 Intravenous infusion for therapy/diagnosis; initiation of prolonged infusion (more than 8 hours), requiring use of portable or implantable pump

Lay Description

Intravenous infusion for therapy/diagnosis; initiation of prolonged infusion (more than 8 hours), requiring use of portable or implantable pump, is a route of administration in pharmacology and toxicology by which a path in a vein is made allowing the administration of a drug, fluid, or other substance for a period of more than 8 hours. An infusion pump is used for such prolonged infusions.

C9025

C9025 Injection, ramucirumab, 5 mg

Lay Description

Ramucirumab is a recombinant human IgG1 monoclonal antibody produced in genetically engineered mammalian cells. It specifically binds to vascular endothelial growth factor (VEGF2) 2 receptor sites. Ramucirumab is indicated for the treatment of advanced or metastatic gastric carcinoma or gastroesophageal junction adenocarcinoma as a single agent after prior fluoropyrimidine or platinum-containing chemotherapy. It is administered as an intravenous infusion over 60 minutes. Recommended dosage is 8 mg per kg every two weeks.

C9026

C9026 Injection, vedolizumab, 1 mg

Lay Description
Vedolizumab is a recombinant human IgG1 monoclonal antibody produced in Chinese hamster ovaries. It binds to a human alpha 4 beta 7 integrin site and blocks the interaction of this integrin with mucosal addressin adhesion molecules. This inhibits the migration of memory T-lymphocytes across the endothelium into the inflamed gastrointestinal tissue. This interaction is thought to be an important contributor to the chronic inflammation of ulcerative colitis and Crohn's disease. Vedolizumab is indicated for adult patients with moderate to severe active ulcerative colitis or Crohn's disease who have lost response or are intolerant of tumor necrosis factor (TNF) blockers, immunomodulation or corticosteroids. Recommended dosage is 300 mg infused intravenously over 30 minutes.

C9027

C9027 Injection, pembrolizumab, 1 mg

Lay Description
Pembrolizumab is a humanized monoclonal antibody that blocks the interaction of PD-1 and its ligands PD-L1 and PD-L2. This releases PD-1 pathway mediated inhibition of the immune response, including antitumor immune response. Pembrolizumab is an IgG4 kappa immunoglobulin. It is indicated for the treatment of unresectable or metastatic melanoma with disease progression following ipilimumab and a BRAF inhibitor (when BRAF V6000 mutation is positive). Recommended dosage is 2 mg/kg as an intravenous infusion over 30 minutes. It is administered every three weeks until disease progression or unacceptable toxicity.

C9113

C9113 Injection, pantoprazole sodium, per vial

Lay Description
Pantoprazole sodium is a compound that inhibits gastric secretions. Pantoprazole is a proton pump inhibitor (PPI) that suppresses the final step in gastric acid production by forming a covalent bond to two sites of the ATPase enzyme system at the secretory surface of the gastric parietal cell. This effect is dose-related and leads to inhibition of both basal and stimulated gastric acid secretion irrespective of the stimulus. This binding results in a period of antisecretory effect that persists longer than 24 hours for all doses tested. This drug is indicated for

short-term treatment (seven to 10 days) for patients with gastroesophageal reflux disease (GERD) and a history of erosive esophagitis, and the hypersecretory conditions that may be associated with Zollinger-Ellison syndrome or other neoplastic conditions.

C9121

C9121 Injection, argatroban, per 5 mg

Lay Description
Argatroban is a synthetic direct thrombin inhibitor derived from the amino acid L-arginine. It binds to the active thrombin site and inhibits coagulation including fibrin formation, activation of coagulation factors and protein C, and platelet aggregation. Argatroban is indicated for use as an anticoagulant for prophylaxis and treatment of thrombosis in patients with heparin-induced thrombocytopenia. It is also indicated as an anticoagulant in patients with or at risk for heparin-induced thrombocytopenia undergoing percutaneous coronary interventions. Argatroban is supplied as a concentrate that must be diluted and administered via intravenous infusion.

C9132

C9132 Prothrombin complex concentrate (human), Kcentra, per IU of Factor IX activity

Lay Description
Kcentra is a concentrate of human prothrombin complex derived from pooled plasma that has been purified, heat-treated, and nanofiltered. It is indicated for the urgent reversal of acquired coagulation factor deficiency induced by vitamin K antagonists (e.g., warfarin). It is indicated only for adult patients with acute major bleeding. It is NOT indicated for use in patients who do not have an acute major bleeding. Kcentra contains factors II, VII, IX, and X, and antithrombin proteins C and S. The actual potency in each vial is listed on the carton. Actual dosage is dependent on the patient's body weight and the predose internal normalized ratio (INR) value. Vitamin K should be administered concurrently with Kcentra. Repeat dosing is not recommended. Kcentra is available as a single use vial of lyophilized concentrate. The potency is derived from the factor IX content. When reconstituted, the final factor IX concentration is from 20 to 31 units per mL.

C9136

C9136 Injection, factor VIII, Fc fusion protein, (recombinant), per IU

Lay Description
Recombinant antihemophiliac factor, Fc Fusion protein is DNA derived Factor VIII produced from a human embryonic kidney cell line. No human or animal derived proteins are used in the purification or formulation processes. It is indicated for use as a treatment for adults and children with hemophilia A

(congenital Factor VIII deficient). It is used as a control and prevention of bleeding episodes, perioperative management, and the routine prophylaxis to prevent or reduce the frequency of bleeding episodes. It is not indicated for the treatment of Von Willebrand's disease. Routine prophylaxis dosage is 50 IU/kg every four days and may be adjusted based on patient response to a range of 25-65 IU/kg at three to five day intervals. Children younger than 6 years of age may require higher doses up to 80 IU/kg. Each vile is labeled with the actual content in IU.

C9248
C9248   Injection, clevidipine butyrate, 1 mg

Lay Description
Clevidipine butyrate is a channel blocker used to treat high blood pressure when other treatments are contraindicated. Channel blockers relax the blood vessels and allow more blood and oxygen to get to the heart. The dose varies depending on the patient's condition and blood pressure. Clevidipine butyrate is administered as an IV infusion.

C9250
C9250   Human plasma fibrin sealant, vapor-heated, solvent-detergent (Artiss), 2 ml

Lay Description
Human plasma fibrin sealant, vapor-heated, solvent-detergent (Artiss) is a two-component fibrin sealant used to adhere autologous skin grafts to surgically prepared wounds in burn patients. It is comprised of human sealer protein concentrate and human fibrin. When these two components are combined, the result is a fibrin that seals the graft to the prepared wound site. The solution is applied in a thin layer to the site and the graft is placed. A 2 ml package covers approximately 100 square centimeter surface area.

C9254
C9254   Injection, lacosamide, 1 mg

Lay Description
Lacosamide is a functional amino acid used as an adjunctive therapy in treating partial-onset seizures for patients 17 years of age or older who are diagnosed with epilepsy. The exact mechanism by which this drug controls seizures is unknown. The lacosamide is believed to act through voltage-gated sodium channels. Voltage-gated sodium channels help control the electrical activity of the neurons. Lacosamide targets neurons that are depolarized or active for long periods of time, typical of neurons at the focus of an epileptic seizure. The recommended dosage is from 100 mg to 400 mg per day, depending on the patient's response. The drug is administered as an IV infusion over 30 to 60 minutes.

C9257
C9257   Injection, bevacizumab, 0.25 mg

Lay Description
Bevacizumab is a monoclonal antibody produced by recombinant DNA technology in Chinese hamster ovaries. This monoclonal antibody binds to and inhibits the biologic activity of human vascular endothelial growth factor preventing the formation of new blood vessels. Bevacizumab, used in combination with intravenous 5-fluorouracil, is indicated for first-line treatment of patients with metastatic carcinoma of the colon or rectum. The recommended dose is 5 mg per kg of body weight administered once every 14 days disease progression is detected. Bevacizumab is administered by intravenous infusion. The initial dose infusion should be delivered over 90 minutes. If the first infusion is well tolerated, the second infusion may be administered over 60 minutes. If the 60-minute infusion is well tolerated, all subsequent infusions may be administered over 30 minutes.

C9275
C9275   Injection, hexaminolevulinate HCl, 100 mg, per study dose

Lay Description
Hexaminolevulinate is an imaging drug that is used to identify bladder cancer. The medication is administered into the bladder where it collects in the neoplastic cells. A blue light cystoscope is used to view the areas of fluorescence. The abnormal cells appear bright red and the surrounding normal tissue appears blue. A blue light cystoscopy is in addition to the regular white light cystoscopy. The recommended dose is 50 mL administered into the bladder through a urinary catheter. The medication is instilled into the bladder approximately one hour before the start of the procedure.

C9285
C9285   Lidocaine 70 mg/tetracaine 70 mg, per patch

Lay Description
A lidocaine 70 mg/tetracaine 70 mg patch is a single-use topical anesthetic patch that delivers equal parts of lidocaine and tetracaine. The patch has a heat-assisted drug delivery device that enhances the delivery of the local anesthetic. The patch is indicated for use on intact skin to provide local dermal analgesia prior to painful procedures such as needle punctures and superficial dermatological procedures in adults and children 3 years of age or older. The patch should be applied 20 to 30 minutes prior to venipuncture or intravenous cannulation and 30 minutes prior to a superficial dermatological procedure.

C9290

C9290   Injection, bupivacaine liposome, 1 mg

Lay Description
Bupivacaine liposome is an amide-type local anesthetic used for postoperative surgical site pain relief. Liposomal encapsulated bupivacaine blocks the production and conduction of the nerve impulses to the brain. Bupivacaine liposome is injected into the soft tissue of the surgical site. Recommended dose varies depending on the surface area to be covered and the surgical site. The maximum dose should not exceed 266 mg.

C9293

C9293   Injection, glucarpidase, 10 units

Lay Description
Glucarpidase is an orphan drug that is an exogenous enzyme produced by recombinant DNA technology in *E. coli*. The enzyme is indicated as a treatment for toxic plasma methotrexate concentrations in patients with delayed clearance due to impaired kidney function. Glucarpidase converts methotrexate into its inactive components and provides a nonrenal path of elimination in patients with renal dysfunction. Recommended dose is a single injection of 50 units per kg. Glucarpidase is administered as an intravenous bolus over five minutes.

C9349

C9349   FortaDerm, and FortaDerm Antimicrobial, any type, per sq cm

Lay Description
FortaDerm Antimicrobial PHMB is a sterile single-use sheet dressing made of collagen matrix that is coated with polyhexamethylene biguanide hydrochloride (PHMB). FortaDerm Antimicrobial PHMB consists of two layers of porcine intestinal collagen coated with PHMB. It is intended for the management of wounds and as an effective barrier to resist microbial colonization within the dressings and reduce microbes penetrating through the dressing. Antimicrobial PHMB wound dressing is supplied dry in sheet form in sizes ranging from 4x4 cm to 12x36 cm. It is intended as a skin substitute designed for use on acute and chronic and partial and full-thickness wounds. It is surgically applied and fixed to a wound using sutures or other fixation methods based on the size of the wound being treated.

C9352

C9352   Microporous collagen implantable tube (NeuraGen Nerve Guide), per cm length

Lay Description
A microporous collagen implantable tube, trade name NeuraGen Nerve Guide, is an absorbable collagen tube intended to serve as an interface between a nerve and the tissue around it. The tube creates a channel for axonal growth across a nerve gap. This code specifies a size of per centimeter length.

C9353

C9353   Microporous collagen implantable slit tube (NeuraWrap Nerve Protector), per cm length

Lay Description
A microporous collagen implantable slit tube, trade name NeuraWrap Nerve Protector, is an absorbable collagen implant that provides a nontightening cover for peripheral nerves that are injure. This code specifies a size of per centimeter length.

C9354

C9354   Acellular pericardial tissue matrix of nonhuman origin (Veritas), per sq cm

Lay Description
Acellular pericardial tissue matrix of nonhuman origin, trade name Veritas, is a strong implantable tissue consisting of noncross linked bovine pericardium. This product is acellular meaning all cells have been removed leaving only a collagen matrix. The acellular pericardial tissue matrix is used as a scaffold for tissue repair. This code specifies a size of per square centimeter.

C9355

C9355   Collagen nerve cuff (NeuroMatrix), per 0.5 cm length

Lay Description
A collagen nerve cuff, trade name NeuroMatrix, is a resorbable, semipermeable, collagen tube intended to create a conduit for axon growth across a nerve gap of 2.5 cm or less. This code specifies a size of 0.5 centimeter length.

C9356

C9356   Tendon, porous matrix of cross-linked collagen and glycosaminoglycan matrix (TenoGlide Tendon Protector Sheet), per sq cm

Lay Description
A tendon, porous matrix of cross-linked collagen and glycosaminoglycan matrix, trade name TenoGlide Tendon Protector Sheet, is an absorbable implant made of a porous matrix of cross linked bovine collagen and glycosaminoglycan. This provides a nonconstricting, protective encasement for injured tendons. This item is intended to serve as an interface between the tendon and the tendon sheath or surrounding tissue. This code specifies a size of per square centimeter.

C9358

C9358   Dermal substitute, native, nondenatured collagen, fetal bovine origin (SurgiMend Collagen Matrix), per 0.5 sq cm

Lay Description
A dermal substitute, native, nondenatured collagen, fetal bovine origin, trade name SurgiMend Collagen

Matrix, is an oval or square shaped, biocompatible, soft material made of an acellular collagen matrix. All cellular components are removed from fetal bovine dermis leaving a collagen matrix. This material is intended for soft tissue repair and reconstructive applications. This code specifies the size of 0.5 square centimeters. In 2014, OPPS considers this product a low cost skin substitute.

C9359

C9359   Porous purified collagen matrix bone void filler (Integra Mozaik Osteoconductive Scaffold Putty, Integra OS Osteoconductive Scaffold Putty), per 0.5 cc

Lay Description
Porous purified collagen matrix is a synthetic type of bone void filler that is used for the treatment of gaps or osseous defects of the skeletal system in the extremities, spine, and pelvis. This filler is made from a purified collage matrix, and its chemical composition allows it to be absorbed and replaced with growing host bone during the healing process. The filler is supplied in powder form and mixed with the bone marrow of the host to form a putty-like substance. This putty is often used as a substitute for harvesting bone graft material from the patient's iliac crest.

C9360

C9360   Dermal substitute, native, nondenatured collagen, neonatal bovine origin (SurgiMend Collagen Matrix), per 0.5 sq cm

Lay Description
A dermal substitute, native, nondenatured collagen, neonatal bovine origin, trade name SurgiMend Collagen Matrix, is an oval or square shaped, biocompatible, soft material made of an acellular collagen matrix. All cellular components are removed from neonatal bovine dermis leaving a collagen matrix. This material is intended for soft tissue repair and reconstructive applications. This code specifies the size of 0.5 square centimeters. In 2014, OPPS considers this product a low cost skin substitute.

C9361

C9361   Collagen matrix nerve wrap (NeuroMend Collagen Nerve Wrap), per 0.5 cm length

Lay Description
Collagen matrix nerve wrap (trade name NeuroMend Collagen Nerve Wrap) is a resorbable, collagen-based membrane matrix for use in the repair of crushed or severed peripheral nerves. The collagen wrap is designed to unroll and self-curl around the injured nerve. NeuroMend provides a protective setting to help the regeneration of the nerve across the injury or gap.

C9362

C9362   Porous purified collagen matrix bone void filler (Integra Mozaik Osteoconductive Scaffold Strip), per 0.5 cc

Lay Description
Porous purified collagen matrix bone void filler (trade name Integra Mozaik Osteoconductive Scaffold Strip and Scaffold Putty) is a resorbable bone filler designed to mimic the structure and composition of natural human bone. It is a highly purified bovine collagen that contains minerals and osteogenic protein-1. The bone filler is indicated as an alternative to autograft in long-bone nonunions, for spinal fusion where autograft is not possible, and for nonunions where alternative treatments failed.

C9363

C9363   Skin substitute (Integra Meshed Bilayer Wound Matrix), per square cm

Lay Description
Integra Meshed Bilayer Wound Matrix is a biologic matrix that provides coverage for partial- and full-thickness wounds. It is used to treat chronic and traumatic wounds including pressure ulcers, venous ulcers, diabetic ulcers, chronic and vascular ulcers, tunneled or undermined wounds, surgical wounds, traumatic wounds abrasions, lacerations, and draining wounds. It is a two-layer material. It has a silicone outer layer and a second layer created of three-dimensional porous material made from the fibers of a cross-linked bovine tendon collagen. The silicone layer provides protection and moisture control. The matrix provides the framework for tissue and capillary growth. The physician completely debrides the wound site, and the wound matrix is applied. It is affixed to the wound site with sutures or staples. Within 14 to 21 days, the tissue is remodeled with the patient's own cells, and the silicone layer is removed. In 2014, OPPS considers this product a low cost skin substitute.

C9364

C9364   Porcine implant, Permacol, per sq cm

Lay Description
A porcine collagen implant (trade name Permacol) is a dermal matrix from which cells, cell debris, DNA, and RNA are removed in a process that does not damage the 3D collagen matrix. This acellular collagen matrix is then cross-linked reportedly for better durability. A porcine collagen implant is indicated for abdominal wall repair.

C9399

C9399   Unclassified drugs or biologicals

Lay Description
This code should be used to report drugs and biologicals that have been approved by the FDA, but

do not have a product-specific, drug/biological HCPCS Level II code assigned.

C9442

C9442   Injection, belinostat, 10 mg

Lay Description

Belinostat is a histone (any of a group of small basic proteins present in cell nuclei that organizes DNA strands by forming molecular complexes around which the DNA winds) deacetylase inhibitor indicated for the treatment of patients with relapsed or refractory peripheral T-cell lymphoma. Histone deacetylase are a class of enzymes that remove acetyl groups from an amino acid on a histone, allowing the histone to wrap the DNA more tightly. The accumulation of acetylated histones and other proteins disrupts the cell cycle and causes cell death. Belinostat shows preferred cytotoxicity toward tumor cells compared to normal cells. Recommended dosage is 10,000 mg/m2 over a 30-minute intravenous infusion, once a day on days one to five of a 21-day cycle. Repeat the cycle until the disease progresses or unacceptable toxicity.

C9443

C9443   Injection, dalbavancin, 10 mg

Lay Description

Dalbavancin is a glycopeptide antibiotic indicated for acute bacterial skin and skin structure infections caused by designated susceptible strains of gram-positive bacteria, specifically *Staphylococcus aureus* (including methicillin susceptible and methicillin resistant strains), *Streptococcus pyogenes, Streptococcus agalactiae,* and the *Streptococcus anginosus* group. Recommended dosage is 1,000 mg followed by 500 mg one week later. Drug is administered via intravenous infusion over 30 minutes.

C9444

C9444   Injection, oritavancin, 10 mg

Lay Description

Oritavancin is a lipoglycopeptide antibiotic indicated for the treatment of adult patients with acute bacterial skin and skin structure infections caused by designated susceptible strains of gram-positive bacteria, specifically *Staphylococcus aureus* (including methicillin susceptible and methicillin resistant strains), *Streptococcus pyogenes, Streptococcus agalactiae,* the *Streptococcus anginosus* group, *Streptococcus dysgalactiae,* and *Enterococcus faecalis* (vancomycin-susceptible only). Recommended dosage is a 1,200 mg single dose administered by intravenous infusion over three hours. It is recommended for patients 18 years of age and older.

C9446

C9446   Injection, tedizolid phosphate, 1 mg

Lay Description

Tedizolid phosphate is an oxazolidinone-class antibiotic that is a phosphate prodrug that is converted to tedizolid in the presence of phosphates. Oxazolidine is an organic compound containing nitrogen and oxygen in a five-membered ring. The antibacterial effect of oxazolidinones works as a protein synthesis inhibitor. It is indicated for the treatment of acute bacterial skin and skin structure infections caused by designated gram-positive susceptible bacteria, specifically *Staphylococcus aureus* (including methicillin susceptible and methicillin resistant strains), *Streptococcus pyogenes, Streptococcus agalactiae,* the *Streptococcus anginosus* group, and *Enterococcus faecalis.* This drug is recommended for adult patients, 18 years of age or older. This drug is not to be administered by push or bolus. Recommended dosage is 200 mg as an intravenous infusion over one hour, administered once daily for a period of six days.

C9447

C9447   Injection, phenylephrine and ketorolac, 4 ml vial

Lay Description

Phenylephrine ketorolac is an alpha-1 adrenergic receptor agonist and nonselective cyclooxygenase inhibitor. It is used to maintain pupil size by preventing intraoperative miosis and for reducing postoperative pain. The drug is added to irrigation solution used during cataract surgery or intraocular lens replacement. For irrigation purposes, 4 ml of the drug is diluted in 500 ml of ophthalmic irrigating solution.

C9497

C9497   Loxapine, inhalation powder, 10 mg

Lay Description

Loxapine inhalation powder is an inhaled form of a typical antipsychotic drug. It is indicated for the acute treatment of agitation associated with schizophrenia or bipolar I disorder in adults. Loxapine inhalation powder is a subclass of tricyclic agents whose mechanism of action is unknown. It is believed that it antagonizes central dopamine D2 and serotonin 5-HT2A receptors. Recommended dosage is 10 mg once in a 24-hour period. Loxapine inhalation powder is available only through a restricted program under a risk evaluation and mitigation strategy and must be administered in an enrolled facility.

C9600-C9601

C9600 Percutaneous transcatheter placement of drug eluting intracoronary stent(s), with coronary angioplasty when performed; single major coronary artery or branch

C9601 Percutaneous transcatheter placement of drug-eluting intracoronary stent(s), with coronary angioplasty when performed; each additional branch of a major coronary artery (list separately in addition to code for primary procedure)

Lay Description

A drug-eluting stent is coated with medication and used to hold open a blocked or collapsed native artery in the heart. The physician makes a small incision in the arm or leg to access the artery for placement of two catheters. A central venous catheter is inserted through the femoral or brachial artery and a second catheter is threaded up to the affected coronary artery. An obstruction may be treated first by inflating a balloon at the tip of the second catheter (PTCA) to flatten the obstruction. A stent is introduced through a catheter, placed under radiographic guidance, and expanded to fit the lumen of the artery by inflating the balloon on the second catheter. The catheters are removed. Pressure is placed over the incision for 20 to 30 minutes to stop the bleeding.

C9602-C9603

C9602 Percutaneous transluminal coronary atherectomy, with drug eluting intracoronary stent, with coronary angioplasty when performed; single major coronary artery or branch

C9603 Percutaneous transluminal coronary atherectomy, with drug-eluting intracoronary stent, with coronary angioplasty when performed; each additional branch of a major coronary artery (list separately in addition to code for primary procedure)

Lay Description

A drug-eluting stent is coated with medication and used to hold open a blocked or collapsed native artery in the heart. The physician makes a small incision in the arm or leg to access the artery for placement of two catheters. A central venous catheter is inserted through the femoral or brachial artery and a second catheter is threaded up to the affected coronary artery. Any obstruction is treated first by using a rotary cutter (atherectomy) to flatten or remove the obstruction. The obstruction may also be treated by inflating a balloon at the tip of the second catheter (PTCA). A stent is introduced through a catheter, placed under radiographic guidance, and expanded to fit the lumen of the artery by inflating the balloon on the second catheter. The catheters are removed. Pressure is placed over the incision for 20 to 30 minutes to stop the bleeding.

C9604-C9605

C9604 Percutaneous transluminal revascularization of or through coronary artery bypass graft (internal mammary, free arterial, venous), any combination of drug-eluting intracoronary stent, atherectomy and angioplasty, including distal protection when performed; single vessel

C9605 Percutaneous transluminal revascularization of or through coronary artery bypass graft (internal mammary, free arterial, venous), any combination of drug-eluting intracoronary stent, atherectomy and angioplasty, including distal protection when performed; each additional branch subtended by the bypass graft (list separately in addition to code for primary procedure)

Lay Description

The use of one or any combination of angioplasty, atherectomy, or drug-eluting stent placement is performed to restore a blocked coronary artery bypass graft (CABG). The physician makes a small incision in the arm or leg to access the artery for placement of two catheters. A central venous catheter is inserted through the femoral or brachial artery and a second catheter is threaded up to the affected graft. The obstruction may be treated by using a rotary cutter (atherectomy) to flatten or remove the obstruction, inflating a balloon at the tip of the second catheter (PTCA), or introducing a drug-eluting stent that is expanded to fit the lumen of the artery. The catheters are removed. Pressure is placed over the incision for 20 to 30 minutes to stop the bleeding.

C9606

C9606 Percutaneous transluminal revascularization of acute total/subtotal occlusion during acute myocardial infarction, coronary artery or coronary artery bypass graft, any combination of drug-eluting intracoronary stent, atherectomy and angioplasty, including aspiration thrombectomy when performed, single vessel

Lay Description

The use of one or any combination of angioplasty, atherectomy, or drug-eluting stent placement is performed to restore an acutely blocked coronary artery bypass graft (CABG) or native coronary artery during an acute myocardial infarction. The physician makes a small incision in the arm or leg to access the artery for placement of two catheters. A central venous catheter is inserted through the femoral or brachial artery and a second catheter is threaded up to the affected vessel or graft. The obstruction may be treated by using a rotary cutter (atherectomy) to flatten or remove the obstruction, inflating a balloon at the tip of the second catheter (PTCA), or introducing a drug-eluting stent that is expanded to fit the lumen of the artery. The catheters are removed. Pressure is placed over the incision for 20 to 30 minutes to stop the bleeding.

C9607-C9608

C9607 Percutaneous transluminal revascularization of chronic total occlusion, coronary artery, coronary artery branch, or coronary artery bypass graft, any combination of drug-eluting intracoronary stent, atherectomy and angioplasty; single vessel

C9608 Percutaneous transluminal revascularization of chronic total occlusion, coronary artery, coronary artery branch, or coronary artery bypass graft, any combination of drug-eluting intracoronary stent, atherectomy and angioplasty; each additional coronary artery, coronary artery branch, or bypass graft (list separately in addition to code for primary procedure)

Lay Description

The use of one or any combination of angioplasty, atherectomy, or drug-eluting stent placement is performed to restore a chronic totally blocked coronary artery bypass graft (CABG) or native coronary artery. The physician makes a small incision in the arm or leg to access the artery for placement of two catheters. A central venous catheter is inserted through the femoral or brachial artery and a second catheter is threaded up to the affected vessel or graft. The obstruction may be treated by using a rotary cutter (atherectomy) to flatten or remove the obstruction, inflating a balloon at the tip of the second catheter (PTCA), or introducing a drug-eluting stent that is expanded to fit the lumen of the artery. The catheters are removed. Pressure is placed over the incision for 20 to 30 minutes to stop the bleeding.

C9724

C9724 Endoscopic full-thickness plication of the stomach using endoscopic plication system (EPS); includes endoscopy

Lay Description

Full-thickness endoscopic plication is the process of creating folds in the stomach near the gastroesophageal junction. Sutures are placed through all layers of the stomach wall to hold the folds in place creating a barrier that blocks gastric acid from reaching the esophagus. This procedure is done under direct endoscopic visualization. The device used to perform this procedure is called an endoscopic plication system (EPS). The full-thickness endoscopic plication is indicated for the treatment of chronic gastroesophageal reflux disease (GERD).

C9725

C9725 Placement of endorectal intracavitary applicator for high intensity brachytherapy

Lay Description

An endorectal intracavitary applicator for high intensity brachytherapy is a disposable, flexible silicone tube developed to meet the criteria of the high dose rate of endorectal brachytherapy. This sphincter preservation surgery modality reduces treatment related toxicity associated with patients with locally advanced resectable rectal cancer. This possible complete sparing of the sphincter and surrounding healthy structures leads to a high sphincter preservation surgery rate and can decrease postoperative complication rates.

C9726

C9726 Placement and removal (if performed) of applicator into breast for intraoperative radiation therapy, add-on to primary breast procedure

Lay Description

An applicator for breast radiation therapy is a device for delivering high dose radiation to the tumor site while minimizing radiation exposure to surrounding tissue. Special catheters are used to deliver needles or a small sphere to the postsurgery cavity. This delivers radiation from the inside out and can save most of the normal breast tissue.

C9727

C9727 Insertion of implants into the soft palate; minimum of 3 implants

Lay Description

Vibrations and collapse of the soft palate contribute to snoring and sleep apnea. To prevent the collapse, implants are placed into the muscles of the soft palate. These implants stimulate fibrosis and overgrowth of fibrous tissue around the implant, which leads to a reduction in the soft palate leaving less to obstruct the airway.

C9728

C9728 Placement of interstitial device(s) for radiation therapy/surgery guidance (e.g., fiducial markers, dosimeter), for other than the following sites (any approach): abdomen, pelvis, prostate, retroperitoneum, thorax, single or multiple

Lay Description

The physician places one or more interstitial devices such as gold seeds (fiducial markers) for radiation therapy guidance or a dosimeter to gauge the amount of radiation received into the targeted soft tissue tumor. Allowing for precision in targeting radiation and/or for measuring the radiation doses received, a fiducial marker is visible by ultrasound and fluoroscopy and permits accurate triangulation of the tissue to be treated. A capsule dosimeter relays radiation dose information so that the clinical team can monitor for any deviation between the radiation plan and the actual radiation received. This code is used to report placement of the devices by any approach to areas other than abdomen, pelvis, prostate, retroperitoneum, or thorax.

C9733

C9733 Nonophthalmic fluorescent vascular angiography

Lay Description
Nonophthalmic fluorescent vascular angiography is an imaging procedure that uses a florescent agent, such as indocyanine green, and a low-power laser to visualize blood perfusion and/or flow. The technique is usually used as intraoperative imaging in conjunction with a surgical procedure that needs confirmation of site perfusion or blood flow.

C9734

C9734 Focused ultrasound ablation/therapeutic intervention, other than uterine leiomyomata, with magnetic resonance (MR) guidance

Lay Description
A focused ultrasound ablation or therapeutic intervention is a noninvasive procedure that uses high-intensity ultrasound waves targeted to a specific tissue. This heats the targeted tissue to temperatures of 65 to 100 degrees Celsius and creates local cavitation. Unlike other thermal therapies, high-intensity ultrasound waves heat only the targeted tissue with little heating of adjacent tissue. This code is to be used for procedures on other than uterine leiomyomata, with or without magnetic resonance (MR) guidance.

C9735

Lay Description
An anoscopy with directed submucosal injection(s) of any substance is a procedure involving injection of a bulking agent into the anal canal for patients with bowel incontinence. The physician advances the anoscope about 5 mm into the submucosal layer of the anal canal. Four 1 mL injections of dextranomer/hyaluronic acid copolymer implant are administered in the anal canal beginning at the posterior, left-lateral, anterior, and right-lateral sites. The needle is left in each site for 15 to 30 seconds. In transmittal R2664-CP dated March 1, 2013, CMS advised OPPS hospitals that HCPCS Level II code C9735 describes the administration/injection procedure for Solesta® and states that C9735 should only be reported with HCPCS Level II code L8605, which describes the Solesta®.

C9737

C9737 Laparoscopy, surgical, esophageal sphincter augmentation with device (e.g., magnetic band)

Lay Description
Laparoscopy, surgical, esophageal sphincter augmentation with device (eg, magnetic band) is a treatment for gastroesophageal reflux. A laparoscope is used to implant a device, for example, magnetic iron beads, around the esophageal sphincter. The devices expand with the passage of food or with intragastric pressure. The expansion inhibits the backflow of gastric fluids into the esophagus.

C9739-C9740

C9739 Cystourethroscopy, with insertion of transprostatic implant; 1 to 3 implants

C9740 Cystourethroscopy, with insertion of transprostatic implant; 4 or more implants

Lay Description
These procedures are used to treat benign prostatic hypertrophy (BPH). A cystourethroscope is inserted and advanced to the area of the obstruction. The obstructing prostatic lobes are retracted away from the urethra. A portion of the lobe is compressed using the implant and with the prostate held way from the urethra, flow is unobstructed. Trade name UroLift®, these implants are permanent and are composed of nitinol, stainless steel, and PET suture.

C9741

C9741 Right heart catheterization with implantation of wireless pressure sensor in the pulmonary artery, including any type of measurement, angiography, imaging supervision, interpretation, and report

Lay Description
An image is taken of the heart and its vessels. A wireless acoustic implant is placed in the pulmonary artery. The device records and transmits tracings of the pulmonary artery pressure. These tracings allow greater management of heart failure.

C9800

C9800 Dermal injection procedure(s) for facial lipodystrophy syndrome (LDS) and provision of Radiesse or Sculptra dermal filler, including all items and supplies

Lay Description
Facial lipodystrophy syndrome (LDS) is a condition that is characterized by localized loss of fat in the face. This loss of fat results in a facial abnormality, such as severely sunken cheeks. Patients with HIV can suffer from this condition due to antiviral treatment or the disease itself. Due to appearance, patients with LDS may discontinue treatment and feel depressed and

E

stigmatized. Dermal filler injection gradually increases the fullness in the face to provide a more normal appearance. The treatment area is sterilely prepped and a series of injections are administered into the deep dermal, subcutaneous areas, or by depot technique. The areas are massaged periodically during the treatment to distribute the medication evenly. The patient may need additional injection sessions to obtain the desired result. This code includes the medication.

C9898

C9898   Radiolabeled product provided during a hospital inpatient stay

Lay Description
Hospitals are to report this code on outpatient claims for nuclear medicine procedures to indicate that a radiolabeled product that provides the radioactivity necessary for the reported diagnostic nuclear medicine procedure was provided during a hospital inpatient stay.

C9899

C9899   Implanted prosthetic device, payable only for inpatients who do not have inpatient coverage

Lay Description
This code is reported when an inpatient who does not have inpatient Part A coverage receives an implanted prosthetic device.

E

E0100-E0105

E0100   Cane, includes canes of all materials, adjustable or fixed, with tip

E0105   Cane, quad or 3-prong, includes canes of all materials, adjustable or fixed, with tips

Lay Description
Walking canes provide the legs with some relief for weight bearing in conditions of impaired ambulation. Canes can be single, three, or four prongs and add another point or points of ground contact that alter the biomechanics of walking to affect balance, relieve pain, and provide stability. Canes are used on the opposite side of the injury or weakness, regardless of which hand is dominant. The patient puts all of their weight on the unaffected leg, then steps with the affected leg and cane at the same time. Tips provide traction.

E0110-E0117

E0110   Crutches, forearm, includes crutches of various materials, adjustable or fixed, pair, complete with tips and handgrips

E0111   Crutch, forearm, includes crutches of various materials, adjustable or fixed, each, with tip and handgrips

E0112   Crutches, underarm, wood, adjustable or fixed, pair, with pads, tips, and handgrips

E0113   Crutch, underarm, wood, adjustable or fixed, each, with pad, tip, and handgrip

E0114   Crutches, underarm, other than wood, adjustable or fixed, pair, with pads, tips, and handgrips

E0116   Crutch, underarm, other than wood, adjustable or fixed, with pad, tip, handgrip, with or without shock absorber, each

E0117   Crutch, underarm, articulating, spring assisted, each

Lay Description
Crutches (wood or aluminum), both standard underarm and forearm crutches that have cuffs encircling the lower portion of the arms, support the body during walking and help protect the injured body limb for patients with impaired ambulation.

E0118

E0118   Crutch substitute, lower leg platform, with or without wheels, each

Lay Description
A crutch substitute is a hands-free device that consists of a long metal bar with a platform attached at knee height at a 90-degree angle. The device has pads on the platform and straps to hold the leg. The patient places the bent knee on the platform and secures the upper leg to the metal bar and the knee to the platform. The device can have a rounded rubber foot or can have wheels attached to the distal end. The device can be used to replace a missing lower leg or to remove weight bearing from an injured lower leg.

E0130-E0144

E0130   Walker, rigid (pickup), adjustable or fixed height

E0135   Walker, folding (pickup), adjustable or fixed height

E0140   Walker, with trunk support, adjustable or fixed height, any type

E0141   Walker, rigid, wheeled, adjustable or fixed height

E0143   Walker, folding, wheeled, adjustable or fixed height

E0144   Walker, enclosed, 4 sided framed, rigid or folding, wheeled with posterior seat

Lay Description
Walkers are used by patients with impaired ambulation when there is a need for greater stability

and security than can be provided by a cane or crutches. Some walkers are simple "semi-cages," which look like two canes with supporting bars between them. Others are more complicated, and can be rigid or folding, with or without seating, with or without wheels, etc. Walkers may also include a device attached to the walker that provides trunk support. A trunk support device holds the patient upright in a standing position. The device may be flexible and soft padded or may be more rigid. The type of device depends upon the patient's medical condition. For example, a patient with cerebral palsy who has diminished muscle control of the trunk may need a rigid trunk support.

E0147-E0149

E0147   Walker, heavy-duty, multiple braking system, variable wheel resistance

E0148   Walker, heavy-duty, without wheels, rigid or folding, any type, each

E0149   Walker, heavy-duty, wheeled, rigid or folding, any type

Lay Description
Walkers are used by patients with impaired ambulation when there is a need for greater stability and security than can be provided by a cane or crutches. Some walkers are simple "semi-cages," which look like two canes with supporting bars between them. Others are more complicated, and can be rigid or folding, with or without seating, with or without wheels, etc. Heavy duty walkers are used by patients with severe neurological disorders or restricted use of one hand and those who exceed the weight limits of a standard wheeled walker.

E0148

E0148   Walker, heavy-duty, without wheels, rigid or folding, any type, each

Lay Description
This code is used to report the hardware that is used to attach a joystick or other device to a wheelchair. This hardware provides the ability to remove or reposition the device.

E0153-E0159

E0153   Platform attachment, forearm crutch, each

E0154   Platform attachment, walker, each

E0155   Wheel attachment, rigid pick-up walker, per pair

E0156   Seat attachment, walker

E0157   Crutch attachment, walker, each

E0158   Leg extensions for walker, per set of 4

E0159   Brake attachment for wheeled walker, replacement, each

Lay Description
These codes report the various attachments used with walkers and crutches.

E0160-E0175

E0160   Sitz type bath or equipment, portable, used with or without commode

E0161   Sitz type bath or equipment, portable, used with or without commode, with faucet attachment(s)

E0162   Sitz bath chair

E0163   Commode chair, mobile or stationary, with fixed arms

E0165   Commode chair, mobile or stationary, with detachable arms

E0167   Pail or pan for use with commode chair, replacement only

E0168   Commode chair, extra wide and/or heavy-duty, stationary or mobile, with or without arms, any type, each

E0170   Commode chair with integrated seat lift mechanism, electric, any type

E0171   Commode chair with integrated seat lift mechanism, nonelectric, any type

E0172   Seat lift mechanism placed over or on top of toilet, any type

E0175   Footrest, for use with commode chair, each

Lay Description
Commodes are generally portable toilets in a chair form that hold a pot under an open toilet seat. Some commodes, known as sitz baths, have large deep pans that also serve as a hip bath to soak the hips, buttocks, or perineal area wounds. There are many types/styles of commodes available on the market.

E0181-E0182

E0181   Powered pressure reducing mattress overlay/pad, alternating, with pump, includes heavy-duty

E0182   Pump for alternating pressure pad, for replacement only

Lay Description
These codes describe power pressure-reducing mattress overlays of alternating pressure or low air loss. These pressure reducing support devices consist of various pads that reduce the pressure of the patient's body weight on any particular area of the body. They are characterized by an air pump or blower that provides sequential inflation or deflation of air cells or a low interface pressure throughout the overlay. They have inflated cell height of the air cells through which air is being circulated of 2.5 inches or greater. The height of the air chambers, proximity of the air chambers to one another, frequency of air cycling (for alternating pressure overlays), and air pressure provide adequate patient lift, pressure reduction, and prevention of bottoming out. Typically used for patients who are fully or partially immobile (e.g., paraplegic patient), they assist in reducing the pressure on skin and tissues, allowing blood flow to the focal points in question, to prevent and/or treat pressure ulcers and lesions, such as decubitus ulcers.

E0184, E0186-E0187

E0184   Dry pressure mattress
E0186   Air pressure mattress
E0187   Water pressure mattress

Lay Description
These codes report special mattresses that reduce the pressure of the patient's body weight on any particular area of the body. Generally used for patients who are fully or partially immobile (e.g., paraplegic patient), they assist in reducing the pressure on skin and tissues, allowing blood flow to the focal points in question, to prevent and/or treat pressure ulcers and lesions, such as decubitus ulcers. These codes describe non-powered pressure-reducing mattresses. A foam or dry pressure mattress is characterized by a height of 5 inches or greater, with a density and other qualities that provide adequate pressure reduction. It is durable, has a waterproof cover, and can be placed directly on a hospital bed frame. An air pressure or water pressure mattress is characterized by a height of 5 inches or greater of the air or water contained inside, has a durable, waterproof cover, and can be placed directly on a hospital bed frame.

E0185, E0197-E0199

E0185   Gel or gel-like pressure pad for mattress, standard mattress length and width
E0197   Air pressure pad for mattress, standard mattress length and width
E0198   Water pressure pad for mattress, standard mattress length and width
E0199   Dry pressure pad for mattress, standard mattress length and width

Lay Description
These codes, identified as "pressure pad for mattress," describe nonpowered pressure reducing mattress overlays. These devices are designed to be placed on top of a hospital or home mattress of standard length and width. Pressure reducing support services consist of various pads for mattresses that reduce the pressure of the patient's body weight on any particular area of the body. Typically used for patient's that are fully or partially immobile (e.g., paraplegic patient), they assist in reducing the pressure on skin and tissues, allowing blood flow to the focal points in question, to prevent and/or treat pressure ulcers and lesions, such as decubitus ulcers. A gel or gel-like mattress overlay is characterized by a gel or gel-like layer contained within the pad reaching a height of 2 inches or greater. An air pressure pad is characterized by interconnected air cells having a cell height of 3 inches or greater. A water pressure mattress overlay (E0198) is characterized by a filled height of 3 inches or greater of water contained within the pads cells. A foam mattress overlay, or dry pressure pad, is characterized by a base thickness of 2 inches or greater and peak height of 3 inches or greater if it is a convoluted overlay (e.g., egg crate-type) or an overall height of at least 3 inches if it is a non-convoluted overlay.

E0186-E0187

E0186   Air pressure mattress
E0187   Water pressure mattress

Lay Description
Please refer to code E0184 for the description, coding, and billing information.

E0188-E0189, E0191-E0194

E0188   Synthetic sheepskin pad
E0189   Lambswool sheepskin pad, any size
E0191   Heel or elbow protector, each
E0193   Powered air flotation bed (low air loss therapy)
E0194   Air fluidized bed

Lay Description
A decubitus ulcer is also known as a pressure ulcer, pressure sore, or bedsore. Bedsores can range from a mild erythema of the skin to a deep wound extending through bone. Pressure ulcers occur when an incapacitated, bedridden person has constant pressure against the skin, usually over a bony area, which decreases the blood supply, causing tissue death. Use of special pads or beds relieves pressure on the skin. Pads made of synthetic sheepskin or lambs wool with heel or elbow protectors prevent friction against thin fragile skin. Specialized beds, such as a powered air flotation bed or an air-fluidized bed, are often used for patients with stage three or four pressure sores that would otherwise require institutionalization.

E0190

E0190   Positioning cushion/pillow/wedge, any shape or size, includes all components and accessories

Lay Description
Positioning cushions/pillows/wedges are typically made of foam or foam-like materials, and come in a variety of densities, shapes, and designs depending on the manufacturer. Most have anatomic-oriented designs so as to provide as much support as possible, although they somewhat limit range of motion. These cushions/pillows/wedges relieve and/or prevent neck tension and may protect against inadvertent reinjury during sleep.

E0191-E0194

E0191   Heel or elbow protector, each
E0193   Powered air flotation bed (low air loss therapy)
E0194   Air fluidized bed

Lay Description
Please refer to codes E0188-E0189 for the description, coding, and billing information.

E0196

E0196   Gel pressure mattress

Lay Description
A gel pressure mattress is a mattress with a top layer of gel that is enclosed in a durable, waterproof bladder. The gel layer must be at least a height of 5 inches. Some gel mattresses have a layer of soft or pillow-top material directly under the gel layer. This is a full mattress that can be placed directly on a bed frame. A gel pressure mattress is designed to distribute weight more evenly across the surface of the mattress and eliminate pressure points. When there is decreased pressure on skin at contact points, such as buttocks and ankles, skin and soft tissue is less likely to break down and form ulcers or other types of open wounds.

E0197-E0199

E0197   Air pressure pad for mattress, standard mattress length and width

E0198   Water pressure pad for mattress, standard mattress length and width

E0199   Dry pressure pad for mattress, standard mattress length and width

Lay Description
Please refer to code E0185 for the description, coding, and billing information.

E0200, E0205

E0200   Heat lamp, without stand (table model), includes bulb, or infrared element

E0205   Heat lamp, with stand, includes bulb, or infrared element

Lay Description
Heat causes blood vessels to open, creating increased blood flow and allowing tissue purging of debris and by-products of injury. Heat therapy promotes relaxation of collagen tissues within muscle, tendons, and ligaments, which allow them to be stretched. Heat lamps provide dry heat to patients who cannot tolerate pressure of a directly applied heat source, or who may have positioning needs. The heat from a lamp is controlled by the distance between the lamp and the patient.

E0202

E0202   Phototherapy (bilirubin) light with photometer

Lay Description
A phototherapy (bilirubin) light with photometer is used to treat infants with jaundice caused by elevated levels of bilirubin in the blood. Phototherapy lights provide a specific wavelength of blue fluorescent light that breaks down bilirubin into nontoxic water-soluble components that are excreted by the infant. The photometer or "blue meter" on the lamp measures the intensity of the light emission. Phototherapy lights are available in the form of a lamp, light panel, or special light blanket (wallaby blanket) and all are reported with this code.

E0203

E0203   Therapeutic lightbox, minimum 10,000 lux, table top model

Lay Description
A therapeutic lightbox with a minimum of 10,000 lux is used to treat seasonal affective disorder (SAD), which is a form of depression; diurnal disorders; or sometimes to mitigate the effects of medications. SAD occurs most frequently in the fall or winter as the daylight hours become shorter and shorter. Therapeutic lightboxes provide cool-white or full spectrum fluorescent light to treat this disorder. The light boxes deliver strong light near the intensity and wavelength of noontime during high summer. Patients expose themselves to the light for a prescribed amount of time per day at set times. Tabletop or desktop lightboxes that emit a minimum of 10,000 lux, which is a measurement of the light intensity, are reported with this code. Lightboxes that emit lower levels of lux (5,000 or 2,500) should not be reported.

E0205

E0205   Heat lamp, with stand, includes bulb, or infrared element

Lay Description
Please refer to code E0200 for description, coding, and billing information.

E0210-E0215

E0210   Electric heat pad, standard

E0215   Electric heat pad, moist

Lay Description
Heat causes blood vessels to open, creating increased blood flow and allowing tissue purging of debris and by-products of injury. Heat therapy promotes relaxation of collagen tissues within muscle, tendons, and ligaments, which allow them to be stretched. Electric heating pads are alternatives to hot packs. Because electric heating pads do not cool spontaneously, use should be limited to 20 minutes to avoid the risk of burns.

E0217-E0218, E0236-E0218, E0249

E0217   Water circulating heat pad with pump

E0218   Water circulating cold pad with pump

E0236   Pump for water circulating pad

E0249   Pad for water circulating heat unit, for replacement only

Lay Description
Heat causes blood vessels to open, creating increased blood flow and allowing tissue purging of debris and by-products of injury. Heat therapy promotes relaxation of collagen tissues within muscle, tendons,

and ligaments, which allow them to be stretched. A water circulating heating pad with pump is a device that circulates heated water through the pad using a mechanical pump. Cold therapy is the application of cold treatment to affected tissues, generally used in the immediate postoperative or post-trauma period to reduce edema and enhance pain control. Pain sensations are inhibited by cold by reducing the speed of impulses conducted by nerve fibers. Cold therapy reduces muscle spasms and causes constriction of small arteries and veins, which reduces hemorrhage and swelling within injured tissues. A water circulating cold pad with pump consists of ice water placed into a reservoir that is circulated through a pad using a mechanical pump.

E0221

E0221   Infrared heating pad system

Lay Description
An infrared heating pad system consists of a pad or pads containing mechanisms, such as luminous gallium aluminum arsenide diodes, that generate infrared (or near infrared) light and a power source.

E0225, E0239

E0225   Hydrocollator unit, includes pads
E0239   Hydrocollator unit, portable

Lay Description
Hydrocollator packs are also known as hot packs and warm tissue by conduction. Usually made of canvas bags filled with silicon dioxide, which absorbs many times its own weight in water, hydrocollator packs are immersed in a hot water bath, removed as needed, then wrapped in layered toweling or padding, or some kind of insulating cover, and applied to the patient. The packs cool slowly and can remain warm for around 30 minutes.

E0231-E0232

E0231   Noncontact wound-warming device (temperature control unit, AC adapter and power cord) for use with warming card and wound cover
E0232   Warming card for use with the noncontact wound-warming device and noncontact wound-warming wound cover

Lay Description
Wound healing occurs best in a warm, moist environment that enhances subcutaneous oxygen tension and increases blood flow to the wound. A noncontact wound warming device, also referred to as noncontact normothermic wound therapy (NNWT), is a wound treatment device designed to create an optimal environment to promote wound healing. A noncontact wound warming device includes a noncontact bandage and a warming unit designed to maintain 100 percent relative humidity and to produce optimal temperatures in the wound and

surrounding tissues. The bandage consists of a sterile foam collar that adheres to the skin surrounding the wound and a sterile, transparent film that covers the top of the wound without touching it. An infrared warming card or flexible heat unit is inserted into a pocket in the film covering.

E0235

E0235   Paraffin bath unit, portable (see medical supply code A4265 for paraffin)

Lay Description
Paraffin baths are used mainly for treating contractures, occurring in patients with rheumatoid arthritis or scleroderma. The typical paraffin bath is a container that holds and heats a 1:7 mixture of mineral oil and paraffin, maintaining it at around 53¡C into which the patient may either continuously immerse the treated part, such as the hand, for 20-30 minutes, or repetitively dip and remove the treated area from the paraffin. This code is for a portable paraffin bath unit, excluding the paraffin.

E0236

E0236   Pump for water circulating pad

Lay Description
Please refer to codes E0217-E0218 for the description, coding, and billing information.

E0239

E0239   Hydrocollator unit, portable

Lay Description
Please refer to code E0225 for the description, coding, and billing information.

E0240

E0240   Bath/shower chair, with or without wheels, any size

Lay Description
A bath or shower chair is a seat designed to fit into a standard bathtub or walk-in shower that provides stable seating while bathing or showering for those people unsteady on their feet or those unable to stand.

E0241-E0246

E0241   Bathtub wall rail, each
E0242   Bathtub rail, floor base
E0243   Toilet rail, each
E0244   Raised toilet seat
E0245   Tub stool or bench
E0246   Transfer tub rail attachment

Lay Description
Rails are safety items for home use to help a person get in and out of the bathtub or up and down from the toilet by providing a strong hold while securely stepping into the tub, or lowering or raising body weight.

E0247-E0248

E0247 Transfer bench for tub or toilet with or without commode opening

E0248 Transfer bench, heavy-duty, for tub or toilet with or without commode opening

Lay Description

A transfer bench for tub or toilet is a flat expanded surface without a back that provides stable seating while the person is bathing or showering. These benches may have a commode opening that allows the person to more comfortably maneuver and use a toilet. The benches may be freestanding with legs or attachable to wall or tub. Transfer benches are intended for those people unsteady on their feet or those unable to stand. Heavy-duty benches are generally designed for people who weigh more than 300 pounds.

E0249

E0249 Pad for water circulating heat unit, for replacement only

Lay Description

Please refer to codes E0217–E0218 for the description, coding, and billing information.

E0250-E0256, E0290-E0293

E0250 Hospital bed, fixed height, with any type side rails, with mattress

E0251 Hospital bed, fixed height, with any type side rails, without mattress

E0255 Hospital bed, variable height, hi-lo, with any type side rails, with mattress

E0256 Hospital bed, variable height, hi-lo, with any type side rails, without mattress

E0290 Hospital bed, fixed height, without side rails, with mattress

E0291 Hospital bed, fixed height, without side rails, without mattress

E0292 Hospital bed, variable height, hi-lo, without side rails, with mattress

E0293 Hospital bed, variable height, hi-lo, without side rails, without mattress

Lay Description

Hospital beds for patient home use come in a variety of designs, with a multitude of features and accessories to assist and protect the patient. A hospital bed is generally needed when an ordinary (regular) bed is not suitable for the patient's medical needs. Hospital beds provide features such as head and leg elevation and height adjustment. Clinical cases generally requiring variable-height hospital bed use include severe arthritis and other injuries to lower extremities (e.g., fractured hip). Variable-height (hi-lo) feature beds assist patients to ambulate by enabling them to place their feet on the floor while sitting on the edge of the bed.

E0260-E0266, E0294-E0297

E0260 Hospital bed, semi-electric (head and foot adjustment), with any type side rails, with mattress

E0261 Hospital bed, semi-electric (head and foot adjustment), with any type side rails, without mattress

E0265 Hospital bed, total electric (head, foot, and height adjustments), with any type side rails, with mattress

E0266 Hospital bed, total electric (head, foot, and height adjustments), with any type side rails, without mattress

E0294 Hospital bed, semi-electric (head and foot adjustment), without side rails, with mattress

E0295 Hospital bed, semi-electric (head and foot adjustment), without side rails, without mattress

E0296 Hospital bed, total electric (head, foot, and height adjustments), without side rails, with mattress

E0297 Hospital bed, total electric (head, foot, and height adjustments), without side rails, without mattress

Lay Description

Hospital beds for patient home use come in a variety of designs, with a multitude of features and accessories to assist and protect the patient. A hospital bed is generally needed when an ordinary, regular bed, is not suitable for the patient's medical needs. Hospital beds provide features such as head and leg elevation and height adjustment. Hospital beds with the semi-electric feature allow for head and foot adjustment, and are used by patients with congestive heart failure, chronic pulmonary disease, or problems with aspiration who require positioning of the body in ways not feasible with an ordinary flat bed.

E0270

E0270 Hospital bed, institutional type includes: oscillating, circulating and Stryker frame, with mattress

Lay Description

Standard institutional hospital beds typically include a frame for oscillating on a longitudinally extending axis and a patient support which is mounted on the oscillating frame, providing controlled pivoting of the patient support on a transverse axis. A Stryker bed consists of a bed frame that holds the patient and permits turning in various planes without individual motion of parts, allowing medical staff to turn a patient easily. These beds also include securing devices provided on the patient support to hold a patient in place. The mattress is typically made of water resistant vinyl and is durable for long term use while also being fire retardant.

E0271-E0272

E0271   Mattress, innerspring

E0272   Mattress, foam rubber

Lay Description

A foam rubber mattress is used to add comfort to a hospital bed. This device is commonly used in conjunction with other hospital bed components, such as bed boards and inner springs.

E0273

E0273   Bed board

Lay Description

A bed board is a device placed under a mattress to support the mattress and keep it firm by preventing the mattress from sagging. Bed boards usually consist of wood slats inside a canvas cover or are made of wood with hinges allowing the board to bend with the position of the bed.

E0274, E0315

E0274   Over-bed table

E0315   Bed accessory: board, table, or support device, any type

Lay Description

An over-bed table, board, or support device is a functional convenience item, adjustable in height, or angle, to allow the patient more comfort and ease while writing or eating in bed. An over-the-bed table has a laminate top affixed to a chrome-plated, height-adjustable bar, and casters to ease mobility of the table in any direction.

E0275-E0276

E0275   Bed pan, standard, metal or plastic

E0276   Bed pan, fracture, metal or plastic

Lay Description

Bedpans are used by patients whose conditions require them to remain in bed and not ambulate, even for the purpose of getting to the bathroom.

E0277

E0277   Powered pressure-reducing air mattress

Lay Description

This code describes a powered pressure-reducing mattress (alternating pressure, low air loss, or powered flotation without low air loss) that is characterized by the following: an air pump or blower that provides either sequential inflation and deflation of the air cells or a low interface pressure throughout the mattress; an inflated cell height of the air cells through which air is being circulated of 5 inches or greater; air chamber height and proximity and frequency of air circulation (for alternating pressure mattresses), which provides adequate patient lift and pressure reduction to prevent bottoming out; a surface designed to reduce friction; and the ability to be placed directly on a hospital bed frame.

E0280

E0280   Bed cradle, any type

Lay Description

A bed cradle is used for patients with acute gouty arthritis or burns for whom it is necessary to prevent contact with the bed coverings and any pressure applied to the area. Report this code for any type of bed cradle.

E0290-E0293

E0290   Hospital bed, fixed height, without side rails, with mattress

E0291   Hospital bed, fixed height, without side rails, without mattress

E0292   Hospital bed, variable height, hi-lo, without side rails, with mattress

E0293   Hospital bed, variable height, hi-lo, without side rails, without mattress

Lay Description

Please refer to codes E0250-E0256 for the description, coding, and billing information.

E0294-E0297

E0294   Hospital bed, semi-electric (head and foot adjustment), without side rails, with mattress

E0295   Hospital bed, semi-electric (head and foot adjustment), without side rails, without mattress

E0296   Hospital bed, total electric (head, foot, and height adjustments), without side rails, with mattress

E0297   Hospital bed, total electric (head, foot, and height adjustments), without side rails, without mattress

Lay Description

Please refer to codes E0260-E0266 for the description.

E0300

E0300   Pediatric crib, hospital grade, fully enclosed, with or without top enclosure

Lay Description

A pediatric enclosed crib is an alternative bed for the pediatric patient. It allows the patient full range of motion with no traditional restraints. The crib consists of a mesh like screen that gently contains the patient and prevents wandering. Typically these cribs are available in different sizes and materials.

E0301-E0302

E0301   Hospital bed, heavy-duty, extra wide, with weight capacity greater than 350 pounds, but less than or equal to 600 pounds, with any type side rails, without mattress

E0302 Hospital bed, extra heavy-duty, extra wide, with weight capacity greater than 600 pounds, with any type side rails, without mattress

Lay Description
A hospital bed is generally needed when a home bed, sold as furniture, is not suitable for the patient's medical needs. Heavy duty, extra wide beds are available for individuals weighing more than 350 pounds. These beds have additional support in all parts, including the frame and legs. These beds include side rails as a safety feature.

E0303-E0304

E0303 Hospital bed, heavy-duty, extra wide, with weight capacity greater than 350 pounds, but less than or equal to 600 pounds, with any type side rails, with mattress
E0304 Hospital bed, extra heavy-duty, extra wide, with weight capacity greater than 600 pounds, with any type side rails, with mattress

Lay Description
A hospital bed is generally needed when a home bed, sold as furniture, is not suitable for the patient's medical needs. Extra-wide, heavy-duty hospital beds have side rails and a mattress that has additional support in all parts (e.g., legs) for an individual who weighs anywhere from 350-600 pounds or for an individual who weighs more than 600 pounds.

E0305-E0310

E0305 Bedside rails, half-length
E0310 Bedside rails, full-length

Lay Description
Bedside rails are used to protect the patient from injury. Full-length bedside rails, which run the entire length of the bed, are used when the patient has a higher risk of falling out of bed.

E0315

E0315 Bed accessory: board, table, or support device, any type

Lay Description
Please refer to code E0274 for the description.

E0316

E0316 Safety enclosure frame/canopy for use with hospital bed, any type

Lay Description
A safety enclosure such as a frame or canopy is used to prevent a patient from leaving the bed. This item encloses the standard hospital bed with a netting attached to a frame and is designed for patients who would need to be restrained. This allows the patient to remain in a safe environment without the need for leg or wrist restraints.

E0325-E0326

E0325 Urinal; male, jug-type, any material
E0326 Urinal; female, jug-type, any material

Lay Description
A urinal is a hand-held container used to collect urine. Some urinals have handles. Urinals are usable in a variety of positions. Jug type urinals generally have a lid and can be used multiple times. Urinals provide an option for bed-confined people who cannot use a bedpan. Male urinals are designed to accommodate a penis. Female urinals have various designs that can be used by women to collect urine.

E0328-E0329

E0328 Hospital bed, pediatric, manual, 360 degree side enclosures, top of headboard, footboard and side rails up to 24 in above the spring, includes mattress
E0329 Hospital bed, pediatric, electric or semi-electric, 360 degree side enclosures, top of headboard, footboard and side rails up to 24 in above the spring, includes mattress

Lay Description
Pediatric hospital beds are surfaces for sleep or rest that are designed for non-adult patients. Different parts of the bed can be adjusted to different levels, angles, and configurations to provide physical relief or ease in comfort. Manual pediatric beds typically include manual cranks by which the patient can be raised or lowered in bed. Electric or semi-electric pediatric beds typically allow back and foot adjustment electronically. Some semi-electric beds allow manual height adjustment. Each type of bed usually includes removable bedside rails. The mattress used for these beds is typically made with a water resistant vinyl cover and is durable for long-term use while also being fire retardant.

E0350-E0352

E0350 Control unit for electronic bowel irrigation/evacuation system
E0352 Disposable pack (water reservoir bag, speculum, valving mechanism, and collection bag/box) for use with the electronic bowel irrigation/evacuation system

Lay Description
Pulsed irrigation bowel evacuation is used for bowel management of chronic constipation and fecal impaction in patients with neurogenic bowel dysfunction. Neurogenic bowel dysfunction may be present in patients with spinal cord injury, amyotrophic lateral sclerosis, spina bifida, multiple sclerosis, and diabetes mellitus. Pulsed irrigation bowel evacuation system is an electronic device that delivers small pulses of warm tap water into the rectum to rehydrate feces and promote peristalsis. The system consists of a speculum, tubing, water reservoir

bag, valve, a disposable collection container, and an electrical unit that delivers positive and negative air pressure through the tubing.

E0370

E0370   Air pressure elevator for heel

Lay Description

Lower extremities are susceptible to pressure ulcers. The heel is a small area that receives a great deal of pressure as it rests on a surface. An air pressure elevator for a heel is a device consisting of one or more air filled chambers that surround the heel and raise it above a hard surface. It may be used with wheelchairs, day chairs, and in bed.

E0371

E0371   Nonpowered advanced pressure reducing overlay for mattress, standard mattress length and width

Lay Description

A nonpowered advanced pressure-reducing mattress overlay is a device composed of separate cells filled with air or fluid that is attached or laid on the top of a mattress. It generally has a height of three inches or more and is covered in a surface that reduces friction. This overlay is designed to raise pressure points. When there is decreased pressure on skin at contact points, such as buttocks and ankles, skin and soft tissue is less likely to break down and form ulcers or other types of open wounds.

E0372

E0372   Powered air overlay for mattress, standard mattress length and width

Lay Description

A powered pressure-reducing mattress overlay is a device filled with air or fluid that is attached to an electronic device that alternately raises and lowers the air pressure or circulates the air or fluid. The overlay is attached to or laid on top of a mattress. It generally has a height of 3 inches or more and is covered in a surface that reduces friction. This overlay is designed to raise pressure points. When there is decreased pressure on skin at contact points, such as buttocks and ankles, skin and soft tissue is less likely to break down and form ulcers or other types of open wounds.

E0373

E0373   Nonpowered advanced pressure reducing mattress

Lay Description

A nonpowered, advanced pressure-reducing mattress is a mattress composed of separate cells filled with air or fluid. It generally has a height of 5 inches or more and is covered in a surface that reduces friction. The mattress is designed to raise pressure points. When there is decreased pressure on skin at contact points, such as buttocks and ankles, skin and soft tissue is less

likely to break down and form ulcers or other types of open wounds.

E0424-E0425

E0424   Stationary compressed gaseous oxygen system, rental; includes container, contents, regulator, flowmeter, humidifier, nebulizer, cannula or mask, and tubing

E0425   Stationary compressed gas system, purchase; includes regulator, flowmeter, humidifier, nebulizer, cannula or mask, and tubing

Lay Description

Oxygen is stored in several manners, one of which is as a compressed gas. The compression mandates use of heavy, reinforced tanks that constitute a stationary system. A regulator fits on top of the tank and is an adjustment device to control the flow of oxygen at the prescribed rate. A flow meter conserves the release of oxygen by turning on and shutting off the regulated flow as the patient inhales and exhales. A nasal cannula is common for lower delivery rates. A mask and/or nebulizer may be used for higher delivery rates and a catheter directly to the trachea is sometimes required. An in-line humidification system may also be used to modulate effects of higher flows.

E0430-E0431

E0430   Portable gaseous oxygen system, purchase; includes regulator, flowmeter, humidifier, cannula or mask, and tubing

E0431   Portable gaseous oxygen system, rental; includes portable container, regulator, flowmeter, humidifier, cannula or mask, and tubing

Lay Description

Portable gaseous oxygen systems are typically lightweight aluminum tanks (usually designated as C tanks) containing pressurized gaseous oxygen. The pressurized systems are stable and the product stores well up to time of use. In some instances, these units may be refilled from large stationary gas oxygen tanks. These systems are generally designed for emergency or occasional use. These codes include all delivery hardware associated with use of the system (regulator, flowmeter, mask, tubing, etc.).

E0433

E0433   Portable liquid oxygen system, rental; home liquefier used to fill portable liquid oxygen containers, includes portable containers, regulator, flowmeter, humidifier, cannula or mask and tubing, with or without supply reservoir and contents gauge

Lay Description

A portable liquid oxygen system is a cooling device that converts air into liquid oxygen by cooling it to

-279 degrees Fahrenheit. The device is designed to store the liquid oxygen and allow patients to refill their portable oxygen containers.

E0434-E0435

E0434 Portable liquid oxygen system, rental; includes portable container, supply reservoir, humidifier, flowmeter, refill adaptor, contents gauge, cannula or mask, and tubing

E0435 Portable liquid oxygen system, purchase; includes portable container, supply reservoir, flowmeter, humidifier, contents gauge, cannula or mask, tubing and refill adaptor

Lay Description
Portable liquid oxygen tanks are insulated thermos-like units that store comparatively large quantities of oxygen at lower pressures than gaseous systems. Several hundred times more oxygen can be stored as liquid in the same amount of space than in its gaseous form. The liquid oxygen is stored cold and converted to gas as it is warmed through an apparatus at the reservoir. Portable units typically weigh eight to 10 pounds and are designed to be refillable from larger, stationary tanks. Portable liquid systems are prone to evaporation loss and the product should be used shortly after decanting. These codes include all oxygen delivery hardware associated with use of the system (regulator, flowmeter, mask, tubing, etc.), including refill adapters.

E0439-E0440

E0439 Stationary liquid oxygen system, rental; includes container, contents, regulator, flowmeter, humidifier, nebulizer, cannula or mask, & tubing

E0440 Stationary liquid oxygen system, purchase; includes use of reservoir, contents indicator, regulator, flowmeter, humidifier, nebulizer, cannula or mask, and tubing

Lay Description
Stationary liquid oxygen systems are insulated thermos-like units that store comparatively large quantities of oxygen at lower pressures than gaseous systems. (Several hundred times more oxygen can be stored as liquid in the same amount of space than in its gaseous form.) The liquid oxygen is stored cold and converted to gas as it is warmed through an apparatus at the reservoir. Stationary units may weigh 75 to 100 pounds and can contain enough liquid oxygen to last patients up to eight days, depending on level of use. In many instances, the stationary system is also used to decant liquid oxygen into smaller, portable systems. These codes include all oxygen delivery hardware associated with use of the stationary system (regulator, flowmeter, mask, tubing, etc.).

E0441-E0442

E0441 Stationary oxygen contents, gaseous, 1 month's supply = 1 unit

E0442 Stationary oxygen contents, liquid, 1 month's supply = 1 unit

Lay Description
Traditional oxygen systems are of two general varieties. Compressed gaseous systems, commonly known as "green tanks" or H tanks, are large stationary units that must be secured in place during use. These tanks may be steel, aluminum, or reinforced synthetic material. Smaller units, designated as E tanks and D tanks, are semi-portable units and, in some instances, may be refilled from a larger unit. Gaseous oxygen for stationary systems is typically sold in increments of 50 cubic feet. Report E0441 for a one-month supply of gaseous oxygen product for a purchased system, with or without refillable portable tanks. The second variety consists of liquid oxygen systems. Stationary liquid oxygen systems are insulated thermos-like units that store comparatively large quantities of oxygen at lower pressures than gaseous systems. (Several hundred times more oxygen can be stored as liquid in the same amount of space than in its gaseous form.) The liquid oxygen is stored cold and converted to gas as it is warmed through an apparatus at the reservoir. Stationary units may weigh 75 to 100 pounds and can contain enough liquid oxygen to last patients up to eight days, depending on level of use. In many instances, the stationary system is also used to decant liquid oxygen into smaller, portable systems. Liquid oxygen for stationary systems is typically sold in 10-pound increments.

E0443-E0444

E0443 Portable oxygen contents, gaseous, 1 month's supply = 1 unit

E0444 Portable oxygen contents, liquid, 1 month's supply = 1 unit

Lay Description
Traditional portable oxygen systems are of two general varieties. Smaller compressed gaseous systems are designated as E tanks and D tanks and are semi-portable reinforced tanks. Fully portable gaseous oxygen systems are typically lightweight aluminum tanks (usually designated as C tanks) containing the pressurized gaseous oxygen. These pressurized systems are stable and the oxygen product stores well up to time of use. These systems are generally designed for emergency or occasional use. Gaseous oxygen for portable systems is typically sold in increments of five cubic feet. Report E0443 for a one-month supply of gaseous oxygen product for a portable system not refillable from a stationary tank. The second variety consists of liquid oxygen systems. Liquid oxygen is stored cold in low-pressure insulated tanks and converted to gas as it is warmed through an apparatus at the reservoir. Portable units may weigh eight to 10 pounds and can contain enough liquid oxygen to last patients up to four hours, depending

on level of use. Liquid oxygen for portable systems is typically sold in one-pound increments.

E0445

E0445   Oximeter device for measuring blood oxygen levels noninvasively

Lay Description
Oximetry is a noninvasive method to measure blood hemoglobin (Hb) oxygen saturation. A probe is attached to the patient's earlobe or a fingertip. The probe emits a light source. The hemoglobin absorbs a percentage of the light, depending upon its oxygen saturation level, and the results are digitally recorded and displayed on a hand-held unit. Additional data, such as pulse, are sometimes recorded and displayed. This code reports supply of the oximeter unit itself.

E0446

E0446   Topical oxygen delivery system, not otherwise specified, includes all supplies and accessories

Lay Description
A topical oxygen delivery system supplies continuous oxygen therapy to wounds. The device converts room air to concentrated oxygen that is delivered directly to the wound. Components of the system include the oxygenation system, the battery charger, the protective covering, the oxygen delivery extension set, and the wound oxygen delivery cannula. This is used in conjunction with a moist dressing system.

E0450, E0461

E0450   Volume control ventilator, without pressure support mode, may include pressure control mode, used with invasive interface (e.g., tracheostomy tube)

E0461   Volume control ventilator, without pressure support mode, may include pressure control mode, used with noninvasive interface (e.g., mask)

Lay Description
Volume control ventilators are typically used to transition patients from fully assisted critical care mechanical ventilation to normal respiration of room air. These systems may fall under the general heading of intermittent positive pressure breathing (IPPB) treatment. Typically, the patient initiates spontaneous breathing activity that is machine assisted by volume and pressure control. Airflow may be terminated when the airway pressure raises a certain amount above the set pressure criteria. The tidal volume may be controlled by determining the length of inspired breaths. A backup rate feature sounds an alarm should the patient become unable to initiate breathing activity. The machine then automatically takes over breathing functions until the patient once again initiates spontaneous respiratory activity. Numerous

settings and alarms are typically featured to monitor respiratory activity and effectiveness.

E0455

E0455   Oxygen tent, excluding croup or pediatric tents

Lay Description
An oxygen tent is a canopy placed over the head and shoulders or over the entire body of a patient to provide oxygen at a higher level than normal. They are made of plastic or other material through which oxygen cannot pass. Oxygen enters the tent through a hose. Physicians seldom use oxygen tents today as newer methods of oxygen delivery provide a better environment and easier patient access.

E0457-E0459

E0457   Chest shell (cuirass)
E0459   Chest wrap

Lay Description
A chest shell or cuirass is a rigid plastic or metal dome, similar to a tortoise shell, that surrounds the chest and abdomen. The shell has a rubber or foam seal that is attached to the edges of the shell to create a tight seal. A chest wrap is an impermeable nylon jacket suspended by a rigid chest piece that fits over the chest and abdomen. A hose is attached to the center or side of the shell or wrap. The other end of the hose is attached to the ventilator. The ventilator cycles air in and out, creating a vacuum. This causes the chest to raise and air to enter the nose and mouth. A cuirass and a chest wrap are non-invasive methods of negative pressure mechanical ventilation that assist people with paralyzed or weakened diaphragm or intercostal muscles. People with stable or slowly progressing neuromuscular diseases (such as polio or multiple sclerosis), central hypoventilation (e.g., apnea not due to airway obstruction), or chest wall deformities are candidates for the use of negative pressure ventilation.

E0460

E0460   Negative pressure ventilator; portable or stationary

Lay Description
The "iron lung" was the prototypical negative pressure ventilator device. Fully natural respiration is largely a function of the broad diaphragm muscle that separates the thoracic and abdominal cavities working with intercostals (rib) muscles. Mechanical ventilation may be required when these muscles are paralyzed or otherwise underperforming, as occurs in polio. A patient's thorax is placed in a closed container that can be negatively pressurized and released. As the air pressure surrounding the chest becomes less than atmospheric, the chest expands and the lungs inflate. When the pressure surrounding the chest returns to atmospheric pressure, exhalation occurs as it would naturally. This push-pull action of a negative

pressure ventilator can mechanically breathe for the patient. The large stationary iron lung systems are rarely used today. More portable models are still used, however, and E0460 reports the supply of this type of negative pressure ventilator.

E0461

E0461 Volume control ventilator, without pressure support mode, may include pressure control mode, used with noninvasive interface (e.g., mask)

Lay Description
Please refer to code E0450 for the description.

E0462

E0462 Rocking bed, with or without side rails

Lay Description
A rocking bed is a bed mounted on a mechanized platform that moves the patient's upper body up and down. This change of positions promotes movement of the diaphragm and thus breathing, particularly for patients who are quadriplegic or have paralysis of the diaphragm. A rocking bed may also be used to improve blood circulation in the treatment of chronic occlusive arterial disease.

E0463-E0464

E0463 Pressure support ventilator with volume control mode, may include pressure control mode, used with invasive interface (e.g., tracheostomy tube)

E0464 Pressure support ventilator with volume control mode, may include pressure control mode, used with noninvasive interface (e.g., mask)

Lay Description
These codes report a pressure support ventilator used to provide breathing assistance and help maintain open airways. This type of ventilator monitors the patient's breathing efforts and provides the required inspiratory or expiratory airway pressure set by the physician or therapist when the patient's own breathing efforts fall short of the prescribed levels. Airflow may also be terminated when the airway pressure raises a certain amount above the set pressure support level (pressure criteria). The tidal volume may be controlled by the patient when the machine is set in a certain mode by allowing the user to determine the length of inspired breaths.

E0470-E0472

E0470 Respiratory assist device, bi-level pressure capability, without backup rate feature, used with noninvasive interface, e.g., nasal or facial mask (intermittent assist device with continuous positive airway pressure device)

E0471 Respiratory assist device, bi-level pressure capability, with back-up rate feature, used with noninvasive interface, e.g., nasal or facial mask (intermittent assist device with continuous positive airway pressure device)

E0472 Respiratory assist device, bi-level pressure capability, with backup rate feature, used with invasive interface, e.g., tracheostomy tube (intermittent assist device with continuous positive airway pressure device)

Lay Description
RADs are noninvasive, spontaneous respiratory assistance devices with positive pressure that use a nasal or facial mask interface, creating a seal. Some of these devices enable the treating physician to avoid the use of more invasive airway access, such as a tracheostomy, and some of these devices are used in conjunction with invasive therapies. A RAD without backup rate delivers adjustable, variable levels (within a single respiratory cycle) of positive air pressure by way of tubing and a nasal or oral facial mask to assist in the spontaneous respiratory efforts of the patient, and to supplement the volume of inspired air into the lungs. This is also called noninvasive positive pressure respiratory assistance or NPPRA. A RAD with backup rate has, in addition, a timed backup feature to deliver the air pressure whenever sufficient spontaneous patient respiratory efforts fail to occur (i.e., it has a trigger device to deliver a quantity of air into the patient's lungs whenever the patient's spontaneous respiration is insufficient). A RAD with backup rate used in conjunction with invasive therapy versus a noninvasive regimen, delivers adjustable, variable levels (within a single respiratory cycle) of positive air pressure to assist in the spontaneous respiratory efforts of the patient following invasive therapy or surgery, and to supplement the volume of inspired air into the lungs. Noninvasive RADs are different from invasive ventilation, which is administered through a securely intubated airway, generally in patients for whom interruption or failure of the ventilation support would lead to their imminent demise. These devices are not the same as the continuous positive airway pressure (CPAP) devices that are used primarily in the conservative therapy approach (versus surgery) for patients with documented sleep apnea. CPAP devices provide for continuous amounts of air pressure throughout the oropharynx to prevent the collapse of the oropharyngeal tissues during sleep.

E0480

E0480 Percussor, electric or pneumatic, home model

Lay Description
A pneumatic or electric percussor is typically a hand-held unit that mimics the hand percussion of the chest traditionally exercised by respiratory therapists to loosen and clear a patient's lungs of

E

mucous and phlegm. Pneumatic models employ a gas driven cylinder to create pulses that reverberate into lung tissues. Electric models create a similar effect through vibration. Either variety will feature adjustments for pulse speed and intensity. Report E0480 for models designed for home use.

E0481

E0481 Intrapulmonary percussive ventilation system and related accessories

Lay Description
An intrapulmonary percussive ventilation system (IPV) is a device that delivers a series of very small bursts of pressurized gas at rates greater than 100 cycles per minute to the respiratory tract. IPV is a mechanized form of chest physical therapy. Instead of a therapist clapping or slapping the patient's chest wall, the IPV delivers small bursts of respiratory gases to the lungs via a mouthpiece. It is intended to mobilize endobronchial secretions and diffuse patchy atelectasis. The patient controls variables such as inspiratory time, peak pressure, and delivery rates. Code E0481 includes the compressor, hand held units, tubing, and all related accessories. This includes both systems in which the very small bursts of air are generated by the compressor and systems in which the very small bursts of air are generated by a hand-held percussive nebulizer used with a standard high-pressure compressor.

E0482

E0482 Cough stimulating device, alternating positive and negative airway pressure

Lay Description
This code reports supply of a specific variety of cough stimulating device. This type of device stimulates the cough reflex by providing alternating positive and negative airway pressure to loosen and clear a patient's lungs of mucous and phlegm. Peak cough ability is important to maintain in patients with diminished pulmonary function. These types of devices are designed to stimulate natural inspiratory and expiratory lung-clearing action. The units are non-invasive, using a mouthpiece or face mask.

E0483

E0483 High frequency chest wall oscillation air-pulse generator system, (includes hoses and vest), each

Lay Description
High frequency chest wall oscillation (HFCWO) is a therapy strategy to treat patients who suffer from excessive bronchial secretions. It may be used to treat patients with cystic fibrosis and other lung diseases where bronchial secretions can obstruct the airways. Treatments typically involve use of a vest, which is worn while the patient is in an upright position. Tubes connecting the vest to an air-pulse generator provide oscillations, which may be adjustable for intensity and

duration. A patient can operate the equipment by use of hand or sometimes foot controls. Treatment intervals last about 10 minutes and may be repeated. The patient clears mobilized bronchial secretions by coughing.

E0484

E0484 Oscillatory positive expiratory pressure device, nonelectric, any type, each

Lay Description
Oscillatory positive expiratory pressure devices create air vibrations to assist the patient in clearing the airway of mucous and secretions. Nonelectric devices are typically hand held units. They manipulate expired air by passing it through or over a vibration-creating apparatus. A vibrating metal ball within a cone is one method. Another involves use of a magnet and counterweight. The oscillation, or flutter, occurs as back pressure is created in the bronchial tract. The natural movement of secretions from the lungs and bronchial tract is assisted, similar to many tiny coughs.

E0485-E0486

E0485 Oral device/appliance used to reduce upper airway collapsibility, adjustable or nonadjustable, prefabricated, includes fitting and adjustment

E0486 Oral device/appliance used to reduce upper airway collapsibility, adjustable or nonadjustable, custom fabricated, includes fitting and adjustment

Lay Description
An oral device or appliance designed to reduce upper airway soft tissue collapse may be used to treat snoring and/or apnea during sleep. These devices increase the cross-sectional area of the upper airways by moving the mandible and/or the tongue forward. This helps to stabilize the upper airway in patients with obstructive sleep apnea syndrome (OSAS).

E0487

E0487 Spirometer, electronic, includes all accessories

Lay Description
A spirometer is a device used to measure pulmonary function. It measures the lung output on both inspiration and expiration. This is used to track and diagnose a number of respiratory and cardiac conditions. It may also be used to keep the lungs clear and functioning.

E0500

E0500 IPPB machine, all types, with built-in nebulization; manual or automatic valves; internal or external power source

Lay Description
This code reports the supply of any type of intermittent positive pressure breathing (IPPB)

machine. These units will have a built-in reservoir for medications and neutral liquids. A nebulizer feature atomizes liquid to aerosol spray, which is inhaled by the patient. Control valves may be manual or automatic. Many units have a port to attach an oxygen supply to the mix. These units may be hand-held with a mouthpiece and are used with the nose occluded by a clip. Batteries, an external AC source, or both may power the unit. Although volume ventilators may deliver intermittent positive pressure treatments, these IPPB units are generally classified for use among patients with spontaneous breathing capabilities. The main use of an IPPB machine is for patients with atelectasis (inability to fully expand the lung) or for the delivery of aerosol medication, usually bronchodilators.

E0550-E0560

E0550 Humidifier, durable for extensive supplemental humidification during IPPB treatments or oxygen delivery

E0555 Humidifier, durable, glass or autoclavable plastic bottle type, for use with regulator or flowmeter

E0560 Humidifier, durable for supplemental humidification during IPPB treatment or oxygen delivery

Lay Description

Intermittent positive pressure breathing (IPPB) treatments may be used for a variety of respiratory conditions. During treatment, machine assisted pressure is delivered upon inspiration to help the patient take large, deep breaths. The IPPB unit features pressurized gas in tanks or an electric air compressor. Respiratory therapists usually provide treatments. The treatment may be used to deliver medication, to open air passages and loosen mucous, or to increase lung capacity. Humidification is often required for IPPB treatments, particularly when oxygen delivery is involved. Humidifiers reported by this range are durable, reusable containers and the connection devices for an IPPB treatment unit or oxygen system. The containers can be cleaned or autoclaved before refilling with distilled water.

E0561-E0562

E0561 Humidifier, nonheated, used with positive airway pressure device

E0562 Humidifier, heated, used with positive airway pressure device

Lay Description

A humidifier is a device that increases the amount of moisture in indoor air or in a stream of air. It operates by circulating air over a water-filled pan or wet surface. The water then evaporates and is incorporated into the air stream. Heated humidifiers gently heat the water and the air stream as it comes in contact with the device. This device is used in connection with a continuous positive airway pressure (CPAP) system.

E0565-E0585

E0565 Compressor, air power source for equipment which is not self-contained or cylinder driven

E0570 Nebulizer, with compressor

E0572 Aerosol compressor, adjustable pressure, light duty for intermittent use

E0574 Ultrasonic/electronic aerosol generator with small volume nebulizer

E0575 Nebulizer, ultrasonic, large volume

E0580 Nebulizer, durable, glass or autoclavable plastic, bottle type, for use with regulator or flowmeter

E0585 Nebulizer, with compressor and heater

Lay Description

Nebulizer base equipment is comprised of an air compressor for airflow nebulization or a generator for nebulization of liquid by means of ultrasonic vibrations. The actual nebulizer is the chamber in which the nebulization of the liquid (usually medication) occurs and is considered an accessory to the base equipment. The nebulizing chamber is attached to the aerosol compressor or an ultrasonic generator. Specific accessories, supplies, and medications are used with this equipment. Nebulization therapy is considered beneficial to patients with a variety of respiratory and/or pulmonary conditions and diseases, including cystic fibrosis, bronchiectasis, chronic obstructive pulmonary disease, emphysema, severe asthma (when metered dose inhalers are ineffective), as well as other conditions such as AIDS, which requires the administration of medications like pentamidine. Nebulization occurs when the medication and/or solution to be administered is vaporized and subsequently inspired by the patient via the lungs, through which the medication enters the patient's system, or the medication has a direct effect on mucus retained by the lungs and bronchi (known as mucolytic action). An aerosol compressor can be set for pressures above 30 pounds per sq inch (psi) at a flow of 6-8 L/m and is capable of continuous operation. A nebulizer with compressor is an aerosol compressor delivering a fixed low pressure, typically used with a small volume nebulizer. A portable compressor is an aerosol compressor that delivers a fixed low pressure, used with a small volume nebulizer. It must have battery or DC power capability, but may have an AC power option. The light duty adjustable pressure compressor is a pneumatic aerosol compressor that can be set for pressures above 30 psi at a flow of 6-8 L/m, but is only capable of intermittent operation.

E

E0600

E0600   Respiratory suction pump, home model, portable or stationary, electric

Lay Description

A portable home model respiratory suction pump is a lightweight, compact, electric aspirator designed for upper respiratory oral pharyngeal and tracheal suction to be used in the home. Use of the device does not require technical or professional supervision. Units are equipped with vacuum regulators to allow variation of vacuum values, varying lamp flow, overflow safety devices, and battery or AC power.

E0601

E0601   Continuous positive airway pressure (CPAP) device

Lay Description

A continuous airway pressure (CPAP) device is a noninvasive method of providing air pressure through the patient's nostrils, usually through a nasal mask or flow generator system. A CPAP device delivers single pressure continuously and assists the patient in nocturnal respiration (breathing during sleep), particularly when the patient's oropharyngeal tissues relax, collapse, and/or otherwise obstruct the normal airflow, causing a variety of symptoms including hypersomnolence during the day, loss of concentration, headache, agitation, depression, fatigue, and many others. These devices are used primarily in conservative therapy (vs. surgery) for patients with documented sleep apnea.

E0602-E0604

E0602   Breast pump, manual, any type

E0603   Breast pump, electric (AC and/or DC), any type

E0604   Breast pump, hospital grade, electric (AC and/or DC), any type

Lay Description

Breast pumps are available in a variety of configurations, all of which are designed to pump human breast milk for short- or long-term storage. Some models are simple cylinders that interface with a plastic cone that fits over the areola. A syringe-type piston can then be manually retracted by the user to create and release suction on the nipple. The pumped milk drains by gravity into an attached container. The milk can be decanted into plastic bags for refrigerated storage or freezing. Electric models work by creating pulsating suction, usually by pneumatic action against a diaphragm. Larger facilities may use hospital grade piston operated electric pumps. With the exception of disposable plastic storage containers, components to all models are generally cleanable and reusable.

E0605

E0605   Vaporizer, room type

Lay Description

This code reports the supply of a room type vaporizer. Humidifiers and moisturizers typically work by absorbing cool water through a wick, which is exposed to a fan. Some models vibrate the cool water (ultrasonic). These devices can effectively raise humidity to larger rooms. Vaporizers heat water to create steam and are usually used for individual treatment of respiratory illness. Extracts can be added to the heated water or steam. Vaporizers are not usually effective to humidify large cubic footage, although room-size models are available and are reported by this code.

E0606

E0606   Postural drainage board

Lay Description

Postural drainage uses the force of gravity to assist in effectively draining secretions from the lungs and into the central airway where they can be coughed up or suctioned out. The patient is placed in a head or chest down position and turned so that each lung segment can be drained. Percussion and vibration may be performed in conjunction with postural drainage. Postural drainage is used to assist patients with chronic pulmonary conditions or diseases that limit the ability to cough and eliminate secretions, such as cystic fibrosis. A postural drainage board is a smooth, flat, hard surface that supports the patient during postural drainage. Some boards may have foam or other padding that raises the patient's torso above the upper chest.

E0607, E2100-E2101

E0607   Home blood glucose monitor

E2100   Blood glucose monitor with integrated voice synthesizer

E2101   Blood glucose monitor with integrated lancing/blood sample

Lay Description

Glucometers are used for patients with all types of diabetes mellitus to monitor blood glucose and are available in a variety of models with various features, including digital read-out, memory, result print-out, easy specimen capture, and many others. Glucometers with special features, such as voice-activated or voice-synthesized capabilities, are needed for patients with other concurrent conditions, such as patients with impaired vision. Whether or not the patient is on insulin, many diabetics require frequent, if not daily, blood glucose monitoring. For Type I diabetes mellitus patients who require insulin (the patient's body does not manufacture insulin and therefore it must come from an external source, such as injections), blood glucose monitoring is a life-sustaining requirement.

E0610-E0615

E0610 Pacemaker monitor, self-contained, (checks battery depletion, includes audible and visible check systems)

E0615 Pacemaker monitor, self-contained, checks battery depletion and other pacemaker components, includes digital/visible check systems

Lay Description
These codes report the supply of self-contained pacemaker monitors. A pacemaker is a device to control cardiac arrhythmias by programmed electrical stimulation of the heart. Pacemaker monitoring equipment detects impending battery failure and checks the overall performance of the pacemaker. Patients with pacemakers, whether permanent or temporary, require periodic examination of battery life and electrical functions. Self-contained units allow patients to perform the evaluation themselves. Some devices collect data that can be transmitted to a provider over a phone line. Battery life is a major factor in many pacemaker malfunctions and is monitored by these units. The conductivity of the pacemaker leads is another major consideration in monitoring.

E0616

E0616 Implantable cardiac event recorder with memory, activator, and programmer

Lay Description
Implantable event recorders are implanted in the left front of the chest in a pocket created in the skin. Once implanted, the patient's cardiac events are recorded. Implantable cardiac event monitors are used for long periods of time, which enables the recorder to capture more infrequent heart rhythms. The device can have autoactivation or manual activation depending upon the needs of the patient. If the patient experiences syncopal episodes, the manual activation button can be pressed after the patient is conscious again. If the device has an autoactivation, the device records rhythms automatically when the heart rate is in excess or under a preset limit.

E0617

E0617 External defibrillator with integrated electrocardiogram analysis

Lay Description
Automatic external defibrillators are compact and portable devices that deliver electrical shock to a person who has a sudden cardiac arrest. Automatic external defibrillator units use a microprocessor inside of a portable defibrillator to interpret a person's heart rhythm through electrodes. The computer recognizes ventricular fibrillation or ventricular tachycardia. Once recognized, the computer advises the operator/user that electrical defibrillation is needed or it will automatically deliver a countershock.

E0618-E0619

E0618 Apnea monitor, without recording feature

E0619 Apnea monitor, with recording feature

Lay Description
An apnea monitor is a device designed to detect cessation of breathing, either directly through measurement of respiration and/or indirectly through monitoring of physiological signs such as heart rate, pulse, or blood oxygen concentration. Devices typically feature both visual and audio alarm systems. Some models may differentiate between detection of obstructive apnea (such as is caused by mucous or oropharyngeal membrane) and central apnea (as may be caused by organ system failure). Models are typically connected to AC circuitry with battery power backup. Some may feature remote alarm systems, programmed software, and a monitor. An internal and/or hard copy recording system may also be featured.

E0620

E0620 Skin piercing device for collection of capillary blood, laser, each

Lay Description
A laser skin-piercing device is a low strength laser that is directed to one area, usually on a finger, and pierces the skin and subcutaneous tissue, allowing blood to be drawn from a capillary or surface blood vessel. This device is used in place of a lancet to draw blood for blood glucose monitoring or similar home blood testing.

E0621-E0625, E0630-E0635

E0621 Sling or seat, patient lift, canvas or nylon

E0625 Patient lift, bathroom or toilet, not otherwise classified

E0630 Patient lift, hydraulic or mechanical, includes any seat, sling, strap(s), or pad(s)

E0635 Patient lift, electric, with seat or sling

Lay Description
Patient lift mechanisms are hydraulic or motorized (electric) lifts that enable the patient to transfer from the bed to a chair or other sitting device, or vice versa. The electric patient lifts can be electric (AC) or battery powered (DC). These lift mechanisms assist patients with varying abnormalities that prevent them from being able to change, unassisted, from a lying down position (in a bed) to a seated position (in a chair, wheelchair, etc.), and vice versa. Trauma, stroke, and chronic diseases are the usual etiologies for the patient's inability to change in these positions. These devices can help during the convalescence period in posttraumatic or postoperative cases, and act as prevention against patient injury or reinjury. A seat or sling for a patient lift is a reinforced width of nylon or cloth that replaces a similar device used in a patient lift. A seat or sling is considered an accessory item. One type of device uses a manual pumping action to

E

compress a cylinder filled with a fluid, usually oil. Since the oil is thick and molecule dense, it does not absorb the energy or force generated by the pumping action. Instead, the oil amplifies and transfers the energy to the lever used to raise the patient. The hydraulic action allows less energy to be used in the pumping action. Another type of device uses electricity to run a motor that raises and moves the patient from one surface (e.g., a bed, chair, or toilet) to another surface. The patient is positioned in a seat or sling and the device performs the work. Electric lifts can be freestanding or ceiling and wall mounted. One system raises and moves the patient using a hinged platform that can be manipulated into various positions. When laid flat and positioned close to the bed, the patient can roll or be lifted onto the platform. The platform can then be positioned so the patient is standing upright or in a seated position. The system can contain both hydraulic and electronic driven mechanisms. The system is padded or cushioned for patient comfort and may contain side rails or straps to securely hold the patient during transfer.

E0627-E0629

E0627   Seat lift mechanism incorporated into a combination lift-chair mechanism

E0628   Separate seat lift mechanism for use with patient-owned furniture, electric

E0629   Separate seat lift mechanism for use with patient-owned furniture, nonelectric

Lay Description

Seat lift mechanisms are motorized seat lifts that enable the patient to change from a seated position to a standing position. The lifting mechanism is graded and not based on a catapult or other type of spring system. These mechanisms can be electric or battery powered. Some mechanisms can be used with the patient's own furniture; others are already built into specially designed chairs, sometimes incorporating the seat lift action with a more total patient lift action, including elevating and pushing the back and arms. Seat lift mechanisms assist patients with varying abnormalities that prevent them from being able to change, unassisted, from a seated to a standing position. Trauma and chronic diseases are the usual etiologies for the patient's inability to change in these positions. These devices can help in posttraumatic or postoperative convalescence, act as adjunctive treatment for chronic diseases, and act as prevention against patient injury or reinjury.

E0630-E0635

E0630   Patient lift, hydraulic or mechanical, includes any seat, sling, strap(s), or pad(s)

E0635   Patient lift, electric, with seat or sling

Lay Description

Please refer to codes E0621-E0625 for the description.

E0636-E0638, E0641-E0642

E0636   Multipositional patient support system, with integrated lift, patient accessible controls

E0637   Combination sit-to-stand frame/table system, any size including pediatric, with seat lift feature, with or without wheels

E0638   Standing frame/table system, one position (e.g., upright, supine or prone stander), any size including pediatric, with or without wheels

E0641   Standing frame/table system, multi-position (e.g., 3-way stander), any size including pediatric, with or without wheels

E0642   Standing frame/table system, mobile (dynamic stander), any size including pediatric

Lay Description

A standing frame system is an assistive device that provides musculoskeletal support for disabled or injured individuals. This device allows an individual to move from a sitting to standing position and provides support when standing. Standing frame systems may include lift devices that assist the patient in moving from a sitting to standing position. Multi-position standing frames allow progressive levels of standing that gradually relieve contractures and spasticity. A standing frame system may be stationary or mobile.

E0639-E0640

E0639   Patient lift, moveable from room to room with disassembly and reassembly, includes all components/accessories

E0640   Patient lift, fixed system, includes all components/accessories

Lay Description

Patient lifts are mechanical devices that elevate and transfer patients from one point to another. The devices may be powered or manual. There are various designs based on the condition of the patient. The lift may be a flat litter, a chair, or other configuration. It usually has straps or restraints to hold the patient in place during the transfer. The lift may be fixed, such as a lift permanently anchored in the ceiling or on a wall, or may be moveable from one room to another with some disassembly and reassembly at each point.

E0650-E0673

E0650 Pneumatic compressor, nonsegmental home model

E0651 Pneumatic compressor, segmental home model without calibrated gradient pressure

E0652 Pneumatic compressor, segmental home model with calibrated gradient pressure

E0655 Nonsegmental pneumatic appliance for use with pneumatic compressor, half arm

E0656 Segmental pneumatic appliance for use with pneumatic compressor, trunk

E0657 Segmental pneumatic appliance for use with pneumatic compressor, chest

E0660 Nonsegmental pneumatic appliance for use with pneumatic compressor, full leg

E0665 Nonsegmental pneumatic appliance for use with pneumatic compressor, full arm

E0666 Nonsegmental pneumatic appliance for use with pneumatic compressor, half leg

E0667 Segmental pneumatic appliance for use with pneumatic compressor, full leg

E0668 Segmental pneumatic appliance for use with pneumatic compressor, full arm

E0669 Segmental pneumatic appliance for use with pneumatic compressor, half leg

E0671 Segmental gradient pressure pneumatic appliance, full leg

E0672 Segmental gradient pressure pneumatic appliance, full arm

E0673 Segmental gradient pressure pneumatic appliance, half leg

Lay Description
Lymphedema is the swelling of subcutaneous tissue due to the accumulation of excessive lymph fluid from impairment in the normal clearing function of the lymphatic system and/or from excessive lymph production. Lymphedema pumps are segmental or nonsegmental long arm or leg sleeves (similar to a blood pressure cuff) that are placed up around the area of swelling. The device is turned on and the sleeve is periodically inflated to compress the tissues (in segments or in total length), and then deflated. A tube from the compression device (pump) that is attached to the sleeve allows air to be pumped into the sleeve (compression) or air to be removed from the sleeve (decompression). Pneumatic pumps mechanically assist blood and lymph flow through the extremities. This assistance lessens the accumulation of fluids in the affected limb and reduces associated complications such as thrombosis or vessel damage.

E0670

E0670 Segmental pneumatic appliance for use with pneumatic compressor, integrated, 2 full legs and trunk

Lay Description
Pneumatic compression therapy is used to treat lymphedema or other venous and/or muscle disorders of the trunk, torso, legs, genitals, abdomen, hips, buttocks, or high upper thighs. The device includes the garment and hoses and fits over the patient's legs and trunk. The physician orders the appropriate treatment pressure, time, and duration. Treatment sessions are usually one to two times a day for about one hour each.

E0675

E0675 Pneumatic compression device, high pressure, rapid inflation/deflation cycle, for arterial insufficiency (unilateral or bilateral system)

Lay Description
Pneumatic compression devices, along with an electrical pneumatic pump, are used to pump compressed air into a garment placed on upper or lower extremities (including feet). The garment is intermittently inflated and deflated with pressure and various time cycles. The use of the pneumatic compression device can greatly reduce the risk of deep venous thrombosis (DVT) and pulmonary embolism (PE) by limiting venous stasis and increasing fibrinolytic activity at both the local and systemic levels.

E0676

E0676 Intermittent limb compression device (includes all accessories), not otherwise specified

Lay Description
An intermittent limb compression device inflates and deflates a compression sleeve that has multiple compression chambers encircling the limb of the patient. The sleeve inflates to apply compressive pressure gradient against the limb of the patient, which decreases from the lower to the upper portion of the limb to enhance the acceleration of blood flow through the limb.

E0691-E0694

E0691 Ultraviolet light therapy system, includes bulbs/lamps, timer and eye protection; treatment area 2 sq ft or less

E0692 Ultraviolet light therapy system panel, includes bulbs/lamps, timer and eye protection, 4 ft panel

E0693 Ultraviolet light therapy system panel, includes bulbs/lamps, timer and eye protection, 6 ft panel

E0694 Ultraviolet multidirectional light therapy system in 6 ft cabinet, includes bulbs/lamps, timer, and eye protection

Lay Description
An ultraviolet light therapy system is considered durable medical equipment typically consisting of a system panel, ultraviolet bulbs/lamp that emit UVB rays, a timer, and eye protection. It is commonly used

for the treatment of skin conditions including psoriasis, pruritic eruptions of HIV, and acne.

E0700

E0700   Safety equipment, device or accessory, any type

Lay Description
Safety equipment such as a belts, harnesses, or vests are used to secure a patient's positioning when the patient is at risk for a fall that could lead to harm or injury. The equipment is comfortably secured around the patient and fastened to a bed or chair to prevent sliding or falling.

E0705

E0705   Transfer device, any type, each

Lay Description
A transfer board is used for ease of moving patients from one stable surface to another (i.e. bed to wheelchair, bed to portable toilet, wheelchair to toilet) and is primarily for seated type transports.

E0710

E0710   Restraints, any type (body, chest, wrist, or ankle)

Lay Description
Restraints are used to contain and control an individual who exhibits behavior that may be harmful to self or others, such as violent behavior or pulling at lifesaving treatments. This code includes body, chest, wrist, or ankle restraints. Each strap is designed with a cuff to be placed around the patient, and a strap that can be threaded through a U bar and secured. Report this code for any type of restraint.

E0720-E0730

E0720   Transcutaneous electrical nerve stimulation (TENS) device, 2 lead, localized stimulation

E0730   Transcutaneous electrical nerve stimulation (TENS) device, 4 or more leads, for multiple nerve stimulation

Lay Description
A transcutaneous electrical nerve stimulator (TENS) is a device that uses electrical current delivered through electrodes placed on the surface of the skin to decrease the patient's perception of pain, by inhibiting the transmission of afferent pain nerve impulses and/or by stimulating the release of endorphins. The TENS unit can be applied in a variety of settings (in the patient's home, a physician's office, or in an outpatient clinic). This device alleviates or palliates acute postoperative pain, as well as chronic or intractable pain, depending on the etiology of the patient's condition. TENS therapy is typically not used for patients with visceral pain or headache, female patients with pelvic pain, and other types of pain considered unresponsive to TENS therapy.

E0731

E0731   Form-fitting conductive garment for delivery of TENS or NMES (with conductive fibers separated from the patient's skin by layers of fabric)

Lay Description
A form-fitting conductive garment has tiny electro-conductive leads and electrodes woven into a stretch fabric. The system offers a great many of easily accessible and interchangeable electrode sites throughout the fabric area. A second layer of conventional fabric lines the garment against the skin. The garment may be worn on an extremity alone or on part or the entire torso. The garment is designed to interface with a transcutaneous electrical nerve stimulation (TENS) generator. The system may be used for patients with conditions that require a great many TENS electrodes for effective therapy and for those with sensitive skin. The system is also sometimes used underneath plaster casting where conventional TENS therapy cannot reach.

E0740

E0740   Incontinence treatment system, pelvic floor stimulator, monitor, sensor, and/or trainer

Lay Description
Pelvic floor stimulators are used for the treatment of urinary incontinence to strengthen and exercise the muscles of the pelvic floor. Electrical stimulations targeting the muscles involved are delivered via probes connected to an external pulse generator. The frequency and intensity of the electrical pulse varies based on the patient's needs. Report this code for a pelvic floor stimulator with a monitor, sensor, and/or trainer.

E0744

E0744   Neuromuscular stimulator for scoliosis

Lay Description
Neuromuscular stimulators are used to stimulate muscles into activity through an electrical impulse. These devices consist of superficial or implantable electrodes, a modulating output and control circuit, a signal generator, and a battery power supply.

E0745

E0745   Neuromuscular stimulator, electronic shock unit

Lay Description
Neuromuscular stimulation artificially stimulates muscles that may have atrophied because of damaged nerve pathways, often due to injury, surgery, or infarction. Computer-controlled sequential electrical stimulation of muscles simulates actual use, even when actual muscle contraction is not attained, and may result in a level of muscle tone and strength.

E0746

E0746   Electromyography (EMG), biofeedback device

Lay Description
An electromyography (EMG) biofeedback device consists of electrodes that are placed over specific muscles, and a recording unit that stores and displays the information from the physiological responses being monitored. Muscle activity can be displayed in real-time or an average over a period of time.

E0747-E0749, E0760

E0747   Osteogenesis stimulator, electrical, noninvasive, other than spinal applications

E0748   Osteogenesis stimulator, electrical, noninvasive, spinal applications

E0749   Osteogenesis stimulator, electrical, surgically implanted

E0760   Osteogenesis stimulator, low intensity ultrasound, noninvasive

Lay Description
An electrical osteogenesis stimulator is a device that provides electrical stimulation to augment bone repair by stimulating the production of osteocytes (bone cells) and can be invasive or noninvasive. A noninvasive electrical stimulator is characterized by an external power source, which is attached to a coil or electrodes placed on the skin, or placed on a cast or brace over a fracture or surgical bone fusion site. Invasive devices provide electrical stimulation directly at the fracture site, through percutaneous placement of cathodes or by implantation of a coiled cathode wire into the fracture site. The power pack is implanted into soft tissue near the fracture site and subcutaneously connected to the cathode, creating a self-contained system with no external components. With the noninvasive device, opposing pads, wired to an external power supply, are placed over the cast. An electromagnetic field is created between the pads at the fracture site. An ultrasonic osteogenic stimulator emits low intensity, pulsed ultrasound (as opposed to electricity) to stimulate bone repair. The ultrasound signal is applied to the skin surface at the fracture location via ultrasound conductive coupling gel to accelerate the healing time of the fracture. The device is intended for use with cast immobilization.

E0755

E0755   Electronic salivary reflex stimulator (intraoral/noninvasive)

Lay Description
An electronic salivary reflex stimulator is used to treat xerostomia (dry mouth). Chronic xerostomia may be caused by a number of conditions, including Sjögren's syndrome, certain medications, and radiation therapy. Xerostomia can cause difficulty in eating and swallowing. An electronic salivary reflex stimulator is an intraoral, noninvasive device that emits electrical impulses to the tongue and roof of the mouth. These electrical impulses are distributed to all residual salivary tissues in the oral and pharyngeal regions stimulating salivation.

E0760

E0760   Osteogenesis stimulator, low intensity ultrasound, noninvasive

Lay Description
Please refer to codes E0747-E0749 for the description.

E0761

E0761   Nonthermal pulsed high frequency radiowaves, high peak power electromagnetic energy treatment device

Lay Description
A nonthermal pulsed high frequency radiowave, high peak power electromagnetic energy treatment device produces the energy used in electromagnetic therapy. The pulsed methodology allows treatment while allowing associated heat production to dissipate. Electromagnetic therapy is a distinct form of treatment using application of electromagnetic fields rather than direct electrical current for wound treatment.

E0762

E0762   Transcutaneous electrical joint stimulation device system, includes all accessories

Lay Description
A transcutaneous electrical joint stimulation device used to treat osteoarthritis of the knee and rheumatoid arthritis of the hands. This battery powered device consists of an electrical stimulator with electrical leads that are placed over the affected area. The leads are held in place with a lightweight, flexible wrap and Velcro fasteners. The device delivers electrical impulses of 0.0 to 12.0 volt output to the joint. The device is typically worn for at least six hours per day. The device appears to stimulate development of new hyaline cartilage. Patients using transcutaneous electrical joint stimulation devices report reduced pain and stiffness and improved range of motion and function of the treated joints. This code reports the electrical joint stimulation device and all accessories (wrap, fasteners) needed to use the device.

E0764

E0764   Functional neuromuscular stimulation, transcutaneous stimulation of sequential muscle groups of ambulation with computer control, used for walking by spinal cord injured, entire system, after completion of training program

Lay Description
This code reports a transcutaneous, functional neuromuscular stimulator with computer control

E

used to stimulate muscles of ambulation, which aids patients with spinal cord injuries in walking. A functional neuromuscular stimulator provides sequential electrical stimulation of muscles in the spinal cord injured patient. Use of electrical stimulation to replace stimuli when the nerve pathway has been injured or destroyed may assist in maintaining healthy muscle tone and strength and may enable the spinal cord injured patient to stand or walk independently. Patients are required to complete a training program prior to receiving the device.

E0765

E0765   FDA approved nerve stimulator, with replaceable batteries, for treatment of nausea and vomiting

Lay Description
The FDA approved nerve stimulator for treatment of nausea and vomiting is a battery-powered, noninvasive, portable, stimulation device. It is a small, watch-like device with two metal electrodes that are placed in contact with the skin on the volar aspect of the wrist over the median nerve following application of a hypoallergenic conductive gel to the skin contact site. The device is held in place with a Velcro band. Nerve stimulation therapy is administered by direct skin contact via two metal electrodes. The device has five intensity levels that are controlled by the patient by means of a rotary dial. This device may be used to treat nausea and vomiting secondary to pregnancy, chemotherapy, anesthesia, and motion sickness.

E0766

E0766   Electrical stimulation device used for cancer treatment, includes all accessories, any type

Lay Description
Novo TTF-100A is a portable battery or power-supply operated system that produces changing electrical fields, called tumor treatment fields, within the human body. The complete system includes a portable electric field generator, transducer arrays, rechargeable batteries, and more. Electric fields are delivered through four transducer arrays that are placed directly on the scalp to target the tumor. The transducer array placement is determined based on each patient's MRI results to maximize the therapy's effect on the tumor. The electric fields stop the growth of tumor cells resulting in cell death of the rapidly dividing cancer cells. The geometrical shape and scattering of the electrical charges within the dividing tumor cells allows the electrical fields to physically break up the tumor cell membrane. The frequency of the fields used for a particular treatment is specific to the size of the cell type being treated. The system is intended as a treatment for adult patients (22 years of age or older) with confirmed glioblastoma multiforme (GBM), following confirmed recurrence in an upper region of the brain (supratentorial) after receiving chemotherapy. The device is intended to be used as a

stand-alone treatment, and is an alternative to standard medical therapy for recurrent GBM after surgical and radiation options have been exhausted.

E0769

E0769   Electrical stimulation or electromagnetic wound treatment device, not otherwise classified

Lay Description
This code reports two different types of wound treatment devices that are not otherwise classified. The first type is an electrical stimulation wound treatment device. This type of device uses the application of electrical current through electrodes placed directly on the skin in close proximity to the wound. There are four categories of electrical stimulation devices used for wound healing, including low intensity direct current (LIDC), high voltage pulsed current (HVPC), alternative current (AC), and transcutaneous electrical nerve stimulation (TENS). The second type of device described by this code is an electromagnetic wound treatment device. This type of device employs electromagnetic fields rather than a direct electrical current.

E0770

E0770   Functional electrical stimulator, transcutaneous stimulation of nerve and/or muscle groups, any type, complete system, not otherwise specified

Lay Description
This code reports a transcutaneous, functional electric stimulator for muscles or nerves not otherwise specified. A functional neuromuscular stimulator provides sequential electrical stimulation of muscles or nerves to help regain some function. Transcutaneous stimulation therapy is administered by direct skin contact via metal electrodes. Use of electrical stimulation to replace stimuli when the nerve pathway has been injured or destroyed may assist in maintaining healthy muscle tone and strength. This code should only be used if there is not a more specific code to report the device.

E0776

E0776   IV pole

Lay Description
An intravenous (IV) pole is generally a portable, adjustable stand designed primarily to hang IV solution bags. Most models are mounted on rollers and are adjustable from a base height of about 56 inches up to about 96 inches. Many also feature optional attachments such as urinary bag hooks and clamps to secure oxygen tanks.

E0779-E0781

E0779 Ambulatory infusion pump, mechanical, reusable, for infusion 8 hours or greater

E0780 Ambulatory infusion pump, mechanical, reusable, for infusion less than 8 hours

E0781 Ambulatory infusion pump, single or multiple channels, electric or battery operated, with administrative equipment, worn by patient

Lay Description
Ambulatory infusion pumps are portable devices that are typically carried or worn by the patient, often on a belt or strap, to directly infuse medications. The pumps reported by this code range may be electric or mechanical devices that feature reservoirs to hold liquid medication. Pressure is created, mechanically or electrically, to infuse a regulated flow of medication into the patient over a set period of time. Routes of administration are by cannula and may include intravenous, intra-arterial, intrathecal, or intraperitoneal, among others; however, subcutaneous delivery is perhaps most common. A multiple channel pump allows for several different infusions at one time and features a programmable display to enter the prescribed rates.

E0782

E0782 Infusion pump, implantable, nonprogrammable (includes all components, e.g., pump, catheter, connectors, etc.)

Lay Description
An implantable infusion pump is a device carried by the patient in a surgically created subcutaneous pocket to directly infuse medications. Implanted pumps contain a refillable reservoir to hold liquid medication. The units may be used to deliver chemotherapy medications, drugs to address chronic pain, anti-spasmodics, or heparin, among others. Routes may include intravenous, intra-arterial, intrathecal, or intraperitoneal, among others. The reservoir is refilled by needle injection through a self-sealing membrane.

E0783, E0785-E0786

E0783 Infusion pump system, implantable, programmable (includes all components, e.g., pump, catheter, connectors, etc.)

E0785 Implantable intraspinal (epidural/intrathecal) catheter used with implantable infusion pump, replacement

E0786 Implantable programmable infusion pump, replacement (excludes implantable intraspinal catheter)

Lay Description
This code reports the supply of an implantable, programmable infusion pump system. These devices are subcutaneously implanted near the site where the infusion is needed. The system is designed for patients requiring regular or continuous intravenous or intra-arterial infusions of drugs. The system may be used to deliver any of a variety of medicines, particularly those for oncology therapy. Implantable infusion pumps are typically small, biocompatible stainless steel units that are surgically placed subcutaneously near the site of optimal drug delivery. The port and reservoir can be smaller in diameter than a nickel coin. A refillable reservoir delivers a constant, prescribed rate of liquid drug to the target site. Typically, the reservoir features a rubber diaphragm that can be penetrated by a non-coring needle to refill the drug. This code reports the supply of a system that can be programmed to deliver a prescribed quantity of medicine over a given period of time.

E0784

E0784 External ambulatory infusion pump, insulin

Lay Description
An external ambulatory infusion pump, also known as continuous subcutaneous insulin infusion (CSII), is a portable battery-powered device typically worn on a belt or strap. The device contains a reservoir to hold insulin. An infusion set comprising catheter tubing and a needle delivers microdoses of insulin, usually into subcutaneous tissues of the abdomen. Delivery rates can be closely adjusted to meet changing background needs, such as during strenuous exercise or around meals.

E0791

E0791 Parenteral infusion pump, stationary, single, or multichannel

Lay Description
A stationary parenteral infusion pump is used to deliver liquid nutritional emulsions to patients whose normal gastrointestinal functions are compromised, and for the delivery of certain medications such as chemotherapies and pain management drugs. Proteins, carbohydrates, lipids, and electrolytes are the main components of parenteral nutrition, usually in carefully balanced combinations. The pumps are programmable and multi-channel units allow for several different infusions at one time. Lipids may be introduced separately, for example. Routes of administration include the subclavian, jugular, and femoral veins, as well as smaller vessels and, in some instances, arterial vessels.

E0830

E0830 Ambulatory traction device, all types, each

Lay Description
An ambulatory traction device uses two supports positioned on the body in such a way that they can lift and provide a decompressive force to the affected body part. In addition to the two supports, a lifting or stretching mechanism must be employed to provide

the traction. This code reports any type of ambulatory traction device. If multiple traction devices are employed, each device is reported separately.

E0840-E0860

E0840   Traction frame, attached to headboard, cervical traction

E0849   Traction equipment, cervical, free-standing stand/frame, pneumatic, applying traction force to other than mandible

E0850   Traction stand, freestanding, cervical traction

E0855   Cervical traction equipment not requiring additional stand or frame

E0860   Traction equipment, overdoor, cervical

Lay Description

Cervical traction equipment extends the neck muscles, tissue, and ligaments of the upper portion of the spinal column through a gentle pulling action. Code E0840 reports a cervical traction frame designed to be attached to a headboard. Code E0849 reports cervical traction equipment inclusive of a freestanding stand or frame and pneumatic pump designed to apply traction force to the occiput or any site other than the mandible. Code E0850 reports a freestanding cervical traction stand. Code E0855 reports cervical traction equipment not requiring an additional stand or frame, which typically consists of a foam roll for under the neck, an adjustable head harness, and a weight bag. Code E0860 reports overhead cervical traction, which typically consists of a water-weighted bag suspended from a frame mounted on an overhead door. A cord is threaded through a pulley and attached to a stabilization harness on the patient's head. The traction is designed to relieve gravity pressure on a cervical injury.

E0856

E0856   Cervical traction device, with inflatable air bladder(s)

Lay Description

A cervical collar with inflatable air bladder is a bracing device made from plastic or another rigid material that surrounds and immobilizes the cervical spine and neck. The inflated air bladder assists in supporting the head, provides spacing between the cervical vertebrae, and helps to reduce intradiscal pressure. A cervical collar with an inflatable air bladder is indicated for short-term treatment of neck pain.

E0870-E0900

E0870   Traction frame, attached to footboard, extremity traction (e.g., Buck's)

E0880   Traction stand, freestanding, extremity traction (e.g., Buck's)

E0890   Traction frame, attached to footboard, pelvic traction

E0900   Traction stand, freestanding, pelvic traction (e.g., Buck's)

Lay Description

Traction stands and frames are available in a variety of configurations, depending on the treatment desired. Perhaps most recognizable is the Buck's traction system, which applies gentle, but firm traction (pulling action) to the affected extremity to stabilize the injury. A floor stand or hospital bed is mounted with a frame that curves over the injured arm or leg like a gallows frame. The frame may be fitted with counterweights, pulleys, and cable that connect to traction pins transfixed to the fractured bone or to the casting. It can be a freestanding, floor mechanism or one that is attached using the support of another object for traction. Pelvic fractures may require supports at both ends of the bed or two floor stands at either end. These mechanisms usually comprise a padded sleeve or splint-type product that is applied to the affected extremity, as well as a metal or durable frame affixed to both the sleeve or splint and to the traction-exerting rope and pulley or other system. The benefits from traction use include better extremity circulation, pressure release, separation of bony components, support and protection, and prevention of surrounding ligament and myofascial contracture.

E0910-E0912, E0940

E0910   Trapeze bars, also known as Patient Helper, attached to bed, with grab bar

E0911   Trapeze bar, heavy-duty, for patient weight capacity greater than 250 pounds, attached to bed, with grab bar

E0912   Trapeze bar, heavy-duty, for patient weight capacity greater than 250 pounds, freestanding, complete with grab bar

E0940   Trapeze bar, freestanding, complete with grab bar

Lay Description

A trapeze bar with a grab bar, also referred to as a Patient Helper, is used when a patient needs a device to assist with movement because of a respiratory condition, fracture, or other medical condition. The patient holds onto the bar to maintain control while lifting the body or changing position. Trapeze bars may be attached to the bed or freestanding.

E0920-E0930

E0920 Fracture frame, attached to bed, includes weights

E0930 Fracture frame, freestanding, includes weights

Lay Description

Fracture frames are over-the-bed support structures from which traction weights and pulley can be mounted for the treatment of serious fractures. The units are available in several configurations. One style attaches to brackets at either end of the bed and another is a freestanding unit, mounting on legged supports. Both feature a strong bar that bridges over the bed and connects to the brackets. Traction weights and pulleys are arrayed along the bar as needed. Most models are modular and can accommodate variations in prescribed traction and weights. Traction counterweights are suspended from an array of cables and pulleys and rarely exceed eight pounds. Fixed, balanced, and sliding traction may be prescribed for treatment.

E0935

E0935 Continuous passive motion exercise device for use on knee only

Lay Description

Passive motion exercise devices (also known as continuous passive motion or CPM) are rehabilitation treatment strategies that usually follow orthopedic surgery. The knee joint is treated to sessions of continuous motion provided by a mechanical device.

E0936

E0936 Continuous passive motion exercise device for use other than knee

Lay Description

A continuous passive motion (CPM) device is attached to the patient and moves the affected joint for flexion and/or extension continuously for extended periods of time without patient assistance. The power unit is used to set the variable range of motion and speed. The initial setting for range of motion is based on the patient's comfort level. There may also be other factors used to set motion and speed. Motion and stress play a key role in healing connective tissue. Motion enhances blood flow and decreases pain. CPM can used in postoperative patients to enhance pain relief, improve the circulation of the extremity, reduce edema, improve the cartilage of synovial joints, retard muscular atrophy, reduce stiffness, and prevent contractures and adhesions.

E0940

E0940 Trapeze bar, freestanding, complete with grab bar

Lay Description

Please refer to codes E0910-E0912 for the description.

E0941

E0941 Gravity assisted traction device, any type

Lay Description

This code reports the supply of a specialized traction device. Gravity traction devices can range from so-called "tilt tables" to inversion racks and "gravity boots." All of the systems promote spinal or other orthopedic therapy by reversing gravitational forces. Inversion tables and racks turn the user upside-down for a period of time. Gravity boots work in a similar fashion to allow the user to stretch the spine and hips by hanging upside-down from specialized boots. Other gravity traction devices work in a similar fashion. Gravity traction devices may be used to relieve chronic back pain by offering the user a period of suspension from gravitational pressures on the vertebral disk spaces.

E0942

E0942 Cervical head harness/halter

Lay Description

This code reports the supply of a specialized head harness for rehabilitation therapy, usually for cervical injuries or disorders. A halo-type apparatus is fitted to the patient's head, sometimes in combination with a chinstrap. This halo is connected to a larger ring attached to a wall surface. Elastic resistance straps or springs connect the patient's halo apparatus to the larger, fixed ring. The patient goes through a variety of range of motion exercises designed to build strength and flexibility in the cervical spine and its supporting musculature.

E0944

E0944 Pelvic belt/harness/boot

Lay Description

This code reports the supply of a specialized orthopedic device known as a pelvic belt. This is a traction device that may be used intermittently by the patient, usually to relieve chronic pain of the lower back, sacrum, or pelvic regions, or to treat the effects of spondylosis. A wide, padded, form-fitting belt or harness is worn around the lower waist, often with Velcro closures. The belt is connected by elastic resistance straps to provide traction on the belt, relieving lumbosacral pressures.

E0945

E0945 Extremity belt/harness

Lay Description

This code reports supply of a specialized orthopedic device known as an extremity belt or harness. Extremity belts or harnesses are used with other traction devices to treat fractures of the extremities. The belt or harness is applied distal to the fracture site and is used to suspend the extremity so traction can be applied.

E

E0946

E0946   Fracture, frame, dual with cross bars, attached to bed, (e.g., Balken, 4 Poster)

Lay Description

A fracture frame with cross bars attached to a bed that consists of an overhead frame supported by upright bars attached to the bedposts or to a separate stand. The fractured limb may be splinted and suspended in a harness that is attached to a rope and pulley with a weight to provide the traction. This type of fracture frame may be referred to as a Balkan or four poster frame. This code reports the frame only.

E0947

E0947   Fracture frame, attachments for complex pelvic traction

Lay Description

Fracture and/or traction frames and related equipment are devices usually attached to a hospital bed. The unit uses free weights and/or pulleys to pull the injured body part by immobilizing, aligning, and reducing pain, inflammation, and muscle spasms. This code is used for attachments for complex pelvic traction for fractures.

E0948

E0948   Fracture frame, attachments for complex cervical traction

Lay Description

A fracture frame for complex cervical traction describes cervical traction devices that provide traction for the cervical spine by the use of a free-standing frame or a headboard. Traction force is applied by means of pneumonic displacement to anatomical areas other than the mandible. The devices must be capable of generating traction forces greater than 20 pounds and the device permits traction to be applied with alternative vectors of force. This code is used for attachments for complex cervical traction for fractures.

E0950

E0950   Wheelchair accessory, tray, each

Lay Description

Wheelchair accessory trays are attached securely to the side surface of a conventional wheelchair. There are different tray styles with different functionality, including concealed compartments beneath an extension of an armrest for holding personal items, a cane holder, and a table tray (usually a standard feature).

E0951

E0951   Heel loop/holder, any type, with or without ankle strap, each

Lay Description

A heel loop/holder is a wheelchair accessory used to position and hold the heel of the foot safely on the footrest and assist with maintaining proper foot alignment.

E0952

E0952   Toe loop/holder, any type, each

Lay Description

A toe loop/holder is a wheelchair accessory used to position and hold the toes of the foot safely on the footrest and assist with maintaining proper foot alignment.

E0955

E0955   Wheelchair accessory, headrest, cushioned, any type, including fixed mounting hardware, each

Lay Description

A head rest is a wheelchair accessory that supports the head and neck muscles. This code represents any cushioned headrest of any type. It includes any fixed mounting hardware.

E0956

E0956   Wheelchair accessory, lateral trunk or hip support, any type, including fixed mounting hardware, each

Lay Description

A lateral trunk or a hip support is a wheelchair accessory used to position a patient who is not able to shift weight or that has any significant postural asymmetries that are due to an absent or impaired sensation in the area of contact with the seating surface. It provides positioning for proper body alignment.

E0957

E0957   Wheelchair accessory, medial thigh support, any type, including fixed mounting hardware, each

Lay Description

A medial thigh support is a wheelchair accessory used to position a patient who is not able to shift weight or that has any significant postural asymmetries that are due to an absent or impaired sensation in the area of contact with the seating surface. The medial thigh support separates the thighs for improved hip alignment.

E0958

E0958   Manual wheelchair accessory, one-arm drive attachment, each

Lay Description

A one-arm drive attachment is a manual wheelchair accessory that allows the patient to propel the wheelchair with only one hand. A patient with hemiplegia or an injury to one extremity might require this option.

E0959

E0959   Manual wheelchair accessory, adapter for amputee, each

Lay Description
This code is reported for any amputee adapter accessory that can be used on a manual wheelchair.

E0960

E0960   Wheelchair accessory, shoulder harness/straps or chest strap, including any type mounting hardware

Lay Description
This code is used to report a positioning accessory for the upper torso. The chest and shoulder harness/strap provides positioning for proper body alignment.

E0961

E0961   Manual wheelchair accessory, wheel lock brake extension (handle), each

Lay Description
This code is reported for an accessory for the rear wheel brakes in a manual wheelchair. The extension brake handle provides easier access to applying the brakes.

E0966

E0966   Manual wheelchair accessory, headrest extension, each

Lay Description
A headrest extension is an accessory for a manual wheelchair that allows the headrest to be raised to a higher position than standard headrest height. Patients requiring a headrest for support due to weak neck muscles and patients who require reclining back wheelchairs may also require a headrest extension for proper positioning of the headrest.

E0967

E0967   Manual wheelchair accessory, hand rim with projections, any type, each

Lay Description
Hand rims are wheel attachments that allow the user to independently move the wheelchair. Hand rims have been found to reduce fatigue, stress in wrists and shoulders, and carpal tunnel syndrome. These rims are also known as push rims. Some have projections attached to the side for better grip. Report this code for a hand rim, with projections, for a manual wheelchair.

E0968

E0968   Commode seat, wheelchair

Lay Description
A wheelchair commode seat is a specialized seat that has cutouts that mimic a toilet seat. The entire wheelchair with the commode seat and a commode pail can be used as a bedside commode. It may also be positioned over an existing toilet for added user support or it can be used as a transport wheelchair inside the house.

E0969

E0969   Narrowing device, wheelchair

Lay Description
This code is used to report a wheelchair accessory device that permits a wheelchair to be made narrower temporarily by a few inches by using a crank and gear mechanism providing the force to begin the folding process. The narrowing device is usually left in place but the crank handle is removable for storage.

E0970

E0970   No. 2 footplates, except for elevating legrest

Lay Description
Footplates provide a flat surface on which to rest the foot. Footplates are generally a standard feature on a wheelchair. If a user has problems with the standard plates, an angle adjustable footplate may be used. Adjustability is limited to front to back and side to side. Footrests should not be lower than 2 1/2 inches from the ground to safeguard clearance.

E0971

E0971   Manual wheelchair accessory, antitipping device, each

Lay Description
Anti-tipping devices are common wheelchair accessory options, particularly for pediatric patients. The devices may be paired and clamped onto the front of the chair to prevent forward spills.

E0973

E0973   Wheelchair accessory, adjustable height, detachable armrest, complete assembly, each

Lay Description
An adjustable height, detachable armrest is a wheelchair accessory designed for patients who require an armrest height that is not available in standard nonadjustable armrests. This code reports a single armrest and all hardware required for complete assembly. For patients who require adjustable height, detachable armrests for both the right and left arms, the code is reported separately for each side.

E0974

E0974   Manual wheelchair accessory, antirollback device, each

Lay Description
Wheelchair anti-rollback devices prevent a manual wheelchair from rolling away when a person stands or lowers themselves into the chair. Most devices consist of breaking systems that automatically engage the tires when weight is removed from the wheelchair

seat. One type uses a lever that makes direct contact with the seat. When the lever senses the patient's weight is removed from the seat, the brake arms automatically clamp down. The chair can be moved forwarded even with the device engaged, but cannot be rolled backward. The device is disengaged by weight placed on the seat.

E0978

E0978   Wheelchair accessory, positioning belt/safety belt/pelvic strap, each

Lay Description
A positioning belt, safety belt, or pelvic strap is a wheelchair accessory that helps maintain proper positioning in the wheelchair. One or more of these items may be required for a patient with weak upper body muscles, upper body instability, or muscle spasticity. If more than one positioning/safety belt/strap is required, each one is reported separately.

E0980

E0980   Safety vest, wheelchair

Lay Description
A safety vest is a restraint designed to securely hold a person in an upright position in a wheelchair. The vest prevents the patient from leaning forward or laterally. A patient that has weak upper body muscles, upper body instability, or muscle spasticity might need the safety vest for proper positioning.

E0981-E0982

E0981   Wheelchair accessory, seat upholstery, replacement only, each

E0982   Wheelchair accessory, back upholstery, replacement only, each

Lay Description
The life of a wheelchair seat cushion or back is usually five years or more. Upholstery is the covering and any underlying padding.

E0983-E0984

E0983   Manual wheelchair accessory, power add-on to convert manual wheelchair to motorized wheelchair, joystick control

E0984   Manual wheelchair accessory, power add-on to convert manual wheelchair to motorized wheelchair, tiller control

Lay Description
A wheelchair is a chair-like device that can be categorized as manual or as a power mobility device (e.g., power wheelchair [PWC] or power operated vehicle [POV]/scooter). There are options and accessories for wheelchairs that allow patients to function successfully in the home or to perform the usual activities of daily living. There are various types of power add-on attachments that convert a manual wheelchair into a power chair, including a master power switch that can be turned on and off. The

majority of PWCs are controlled through a side-mounted joystick. The joystick can adjust up to five specific speed programs. A tiller is a lever that is pushed or pulled to control the PWC.

E0985

E0985   Wheelchair accessory, seat lift mechanism

Lay Description
Seat lifts are mechanisms that enable the patient to increase the seat height in their wheelchair. Some wheelchair seat lifts enable the patient to go from a sitting to standing position, allowing the patient to be in the most comfortable and functional position for his or her needs. The lifting mechanism is graded and not based on a catapult or other type of spring system. These mechanisms can be manual, electric, or battery powered. These devices can help disabled patient's functionality and help with patient transfer.

E0986

E0986   Manual wheelchair accessory, push-rim activated power assist system

Lay Description
A push activated power assist accessory for a manual wheelchair is a device fitted to a rear wheel to sense the force exerted on the wheels. A battery-powered brake and/or propulsion system may then be activated to assist the patient in stopping or advancing the chair.

E0988

E0988   Manual wheelchair accessory, lever-activated, wheel drive, pair

Lay Description
A manual wheelchair is a chair-like device that grants the user some mobility when the user has limited or no control over the legs and/or spine. Manual wheelchairs are usually propelled by the use of a large wheel rotated by user movements. These movements put a great deal of stress and strain on the shoulder muscles. Lever activated wheel drives use pushing and pulling motion on the levers to move gears that propel the wheelchair.

E0990

E0990   Wheelchair accessory, elevating legrest, complete assembly, each

Lay Description
An elevating legrest is a wheelchair accessory required by patients who have musculoskeletal conditions, casts, or braces that prevent 90-degree flexion at the knee. It may also be required for patients with significant edema of the lower extremities requiring elevation of the legs and for patients who require a reclining back on the wheelchair. This code reports a single elevating legrest and all hardware required for complete assembly. For patients who

require elevating legrests for both the right and left legs, the code is reported separately for each side.

E0992

E0992 Manual wheelchair accessory, solid seat insert

Lay Description
A solid seat insert is a wooden or plastic device to bridge the suspension-style seat that comes standard on collapsible wheelchairs.

E0994-E0995

E0994 Armrest, each

E0995 Wheelchair accessory, calf rest/pad, each

Lay Description
Armrests are components of a wheelchair that support the arms and take the pull of gravity off user arms and shoulders. This straightens the spine and aids in keeping a person more upright in a wheelchair. The calf rests/pads are components of a wheelchair that support a person's calves when extended outward from the wheelchair.

E1002

E1002 Wheelchair accessory, power seating system, tilt only

Lay Description
This code reports a tilt power seating system, a wheelchair accessory that can be added to a power wheelchair. The tilt feature allows the wheelchair to be tilted backward to at least 45 degrees from horizontal. Tilting the chair can increase comfort, reduce fatigue, and relieve pressure points caused by sitting in the same position for long periods of time. Power tilt seating systems include a solid seat platform and solid back; any frame width and depth; armrests; fixed or swing-away detachable legrests; fixed or flip-up footplates; a motor and related electronics, with or without variable speed programmability; a switch control that is independent of the power wheelchair drive control interface; and any hardware required to attach the seating system to the wheelchair base. In addition to the tilt specifications, tilt systems must have a back height of at least 20 inches, the ability for the supplier to adjust the seat to back angle, and the ability to support a patient weighing up to 250 pounds.

E1003-E1008

E1003 Wheelchair accessory, power seating system, recline only, without shear reduction

E1004 Wheelchair accessory, power seating system, recline only, with mechanical shear reduction

E1005 Wheelchair accessory, power seating system, recline only, with power shear reduction

E1006 Wheelchair accessory, power seating system, combination tilt and recline, without shear reduction

E1007 Wheelchair accessory, power seating system, combination tilt and recline, with mechanical shear reduction

E1008 Wheelchair accessory, power seating system, combination tilt and recline, with power shear reduction

Lay Description
These codes report a recline power seating system and a combination tilt and recline power seating system, accessories that can be added to a power wheelchair. The tilt feature allows the wheelchair to be tilted to at least 45 degrees from horizontal. The recline feature allows the chair to recline to at least 150 degrees from horizontal. There are several types of systems, differing primarily in their ability to reduce the shearing forces that occur when the wheelchair is reclined. Shearing refers to the shifting of the torso in the chair as it is reclined or raised, causing the patient to slide along the back of the chair. Recline systems that reduce the shearing forces allow the patient's back to stay in contact with the chair without sliding. Wheelchair reclining systems that do not have shear reduction capabilities require that the wheelchair user be able to shift position to compensate for the 2- to 3-inch shear that occurs when the wheelchair is reclined or raised. Reclining wheelchairs are categorized as those that do not provide shear reduction, those that provide mechanical shear reduction, and those that provide power shear reduction. A mechanical shear reduction feature consists of two separate back panels. As the posterior back panel reclines or rises, there is a mechanical linkage between the two panels that allows the patient's back to stay in contact with the anterior panel without sliding along that panel. A power shear reduction feature also consists of two back panels. As the posterior back panel reclines or rises, a separate motor controls the linkage between the two panels that allows the patient's back to stay in contact with the anterior panel without sliding along that panel. Power recline seating systems include a solid seat platform and solid back; any frame width and depth; arm rests; fixed or swing-away detachable leg rests; fixed or flip-up footplates; a motor and related electronics, with or without variable speed programmability; a switch control independent of the power wheelchair drive control interface; and any

hardware required to attach the seating system to the wheelchair base. In addition to the recline specifications, recline systems must have a back height of at least 20 inches and the ability to support a patient weighing up to 250 pounds.

E1009-E1010

E1009　Wheelchair accessory, addition to power seating system, mechanically linked leg elevation system, including pushrod and legrest, each

E1010　Wheelchair accessory, addition to power seating system, power leg elevation system, including legrest, pair

Lay Description
A leg elevation system is a wheelchair accessory that can be added to a power seating system. Two types are available: a mechanically linked leg elevation system and a power leg elevation system. A mechanically linked system uses a pushrod that connects the leg rest to a power recline seating system. With such a leg elevation system, when the back reclines, the leg rest rises; when the back is raised, the leg rest lowers. A power leg elevation system uses a dedicated motor and related electronics, with or without variable speed programmability, that allows the leg rest to be raised and lowered independently of the recline and/or tilt of the seating system. It includes a switch control that may or may not be integrated with the power tilt or recline controls.

E1011

E1011　Modification to pediatric size wheelchair, width adjustment package (not to be dispensed with initial chair)

Lay Description
Some wheelchair companies offer "growth options" on pediatric wheelchairs since buying a new wheelchair each year would be very expensive. Growth kits or growth chairs allow adjustments to be made to the wheelchair. These replaceable components can be adjusted from smaller to larger to accommodate a growing child.

E1014

E1014　Reclining back, addition to pediatric size wheelchair

Lay Description
Reclining wheelchair backs are options that may be required for pediatric patients with certain medical conditions including quadriplegia, fixed hip angle, trunk or lower extremity casts/braces, excess extensor tone of the trunk muscles, or the need to rest in a recumbent position periodically during the day. A semi-reclining back is defined as one with a recline capability of greater than 15 degrees, but less than 80 degrees. A fully reclining back is one that can recline to greater than 80 degrees.

E1015-E1018

E1015　Shock absorber for manual wheelchair, each

E1016　Shock absorber for power wheelchair, each

E1017　Heavy-duty shock absorber for heavy-duty or extra heavy-duty manual wheelchair, each

E1018　Heavy-duty shock absorber for heavy-duty or extra heavy-duty power wheelchair, each

Lay Description
Wheelchair shock absorbers provide a smoother, less jarring ride for disabled patients. The shock absorbers are attached to the front wheels and include a suspension system with a hinge damper or a spring coil to absorb the impact of rough surfaces. The shock absorbers can be fit for manual or electric wheelchairs.

E1020

E1020　Residual limb support system for wheelchair, any type

Lay Description
A wheelchair residual limb support system is an attachment that provides a wheelchair patient a place to rest the stump of an amputated leg. This additional support allows the patient proper and comfortable positioning when seated in the wheelchair. The residual support device is similar to a leg rest but is shorter. It can be adjustable to allow for differences in the residual limb length and allow different positions.

E1028

E1028　Wheelchair accessory, manual swingaway, retractable or removable mounting hardware for joystick, other control interface or positioning accessory

Lay Description
Retractable or removable mounting hardware devices are used to attach wheelchair accessories that allow the accessory to be manually moved, either to the side or up and down, or removed from the wheelchair mount. This hardware is specific for a joystick, other control interface, or positioning accessory.

E1029-E1030

E1029　Wheelchair accessory, ventilator tray, fixed

E1030　Wheelchair accessory, ventilator tray, gimbaled

Lay Description
A ventilator tray is a platform attached to the wheelchair back that allows the patient's ventilator to be transported with the patient. A gimbaled tray remains horizontal when the seat back is raised or lowered.

E1031

E1031   Rollabout chair, any and all types with castors 5 in or greater

Lay Description

Rollabout chairs, any and all types that have casters of 5 inches or larger, are prescribed for ill, injured, or impaired individuals who require a level of mobility without standing and walking that may be met by the rollabout chair in lieu of a wheelchair. Rollabout chairs are not general use home or office chairs. Rollabout chairs are also referred to as mobile geriatric chairs and geri-chairs.

E1035-E1036

E1035   Multi-positional patient transfer system, with integrated seat, operated by care giver, patient weight capacity up to and including 300 lbs

E1036   Multi-positional patient transfer system, extra-wide, with integrated seat, operated by caregiver, patient weight capacity greater than 300 lbs

Lay Description

A multi-positional patient transfer system is a medical device, with an integrated seat, that allows positioning and adjustment of bed-bound people. The person can be transferred onto the device in a supine position. Once positioned, the device can be adjusted into chair-like positions. This device is not electric. It is operated by a care giver.

E1037-E1039

E1037   Transport chair, pediatric size

E1038   Transport chair, adult size, patient weight capacity up to and including 300 pounds

E1039   Transport chair, adult size, heavy-duty, patient weight capacity greater than 300 pounds

Lay Description

Transport chairs come in a variety of sizes with multiple functions, also referred to as a companion wheelchair. Transport chairs are convenient for any type of travel. Transport chairs are usually light weight and can fit into the patient's back seat or trunk.

E1050-E1070

E1050   Fully-reclining wheelchair, fixed full-length arms, swing-away detachable elevating legrests

E1060   Fully-reclining wheelchair, detachable arms, desk or full-length, swing-away detachable elevating legrests

E1070   Fully-reclining wheelchair, detachable arms (desk or full-length) swing-away detachable footrest

Lay Description

Fully reclining wheelchairs are indicated for patients who are quadriplegic, have a fixed hip angle, may be currently wearing body or extremity casts or braces that necessitate a reclining position, and for patients who need to rest in their wheelchair in a recumbent position two or more times per day because transfer between wheelchair and bed is difficult. These wheelchairs include a fully reclining backrest with detachable armrests (desk arm or full-length) or fixed full-length armrests, and swing-away, detachable, elevating legrests with a pad used to support the calf when the legrest is in an elevated position.

E1083-E1086

E1083   Hemi-wheelchair, fixed full-length arms, swing-away detachable elevating legrest

E1084   Hemi-wheelchair, detachable arms desk or full-length arms, swing-away detachable elevating legrests

E1085   Hemi-wheelchair, fixed full-length arms, swing-away detachable footrests

E1086   Hemi-wheelchair, detachable arms, desk or full-length, swing-away detachable footrests

Lay Description

The hemi-wheelchair is indicated for patients requiring a lower seat height (17 to 18 inches) than the standard 19 to 21 inches from seat to floor because of short stature or the inability to place the feet on the ground for propulsion due to amputation, paralysis, or stroke. Hemi-wheelchairs have a fully reclining backrest.

E1087-E1090

E1087   High strength lightweight wheelchair, fixed full-length arms, swing-away detachable elevating legrests

E1088   High strength lightweight wheelchair, detachable arms desk or full-length, swing-away detachable elevating legrests

E1089   High-strength lightweight wheelchair, fixed-length arms, swing-away detachable footrest

E1090   High-strength lightweight wheelchair, detachable arms, desk or full-length, swing-away detachable footrests

Lay Description

The high-strength lightweight wheelchair is indicated for patients requiring a chair for self-propulsion and/or when the seat height, width, or depth measurements required cannot be accommodated by a standard, hemi, or lightweight wheelchair. This device weighs less than 34 pounds, is fully reclining, and has high-strength side frames and cross braces.

E1092-E1093

E1092   Wide heavy-duty wheel chair, detachable arms (desk or full-length), swing-away detachable elevating legrests

E1093   Wide heavy-duty wheelchair, detachable arms, desk or full-length arms, swing-away detachable footrests

Lay Description

A wide, heavy-duty wheelchair is indicated for obese patients when the seat measurements required cannot be accommodated by a standard wheelchair. This device is fully reclining and includes detachable desk or full-length arms.

E1100-E1110

E1100   Semi-reclining wheelchair, fixed full-length arms, swing-away detachable elevating legrests

E1110   Semi-reclining wheelchair, detachable arms (desk or full-length) elevating legrest

Lay Description

A semi-reclining wheelchair provides a backrest that tilts back from the upright position but not into a full-recumbent posture and swing-away, detachable elevating legrests that have a pad used to support the calf when the legrest is in an elevated position.

E1130-E1160

E1130   Standard wheelchair, fixed full-length arms, fixed or swing-away detachable footrests

E1140   Wheelchair, detachable arms, desk or full-length, swing-away detachable footrests

E1150   Wheelchair, detachable arms, desk or full-length swing-away detachable elevating legrests

E1160   Wheelchair, fixed full-length arms, swing-away detachable elevating legrests

Lay Description

A standard wheelchair generally has a seat width of 16, 18, or 20 inches, is 16 inches in depth, and 21 inches from seat to floor. It comes with a chrome-plated frame, 24 inch molded rear wheels, 8 inch molded casters, nylon or vinyl upholstery, and arm and footrests.

E1161

E1161   Manual adult size wheelchair, includes tilt in space

Lay Description

A tilt-in-space system in a standard wheelchair that changes a person's orientation in space while maintaining fixed hip, knee, and ankle angles. The system redistributes pressure from one area to another and maintains physical angles at the hips, knees, and ankles.

E1170-E1190

E1170   Amputee wheelchair, fixed full-length arms, swing-away detachable elevating legrests

E1171   Amputee wheelchair, fixed full-length arms, without footrests or legrest

E1172   Amputee wheelchair, detachable arms (desk or full-length) without footrests or legrest

E1180   Amputee wheelchair, detachable arms (desk or full-length) swing-away detachable footrests

E1190   Amputee wheelchair, detachable arms (desk or full-length) swing-away detachable elevating legrests

Lay Description

An amputee wheelchair is specially designed for patients missing one or both legs. When a patient has one or both legs amputated, the center of gravity and weight distribution changes. An amputee wheelchair is designed with large wheels and the rear axle placed further back on the chair to compensate for less weight at the front of the chair from the missing limb(s). Amputee wheelchairs are available with different options for patient need and comfort.

E1195

E1195   Heavy-duty wheelchair, fixed full-length arms, swing-away detachable elevating legrests

Lay Description

A heavy-duty wheelchair is designed to support larger people with weight capacities that begin at 500 pounds. Frames are usually reinforced. Seats are usually wider and deeper than non-heavy duty chairs.

E1200

E1200   Amputee wheelchair, fixed full-length arms, swing-away detachable footrest

Lay Description

An amputee wheelchair is specially designed for patients missing one or both legs. When a patient has one or both legs amputated, the center of gravity and weight distribution changes. An amputee wheelchair is designed with large wheels and the rear axle placed further back on the chair to compensate for less weight at the front of the chair from the missing limb(s). The swing away feature gets the attachment out of the way, allowing patients to be transferred in and out of the wheelchair and provides patients a fully adjustable amputee support.

E1220

E1220 Wheelchair; specially sized or constructed, (indicate brand name, model number, if any) and justification

Lay Description
A specially sized or constructed wheelchair is indicated for patients in cases when the measurements of a standard wheelchair will not accommodate the patient's needs. This wheelchair must be justified by reasons such as a patient's physical size or the specific requirements for wheelchair usage in the patient's place of residence, such as narrow doorways that prevent the passage of a standard wheelchair. Report the brand name and model number.

E1221-E1224

E1221 Wheelchair with fixed arm, footrests
E1222 Wheelchair with fixed arm, elevating legrests
E1223 Wheelchair with detachable arms, footrests
E1224 Wheelchair with detachable arms, elevating legrests

Lay Description
A wheelchair is a chair with wheels designed to provide mobility to people for whom walking is difficult or impossible. Armrests can be fixed to the chair or detachable. Footrests are usually attached to the chair. Elevating leg rests attach to the lower front of the chair and are used to support the legs. The elevating leg rest can be positioned to maintain the leg in an extended position or at varying angles.

E1225-E1226

E1225 Wheelchair accessory, manual semi-reclining back, (recline greater than 15 degrees, but less than 80 degrees), each
E1226 Wheelchair accessory, manual fully reclining back, (recline greater than 80 degrees), each

Lay Description
Manual semi-reclining or fully reclining wheelchair backs are options that may be required for patients with certain medical conditions including quadriplegia, fixed hip angle, trunk or lower extremity casts/braces, excess extensor tone of the trunk muscles, or the need to rest in a recumbent position periodically during the day. A semi-reclining back is defined as one with a recline capability of greater than 15 degrees, but less than 80 degrees. A fully reclining back is one that can recline to greater than 80 degrees.

E1227-E1228

E1227 Special height arms for wheelchair
E1228 Special back height for wheelchair

Lay Description
A specially sized or constructed wheelchair is indicated in cases where the measurements of a standard wheelchair do not accommodate the patient's needs. This wheelchair must be justified by reasons such as a patient's physical size or the specific requirements for wheelchair usage in the patient's place of residence, such as narrow doorways that prevent the passage of a standard wheelchair.

E1229

E1229 Wheelchair, pediatric size, not otherwise specified

Lay Description
Report this code for a pediatric sized wheelchair that is not otherwise specified in other HCPCS Level II codes.

E1230

E1230 Power operated vehicle (3- or 4-wheel nonhighway), specify brand name and model number

Lay Description
A POV is a power-operated vehicle with three to four wheels. These may be indoor, outdoor, or both indoor/outdoor models. Indoor models are generally slow-speed with highly maneuverable mechanisms that assist the patient with mobility inside the home. Outdoor models can reach greater speeds and are more durable. POVs usually work from a battery power source. An indoor POV assists patients for whom a wheelchair is unsuitable in the activities of daily living, but POVs are not suited to all types of patients such as stroke victims or some quadriplegic and/or hemiplegic patients who cannot operate the controls nor be left alone while the vehicle is in operation. This code requires specifying the brand name and model number when reporting.

E1231-E1234

E1231 Wheelchair, pediatric size, tilt-in-space, rigid, adjustable, with seating system
E1232 Wheelchair, pediatric size, tilt-in-space, folding, adjustable, with seating system
E1233 Wheelchair, pediatric size, tilt-in-space, rigid, adjustable, without seating system
E1234 Wheelchair, pediatric size, tilt-in-space, folding, adjustable, without seating system

Lay Description
A tilt-in-space system in a standard wheelchair that changes a person's orientation in space while maintaining fixed hip, knee, and ankle angles. The system redistributes pressure from one area to another and maintains physical angles at the hips,

knees, and ankles. This wheelchair provides positioning and is perfect for individuals who require tilt adjustment for pressure relief, digestion, and respiratory assistance. Pediatric wheelchairs are smaller in size to accommodate the smaller stature of a child. Rigid wheelchairs do not fold or collapse. Folding wheelchairs allow the chair to be folded for travel purposes. Seating systems include seat pads and back rests that can be customized to the user's needs.

E1235-E1238

E1235 Wheelchair, pediatric size, rigid, adjustable, with seating system

E1236 Wheelchair, pediatric size, folding, adjustable, with seating system

E1237 Wheelchair, pediatric size, rigid, adjustable, without seating system

E1238 Wheelchair, pediatric size, folding, adjustable, without seating system

Lay Description

Pediatric wheelchairs are smaller in size to accommodate the smaller stature of a child. Rigid wheelchairs do not fold or collapse. Folding wheelchairs allow the chair to be folded or collapsed for travel purposes. Seating systems include seat pads and back rests that can be customized to the user's needs.

E1239

E1239 Power wheelchair, pediatric size, not otherwise specified

Lay Description

A power wheelchair is a power-operated wheelchair with three to four wheels. These may be indoor, outdoor, or both indoor/outdoor models. Indoor models are generally slow-speed with highly maneuverable mechanisms that assist the patient with mobility inside the home. Outdoor models can reach greater speeds and are more durable. Power wheelchairs usually work from a battery power source. Pediatric wheelchairs are smaller in size to accommodate the smaller stature of a child. Report this code for a pediatric sized power wheelchair that is not otherwise specified by other HCPCS Level II codes.

E1240-E1270

E1240 Lightweight wheelchair, detachable arms, (desk or full-length) swing-away detachable, elevating legrest

E1250 Lightweight wheelchair, fixed full-length arms, swing-away detachable footrest

E1260 Lightweight wheelchair, detachable arms (desk or full-length) swing-away detachable footrest

E1270 Lightweight wheelchair, fixed full-length arms, swing-away detachable elevating legrests

Lay Description

Lightweight wheelchairs are designed for patients who spend a great deal of time in the unit and can take full advantage of the increased mobility a lighter chair offers. Most models weigh 26 to 34 pounds and the patient can mobilize it more effectively than conventional wheelchairs.

E1280-E1295

E1280 Heavy-duty wheelchair, detachable arms (desk or full-length) elevating legrests

E1285 Heavy-duty wheelchair, fixed full-length arms, swing-away detachable footrest

E1290 Heavy-duty wheelchair, detachable arms (desk or full-length) swing-away detachable footrest

E1295 Heavy-duty wheelchair, fixed full-length arms, elevating legrest

Lay Description

Heavy-duty wheelchairs may be called for to supply patients of extreme size or weight. Most models feature reinforced frames and wheels and can seat patients from 300 to 400 pounds or greater. Some models can accommodate up to 700 pounds. The unit itself may weigh up to 58 pounds.

E1296-E1298

E1296 Special wheelchair seat height from floor

E1297 Special wheelchair seat depth, by upholstery

E1298 Special wheelchair seat depth and/or width, by construction

Lay Description

A specially sized or constructed wheelchair component is indicated when the measurements of a standard wheelchair do not accommodate the patient's needs. This wheelchair must be justified by reasons such as a patient's physical size or the specific requirements for wheelchair usage in the patient's place of residence, such as narrow doorways that prevent the passage of a standard wheelchair. The standard seat height from the floor is 18 to 20 inches. The standard seat width and depth is 15 to 19 inches. When a deviation is more than 2 inches from the standard, the sizing is labeled "special."

E1300-E1310

E1300 Whirlpool, portable (overtub type)

E1310 Whirlpool, nonportable (built-in type)

Lay Description

A therapeutic bath device that uses circulating water and water jets to stimulate circulation, relieve pain, and massage the body. Whirlpools may have a single pump that circulates the water or multiple pumps—one to circulate the water and the others to drive the hydrotherapy jets.

E1352

E1352 Oxygen accessory, flow regulator capable of positive inspiratory pressure

Lay Description
The Noninvasive OPEN Ventilation System (NIOV™) by Breathe Technologies, Inc. provides positive pressure inspiratory support for patients using oxygen. This product consists of multiple components, including a control unit, flow regulator, connecting hose, and nasal interface (pillows).

E1353

E1353 Regulator

Lay Description
An oxygen regulator is a brass (or sometimes aluminum) device that governs the flow of gaseous oxygen from the tank. Some devices may feature an integrated pressure gauge and additional flow ports and safety relief valves.

E1354-E1355

E1354 Oxygen accessory, wheeled cart for portable cylinder or portable concentrator, any type, replacement only, each

E1355 Stand/rack

Lay Description
A wheeled cart is a device with a platform, straps, or hooks to secure the oxygen cylinder or concentrator and wheels. Using a wheeled cart while traveling with oxygen. This cart falls into the category of additional oxygen related equipment. A stand or rack is a device with a platform, straps, or hooks to secure the oxygen cylinder or concentrator. Racks or stands can hold one or multiple cylinders. Some may attach to wheelchairs while others are freestanding. Stands and racks allow for easier movement of the oxygen equipment. This cart falls in the category of additional oxygen related equipment.

E1356

E1356 Oxygen accessory, battery pack/cartridge for portable concentrator, any type, replacement only, each

Lay Description
A battery pack or cartridge is an oxygen accessory that supplies power to a portable oxygen concentrator using AC/DC or lithium power cartridges. Batteries automatically charge if the units plugged into an AC source. These ambulatory systems make it easy for patients to go just about anywhere without the concern of running out of oxygen.

E1357

E1357 Oxygen accessory, battery charger for portable concentrator, any type, replacement only, each

Lay Description
A battery charger is a device used to put energy into rechargeable batteries by forcing an electric current through it. Simply insert the battery into the charger and it stops charging when the battery is fully charged.

E1358

E1358 Oxygen accessory, DC power adapter for portable concentrator, any type, replacement only, each

Lay Description
A direct current (DC) power adapter converts DC into the alternating current (AC) that a portable concentrator needs. Many DC adapters can power an oxygen concentrator from the "cigarette lighter" style sockets found in most vehicles.

E1372

E1372 Immersion external heater for nebulizer

Lay Description
An immersion external heater for a nebulizer is an accessory for a pneumatic nebulizer. It is an external slip-on heater that heats the aerosol mixture before inhalation. It is believed that the heating reduces the possibility of contamination.

E1390-E1392

E1390 Oxygen concentrator, single delivery port, capable of delivering 85 percent or greater oxygen concentration at the prescribed flow rate

E1391 Oxygen concentrator, dual delivery port, capable of delivering 85 percent or greater oxygen concentration at the prescribed flow rate, each

E1392 Portable oxygen concentrator, rental

Lay Description
An oxygen concentrator takes oxygen from room air and removes nitrogen, which comprises about 80 percent of room air. These units alternately compress ambient air through chambers containing zeolite granules, which absorb nitrogen. While one chamber is pressurized, the second rests and the zeolite release the absorbed nitrogen back into the room air. The concentrated oxygen is filtered and delivered at levels of about 5 liters per minute at levels approaching 95 percent pure oxygen.

E1399

E1399 Durable medical equipment, miscellaneous

Lay Description

Durable medical equipment is a diverse term used to describe any medical equipment used in the home to aid in a better quality of living where people can be more mobile and independent. The term "durable medical equipment" includes iron lungs, oxygen tents, nebulizers, continuous positive airway pressure devices, catheters, hospital beds, and wheelchairs, whether furnished on a rental basis or purchased. There are also other simple tools such as ramps that can help wheelchair users access steps and vehicles and highly specialized devices, such as hearing aids and a breathing apparatus. Report this code when a more specific HCPCS Level II code is not available for durable medical equipment.

E1405-E1406

E1405 Oxygen and water vapor enriching system with heated delivery

E1406 Oxygen and water vapor enriching system without heated delivery

Lay Description

Oxygen delivery systems are units of compressed gaseous, liquid, or concentrated O2 for home use, which are stationary or portable. In many cases, the units also include the system components required to administer the O2, such as the regulator, flowmeter, contents indicator, nebulizer, humidifier, cannula or mask, and the O2 tubing. The administration of O2 assists in oxygenation of tissues when the patient's cardiopulmonary system is unable to intake sufficient quantities of O2 or is unable to process outside or room air into its elemental components to use the O2 content. For instance, patients with severe chronic obstructive pulmonary disease and emphysema may require O2 therapy. Oxygen also aids in and/or expedites the healing of injured or diseased tissues or organs.

E1500-E1699

E1500 Centrifuge, for dialysis

E1510 Kidney, dialysate delivery system kidney machine, pump recirculating, air removal system, flowrate meter, power off, heater and temperature control with alarm, IV poles, pressure gauge, concentrate container

E1520 Heparin infusion pump for hemodialysis

E1530 Air bubble detector for hemodialysis, each, replacement

E1540 Pressure alarm for hemodialysis, each, replacement

E1550 Bath conductivity meter for hemodialysis, each

E1560 Blood leak detector for hemodialysis, each, replacement

E1570 Adjustable chair, for ESRD patients

E1575 Transducer protectors/fluid barriers, for hemodialysis, any size, per 10

E1580 Unipuncture control system for hemodialysis

E1590 Hemodialysis machine

E1592 Automatic intermittent peritoneal dialysis system

E1594 Cycler dialysis machine for peritoneal dialysis

E1600 Delivery and/or installation charges for hemodialysis equipment

E1610 Reverse osmosis water purification system, for hemodialysis

E1615 Deionizer water purification system, for hemodialysis

E1620 Blood pump for hemodialysis, replacement

E1625 Water softening system, for hemodialysis

E1630 Reciprocating peritoneal dialysis system

E1632 Wearable artificial kidney, each

E1634 Peritoneal dialysis clamps, each

E1635 Compact (portable) travel hemodialyzer system

E1636 Sorbent cartridges, for hemodialysis, per 10

E1637 Hemostats, each

E1639 Scale, each

E1699 Dialysis equipment, not otherwise specified

Lay Description

These codes describe miscellaneous supplies and equipment needed to accomplish home dialysis. Dialysis is a filtration process that filters impurities from the blood. Dialysis assists malfunctioning kidneys and can replace nonfunctioning kidneys. The functioning of all body parts requires the removal of the various toxins and metabolic byproducts from the blood. If these impurities are allowed to accumulate, death will occur within days. Home dialysis allows the patient to perform this function in home rather than at a facility.

E1700

E1700   Jaw motion rehabilitation system

Lay Description
This code reports the supply of a rehabilitative device for disorders of the temporomandibular joint (TMJ) and restrictive jaw motion. These devices may feature a cushioned mouthpiece that the patient bites against. The patient then squeezes a lever that forces open the mouthpiece and the jaw. Adjustments on the device control the leverage action. The therapy works to improve the range of the TMJ. Patients who have undergone certain radiation treatments often suffer a restrictive and spastic jaw movement known as trismus. Rehabilitation for surgery of the jaw and treatment of conditions that cause "lockjaw" may also warrant use of this type of device.

E1701

E1701   Replacement cushions for jaw motion rehabilitation system, package of 6

Lay Description
Replacement cushions for a jaw motion rehabilitation system are padded bite plates attached to a scissor-like device that are intended to prevent hypomobility and gradually increase the range of jaw motion.

E1702

E1702   Replacement measuring scales for jaw motion rehabilitation system, package of 200

Lay Description
Replacement scales used in a jaw motion rehabilitation system are special disposable paper scale (measuring) devices that measure the opening, movement, and function of the mouth and jaw.

E1800-E1841

E1800   Dynamic adjustable elbow extension/flexion device, includes soft interface material

E1801   Static progressive stretch elbow device, extension and/or flexion, with or without range of motion adjustment, includes all components and accessories

E1802   Dynamic adjustable forearm pronation/supination device, includes soft interface material

E1805   Dynamic adjustable wrist extension/flexion device, includes soft interface material

E1806   Static progressive stretch wrist device, flexion and/or extension, with or without range of motion adjustment, includes all components and accessories

E1810   Dynamic adjustable knee extension/flexion device, includes soft interface material

E1811   Static progressive stretch knee device, extension and/or flexion, with or without range of motion adjustment, includes all components and accessories

E1812   Dynamic knee, extension/flexion device with active resistance control

E1815   Dynamic adjustable ankle extension/flexion device, includes soft interface material

E1816   Static progressive stretch ankle device, flexion and/or extension, with or without range of motion adjustment, includes all components and accessories

E1818   Static progressive stretch forearm pronation/supination device, with or without range of motion adjustment, includes all components and accessories

E1820   Replacement soft interface material, dynamic adjustable extension/flexion device

E1821   Replacement soft interface material/cuffs for bi-directional static progressive stretch device

E1825   Dynamic adjustable finger extension/flexion device, includes soft interface material

E1830   Dynamic adjustable toe extension/flexion device, includes soft interface material

E1831   Static progressive stretch toe device, extension and/or flexion, with or without range of motion adjustment, includes all components and accessories

E1840   Dynamic adjustable shoulder flexion/abduction/rotation device, includes soft interface material

E1841   Static progressive stretch shoulder device, with or without range of motion adjustment, includes all components and accessories

Lay Description
These codes report the supply of specific rehabilitation devices for the upper or lower limb. These devices are designed to be strapped onto the affected joint. The device may be dynamic, which allows a constant, slow stretch of the joint, or static, which is operated by the patient for intermittent use. The devices may include range of motion adjustment. Adjustable pads and cuffs are positioned to maximize function. The codes include supply of the soft material that interfaces between the skin and the hard structure of the device.

E

E1902

E1902 Communication board, nonelectronic augmentative or alternative communication device

Lay Description

An augmentative or alternative communication board is an umbrella term that encompasses methods of communication for people with impairments or restrictions on the production or comprehension of the spoken or written language. Augmentative or alternative communication board devices are therapeutically used to establish, develop, or maintain the ability to communicate functional needs. Low technology, non-electronic augmentative communication devices include boards that use letters, words, phrases, and/or symbols (communication boards); mini boards; schedule boards; and conversation books.

E2000

E2000 Gastric suction pump, home model, portable or stationary, electric

Lay Description

A gastric suction pump is an aspiration device used to remove gastrointestinal fluids under continuous or intermittent suction through a tube. It is generally used for patients who are unable to empty gastric secretions normally. This is a home model, portable or stationary, that is lightweight, compact and has an electric aspirator. Use of the device does not require technical or professional supervision.

E2000

E2000 Gastric suction pump, home model, portable or stationary, electric

Lay Description

Please refer to code E0600 for the description.

E2100-E2101

E2100 Blood glucose monitor with integrated voice synthesizer

E2101 Blood glucose monitor with integrated lancing/blood sample

Lay Description

Please refer to code E0607 for the description.

E2100-E2101

E2100 Blood glucose monitor with integrated voice synthesizer

E2101 Blood glucose monitor with integrated lancing/blood sample

Lay Description

Please refer to code E0607 for the description, coding, and billing information.

E2120

E2120 Pulse generator system for tympanic treatment of inner ear endolymphatic fluid

Lay Description

A portable, low-pressure pulse generator system for tympanic treatment of inner ear endolymphatic fluid, also known as Ménière's disease, is reported with this code. Prior to application of the pulse generator, the patient undergoes a tympanostomy with ventilation tube insertion. The patient must then wait approximately two weeks before treatment with the pressure pulse generator can begin. The device delivers repeated pressure pulses to the ear canal using an air pressure generator and a close-fitting cuff in the ear canal. The treatment is performed several times a day for short intervals (approximately five minutes per treatment session).

E2201-E2204

E2201 Manual wheelchair accessory, nonstandard seat frame, width greater than or equal to 20 in and less than 24 in

E2202 Manual wheelchair accessory, nonstandard seat frame width, 24-27 in

E2203 Manual wheelchair accessory, nonstandard seat frame depth, 20 to less than 22 in

E2204 Manual wheelchair accessory, nonstandard seat frame depth, 22 to 25 in

Lay Description

A nonstandard seat frame for a manual wheelchair identifies seat supports that are different sizes. Such seats are required if the patient's physical dimensions justify the need for a nonstandard size.

E2205

E2205 Manual wheelchair accessory, handrim without projections (includes ergonomic or contoured), any type, replacement only, each

Lay Description

Handrims, also known as pushrims, are metal devices that attach to the wheels of a manual wheelchair. The user grips the handrim and turns the wheel, which propels the wheelchair. There are many types of handrims, including chrome, aluminium anodized, composite, vinyl coated, foam covered, projection, oblique projection, and natural fit.

E2206

E2206 Manual wheelchair accessory, wheel Lock assembly, complete, each

Lay Description

A wheel lock is a safety device that stops a wheelchair from moving. There are several different types of wheel locks, including push to lock, pull to lock, and an automatic wheel lock system. The automatic wheel lock system helps prevent falls for people who cannot or do not consistently lock the manual brakes on their wheelchairs.

E2207

E2207 **Wheelchair accessory, crutch and cane holder, each**

Lay Description

A crutch and cane holder for a wheelchair is a clip device that attaches to a wheelchair to hold a crutch or a cane. This allows users to keep a cane or crutch handy. Gripping surfaces of the holder are soft plastic rollers and do not damage canes or crutches.

E2208

E2208 **Wheelchair accessory, cylinder tank carrier, each**

Lay Description

A cylinder tank carrier is a devise that attaches to a wheelchair to hold an oxygen tank. It offers increased mobility and freedom for individuals who are required to use oxygen and a wheelchair.

E2209

E2209 **Accessory, arm trough, with or without hand support, each**

Lay Description

An arm trough for a manual wheelchair is an accessory designed to support the arm in patients with quadriplegia, hemiplegia, or spasticity of the arms. The arm trough replaces the standard armrest.

E2210

E2210 **Wheelchair accessory, bearings, any type, replacement only, each**

Lay Description

A wheelchair bearing is a device that allows constrained motion between two parts of the wheelchair. There are three types. Stem bearings are located where the front fork attaches to the wheelchair frame. Caster bearings are located in the caster wheels. Rear bearings are located in the rear wheels.

E2211-E2212

E2211 **Manual wheelchair accessory, pneumatic propulsion tire, any size, each**

E2212 **Manual wheelchair accessory, tube for pneumatic propulsion tire, any size, each**

Lay Description

A pneumatic tire is a ring-shaped covering that fits around a wheel rim to protect it and to provide a cushion. These are commonly made of rubber and require an inner tube that is filled with air. Pneumatic tires are on most manual and power wheelchairs because they are lighter, shock-absorbing, and offer good traction. A propulsion tire is a large wheel that

can be used by a person to propel the wheelchair with his/her arms.

E2213

E2213 **Manual wheelchair accessory, insert for pneumatic propulsion tire (removable), any type, any size, each**

Lay Description

A pneumatic tire is a ring-shaped covering that fits around a wheel rim to protect it and to provide a cushion. A pneumonic tire may come with an airless insert that is soft rubber or a latex gel that replaces the inner tube. This removable ring of firm material placed inside of a pneumatic tire allows a wheelchair to continue to move if the pneumatic tire is punctured. This type of tire insert is sometimes referred to as a flat free insert or a zero pressure tube. The ride is cushioned but it is a little heavier than the basic pneumonic tire. A propulsion wheel is a large wheel that can be used by a person to propel the wheelchair with his/her arms.

E2214-E2215

E2214 **Manual wheelchair accessory, pneumatic caster tire, any size, each**

E2215 **Manual wheelchair accessory, tube for pneumatic caster tire, any size, each**

Lay Description

A pneumatic caster tire is a ring-shaped device made of flexible fabric, such as India rubber, that contains an inner tube filled with compressed air. Pneumatic caster tires on a wheelchair are shock absorbing wheels that absorb vibrations thus providing a smooth cushioned ride and quiet operation. A caster tire is a small wheel that is in contact with the ground during normal operation of the wheelchair and cannot be used for arm propulsion.

E2216-E2219

E2216 **Manual wheelchair accessory, foam filled propulsion tire, any size, each**

E2217 **Manual wheelchair accessory, foam filled caster tire, any size, each**

E2218 **Manual wheelchair accessory, foam propulsion tire, any size, each**

E2219 **Manual wheelchair accessory, foam caster tire, any size, each**

Lay Description

A propulsion tire is a large wheel that allows the person in the wheelchair to move the chair with his or her arms. A caster tire is a small wheel that is in contact with the ground during normal operation of the wheelchair and cannot be used for arm propulsion. A foam tire made entirely of polyurethane. A foam filled tire is a rubber tire injected with polyurethane. These codes are reported for each tire.

E

E2220

E2220 Manual wheelchair accessory, solid (rubber/plastic) propulsion tire, any size, each

Lay Description
A propulsion tire is a large wheel that allows the person in the wheelchair to move the chair with his or her arms. This code represents a propulsion tire made of hard plastic or rubber.

E2221

E2221 Manual wheelchair accessory, solid (rubber/plastic) caster tire (removable), any size, each

Lay Description
A caster tire is a small wheel that is in contact with the ground during normal operation of the wheelchair and cannot be used for arm propulsion. This code is for a caster tire made of hard plastic or rubber.

E2222

E2222 Manual wheelchair accessory, solid (rubber/plastic) caster tire with integrated wheel, any size, each

Lay Description
A caster tire is a smaller wheel that is in contact with the ground during normal operation of the wheelchair and cannot be used for arm propulsion. The integrated caster has the tire attached to the wheel as one unit. Report this code for an integrated caster tire made of hard plastic or rubber.

E2224

E2224 Manual wheelchair accessory, propulsion wheel excludes tire, any size, each

Lay Description
A propulsion wheel is a large wheel that can be used by a person in a wheelchair to propel the chair with his or her arms. This code is for a propulsion wheel, excluding the tire.

E2225

E2225 Manual wheelchair accessory, caster wheel excludes tire, any size, replacement only, each

Lay Description
A caster wheel is a single, double, or compound wheel that is designed to be mounted to the bottom of a larger object to enable the object to be easily moved. Report this code for any size replacement caster wheel, tire not included.

E2226

E2226 Manual wheelchair accessory, caster fork, any size, replacement only, each

Lay Description
Wheelchair caster wheels are mounted using a caster fork assembly. A caster fork assembly consists of the fork, the caster stem bolt (the long bolt coming up from the top of the fork), caster stem bearings, and sometimes a spacer or spacers. This code is for any size replacement caster fork.

E2227

E2227 Manual wheelchair accessory, gear reduction drive wheel, each

Lay Description
A gear reduction drive wheel is a mechanical device that propels a manual wheelchair. The gear reduction device allows the user to slow down or speed up the motion. It provides a user with additional assistance by providing "leverage" through gearing (like a bicycle).

E2228

E2228 Manual wheelchair accessory, wheel braking system and lock, complete, each

Lay Description
Wheelchair locks prohibit motion of the wheels, keeping the wheelchair in "park" while the user transfers in or out of the chair. Wheelchair brakes help to slow or stop a wheelchair when descending or turning. There are different types of wheelchair brakes/locks, including manual, auto-lock, and disc brake systems. The push/pull style of lock is standard. The basic wheel lock is commonly known as a wheelchair brake.

E2230

E2230 Manual wheelchair accessory, manual standing system

Lay Description
A wheelchair standing system, also known as a standing chair or frame, is a mechanical device that allows the chair and the user to be moved into an upright standing position. A person can stand anywhere anytime.

E2231

E2231 Manual wheelchair accessory, solid seat support base (replaces sling seat), includes any type mounting hardware

Lay Description
Sling support seats are pieces of leather, plastic, or other material that are suspended loosely between two supports. The user sits in the sling, which conforms to his or her body. A solid seat support base provides a sturdy stiff pillow base that can improve posture and increase comfort.

E2291-E2292

E2291 Back, planar, for pediatric size wheelchair including fixed attaching hardware

E2292 Seat, planar, for pediatric size wheelchair including fixed attaching hardware

Lay Description
Planar systems are flat positioning components that allow a person to move. The planar system is composed of foam interfaced with a wood or plastic base. The simplest form of seating system is a linear seating system. A linear seating system refers to a planar seat and back with fixed angles and orientations. This solid base of support enhances posture and provides comfort for longer periods of sitting.

E2293-E2294

E2293 Back, contoured, for pediatric size wheelchair including fixed attaching hardware

E2294 Seat, contoured, for pediatric size wheelchair including fixed attaching hardware

Lay Description
A contoured cushion is shaped to the user's body helping bring the body back to the same place every time. The cushion helps support the correct positioning of the user's body.

E2295

E2295 Manual wheelchair accessory, for pediatric size wheelchair, dynamic seating frame, allows coordinated movement of multiple positioning features

Lay Description
A dynamic seating frame is a device that allows the wheelchair user's own body to initiate and control the level of seating movements. Benefits of such a system include relaxed overall muscle tone, increased muscle control, and the end or lessening of back/buttock pain and discomfort. This seat, which pivots, is connected to the wheelchair's frame and is attached to resilient supports. By various supports and attachments, a spring biases attaches to other components that enables the force of the spring to vary to alter resiliency of the support.

E2300

E2300 Wheelchair accessory, power seat elevation system, any type

Lay Description
A power seat elevation system allows the seat to be raised and lowered. The system should be able to raise the seat a minimum of 6 inches from its lowest point. A power seat elevation system consists of a motor and related electronics, with or without variable speed programmability; a switch control that is independent of the power wheelchair drive control interface; and hardware needed to attach the seating system to the wheelchair base.

E2301

E2301 Wheelchair accessory, power standing system, any type

Lay Description
A power standing system wheelchair accessory assists the patient in moving from a sitting to standing position. Power standing systems must have the ability to support a patient weight of at least 250 pounds. A power standing system consists of a solid seat platform and solid back; detachable or flip-up fixed height armrests; hinged legrests; anterior knee supports; fixed or flip-up foot plates; a motor and related electronics, with or without variable speed programmability; a basic switch control that is independent of the power wheelchair drive control interface; and any hardware that is needed to attach the seating system to the wheelchair base. A headrest is not included and should be reported additionally if supplied.

E2310-E2311

E2310 Power wheelchair accessory, electronic connection between wheelchair controller and one power seating system motor, including all related electronics, indicator feature, mechanical function selection switch, and fixed mounting hardware

E2311 Power wheelchair accessory, electronic connection between wheelchair controller and 2 or more power seating system motors, including all related electronics, indicator feature, mechanical function selection switch, and fixed mounting hardware

Lay Description
These codes describe electronic components that allow the patient to control two or more motors from a single interface using a proportional joystick, touchpad, or nonproportional interface. The motors that can be controlled from the electronic connection include power wheelchair drive, power tilt, power recline, power shear reduction, power leg elevation, power seat elevation, and power standing system. This type of wheelchair accessory includes a function selection switch that allows the patient to select the motor being controlled and an indicator feature to visually show which function has been selected. The indicator feature may also show the direction that has been selected (forward, reverse, left, right). The indicator feature may be in a separate display box or may be integrated into the wheelchair interface.

E

E2312

E2312 **Power wheelchair accessory, hand or chin control interface, mini-proportional remote joystick, proportional, including fixed mounting hardware**

Lay Description

A proportional interface is one in which the direction and amount of movement by the patient controls the direction and speed of the wheelchair. Mini proportional joysticks are small joysticks that require significantly less force and travel distance than a standard joystick. Joystick placement is typically by the hand, in line with an arm pad and parallel with the floor. When controlled by the chin, the gimbal is mounted on a swing-away mount of some sort and positioned slightly below and forward of the chin. Chin controls work much the same as conventional joysticks in that the user simply pushes the gimbal the direction he or she wants to go and controls speed by the distance the gimbal is pushed.

E2313

E2313 **Power wheelchair accessory, harness for upgrade to expandable controller, including all fasteners, connectors and mounting hardware, each**

Lay Description

A controller describes the microprocessor and related electronics that receive and interpret input from the drive control interface and converts that input into power output that controls speed and direction. The separate controller connects directly to the motors and batteries through a high power wire harness. An expandable controller is capable of accommodating one or more of the following additional functions: other types of proportional input devices, non-proportional input devices, and operate three or more powered seating actuators through the drive control. It may also operate a separate display (i.e., for alternate control devices), some other electronic devices, and an attendant control. This code is used to report the harness, including wires, fuses, fuse boxes, circuits, switches, and similar items that is required for the operation of the expandable controller.

E2321-E2322

E2321 **Power wheelchair accessory, hand control interface, remote joystick, nonproportional, including all related electronics, mechanical stop switch, and fixed mounting hardware**

E2322 **Power wheelchair accessory, hand control interface, multiple mechanical switches, nonproportional, including all related electronics, mechanical stop switch, and fixed mounting hardware**

Lay Description

An interface is the mechanism for controlling the movement of the power wheelchair of which there are a number of different types. These codes describe a nonproportional hand control interface that uses a remote joystick (E2321) or multiple mechanical switches (E2322). A remote joystick is one that is separate from the box containing the electronics that connects the interface to the motor and gears (controller box). A mechanical switch system describes a system with three to five mechanical switches that require physical contact to be activated. The switch selected determines the direction of the wheelchair. A mechanical direction change switch, if provided, is included in E2322. A nonproportional interface is a type of interface that allows the patient to control the direction of the wheelchair, but the speed is pre-programmed and cannot be affected by the user. The two nonproportional interface mechanisms described by E2321 and E2322 include all related electronics, mechanical stop switch, and the fixed mounting hardware.

E2323

E2323 **Power wheelchair accessory, specialty joystick handle for hand control interface, prefabricated**

Lay Description

A prefabricated specialty joystick handle has a shape other than a straight stick. U-shaped and T-shaped handles are reported with this code. Joysticks that have some other nonstandard feature such as a flexible shaft are also reported with E2323.

E2324

E2324 **Power wheelchair accessory, chin cup for chin control interface**

Lay Description

Wheelchair users who do not have the ability to control a joystick using hand or upper extremity motion can have the joystick modified with a chin cup that allows movement of the wheelchair to be controlled with the chin. The chin cup is attached to the joystick and reported additionally with E2324.

E2325-E2326

E2325 **Power wheelchair accessory, sip and puff interface, nonproportional, including all related electronics, mechanical stop switch, and manual swingaway mounting hardware**

E2326 **Power wheelchair accessory, breath tube kit for sip and puff interface**

Lay Description

A sip and puff interface is a nonproportional interface in which the patient holds a tube in the mouth and controls the wheelchair by sucking in (sip) or blowing out (puff). A nonproportional interface is a type of interface that allows the patient to control the direction of the wheelchair, but the speed is pre-programmed and cannot be affected by the user. Code E2325 reports the nonproportional sip and puff interface, all related electronics, a mechanical stop switch, and manual swing-away mounting hardware. The breath tube kit for the sip and puff interface is reported additionally with E2326.

E2327-E2328

E2327   **Power wheelchair accessory, head control interface, mechanical, proportional, including all related electronics, mechanical direction change switch, and fixed mounting hardware**

E2328   **Power wheelchair accessory, head control or extremity control interface, electronic, proportional, including all related electronics and fixed mounting hardware**

Lay Description
An interface is the mechanism for controlling the movement of the power wheelchair of which there are a number of different types. Code E2327 describes a mechanical, proportional, head control interface, and E2328 describes an electronic, proportional, head or extremity control interface. A proportional interface is directly controlled by the patient such that both direction and speed is controlled by the patient. A mechanical, proportional, head control interface (E2327) is one in which a headrest is attached to a joystick-like device. The direction and amount of movement of the patient's head pressing on the headrest controls the direction and speed of the wheelchair. An electronic, proportional, head control interface (E2328) is one in which a patient's head movements are sensed by a box placed behind the patient's head, and the direction and speed of the wheelchair are controlled by the sensors. The box does not come into direct contact with the patient's head. An electronic, proportional, extremity control interface, also reported with E2328, is one in which the direction and amount of movement of the patient's arm or leg control the direction and speed of the wheelchair. Interface mechanisms include all related electronics and the fixed mounting hardware. A mechanical direction control switch is included in E2327.

E2329-E2330

E2329   **Power wheelchair accessory, head control interface, contact switch mechanism, nonproportional, including all related electronics, mechanical stop switch, mechanical direction change switch, head array, and fixed mounting hardware**

E2330   **Power wheelchair accessory, head control interface, proximity switch mechanism, nonproportional, including all related electronics, mechanical stop switch, mechanical direction change switch, head array, and fixed mounting hardware**

Lay Description
An interface is the mechanism for controlling the movement of the power wheelchair of which there

are a number of different types. Code E2329 describes a nonproportional, contact switch, head control interface, and E2330 describes a nonproportional, proximity switch, head control interface. A nonproportional interface is a type of interface that allows the patient to control the direction of the wheelchair, but the speed is preprogrammed and cannot be affected by the user. A nonproportional, contact switch, head control interface (E2329) is one in which the patient activates one of three mechanical switches placed around the back and sides of the head. These switches are activated by pressure of the head against the switch. The switch that is selected determines the direction of the wheelchair. A nonproportional, proximity switch, head control interface (E2330) is one in which the patient activates one of three switches placed around the back and sides of the head. These switches are activated by movement of the head toward the switch, though the head does not touch the switch. The switch that is selected determines the direction of the wheelchair. Both interface mechanisms include all related electronics, mechanical stop switch, mechanical direction change switch, head array, and the fixed mounting hardware.

E2331

E2331   **Power wheelchair accessory, attendant control, proportional, including all related electronics and fixed mounting hardware**

Lay Description
An attendant control for a power wheelchair allows a caregiver to drive the wheelchair instead of the patient. The attendant control is usually mounted on one of the rear canes of the wheelchair. Attendant control devices are proportional controls, allowing the attendant to control both the direction and the speed of the wheelchair, usually by means of a joystick. All related electronics and fixed mounting hardware are included.

E2340-E2343

E2340   **Power wheelchair accessory, nonstandard seat frame width, 20-23 in**

E2341   **Power wheelchair accessory, nonstandard seat frame width, 24-27 in**

E2342   **Power wheelchair accessory, nonstandard seat frame depth, 20 or 21 in**

E2343   **Power wheelchair accessory, nonstandard seat frame depth, 22-25 in**

Lay Description
A specially sized or constructed wheelchair component is indicated for patients when the measurements of a standard wheelchair do not accommodate the patient's needs. This wheelchair must be justified by reasons such as a patient's physical size or the specific requirements for wheelchair usage in the patient's place of residence, such as narrow doorways that prevent the passage of

a standard wheelchair. The standard seat height from the floor is 18 to 20 inches. The standard seat width and depth is 15 to 19 inches. When a deviation is more than 2 inches from the standard, the sizing is nonstandard.

E2351

E2351 **Power wheelchair accessory, electronic interface to operate speech generating device using power wheelchair control interface**

Lay Description

An electronic interface is a device that allows the power wheelchair controls to operate a speech generating device. Speech generating devices are electronic systems that enable individuals with severe speech impairment to verbally communicate their needs. There are multiple methods of accessing messages on devices, which can be done directly, indirectly, and with specialized access devices. The method depends on the skills and abilities of the communicator.

E2358-E2365, E2371-E2372

E2358 **Power wheelchair accessory, group 34 nonsealed lead acid battery, each**

E2359 **Power wheelchair accessory, group 34 sealed lead acid battery, each (e.g., gel cell, absorbed glass mat)**

E2360 **Power wheelchair accessory, 22 NF nonsealed lead acid battery, each**

E2361 **Power wheelchair accessory, 22 NF sealed lead acid battery, each (e.g., gel cell, absorbed glassmat)**

E2362 **Power wheelchair accessory, group 24 nonsealed lead acid battery, each**

E2363 **Power wheelchair accessory, group 24 sealed lead acid battery, each (e.g., gel cell, absorbed glassmat)**

E2364 **Power wheelchair accessory, U-1 nonsealed lead acid battery, each**

E2365 **Power wheelchair accessory, U-1 sealed lead acid battery, each (e.g., gel cell, absorbed glassmat)**

E2371 **Power wheelchair accessory, group 27 sealed lead acid battery, (e.g., gel cell, absorbed glassmat), each**

E2372 **Power wheelchair accessory, group 27 nonsealed lead acid battery, each**

Lay Description

Lead-acid batteries are physically large batteries that contain lead plates in a solution of acid to create electricity. During normal operation, water is lost from a non-sealed (or flooded) battery due to evaporation. They are also known as flooded, vented, or wet-cell batteries. Since they are not sealed, water must be frequently added. If inverted, the contents can spill out. These used to be the most common type of battery, but now they are seen as old fashioned and

are becoming less common. Sealed batteries are known as maintenance free batteries. Sealed lead acid (SLA) batteries are valve-regulated, which fixes the acid electrolyte in a gel or in an absorptive fiberglass mat. The advantages of this design are that the battery needs no added water, can be operated in any position, and can be used in close proximity to people and sensitive equipment. Gelled batteries contain acid that has been "gelled" by the addition of Silica Gel, turning the acid into a solid mass that looks like gooey Jell-O. The advantage of these batteries is that it is impossible to spill acid even if they are broken. Absorbed glass mat is a very fine fiber Boron-Silicate glass mat. These type of batteries have all the advantages of gelled, but can take much more abuse.

E2366-E2367

E2366 **Power wheelchair accessory, battery charger, single mode, for use with only one battery type, sealed or nonsealed, each**

E2367 **Power wheelchair accessory, battery charger, dual mode, for use with either battery type, sealed or nonsealed, each**

Lay Description

A battery charger is a device that replenishes battery energy by forcing an electric current through it. There are three different main types of batteries: wet battery, gel battery, and the absorbed glass mat battery. A different battery charger is required for each model.

E2368

E2368 **Power wheelchair component, drive wheel motor, replacement only**

Lay Description

A motor is a machine that converts energy into useful mechanical motion. In a power wheelchair, motors provide the energy needed to propel the chair. Normally a motor is included in the purchase of a motored wheelchair.

E2369

E2369 **Power wheelchair component, drive wheel gear box, replacement only**

Lay Description

A gearbox is a protective casing for a system consisting of a collection of mechanical components that deliver maximum power from a motor by managing a series of gear ratios that in turn operate a transmission. These components include a gear selector, fork, collar, dog teeth, and a gear set.

E2370

E2370 Power wheelchair component, integrated drive wheel motor and gear box combination, replacement only

Lay Description
A motor is a machine that converts energy into useful mechanical motion. In a power wheelchair, motors provide the energy needed to propel the chair. A gearbox is a protective casing for a system consisting of a collection of mechanical components that deliver maximum power from a motor by managing a series of gear ratios that in turn operate a transmission. These components include a gear selector, fork, collar, dog teeth, and a gear set. Normally a motor and gearbox are included in the purchase of a motored wheelchair.

E2371-E2372

E2371 Power wheelchair accessory, group 27 sealed lead acid battery, (e.g., gel cell, absorbed glassmat), each

E2372 Power wheelchair accessory, group 27 nonsealed lead acid battery, each

Lay Description
Please refer to codes E2358-E2372 for the description.

E2373-E2374

E2373 Power wheelchair accessory, hand or chin control interface, compact remote joystick, proportional, including fixed mounting hardware

E2374 Power wheelchair accessory, hand or chin control interface, standard remote joystick (not including controller), proportional, including all related electronics and fixed mounting hardware, replacement only

Lay Description
An interface is the mechanism for controlling the movement of the power wheelchair of which there are a number of different types. This code describes a proportional hand or chin control interface that uses a remote joystick or touchpad. A proportional interface is directly controlled by the patient such that both direction and speed is controlled by the patient moving the joystick or using the touchpad. A remote joystick is separate from the box containing the electronics that connects the interface to the motor and gears (controller box), and encompasses a standard joystick or one that can be controlled by small movements. The latter type may be mini-proportional, compact, or short throw joystick. The second type of interface described by this code is a touchpad similar to the pad-type mouse found on laptop computers. Interface mechanisms include all related electronics and the fixed mounting hardware. The chin cup is reported separately with E2324.

E2375-E2378

E2375 Power wheelchair accessory, nonexpandable controller, including all related electronics and mounting hardware, replacement only

E2376 Power wheelchair accessory, expandable controller, including all related electronics and mounting hardware, replacement only

E2377 Power wheelchair accessory, expandable controller, including all related electronics and mounting hardware, upgrade provided at initial issue

E2378 Power wheelchair component, actuator, replacement only

Lay Description
A controller describes the microprocessor and related electronics that receive and interpret input from the joystick (or some other drive control interface) and converts that input into power output that controls speed and direction. The separate controller connects directly to the motors and batteries through a high-power wire harness. A nonexpandable controller may have the ability to control up to two power seating actuators through the drive control and may allow for the incorporation of an attendant control. It is also capable of accommodating one or more other types of proportional input devices, nonproportional input devices, and operating three or more powered seating actuators through the drive control. A nonexpandable controller may also operate a separate display (i.e., for alternate control devices), some other electronic devices, and an attendant control.

E2381-E2382

E2381 Power wheelchair accessory, pneumatic drive wheel tire, any size, replacement only, each

E2382 Power wheelchair accessory, tube for pneumatic drive wheel tire, any size, replacement only, each

Lay Description
Drive wheels come in three positions on a power wheelchair: rear-wheel drive, mid-wheel drive, and front-wheel drive. A pneumatic tire is a rubber tire used in conjunction with a separate tube that is filled with air.

E2383

E2383 Power wheelchair accessory, insert for pneumatic drive wheel tire (removable), any type, any size, replacement only, each

Lay Description
A pneumonic tire comes with an airless insert that is soft rubber or a latex gel that replaces the inner tube. This is also known as a flat free insert. This removable ring of firm material placed inside of a pneumatic tire allows a wheelchair to continue to move if the

pneumatic tire is punctured. This type of tire insert is sometimes referred to as a flat free insert or a zero pressure tube.

E2384

E2384   Power wheelchair accessory, pneumatic caster tire, any size, replacement only, each

Lay Description

A pneumatic caster tire is made of an annular tube of flexible fabric, such as India rubber, and filled with compressed air. A pneumatic caster tire is a shock absorbing wheel that absorbs vibrations thus providing a smooth cushioned ride and quiet operation. A caster is a smaller wheel that is in contact with the ground during normal operation of the wheelchair and that is not directly controlled by the motor. It may be in the front and/or rear, depending on the location of the drive wheel.

E2385

E2385   Power wheelchair accessory, tube for pneumatic caster tire, any size, replacement only, each

Lay Description

A caster is a smaller wheel that is in contact with the ground during normal operation of the wheelchair and is not directly controlled by the motor. It may be in the front and/or rear, depending on the location of the drive wheel. A pneumatic caster tire is formed of an annular tube of flexible fabric, such as India rubber, suitable to be inflated with air. A tube for a pneumatic tire is an inflatable rubber tube that fits inside the casing of a pneumatic tire. This inner tube keeps the tire airtight.

E2386

E2386   Power wheelchair accessory, foam filled drive wheel tire, any size, replacement only, each

Lay Description

Drive wheels come in three positions: rear-wheel drive, mid-wheel drive, and front-wheel drive on a power wheelchair. A foam filled drive wheel tire is a rubber tire shell that has been filled with foam that is nonremovable.

E2387

E2387   Power wheelchair accessory, foam filled caster tire, any size, replacement only, each

Lay Description

A caster tire is a smaller wheel that is in contact with the ground during normal operation of the wheelchair and is not directly controlled by the motor. It may be in the front and/or rear, depending on the location of the drive wheel. A foam filled caster tire is a rubber tire shell filled with foam that is nonremovable.

E2388

E2388   Power wheelchair accessory, foam drive wheel tire, any size, replacement only, each

Lay Description

Drive wheels come in three positions: rear-wheel drive, mid-wheel drive, and front-wheel drive on a power wheelchair. A foam tire is made entirely of self-skinning urethane.

E2389

E2389   Power wheelchair accessory, foam caster tire, any size, replacement only, each

Lay Description

A caster tire is a smaller wheel that is in contact with the ground during normal operation of the wheelchair and is not directly controlled by the motor. It may be in the front and/or rear, depending on the location of the drive wheel. A foam tire is made entirely of self-skinning urethane.

E2390

E2390   Power wheelchair accessory, solid (rubber/plastic) drive wheel tire, any size, replacement only, each

Lay Description

Drive wheels come in three positions: rear-wheel drive, mid-wheel drive, and front-wheel drive on a power wheelchair. This solid tire is made of hard plastic or rubber.

E2391

E2391   Power wheelchair accessory, solid (rubber/plastic) caster tire (removable), any size, replacement only, each

Lay Description

A caster is a smaller wheel that is in contact with the ground during normal operation of the wheelchair and is not directly controlled by the motor. It may be in the front and/or rear, depending on the location of the drive wheel. This solid tire is made of hard plastic or rubber. This code is for replacement of a solid (rubber/plastic) caster tire.

E2392

E2392   Power wheelchair accessory, solid (rubber/plastic) caster tire with integrated wheel, any size, replacement only, each

Lay Description

A caster is a smaller wheel that is in contact with the ground during normal operation of the wheelchair and is not directly controlled by the motor. It may be in the front and/or rear, depending on the location of the drive wheel. This solid caster tire is made of hard plastic or rubber. The integrated caster has the tire attached to the wheel as one unit. This code is for replacement of a solid (rubber/plastic) caster tire with an integrated wheel.

E2394

E2394 **Power wheelchair accessory, drive wheel excludes tire, any size, replacement only, each**

Lay Description
Drive wheel refers to the position of the wheels to which the motors are attached. In rear wheel drives wheelchairs, the drive wheels are located at the very back of the chair. In mid wheel drive wheelchairs, the drive wheels are located under the chair toward the center with smaller wheels (casters) in the front and behind. In front wheel drive wheelchairs, the drive wheels are located at the front of the chair with casters behind.

E2395

E2395 **Power wheelchair accessory, caster wheel excludes tire, any size, replacement only, each**

Lay Description
A caster wheel is a small wheel that is in contact with the ground during normal operation of the wheelchair and cannot be used for arm propulsion.

E2396

E2396 **Power wheelchair accessory, caster fork, any size, replacement only, each**

Lay Description
Wheelchair caster wheels are mounted to a caster fork assembly. A caster fork assembly consists of the fork, the caster stem bolt (the long bolt coming up from the top of the fork), caster stem bearings, and sometimes a spacer or spacers.

E2397

E2397 **Power wheelchair accessory, lithium-based battery, each**

Lay Description
Lithium-ion is a low maintenance battery made from chemicals. Lithium-ion batteries have no memory effect and do not use poisonous metals, such as lead, mercury, or cadmium. They require little to no maintenance, and can pack a lot of voltage into a small area. However, they are particularly fragile in nature and need to be protected from extreme temperatures.

E2402

E2402 **Negative pressure wound therapy electrical pump, stationary or portable**

Lay Description
Negative pressure wound therapy (NPWT) is controlled application of subatmospheric pressure to wounds. A pump continuously or intermittently carries subatmospheric pressure through connected tubes directly to a specialized wound dressing. A canister collects the drainage from the wound. NPWT promotes healing of chronic wounds and decubitus ulcers. Controlled pressure of the wound increases vascularity and oxygenation of the wound bed thus reducing edema by getting rid of the wound fluid and removing exudate and bacteria.

E2500-E2510

E2500 **Speech generating device, digitized speech, using prerecorded messages, less than or equal to 8 minutes recording time**

E2502 **Speech generating device, digitized speech, using prerecorded messages, greater than 8 minutes but less than or equal to 20 minutes recording time**

E2504 **Speech generating device, digitized speech, using prerecorded messages, greater than 20 minutes but less than or equal to 40 minutes recording time**

E2506 **Speech generating device, digitized speech, using prerecorded messages, greater than 40 minutes recording time**

E2508 **Speech generating device, synthesized speech, requiring message formulation by spelling and access by physical contact with the device**

E2510 **Speech generating device, synthesized speech, permitting multiple methods of message formulation and multiple methods of device access**

Lay Description
Speech generating devices, also called communication devices, enable an individual to communicate with others more effectively. There are many devices that assist individuals by using speech or voice output and other combinations of assistance. Speech generating devices have been created for individuals who cannot speak, are difficult to understand, or have language retrieval issues. Digitized speech devices are referred to as devices with "whole message" speech output. Digitized speech devices utilize words and phrases that have been pre-recorded by someone other than the user and used for playback by the user. Synthesized speech devices translate a user's input into device-generated speech. Users of synthesized speech devices are not limited to prerecorded messages but can independently create messages as their own communication needs arise. These devices require the user to use a keyboard, touch screen, or other display containing an alphanumeric display. Synthesized speech devices allow the user different methods of message formulation and many methods of access. These methods of message formulation must include the capability for message selection by two or more of the following methods: letters, words, pictures, or symbols. Multiple methods of access must include the capability to access the device by two or more of the following methods: entering information by a

E

keyboard, touch screen, or indirect selection techniques via a specialized access device such as a joystick, a head-mouse, an optical head-pointer, a switch, a light pointer, an infrared pointer, a scanning device, or Morse code.

E2511

E2511 Speech generating software program, for personal computer or personal digital assistant

Lay Description
Speech generating software allows laptops and/or desktop computers or personal digital assistant (PDA) devices to function as a speech generating device. The information can be entered with a pen based system using a stylus and handwriting recognition software, keyboard, downloaded from a computer using special cables, and software.

E2512

E2512 Accessory for speech generating device, mounting system

Lay Description
A mounting system for a speech generating device is a mechanism for fastening the speech generating device to the wheelchair. Generally mounting systems consist of three parts: a mounting block, which attaches to the wheelchair frame; a tubing system, which provides the majority of positioning; and a mounting plate, which attaches to the device.

E2599

E2599 Accessory for speech generating device, not otherwise classified

Lay Description
Report this code for any accessory for a speech generating device that is not described in other HCPCS Level II codes.

E2601-E2602

E2601 General use wheelchair seat cushion, width less than 22 in, any depth

E2602 General use wheelchair seat cushion, width 22 in or greater, any depth

Lay Description
A general use wheelchair seat cushion is a static, prefabricated cushion. Several cushion types exist: planar, contoured, and molded. A planar surface offers the least support and pressure relief, but may require the least experience and is simplest to maintain. A contoured surface assumes contour with pressure through the use of foam, air, or gel within the cushion, or it may be preformed. It provides more support than the planar surface, and is more adjustable than the molded surface. A molded seat is created from liquid foam that follows the direct contours of the specific user. It offers the most support for an individual with reduced trunk control and may be formed to accommodate fixed deformities. Wheelchair seat cushions can provide leg positioning, pelvic stability, and pressure management for patients with postural asymmetry. A cushion may provide high-end protection for individuals considered prone to developing skin breakdown. The size of a standard adult wheelchair seat has a seat width of 18 inches, seat depth of 16 inches, and seat height of 20 inches.

E2603-E2604

E2603 Skin protection wheelchair seat cushion, width less than 22 in, any depth

E2604 Skin protection wheelchair seat cushion, width 22 in or greater, any depth

Lay Description
A skin protection wheelchair seat cushion is a static, prefabricated cushion. A skin protection seat cushion usually uses high-grade polyurethane foam and a gel solution or puffed layer to provide high-end protection for individuals considered prone to developing skin breakdown. A skin protection seat cushion is beneficial if a person has a past history of or current pressure ulcer on the area of contact with the seating surface, absent or impaired sensation in the area of contact with the seating surface, or significant postural asymmetries.

E2605-E2606

E2605 Positioning wheelchair seat cushion, width less than 22 in, any depth

E2606 Positioning wheelchair seat cushion, width 22 in or greater, any depth

Lay Description
A positioning seat cushion is a static, prefabricated cushion. Positioning seat cushions provide leg, hip, and pelvic positioning and stability, and pressure management for patients with postural asymmetry. A positioning seat cushion is beneficial to a person who has significant postural asymmetries, providing seat stabilization, positioning, pressure reduction, and correct seating posture.

E2607-E2608

E2607 Skin protection and positioning wheelchair seat cushion, width less than 22 in, any depth

E2608 Skin protection and positioning wheelchair seat cushion, width 22 in or greater, any depth

Lay Description
A skin protection positioning wheelchair seat cushion is a static, prefabricated cushion. A skin protection seat cushion usually uses high-grade polyurethane foam and a gel solution or puffed layer to provide high-end protection for individuals considered prone to developing skin breakdown while affording the positioning and stability necessary for the leg, hip, and pelvis. A skin protection positioning seat cushion is beneficial if a person has a past history of or current

pressure ulcer on the area of contact with the seating surface, absent or impaired sensation in the area of contact with the seating surface, or significant postural asymmetries.

E2609

E2609   Custom fabricated wheelchair seat cushion, any size

Lay Description

Custom made seats for a wheelchair (e.g., custom fabricated from an impression or digital image of a specific body part) are indicated when the user has gross spinal deformities and/or severely impaired sitting ability.

E2610

E2610   Wheelchair seat cushion, powered

Lay Description

A powered wheelchair seat cushion is a prefabricated, battery-powered cushion in which an air pump provides sequential inflation and deflation of the air cells or a low interface pressure throughout the cushion. An alternating pressure cushion is one type of powered seat cushion.

E2611-E2612

E2611   General use wheelchair back cushion, width less than 22 in, any height, including any type mounting hardware

E2612   General use wheelchair back cushion, width 22 in or greater, any height, including any type mounting hardware

Lay Description

A general use wheelchair back is a static, prefabricated cushion that functions as a comfortable, supportive positioning device and provides pressure relief to the wheelchair user.

E2613-E2614

E2613   Positioning wheelchair back cushion, posterior, width less than 22 in, any height, including any type mounting hardware

E2614   Positioning wheelchair back cushion, posterior, width 22 in or greater, any height, including any type mounting hardware

Lay Description

A posterior positioning wheelchair back cushion aids in back support and is designed to provide posterior lateral pelvic stabilization, along with better trunk stability.

E2615-E2616

E2615   Positioning wheelchair back cushion, posterior-lateral, width less than 22 in, any height, including any type mounting hardware

E2616   Positioning wheelchair back cushion, posterior-lateral, width 22 in or greater, any height, including any type mounting hardware

Lay Description

A posterior-lateral positioning wheelchair back cushion aids in back support and is designed to provide posterior lateral pelvic stabilization, along with better trunk stability.

E2617

E2617   Custom fabricated wheelchair back cushion, any size, including any type mounting hardware

Lay Description

Custom-fabricated wheelchair back cushions provide positioning and/or pressure relief that cannot be met with a prefabricated cushion. They are fabricated using molded-to-patient-model techniques to create a configured cushion.

E2619

E2619   Replacement cover for wheelchair seat cushion or back cushion, each

Lay Description

A universal wheelchair cushion cover is made of durable material that is soft to the touch and is fluid-proof with a non-skid base material. A heavy duty cushion cover is made to protect the cushion from rough wear and tear and incontinence with fluid-resisting material and durable construction.

E2620-E2621

E2620   Positioning wheelchair back cushion, planar back with lateral supports, width less than 22 in, any height, including any type mounting hardware

E2621   Positioning wheelchair back cushion, planar back with lateral supports, width 22 in or greater, any height, including any type mounting hardware

Lay Description

A planar back with lateral supports on a positioning wheelchair refers to a modification in the back support to allow various lateral supports to be mounted.

E2622-E2623

E2622 Skin protection wheelchair seat cushion, adjustable, width less than 22 in, any depth

E2623 Skin protection wheelchair seat cushion, adjustable, width 22 in or greater, any depth

Lay Description

Adjustable wheelchair seat cushions provide skin protection and comfort for individuals who must sit for long periods of time. Adjustable cushions are those that can be adapted to conform to the specific requirements of the individual. Cushions can be constructed of a variety of materials including rubber, foam, gel-foam, and polyester fiber-filled cores with adjustable air pads that allow the user to control the cushion fit. Some cushions have dual air controls that allow the side and center to be inflated to differing levels.

E2624-E2625

E2624 Skin protection and positioning wheelchair seat cushion, adjustable, width less than 22 in, any depth

E2625 Skin protection and positioning wheelchair seat cushion, adjustable, width 22 in or greater, any depth

Lay Description

Adjustable positioning wheelchair seat cushions provide skin protection and positioning for individuals with paralysis, deformities, scoliosis, poor muscle control, or other conditions. Positioning seat cushions can aid in manipulation or control of objects, can assist in the performance of specific activities, and can provide added balance and support. Adjustable cushions are those that can be adapted to conform to the specific requirements of the individual. Cushions can be constructed of a variety of materials including rubber, foam, gel-foam, and polyester fiber-filled cores with adjustable air pads that allow the user to control the cushion fit. Some cushions have dual air controls that allow the sides and center to be inflated to differing levels.

E2626-E2632

E2626 Wheelchair accessory, shoulder elbow, mobile arm support attached to wheelchair, balanced, adjustable

E2627 Wheelchair accessory, shoulder elbow, mobile arm support attached to wheelchair, balanced, adjustable Rancho type

E2628 Wheelchair accessory, shoulder elbow, mobile arm support attached to wheelchair, balanced, reclining

E2629 Wheelchair accessory, shoulder elbow, mobile arm support attached to wheelchair, balanced, friction arm support (friction dampening to proximal and distal joints)

E2630 Wheelchair accessory, shoulder elbow, mobile arm support, monosuspension arm and hand support, overhead elbow forearm hand sling support, yoke type suspension support

E2631 Wheelchair accessory, addition to mobile arm support, elevating proximal arm

E2632 Wheelchair accessory, addition to mobile arm support, offset or lateral rocker arm with elastic balance control

Lay Description

A shoulder-elbow-wrist-hand orthosis (SEWHO) is used for the purpose of supporting injured, post-surgical, and/or weak or deformed areas of the shoulder, elbow, wrist, or hand. These codes may be similar in design, depending on the manufacturer and the intended application. These bracing devices are attached to wheelchairs, typically containing hardware such as aluminum or other lightweight arm supports for the desired degree of abduction, as well as plastic, polyethylene, or foam. These devices may use the patient torso or neck as an anchor, as well as the phalanges. There may be hinges at certain points in the device to allow for a certain degree of elbow or wrist motion. The treating provider must initially apply these items, but a person other than the patient can be instructed in the proper application when/if the patient removes the device during specified intervals. Sizes can vary according to the manufacturer (there may be pediatric sizes as well). The items are generally manufactured in right and left models. Shoulder braces with arm, elbow, and wrist immobilization support and control the range of motion of the upper extremity, including the upper arm, scapula, clavicle, elbow, forearm, and/or wrist. They also support most muscles and ligamentous tissues related to the movement of the upper extremity. They maintain a degree of abduction between the patient's torso and the affected upper limb, at the degree desired (usually 45-90 degrees). Each of these devices typically leaves the fingers free, but grasping heavy items is usually unable to be accomplished and is not advised. They are used posttraumatically for severe fractures and for certain types of surgical procedures, such as partial or total shoulder replacement. A prefabricated or custom fitted orthosis is one that the manufacturer has produced in quantity, without a specific patient in mind. A prefabricated orthosis may be trimmed, bent, molded (with or without heat), or otherwise modified for use by a specific patient (i.e., custom fitted). An orthosis that is assembled from prefabricated components is considered prefabricated. Any orthosis that does not meet the definition of a custom fabricated orthosis is considered prefabricated. A custom fabricated orthosis is one that is individually made for a specific patient, starting with basic materials including, but not limited to, plastic, metal, leather, or cloth in the form of sheets, bars, and so forth. It involves substantial work, such as cutting, bending, molding, sewing, and so forth. It may involve the incorporation of some prefabricated components. It involves more than trimming, bending, or making other modifications to a substantially prefabricated item. A molded-to-patient-model orthosis is a particular type of custom fabricated orthosis in which an impression of the specific body part is made (by means of a plaster cast, CAD-CAM technology, etc.). These codes describe shoulder-elbow-wrist-hand orthoses that are supports attached to a wheelchair.

E2633

E2633   Wheelchair accessory, addition to mobile arm support, supinator

Lay Description
An arm supinator is an accessory that attaches to a wheelchair and replaces the forearm swivel. It allows the patient's arm to be rotated to a palm up position.

E8000-E8002

E8000   Gait trainer, pediatric size, posterior support, includes all accessories and components

E8001   Gait trainer, pediatric size, upright support, includes all accessories and components

E8002   Gait trainer, pediatric size, anterior support, includes all accessories and components

Lay Description
A gait trainer is a device that allows patients to move about freely using their own legs. Each gait trainer should be specifically sized for the individual patient and is used in different therapy modalities for gait restoration. A gait trainer supports each patient according to ability and controls the center of mass in the vertical and horizontal directions.

G

G0008

G0008   Administration of influenza virus vaccine

Lay Description
Use this code to report the administration of an influenza virus vaccine. Do not bill an office visit if the only reason for the visit was to receive a vaccination.

G0009

G0009   Administration of pneumococcal vaccine

Lay Description
Use this code to report the administration of a pneumococcal vaccine. Do not bill an office visit if the only reason for the visit was to receive a vaccination.

G0010

G0010   Administration of hepatitis B vaccine

Lay Description
Use this code to report the administration of a hepatitis B vaccine on a day when no other service is performed for which there is a physician fee schedule set.

G0027

G0027   Semen analysis; presence and/or motility of sperm excluding Huhner

Lay Description
Semen analysis is the microscopic examination of semen for the presence, quality, and mobility of the sperm contained within the semen. This is usually performed to determine if this is the source of infertility.

G0101

G0101   Cervical or vaginal cancer screening; pelvic and clinical breast examination

Lay Description
This code reports a cervical or vaginal cancer screening and a pelvic and clinical breast examination. The specimen for cancer screening is collected by cervical, endocervical, or vaginal scrapings or by aspiration of vaginal fluid and cells. The pelvic and breast exams are done manually by the physician to check for abnormalities, pain, and/or any palpable lumps or masses.

G0102

G0102   Prostate cancer screening; digital rectal examination

Lay Description
This code reports a prostate cancer screening performed manually by the physician as a digital rectal exam in order to palpate the prostate and check for abnormalities.

G0103

G0103   Prostate cancer screening; prostate specific antigen test (PSA)

Lay Description
This code reports a total prostate specific antigen (PSA) test for cancer screening. The specimen collection is by venipuncture. Methods may include radioimmunoassay (RIA) and monoclonal two-site immunoradiometric assay. There are several forms of PSA present in serum. PSA may be complexed with the protease inhibitor alpha-1 antichymotrypsin (PSA-ACT) or found in a free form. Higher levels of free PSA are more often associated with benign conditions than with cancer. Total PSA measures both complexed and free levels to provide a total amount present in the serum. A percentage of each form is sometimes calculated to help distinguish benign from malignant conditions.

G

G0104

G0104 Colorectal cancer screening; flexible sigmoidoscopy

Lay Description
A flexible sigmoidoscopy is performed for colorectal cancer screening. After the patient's bowel has been prepped, the physician inserts the flexible sigmoidoscope through the anus and advances the scope into the sigmoid colon. The lumen of the sigmoid colon and rectum are visualized and brushings or washings may be obtained. The sigmoidoscope is withdrawn.

G0105

G0105 Colorectal cancer screening; colonoscopy on individual at high risk

Lay Description
A colonoscopy is performed on a high-risk patient for colorectal cancer screening. A high-risk patient is one with ulcerative enteritis or a history of malignant neoplasm of the lower gastrointestinal tract. After the patient's bowel has been prepped, the physician inserts the colonoscope through the anus and advances the scope through the colon past the splenic flexure. The lumen of the colon and rectum is visualized. Brushings or washings may be obtained. The colonoscope is withdrawn.

G0106

G0106 Colorectal cancer screening; alternative to G0104, screening sigmoidoscopy, barium enema

Lay Description
A colorectal screening for cancer is performed via barium enema as an alternative to a screening sigmoidoscopy (G0104). This is a radiological exam of the large intestine carried out after the administration of a barium enema to instill the contrast medium into the colon. Fluoroscopy and x-rays are used to observe the images as the contrast fills the colon and helps the physician to diagnose cancer, even colitis, and other diseases. After the patient has emptied the colon, more films are taken.

G0108-G0109

G0108 Diabetes outpatient self-management training services, individual, per 30 minutes

G0109 Diabetes outpatient self-management training services, group session (2 or more), per 30 minutes

Lay Description
These codes are for diabetes self-management training services, either individually or in a group of two or more. Diabetes self-management training is done to teach the diabetic how to control and monitor blood glucose levels with the proper use of the monitoring device, dietary calculations and restrictions, and correct administration of diabetic medications. These codes are reported per 30 minute intervals.

G0117-G0118

G0117 Glaucoma screening for high risk patients furnished by an optometrist or ophthalmologist

G0118 Glaucoma screening for high risk patient furnished under the direct supervision of an optometrist or ophthalmologist

Lay Description
Glaucoma screening is performed on a high-risk patient. Glaucoma is a progressive eye disorder, without signs or symptoms in its earlier stages, that leads to irreversible vision loss. Aqueous pressure in the anterior chamber of a healthy eye remains constant even though it is continually being flushed and renewed. Too little or too much fluid can cause permanent damage. In a test for glaucoma, the patient drinks one quart of water after fasting and then the intraocular pressure of the eye is measured. The patient may also be placed in a dark room, where the eyes are rechecked once they have sufficiently dilated. This determines if fluids in the eyes are at proper levels. High risk factors are related to age, family history, and personal medical history, such as diabetes, previous eye injury, and use of certain medications such as steroids.

G0120

G0120 Colorectal cancer screening; alternative to G0105, screening colonoscopy, barium enema

Lay Description
A colorectal screening for cancer is performed via barium enema as an alternative to a screening colonoscopy on a high-risk individual (G0105). This is a radiological exam of the large intestine carried out after the administration of a barium enema to instill the contrast medium into the colon. Fluoroscopy and x-rays are used to observe the images as the contrast fills the colon and helps the physician to diagnose cancer, even colitis, and other diseases. After the patient has emptied the colon, more films are taken.

G0121

G0121 Colorectal cancer screening; colonoscopy on individual not meeting criteria for high risk

Lay Description
A colonoscopy is performed for colorectal cancer screening on a patient who does not meet high-risk criteria. This would be a patient without a diagnosis of ulcerative enteritis or without a history of malignant neoplasm of the lower gastrointestinal tract. After the patient's bowel has been prepped, the physician inserts the colonoscope through the anus and advances the scope through the colon past the

splenic flexure. The lumen of the colon and rectum is visualized. Brushings or washings may be obtained. The colonoscope is withdrawn.

G0122

G0122 Colorectal cancer screening; barium enema

Lay Description
A colorectal screening for cancer is done via barium enema. This is a radiological exam of the large intestine carried out after the administration of a barium enema to instill the contrast medium into the colon. Fluoroscopy and x-rays are used to observe the images as the contrast fills the colon and helps the physician to diagnose cancer, even colitis, and other diseases. After the patient has emptied the colon, more films are taken.

G0123-G0124

G0123 Screening cytopathology, cervical or vaginal (any reporting system), collected in preservative fluid, automated thin layer preparation, screening by cytotechnologist under physician supervision

G0124 Screening cytopathology, cervical or vaginal (any reporting system), collected in preservative fluid, automated thin layer preparation, requiring interpretation by physician

Lay Description
These cervical or vaginal cytopathology screenings (any reporting system) of specimens collected in preservative fluid may be identified as "thin prep." The specimen is collected by cervical, endocervical, or vaginal scrapings or by aspiration of vaginal fluid and cells. This method saves time by eliminating the need for the physician to prepare a smear; the specimen is placed in a preservative suspension instead. At the laboratory, special instruments take the cells in the preservative suspension and "plate-out" a monolayer for screening, which will carefully review the specimen for abnormal cells.

G0127

G0127 Trimming of dystrophic nails, any number

Lay Description
A physician trims fingernails or toenails usually with scissors, nail cutters, or other instruments when the nails are defective and dystrophic from nutritional or metabolic abnormalities. Report this code for any number of nails trimmed.

G0128

G0128 Direct (face-to-face with patient) skilled nursing services of a registered nurse provided in a comprehensive outpatient rehabilitation facility, each 10 minutes beyond the first 5 minutes

Lay Description
This code reports direct one-on-one skilled nursing services provided to the patient by a registered nurse in a comprehensive outpatient rehabilitation facility. Report this code as a unit of 10 minutes, for each 10 minutes beyond the initial 5 minutes.

G0129

G0129 Occupational therapy services requiring the skills of a qualified occupational therapist, furnished as a component of a partial hospitalization treatment program, per session (45 minutes or more)

Lay Description
Occupational therapy focuses on helping a person recovering from a serious illness or injury retain movement capabilities for independently managing the activities of daily life. Report this code per day that treatment was given.

G0130

G0130 Single energy x-ray absorptiometry (SEXA) bone density study, one or more sites; appendicular skeleton (peripheral) (e.g., radius, wrist, heel)

Lay Description
Bone mineral density studies are used to evaluate diseases of bone and/or the responses of bone disease to treatment. Densities are measured at the wrist, radius, hip, pelvis, spine, or heel. The studies assess bone mass or density associated with such diseases as osteoporosis, osteomalacia, and renal osteodystrophy. Single energy x-ray absorptiometry (SEXA) utilizes an x-ray tube as the radiation source that is pulsed at a certain energy level. SEXA is used to scan bone that is in a superficial location with little adjacent soft tissue, such as the wrist or heel. There is a differential attenuation between bone and soft tissue for the energy beam. Excessive soft tissue renders the measurement incorrect. An attenuation profile of the bony components is calculated and the results are given in two scores, which are reported as standard deviations from the normal bone density of a person the same sex, 30 years old, which is the age of peak bone mass, and from the normal bone density of an "age matched" that compares the patient's bone density to what is expected in someone the same age, sex, and size.

G

G0141, G0147-G0148

G0141   Screening cytopathology smears, cervical or vaginal, performed by automated system, with manual rescreening, requiring interpretation by physician

G0147   Screening cytopathology smears, cervical or vaginal, performed by automated system under physician supervision

G0148   Screening cytopathology smears, cervical or vaginal, performed by automated system with manual rescreening

Lay Description

These cervical or vaginal cytopathology screenings are done on specimens prepared in a smear. The specimen is collected by cervical, endocervical, or vaginal scrapings or by aspiration of vaginal fluid and cells. The screening method is microscopy examination of a spray or liquid fixated smear prepared by the physician collecting the specimen. Screening, defined as the careful review of the specimen for abnormal cells, may then be accomplished by different methods that involve the use of automated systems.

G0143-G0145

G0143   Screening cytopathology, cervical or vaginal (any reporting system), collected in preservative fluid, automated thin layer preparation, with manual screening and rescreening by cytotechnologist under physician supervision

G0144   Screening cytopathology, cervical or vaginal (any reporting system), collected in preservative fluid, automated thin layer preparation, with screening by automated system, under physician supervision

G0145   Screening cytopathology, cervical or vaginal (any reporting system), collected in preservative fluid, automated thin layer preparation, with screening by automated system and manual rescreening under physician supervision

Lay Description

These cervical or vaginal cytopathology screenings (any reporting system) of specimens collected in preservative fluid may be identified as "thin prep." The specimen is collected by cervical, endocervical, or vaginal scrapings or by aspiration of vaginal fluid and cells. This method saves time by eliminating the need for the physician to prepare a smear; the specimen is placed in a preservative suspension instead. At the laboratory, special instruments take the cells in the preservative suspension and "plate-out" a monolayer for screening, which will carefully review the specimen for abnormal cells.

G0147-G0148

G0147   Screening cytopathology smears, cervical or vaginal, performed by automated system under physician supervision

G0148   Screening cytopathology smears, cervical or vaginal, performed by automated system with manual rescreening

Lay Description

Please refer to code G0141 for the description.

G0151-G0161

G0151   Services performed by a qualified physical therapist in the home health or hospice setting, each 15 minutes

G0152   Services performed by a qualified occupational therapist in the home health or hospice setting, each 15 minutes

G0153   Services performed by a qualified speech-language pathologist in the home health or hospice setting, each 15 minutes

G0154   Direct skilled nursing services of a licensed nurse (LPN or RN) in the home health or hospice setting, each 15 minutes

G0155   Services of clinical social worker in home health or hospice settings, each 15 minutes

G0156   Services of home health/hospice aide in home health or hospice settings, each 15 minutes

G0157   Services performed by a qualified physical therapist assistant in the home health or hospice setting, each 15 minutes

G0158   Services performed by a qualified occupational therapist assistant in the home health or hospice setting, each 15 minutes

G0159   Services performed by a qualified physical therapist, in the home health setting, in the establishment or delivery of a safe and effective physical therapy maintenance program, each 15 minutes

G0160   Services performed by a qualified occupational therapist, in the home health setting, in the establishment or delivery of a safe and effective occupational therapy maintenance program, each 15 minutes

G0161 **Services performed by a qualified speech-language pathologist, in the home health setting, in the establishment or delivery of a safe and effective speech-language pathology maintenance program, each 15 minutes**

Lay Description
These codes report various services provided by different types of qualified professionals in a home health setting in units of 15 minute increments. Home health includes not only traditional private home settings, but also assisted living quarters, group homes, custodial care facilities, or similar type settings that constitute the patient's place of residence. Medicare requires that the discipline of the home health staff be reported using these codes. Check other payer requirements before using these codes on non-Medicare claims.

G0162-G0164

G0162 **Skilled services by a registered nurse (RN) for management and evaluation of the plan of care; each 15 minutes (the patient's underlying condition or complication requires an RN to ensure that essential nonskilled care achieves its purpose in the home health or hospice setting)**

G0163 **Skilled services of a licensed nurse (LPN or RN) for the observation and assessment of the patient's condition, each 15 minutes (the change in the patient's condition requires skilled nursing personnel to identify and evaluate the patient's need for possible modification of treatment in the home health or hospice setting)**

G0164 **Skilled services of a licensed nurse (LPN or RN), in the training and/or education of a patient or family member, in the home health or hospice setting, each 15 minutes**

Lay Description
These codes report various services provided by a licensed nurse in a home health setting in units of 15 minute increments. Home health includes not only traditional private home settings, but also assisted living quarters, group homes, custodial care facilities, or similar type settings that constitute the patient's place of residence. Per code description, these services include skilled services of a licensed nurse in the evaluation and management of the care plan; the observation and assessment of the patient's condition when the specialized skills of a licensed nurse are required to determine the status of the patient until such time as the treatment regimen is stabilized; and the reporting of the education or training of the patient, the patient's caregiver, or the patient's family. Medicare requires that the type of home health service be reported using these codes. Check other payer requirements before using these codes on non-Medicare claims

G0166

G0166 **External counterpulsation, per treatment session**

Lay Description
External counterpulsation is a therapy for relieving angina and is also beneficial for congestive heart failure patients. The treatment increases blood flow into the arteries and decreases the workload of the heart. The therapy is believed to work by stimulating the growth of new blood vessels around the arteries in the heart that are blocked. The patient has compressive cuffs wrapped around his/her calves and upper and lower thighs. The cuffs inflate when the heart is filling with blood and deflate when the heart is ejecting blood. Treatment sessions last one hour and are usually for a period of five times a week for seven weeks. This code reports one treatment session.

G0168

G0168 **Wound closure utilizing tissue adhesive(s) only**

Lay Description
Wound closure done by using tissue adhesive only, not any kind of suturing or stapling, is reported with this code. Tissue adhesives, such as Dermabond, are materials that are applied directly to the skin or tissue of an open wound to hold the margins closed for healing.

G0173

Lay Description
Stereotactic radiosurgery is a form of computer-assisted radiation therapy for treating tumors or lesions, mainly intracranial, that are not accessible or suitable for open surgery, by high dosage radiation that employs exact three-dimensional location planning. This code reports linear accelerator based stereotactic radiosurgery that directs an extremely narrow x-ray beam from a machine that remains focused on the tumor volume of the lesion while the movement of the machine is carefully coordinated to distribute the beam entry points over a wider radius. Linear accelerators can deliver x-rays (photons) or electrons to a targeted area. Photons can target deeper lying tumor tissue, while electrons are used for the maximum dose of radiation near the skin surface, making the method suitable to treat skin, superficial lesions, and shallow tumor volumes where underlying tissues need to be protected. Use this code for a complete course of linear accelerator based stereotactic radiosurgery therapy in one session.

G

G0175

G0175 Scheduled interdisciplinary team conference (minimum of 3 exclusive of patient care nursing staff) with patient present

Lay Description
Use this code to report an interdisciplinary team conference with a minimum of three care giving professionals present, not counting the patient care nursing staff. The patient is also present. An interdisciplinary team is composed of professionals who are specialists in different areas and who work together to coordinate the care of patients whose medical condition has multiple diagnoses that require more than one focus of care from different or related fields.

G0176

G0176 Activity therapy, such as music, dance, art or play therapies not for recreation, related to the care and treatment of patient's disabling mental health problems, per session (45 minutes or more)

Lay Description
Activity therapy is therapeutic activity such as music, dance, art, or play therapies not for recreation. The activities are related to the care and treatment of patient's disabling mental health problems and are intended to alter the thought process of a patient in a positive way. Each session should last 45 minutes or more.

G0177

G0177 Training and educational services related to the care and treatment of patient's disabling mental health problems per session (45 minutes or more)

Lay Description
Training and educational services are therapeutic procedures related to the care and treatment of a patient's disabling mental health problems. The goal is to alleviate patient discomfort and allow the patient to cope or control mental health issues. Each session should be 45 minutes or more.

G0179-G0180

G0179 Physician re-certification for Medicare-covered home health services under a home health plan of care (patient not present), including contacts with home health agency and review of reports of patient status required by physicians to affirm the initial implementation of the plan of care that meets patient's needs, per re-certification period

G0180 Physician certification for Medicare-covered home health services under a home health plan of care (patient not present), including contacts with home health agency and review of reports of patient status required by physicians to affirm the initial implementation of the plan of care that meets patient's needs, per certification period

Lay Description
These codes report one period of certification or recertification of a patient's qualifying status for Medicare-covered home health services under a home health plan of care by a physician, without the patient present. This includes all contacts made with the home health agency and reviewing of patient status reports required by physicians to affirm the initial implementation of the care plan designed to meet the patient's needs.

G0181-G0182

G0181 Physician supervision of a patient receiving Medicare-covered services provided by a participating home health agency (patient not present) requiring complex and multidisciplinary care modalities involving regular physician development and/or revision of care plans, review of subsequent reports of patient status, review of laboratory and other studies, communication (including telephone calls) with other health care professionals involved in the patient's care, integration of new information into the medical treatment plan and/or adjustment of medical therapy, within a calendar month, 30 minutes or more

G0182 Physician supervision of a patient under a Medicare-approved hospice (patient not present) requiring complex and multidisciplinary care modalities involving regular physician development and/or revision of care plans, review of subsequent reports of patient status, review of laboratory and other studies, communication (including telephone calls) with other health care professionals involved in the patient's care, integration of new information into the medical treatment plan and/or adjustment of medical therapy, within a calendar month, 30 minutes or more

Lay Description
These codes represent physician supervision of a patient receiving Medicare-covered services provided by a participating home health agency or of a patient under a Medicare-approved hospice. This includes complex and multidisciplinary care modalities involving regular physician development and/or

revision of care plans, review of subsequent reports of patient status, review of laboratory and other studies, communication with other health care professionals involved in the patient's care, including all telephone calls, and integration of new information into the medical treatment plan and/or adjustment of medical therapy, within a calendar month. The patient is not present for the physician supervision.

G0186

G0186   Destruction of localized lesion of choroid (for example, choroidal neovascularization); photocoagulation, feeder vessel technique (one or more sessions)

Lay Description
The physician destroys a localized lesion of the choroid, such as choroidal neovascularization (CNV) due to age related macular degeneration, using extrafoveal laser photocoagulation of the feeder vessel providing blood supply to the CNV. The feeder vessel is identified by indocyanine green angiography and looks like a spot in the choroid that is seen to branch off into the CNV as a distinct blood vessel. The physician directs short spots of a laser's beam in a racquet-like pattern at the feeder vessel(s) that have grown beneath the macula to occlude or obliterate the vessel supplying blood flow to the lesion. One or two treatments may be necessary. The patient is followed-up with another angiography to determine that there has been closure of the feeder vessel after treatment.

G0202-G0206

G0202   Screening mammography, producing direct digital image, bilateral, all views

G0204   Diagnostic mammography, producing direct 2D digital image, bilateral, all views

G0206   Diagnostic mammography, producing direct 2D digital image, unilateral, all views

Lay Description
Mammography is a radiographic technique used to diagnose breast cysts or tumors in women with current symptoms of breast disease or screen for lumps or masses before they are palpable in asymptomatic women. Mammography is done using a different type of x-ray than is used for routine exams that do not penetrate tissue as easily. The breast is compressed firmly between two planes and pictures are taken. This spreads the tissue and allows for a lower x-ray dose. Digital mammography stores the electronic image directly on a computer. Images are recorded digitally, without film, and can be magnified and enhanced, providing better images of the breast tissues. Small tumors and other early signs of cancer can be detected when treatment may be more effective.

G0219

G0219   PET imaging whole body; melanoma for noncovered indications

Lay Description
The whole body is imaged using data received from positron-emitting radionuclides administered to the patient in positron emission tomography (PET) imaging. The imaging relies upon capturing the gamma rays or the positively charged particles and photons, emitted by the decaying radionuclide. The collision of the positrons emitted by the radionuclide with the negatively-charged electrons normally present in body tissue is computer synthesized to produce an image, usually in vivid color, that shows the presence of cancer in tissue through the altered cell function caused by the disease and not simply from anatomical structure changes. PET imaging produces real time functional images of the metabolic processes of body tissue, such as glucose metabolism, and shows precisely where changes induced by a disease are taking place. This code is reported for whole body imaging of the entire body seeking regional lymph nodes with increased activity that may indicate that a diagnosed melanoma has metastasized.

G0235

G0235   PET imaging, any site, not otherwise specified

Lay Description
The whole body or body region is imaged using data received from positron-emitting radionuclides administered to the patient in positron emission tomography (PET) imaging. The imaging relies upon capturing the gamma rays or the positively charged particles, photons, emitted by the decaying radionuclide. This detection can be done by using stationary single or double-headed gamma cameras or by rotating a detector, or scanner, around the patient as is done with full and partial-ring bismuth germinate (BGO), sodium iodide (NAI), or crystal detector PET scanner systems. The collision of the positrons emitted by the radionuclide with the negatively-charged electrons normally present in body tissue is computer synthesized to produce an image, usually in vivid color, that will show the presence of cancer in tissue through the altered cell function caused by the disease and not simply from anatomical structure changes. PET imaging produces real time functional images of the metabolic processes of body tissue, such as glucose metabolism, and shows precisely where changes induced by a disease are taking place. This code is for PET imaging of any site not otherwise specified. Not otherwise specified codes are used only when a more specific code is not available to report the service.

G

G0237-G0239

G0237 Therapeutic procedures to increase strength or endurance of respiratory muscles, face-to-face, one-on-one, each 15 minutes (includes monitoring)

G0238 Therapeutic procedures to improve respiratory function, other than described by G0237, one-on-one, face-to-face, per 15 minutes (includes monitoring)

G0239 Therapeutic procedures to improve respiratory function or increase strength or endurance of respiratory muscles, 2 or more individuals (includes monitoring)

Lay Description
These codes are for therapeutic procedures such as special breathing exercises, performed under the supervision of a therapist, intended to increase the strength or endurance of the respiratory muscles, and to improve overall respiratory functioning in the patient. These two codes are reported once for each 15 minutes of individual, one-on-one, face-to-face, therapy time. Special therapeutic exercises are intended to increase the strength or endurance of respiratory muscles or improve overall respiratory functioning done under the supervision of a therapist in a group setting of two or more individuals. All codes include monitoring.

G0245-G0246

G0245 Initial physician evaluation and management of a diabetic patient with diabetic sensory neuropathy resulting in a loss of protective sensation (LOPS) which must include: (1) the diagnosis of LOPS, (2) a patient history, (3) a physical examination that consists of at least the following elements: (a) visual inspection of the forefoot, hindfoot, and toe web spaces, (b) evaluation of a protective sensation, (c) evaluation of foot structure and biomechanics, (d) evaluation of vascular status and skin integrity, and (e) evaluation and recommendation of footwear, and (4) patient education

G0246 Follow-up physician evaluation and management of a diabetic patient with diabetic sensory neuropathy resulting in a loss of protective sensation (LOPS) to include at least the following: (1) a patient history, (2) a physical examination that includes: (a) visual inspection of the forefoot, hindfoot, and toe web spaces, (b) evaluation of protective sensation, (c) evaluation of foot structure and biomechanics, (d) evaluation of vascular status and skin integrity, and (e) evaluation and recommendation of footwear, and (3) patient education

Lay Description
Physician evaluation and management is given to a diabetic patient with diabetic sensory neuropathy resulting in a loss of protective sensation, including all of the following in addition to the initial diagnosis of lops: a patient history; patient education; and a physical examination consisting of at least visual inspection of the forefoot, hindfoot, and toe web spaces, evaluation of protective sensation, foot structure, and biomechanics, as well as vascular status and skin integrity, and evaluation and recommendation of footwear.

G0247

G0247 Routine foot care by a physician of a diabetic patient with diabetic sensory neuropathy resulting in a loss of protective sensation (LOPS) to include the local care of superficial wounds (i.e., superficial to muscle and fascia) and at least the following, if present: (1) local care of superficial wounds, (2) debridement of corns and calluses, and (3) trimming and debridement of nails

Lay Description
Routine foot care is provided by a physician to a diabetic patient with diabetic sensory neuropathy resulting in a loss of protective sensation and must include, when present, all of the following: local care of superficial wounds, debridement of corns and calluses, and trimming and debridement of nails.

G0248-G0250

G0248 Demonstration, prior to initiation of home INR monitoring, for patient with either mechanical heart valve(s), chronic atrial fibrillation, or venous thromboembolism who meets Medicare coverage criteria, under the direction of a physician; includes: face-to-face demonstration of use and care of the INR monitor, obtaining at least one blood sample, provision of instructions for reporting home INR test results, and documentation of patient's ability to perform testing and report results

G0249 Provision of test materials and equipment for home INR monitoring of patient with either mechanical heart valve(s), chronic atrial fibrillation, or venous thromboembolism who meets Medicare coverage criteria; includes: provision of materials for use in the home and reporting of test results to physician; testing not occurring more frequently than once a week; testing materials, billing units of service include 4 tests

G0250 Physician review, interpretation, and patient management of home INR testing for patient with either mechanical heart valve(s), chronic atrial fibrillation, or venous thromboembolism who meets Medicare coverage criteria; testing not occurring more frequently than once a week; billing units of service include 4 tests

Lay Description

Patients with a mechanical heart valve, chronic atrial fibrillation, or venous thromboembolism are at risk of developing intracardiac or intravascular thrombi and are frequently managed with long-term use of warfarin anticoagulation. Periodic monitoring is necessary to maintain a therapeutic effect of the anticoagulation treatment and reduce thromboembolic and hemorrhagic events. The use of the internationalized normalized ratio (INR) (rather than the prothrombin time) provides a result that is independent of the laboratory reagents used. The INR is the ratio of the patient's prothrombin time compared to the mean prothrombin time for a group of normal individuals. Patient self-testing and self-management through the use of a home INR monitor improve the time in therapeutic rate and hence clinical outcomes. Portable coagulometers that measure the prothrombin time and calculate the INR with the use of a drop of whole blood allow the patient to do self-testing.

G0251

Lay Description

Linear accelerator based stereotactic radiosurgery is a form of computer-assisted radiation therapy for treating tumors or lesions that are not accessible or suitable for open surgery by high dosage radiation that employs exact three-dimensional location planning. Narrow beams of radiation are directed through a guiding device attached to the patient's head to destroy the appropriate area. When a linear accelerator is used, the extremely narrow x-ray beam from the machine remains focused on the tumor volume of the lesion while the movement of the machine is carefully coordinated to distribute the beam entry points over a wider radius. Linear accelerators can deliver x-rays (photons) or electrons to a targeted area. Photons can target deeper lying tumor tissue, while electrons are used for the maximum dose of radiation near the skin surface, making the method suitable to treat skin, superficial lesions, and shallow tumor volumes where underlying tissues need to be protected. This code is for the delivery of such treatment including collimator changes and custom plugging or blocking, which is a form of shield made from a special energy-absorbing material calculated to protect healthy tissue surrounding the treatment area. Use this code for fractionated treatment, per session, all lesions, up to five sessions for the entire course of treatment.

G0252

G0252 PET imaging, full and partial-ring PET scanners only, for initial diagnosis of breast cancer and/or surgical planning for breast cancer (e.g., initial staging of axillary lymph nodes)

Lay Description

Positron emission tomography (PET) is a noninvasive diagnostic imaging procedure that assesses the level of metabolic activity and perfusion in various organ systems. Initial staging is when a cancer's stage remains in question after a standard diagnostic workup, including conventional imaging (computed tomography, magnetic resonance imaging, or ultrasound). PET is used to diagnose cancer when it is expected that conventional imaging is not sufficient for the patient's clinical management and when the patient's clinical management could differ depending on the cancer's stage. Report this code for PET imaging used for the initial diagnosis of breast cancer and/or surgical planning for breast cancer (e.g., initial staging of axillary lymph nodes).

G0255

G0255 Current perception threshold/sensory nerve conduction test, (SNCT) per limb, any nerve

Lay Description

A current perception threshold/sensory nerve conduction test (CPT/SNCT) is used to diagnose sensory neurological impairments caused by various pathological conditions or toxic substance exposures. It is a noninvasive test that uses transcutaneous electrical stimulus to evoke a sensation. CPT/SNCT methods quantitate the level of sensory deficit by comparing current output to the nerve conduction threshold. Sensory nerve conduction testing is based on the concept that nerves are voltage sensitive. It can be done to quantitate sensory function with an instrument that provides voltage mediated testing (V-SNCT). It painlessly gathers enough objective data so measurements of subtle changes preceding gross morbidity can be detected. This method measures the actual instigator of nerve conduction voltage and the results are independent of changes in skin resistance.

G0257

G0257 Unscheduled or emergency dialysis treatment for an ESRD patient in a hospital outpatient department that is not certified as an ESRD facility

Lay Description

Dialysis is a process to remove toxins from the blood and to maintain fluid and electrolyte balance when the kidneys no longer function. The patient's blood is removed through a previously placed catheter, pumped through a dialysis machine, and returned to the patient through a second catheter. This code is for an unscheduled or emergency dialysis treatment for a

G

patient with end stage renal disease (ESRD) in a hospital outpatient department that has not been certified as an ESRD facility.

G0259-G0260

G0259   Injection procedure for sacroiliac joint; arthrography

G0260   Injection procedure for sacroiliac joint; provision of anesthetic, steroid and/or other therapeutic agent, with or without arthrography

Lay Description
The physician injects the sacroiliac joint for the purpose of arthrography, which is taking radiographic pictures of the joint internally to visualize the cartilage and ligaments. The contrast material, or gas, is drawn into a syringe and the target structure is localized. Through a posterior approach, the needle is inserted and advanced into the sacroiliac joint, the articulation between the sacrum and ilium in the pelvis, and the contrast injection is visualized under the aid of separately reportable computerized tomography (CT) or fluoroscopic guidance.

G0268

G0268   Removal of impacted cerumen (one or both ears) by physician on same date of service as audiologic function testing

Lay Description
Under direct visualization, the physician removes impacted cerumen (earwax) using suction, a cerumen spoon, or delicate forceps. If no infection is present, the ear canal may be irrigated. This is done on the same day that the physician performs an audiologic function test.

G0269

G0269   Placement of occlusive device into either a venous or arterial access site, postsurgical or interventional procedure (e.g., angioseal plug, vascular plug)

Lay Description
Incisions into arteries and veins must be closed by suture or a device to stem the loss of blood. Such incisions are frequently made during angioplasties and diagnostic radiological procedures. An occlusive device is a plug or stopper used to close an incision into an artery or vein. This code is intended only for devices such as an Angio-Seal or vascular plug. It should not be used for procedures such as vascular or pseudoaneurysm repair.

G0270-G0271

G0270   Medical nutrition therapy; reassessment and subsequent intervention(s) following second referral in same year for change in diagnosis, medical condition or treatment regimen (including additional hours needed for renal disease), individual, face-to-face with the patient, each 15 minutes

G0271   Medical nutrition therapy, reassessment and subsequent intervention(s) following second referral in same year for change in diagnosis, medical condition, or treatment regimen (including additional hours needed for renal disease), group (2 or more individuals), each 30 minutes

Lay Description
These codes report reassessment and interventions in a patient's medical nutrition therapy when a person has had a change in diagnosis or his/her medical condition and/or treatment regimen, following a second referral in the same year because of the change. Additional hours needed for renal disease cases are included.

G0277

G0277   Hyperbaric oxygen under pressure, full body chamber, per 30 minute interval

Lay Description
In hyperbaric oxygen (HBO) therapy, the patient is enclosed in a pressure chamber breathing oxygen at a pressure greater than one's atmosphere. The therapeutic result is hyperoxygenation, with extra oxygen dissolved into the blood plasma. Breathing pure oxygen at three times the normal pressure delivers 15 times as much dissolved oxygen to tissues than room air. This promotes formation of new capillaries into wound areas and sufficient oxygen tensions to meet the needs of the ischemic tissues. Anemias, ischemias, and certain poisonings are effectively treated using hyperoxygenation. HBO therapy also helps free gas bubbles that are trapped in the body. Hyperoxygenation reduces the size of gas bubbles by two-thirds and aids in successful reduction in gas volume to air embolisms and decompression sickness. There is also a "gas wash out" or mass action of gases. This is the flooding of the body with any one gas to wash out all other gases. This treatment occurs quickly under pressure and is excellent as a treatment for carbon monoxide poisoning/intoxication and acute cyanide poisoning. Vasoconstriction is also treated with HBO. High pressure oxygen causes the blood vessels to constrict without creating hypoxia, therefore decreasing edema in affected or injured tissues and decreasing intracranial pressure. This treatment is useful for interstitial bleeding, burns, and crash victims. HBO also restrains the growth of anaerobic and aerobic organisms called Bacteriosis and is useful in conditions where resistant elements are compromised, as in dysvascular conditions. This

effect complements the improved action of host disease fighting components.

G0278

G0278 Iliac and/or femoral artery angiography, nonselective, bilateral or ipsilateral to catheter insertion, performed at the same time as cardiac catheterization and/or coronary angiography, includes positioning or placement of the catheter in the distal aorta or ipsilateral femoral or iliac artery, injection of dye, production of permanent images, and radiologic supervision and interpretation (List separately in addition to primary procedure)

Lay Description
An iliac artery is radiologically examined using contrast material at the same time as cardiac catheterization. The catheter that has been threaded over the guidewire from the access site is positioned nonselectively in the distal aorta or iliac artery. Contrast medium is injected and a series of permanent images are taken to visualize the vessels and evaluate any abnormalities. The catheter is removed and pressure applied to the site. Radiological supervision and interpretation is included. List this code separately in addition to the code for the main cardiac catheterization procedure.

G0279

Lay Description
Digital breast tomosynthesis is an imaging modality that uses a limited number of projections from a narrow angular range that are combined to present a three-dimensional image of the breast.

G0281-G0283

G0281 Electrical stimulation, (unattended), to one or more areas, for chronic Stage III and Stage IV pressure ulcers, arterial ulcers, diabetic ulcers, and venous stasis ulcers not demonstrating measurable signs of healing after 30 days of conventional care, as part of a therapy plan of care

G0282 Electrical stimulation, (unattended), to one or more areas, for wound care other than described in G0281

G0283 Electrical stimulation (unattended), to one or more areas for indication(s) other than wound care, as part of a therapy plan of care

Lay Description
Electrical stimulation is the use of electric current that mimics the body's own natural bioelectric system's current when injured and jump starts or accelerates the wound healing process by attracting the body's repair cells, changing cell membrane permeability

and hence cellular secretion, and orientating cell structures. A current is generated between the skin and inner tissues when there is a break in the skin. The current is kept flowing until the open skin defect is repaired. There may be different types of electricity used, controlled by different electrical sources. A moist wound environment is required for capacitatively coupled electrical stimulation, which involves using a surface electrode pad in wet contact (capacitatively coupled) with the external skin surface and/or wound bed. Two electrodes are required to complete the electric circuit and are usually placed over a wet conductive medium in the wound bed and on the skin away from the wound. One of the most safe and effective wavelengths used is monophasic twin peaked high voltage pulsed current (HVPC), allowing for selection of polarity, variation in pulse rates, and very short pulse duration. Significant changes in tissue pH and temperature are avoided, which is good for healing.

G0288

G0288 Reconstruction, computed tomographic angiography of aorta for surgical planning for vascular surgery

Lay Description
Report this code for the computer reconstruction of computerized tomography (CT) generated angiographic images of the aorta for the purpose of planning vascular surgery.

G0289

G0289 Arthroscopy, knee, surgical, for removal of loose body, foreign body, debridement/shaving of articular cartilage (chondroplasty) at the time of other surgical knee arthroscopy in a different compartment of the same knee

Lay Description
A surgical knee arthroscopy is done with removal of loose or foreign bodies and debridement of articular cartilage at the same surgical session as other arthroscopy done in a separate compartment of the knee. The physician makes 1.0 cm long portal incisions on either side of the patellar tendon for arthroscopic access into the knee joint. Any loose bodies (fragments of cartilage or bone) encountered are removed through the portal incisions. Small loose bodies are suctioned or irrigated from the joint. Larger loose or foreign bodies are grasped by a clamp and removed. A chondroplasty is done to debride or shave the partially fragmented or unstable articular cartilage with a motorized suction cutter. This smoothes the roughened or damaged cartilage and promotes bleeding and regeneration of cartilage. The joint is thoroughly flushed. A temporary drain may be applied and incisions are closed with sutures.

G0293-G0294

G0293   Noncovered surgical procedure(s) using conscious sedation, regional, general, or spinal anesthesia in a Medicare qualifying clinical trial, per day

G0294   Noncovered procedure(s) using either no anesthesia or local anesthesia only, in a Medicare qualifying clinical trial, per day

Lay Description

Clinical trials are tests of a new procedure or drug using human patients to determine its effectiveness, side effects, and optimal dosage levels. These codes represent the use of the facility, staff time, and related supplies and drugs associated with an experimental procedure performed under regional, general, or spinal anesthesia, and the use of the facility, staff time, and related supplies and drugs associated with an experimental procedure performed without any type of anesthesia or under a local spinal anesthesia. These are daily charges and should not be reported more than once per calendar day.

G0295

G0295   Electromagnetic therapy, to one or more areas, for wound care other than described in G0329 or for other uses

Lay Description

Electromagnetic therapy is the application of low doses of electromagnetic current into the body. It is a form of electrical stimulation that is used for many different applications, including helping to heal wounds that have not been responding to conventional care. This code covers electromagnetic therapy applied for wound care that is not any type of chronic stage III or IV ulcer.

G0302-G0305

G0302   Preoperative pulmonary surgery services for preparation for LVRS, complete course of services, to include a minimum of 16 days of services

G0303   Preoperative pulmonary surgery services for preparation for LVRS, 10 to 15 days of services

G0304   Preoperative pulmonary surgery services for preparation for LVRS, 1 to 9 days of services

G0305   Postdischarge pulmonary surgery services after LVRS, minimum of 6 days of services

Lay Description

Lung volume reduction surgery (LVRS) is an invasive procedure to reduce the volume of a hyperinflated lung, allowing the underlying lung to expand to improve respiratory function. LRVS may also be called reduction pneumoplasty, lung shaving, or lung contouring. The procedure may be performed on patients with severe upper lobe predominant emphysema or those with severe non-upper lobe emphysema with low exercise capacity.

G0306-G0307

G0306   Complete CBC, automated (HgB, HCT, RBC, WBC, without platelet count) and automated WBC differential count

G0307   Complete (CBC), automated (HgB, Hct, RBC, WBC; without platelet count)

Lay Description

A complete blood count (CBC) is a series of tests of peripheral blood that measure the hematocrit, hemoglobulin, red blood cell count (RBC), white blood cell count (WBC), and the proportion of different white cells as they appear on a blood smear. The CBC may or may not include an enumeration of platelets within the specimen. A WBC differential count is an enumeration, expressed as a percentage, of the different types of white blood cells (e.g., leukocytes) that are present in a specific blood specimen. Both assays may be performed manually or automated.

G0328

G0328   Colorectal cancer screening; fecal occult blood test, immunoassay, 1-3 simultaneous determinations

Lay Description

Colorectal cancer screening is a preventive measure to detect precancerous signs in the colon and rectum. A fecal-occult blood test is an examination that detects the presence of blood in the stool that cannot be seen with the naked eye. An immunoassay detects the presence of antigen or antibodies. Several methods of screening may be performed, including colonoscopy, barium enema, and fecal-occult blood tests. This code includes the use of a spatula or special brush to collect the appropriate number of samples.

G0329

G0329   Electromagnetic therapy, to one or more areas for chronic Stage III and Stage IV pressure ulcers, arterial ulcers, diabetic ulcers and venous stasis ulcers not demonstrating measurable signs of healing after 30 days of conventional care as part of a therapy plan of care

Lay Description

Electromagnetic therapy is a distinct form of treatment using application of electromagnetic fields rather than direct electrical current. Electromagnetic therapy is used for wound treatment for stage III and/or stage IV pressure ulcers, arterial ulcers, diabetic ulcers, and venous stasis ulcers. Electromagnetic therapy is only considered appropriate after standard wound therapy has been tried for a minimum of 30 days with documentation showing no measurable signs of healing.

G0333

G0333 Pharmacy dispensing fee for inhalation drug(s); initial 30-day supply as a beneficiary

Lay Description
Medicare pays an initial dispensing fee to a pharmacy for the first 30-day period of inhalation drugs furnished through DME, regardless of the number of shipments or drugs dispensed during that time and regardless of the number of pharmacies a beneficiary uses during that time. This initial 30-day dispensing fee is a one-time fee applicable only to those who are using inhalation drugs for the first time as Medicare beneficiaries.

G0337

G0337 Hospice evaluation and counseling services, preelection

Lay Description
This code reports an evaluation of a terminally ill, Medicare beneficiary by a physician who is either the medical director or an employee of the hospice. This hospice consultation service is available to those who have not made a hospice election, nor received a previous hospice consultation. It includes an assessment of the patient's need for pain and symptom management, counseling regarding hospice and other care options, and may include advice regarding advanced care planning. The beneficiary or his or her physician must request this evaluation.

G0339-G0340

G0339 Image guided robotic linear accelerator-based stereotactic radiosurgery, complete course of therapy in one session or first session of fractionated treatment

G0340 Image guided robotic linear accelerator-based stereotactic radiosurgery, delivery including collimator changes and custom plugging, fractionated treatment, all lesions, per session, second through fifth sessions, maximum 5 sessions per course of treatment

Lay Description
Image-guided robotic linear accelerator-based stereotactic radiosurgery is treatment using a robotic device of a precisely defined area (stereotactic) with radiation generated by a linear accelerator. A linear accelerator is a device that increases the motion of ions to high energy or frequency levels. Electrodes are lined up with very small spaces between them creating very excited molecules that possess high levels of energy. The robotic device is guided by images taken during the course of treatment. This code includes collimator changes and custom plugging. This code represents all lesions treated in

one treatment plan. When reporting fractionated treatments, the maximum number of fractionated treatments allowed is five.

G0341-G0343

G0341 Percutaneous islet cell transplant, includes portal vein catheterization and infusion

G0342 Laparoscopy for islet cell transplant, includes portal vein catheterization and infusion

G0343 Laparotomy for islet cell transplant, includes portal vein catheterization and infusion

Lay Description
Islets cells are found in clusters throughout the pancreas and can be taken from an organ donor and transferred into the pancreas of the patient. Once transplanted, the cells can take over the task of destroyed cells. For example, diabetic Type I patients have a pancreas that no longer makes insulin and must take insulin daily. Once implanted, the islet cells, which contain beta cells, begin to make insulin. Each approach requires access to the portal vein, commonly via a transhepatic approach.

G0364

G0364 Bone marrow aspiration performed with bone marrow biopsy through the same incision on the same date of service

Lay Description
The physician performs a bone marrow aspiration with a bone marrow biopsy through the same incision at the same surgical session. Bone marrow samples are usually taken from the pelvic bone or sternum. The skin over the bone is first cleaned with an antiseptic solution. A local anesthetic is injected. To obtain bone marrow aspirate, the physician inserts a needle beneath the skin and rotates it until the needle penetrates the cortex. At least half a teaspoon of marrow is sucked out of the bone by a syringe attached to the needle. If more marrow is needed, the needle is repositioned slightly, a new syringe is attached, and a second sample is taken. The samples are transferred from the syringes to slides and sent to a laboratory for analysis. To obtain a bone marrow biopsy, the physician inserts the needle, rotates the needle to the right and the left, withdraws the needle, and reinserts the needle at a slightly different angle. The procedure is repeated until a small chip is separated from the bone marrow. The needle is again removed and a piece of fine wire threaded through the tip transfers the specimen onto sterile gauze. The chip contains bone marrow that has not had the structure disturbed or destroyed. The bone marrow biopsy tissue must be decalcified overnight before it can be stained and examined.

G

G0365

G0365   Vessel mapping of vessels for
hemodialysis access (services for
preoperative vessel mapping prior to
creation of hemodialysis access using an
autogenous hemodialysis conduit,
including arterial inflow and venous
outflow)

Lay Description
The physician performs preoperative vessel mapping
prior to creation of an autogenous hemodialysis
conduit to assess suitability of the vessels for creation
of the conduit. Both arterial inflow and venous
outflow are evaluated. The forearm vessels are
evaluated first. Creation of an arteriovenous fistula
(AVF) requires an arterial diameter of at least 2 mm
and a venous diameter of at least 2.5 mm. The arm is
comfortably positioned at a 45-degree angle from the
body. Antegrade radial arterial flow is evaluated at the
wrist level, and the radial arterial diameter is
determined. If the radial arterial diameter is less than
2 mm, the ulnar artery is evaluated. If either artery
measures at least 2 mm, the physician places a
tourniquet at the middle forearm and the distal
forearm is percussed to promote vein distension.
Special attention is paid to the cephalic and dorsal
forearm veins. The cephalic vein is measured. If the
cephalic vein is at least 2.5 mm in diameter, the
cephalic vein is followed to the elbow and the
cephalic vein branches assessed. The tourniquet is
moved to the antecubital area and then to the upper
arm and the veins assessed in the upper arm to the
point of insertion of the cephalic vein into the
subclavian vein. If the cephalic vein is occluded or
measures less than 2.5 mm it may still be possible to
create an AVF using the cephalic vein if the cephalic
vein branches are of sufficient size. If it is determined
that the cephalic vein is not suitable for an AVF, the
physician evaluates veins in the dorsal and volar
aspects to determine if another suitable vein exists. If
blood vessels in the forearm are not suitable, the
physician evaluates vessels in the upper arm. The
brachial artery and the cephalic, basilic, and brachial
veins are evaluated. Veins measuring 2.5 mm in
diameter are followed to the insertion into the
subclavian vein. Outflow in all draining veins is then
assessed to identify any occlusion or stenosis.
Adequate vein diameter is confirmed into the deep
veins and deep vein drainage evaluated.

G0372

G0372   Physician service required to establish
and document the need for a power
mobility device

Lay Description
A physician or treating nonphysician practitioner (a
physician assistant, nurse practitioner, or clinical nurse
specialist) must conduct a face-to-face examination of
the patient and write a written order for a power
mobility device (PMD). The written order must include

the patient's name, the date of the face-to-face
examination, the diagnoses and conditions that the
PMD is expected to modify, a description of the item,
the length of need, the physician or treating
nonphysician practitioner's signature, and the date
the order is written.

G0378

G0378   Hospital observation service, per hour

Lay Description
Observation in a hospital setting is the monitoring,
testing, short term treatment, and assessment of a
patient, to determine if the patient requires further
treatment as a hospital inpatient or can be discharged
from the hospital. Observation status is commonly
assigned to patients who present to the emergency
department and who then require a significant period
of treatment or monitoring in order to make a
decision concerning their admission or discharge.

G0379

G0379   Direct admission of patient for hospital
observation care

Lay Description
Observation is commonly assigned to patients who
present to the emergency department and who then
require a significant period of treatment or
monitoring in order to make a decision concerning
their admission or discharge. The decision to admit a
patient for observation care may sometimes be made
in the physician office or other community setting.
Report this code when a patient is admitted to
observation directly from the community without
being seen in the hospital's clinic or emergency
department.

G0380-G0384

G0380   Level 1 hospital emergency department
visit provided in a type B emergency
department; (the ED must meet at least
one of the following requirements: (1) it is
licensed by the state in which it is located
under applicable state law as an
emergency room or emergency
department; (2) it is held out to the public
(by name, posted signs, advertising, or
other means) as a place that provides care
for emergency medical conditions on an
urgent basis without requiring a
previously scheduled appointment; or (3)
during the calendar year immediately
preceding the calendar year in which a
determination under 42 CFR 489.24 is
being made, based on a representative
sample of patient visits that occurred
during that calendar year, it provides at
least one-third of all of its outpatient
visits for the treatment of emergency
medical conditions on an urgent basis
without requiring a previously scheduled

appointment)

G0381 Level 2 hospital emergency department visit provided in a type B emergency department; (the ED must meet at least one of the following requirements: (1) it is licensed by the state in which it is located under applicable state law as an emergency room or emergency department; (2) it is held out to the public (by name, posted signs, advertising, or other means) as a place that provides care for emergency medical conditions on an urgent basis without requiring a previously scheduled appointment; or (3) during the calendar year immediately preceding the calendar year in which a determination under 42 CFR 489.24 is being made, based on a representative sample of patient visits that occurred during that calendar year, it provides at least one-third of all of its outpatient visits for the treatment of emergency medical conditions on an urgent basis without requiring a previously scheduled appointment)

G0382 Level 3 hospital emergency department visit provided in a type B emergency department; (the ED must meet at least one of the following requirements: (1) it is licensed by the state in which it is located under applicable state law as an emergency room or emergency department; (2) it is held out to the public (by name, posted signs, advertising, or other means) as a place that provides care for emergency medical conditions on an urgent basis without requiring a previously scheduled appointment; or (3) during the calendar year immediately preceding the calendar year in which a determination under 42 CFR 489.24 is being made, based on a representative sample of patient visits that occurred during that calendar year, it provides at least one-third of all of its outpatient visits for the treatment of emergency medical conditions on an urgent basis without requiring a previously scheduled appointment)

G0383 Level 4 hospital emergency department visit provided in a type B emergency department; (the ED must meet at least one of the following requirements: (1) it is licensed by the state in which it is located under applicable state law as an emergency room or emergency department; (2) it is held out to the public (by name, posted signs, advertising, or other means) as a place that provides care for emergency medical conditions on an urgent basis without requiring a

previously scheduled appointment; or (3) during the calendar year immediately preceding the calendar year in which a determination under 42 CFR 489.24 is being made, based on a representative sample of patient visits that occurred during that calendar year, it provides at least one-third of all of its outpatient visits for the treatment of emergency medical conditions on an urgent basis without requiring a previously scheduled appointment)

G0384 Level 5 hospital emergency department visit provided in a type B emergency department; (the ED must meet at least one of the following requirements: (1) it is licensed by the state in which it is located under applicable state law as an emergency room or emergency department; (2) it is held out to the public (by name, posted signs, advertising, or other means) as a place that provides care for emergency medical conditions on an urgent basis without requiring a previously scheduled appointment; or (3) during the calendar year immediately preceding the calendar year in which a determination under 42 CFR 489.24 is being made, based on a representative sample of patient visits that occurred during that calendar year, it provides at least one-third of all of its outpatient visits for the treatment of emergency medical conditions on an urgent basis without requiring a previously scheduled appointment)

Lay Description

Type B emergency departments (ED) are areas within a hospital that provide emergency and urgent care to patients. Type B EDs meet the EMTALA definition of a dedicated ED, but do not meet the CPT definition of an ED. Hospitals that meet the CPT definition are labeled Type A EDs. Type B EDs most likely are not available 24 hours a day, seven days a week as required for the Type A designation. A Type B ED must be licensed by the state in which it is located under applicable state law as an ED, or be held out to the public (by name, posted signs, advertising, or other means) as a place that provides care for emergency medical conditions on an urgent basis without requiring a previously scheduled appointment, or provide one third of all its outpatient visits for the treatment of emergency medical conditions on an urgent basis without requiring a previously scheduled appointment. Hospitals may make their own determination as to the assignment of the various levels of care. Determination should be documented and consistently applied.

G0389

G0389 Ultrasound B-scan and/or real time with image documentation; for abdominal aortic aneurysm (AAA) screening

Lay Description
An abdominal aortic aneurysm (AAA) is a condition in the abdominal aorta characterized by thinning of the vascular wall causing weakness of the structure. A ruptured AAA can cause blood loss, shock, and death. This can happen very quickly and often there are no warning signs of the condition. An ultrasound screening can detect an AAA and allow the patient to get appropriate treatment if needed. An ultrasound uses high-frequency sound waves to create images of the aorta. Measurements of the aorta are taken to determine the presence of an aneurysm. An ultrasound B-scan and/or real time with image documentation as a screening for abdominal aortic aneurysm (AAA) is a one-time only Medicare screening benefit.

G0390

G0390 Trauma response team associated with hospital critical care service

Lay Description
Trauma response teams are specialized teams of key hospital personnel who respond to triage information from prehospital caregivers in advance of the patient's arrival. The trauma team designation may only be used by trauma center/hospitals as licensed or designated by the state or local government authority entitled to do so, or as verified by the American College of Surgeons. Patients can only be billed the trauma activation fee charge if there has been prehospital notification for them; they meet local, state, or American College of Surgeons field triage criteria; or they are delivered by inter-hospital transfers; and if they are given the appropriate team response.

G0396-G0397

G0396 Alcohol and/or substance (other than tobacco) abuse structured assessment (e.g., AUDIT, DAST), and brief intervention 15 to 30 minutes

G0397 Alcohol and/or substance (other than tobacco) abuse structured assessment (e.g., AUDIT, DAST), and intervention, greater than 30 minutes

Lay Description
Alcohol and substance abuse may be assessed by several different methods, including a drug abuse screening test (DAST) and an alcohol use disorder identification test (AUDIT).

G0398-G0400

G0398 Home sleep study test (HST) with type II portable monitor, unattended; minimum of 7 channels: EEG, EOG, EMG, ECG/heart rate, airflow, respiratory effort and oxygen saturation

G0399 Home sleep test (HST) with type III portable monitor, unattended; minimum of 4 channels: 2 respiratory movement/airflow, 1 ECG/heart rate and 1 oxygen saturation

G0400 Home sleep test (HST) with type IV portable monitor, unattended; minimum of 3 channels

Lay Description
Sleep apnea is a serious sleep disorder in which breathing repeatedly stops and starts. There are two main types of sleep apnea. Obstructive sleep apnea is the more common form that occurs when throat muscles relax. Central sleep apnea occurs when the brain doesn't send proper signals to the muscles that control breathing. Some people may have a complex sleep apnea, which is a combination of both. Medicare covers continuous positive airway pressure (CPAP) as a treatment for obstructive sleep apnea. Sleep studies, whether in a facility or performed at home, generally have the following components: electroencephalogram (EEG) to measure brain activity, electrooculogram (EOG) to monitor eye movements, electromyogram (EMG) to monitor muscle movements, electrocardiogram (EKG) to monitor heart rate and rhythm, blood oxygen saturation, breathing effort or respiratory disturbance index (RDI), and airflow monitors. Chest and abdomen movements are also sometimes monitored. Home sleep studies used to diagnose obstructive sleep apnea are reported with these codes.

G0402

G0402 Initial preventive physical examination; face-to-face visit, services limited to new beneficiary during the first 12 months of Medicare enrollment

Lay Description
An initial preventive physical examination is provided to a new beneficiary during the first 12 months of Medicare enrollment. It is also referred to as a "Welcome to Medicare" physical examination. The physician performs a thorough review of the patient's health. The physician takes a medical history on the patient and performs an exam that includes a blood pressure check, height and weight assessment, and a vision screen. Depending on the medical history information provided by the patient and the results of the physical examination, the physician orders or performs additional tests as medically necessary. The physician also provides preventive medicine education and counseling services based on the patient's medical history and examination results. The physician provides a written plan of care to the

patient detailing any follow-up screening or preventive services that the patient should receive.

G0403-G0405

G0403 **Electrocardiogram, routine ECG with 12 leads; performed as a screening for the initial preventive physical examination with interpretation and report**

G0404 **Electrocardiogram, routine ECG with 12 leads; tracing only, without interpretation and report, performed as a screening for the initial preventive physical examination**

G0405 **Electrocardiogram, routine ECG with 12 leads; interpretation and report only, performed as a screening for the initial preventive physical examination**

Lay Description
Electrocardiogram (ECG) services are performed as a component of the initial preventive physical examination provided to a new beneficiary during the first 12 months of Medicare enrollment. Twelve electrodes are placed on a patient's chest to record electrical activity of the heart. A physician interprets the findings.

G0406-G0408

G0406 **Follow-up inpatient consultation, limited, physicians typically spend 15 minutes communicating with the patient via telehealth**

G0407 **Follow-up inpatient consultation, intermediate, physicians typically spend 25 minutes communicating with the patient via telehealth**

G0408 **Follow-up inpatient consultation, complex, physicians typically spend 35 minutes communicating with the patient via telehealth**

Lay Description
These codes are used to report consultative visits or consultations that are furnished via telehealth in response to a request by the attending physician to follow up on an initial consultation or a subsequent consultative visit. Telehealth is the delivery of health-related services via telecommunications equipment. The initial inpatient visit may have also been made via telehealth. These services include following the progress and recommending modifications to the management of care or recommending a new plan of care as a result of changes in the patient's status or absence of changes in the health issue that required the consultation.

G0409

G0409 **Social work and psychological services, directly relating to and/or furthering the patient's rehabilitation goals, each 15 minutes, face-to-face; individual (services provided by a CORF qualified social worker or psychologist in a CORF)**

Lay Description
A comprehensive outpatient rehabilitation facility (CORF) is a facility established and operated at a single fixed location exclusively for the purpose of providing diagnostic, therapeutic, and restorative services to outpatients by or under the supervision of a physician. The CORF must provide at least the following three services: physicians' services, physical therapy, and social or psychological services. Social work and psychological services must be directly related to the patient's rehabilitation goal. .

G0410

G0410 **Group psychotherapy other than of a multiple-family group, in a partial hospitalization setting, approximately 45 to 50 minutes**

Lay Description
The psychiatric treatment provider conducts psychotherapy for a group of patients in one session. Group dynamics are explored. Emotional and rational cognitive interactions between individual persons in the group are facilitated and observed. Personal dynamics of any individual patient may be discussed within the group setting. Processes that help patients move toward emotional healing and modification of thought and behavior are used, such as facilitating improved interpersonal exchanges, group support, and reminiscing. The group may be composed of patients with separate and distinct maladaptive disorders or persons sharing some facet of a disorder. This code should be used for group psychotherapy with other patients, and not members of the patients' families.

G0411

G0411 **Interactive group psychotherapy, in a partial hospitalization setting, approximately 45 to 50 minutes**

Lay Description
A therapist provides therapeutic, interactive psychiatric services in a partial hospitalization setting to a group of individuals. The interactive method is most often used with individuals who are too young, or incapable, of developing expressive communication skills, or individuals who have lost that ability. This type of psychotherapy is often done with children. Toys, physical aids, and non-verbal play and interaction, including the use of interpreter skills, are employed to gain communication with a patient not capable of engaging with the clinician by using adult language skills.

G0412

G0412   Open treatment of iliac spine(s),
tuberosity avulsion, or iliac wing
fracture(s), unilateral or bilateral for
pelvic bone fracture patterns which do
not disrupt the pelvic ring, includes
internal fixation, when performed

Lay Description
The physician performs open treatment of iliac
spine(s), tuberosity avulsion, or iliac wing fracture(s)
by making an incision overlying the site of injury.
Dissection exposes the avulsion and/or fracture. For
an avulsion, a screw(s) is drilled through the bone
fragment, reattaching the tendon and bone fragment
to the original positions. The physician stabilizes an
iliac wing fracture with a plate and screws across the
fracture. The incision is repaired in layers. Suction
drains may be applied. This code reports unilateral or
bilateral treatment for fracture patterns of the pelvic
bone that do not disrupt the pelvic ring and includes
internal fixation when performed.

G0413

G0413   Percutaneous skeletal fixation of
posterior pelvic bone fracture and/or
dislocation, for fracture patterns which
disrupt the pelvic ring, unilateral or
bilateral, (includes ilium, sacroiliac joint
and/or sacrum)

Lay Description
The physician performs unilateral or bilateral
percutaneous skeletal fixation of a posterior pelvic
bone fracture (including ipsilateral ilium, sacroiliac
joint, and/or sacrum) for fracture patterns that disrupt
the pelvic ring. With the patient in a supine position,
the physician inserts two to three pins through the
skin and into the iliac crest. The pins are directed at
specific angles. The physician attaches pin holders to
each ring and curved ring segments to pin holders.
The physician uses the rings to gently reduce
(reposition) an unstable pelvic fracture or dislocation,
if needed. Frame clamps are attached to the rings and
tightened to secure fixation.

G0414

G0414   Open treatment of anterior pelvic bone
fracture and/or dislocation for fracture
patterns which disrupt the pelvic ring,
unilateral or bilateral, includes internal
fixation when performed (includes pubic
symphysis and/or superior/inferior rami)

Lay Description
The physician performs unilateral or bilateral open
treatment of an anterior pelvic bone fracture or
dislocation (includes the pubic symphysis and/or
superior/inferior rami). With the patient in a supine
position, the physician makes a curvilinear, transverse
incision above the superior pubic ramus. Dissection
exposes the pubic symphysis and/or rami. The

separation (fracture and/or dislocation) may be
reduced by the physician by applying manual
ilium-to-ilium compression. For internal fixation, a
plate is applied with screws directed into the bone.
The incision is repaired in layers with suction drains.
This code is reported for fracture patterns that disrupt
the pelvic ring and includes internal fixation when
performed.

G0415

G0415   Open treatment of posterior pelvic bone
fracture and/or dislocation, for fracture
patterns which disrupt the pelvic ring,
unilateral or bilateral, includes internal
fixation, when performed (includes ilium,
sacroiliac joint and/or sacrum)

Lay Description
The physician performs unilateral or bilateral open
treatment of a posterior pelvic bone fracture or
dislocation (includes ilium, sacroiliac joint, and/or
sacrum). With the patient in a supine position, the
physician makes an incision along the anterior iliac
crest. The iliacus muscle is dissected and reflected
medially with the abdominal contents to expose the
injury. If needed, the physician manipulates the pelvis
and leg to reduce (reposition) the fracture or
dislocation. Compression plates and screws achieve
internal fixation. In other approaches, reconstruction
plates, transiliac rod fixators, or screws alone may be
used for internal fixation of the ilium, sacroiliac joint,
and/or sacrum. The incision is repaired in layers with
suction drains. This code reports treatment for
fracture patterns that disrupt the pelvic ring and
include internal fixation when performed.

G0416-G0419

G0416   Surgical pathology, gross and
microscopic examinations, for prostate
needle biopsy, any method

Lay Description
An alternative technique to the transrectal ultrasound
(TRUS) biopsy procedure, the prostate saturation
biopsy (PSB) is used to help identify prostate cancer in
high-risk patients. The procedure is especially helpful
on patients who have high PSA levels and a history of
negative biopsies or abnormal biopsies, or abnormal
rectal exams. The PSB is usually done under general
anesthesia and ultrasonic guidance. The physician is
able to identify each specimen/biopsy and create a
map of the cancer. Several biopsies are obtained,
increasing the chances of detecting cancer. Use these
codes to report the pathology services.

G0420-G0421

G0420 Face-to-face educational services related to the care of chronic kidney disease; individual, per session, per one hour

G0421 Face-to-face educational services related to the care of chronic kidney disease; group, per session, per one hour

Lay Description
Face-to-face kidney disease education services provide patients with chronic kidney disease the information they need to manage concurrent health issues and to prevent complications. These services also include an explanation of the need to delay dialysis, as well as the treatment options available for renal replacement. These educational services may be done on an individual basis or in a group setting.

G0422-G0423

G0422 Intensive cardiac rehabilitation; with or without continuous ECG monitoring with exercise, per session

G0423 Intensive cardiac rehabilitation; with or without continuous ECG monitoring; without exercise, per session

Lay Description
Cardiac rehabilitation is a medically supervised program intended to help people with heart problems. The program includes training and education on the risk factors of heart disease, such as smoking, high blood pressure, and lack of exercise. Encouragement is given to adopt a healthy lifestyle by increasing physical activity, developing stress coping techniques, and adopting a healthy diet. The program may or may not include exercise and continuous ECG monitoring. Intensive cardiac rehabilitation (ICR) sessions are limited to 72 one-hour sessions, up to six sessions per day, over a period of up to 18 weeks.

G0424

G0424 Pulmonary rehabilitation, including exercise (includes monitoring), one hour, per session, up to 2 sessions per day

Lay Description
Pulmonary rehabilitation (PR) is a program to help improve the quality of life for people with chronic breathing problems. PR may include psychological counseling, breathing strategies, exercise training, ways to conserve energy, and education on the patient's lung disease, including how to manage it. This code includes monitoring services and exercise. Medicare covers pulmonary rehabilitation items and services for patients who are diagnosed with moderate to severe COPD, when referred by the physician who is treating the chronic respiratory disease. Pulmonary rehabilitation items and services must be provided in a hospital outpatient setting or in a physician's office. A physician must be immediately available and accessible to provide medical consultations and emergency care in either setting.

G0425-G0427

G0425 Telehealth consultation, emergency department or initial inpatient, typically 30 minutes communicating with the patient via telehealth

G0426 Telehealth consultation, emergency department or initial inpatient, typically 50 minutes communicating with the patient via telehealth

G0427 Telehealth consultation, emergency department or initial inpatient, typically 70 minutes or more communicating with the patient via telehealth

Lay Description
These codes are used to report an initial inpatient or emergency department consultative visit or consultations that are furnished via telehealth in response to a request by the attending physician. Telehealth is the delivery of health-related services via telecommunications equipment. These services include counseling and coordination of patient care with the other providers.

G0428

G0428 Collagen meniscus implant procedure for filling meniscal defects (e.g., CMI, collagen scaffold, Menaflex)

Lay Description
The meniscus collagen implant is designed to fill any meniscal defects that are still present after a partial meniscectomy. It cannot replace the entire meniscus since it requires a meniscal rim for attachment. The collagen implant works as a scaffold for new tissue growth in the meniscus. The implant is placed via arthroscopy and is sutured into position.

G0429

G0429 Dermal filler injection(s) for the treatment of facial lipodystrophy syndrome (LDS) (e.g., as a result of highly active antiretroviral therapy)

Lay Description
Facial lipodystrophy syndrome (LDS) is a condition that is characterized by localized loss of fat in the face. This loss of fat results in a facial abnormality, such as severely sunken cheeks. Patients with HIV can suffer from this condition due to antiviral treatment or the disease itself. Due to appearance, patients with LDS may discontinue treatment and feel depressed and stigmatized. Dermal filler injection gradually increases the fullness in the face to provide a more normal appearance. The treatment area is sterilely prepped and a series of injections are administered into the deep dermal, subcutaneous areas, or by depot technique. The areas are massaged periodically during the treatment to distribute the medication evenly. The patient may need additional injection sessions to obtain the desired result.

G

G0431

G0431 Drug screen, qualitative; multiple drug classes by high complexity test method (e.g., immunoassay, enzyme assay), per patient encounter

Lay Description
This code is used to report complex testing methods, such as multi-channel chemistry analyzers, where a more complex instrumented device is required to perform some or all of the screening tests for the patient. Tests that qualify for this are defined by the Clinical Laboratory Improvement Amendment (CLIA) as high complexity. It may only be used to report tests that are performed using instrumented systems (i.e., durable systems capable of withstanding repeated use). Do not use this code to report any CLIA waived tests or more simple non-waived tests. This code should be reported only once per patient encounter regardless of the number of drug classes tested.

G0432-G0433, G0435

G0432 Infectious agent antibody detection by enzyme immunoassay (EIA) technique, HIV-1 and/or HIV-2, screening

G0433 Infectious agent antibody detection by enzyme-linked immunosorbent assay (ELISA) technique, HIV-1 and/or HIV-2, screening

G0435 Infectious agent antigen detection by rapid antibody test of oral mucosa transudate, HIV-1 or HIV-2, screening

Lay Description
These codes are used to describe the screening tests used for early detection of HIV infection. The enzyme immunoassay (EIA) technique is the conventional test. The analysis is homogenous (no physical separation is done during the analysis). The enzyme-linked immunosorbent assay (ELIASA) is similar to the EIA but is heterogenous (the plate is washed before the reaction is allowed to be completed) and usually produces more accurate results. The HIV rapid antibody test can produce results in about 20 minutes and although it is usually done with oral fluids, it may also be done with blood from a finger stick.

G0434

G0434 Drug screen, other than chromatographic; any number of drug classes, by CLIA waived test or moderate complexity test, per patient encounter

Lay Description
This code is used to report simple testing methods, such as dipsticks, cups, cassettes, and cards that give visual results. It also includes tests that may be read using a scanner or a complex reader. This code should be used to report any other type of drug screening test defined as a CLIA waved test or a moderate complexity test, other than chromatographic. This code is reported per patient encounter regardless of the number of drug classes tested.

G0436-G0437

G0436 Smoking and tobacco cessation counseling visit for the asymptomatic patient; intermediate, greater than 3 minutes, up to 10 minutes

G0437 Smoking and tobacco cessation counseling visit for the asymptomatic patient; intermediate, greater than 10 minutes

Lay Description
Tobacco cessation counseling services provide instruction, assistance, and guidance in the discontinuance of smoking. Nonsymptomatic patients are those who don't have signs or symptoms of tobacco-related disease. Smoking usually refers to tobacco smoking, but may also apply to other substances. The counseling may include educating the patient about tobacco, providing strategies for handling situations that may be difficult for the patient, and relaxation and stress management techniques. Medication may or may not be used.

G0438-G0439

G0438 Annual wellness visit; includes a personalized prevention plan of service (PPS), initial visit

G0439 Annual wellness visit, includes a personalized prevention plan of service (PPS), subsequent visit

Lay Description
The initial annual wellness visit (AWV) includes taking the patient's history; compiling a list of the patient's current providers; taking the patient's vital signs, including height and weight; reviewing the patient's risk factor for depression; identifying any cognitive impairment; reviewing the patient's functional ability and level of safety (based on observation or screening questions); setting up a written patient screening schedule; compiling a list of risk factors, and furnishing personalized health services and referrals, as necessary. Subsequent annual wellness visits (AWV) include updating the patient's medical and family history, updating the current provider list, obtaining the patient's vital signs and weight, identifying cognitive impairment, updating the screening schedule, updating the risk factors list, and providing personalized health advice to the patient.

G0442-G0443

G0442 Annual alcohol misuse screening, 15 minutes

G0443 Brief face-to-face behavioral counseling for alcohol misuse, 15 minutes

Lay Description
Screening and behavioral counseling interventions are used to identify and reduce alcohol misuse.

Alcohol misuse includes risky/hazardous and harmful drinking that puts individuals at risk for future problems. Risky or hazardous drinking is defined by the United States Preventive Services Task Force (USPSTF) as "more than seven standard drinks per week or more than three drinks per occasion for women and anyone over the age of 65; more than 14 standard drinks per week or more than four drinks per occasion for men 65 years of age or younger; and alcohol use by pregnant women." Lower limits are recommended for patients taking medication that may interact with alcohol or who are performing activities that require attention, skill, or coordination, such as driving or operating heavy machinery or someone who has a medical condition that may be worsened by alcohol use. Harmful drinking is defined as anyone that is currently experiencing physical, social, or psychological harm from alcohol use but doesn't meet the criteria for dependence. Alcohol dependence can be defined as at least three of the following: tolerance; withdrawal symptoms; impaired control; preoccupation with acquisition or use; persistent desire or unsuccessful efforts to quit; sustains social, occupational, or recreational disability; used continually despite adverse conditions. The face-to-face counseling code is used to report visits for patients, including pregnant women, who misuse alcohol but don't meet the criteria for alcohol dependence; who are competent and alert at the time the counseling is provided; and whose counseling is furnished by a primary care health care professional in the primary care setting.

G0444

G0444   Annual depression screening, 15 minutes

Lay Description
Annual depression screening services are used to identify depression in patients. There should be staff in place to ensure accurate diagnosis, effective treatment, follow-up, and coordinate referrals. There are various tools that can be used to determine the screening. Depression screening services do not include treatment options for depression or any diseases, complications, or chronic conditions that the patient may have due to the depression. It also doesn't include any therapeutic interventions, such as medication therapy, or a combination of drug and counseling to treat the depression.

G0445

G0445   Semiannual high intensity behavioral counseling to prevent STIs, individual, face-to-face, includes education skills training & guidance on how to change sexual behavior

Lay Description
This code is used to report high intensity behavioral counseling to prevent sexually transmitted infections (STI) for sexually active and at risk patients. Risk reduction includes education, behavior modification,

and skills training. The United States Preventive Services Task Force (USPSTF) considers patients at high or increased risk who have any of the following conducts: multiple sex partners, using barrier protection inconsistently, having sex under the influence of alcohol or drugs, having sex in exchange for money or drugs, age (24 years of age or younger and sexually active for women for chlamydia and gonorrhea), having an STI within the past year, and IV drug use (hepatitis B only). Men having sex with men (MSM) and engaged in high risk sexual behavior are also considered at risk. The health care provider should also determine risk factors not based on individual behavior, such as a high instance of sexually communicable diseases in the community. Behavioral counseling interventions should include the following Five A's approach that has been adopted by the (USPSTF): Assess: Ask about/assess behavioral health risk(s) and factors affecting choice of behavior and change goals/methods; Advise: Give clear, specific, and personalized behavior change advice, including information about personal health harms and benefits; Agree: collaboratively select appropriate treatment goals and methods based on the patient's interest in and willingness to change the behavior; Assist: Using behavior change techniques (self-help and/or counseling), aid the patient in achieving agreed-upon goals by acquiring the skills, confidence, and social/environmental supports for behavior change, supplemented with adjunctive medical treatments when appropriate; Arrange: Schedule follow-up contacts (in person or by telephone) to provide ongoing assistance/support and to adjust the treatment plan as needed, including referral to more intensive or specialized treatment. The appropriate diagnosis code should be reported on the claim to indicate the risk factor.

G0446

G0446   Annual, face-to-face intensive behavioral therapy for cardiovascular disease, individual, 15 minutes

Lay Description
Annual intensive behavioral therapy for cardiovascular disease for risk reduction is reported with this code. Risk reduction includes encouraging aspirin therapy for the primary prevention of cardiovascular disease when the benefits outweigh the risks for men ages 45 to 70 years and women 55 to 79 years; screening for high blood pressure for patients 18 years and older; and intensive behavioral counseling to promote a healthy diet for adults with hyperlipidemia, hypertension, advancing age, and any other risk factors for cardiovascular and diet-related chronic disease. Behavioral counseling interventions should include the following Five A's approach that has been adopted by the United States Preventive Services Task Force (USPSTF): Assess: Ask about/assess behavioral health risk(s) and factors affecting choice of behavior and change goals/methods; Advise: Give clear, specific, and

personalized behavior change advice, including information about personal health harms and benefits; Agree: collaboratively select appropriate treatment goals and methods based on the patient's interest in and willingness to change the behavior; Assist: Using behavior change techniques (self-help and/or counseling), aid the patient in achieving agreed-upon goals by acquiring the skills, confidence, and social/environmental supports for behavior change, supplemented with adjunctive medical treatments when appropriate; Arrange: Schedule follow-up contacts (in person or by telephone) to provide ongoing assistance/support and to adjust the treatment plan as needed, including referral to more intensive or specialized treatment.

G0447

G0447 Face-to-face behavioral counseling for obesity, 15 minutes

Lay Description

Behavioral counseling for obesity is reported with this code. The United States Preventive Services Task Force (USPSTF) considers body mass index (BMI) a good indication of morbidity and mortality as a result of being overweight or obesity. BMI is calculated using the following formula: BMI = (weight in pounds / (height in inches x height in inches)) x 703. Obese adults are considered those that have a BMI >=30 kg/m2. Behavioral counseling and behavior modification can be an effective combination to produce moderate, sustainable weight loss. The patients should have the following services: screening for obesity using BMI, assessment of food and nutritional intake, and counseling to include diet and exercise. Behavioral counseling interventions should include the following Five A's approach that has been developed by the United States Preventive Services Task Force (USPSTF): Assess: Ask about/assess behavioral health risk(s) and factors affecting choice of behavior and change goals/methods; Advise: Give clear, specific, and personalized behavior change advice, including information about personal health harms and benefits; Agree: collaboratively select appropriate treatment goals and methods based on the patient's interest in and willingness to change the behavior; Assist: Using behavior change techniques (self-help and/or counseling), aid the patient in achieving agreed-upon goals by acquiring the skills, confidence, and social/environmental supports for behavior change, supplemented with adjunctive medical treatments when appropriate; Arrange: Schedule follow-up contacts (in person or by telephone) to provide ongoing assistance/support and to adjust the treatment plan as needed, including referral to more intensive or specialized treatment.

G0448

G0448 Insertion or replacement of a permanent pacing cardioverter-defibrillator system with transvenous lead(s), single or dual chamber with insertion of pacing electrode, cardiac venous system, for left ventricular pacing

Lay Description

This code is reported only by an ambulatory surgery center (ASC) when a permanent pacing cardioverter-defibrillator (ICD) system with transvenous lead(s), single or dual chamber, is inserted or replaced on the same date of service and at the same time as insertion of a pacing electrode, cardiac venous system, for left ventricular pacing (including upgrade to dual chamber system and pocket revision). Hospital outpatient departments and physicians continue to report the appropriate CPT codes. The physician inserts or replaces a permanent pacing cardioverter-defibrillator system, including the pulse generator with transvenous electrode placement. Transvenous placement is currently the most common technique for placing implantable cardioverter-defibrillator electrodes. An ICD is a device designed to administer an electric shock to control cardiac arrhythmias and restore a normal heartbeat. Local anesthesia is administered. An incision is made in the infraclavicular area. The subcutaneous tissue is opened and a pocket is created for the pulse generator. Transvenous electrode placement is performed under separately reportable fluoroscopic guidance. The electrode catheter is advanced through the superior vena cava into the heart and placed in the appropriate site in the right ventricle (single chamber system) or in the right ventricle and atrium (dual chamber system). Multiple leads may be required for single and dual chamber systems. When biventricular pacing is required, an additional electrode is placed in the left ventricle. A fluoroscope may be used for guidance and a pacing electrode is inserted in the left ventricular chamber of the heart, usually in the coronary sinus tributary. The electrode is connected to the generator and the generator pocket is closed.

G0451

G0451 Development testing, with interpretation and report, per standardized instrument form

Lay Description

Developmental testing is an assessment of the patient's mastery of developmental milestones. The assessment usually includes observation, interviews, and actual tests. The aim is to assess the person's current skills based on standardized criteria for each age group. This code represents testing using a standardized test form and includes the interpretation and a report prepared by a professional practitioner.

G0452

G0452 Molecular pathology procedure; physician interpretation and report

Lay Description
A molecular pathology procedure physician interpretation and report is used to report a medically necessary interpretation and written report of a molecular pathology test, above and beyond the report of laboratory results. This is a professional component only.

G0453

G0453 Continuous intraoperative neurophysiology monitoring, from outside the operating room (remote or nearby), per patient, (attention directed exclusively to one patient) each 15 minutes (list in addition to primary procedure)

Lay Description
Continuous intraoperative neurophysiology monitoring (IONM) is performed by a qualified health care provider other than the surgeon or anesthesiologist involved in the surgical procedure. IONM may include various electrophysiologic modalities, such as electroencephalography (EEG), electromyography (EMG), and evoked potentials. The provider must be solely dedicated to monitoring the neurophysiological tests and available to intervene if necessary.

G0454

G0454 Physician documentation of face-to-face visit for durable medical equipment determination performed by nurse practitioner, physician assistant or clinical nurse specialist

Lay Description
This HCPCS Level II code allows a physician who documents that a PA, NP, or CNS practitioner has performed a face-to-face encounter for the list of specified DME covered items to be paid for the service.

G0455

G0455 Preparation with instillation of fecal microbiota by any method, including assessment of donor specimen

Lay Description
Fecal microbiota transplantation (FMT) is the process of instilling fecal matter from a donor to a patient to treat a *Clostridium difficile* (*C. diff*) infection, most commonly. The donor stool is thinned using a normal saline solution and filtered for use in a nasogastric tube or an enema application. This code includes the screening protocol of the donor specimen for *C. diff* and other enteric bacterial pathogens and any ova or parasites.

G0456-G0457

Lay Description
Negative pressure wound therapy (NPWT) with vacuum assisted drainage collection is performed to promote healing of a chronic nonhealing wound, including a diabetic or pressure (decubitus) ulcer. This procedure includes topical applications to the wound, wound assessment, and patient or caregiver instruction related to on-going care per session. Negative pressure wound therapy uses controlled application of subatmospheric pressure to a wound. The subatmospheric pressure is generated using a mechanically-powered device, not durable medical equipment. The mechanical pump conveys intermittent or continuous subatmospheric pressure through connecting tubing to a specialized wound dressing. The specialized wound dressing includes a porous foam dressing that covers the wound surface and an airtight adhesive dressing that seals the wound and contains the subatmospheric pressure at the wound site. Negative pressure wound therapy promotes healing by increasing local vascularity and oxygenation of the wound bed, evacuating wound fluid thereby reducing edema, and removing exudates and bacteria. Drainage from the wound(s) is collected in a canister.

G0458

G0458 Low dose rate (LDR) prostate brachytherapy services, composite rate

Lay Description
Low dose rate (LDR) brachytherapy is performed by inserting tiny permanent radioactive iodine (I-125) seeds into the prostate. The seeds are small enough that the patient does not feel their presence. The seeds emit a low dose radiation that is absorbed by the prostate gland. The treatment is customized to the patient based on the shape and size of the prostate. There are normally about 90 to 120 seeds implanted. The seeds deliver a radiation field capable of destroying the prostate cancer cells. The level of radiation gradually decreases over several months.

G0459

G0459 Inpatient telehealth pharmacologic management, including prescription, use, and review of medication with no more than minimal medical psychotherapy

Lay Description
Medication management is furnished via telehealth, which is the delivery of health-related services via telecommunications equipment.

G0460

G0460   Autologous platelet rich plasma for chronic wounds/ulcers, including phlebotomy, centrifugation, and all other preparatory procedures, administration and dressings, per treatment

Lay Description
Autologous platelet rich plasma for chronic wounds/ulcers, including phlebotomy, centrifugation, and all other preparatory procedures, administration and dressings, per treatment is a biological prepared from the patient's blood that is used for nonhealing wounds. CMS covers autologous PRP only for the treatment of chronic, nonhealing diabetic, venous, and/or pressure wounds when PRP is provided as a randomized clinical trial that meets specific requirements to assess the health outcomes of PRP for the treatment of chronic nonhealing diabetic, venous, and/or pressure wounds. See the Medicare National Coverage Determinations Manual, Pub. 100-03, chapter 1, section 270.3, Transmittal 153, May 21, 2013, for the requirements for this clinical research study.

G0463

G0463   Hospital outpatient clinic visit for assessment and management of a patient

Lay Description
OPPS hospitals are to report this code in place of CPT codes 99201–99205 and 99211–99215 for clinic visits. There is no distinction between new and established patients or levels of care.

G0464

G0464   Colorectal cancer screening; stool-based DNA and fecal occult hemoglobin (e.g., KRAS, NDRG4 and BMP3)

Lay Description
This colorectal cancer screening test looks for blood and/or DNA changes (e.g., KRAS, NDRG4, and BMP3i genes) in a stool sample.

G0466-G0467

G0466   Federally qualified health center (FQHC) visit, new patient

G0467   Federally qualified health center (FQHC) visit, established patient

Lay Description
A new patient (G0466) or established patient (G0467) is seen in a federally qualified health center (FQHC). This service is payable under the FQHC prospective payment system (PPS). Code G0466 must be accompanied by qualifying visit code 92002, 92004, 97802, 99201—99205, 99324—99325, 99328, 99341—99345, 99381—99387, G0101, G0102, G0108, G0117, G0118, G0436, G0437, or G0442—G0447. Code G0467 must be accompanied by qualifying visit code 92012, 92014, 97802, 97803,

99211—99215, 99304—99310, 99315, 99316, 99318, 99334—99337, 99347—99350, 99391—99397, 99495, 99496, G0101, G0102, G0108, G0117, G0118, G0270, G0436, G0437, G0442—G0447, or M0064. Medical visit codes G0466—G0468 must be reported with revenue code 052X or 0519.

G0468

G0468   Federally qualified health center (FQHC) visit, initial preventive physical exam (IPPE) or annual wellness visit (AWV)

Lay Description
An initial preventive physical exam (IPPE) or an annual wellness visit (AWV) is performed in a federally qualified health center (FQHC). This service is payable under the FQHC prospective payment system (PPS). Code G0468 must be accompanied by qualifying visit code G0402, G0438, or G0439. Medical visit codes G0466—G0468 must be reported with revenue code 052X or 0519.

G0469-G0470

G0469   Federally qualified health center (FQHC) visit, mental health, new patient

G0470   Federally qualified health center (FQHC) visit, mental health, established patient

Lay Description
A new patient (G0469) or established patient (G0470) is seen for a mental health visit at a federally qualified health center (FQHC). This service is payable under the FQHC prospective payment system (PPS). Codes G0469 and G0470 must be accompanied by qualifying visit code 90791, 90792, 90832—90839, or 90845. Mental health visit codes G0469 and G0470 must be reported with revenue code 0900 or 0519.

G0471

G0471   Collection of venous blood by venipuncture or urine sample by catheterization from an individual in a skilled nursing facility (SNF) or by a laboratory on behalf of a home health agency (HHA)

Lay Description
This code reports the collection of venous blood by venipuncture or a urine sample by catheterization from an individual in a skilled nursing facility (SNF) or by a laboratory on behalf of a home health agency (HHA). This code should only be reported when the following statements apply. The sample is being collected by a laboratory technician that is employed by the laboratory performing the test or the sample is from an individual in an SNF or HHA.

G0472

G0472 Hepatitis C antibody screening for individual at high risk and other covered indication(s)

Lay Description
Hepatitis C virus (HCV) screenings test for HCV antibodies that indicate an infection with the hepatitis C virus. Results are usually reported as reactive or nonreactive. Screening for HCV is covered when ordered by the patient's primary care physician or practitioner within the context of a primary care setting, for the following patients. 1) Patients who are not high risk and are born between 1945 and 1965. A single screening test is covered for adults who do not meet the high risk criteria. HCV screening is limited to once per lifetime. 2) Adults at high risk for HCV infection. High risk is defined as persons with a current or past history of illicit injection drug use and persons who have a history of receiving a blood transfusion prior to 1992. Repeat screening for high-risk persons is covered annually only for persons who have had continued illicit injection drug use since the prior negative screening test. The determination of high risk for HCV is in the hands of the primary care physician or practitioner who assesses the patient's history, which is part of any complete medical history. The medical record should be a reflection of the service provided. 3) Beneficiaries determined to be high-risk. Initially ICD-9-CM diagnosis code V69.8 (Other problems related to life style) or ICD-10-CM diagnosis code Z72.89 (Other problems related to lifestyle) is required. For repeat annual testing, report an additional diagnosis of ICD-9-CM diagnosis code 304.91 (Unspecified drug dependence, continuous) or ICD-10-CM diagnosis code F19.20 (Other psychoactive substance abuse, uncomplicated).

G0473

G0473 Face-to-face behavioral counseling for obesity, group (2-10), 30 minutes

Lay Description
Behavioral counseling for obesity in a group setting is reported with this code. The United States Preventive Services Task Force (USPSTF) considers body mass index (BMI) a good indication of morbidity and mortality. BMI is calculated using the following formula: $BMI = (\text{weight in pounds} / (\text{height in inches} \times \text{height in inches})) \times 703$. Obese adults are considered those that have a BMI $>=30$ kg/m2. Behavioral counseling and behavior modification can be an effective combination to produce moderate, sustainable weight loss. The patients should have the following services: screening for obesity using BMI, assessment of food and nutritional intake, and counseling to include diet and exercise. Behavioral counseling interventions should include the following Five A's approach that has been developed by the United States Preventive Services Task Force (USPSTF): Assess: Ask about/assess behavioral health risk(s) and factors affecting choice of behavior and change goals/methods; Advise: Give clear, specific, and personalized behavior change advice, including information about personal health harms and benefits; Agree: Collaboratively select appropriate treatment goals and methods based on the patient's interest in and willingness to change the behavior; Assist: Using behavior change techniques (self-help and/or counseling), aid the patient in achieving agreed-upon goals by acquiring the skills, confidence, and social/environmental supports for behavior change, supplemented with adjunctive medical treatments when appropriate; Arrange: Schedule follow-up contacts (in person or by telephone) to provide ongoing assistance/support and to adjust the treatment plan as needed, including referral to more intensive or specialized treatment.

G3001

G3001 Administration and supply of tositumomab, 450 mg

Lay Description
Tositumomab (trade name Bexxar) is a murine monoclonal antibody that is directed against the CD20 antigen, which is found on the surface of normal and malignant B lymphocytes. When linked to Iodine I-131, it is used as an anti-neoplastic treatment of patients with CD20 positive, follicular, non-Hodgkin's lymphoma, with and without transformation, whose disease is refractory to rituximab, and whose disease has recurred following chemotherapy. The tositumomab therapeutic regimen is not indicated for the initial treatment of patients with CD20 positive non-Hodgkin's lymphoma. Prior to the administration of the radioactive iodine I-131 tositumomab, non-radioactive tositumomab is given to determine the proper treatment dose for the patient. This code represents the 450 mg of the non-radioactive tositumomab dose used for treatment planning. It includes the intravenous administration of the drug.

G6001

G6001 Ultrasonic guidance for placement of radiation therapy fields

Lay Description
Ultrasound is used to place radiation therapy fields. Ultrasound is an imaging technique bouncing sound waves far above the level of human perception through interior body structures. The sound waves pass through different densities of tissue and reflect back to a receiving unit, which converts the waves to electrical pulses that are immediately displayed in picture form on screen. Images of normal and abnormal tissue structures are obtained and the treatment field area volume is determined. The normal tissues surrounding the treatment area are also defined. Acquiring this data is an important step in planning the patient's radiation treatment.

G

G6002

G6002 Stereoscopic x-ray guidance for localization of target volume for the delivery of radiation therapy

Lay Description

Radiation treatment delivery involves the transfer of a beam of high-energy radiation from a treatment machine distanced from the treatment area. Stereotactic body radiation therapy is a radiation therapy technique that uses special equipment to position a patient and precisely deliver a large radiation dose to discrete tumor sites while minimizing damage to healthy tissue. Stereoscopic x-ray guidance utilizes infrared and/or camera technology to precisely localize targets in conjunction with intensity modulated radiation therapy and stereotactic radiotherapy. This code reports the stereoscopic x-ray guidance only.

G6003-G6006

G6003 Radiation treatment delivery, single treatment area, single port or parallel opposed ports, simple blocks or no blocks: up to 5 mev

G6004 Radiation treatment delivery, single treatment area, single port or parallel opposed ports, simple blocks or no blocks: 6-10 mev

G6005 Radiation treatment delivery, single treatment area, single port or parallel opposed ports, simple blocks or no blocks: 11-19 mev

G6006 Radiation treatment delivery, single treatment area, single port or parallel opposed ports, simple blocks or no blocks: 20 mev or greater

Lay Description

Radiation treatment delivery involves the delivery of a beam of high-energy radiation from an external treatment machine distanced from the treatment area. External radiation is often delivered by linear accelerator, which can deliver x-rays (photons) or electrons to a targeted area. Cobalt teletherapy units and cesium teletherapy units are also used to direct gamma rays from a distance to the targeted area. Photons can target deeper lying tumor tissue, while electrons are used for the maximum dose of radiation near the skin surface, making the method suitable to treat skin, superficial lesions, and shallow tumor volumes where underlying tissues need to be protected. These codes are dependent upon the number and complexity of treatment areas, as well as the energy level, measured in megavolts (MeV). Report G6003 for a single treatment area, single port or parallel opposed ports, simple or no blocks, up to 5 MeV; G6004 for 6-10 MeV; G6005 for 11-19 MeV; and G6006 for 20 MeV or greater.

G6007-G6010

G6007 Radiation treatment delivery, 2 separate treatment areas, 3 or more ports on a single treatment area, use of multiple blocks: up to 5 mev

G6008 Radiation treatment delivery, 2 separate treatment areas, 3 or more ports on a single treatment area, use of multiple blocks: 6-10 mev

G6009 Radiation treatment delivery, 2 separate treatment areas, 3 or more ports on a single treatment area, use of multiple blocks: 11-19 mev

G6010 Radiation treatment delivery, 2 separate treatment areas, 3 or more ports on a single treatment area, use of multiple blocks: 20 mev or greater

Lay Description

Radiation treatment delivery involves the delivery of a beam of high-energy radiation from an external treatment machine distanced from the treatment area. External radiation is often delivered by linear accelerator, which can deliver x-rays (photons) or electrons to a targeted area. Cobalt teletherapy units and cesium teletherapy units are also used to direct gamma rays from a distance to the targeted area. Photons can target deeper lying tumor tissue, while electrons are used for the maximum dose of radiation near the skin surface, making the method suitable to treat skin, superficial lesions, and shallow tumor volumes where underlying tissues need to be protected. These codes are dependent upon the number and complexity of treatment areas, as well as the energy level, measured in megavolts (MeV). Report G6007 for two separate treatment areas, three or more ports on a single treatment area, multiple blocks, up to 5 MeV; G6008 for 6-10 MeV; G6009 for 11-19 MeV; and G6010 for 20 MeV or greater.

G6011-G6014

G6011 Radiation treatment delivery, 3 or more separate treatment areas, custom blocking, tangential ports, wedges, rotational beam, compensators, electron beam; up to 5 mev

G6012 Radiation treatment delivery, 3 or more separate treatment areas, custom blocking, tangential ports, wedges, rotational beam, compensators, electron beam; 6-10 mev

G6013 Radiation treatment delivery, 3 or more separate treatment areas, custom blocking, tangential ports, wedges, rotational beam, compensators, electron beam; 11-19 mev

G6014 Radiation treatment delivery, 3 or more separate treatment areas, custom blocking, tangential ports, wedges, rotational beam, compensators, electron beam; 20 mev or greater

Lay Description
Radiation treatment delivery involves the delivery of a beam of high-energy radiation from an external treatment machine distanced from the treatment area. External radiation is often delivered by linear accelerator, which can deliver x-rays (photons) or electrons to a targeted area. Cobalt teletherapy units and cesium teletherapy units are also used to direct gamma rays from a distance to the targeted area. Photons can target deeper lying tumor tissue, while electrons are used for the maximum dose of radiation near the skin surface, making the method suitable to treat skin, superficial lesions, and shallow tumor volumes where underlying tissues need to be protected. These codes are dependent upon the number and complexity of treatment areas, as well as the energy level, measured in megavolts (MeV). Report G6011 for three or more two separate treatment areas, custom blocking, tangential ports, wedges, rotational beam, compensators, electron beam, up to 5MeV; G6012 for 6-10 MeV; G6013 for 11-19 MeV; and G6014 for 20 MeV or greater.

G6015

G6015 Intensity modulated treatment delivery, single or multiple fields/arcs, via narrow spatially and temporally modulated beams, binary, dynamic MLC, per treatment session

Lay Description
Intensity modulated radiotherapy treatment (IMRT) is the use of varying intensities of radiation. A single dose is shaped by hundreds of beam-shaping devices called collimators. These collimators are calculated to hit tumors with high-dose radiation and sensitive normal tissues with modulated, lower-intensity beams, leaving them mostly unaffected. By dividing the radiation beam into multiple slices, the intensity of the beam in any slice can be varied by computer-controlled dynamic multileaf collimation (MLC) during the radiation exposure. MLC systems consist of multiple narrow leaves that are modulated under computer control and allow custom-shaped beam apertures without fabricated blocks. During IMRT delivery, the leaves of the MLC are adjusted while the beam is on to modify the delivery of radiation across the portal. This code reports IMRT delivery, single or multiple fields/arcs, via narrow spatially and temporally modulated beams, binary, dynamic MLC, per treatment session.

G6016

G6016 Compensator-based beam modulation treatment delivery of inverse planned treatment using 3 or more high resolution (milled or cast) compensator, convergent beam modulated fields, per treatment session

Lay Description
Compensator-based beam modulation treatment delivery of inversed planned treatment using three or more high-resolution (milled or cast) compensator convergent beam modulated fields is a method of delivering intensity modulated radiation therapy (IMRT). Prior to treatment delivery, a computerized planning system is used to calculate dose by inverse treatment planning method for IMRT optimization. The planner chooses beam angles and writes a prescription for targets identifying critical structures. The computerized planning system optimizes beam weights and modulation patterns and generates files for milling or casting of the required high-resolution compensators that are fabricated as prescribed and planned. During treatment delivery, solid filters modulate the beams. This code represents one treatment session.

G6017

G6017 Intra-fraction localization and tracking of target or patient motion during delivery of radiation therapy (e.g., 3D positional tracking, gating, 3D surface tracking), each fraction of treatment

Lay Description
Image-guided radiation therapy is a technique in which frequent imaging occurs during the course of a radiation therapy session (intra-fraction) in order to ensure that the radiation is delivered to the correct target location and spares surrounding tissues. Decisions regarding administration adjustments are made on the basis of the imaging results. Various methods of localization and tracking of patient or tumor motion may be used, including gating or 3D positional or surface tracking technology. In one method, an electromagnetic transponder is implanted into the prostate prior to external beam therapy for prostate cancer. This transponder transmits radiofrequency waves to a computerized system, which provides information regarding position and movement of the prostate. This motion data is used by clinicians to assist in radiation therapy setup and as a positional monitor during delivery of treatment, alerting the clinician if the tumor moves outside the pathway of the radiation beam. Report G0617 for each fraction of treatment.

G6018

G6018   Ileoscopy, through stoma; with transendoscopic stent placement (includes predilation)

Lay Description

The physician inserts an endoscope through an opening into the ileum (ileostomy) to view the ileum and places a transendoscopic stent. The physician places an endoscope into the mouth and advances it into the small intestine. The lumen of the ileum is visualized. The endoscope is removed. The endoscope is placed at the site of an obstruction or stricture and the necessary stent length is determined. The stent (endoprosthesis) is introduced into the site of the obstruction. Using a commercial delivery system, a plastic covering over the stent is removed and the stent self-deploys, shoring-up the walls at a specific site in the ileum. When necessary, a balloon catheter is placed into the stent and gently inflated to more fully deploy the stent. The delivery system and endoscope are removed.

G6019

G6019   Colonoscopy through stoma; with ablation of tumor(s), polyp(s), or other lesion(s) not amenable to removal by hot biopsy forceps, bipolar cautery or snare technique

Lay Description

The physician performs colonoscopy through an abdominal wall colostomy and performs ablation of a tumor, polyp, or other lesion. The physician places the endoscope into the colostomy and advances the endoscope into the colon. The lumen of the colon is visualized and the tumor, polyp, or other lesion is identified and ablated. The endoscope is withdrawn at the completion of the procedure.

G6020

G6020   Colonoscopy through stoma; with transendoscopic stent placement (includes predilation)

Lay Description

The physician uses a colonoscope to examine the colon through an abdominal wall colostomy and places a transendoscopic stent. The physician places the endoscope into the colostomy and advances the endoscope into the colon. The lumen of the colon is visualized. The endoscope is placed at the site of an obstruction or stricture and the necessary stent length is determined. The stent (endoprosthesis) is introduced into the site of the obstruction. Using a commercial delivery system, a plastic covering over the stent is removed and the stent self-deploys, shoring-up the walls at a specific site in the large intestine. When necessary, a balloon catheter is placed into the stent and gently inflated to more fully deploy the stent. The delivery system and colonoscope are removed.

G6021

G6021   Unlisted procedure, intestine

Lay Description

This code reports any type of procedure on the small intestine that is not described by the other codes.

G6022

G6022   Sigmoidoscopy, flexible; with ablation of tumor(s), polyp(s), or other lesions(s) not amenable to removal by hot biopsy forceps, bipolar cautery or snare technique

Lay Description

The physician performs flexible sigmoidoscopy and performs ablation of a tumor, polyp, or other lesion. The physician inserts the sigmoidoscope into the anus and advances the scope into the sigmoid colon. The lumen of the sigmoid colon and rectum are visualized. The tumor, polyp, or other lesions are identified and ablated by laser or other method. The sigmoidoscope is withdrawn at the completion of the procedure.

G6023

G6023   Sigmoidoscopy, flexible; with transendoscopic stent placement (includes predilation)

Lay Description

The physician uses a flexible sigmoidoscope to examine the rectum and sigmoid colon and places a transendoscopic stent. The physician inserts the sigmoidoscopy into the anus and advances the scope into the sigmoid colon. The lumen of the sigmoid colon and rectum are visualized. The endoscope is placed at the site of an obstruction or stricture and the necessary stent length is determined. The stent (endoprosthesis) is introduced into the site of the obstruction. Using a commercial delivery system, a plastic covering over the stent is removed and the stent self-deploys, shoring-up the walls at a specific site in the sigmoid colon. When necessary, a balloon catheter is placed into the stent and gently inflated to more fully deploy the stent. The delivery system and endoscope are removed.

G6024

G6024   Colonoscopy, flexible; proximal to splenic flexure; with ablation of tumor(s), polyp(s), or other lesion(s) not amenable to removal by hot biopsy forceps, bipolar cautery or snare tehnique

Lay Description

The physician performs colonoscopy and performs ablation of a tumor, polyp, or other lesions. The physician inserts the colonoscope into the anus and advances the scope past the splenic flexure. The lumen of the colon and rectum are visualized. The tumor, polyp, or other lesions are identified and ablated by laser or other method. The colonoscope is withdrawn at the completion of the procedure.

G6025

G6025 Colonoscopy, flexible, proximal to splenic flexure; with transendoscopic stent placement (includes predilation)

Lay Description

The physician uses a colonoscope to examine the colon and place a transendoscopic stent. The physician inserts the flexible endoscope into the anus and advances the scope beyond the splenic flexure. The lumen of the colon is visualized. The endoscope is placed at the site of an obstruction or stricture and the necessary stent length is determined. If the area is partially occluded or obstructed, a balloon-tipped catheter is inserted through the scope and the balloon is inflated to dilate the area before stent placement. The stent (endoprosthesis) is introduced to the site of the lesion by a stent-carrying catheter inserted through the scope. The plastic covering over the stent is removed and the stent self-deploys, shoring-up the walls at the target site in the colon, proximal to the splenic flexure. When necessary, a balloon catheter is placed into the stent and gently inflated to more fully deploy the stent. The delivery system and endoscope are removed.

G6027-G6028

G6027 Anoscopy, high resolution (HRA) (with magnification and chemical agent enhancement); diagnostic, including collection of specimen(s) by brushing or washing when performed

G6028 Anoscopy, high resolution (HRA) (with magnification and chemical agent enhancement); with biopsy(ies)

Lay Description

The physician performs a diagnostic examination of the anal canal using high resolution anoscopy (HRA), frequently indicated for patients with abnormal anal cytology. The physician examines the anal canal using a thin round tube (anoscope) and a high resolution magnifying instrument (colposcope). A mild acidic liquid may be applied to the anal canal to enhance any abnormal or dysplastic tissue. Code G6027 includes specimens obtained by brushing or washing, when performed. Report G6028 if the specimens are obtained by biopsy. The anoscope is withdrawn at the completion of the procedure.

G6030-G6038, G6040-G6057

G6030 Assay of amitriptyline

G6031 Assay of benzodiazepines

G6032 Assay of desipramine

G6034 Assay of doxepin

G6035 Assay of gold

G6036 Assay of imipramine

G6037 Assay of nortriptyline

G6038 Assay of salicylate

G6040 Assay of alcohol (ethanol); any specimen except breath

G6041 Alkaloids, urine, quantitative

G6042 Assay of amphetamine or methamphetamine

G6043 Assay of barbiturates, not elsewhere specified

G6044 Assay of cocaine or metabolite

G6045 Assay of dihydrocodeinone

G6046 Assay of dihydromorphinone

G6047 Assay of dihydrotestosterone

G6048 Assay of dimethadione

G6049 Assay of epiandrosterone

G6050 Assay of ethchlorvynol

G6051 Assay of flurazepam

G6052 Assay of meprobamate

G6053 Assay of methadone

G6054 Assay of methsuximide

G6055 Assay of nicotine

G6056 Opiate(s), drug and metabolites, each procedure

G6057 Assay of phenothiazine

Lay Description

Beginning in January 2015, the CPT codes used for drug testing are grouped into drug classes, and further broken down into therapeutic assays, presumptive testing, and definitive testing. Previously a CPT had been assigned to each drug. Medicare is not prepared to accept and process the codes based on drug classes. Providers should report the HCPCS Level II G code that identifies the specific drug in place of the 2015 CPT drug class codes.

G6058

G6058 Drug confirmation, each procedure

Lay Description

This test is performed when the initial drug screen is positive. Confirmatory tests must be sensitive and specific and involve a different technique than the initial screen. For example, if the initial screen is performed by thin layer chromatography identifying a spot on the chromatogram that is the right color and in the right place to be consistent with a particular drug, it is confirmed with a more specific method, like high performance liquid chromatography (HPLC), gas chromatography-mass spectrometry (GC-MS), or immunoassay. If the drug suspected is a barbiturate, for example, a confirmatory HPLC method might be

G

done to prove that the compound had the correct retention time, etc., and to identify it exactly as a particular barbiturate.

G8978-G8995

G8978 Mobility: walking and moving around functional limitation, current status, at therapy episode outset and at reporting intervals

G8979 Mobility: walking and moving around functional limitation, projected goal status, at therapy episode outset, at reporting intervals, and at discharge or to end reporting

G8980 Mobility: walking and moving around functional limitation, discharge status, at discharge from therapy or to end reporting

G8981 Changing and maintaining body position functional limitation, current status, at therapy episode outset and at reporting intervals

G8982 Changing and maintaining body position functional limitation, projected goal status, at therapy episode outset, at reporting intervals, and at discharge or to end reporting

G8983 Changing and maintaining body position functional limitation, discharge status, at discharge from therapy or to end reporting

G8984 Carrying, moving and handling objects functional limitation, current status, at therapy episode outset and at reporting intervals

G8985 Carrying, moving and handling objects, projected goal status, at therapy episode outset, at reporting intervals, and at discharge or to end reporting

G8986 Carrying, moving and handling objects functional limitation, discharge status, at discharge from therapy or to end reporting

G8987 Self care functional limitation, current status, at therapy episode outset and at reporting intervals

G8988 Self care functional limitation, projected goal status, at therapy episode outset, at reporting intervals, and at discharge or to end reporting

G8989 Self care functional limitation, discharge status, at discharge from therapy or to end reporting

G8990 Other physical or occupational therapy primary functional limitation, current status, at therapy episode outset and at reporting intervals

G8991 Other physical or occupational therapy primary functional limitation, projected goal status, at therapy episode outset, at reporting intervals, and at discharge or to end reporting

G8992 Other physical or occupational therapy primary functional limitation, discharge status, at discharge from therapy or to end reporting

G8993 Other physical or occupational therapy subsequent functional limitation, current status, at therapy episode outset and at reporting intervals

G8994 Other physical or occupational therapy subsequent functional limitation, projected goal status, at therapy episode outset, at reporting intervals, and at discharge or to end reporting

G8995 Other physical or occupational therapy subsequent functional limitation, discharge status, at discharge from therapy or to end reporting

Lay Description
These codes represent functional limitations usually assessed by physical and occupational therapists. The codes are reported with HCPCS Level II modifiers CH, CI, CJ, CK, CL, CM, or CN, which indicate the degree of impairment. These codes and modifiers are not payable, but are used to report the patient's type of functional limitation and whether the report is on the current status, projected goal status, or discharge status. The first claim for therapy services also requires the therapist's projected goal for functional status at the end of treatment. This reporting is required on selected claims for all outpatient therapy services, including those for services above the therapy caps and those that include modifier KX for the cap exemption. They apply to all services furnished under the Medicare Part B outpatient therapy benefit and PT, OT, and SLP services under the comprehensive outpatient rehabilitation facilities (CORF) benefit. Therapy services included are those furnished personally and incident to the services of physicians or nonphysician practitioners (NPP). Functional limitations are reported for therapy services furnished in hospitals, critical access hospitals (CAH), skilled nursing facilities (SNF), CORFs, rehabilitation agencies, home health agencies (when the beneficiary is not under a home health plan of care), and in private offices of therapists, physicians, and NPPs.

G8996-G8999

G8996 Swallowing functional limitation, current status at therapy episode outset and at reporting intervals

G8997 Swallowing functional limitation, projected goal status, at therapy episode outset, at reporting intervals, and at discharge or to end reporting

G8998 Swallowing functional limitation, discharge status, at discharge from therapy or to end reporting

G8999 Motor speech functional limitation, current status at therapy episode outset and at reporting intervals

Lay Description
These codes represent functional limitations usually assessed by speech therapists and speech-language pathologists. The codes are reported with HCPCS Level II modifiers CH, CI, CJ, CK, CL, CM, or CN, which indicate the degree of impairment. These codes and modifiers are not payable, but are used to report the patient's type of functional limitation and whether the report is on the current status, projected goal status, or discharge status. The first claim for therapy services also requires the therapist's projected goal for functional status at the end of treatment. This reporting is required on selected claims for all outpatient therapy services, including those for services above the therapy caps and those that include modifier KX for the cap exemption. They apply to all services furnished under the Medicare Part B outpatient therapy benefit and PT, OT, and SLP services under the comprehensive outpatient rehabilitation facilities (CORF) benefit. Therapy services include those furnished personally and incident to the services of physicians or nonphysician practitioners (NPP). Functional limitations are reported for therapy services furnished in hospitals, critical access hospitals (CAH), skilled nursing facilities (SNF), CORFs, rehabilitation agencies, home health agencies (when the beneficiary is not under a home health plan of care), and in private offices of therapists, physicians and NPPs.

G9001-G9012

G9001 Coordinated care fee, initial rate

G9002 Coordinated care fee (Level 1)

G9003 Coordinated care fee, risk adjusted high, initial

G9004 Coordinated care fee, risk adjusted low, initial

G9005 Coordinated care fee risk adjusted maintenance

G9006 Coordinated care fee, home monitoring

G9007 Coordinated care fee, scheduled team conference

G9008 Coordinated care fee, physician coordinated care oversight services

G9009 Coordinated care fee, risk adjusted maintenance, level 3

G9010 Coordinated care fee, risk adjusted maintenance, level 4

G9011 Coordinated care fee, risk adjusted maintenance, Level 5

G9012 Other specified case management service not elsewhere classified

Lay Description
In an effort to improve care and to contain costs, Medicare is testing several coordinated care demonstration projects. There are fifteen sites that manage or coordinate all care delivered to Medicare beneficiaries with certain complex chronic illnesses, including asthma, diabetes, congestive heart failure and related cardiac conditions, hypertension, coronary artery disease, cardiovascular and cerebrovascular conditions, and chronic lung disease. CMS implemented this demonstration to test whether coordinated care programs can improve medical treatment plans, reduce avoidable hospital admissions, and promote other desirable outcomes for chronically ill beneficiaries, without increasing costs. The selected projects include both case and disease management models in urban and rural settings. These codes should be used only by the fifteen approved demonstration projects. The codes correspond to the rates proposed and included in each specific demonstration project.

G9016

G9016 Smoking cessation counseling, individual, in the absence of or in addition to any other evaluation and management service, per session (6-10 minutes) [demo project code only]

Lay Description
CMS had been conducting a demonstration project to test smoking cessation as a Medicare benefit. The project examined the "quit" rates of Medicare beneficiaries receiving three different types of treatment. The three types are counseling only, counseling and an FDA-approved prescription or nicotine replacement drug therapy, and a telephone counseling hotline and nicotine replacement therapy. This code was used to bill individual counseling services when that counseling is the only service provided. It is reported for each session that must total between six and ten minutes in length. This code was used only for services provided by providers and beneficiaries enrolled in the demonstration project. The project has concluded.

G9017

G9017 Amantadine HCl, oral, per 100 mg (for use in a Medicare-approved demonstration project)

Lay Description
Amantadine hydrochloride is a chemical that has pharmacological actions as both an anti-Parkinson and an antiviral drug. Its mechanism of action for either use is unknown. Amantadine hydrochloride is indicated for the treatment of Parkinsonism and drug-induced extrapyramidal reactions, as well as signs and symptoms of infections caused by the influenza Type A virus. The drug is self-administered orally.

G9018

G9018 Zanamivir, inhalation powder, administered through inhaler, per 10 mg (for use in a Medicare-approved demonstration project)

Lay Description
Zanamivir is an antiviral drug that has an effect against the influenza virus. It inhibits the enzyme that the virus uses to separate itself from other cells. Inhibition of this enzyme allows antibodies to attack and destroy the virus. Zanamivir is indicated for treatment of uncomplicated acute infections with influenza A and B virus in patients 7 years of age and older. The patient should be symptomatic for no more than two days. It is not recommended for patients with an underlying airway disease, such as asthma or COPD. The drug is self-administered in an inhaled powder form via a supplied disk inhaler. This code is for use in a Medicare approved demonstration project.

G9019

G9019 Oseltamivir phosphate, oral, per 75 mg (for use in a Medicare-approved demonstration project)

Lay Description
Oseltamivir phosphate is an oral anti-viral drug for the treatment of uncomplicated influenza in patients one year and older whose flu symptoms have not lasted more than two days. Oseltamivir phosphate is approved to treat Type A and B influenza. It is available in a 75 mg capsule form, as well as in a powder form for oral suspension. The oral suspension is reconstituted with water to contain 12 mg/mL oseltamivir base. Oseltamivir phosphate is an ethyl ester prodrug requiring ester hydrolysis for conversion to the active form, oseltamivir carboxylate. The proposed mechanism of action of oseltamivir phosphate is inhibition of influenza virus neuraminidase with the possibility of alteration of virus particle aggregation and release.

G9020

G9020 Rimantadine HCl, oral, per 100 mg (for use in a Medicare-approved demonstration project)

Lay Description
Rimantadine hydrochloride is an oral anti-viral drug for the treatment of influenza type A. The drug affects only certain susceptible strains of the influenza type A virus. It is available in a 100 mg capsule form, as well as in a syrup form. The mechanism of action is not entirely understood, but Rimantadine hydrochloride appears to interfere with the activity of the virus's genetic material, blocking an essential step in the process of viral replication by possibly inhibiting the uncoating of the virus.

G9033

G9033 Amantadine HCl, oral brand, per 100 mg (for use in a Medicare-approved demonstration project)

Lay Description
Amantadine hydrochloride is a chemical that has pharmacological actions as both an anti-Parkinson and an antiviral drug. Its mechanism of action for either use is unknown. Amantadine hydrochloride is indicated for the treatment of Parkinsonism and drug-induced extrapyramidal reactions, as well as signs and symptoms of infections caused by the influenza Type A virus. The drug is self-administered orally.

G9034

G9034 Zanamivir, inhalation powder, administered through inhaler, brand, per 10 mg (for use in a Medicare-approved demonstration project)

Lay Description
Zanamivir is an antiviral drug that has an effect against the influenza virus. It inhibits the enzyme that the virus uses to separate itself from other cells. Inhibition of this enzyme allows antibodies to attack and destroy the virus. Zanamivir is indicated for treatment of uncomplicated acute infections with influenza A and B virus in patients 7 years of age and older. The patient should be symptomatic for no more than two days. It is not recommended for patients with an underlying airway disease, such as asthma or COPD. The drug is self-administered in an inhaled powder form via a supplied disk inhaler.

G9035

G9035 Oseltamivir phosphate, oral, brand, per 75 mg (for use in a Medicare-approved demonstration project)

Lay Description
Oseltamivir phosphate is an oral anti-viral drug for the treatment of uncomplicated influenza in patients 1 year and older whose flu symptoms have not lasted more than two days. Oseltamivir phosphate is

approved to treat Type A and B influenza. It is available in a 75 mg capsule form, as well as in a powder form for oral suspension. The oral suspension is reconstituted with water to contain 12 mg/mL oseltamivir base. Oseltamivir phosphate is an ethyl ester prodrug requiring ester hydrolysis for conversion to the active form, oseltamivir carboxylate. The proposed mechanism of action of oseltamivir phosphate is inhibition of influenza virus neuraminidase with the possibility of alteration of virus particle aggregation and release.

G9036

G9036 Rimantadine HCl, oral, brand, per 100 mg (for use in a Medicare-approved demonstration project)

Lay Description
Rimantadine hydrochloride is an oral anti-viral drug for the treatment of influenza type A. The drug affects only certain susceptible strains of the influenza type A virus. It is available in a 100 mg capsule form, as well as in a syrup form. The mechanism of action is not entirely understood, but Rimantadine hydrochloride appears to interfere with the activity of the virus's genetic material, blocking an essential step in the process of viral replication by possibly inhibiting the uncoating of the virus.

G9050-G9055

G9050 Oncology; primary focus of visit; work-up, evaluation, or staging at the time of cancer diagnosis or recurrence (for use in a Medicare-approved demonstration project)

G9051 Oncology; primary focus of visit; treatment decision-making after disease is staged or restaged, discussion of treatment options, supervising/coordinating active cancer-directed therapy or managing consequences of cancer-directed therapy (for use in a Medicare-approved demonstration project)

G9052 Oncology; primary focus of visit; surveillance for disease recurrence for patient who has completed definitive cancer-directed therapy and currently lacks evidence of recurrent disease; cancer-directed therapy might be considered in the future (for use in a Medicare-approved demonstration project)

G9053 Oncology; primary focus of visit; expectant management of patient with evidence of cancer for whom no cancer-directed therapy is being administered or arranged at present; cancer-directed therapy might be considered in the future (for use in a Medicare-approved demonstration project)

G9054 Oncology; primary focus of visit; supervising, coordinating or managing care of patient with terminal cancer or for whom other medical illness prevents further cancer treatment; includes symptom management, end-of-life care planning, management of palliative therapies (for use in a Medicare-approved demonstration project)

G9055 Oncology; primary focus of visit; other, unspecified service not otherwise listed (for use in a Medicare-approved demonstration project)

Lay Description
Medicare implemented the oncology demonstration project to capture additional information from hematologists and oncologists treating patients with specific types of cancer. The demo requires physicians to report a code from each of three categories: the primary focus of the visit, the status of the disease, and adherence to the guidelines (National Comprehensive Cancer Network, American Society of Clinical Oncology, or no guideline available). Use these codes to report the primary focus of the evaluation and management services for the specified stage of cancer. Since various issues are addressed in a visit, the physician should make the best choice.

G9056-G9062

G9056 Oncology; practice guidelines; management adheres to guidelines (for use in a Medicare-approved demonstration project)

G9057 Oncology; practice guidelines; management differs from guidelines as a result of patient enrollment in an institutional review board-approved clinical trial (for use in a Medicare-approved demonstration project)

G9058 Oncology; practice guidelines; management differs from guidelines because the treating physician disagrees with guideline recommendations (for use in a Medicare-approved demonstration project)

G

G9059 Oncology; practice guidelines; management differs from guidelines because the patient, after being offered treatment consistent with guidelines, has opted for alternative treatment or management, including no treatment (for use in a Medicare-approved demonstration project)

G9060 Oncology; practice guidelines; management differs from guidelines for reason(s) associated with patient comorbid illness or performance status not factored into guidelines (for use in a Medicare-approved demonstration project)

G9061 Oncology; practice guidelines; patient's condition not addressed by available guidelines (for use in a Medicare-approved demonstration project)

G9062 Oncology; practice guidelines; management differs from guidelines for other reason(s) not listed (for use in a Medicare-approved demonstration project)

Lay Description

Medicare implemented the oncology demonstration project to capture additional information from hematologists and oncologists treating patients with specific types of cancer. The demo requires physicians to report a code from each of three categories: the primary focus of the visit, the status of the disease, and adherence to the guidelines (National Comprehensive Cancer Network, American Society of Clinical Oncology, or no guideline available). These codes are used to describe whether or not the patient management adheres to practice guidelines in the Medicare oncology demonstration. If the patient management does not adhere to practice guidelines, report the code that describes the reason why it does not.

G9063-G9139

G9063 Oncology; disease status; limited to nonsmall cell lung cancer; extent of disease initially established as Stage I (prior to neoadjuvant therapy, if any) with no evidence of disease progression, recurrence, or metastases (for use in a Medicare-approved demonstration project)

G9064 Oncology; disease status; limited to nonsmall cell lung cancer; extent of disease initially established as Stage II (prior to neoadjuvant therapy, if any) with no evidence of disease progression, recurrence, or metastases (for use in a Medicare-approved demonstration project)

G9065 Oncology; disease status; limited to nonsmall cell lung cancer; extent of disease initially established as Stage III a (prior to neoadjuvant therapy, if any) with no evidence of disease progression, recurrence, or metastases (for use in a Medicare-approved demonstration project)

G9066 Oncology; disease status; limited to nonsmall cell lung cancer; Stage III B-IV at diagnosis, metastatic, locally recurrent, or progressive (for use in a Medicare-approved demonstration project)

G9067 Oncology; disease status; limited to nonsmall cell lung cancer; extent of disease unknown, staging in progress, or not listed (for use in a Medicare-approved demonstration project)

G9068 Oncology; disease status; limited to small cell and combined small cell/nonsmall cell; extent of disease initially established as limited with no evidence of disease progression, recurrence, or metastases (for use in a Medicare-approved demonstration project)

G9069 Oncology; disease status; small cell lung cancer, limited to small cell and combined small cell/nonsmall cell; extensive Stage at diagnosis, metastatic, locally recurrent, or progressive (for use in a Medicare-approved demonstration project)

G9070 Oncology; disease status; small cell lung cancer, limited to small cell and combined small cell/nonsmall; extent of disease unknown, staging in progress, or not listed (for use in a Medicare-approved demonstration project)

G9071 Oncology; disease status; invasive female breast cancer (does not include ductal carcinoma in situ); adenocarcinoma as predominant cell type; stage I or stage IIA-IIB; or T3, N1, M0; and ER and/or PR positive; with no evidence of disease progression, recurrence, or metastases (for use in a Medicare-approved demonstration project)

G9072 Oncology; disease status; invasive female breast cancer (does not include ductal carcinoma in situ); adenocarcinoma as predominant cell type; stage I, or stage IIA-IIB; or T3, N1, M0; and ER and PR negative; with no evidence of disease progression, recurrence, or metastases (for use in a Medicare-approved demonstration project)

G9073 Oncology; disease status; invasive female breast cancer (does not include ductal carcinoma in situ); adenocarcinoma as predominant cell type; stage IIIA-IIIB; and not T3, N1, M0; and ER and/or PR positive; with no evidence of disease progression, recurrence, or metastases (for use in a Medicare-approved demonstration project)

G9074 Oncology; disease status; invasive female breast cancer (does not include ductal carcinoma in situ); adenocarcinoma as predominant cell type; stage IIIA-IIIB; and not T3, N1, M0; and ER and PR negative; with no evidence of disease progression, recurrence, or metastases (for use in a Medicare-approved demonstration project)

G9075 Oncology; disease status; invasive female breast cancer (does not include ductal carcinoma in situ); adenocarcinoma as predominant cell type; M1 at diagnosis, metastatic, locally recurrent, or progressive (for use in a Medicare-approved demonstration project)

G9077 Oncology; disease status; prostate cancer, limited to adenocarcinoma as predominant cell type; T1-T2C and Gleason 2-7 and PSA < or equal to 20 at diagnosis with no evidence of disease progression, recurrence, or metastases (for use in a Medicare-approved demonstration project)

G9078 Oncology; disease status; prostate cancer, limited to adenocarcinoma as predominant cell type; T2 or T3a Gleason 8-10 or PSA > 20 at diagnosis with no evidence of disease progression, recurrence, or metastases (for use in a Medicare-approved demonstration project)

G9079 Oncology; disease status; prostate cancer, limited to adenocarcinoma as predominant cell type; T3B-T4, any N; any T, N1 at diagnosis with no evidence of disease progression, recurrence, or metastases (for use in a Medicare-approved demonstration project)

G9080 Oncology; disease status; prostate cancer, limited to adenocarcinoma; after initial treatment with rising PSA or failure of PSA decline (for use in a Medicare-approved demonstration project)

G9083 Oncology; disease status; prostate cancer, limited to adenocarcinoma; extent of disease unknown, staging in progress, or not listed (for use in a Medicare-approved demonstration project)

G9084 Oncology; disease status; colon cancer, limited to invasive cancer, adenocarcinoma as predominant cell type; extent of disease initially established as T1-3, N0, M0 with no evidence of disease progression, recurrence or metastases (for use in a Medicare-approved demonstration project)

G9085 Oncology; disease status; colon cancer, limited to invasive cancer, adenocarcinoma as predominant cell type; extent of disease initially established as T4, N0, M0 with no evidence of disease progression, recurrence, or metastases (for use in a Medicare-approved demonstration project)

G9086 Oncology; disease status; colon cancer, limited to invasive cancer, adenocarcinoma as predominant cell type; extent of disease initially established as T1-4, N1-2, M0 with no evidence of disease progression, recurrence, or metastases (for use in a Medicare-approved demonstration project)

G9087 Oncology; disease status; colon cancer, limited to invasive cancer, adenocarcinoma as predominant cell type; M1 at diagnosis, metastatic, locally recurrent, or progressive with current clinical, radiologic, or biochemical evidence of disease (for use in a Medicare-approved demonstration project)

G9088 Oncology; disease status; colon cancer, limited to invasive cancer, adenocarcinoma as predominant cell type; M1 at diagnosis, metastatic, locally recurrent, or progressive without current clinical, radiologic, or biochemical evidence of disease (for use in a Medicare-approved demonstration project)

G9089 Oncology; disease status; colon cancer, limited to invasive cancer, adenocarcinoma as predominant cell type; extent of disease unknown, staging in progress or not listed (for use in a Medicare-approved demonstration project)

G

G9090 Oncology; disease status; rectal cancer, limited to invasive cancer, adenocarcinoma as predominant cell type; extent of disease initially established as T1-2, N0, M0 (prior to neoadjuvant therapy, if any) with no evidence of disease progression, recurrence, or metastases (for use in a Medicare-approved demonstration project)

G9091 Oncology; disease status; rectal cancer, limited to invasive cancer, adenocarcinoma as predominant cell type; extent of disease initially established as T3, N0, M0 (prior to neoadjuvant therapy, if any) with no evidence of disease progression, recurrence, or metastases (for use in a Medicare-approved demonstration project)

G9092 Oncology; disease status; rectal cancer, limited to invasive cancer, adenocarcinoma as predominant cell type; extent of disease initially established as T1-3, N1-2, M0 (prior to neoadjuvant therapy, if any) with no evidence of disease progression, recurrence or metastases (for use in a Medicare-approved demonstration project)

G9093 Oncology; disease status; rectal cancer, limited to invasive cancer, adenocarcinoma as predominant cell type; extent of disease initially established as T4, any N, M0 (prior to neoadjuvant therapy, if any) with no evidence of disease progression, recurrence, or metastases (for use in a Medicare-approved demonstration project)

G9094 Oncology; disease status; rectal cancer, limited to invasive cancer, adenocarcinoma as predominant cell type; M1 at diagnosis, metastatic, locally recurrent, or progressive (for use in a Medicare-approved demonstration project)

G9095 Oncology; disease status; rectal cancer, limited to invasive cancer, adenocarcinoma as predominant cell type; extent of disease unknown, staging in progress or not listed (for use in a Medicare-approved demonstration project)

G9096 Oncology; disease status; esophageal cancer, limited to adenocarcinoma or squamous cell carcinoma as predominant cell type; extent of disease initially established as T1-T3, N0-N1 or NX (prior to neoadjuvant therapy, if any) with no evidence of disease progression, recurrence, or metastases (for use in a Medicare-approved demonstration project)

G9097 Oncology; disease status; esophageal cancer, limited to adenocarcinoma or squamous cell carcinoma as predominant cell type; extent of disease initially established as T4, any N, M0 (prior to neoadjuvant therapy, if any) with no evidence of disease progression, recurrence, or metastases (for use in a Medicare-approved demonstration project)

G9098 Oncology; disease status; esophageal cancer, limited to adenocarcinoma or squamous cell carcinoma as predominant cell type; M1 at diagnosis, metastatic, locally recurrent, or progressive (for use in a Medicare-approved demonstration project)

G9099 Oncology; disease status; esophageal cancer, limited to adenocarcinoma or squamous cell carcinoma as predominant cell type; extent of disease unknown, staging in progress, or not listed (for use in a Medicare-approved demonstration project)

G9100 Oncology; disease status; gastric cancer, limited to adenocarcinoma as predominant cell type; post R0 resection (with or without neoadjuvant therapy) with no evidence of disease recurrence, progression, or metastases (for use in a Medicare-approved demonstration project)

G9101 Oncology; disease status; gastric cancer, limited to adenocarcinoma as predominant cell type; post R1 or R2 resection (with or without neoadjuvant therapy) with no evidence of disease progression, or metastases (for use in a Medicare-approved demonstration project)

G9102 Oncology; disease status; gastric cancer, limited to adenocarcinoma as predominant cell type; clinical or pathologic M0, unresectable with no evidence of disease progression, or metastases (for use in a Medicare-approved demonstration project)

G9103 Oncology; disease status; gastric cancer, limited to adenocarcinoma as predominant cell type; clinical or pathologic M1 at diagnosis, metastatic, locally recurrent, or progressive (for use in a Medicare-approved demonstration project)

G9104 Oncology; disease status; gastric cancer, limited to adenocarcinoma as predominant cell type; extent of disease unknown, staging in progress, or not listed (for use in a Medicare-approved demonstration project)

G9105 Oncology; disease status; pancreatic cancer, limited to adenocarcinoma as predominant cell type; post R0 resection without evidence of disease progression, recurrence, or metastases (for use in a Medicare-approved demonstration project)

G9106 Oncology; disease status; pancreatic cancer, limited to adenocarcinoma; post R1 or R2 resection with no evidence of disease progression, or metastases (for use in a Medicare-approved demonstration project)

G9107 Oncology; disease status; pancreatic cancer, limited to adenocarcinoma; unresectable at diagnosis, M1 at diagnosis, metastatic, locally recurrent, or progressive (for use in a Medicare-approved demonstration project)

G9108 Oncology; disease status; pancreatic cancer, limited to adenocarcinoma; extent of disease unknown, staging in progress, or not listed (for use in a Medicare-approved demonstration project)

G9109 Oncology; disease status; head and neck cancer, limited to cancers of oral cavity, pharynx and larynx with squamous cell as predominant cell type; extent of disease initially established as T1-T2 and N0, M0 (prior to neoadjuvant therapy, if any) with no evidence of disease progression, recurrence, or metastases (for use in a Medicare-approved demonstration project)

G9110 Oncology; disease status; head and neck cancer, limited to cancers of oral cavity, pharynx and larynx with squamous cell as predominant cell type; extent of disease initially established as T3-4 and/or N1-3, M0 (prior to neoadjuvant therapy, if any) with no evidence of disease progression, recurrence, or metastases (for use in a Medicare-approved demonstration project)

G9111 Oncology; disease status; head and neck cancer, limited to cancers of oral cavity, pharynx and larynx with squamous cell as predominant cell type; M1 at diagnosis, metastatic, locally recurrent, or progressive (for use in a Medicare-approved demonstration project)

G9112 Oncology; disease status; head and neck cancer, limited to cancers of oral cavity, pharynx and larynx with squamous cell as predominant cell type; extent of disease unknown, staging in progress, or not listed (for use in a Medicare-approved demonstration project)

G9113 Oncology; disease status; ovarian cancer, limited to epithelial cancer; pathologic stage 1A-B (Grade 1) without evidence of disease progression, recurrence, or metastases (for use in a Medicare-approved demonstration project)

G9114 Oncology; disease status; ovarian cancer, limited to epithelial cancer; pathologic stage IA-B (grade 2-3); or stage IC (all grades); or stage II; without evidence of disease progression, recurrence, or metastases (for use in a Medicare-approved demonstration project)

G9115 Oncology; disease status; ovarian cancer, limited to epithelial cancer; pathologic stage III-IV; without evidence of progression, recurrence, or metastases (for use in a Medicare-approved demonstration project)

G9116 Oncology; disease status; ovarian cancer, limited to epithelial cancer; evidence of disease progression, or recurrence, and/or platinum resistance (for use in a Medicare-approved demonstration project)

G9117 Oncology; disease status; ovarian cancer, limited to epithelial cancer; extent of disease unknown, staging in progress, or not listed (for use in a Medicare-approved demonstration project)

G9123 Oncology; disease status; chronic myelogenous leukemia, limited to Philadelphia chromosome positive and/or BCR-ABL positive; chronic phase not in hematologic, cytogenetic, or molecular remission (for use in a Medicare-approved demonstration project)

G9124 Oncology; disease status; chronic myelogenous leukemia, limited to Philadelphia chromosome positive and /or BCR-ABL positive; accelerated phase not in hematologic cytogenetic, or molecular remission (for use in a Medicare-approved demonstration project)

G9125 Oncology; disease status; chronic myelogenous leukemia, limited to Philadelphia chromosome positive and/or BCR-ABL positive; blast phase not in hematologic, cytogenetic, or molecular remission (for use in a Medicare-approved demonstration project)

G9126 Oncology; disease status; chronic myelogenous leukemia, limited to Philadelphia chromosome positive and/or BCR-ABL positive; in hematologic, cytogenetic, or molecular remission (for use in a Medicare-approved demonstration project)

G9128 Oncology; disease status; limited to multiple myeloma, systemic disease; smoldering, stage I (for use in a Medicare-approved demonstration project)

G9129 Oncology; disease status; limited to multiple myeloma, systemic disease; stage II or higher (for use in a Medicare-approved demonstration project)

G9130 Oncology; disease status; limited to multiple myeloma, systemic disease; extent of disease unknown, staging in progress, or not listed (for use in a Medicare-approved demonstration project)

G9131 Oncology; disease status; invasive female breast cancer (does not include ductal carcinoma in situ); adenocarcinoma as predominant cell type; extent of disease unknown, staging in progress, or not listed (for use in a Medicare-approved demonstration project)

G9132 Oncology; disease status; prostate cancer, limited to adenocarcinoma; hormone-refractory/androgen-independent (e.g., rising PSA on antiandrogen therapy or postorchiectomy); clinical metastases (for use in a Medicare-approved demonstration project)

G9133 Oncology; disease status; prostate cancer, limited to adenocarcinoma; hormone-responsive; clinical metastases or M1 at diagnosis (for use in a Medicare-approved demonstration project)

G9134 Oncology; disease status; non-Hodgkin's lymphoma, any cellular classification; Stage I, II at diagnosis, not relapsed, not refractory (for use in a Medicare-approved demonstration project)

G9135 Oncology; disease status; non-Hodgkin's lymphoma, any cellular classification; Stage III, IV, not relapsed, not refractory (for use in a Medicare-approved demonstration project)

G9136 Oncology; disease status; non-Hodgkin's lymphoma, transformed from original cellular diagnosis to a second cellular classification (for use in a medicare-approved demonstration project)

G9137 Oncology; disease status; non-Hodgkin's lymphoma, any cellular classification; relapsed/refractory (for use in a medicare-approved demonstration project)

G9138 Oncology; disease status; non-Hodgkin's lymphoma, any cellular classification; diagnostic evaluation, stage not determined, evaluation of possible relapse or nonresponse to therapy, or not listed (for use in a Medicare-approved demonstration project)

G9139 Oncology; disease status; chronic myelogenous leukemia, limited to Philadelphia chromosome positive and/or BCR-ABL positive; extent of disease unknown, staging in progress, not listed (for use in a Medicare-approved demonstration project)

Lay Description

Medicare implemented the oncology demonstration project to capture additional information from hematologists and oncologists treating patients with specific types of cancer. The demo requires physicians to report a code from each of three categories: the primary focus of the visit, the status of the disease, and adherence to the guidelines (National Comprehensive Cancer Network, American Society of Clinical Oncology, or no guideline available). These codes are used to describe the disease status for the first listed cancer diagnosis on the claim form for the Medicare oncology demonstration project.

G9140

G9140 Frontier extended stay clinic demonstration; for a patient stay in a clinic approved for the CMS demonstration project; the following measures should be present: the stay must be equal to or greater than 4 hours; weather or other conditions must prevent transfer or the case falls into a category of

monitoring and observation cases that are permitted by the rules of the demonstration; there is a maximum frontier extended stay clinic (FESC) visit of 48 hours, except in the case when weather or other conditions prevent transfer; payment is made on each period up to 4 hours, after the first 4 hours

Lay Description
The frontier extended stay clinic (FESC) demonstration sets up and maintains remotely located facilities that are at least 75 miles from the nearest critical access hospital (CAH) or acute care hospital. FESCs are allowed to treat patients for more extended periods than routine physician services are entitled to, including overnight stays. The FESC serves patients who are injured or seriously ill and who, due to inclement weather or other reasons, are unable to be transferred to an acute care facility. Patients who need observation or monitoring services also qualify for FESC care. Use this code to report FESC services.

G9143

G9143 Warfarin responsiveness testing by genetic technique using any method, any number of specimen(s)

Lay Description
This code was developed as a means of implementing Medicare's coverage policy for warfarin responsiveness testing, which is only covered by Medicare in the context of an approved, clinical study. This test is considered a once-in-a-lifetime procedure, unless there is a reason to think that the patient's genetics would change. Pharmacogenomics is a study of the response to drugs by a specific individual. The testing includes a study of the inherited components and gene variations that dictate the individual's response to drugs/medications. It also explores the ways that these individual variations can be used to predict a good, a bad, or no response to a drug. The influence of CYP2C9 and VKORC1 on warfarin dose, along with many other factors, has been used to partially predict an individual's response to warfarin.

G9147

G9147 Outpatient Intravenous Insulin Treatment (OIVIT) either pulsatile or continuous, by any means, guided by the results of measurements for: respiratory quotient; and/or, urine urea nitrogen (UUN); and/or, arterial, venous or capillary glucose; and/or potassium concentration

Lay Description
Medicare has determined that outpatient intravenous insulin treatment (OIVIT) is not reasonable and necessary since there is no evidence that it improves health outcomes in Medicare patients. The term OIVIT refers to an outpatient regimen that integrates pulsed or continuous intravenous infusion of insulin with the dosage depending on the results of measurement of

respiratory quotient; urine urea nitrogen (UUN); arterial, venous, or capillary glucose; and/or potassium concentration. OIVIT is also known as cellular activation therapy (CAT), chronic intermittent intravenous insulin therapy (CIIT), hepatic activation therapy (HAT), intercellular activation therapy (iCAT), metabolic activation therapy (MAT), pulsatile intravenous insulin treatment (PIVIT), pulse insulin therapy (PIT), and pulsatile therapy (PT). This code is reported for noncovered OIVIT and any related services.

G9148-G9153

G9148 National Committee for Quality Assurance-Level 1 medical home

G9149 National Committee for Quality Assurance-Level 2 medical home

G9150 National Committee for Quality Assurance-Level 3 medical home

G9151 MAPCP Demonstration-state provided services

G9152 MAPCP Demonstration-Community Health Teams

G9153 MAPCP Demonstration-Physician Incentive Pool

Lay Description
Medicare joined Medicaid and private payers in a demonstration project that is based on state health reform initiatives aimed at improving the delivery of primary care. Advanced primary care (APC) practices, or medical homes, use a team approach to provide patient-centric care. APC practices emphasize prevention, health information technology, care coordination, and shared decision making among patients and their providers. The goal is to improve the quality and coordination of health care services. An APC may be a solo practitioner, a group practice, or a federally qualified health center. APC practices may be led by doctors or nurse practitioners. Under this demonstration program, Medicare participates in existing state multi-payer health reform initiatives that currently include participation from Medicaid and private health plans. The demonstration program pays a monthly care management fee for patients receiving primary care from APC practices. The care management fee is intended to cover care coordination, improved access, patient education, and other services to support chronically ill patients. Additionally, each participating state offers APC practices community support and links to state health promotion and disease prevention initiatives. Individual states control project participation criteria, reporting, and reimbursement instructions.

G9156

G9156 Evaluation for wheelchair requiring face-to-face visit with physician

Lay Description
This code is to be reported by Medicare Fee-For-Service (FFS) physicians/treating practitioners

G

who prescribe power mobility devices (PMD) for Medicare beneficiaries who reside in the demonstration states of California, Texas, Florida, Michigan, Illinois, North Carolina, and New York and submit a prior authorization request to DME Medicare Administrative Contractors for a PMD. If the prior authorization request is submitted by the physician/treating practitioner, the physician/treating practitioner may bill this code. The physician/treating practitioner is entitled to a quarterly incentive payment of $10 for each G9156 code that meets all eligibility requirements. This code must be submitted to the Medicare Administrative Contractor (A/B MACs) and/or carriers with the PMD prior authorization number. The $10 incentive payment is issued to the physician/treating practitioner on a quarterly basis. The provider must also show a billed amount of $10 or the claim will be rejected. Providers should submit the G9156 code on an assigned claim with no other codes.

G9157

G9157 Transesophageal Doppler used for cardiac monitoring

Lay Description
Transesophageal Doppler is an ultrasound diagnostic procedure that uses low energy sound waves to provide noninvasive visualization. This code is specific to Medicare coverage of transesophageal Doppler monitoring of cardiac output for ventilated patients in the ICU and operative patients with a need for intraoperative fluid optimization. This service is only covered in a hospital setting or ambulatory surgical center and is included in the Inpatient Prospective Payment System payment.

G9158-G9176

G9158 Motor speech functional limitation, discharge status, at discharge from therapy or to end reporting

G9159 Spoken language comprehension functional limitation, current status at therapy episode outset and at reporting intervals

G9160 Spoken language comprehension functional limitation, projected goal status at therapy episode outset, at reporting intervals, and at discharge or to end reporting

G9161 Spoken language comprehension functional limitation, discharge status, at discharge from therapy or to end reporting

G9162 Spoken language expression functional limitation, current status at therapy episode outset and at reporting intervals

G9163 Spoken language expression functional limitation, projected goal status at therapy episode outset, at reporting intervals, and at discharge or to end reporting

G9164 Spoken language expression functional limitation, discharge status at discharge from therapy or to end reporting

G9165 Attention functional limitation, current status at therapy episode outset and at reporting intervals

G9166 Attention functional limitation, projected goal status at therapy episode outset, at reporting intervals, and at discharge or to end reporting

G9167 Attention functional limitation, discharge status at discharge from therapy or to end reporting

G9168 Memory functional limitation, current status at therapy episode outset and at reporting intervals

G9169 Memory functional limitation, projected goal status at therapy episode outset, at reporting intervals, and at discharge or to end reporting

G9170 Memory functional limitation, discharge status at discharge from therapy or to end reporting

G9171 Voice functional limitation, current status at therapy episode outset and at reporting intervals

G9172 Voice functional limitation, projected goal status at therapy episode outset, at reporting intervals, and at discharge or to end reporting

G9173 Voice functional limitation, discharge status at discharge from therapy or to end reporting

G9174 Other speech language pathology functional limitation, current status at therapy episode outset and at reporting intervals

G9175 Other speech language pathology functional limitation, projected goal status at therapy episode outset, at reporting intervals, and at discharge or to end reporting

G9176 Other speech language pathology functional limitation, discharge status at discharge from therapy or to end reporting

Lay Description
These codes represent functional limitations usually assessed by speech therapists and speech-language pathologists. The codes are reported with HCPCS Level II modifiers CH, CI, CJ, CK, CL, CM, or CN, which indicate the degree of impairment. These codes and modifiers are not payable, but are used to report the patient's type of functional limitation and whether the report is on the current status, projected goal status, or discharge status. The first claim for therapy services also requires the therapist's projected goal for functional status at the end of treatment. This reporting is required on selected claims for all outpatient therapy services, including those for

services above the therapy caps and those that include modifier KX for the cap exemption. They apply to all services furnished under the Medicare Part B outpatient therapy benefit and PT, OT, and SLP services under the comprehensive outpatient rehabilitation facilities (CORF) benefit. Therapy services included are those furnished personally and incident to the services of physicians or nonphysician practitioners (NPP). Functional limitations are reported for therapy services furnished in hospitals, critical access hospitals (CAH), skilled nursing facilities (SNF), CORFs, rehabilitation agencies, home health agencies (when the beneficiary is not under a home health plan of care), and in private offices of therapists, physicians, and NPPs.

G9186

G9186   Motor speech functional limitation, projected goal status at therapy episode outset, at reporting intervals, and at discharge or to end reporting

Lay Description

This code represents a functional limitation usually assessed by speech therapists and speech-language pathologists. The code is reported with HCPCS Level II modifiers CH, CI, CJ, CK, CL, CM, or CN, which indicate the degree of impairment. The code and modifiers are not payable, but are used to report the patient's type of functional limitation and whether the report is on the current status, projected goal status, or discharge status. The first claim for therapy services also requires the therapist's projected goal for functional status at the end of treatment. This reporting is required on selected claims for all outpatient therapy services, including those for services above the therapy caps and those that include modifier KX for the cap exemption. They apply to all services furnished under the Medicare Part B outpatient therapy benefit and PT, OT, and SLP services under the comprehensive outpatient rehabilitation facilities (CORF) benefit. Therapy services included are those furnished personally and incident to the services of physicians or nonphysician practitioners (NPP). Functional limitations are reported for therapy services furnished in hospitals, critical access hospitals (CAH), skilled nursing facilities (SNF), CORFs, rehabilitation agencies, home health agencies (when the beneficiary is not under a home health plan of care), and in private offices of therapists, physicians, and NPPs.

G9187

G9187   Bundled payments for care improvement initiative home visit for patient assessment performed by a qualified health care professional for individuals not considered homebound including, but not limited to, assessment of safety, falls, clinical status, fluid status, medication reconciliation/management,

patient compliance with orders/plan of care, performance of activities of daily living, appropriateness of care setting; (for use only in the Medicare-approved bundled payments for care improvement initiative); may not be billed for a 30-day period covered by a transitional care management code

Lay Description

The Bundled Payments for Care Improvement Initiative (BPCI) will create a new payment model. Currently, separate payments are made to providers for each individual service they render to patients during a single course of treatment or illness. Under BPCI, organizations will enter into payment arrangements based on entire episodes of care. This code is to be used to report the patient assessment home visit for patients not considered homebound, and is to be used only in a Medicare-approved BPCI initiative. It includes an assessment of clinical and fluid status, possibility of the patient falling, patient compliance, medication management, the appropriateness of the care setting, and activities of daily living. This code may not be reported for the same 30-day period covered by a transitional care management code.

H

H0001

H0001   Alcohol and/or drug assessment

Lay Description

This code reports provision of alcohol and/or drug assessment services. A psychiatrist, clinical psychologist, or other specialized health care professional or team of professionals generally provides drug and/or alcohol assessments. Protocols vary, but an assessment is systematic and thorough and addresses all aspects of a patient's encounters with alcohol and/or drugs. A detailed family, social, and legal history is usually solicited and components may be verified independent of the patient interview. Quantity and frequency of alcohol and/or drug use is documented. Physical manifestations associated with alcohol or drug use or abuse may be noted if present, such as depression, mania, anxiety, etc. A physical medical examination may be a component of the assessment. Questionnaires and tests may be used as components of the assessment. A report is generally issued that characterizes the patient's contact with alcohol and/or drugs as casual, dependent, abusive, addictive, etc. Should alcohol or drug use be determined to have caused adverse effects in the life of the patient or others, a report is issued documenting abuse. In addition to a diagnostic status, an assessment of abuse can have legal repercussions. This assessment should be used to devise a plan of care in treating the patient effectively.

H0002

H0002 Behavioral health screening to determine eligibility for admission to treatment program

Lay Description
Behavioral health screening is done to determine a patient's eligibility for admission to a treatment program. Patients are screened for mental health conditions as well as substance use disorders and are medically assessed to ensure appropriate treatment is given.

H0003

H0003 Alcohol and/or drug screening; laboratory analysis of specimens for presence of alcohol and/or drugs

Lay Description
Alcohol and/or drug screening is performed through laboratory analysis of urine, blood, or hair specimens to determine the presence of alcohol and/or drugs in the patient's system.

H0004

H0004 Behavioral health counseling and therapy, per 15 minutes

Lay Description
This code reports provision of behavioral health counseling and therapy services. Behavioral health counseling and therapy provides individual counseling by a clinician for a patient in a private setting and is billed in 15-minute increments.

H0005

H0005 Alcohol and/or drug services; group counseling by a clinician

Lay Description
Alcohol and/or drug group counseling by a clinician provides the patient support in a group setting (two or more individuals) in abstaining from substance abuse and assisting the patient with sobriety maintenance. Group counseling focuses on cognitive or behavioral approaches that typically address triggers and relapse prevention, self evaluation, the process of recovery, and issues pertaining to changes in lifestyle. Group sizes and treatment plans may vary according to the needs of the individual.

H0006

H0006 Alcohol and/or drug services; case management

Lay Description
Case management for patients needing services relating to alcohol or drug abuse provides assistance and care coordination based on the needs of the individual. The case manager assesses the needs of the patient, assists in developing plans to benefit the patient, as well as implementation of the plans, and reviews and evaluates the patient's status.

H0007

H0007 Alcohol and/or drug services; crisis intervention (outpatient)

Lay Description
Crisis intervention for alcohol and/or drug services is an emergency response by a clinician to provide immediate face-to-face support for an individual.

H0008-H0014

H0008 Alcohol and/or drug services; subacute detoxification (hospital inpatient)

H0009 Alcohol and/or drug services; acute detoxification (hospital inpatient)

H0010 Alcohol and/or drug services; subacute detoxification (residential addiction program inpatient)

H0011 Alcohol and/or drug services; acute detoxification (residential addiction program inpatient)

H0012 Alcohol and/or drug services; subacute detoxification (residential addiction program outpatient)

H0013 Alcohol and/or drug services; acute detoxification (residential addiction program outpatient)

H0014 Alcohol and/or drug services; ambulatory detoxification

Lay Description
These codes are for acute and subacute detoxification services in which the differentiating factor is the setting where the patient is monitored for the long-term symptoms associated with the withdrawal from alcohol and/or drugs. Subacute detoxification deals with severe symptoms, such as alcohol and drug cravings, that do not require immediate intervention. Acute detoxification services are those in which the patient is medically managed and stabilized on an inpatient hospitalization basis for severe withdrawal syndrome associated with the withdrawal from alcohol/drugs. Acute withdrawal begins within hours and includes severe physical and psychological symptoms that may require medical management with medications such as methadone.

H0015

H0015 Alcohol and/or drug services; intensive outpatient (treatment program that operates at least 3 hours/day and at least 3 days/week and is based on an individualized treatment plan), including assessment, counseling; crisis intervention, and activity therapies or education

Lay Description
This code reports alcohol and drug related services within an intensive outpatient treatment program requiring the patient to participate at least 3 hours per day for at least 3 days per week. The patient is assessed medically and psychologically, provided

counseling, intervention, and activity therapy or education, according to the needs of the patient and the individual's treatment plan.

H0016

H0016   Alcohol and/or drug services; medical/somatic (medical intervention in ambulatory setting)

Lay Description
This service includes the supervision of medication, physical examinations, or other medical needs required to maintain the physical health of the patient receiving medical intervention treatment for alcohol and drug related problems in an ambulatory setting.

H0017

H0017   Behavioral health; residential (hospital residential treatment program), without room and board, per diem

Lay Description
Residential treatment on a per diem basis for behavior health issues in a hospital residential treatment program is designed to provide a 24-hour group living situation in which the patient receives treatment under the care of a physician. This code does not include daily room and board.

H0018

H0018   Behavioral health; short-term residential (nonhospital residential treatment program), without room and board, per diem

Lay Description
Short-term residential treatment is typically less than 30 days. This code applies to a residential treatment program for behavior health issues that is not part of a hospital but provides a 24-hour group living situation in which the patient receives treatment and does not include daily room and board.

H0019

H0019   Behavioral health; long-term residential (nonmedical, nonacute care in a residential treatment program where stay is typically longer than 30 days), without room and board, per diem

Lay Description
Long-term residential treatment is typically more than 30 days. This code applies to a residential treatment program for behavioral health issues that are neither medical nor acute in nature. This code is per diem, not including daily room and board.

H0020

H0020   Alcohol and/or drug services; methadone administration and/or service (provision of the drug by a licensed program)

Lay Description
Methadone administration and/or service programs provide opioid replacement treatment (ORT) or opioid maintenance treatment (OMT), including the administration of methadone to an individual for detoxification from opioids and/or maintenance treatment. Overall treatment must be delivered, which should include counseling/therapy, case review, and medication monitoring. ORT/OMT is delivered by providers functioning under a defined set of policies and procedures, including admission, discharge, and continued service criteria stipulated by state law and regulations, Substance Abuse and Mental Health Services Administration (SAMHSA) regulations, and Drug Enforcement Agency (DEA) regulations. The ORT must be licensed by the Drug Enforcement Agency. The ORT should also have accreditation from the Joint Commission on the Accreditation of Healthcare Organizations (JCAHO), Committee for Accreditation (COA), and/or the Commission on the Accreditation of Rehabilitation Facilities (CARF). The ORT/OMT must meet the requirements of the Substance Abuse and Mental Health Administration.

H0021

H0021   Alcohol and/or drug training service (for staff and personnel not employed by providers)

Lay Description
This code is used to report developing alcohol and/or drug service skills of staff and personnel that are not employed by an agency, such as training a counselor/clinician on proper techniques and approaches or sessions for clinicians on the effects of various types of drugs.

H0022

H0022   Alcohol and/or drug intervention service (planned facilitation)

Lay Description
Alcohol and drug intervention services provide treatment services and activities that assist the professionally trained interventionalist to pursue and detect alcohol and or drug addictions and to intercede to halt the progress of the addictions. These services also include early interventions.

H0023

H0023   Behavioral health outreach service (planned approach to reach a targeted population)

Lay Description
Behavioral health outreach is a service targeting specific, at-risk individuals in a given population who

H

are in need of assistance with mental health issues. This may include mobile teams that contact at-risk individuals in the home, centers in which individuals can drop-in and obtain information regarding mental heath treatment or social services, or other various methods of contact that are not represented by a more specific code.

H0024-H0025

H0024 **Behavioral health prevention information dissemination service (one-way direct or nondirect contact with service audiences to affect knowledge and attitude)**

H0025 **Behavioral health prevention education service (delivery of services with target population to affect knowledge, attitude and/or behavior)**

Lay Description

A behavioral health prevention information dissemination service is used to provide facts to individuals in the community or in at-risk populations on issues of mental health. This service includes any form of direct or non-direct contact with the targeted audience to increase their awareness and knowledge of the issues and to affect their attitude. A behavioral health prevention education service is used to deliver services to individuals of a target population on issues of mental health education and to affect their knowledge, attitude, and behavior. It may include screenings to assist individuals in obtaining appropriate treatment. Causes and symptoms of disorders are discussed so as to encourage early intervention and reduce severity of mental illness.

H0026

H0026 **Alcohol and/or drug prevention process service, community-based (delivery of services to develop skills of impactors)**

Lay Description

Community-based, alcohol and/or drug prevention process services enhance the ability of a community to provide violence, alcohol, and/or drug abuse prevention services. The activities include planning, interagency collaboration, coalition building, and networking. Examples include multi-agency coordination and collaboration, community and volunteer training, and systemic planning.

H0027

H0027 **Alcohol and/or drug prevention environmental service (broad range of external activities geared toward modifying systems in order to mainstream prevention through policy and law)**

Lay Description

Alcohol and/or drug prevention environmental services (broad range of external activities geared

toward modifying systems in order to mainstream prevention through policy and law) establish or change written and unwritten community standards and postures that influence the incidence and prevalence of violence and/or the abuse of alcohol and/or drugs used in the general population.

H0028

H0028 **Alcohol and/or drug prevention problem identification and referral service (e.g., student assistance and employee assistance programs), does not include assessment**

Lay Description

This code reports alcohol and/or drug prevention problem identification and referral services (e.g., student assistance and employee assistance programs). Prevention strategies aim to identify individuals who have engaged in illegal and age-inappropriate use of tobacco, alcohol, and/or drugs. Services may include employee assistance programs (EAP), student assistance programs, and driving under the influence (DUI) education programs. Append modifier HA for 12 hours of education program within a community-based setting for youth younger than age 18 who are first-time offenders of alcohol or other drugs. Append modifier HB for 10 hours of education/diversion program within the circuit court districts for 19 to 20 year olds who have been referred to the program due to an alcohol-related offense. Append modifier HK for 30 hours of IPP within a community based setting for adolescents who have multiple offenses of alcohol or other drug use.

H0029

H0029 **Alcohol and/or drug prevention alternatives service (services for populations that exclude alcohol and other drug use e.g., alcohol free social events)**

Lay Description

This code reports alcohol and/or drug prevention alternative services (services for populations that exclude alcohol and other drug use e.g., alcohol free social events). Service strategies provide for the participation of specific inhabitants of a community in activities free from violence and/or alcohol/drug use. This strategy is to create attractive, healthy, and safe activities that increase an individual's commitment to abstain from violence and/or alcohol and drugs. These activities provide opportunities for low-risk choices when it comes to alcohol use and/or violent behavior. Examples include leadership camps, chemical free events, social activities, recreational activities, cultural activities, and behavioral activities at local community centers and other like places.

H0030

H0030 Behavioral health hotline service

Lay Description
Behavioral health hotline is a telephone service that provides crisis intervention and emergency management such as mental health referrals, treatment information, and other verbal assistance.

H0031

H0031 Mental health assessment, by nonphysician

Lay Description
Mental health assessment is provided by someone other than a physician who is a trained staff member. The assessment identifies factors of mental illness, functional capacity, and gathers additional information used for the treatment of mental illness.

H0032

H0032 Mental health service plan development by nonphysician

Lay Description
A mental health service plan is developed for treating a patient, including modifying goals, assessing progress, planning transitions, and addressing other needs. This service is provided by someone other than a physician, who is a clinical, professional, or other specialist.

H0033

H0033 Oral medication administration, direct observation

Lay Description
Patients are assisted or observed by professional medical staff during the administration of oral medication. This is often used in the administration of drugs such as methadone when it must be established that the patient has received the medication.

H0034

H0034 Medication training and support, per 15 minutes

Lay Description
Medication training and support is an educational service to assist the patient, family, or other caretaker in the proper management of prescribed medication regimens, drug interactions, and side effects. This code is reported per 15 minutes.

H0035

H0035 Mental health partial hospitalization, treatment, less than 24 hours

Lay Description
Partial hospitalization for mental health services is a treatment period of less than 24 hours care in which the patient is assisted with issues related to the individual's reintegration into society. This code is not considered an inpatient service.

H0036-H0037

H0036 Community psychiatric supportive treatment, face-to-face, per 15 minutes

H0037 Community psychiatric supportive treatment program, per diem

Lay Description
Community psychiatric supportive treatment programs assist individuals with persistent and severe mental illness to gain and maintain independence in the community. This is done with ongoing assessments, crisis intervention, and support. These programs may include advocacy, family education, helping in the development of activities of daily living, and managing basic needs to assist with achieving independence. The treatment/service may be charged per 15 minutes of face-to-face increments or as a daily (per diem) charge.

H0038

H0038 Self-help/peer services, per 15 minutes

Lay Description
Self help/peer services are specialized therapeutic interactions that are performed by individuals who are current or past recipients of behavioral health services. These individuals are trained and certified to provide support and assistance to individuals in their recovery and integration into the community. The goal is to provide understanding and coping skills and empowerment through mentoring and other supports so that individuals with severe and persistent mental disorders can cope with stress and achieve personal wellness.

H0039-H0040

H0039 Assertive community treatment, face-to-face, per 15 minutes

H0040 Assertive community treatment program, per diem

Lay Description
Assertive community treatment uses a team based, multidisciplinary approach. The goal is to reduce the extent of hospital admissions, to improve the individual's quality of life, and to function in social situations by providing focused, proactive treatments. These services are most appropriate for individuals with severe and persistent mental illness and the greatest level of functional impairment.

H

H0041-H0042

H0041 Foster care, child, nontherapeutic, per diem

H0042 Foster care, child, nontherapeutic, per month

Lay Description
Foster care is a service in which custodial care of a child under the age of 18 is assumed by someone outside the individual's family. The child is cared for and nurtured within a family context, nontherapeutically, per diem in H0041 and per month in H0042.

H0043-H0044

H0043 Supported housing, per diem

H0044 Supported housing, per month

Lay Description
Supported housing service provides individuals with assistance for the responsibilities of obtaining and maintaining independent living. Once housing is established, the clients are monitored through periodic visits to confirm the continued appropriateness of the living situation including affordability, and ensure that issues of independent living are addressed. This service does not include therapeutic aspects. Report H0043 for services performed per diem and code H0044 for services per month.

H0045

H0045 Respite care services, not in the home, per diem

Lay Description
Respite care services provided outside the home give assistance to clients in place of primary care givers on a temporary per diem basis so the patient may be maintained at the current level of care required when the primary care givers are temporarily absent.

H0046

H0046 Mental health services, not otherwise specified

Lay Description
Use this code to report mental health services that are not described by any other HCPCS Level II code.

H0047

H0047 Alcohol and/or other drug abuse services, not otherwise specified

Lay Description
Use this code to report alcohol and/or other drug abuse services that are not described by any other HCPCS Level II code.

H0048

H0048 Alcohol and/or other drug testing: collection and handling only, specimens other than blood

Lay Description
Collection of specimens for alcohol/drug analysis is dependent on the type of biological sample obtained. Samples typically include urine or hair. This code represents the collection and handling of specimens other than blood samples. The handling of specimens requires a chain of custody from the point of collection throughout the analysis process to ensure the integrity of the specimen.

H0049

H0049 Alcohol and/or drug screening

Lay Description
Drug and alcohol screening is performed on patients in a drug and alcohol treatment program to detect the presence or absence of drugs or alcohol in the urine, blood, or breath. Screening tests are used to determine if an individual has recently ingested drugs or alcohol. A screening test does not quantify the amount of a drug in the urine, blood, or breath; it identifies only the presence or absence of these substances. If the individual tests positive, the individual may be tested with a more specific drug test to rule out any false positive results and to identify the specific substance ingested and the amount of the substance ingested.

H0050

H0050 Alcohol and/or drug services, brief intervention, per 15 minutes

Lay Description
A brief intervention for a patient in a drug and/or alcohol treatment program is performed. Professionally trained interventionists who are experts in chemical dependency meet briefly with the patient and/or family members to discuss a current treatment issue. The service may be initiated by the patient or the interventionist in response to a specific issue. The purpose of the intervention is to provide support and feedback related to chemical dependency issues that are currently affecting the patient and/or family members. This code is reported per 15 minute time increment spent in the intervention service.

H1000

H1000 Prenatal care, at-risk assessment

Lay Description
A pregnancy is considered high risk when there are conditions that could affect the baby, the mother, or the baby and mother. Examples of risk factors for a high-risk pregnancy include the age of the mother (younger than 17 or older than 35 years of age when the baby is due); pre-pregnancy medical conditions such as STD, diabetes, HIV or other chronic infection;

family history of genetic disorders; and a history of miscarriages. Medical conditions may occur during the pregnancy, including gestational diabetes and preeclampsia. Other pregnancy-related issues can classify a patient as high risk, including placenta previa, fetal problems, multiple births, and premature labor. Use this code to report the at-risk assessment. This is usually done during the first trimester but may be done later if problems develop later in the pregnancy.

H1001-H1005

H1001 Prenatal care, at-risk enhanced service; antepartum management

H1002 Prenatal care, at risk enhanced service; care coordination

H1003 Prenatal care, at-risk enhanced service; education

H1004 Prenatal care, at-risk enhanced service; follow-up home visit

H1005 Prenatal care, at-risk enhanced service package (includes H1001-H1004)

Lay Description
A pregnancy is considered high risk when there are conditions that could affect the baby, the mother, or the baby and the mother. Examples of risk factors for a high-risk pregnancy include the age of the mother (younger than 17 or older than 35 years of age when the baby is due); pre-pregnancy medical conditions such as STD, diabetes, HIV, or other chronic infection; family history of genetic disorders; and a history of miscarriages. Medical conditions may occur during the pregnancy, including gestational diabetes and preeclampsia. Other pregnancy-related issues can classify a patient as high risk, including placenta previa, fetal problems, multiple births, and premature labor. These codes report additional or enhanced services rendered that are required by the at-risk pregnancy. The physician in charge of the patient's care determines what additional services are required. These services can include the development and implementation of the plan of care for the specific patient, making referrals, monitoring the patient's progress, and assuring access to services required for a healthy pregnancy and birth. Enhanced education services include information to prepare the patient for the birth process, information to help the patient identify and try to prevent preterm labor, guidance for prenatal nutrition, and education on lifestyle and parenting support. The postpartum follow-up home visit is an additional and separate visit from the six week postpartum visit. It is usually done within the first two weeks post discharge of the mother. This visit is intended to provide special support by following up on the identified "at risk" medical conditions and addressing the stress involved with caring for the new baby.

H1010

H1010 Nonmedical family planning education, per session

Lay Description
Use this code to report education of an individual or a couple in the methods of natural family planning.

H1011

H1011 Family assessment by licensed behavioral health professional for state defined purposes

Lay Description
This code is used for Medicaid purposes to report the assessment of a patient's family by a licensed behavioral health professional. Note that both the description of the service and the type of licensed professional are specific to each state.

H2000

H2000 Comprehensive multidisciplinary evaluation

Lay Description
A comprehensive multidisciplinary evaluation consists of a thorough investigation in several areas to provide an accurate representation of the individual's needs and strengths. This evaluates areas such as psychiatric, physical, psychosocial, family, recreational, and occupational therapy.

H2001

H2001 Rehabilitation program, per 1/2 day

Lay Description
The goal of a rehabilitation program is to enhance independent living, along with communication and social skills. The program may include training to develop skills in conflict resolution, problem solving, employment, and social interaction. Use this code to report each half day of a rehabilitation program.

H2010

H2010 Comprehensive medication services, per 15 minutes

Lay Description
Comprehensive medication services are patient centered. They are provided by specially trained pharmacists who work with the patient to make sure that all drug therapies are effective for the intended use, appropriate for the patient's medical condition, able to be taken by the patient as intended, and are safe. The actual outcomes are recorded. These services are intended to improve the quality of patient care, reduce health care costs, and identify and resolve any problems with the drug therapy.

H

H2011

H2011 Crisis intervention service, per 15 minutes

Lay Description

Mental health crisis intervention provides immediate support for an individual in personal crisis with outpatient status. The aim of this service is to stabilize the individual during a psychiatric emergency and is billed in 15-minute increments.

H2012

H2012 Behavioral health day treatment, per hour

Lay Description

Day treatment for behavior health focuses on maintaining and improving functional abilities for the individual. Clients may participate in activities in a therapeutic and social environment several times per week for several hours per day to improve personal skills. This code is reported per hour of daytime behavioral health treatment.

H2013

H2013 Psychiatric health facility service, per diem

Lay Description

A psychiatric health facility is specifically licensed as such and is differentiated from a hospital with an inpatient psychiatric ward, psychiatric hospital, or crisis residential services. This facility provides services in an acute non-hospital inpatient setting, and includes appropriate care in psychiatry, clinical psychology, social work, rehabilitation, drug administration, and other basic needs, per diem.

H2014

H2014 Skills training and development, per 15 minutes

Lay Description

Skills training and development provides the patient with necessary abilities that will enable the individual to live independently and manage his/her illness and treatment. Training focuses on skills for daily living and community integration for patients with functional limitations due to psychiatric disorders, per 15 minutes.

H2015-H2016

H2015 Comprehensive community support services, per 15 minutes
H2016 Comprehensive community support services, per diem

Lay Description

Comprehensive community support services consist of mental health and substance abuse services. These services assist individuals in achieving their recovery and rehabilitation goals. The program aims to reduce psychiatric and addiction symptoms and to assist in developing community living skills. The services may include coordination of services, support during a crisis, development of system monitoring and management skills, monitoring medications, and help in developing independent living skills. Use these codes to report comprehensive community support services per 15 minutes or per diem.

H2017-H2018

H2017 Psychosocial rehabilitation services, per 15 minutes
H2018 Psychosocial rehabilitation services, per diem

Lay Description

Psychosocial rehabilitation services are intended to help individuals to compensate for or to eliminate functional deficits and environmental and interpersonal barriers associated with their mental illness. The goal of the program is to help individuals achieve the fullest possible integration as an active and productive member of their family and community with the least possible ongoing professional intervention. Activities are done to achieve the goals for the individual. This is a face-to-face intervention and the services may be provided in a group or an individual setting. Use these codes to report these services in 15 minutes increments or a per diem charge.

H2019-H2020

H2019 Therapeutic behavioral services, per 15 minutes
H2020 Therapeutic behavioral services, per diem

Lay Description

Therapeutic behavioral services are treatments that attempt to change unhealthy, potentially dangerous, or self-destructive behaviors. It focuses on helping an individual understand how the behavior affects life and emotions. Behavioral therapy is usually action-based, using techniques of classical conditioning and operant conditioning. The behavior itself is the problem and the goal is to minimize or eliminate the problem. Each payer, agency, or organization has their own definition and categorization of therapeutic behavioral services. Consult the appropriate party for addition information.

H2021-H2022

H2021 Community-based wrap-around services, per 15 minutes
H2022 Community-based wrap-around services, per diem

Lay Description

Wrap-around community services are provided for a short period of time for seriously emotionally disabled youth. These services are provided for children/adolescents with a rate classification level (RCL) placement higher than 12. These codes include support and training for family members as an integral part of services provided.

H2023-H2024

H2023 **Supported employment, per 15 minutes**
H2024 **Supported employment, per diem**

Lay Description
Supported employment services are available to individuals with serious mental illness. Employment specialists assist in obtaining and maintaining employment in the community and in continuing treatment for the client to ensure rehabilitation and productive employment.

H2025-H2026

H2025 **Ongoing support to maintain employment, per 15 minutes**
H2026 **Ongoing support to maintain employment, per diem**

Lay Description
Ongoing support to maintain employment services are available to individuals with serious mental illness. Employment specialists provide supportive counseling and interventions within the work environment when needed to ensure the continued employment and self-sufficiency of the client.

H2027

H2027 **Psychoeducational service, per 15 minutes**

Lay Description
The National Library of Medicine, within the National Institutes of Health, defines a psychoeducational service as an item, action, or procedure "of or relating to the psychological aspects of education; specifically: relating to or used in the education of children with behavioral disorders or learning disabilities." Each payer, agency, or organization has its own definition and categorization of psychoeducational services. Consult the appropriate party for addition information.

H2028-H2029

H2028 **Sexual offender treatment service, per 15 minutes**
H2029 **Sexual offender treatment service, per diem**

Lay Description
Sexual offender treatment services provide rehabilitation services that vary depending on the type of treatment facility, security level, and staffing ratios available.

H2030-H2031

H2030 **Mental health clubhouse services, per 15 minutes**
H2031 **Mental health clubhouse services, per diem**

Lay Description
Mental health clubhouse is a community service provided for people with mental illness and promotes a structured environment in which individuals can improve interpersonal skills, and develop personal goals that will assist with success in the community. Participants are required to take part in the operations of the clubhouse.

H2032

H2032 **Activity therapy, per 15 minutes**

Lay Description
Activity therapy such as music, dance, creative art, or any type of play, not for recreation, but related to the care and treatment of the patient's disabling mental health problems is reported for services per 15 minutes.

H2033

H2033 **Multisystemic therapy for juveniles, per 15 minutes**

Lay Description
Multisystemic therapy uses the strengths found in key environmental settings of juveniles to promote and maintain positive behavioral changes. These services focus on individual, family, and extrafamilial (such as peer, school, and neighborhood) influences, reported in 15 minute increments.

H2034-H2036

H2034 **Alcohol and/or drug abuse halfway house services, per diem**
H2035 **Alcohol and/or other drug treatment program, per hour**
H2036 **Alcohol and/or other drug treatment program, per diem**

Lay Description
Halfway house services for alcohol and chemical dependency provide a transitional living environment. These services are structured to promote sobriety and independent living, and assist with continued treatment. Patients are free to work or attend classes during the day, and return to the facility at night.

H2037

H2037 **Developmental delay prevention activities, dependent child of client, per 15 minutes**

Lay Description
Developmental delay prevention activities are designed to reduce the occurrence of problems

H

stemming from inhibited or suppressed development in children that can have effects carrying over into later years. The developmental activities promote the physical and mental well being of dependent children of patients in treatment for alcohol/drug abuse. These services focus on overall healthy development of the child, reported in 15-minute blocks.

J

J0120

J0120   Injection, tetracycline, up to 250 mg

Lay Description
Tetracycline is a broad-spectrum antibiotic prepared from cultures of certain species of streptomyces bacteria. It is thought to inhibit protein synthesis in bacteria, causing cell death. Many microorganisms have developed a resistance to tetracycline and related antibiotics. Susceptibility studies should be performed prior to administration. Tetracycline can be effective against gram-negative and gram-positive organisms. Susceptible organisms include *Rickettsiae, Mycoplasma pneumoniae, Borrelia recurrentis, Haemophilus ducreyi, Pasteurella pestis, Pasteurella tularensis, Bartonella bacilliformis, Bacteroides species, Vibrio comma, Vibrio fetus, Brucella* species (in conjunction with streptomycin), *Escherichia coli, Enterobacter aerogenes, Shigella* species, *Mima* species, *Herellea* species, *Haemophilus influenzae*, and *Klebsiella* species.

J0129

J0129   Injection, abatacept, 10 mg (code may be used for Medicare when drug administered under the direct supervision of a physician, not for use when drug is self-administered)

Lay Description
Abatacept is a protein combination of human cytotoxic T-lymphocyte-associated antigen 4 (CTLA-4) linked to a modified portion of human immunoglobulin G1 (IgG1). It is produced by recombinant DNA technology. Abatacept binds to specific receptor sites of T lymphocyte cells and inhibits their activation. Activated T lymphocytes are found in joint fluid of patients with rheumatoid arthritis. Abatacept is indicated for reducing signs and symptoms, slowing the progression of structural damage, and improving physical function of adult patients with moderately to severely active rheumatoid arthritis who have had an inadequate response to other drugs. The drug can be used singularly or in combination with other disease-modifying, anti-rheumatic drugs. The drug is administered by intravenous infusion over a 30-minute period. Dosage varies from 500 mg to 1 g depending on body weight.

J0130

J0130   Injection abciximab, 10 mg

Lay Description
Abciximab is a murine monoclonal antibody. It blocks certain glycoprotein receptors on platelets and prevents them from aggregating or sticking together. Abciximab also blocks receptors on vessel walls and smooth muscle cells preventing the platelets from aggregating in those sites. It is used as an adjunct with percutaneous transluminal coronary angioplasty (PTCA). Abciximab may be used to treat unstable angina when the patient is not responding to conventional therapy and PTCA is planned within 24 hours. The recommended dosage is 0.25 mg per kg of body weight. The drug is administered as an intravenous bolus 10 to 60 minutes prior to the PTCA, followed by continuous intravenous infusion for 12 hours. When given to unstable angina patients for whom PTCA is planned, a 0.25 mg bolus is administered followed by an 18 to 24 hour intravenous infusion.

J0131

J0131   Injection, acetaminophen, 10 mg

Lay Description
Acetaminophen is a non-opioid, non-steroidal anti-inflammatory drug (NSAID). This code represents the intravenous formulation of acetaminophen. This drug is indicated for the management of mild to moderate pain, the management of moderate to severe pain with adjunctive opioid analgesics, and for fever reduction in adults and children 2 years of age or older. It is administered only as a 15-minute IV infusion and may be given as a single or repeated dose. The recommended adult dosage is 650 to 1,000 mg to a maximum dose of 4,000 mg per 24 hours with intervals of four hours.

J0132

J0132   Injection, acetylcysteine, 100 mg

Lay Description
Acetylcysteine is a derivative of the naturally occurring amino acid L-cysteine. It is used as an antidote for acetaminophen overdose to prevent life-threatening liver damage. Acetylcysteine reacts with the acetaminophen rendering some of the acetaminophen harmless. As an antidote for acetaminophen poisoning, acetylcysteine should be administered as soon as possible but within 24 hours after the overdose. Acetylcysteine is administered by intravenous infusion over 60 minutes.

J0133

J0133   Injection, acyclovir, 5 mg

Lay Description
Acyclovir injection is used to treat herpes infections, including herpes zoster and varicella (chickenpox). It does not cure the infection but does reduce pain and may promote faster healing. Acyclovir is given

intravenously over at least an hour. This code reports a 5 mg injection.

J0135

J0135   Injection, adalimumab, 20 mg

Lay Description
Adalimumab is a human IgG1 monoclonal antibody that is specific for human tumor necrosis factor (TNF). It is produced by recombinant DNA technology. Adalimumab binds specifically to TNF-alpha, blocks its interaction with cell surface TNF receptors and lyses surface TNF expressing cells. Adalimumab also modulates biological responses that are induced or regulated by TNF, including changes in the levels of adhesion molecules responsible for leukocyte migration. Adalimumab is indicated for reducing signs and symptoms and inhibiting the progression of structural damage in adult patients with moderately to severely active rheumatoid arthritis who have had an inadequate response to one or more disease modifying antirheumatic drugs and patients with active arthritis with psoriatic arthritis. Adalimumab can be used alone or in combination with methotrexate or other disease modifying antirheumatic drugs. Adalimumab is administered by subcutaneous injection and can be self-administered.

J0153

J0153   Injection, adenosine, 1 mg (not to be used to report any adenosine phosphate compounds)

Lay Description
Adenosine is a nucleoside that is a component of RNA. Its nucleotides play major roles in the reactions and regulation of metabolism. Preparations of adenosine act as cardiac depressants, antiarrhythmics, and vasodilators. Adenosine is administered to convert paroxysmal supraventricular tachycardia (PSVT) to normal sinus rhythm. Diagnostic adenosine is administered to patients as an adjunct to a thallium myocardial perfusion scan for patients who are unable to adequately exercise. Recommended dose for therapeutic use is an initial 6 mg followed by 12 mg if the arrhythmia continues. Adenosine is administered via intravenous push injection.

J0171

J0171   Injection, Adrenalin, epinephrine, 0.1 mg

Lay Description
Epinephrine hydrochloride (HCl), also known as adrenalin, is a synthetic version of a hormone secreted by the adrenal gland. Epinephrine is a potent stimulator of the sympathetic nervous system that increases blood pressure, stimulates the heart, and increases metabolic functions. Exogenous epinephrine is used as a cardiac stimulant, to increase blood pressure, and to relax bronchial smooth muscles. The injectable version of epinephrine HCl is administered subcutaneously or intramuscularly and

is used to treat serious hypersensitivity (allergic) reactions and anaphylaxis, and to restore cardiac rhythm in cardiac arrest.

J0178

J0178   Injection, aflibercept, 1 mg

Lay Description
Aflibercept is a recombinant protein produced in Chinese hamster cells. The fused protein consists of portions of human vascular endothelial growth factor-A (VEGF) and placental growth factor (P1GF) receptors fused to human IgG1. VEGF and P1GF act on receptor sites to stimulate neovascularization and vascular permeability. Aflibercept is indicated as a treatment for neovascular (or wet) age-related macular degeneration (AMD). The recommended dose for aflibercept is 2 mg every four weeks for the first 12 weeks followed by 2 mg once every eight weeks. The drug is for intravitreal administration only.

J0180

J0180   Injection, agalsidase beta, 1 mg

Lay Description
Agalsidase beta is a recombinant human a-galactosidase A enzyme with the same amino acid sequence as the naturally occurring enzyme. It is produced by recombinant DNA technology in a Chinese hamster ovary. Agalsidase beta is an orphan drug specifically targeted to Fabry disease. Fabry disease is an X-linked genetic disorder of glycosphingolipid metabolism. A deficiency of enzyme a-galactosidase A leads to progressive accumulation of glycosphingolipids, predominantly GL-3, in many body tissues, occurring over a period of years or decades. Clinical manifestations of Fabry disease include renal failure, cardiomyopathy, and cerebrovascular accidents. Recommended dose is 1.0 mg per kg of body weight. Agalsidase beta is administered by intravenous infusion.

J0190

J0190   Injection, biperiden lactate, per 5 mg

Lay Description
The injectable form of biperiden lactate has been discontinued.

J0200

J0200   Injection, alatrofloxacin mesylate, 100 mg

Lay Description
Per the FDA, this drug is no longer available in the United States.

J0205

J0205   Injection, alglucerase, per 10 units

Lay Description
Alglucerase is a modified form of beta-glucocerebrosidase prepared from pooled

human placental tissue. It is an orphan drug used to treat Gaucher's disease caused by the lack of the enzyme glucocerebrosidase, which is crucial to the metabolism of fats. Alglucerase normalizes the pathway for membrane lipids. Dose is based on disease severity and individual patient response to treatment. Initial dosage may be as little as 2.5 units per kg of body weight three times a week up to as much as 60 units per kg administered as often as once a week or as infrequently as every four weeks. Alglucerase is administered by intravenous infusion over one to two hours.

J0207

J0207   Injection, amifostine, 500 mg

Lay Description

Amifostine is dephosphorylated in living tissue by an alkaline phosphate enzyme to become a biologically active form of free thiol in the body. Free thiol will bind to and detoxify the reactive metabolites of cisplatin, scavenges free radicals from tissues exposed to cisplatin. Amifostine is used to reduce the cumulative nephrotoxicity in patients who have received repeated doses of cisplatin because of advanced ovarian cancer, bladder cancer, testicular cancer, or non-small cell lung cancer. It is also newly used to reduce xerostomia in patients with head and neck cancer receiving postoperative radiation treatment. For patients on chemotherapy, it is injected over a 15-minute period one half hour before chemotherapy. For patients receiving radiation treatment, it is injected over a three minute period 15 to 30 minutes prior to radiation.

J0210

J0210   Injection, methyldopate HCl, up to 250 mg

Lay Description

Methyldopate hydrochloride is an aromatic-amino-acid decarboxylase inhibitor used primarily to treat hypertension or during a hypertensive crisis. It decreases the sympathetic outflow to the heart, kidneys, and peripheral vasculature. Decreased blood pressure may occur four to six hours after the administration of methyldopate hydrochloride and last 10 to 16 hours. The usual dose is 250 to 500 mg intravenously at six-hour intervals as required. The maximum recommended intravenous dose is 1 gram every six hours. Methyldopate hydrochloride is administered via intravenous infusion over 30 to 60 minutes.

J0215

J0215   Injection, alefacept, 0.5 mg

Lay Description

Alefacept is an injectable drug that suppresses the immune system and is used for the treatment of moderate to severe chronic plaque psoriasis. It interferes with lymphocyte activation by binding to the lymphocyte antigen and interfering with the human leukocyte function antigen-3 and the CD2 binding interaction. It is produced by recombinant DNA technology in a Chinese hamster ovary (CHO) mammalian cell expression system. The recommended dose is 7.5 mg given once weekly as an intravenous injection or 15 mg given once weekly as an intramuscular injection. The recommended regimen is a course of 12 weekly injections.

J0220

J0220   Injection, alglucosidase alfa, 10 mg, not otherwise specified

Lay Description

Alglucosidase alfa is an exogenous source of the human enzyme alpha-glucosidase (GAA) made from recombinant DNA technology using Chinese hamster ovaries. It is an orphan drug used to treat infantile onset Pompe disease (GAA deficiency). Pompe disease is caused by the lack of the enzyme alpha-glucosidase, which is crucial to the metabolism of glycogen. A deficiency of GAA leads to a build up of intralysosomal glycogen resulting in progressive muscle weakness. In infantile onset, Pompe disease may also lead to cardiomyopathy and impairment of respiratory function. . The recommended dosage is 20 mg per kg of patient body weight. Alglucosidase alfa is administered by intravenous infusion, using an infusion pump, over four hours, every two weeks.

J0221

J0221   Injection, alglucosidase alfa, (Lumizyme), 10 mg

Lay Description

Alglucosidase alfa is an exogenous source of the human enzyme alpha-glucosidase made from recombinant DNA technology using Chinese hamster ovaries. It is an orphan drug used to treat non-infantile onset glycogen storage disease (GSD), type II or Pompe disease in patients 8 years of age and older who do not have cardiac hypertrophy. On August 1, 2014, Lumizyme was approved to also treat infantile onset Pompe's disease, including patients who are younger than 8 years of age. GSD II is caused by the lack of the enzyme alpha-glucosidase, which is crucial to the metabolism of glycogen. GSD II leads to a buildup of intralysosomal glycogen, resulting in progressive muscle weakness. In infantile onset, GSD II may also lead to cardiomyopathy and impairment of respiratory function. This code represents 1 mg of Lumizyme. The recommended dosage is 20 mg per kg of patient body weight. Alglucosidase alfa is administered by intravenous infusion, using an infusion pump, over four hours, every two weeks.

J0256

J0256   Injection, alpha 1-proteinase inhibitor (human), not otherwise specified, 10 mg

Lay Description

Alpha 1-proteinase inhibitor, human is a plasma product prepared from pooled human plasma of normal donors that contains high levels of purified human alpha 1-proteinase inhibitor (alpha1-PI) also known as alpha 1-antitrypsin. This is used to treat patients with alpha 1 antitrypsin deficiency (A1AD), a genetic protein deficiency that results in advanced emphysema showing up in young patients as an inherited disease, not related to smoking or environmental factors. It mimics COPD, asthma, and acquired emphysema and is therefore difficult to diagnose and rated as rare. Replacing the protein helps prevent the continued lung destruction caused by this deficiency. Recommended dose is 60 mg per kg of body weight once a week. Alpha 1-proteinase inhibitor is administered via intravenous infusion over 15 to 30 minutes.

J0257

J0257   Injection, alpha 1 proteinase inhibitor (human), (GLASSIA), 10 mg

Lay Description

Alpha 1-proteinase inhibitor (GLASSIA) human is a plasma product prepared from pooled human plasma of normal donors that contains high levels of purified human alpha 1-proteinase inhibitor (alpha1-PI), also known as alpha 1-antitrypsin. This is used to treat patients with alpha 1 antitrypsin deficiency (A1AD), also known as alpha1-antitrypsin (AAT) deficiency, a genetic protein deficiency that results in advanced emphysema showing up in young patients as an inherited disease, not related to smoking or environmental factors. It mimics COPD, asthma, and acquired emphysema and is therefore difficult to diagnose and rated as rare. Replacing the Alpha1-PI protein helps prevent the continued lung destruction caused by this deficiency. GLASSIA contains 2% active Alpha1-PI in a phosphate-buffered saline solution. Recommended dose is 60 mg per kg of body weight once a week. Alpha 1-proteinase inhibitor is administered via intravenous infusion over 60 to 80 minutes.

J0270-J0275

J0270   Injection, alprostadil, 1.25 mcg (code may be used for Medicare when drug administered under the direct supervision of a physician, not for use when drug is self-administered)

J0275   Alprostadil urethral suppository (code may be used for Medicare when drug administered under the direct supervision of a physician, not for use when drug is self-administered)

Lay Description

Alprostadil is a naturally occurring form of prostaglandin. It is a vasodilator that increases blood flow by expanding blood vessels. It is used for patients in need of palliative therapy for the temporary maintenance of patency of ductus arteriosus who have congenital heart defects and who depend upon the patent ductus for survival. Studies have shown that alprostadil reopens a closing ductus arteriosus. It is also indicated in the treatment of erectile dysfunction. Alprostadil increases cavernous arterial blood flow and inhibits platelet aggregation. It induces erection by relaxing the trabecular smooth muscle and dilating the cavernosal arteries. This leads to expansion of lacunar spaces and entrapment of blood by compressing the venules against the tunica. This is also known as the corporal veno-occlusive mechanism. It also lowers the blood pressure and increases cardiac output. Alprostadil can be administered into a large vein or umbilical artery for infants with congenital heart defects. It is administered via injection into the corpora cavernosa or as a urethral suppository for erectile dysfunction. Both of the methods for treatment of erectile dysfunction can be self-administered.

J0278

J0278   Injection, amikacin sulfate, 100 mg

Lay Description

Amikacin sulfate is an antibiotic used to treat susceptible strains of Gram-negative bacteria. It binds to the RNA and will not allow the bacteria to synthesize protein that is essential to its growth. It is effective against *Pseudomonas* species, *E. coli*, *Proteus* species, *Klebsiella-Enterobacter-Serratia* species, *Providencia* species, *Salmonella* species, *Citrobacter* species, and *S. aureus*. Amikacin sulfate may be used to treat bacteremia, septicemia (including neonatal sepsis), osteomyelitis, septic arthritis, respiratory tract, urinary tract, intra-abdominal (including peritonitis) infections, and soft tissue abscesses. This medication is administered via intramuscular injection or intravenous infusion.

J0280

J0280   Injection, aminophyllin, up to 250 mg

Lay Description

Aminophylline is a bronchodilator that is used to treat breathing problems such as asthma, emphysema, and chronic bronchitis. It relaxes the smooth muscle in the bronchial airways and pulmonary blood vessels by interfering with phosphodiesterase, which is the enzyme that corrupts adenosine 3', 5'-cyclic monophosphate (cAMP).

J0282

J0282   Injection, amiodarone HCl, 30 mg

Lay Description

Amiodarone hydrochloride is an antiarrhythmic used in the treatment of ventricular fibrillation and hemodynamically unstable atrial fibrillation that do not respond to other treatment. It blocks the calcium channels and potassium channels and lengthens the cardiac action potential and slows the conduction and prolongation of refractoriness. It decreases the workload of the heart and the amount of oxygen it requires. Amiodarone hydrochloride can be administered orally or by intravenous push followed by intravenous infusion that may be continuous for several days.

J0285-J0289

J0285   Injection, amphotericin B, 50 mg

J0287   Injection, amphotericin B lipid complex, 10 mg

J0288   Injection, amphotericin B cholesteryl sulfate complex, 10 mg

J0289   Injection, amphotericin B liposome, 10 mg

Lay Description

Amphotericin B is an antibiotic derived from a strain of *Streptomyces nodosus* that has antifungal properties. The drug is effective against a wide variety of fungi and some species of *Leishmania*. It binds to the fungus cell membrane and changes the permeability causing the cell contents to leak out, which causes cell death. Amphotericin B may be administered by intravenous infusion or intracavitary instillation over two to six hours. A topical version is used to treat superficial candidiasis. The cholesteryl complex version is administered by intravenous infusion to treat disseminated aspergillosis in patients refractory to or intolerant of conventional amphotericin B. The lipid complex is administered by intravenous infusion to treat invasive fungal infections in patients refractory to or intolerant of conventional amphotericin B. The liposome complex is administered by intravenous infusion to treat sever fungal infections and visceral leishmaniasis in patients refractory to or intolerant of conventional amphotericin B.

J0290

J0290   Injection, ampicillin sodium, 500 mg

Lay Description

Ampicillin is a form of penicillin used to treat respiratory or skin infections, urinary tract infections, bacterial meningitis, septicemia, and as a prophylaxis in dental procedures. It inhibits the formation of a cell wall during replication. It is effective against *E. coli, P. mirabilis*, enterococci, *Shigella, S. typhosa* and other Salmonella, non-penicillinase-producing *N. gonorrhoeae*, non-penicillinase-producing *H. influenzae* and staphylococci, and streptococci including *streptococcus pneumoniae, Shigella, S. typhosa* and other *Salmonella, E. coli, P. mirabilis*, and enterococci, and *O. Meningitides*. This drug may decrease the efficacy of oral contraceptives.

J0295

J0295   Injection, ampicillin sodium/sulbactam sodium, per 1.5 g

Lay Description

Ampicillin sodium and sulbactam sodium are used to treat gynecologic, intra-abdominal, and skin infections. Ampicillin inhibits the formation of a cell wall during replication and sulbactam inactivates the enzyme produced by the bacteria to make them resistant to the ampicillin. It is effective against *Staphylococcus aureus, Staphylococcus epidermidis, Staphylococcus saprophyticus, Streptococcus faecalis, Streptococcus pneumoniae, Streptococcus pyogenes, Streptococcus viridans, Haemophilus influenzae, Moraxella (Branhamella) catarrhalis, Escherichia coli, Klebsiella species, Proteus mirabilis, Proteus vulgaris, Providencia rettgeri, Providencia stuartii, Morganella morganii, Neisseria gonorrhoeae, Clostridium* species, *Peptococcus* species, *Peptostreptococcus* species, and *Bacteroides* species, including *B. fragilis*. Ampicillin sodium and sulbactam sodium are administered via intramuscular injection, which is given only to adults, and intravenous injection, which is given by slow infusion over 10 to 15 minutes.

J0300

J0300   Injection, amobarbital, up to 125 mg

Lay Description

Amobarbital is a barbiturate derivative that activates one of the major inhibitory neurotransmitters in the body, which reduces input resistance, depresses the electrical discharge along the cell and increases the conduction at the chloride channels, and increases the amplitude and decay time of inhibitory postsynaptic currents. Amobarbital, also known as truth serum, is indicated as a treatment for convulsions, anxiety, epilepsy, and as a short-term treatment of insomnia. The drug is also used for preoperative sedation. It is a schedule II drug with the suppository being a schedule III drug. This medication is administered orally, rectally, via intramuscular injection, and via intravenous push injection.

J0330

J0330   Injection, succinylcholine chloride, up to 20 mg

Lay Description

Succinylcholine chloride is skeletal muscle relaxant. It is used in combination with anesthesia to relax skeletal muscles for surgery, intubation, seizure control, and orthopedic manipulations. It reacts with cholinergic receptors of the motor end plates to create depolarization. Flaccid paralysis begins within one minute after administration and lasts approximately four to six minutes.

J0348

J0348   Injection, anidulafungin, 1 mg

Lay Description

Anidulafungin is a semisynthetic lipopeptide derived from the fungus *Aspergillus nidulans*. It is used as an antifungal drug. Anidulafungin disrupts the synthesis of a component of the fungal cell membrane. This component is not present in mammalian cells. Anidulafungin is indicated for the treatment of candidemia, intra-abdominal, peritoneal, and esophageal *Candida* infections. The drug may cause allergic reactions. Anidulafungin must be administered by intravenous infusion. Recommended dosage for esophageal candidiasis is an initial dose of 100 mg followed by 50 mg daily. The duration of treatment depends upon the patient's response, but should be for a minimum of 14 days or for at least seven days following resolution of symptoms. Recommended dosage for candidemia, intra-abdominal and peritoneal *Candida* infections is an initial dose of 200 mg followed by 100 mg daily. The duration of treatment depends upon the patient's response, but should continue for at least 14 days after the last positive culture.

J0350

J0350   Injection, anistreplase, per 30 units

Lay Description

Anistreplase is a complex composed of streptokinase and lys-plasminogen. It is also known as anisoylated plasminogen-streptokinase activator complex (APSAC). It is a thrombolytic agent used to dissolve blood clots that have formed in certain blood vessels. It binds to fibrin, converts plasminogen into plasmin, and breaks down the thrombus into smaller components. Anistreplase is used primarily in the management of an acute myocardial infarction and should be administered as soon as possible after the onset of the heart attack symptoms. Anistreplase is administered via intravenous infusion.

J0360

J0360   Injection, hydralazine HCl, up to 20 mg

Lay Description

Hydralazine hydrochloride falls into a category of drugs known as antihypertensives. It works by exerting a vasodilating effect on vascular smooth muscle. It is used in combination with other drugs in treating a hypertensive crisis and eclampsia. Hydralazine hydrochloride can be administered by intramuscular injection, intravenous injection, or intravenous infusion.

J0364

J0364   Injection, apomorphine HCl, 1 mg

Lay Description

Apomorphine hydrochloride is a non-ergoline dopamine agonist. It is used for the acute, intermittent treatment of hypomobility, "off" episodes ("end-of-dose wearing off" and unpredictable "on/off" episodes) associated with advanced Parkinson's disease. Apomorphine should not be started without use of an associated antiemetic. Trimethobenzamide should be started three days prior to the initial dose of apomorphine and continued at least during the first two months of therapy. Ondansetron, granisetron, dolasetron, palonosetron, and alosetron should not be used as antiemetics due to reports of hypotension and loss of consciousness when given with apomorphine. The maximum recommended dose is 6 mg. Apomorphine is administered via subcutaneous injection.

J0365

J0365   Injection, aprotinin, 10,000 kiu

Lay Description

Aprotinin is broad-spectrum protease inhibitor obtained from a bovine lung that diminishes the inflammatory response in cardiopulmonary bypass surgery. It preserves glycoprotein in platelets. This reduces bleeding and decreases the need for allogenic blood transfusions. Patients receive a 1 milliliter test dose, for allergic reaction, intravenously at least 10 minutes prior to the loading dose. The loading dose is administered via intravenous infusion over 20 to 30 minutes after induction of anesthesia but prior to sternotomy. A dose is also added to the cardiopulmonary bypass circuit and a constant infusion is maintained until the end of surgery.

J0380

J0380   Injection, metaraminol bitartrate, per 10 mg

Lay Description

Metaraminol bitartrate is classified as an adrenergic agent, direct-acting vasopressor. It releases norepinephrine from storage sites and stimulates alpha-receptors, which causes an increase in blood pressure, venous tone, and pulmonary pressure. Metaraminol bitartrate is used in treating surgery related hypotension, trauma, adverse drug reactions, and spinal anesthesia. Metaraminol bitartrate can be administered via subcutaneous injection, intramuscular injection, intravenous push, or intravenous infusion.

J0390

J0390 Injection, chloroquine HCl, up to 250 mg

Lay Description
Chloroquine is an anti-infective used primarily in treating malaria and extraintestinal amebiasis. The mechanism of action is not fully understood but the drug does interfere with certain enzymes. It is effective against *Plasmodium vivax, Plasmodium malariae, P. ovale*, and susceptible strains of *Plasmodium falciparum* (but not the gametocytes of *P. falciparum*). It is not effective against exoerythrocytic forms of the parasite. Chloroquine is administered orally. The injectable form has been discontinued.

J0395

J0395 Injection, arbutamine HCl, 1 mg

Lay Description
Per the FDA, this drug is no longer available in the United States.

J0400-J0401

J0400 Injection, aripiprazole, intramuscular, 0.25 mg

J0401 Injection, aripiprazole, extended release, 1 mg

Lay Description
Aripiprazole is an antipsychotic medication used to treat schizophrenia and bipolar disorder. The precise mechanism of action of aripiprazole is not known. The drug has a strong attraction to dopamine and serotonin receptor sites and acts as an agonist to various dopamine and serotonin subtypes. Aripiprazole is indicated for: treatment of schizophrenia in patients age 13 years or older; acute and maintenance treatment of manic and mixed episodes of bipolar I disorder with or without psychotic features; adjunctive treatment of major depressive disorders; and treatment of agitation associated with schizophrenia or bipolar disorder, manic, or mixed. Aripiprazole is available in oral and injectable forms. The recommended oral dosage is 10 to 15 mg per day for schizophrenia, and 30 mg per day to treat bipolar disorder. When administered with an antidepressant, dosages may be as low as 2 mg per day. When aripiprazole is used to treat agitation associated with schizophrenia or bipolar mania, the dosage is usually 9.75 mg administered by intramuscular injection. The maximum daily dose is 30 mg/day.

J0456

J0456 Injection, azithromycin, 500 mg

Lay Description
Azithromycin is an antibiotic used in treating a wide range of bacterial infections including community acquired pneumonia, urethritis, and tonsillitis. It binds to the ribosomal subunit and disrupts microbial protein synthesis. It is effective against S*taphylococcus aureus, Streptococcus pneumoniae, Haemophilus influenzae, Moraxella catarrhalis, Neisseria gonorrhoeae, Chlamydia pneumoniae, Chlamydia trachomatis, Legionella pneumophila, Mycoplasma hominis, Mycoplasma pneumoniae, Streptococcus agalactiae, Streptococcus pyogenes*, and *Haemophilus ducreyi*. Recommended intravenous dose is 500 mg once a day for one or two days followed by an oral regimen. Azithromycin is administered orally or via intravenous infusion over one to three hours.

J0461

J0461 Injection, atropine sulfate, 0.01 mg

Lay Description
Atropine is an extract of an alkaloid from the plants belladonna, hyoscyamus, or stramonium. It is also made synthetically. Atropine sulfate is a highly toxic compound of atropine and sulfuric acid that has the same uses and effects as atropine. It blocks the neurotransmitter acetylcholine in muscarinic receptors of the parasympathetic system. Muscarinic receptors occur throughout the nervous system, including in the heart, smooth muscles of the blood vessels, lungs, salivary glands, gastrointestinal tract, and eye. Atropine sulfate in clinical doses counteracts the peripheral vessel dilatation and abrupt decrease in blood pressure produced by other drugs or biologicals. Systemic doses slightly raise systolic and lower diastolic pressures, slightly increase cardiac output, and decrease central venous pressure. Atropine is used as an antispasmodic to relax smooth muscles, to reduce secretions in the respiratory tract, and to temporarily increase heart rate or decrease AV-block until definitive treatment can take place, and as an antidote for cholinergic drugs toxins, poisoning from organophosphorus insecticides or certain toxic mushrooms. Since it counteracts the side effects of neuromuscular blockers and gases used in anesthesia, it may also be administered as a preanesthesia medication.

J0470

J0470 Injection, dimercaprol, per 100 mg

Lay Description
Dimercaprol, also known as BAL in oil, is a chemical compound dispersed in peanut oil used as a chelating agent. Certain heavy metals, especially arsenic, gold, lead, and mercury, bind with some of the pyruvate-oxidase enzymes and inhibit their normal functioning. Dimercaprol has a stronger attraction to the metal than the protein. It binds to the metal in a stable complex and carries it out of the body. It is indicated as a treatment for arsenic, gold, and mercury (soluble inorganic compounds) poisoning following ingestion, inhalation, or absorption through the skin of these metals or their salts, or following overdose of therapeutic agents containing these metals. Dimercaprol, in conjunction with edetate calcium disodium (calcium EDTA), is also used as a treatment for lead poisoning. Treatment should begin

immediately after exposure. It is administered by intramuscular injection only and the drug needs to be administered repeatedly for several days. Dosages vary from 2.5 to 5 mg/kg of body weight every four to six hours depending on the metal that caused the poisoning. Pediatric dosages for lead poisoning vary from 50 to 75 mg per square meter of body surface area every four hours followed by calcium EDTA.

J0475-J0476

J0475   Injection, baclofen, 10 mg
J0476   Injection, baclofen, 50 mcg for intrathecal trial

Lay Description
Baclofen is a chemical analogue of y-aminobutyric acid, an amino acid also known as GABA that is used as a muscle relaxant and antispastic. GABA is the principal inhibitory neurotransmitter in the brain, but is also found in several extraneural tissues, including kidney and pancreatic islet cells. GABA modulates membrane chloride permeability and inhibits postsynaptic cell firing. Although baclofen is an analogue of GABA, its exact mechanism of action is not fully understood. It inhibits both monosynaptic and polysynaptic reflexes at the spinal level, possibly by decreasing excitatory neurotransmitter release. Baclofen is available in an oral self-administered version and in an intrathecal version. It is used intrathecally to treat spasticity of cerebral origin, including trauma to the brain or cerebral palsy. The intrathecal administration is a long-term infusion delivered by an implantable pump. Prior to the pump implantation, patients usually receive a test or trial dose of 50 mcg administered via an intrathecal injection.

J0480

J0480   Injection, basiliximab, 20 mg

Lay Description
Basiliximab is a chimeric (murine/human) monoclonal antibody produced by recombinant DNA technology that is an immunosuppressive agent. Basiliximab binds to certain interleukin-2, also as CD25 antigen, receptor sites on activated T lymphocytes. By blocking these receptor sites, it prevents the interleukin-2 from activating the immune response, preventing rejection of allogenic transplants. Basiliximab in combination with cyclosporine and corticosteroids is indicated for the prophylaxis of acute organ rejection in patients receiving renal transplants. It is administered by intravenous bolus or by infusion over a 20-30 minute period. The dosage varies from 10 -20 mg. Basiliximab should only be administered once prior to the transplant when it has been determined that the patient will have the transplant with the concomitant immunosuppression.

J0485

J0485   Injection, belatacept, 1 mg

Lay Description
Belatacept is an immunosuppressive drug that is a selective T-cell costimulation blocker. It is indicated for the prophylaxis of kidney transplant rejection in adult patients. Belatacept is used in combination with basiliximab induction, mycophenolate mofetil, and corticosteroids. The drug increases the risk for developing post-transplant lymphoproliferative disorder, mainly affecting the central nervous system. It has been found that patients without immunity to the Epstein-Barr virus (EBV) are at a increased risk and the manufacturer warns that belatacept should be used only in patients who are EBV seropositive. Belatacept is administered as an intravenous infusion with the total dosage dependent upon the patient's body weight.

J0490

J0490   Injection, belimumab, 10 mg

Lay Description
Belimumab is a human monoclonal antibody used to treat systemic lupus erythematosus (SLE). Lupus is an autoimmune disease in which a person's immune system attacks its own body systems. Belimumab is developed by recombinant DNA technology. Recombinant DNA technology combines two segments of DNA sections to create two or more DNA molecules. These newly created DNA molecules can be reproduced in mammal cells. In this type of technology, large quantities of a specific antibody component can be generated without creating the whole antibody. Recommended dose of belimumab is 10 mg/kg at two-week intervals for the first three doses and every four weeks after that. Administration is by IV infusion over a one-hour period.

J0500

J0500   Injection, dicyclomine HCl, up to 20 mg

Lay Description
Dicyclomine is a chemical compound that is an antispasmodic and anticholinergic (antimuscarinic) agent. It relieves smooth muscle spasms of the gastrointestinal tract. Dicyclomine appears to achieve this effect by inhibiting acetylcholine and by a direct effect on the smooth muscles. It is indicated for the treatment of irritable bowel syndrome. The injectable form is administered by intramuscular injection. Dosages are individualized to the patient depending upon response.

J0515

J0515   Injection, benztropine mesylate, per 1 mg

Lay Description
Benztropine mesylate is a chemical compound containing atropine and diphenhydramine. The drug has anticholinergic and antihistamine effects. Benztropine mesylate is indicated as an adjunct

treatment of Parkinson's disease and as a treatment for extrapyramidal disorders except tardive dyskinesia due to neuroleptic drugs. The drug is available in injectable and oral forms. The injectable form is recommended when a rapid response is desired and is useful for psychotic patients with acute dystonic reactions or other reactions that make oral medication difficult or impossible. The injectable form is administered by intramuscular on intravenous injection. Dosages vary from 0.5 to 6 mg depending upon response.

J0520

J0520 Injection, bethanechol chloride, Myotonachol or Urecholine, up to 5 mg

Lay Description
Bethanechol chloride is a chemical compound that selectively stimulates the parasympathetic nervous system to release acetylcholine, a neurotransmitter. It stimulates the bladder muscles to contract and the motility of the gastric system. Bethanechol chloride is indicated for the treatment of acute postoperative and postpartum nonobstructive urinary retention and for neurogenic bladders with urinary retention. It is administered by subcutaneous injection. Dosages vary depending upon type and severity of the condition.

J0558

J0558 Injection, penicillin G benzathine and penicillin G procaine, 100,000 units

Lay Description
Penicillin G benzathine and penicillin G procaine is a suspension of equal amounts of each penicillin formulation. See the separate entries for penicillin G benzathine and penicillin G procaine for additional information. Penicillin G benzathine and penicillin G procaine is administered by deep intramuscular injection to the buttocks or thigh. The drug is slowly absorbed, released from the injection site. Once in the body, penicillin G benzathine and penicillin G procaine is hydrolyzed to penicillin G. The hydrolysis and slow absorption provide sustained, but lower blood levels of penicillin. Antibiotic action can be present for two to four weeks after a single injection. Susceptibility studies should be performed prior to the administration of this drug. Indications include severe upper respiratory tract infections of susceptible streptococci, scarlet fever, erysipelas, skin and soft tissue infections of susceptible streptococci, and severe pneumonia and otitis media due to susceptible pneumococci.

J0561

J0561 Injection, penicillin G benzathine, 100,000 units

Lay Description
Penicillin G benzathine, also known as benzathine benzylpenicillin, is a version of penicillin that contains dibenzylethylene diamine. Penicillins block the actions of transpeptidase, an enzyme needed to create the cell wall. This weakens the bacterial cell wall causing cellular death. This formulation is administered by deep intramuscular injection to the buttocks or thigh. The drug is slowly absorbed released from the injection site. Once in the body, penicillin G benzathine is hydrolyzed to penicillin G. The hydrolysis and slow absorption provide sustained, but lower blood levels of penicillin. Antibiotic action can be present for two to four weeks after a single injection. Susceptibility studies should be performed prior to the administration of penicillin G benzathine. Indications include mild to moderate upper respiratory tract infections of susceptible streptococci, syphilis, yaws, pinta, as a prophylaxis for rheumatic fever and chorea, and as a prophylactic follow-up for rheumatic heart disease and acute glomerulonephritis. Dosages vary from 300,000 units to 2,400,000 units depending upon the age of the patient and the disease being treated.

J0583

J0583 Injection, bivalirudin, 1 mg

Lay Description
Bivalirudin is a synthetic, 20 amino acid peptide that is a specific and reversible direct thrombin inhibitor. It binds to both circulating and clot-bound thrombin, which in turn prevents the thrombin from activating the coagulant cycle. Bivalirudin is indicated for use in conjunction with aspirin therapy as an anticoagulant in patients with unstable angina undergoing percutaneous transluminal coronary angioplasty (PTCA). The use of bivalirudin in conjunction with glycoprotein IIb/IIIa inhibitor is currently in clinical trials. Bivalirudin is also indicated for patients with or at risk for heparin-induced thrombocytopenia or heparin-induced thrombocytopenia with thrombosis syndrome who are undergoing percutaneous coronary interventions (PCI). Bivalirudin is not recommended for patients with acute coronary syndromes who are not undergoing PTCA or PCI. The drug is administered by intravenous injection and infusion. The recommended initial dosage is an intravenous bolus of 0.75 mg per kg of body weight. This is followed by an infusion of 1.75 mg per kg of body weight per hour for the duration of the procedure. Continued infusion of the drug after the procedure is left to the discretion of the treating physician.

J0585

J0585 Injection, onabotulinumtoxinA, 1 unit

Lay Description
Toxins are poisons, usually proteins produced by some higher plants, certain animals, and pathogenic bacteria, which are highly toxic for other living organisms. OnabotulinumtoxinA is a potent neurotoxin produced by the bacterium *Clostridium botulinum* type A. The toxin binds to sites on motor

and sympathetic nerves and inhibits the release of acetylcholine. Injection of onabotulinumtoxinA produces partial chemical denervation at the injection site resulting in a localized reduction in muscular activity. OnabotulinumtoxinA is indicated as a cosmetic agent to provide temporary improvement in the appearance of moderate to severe glabellar lines associated with corrugator and/or procerus muscle activity. It may also be used as treatment for cervical dystonia in adults to decrease the severity of an abnormal head position and neck pain, severe primary axillary hyperhidrosis that is inadequately managed with topical agents, and strabismus and blepharospasm associated with dystonia in patients 12 years of age or older. OnabotulinumtoxinA is injected intramuscularly.

J0586

J0586   Injection, abobotulinumtoxinA, 5 units

Lay Description
AbobotulinumtoxinA is an acetylcholine release inhibitor and a neuromuscular blocker. It is used to treat adult cervical dystonia and the temporary treatment of glabellar lines in adults age 65 and over. It is a purified form of the Clostridium botulinum type A bacteria. The medication is injected into the affected muscles. The recommended dose is 500 units for patients who have not been treated before. They should be divided between the muscles being treated. The injections may be done with EMG guidance. In clinical studies, it appears that the peak affect is about two to four weeks. If any retreatments are need, there should be a span of at least twelve weeks. Retreatment dosage is between 250 and 1,000 units. The recommended dose for patients with glabellar lines is 50 units divided equally into the five areas. Retreatment should not be any more frequently than every three months.

J0587

J0587   Injection, rimabotulinumtoxinB, 100 units

Lay Description
Botulinum toxin type B is a purified form of the neurotoxin produced from fermentation of *Clostridium botulinum* type B. It inhibits acetylcholine release at the nerve and is used as a neuromuscular blocking agent. Botulinum toxin type B is indicated for the treatment of cervical dystonia to reduce the severity of abnormal head position and associated neck pain caused by cervical dystonia. Botulinum toxin type B is administered by injection directly into the muscles that are affected. The average dose of botulinum toxin type B in adults for the treatment of cervical dystonia and associated abnormal head position and neck pain is one or more injections up to a total of 2,500 to 5,000 units.

J0588

J0588   Injection, incobotulinumtoxinA, 1 unit

Lay Description
IncobotulinumtoxinA is a type of botulinum toxin that is purified and separated from other proteins, leaving a neurotoxin behind. It is used to treat adults with cervical dystonia to help alleviate the abnormal neck position. This may also be used to treat blepharospasm in patients who have previously received onabotulinumtoxinA. IncobotulinumtoxinA is administered by injection into the affected muscle. The recommended dose can vary from 1.25 units up to 150 units depending on the area being treated and the severity of the muscle spasm.

J0592

J0592   Injection, buprenorphine HCl, 0.1 mg

Lay Description
Buprenorphine hydrochloride is a schedule V controlled substance. It is indicated for moderate to severe pain including postoperative pain and chronic pain of patients with terminal diseases. It is also used adjunctively with anesthesia as a means of providing postoperative pain relief. Although the action of the drug is not known, it binds with opiate receptors in the central nervous system and alters not only the perception of pain, but the emotional response as well. Buprenorphine hydrochloride is an injectable solution. It is administered by intramuscular, intravenous, or epidural injection. It may be administered by continuous intravenous infusion.

J0594

J0594   Injection, busulfan, 1 mg

Lay Description
Busulfan is a chemotherapeutic drug classified as a bifunctional alkylating agent that suppresses bone marrow function. Busulfan is used in combination with cyclophosphamide as a conditioning regiment prior to allogenic bone marrow or stem cell transplantation for chronic myelogenous leukemia. Injectable busulfan is administered as an intravenous infusion over two hours via a central venous catheter. The drug should be administered every six hours for four consecutive days for a total of 16 doses. The recommended dose is 0.8 mg per kg of adjusted ideal body weight.

J0595

J0595   Injection, butorphanol tartrate, 1 mg

Lay Description
Butorphanol tartrate is a schedule IV controlled substance. It is indicated for moderate to severe pain, including postoperative pain and labor. It is also used prior to the administration of anesthesia and adjunctively with anesthesia. Although the action of the drug is not known, it binds with opiate receptors in the central nervous system and alters not only the perception of pain, but the emotional response as

well. Butorphanol tartrate is administered by intramuscular and intravenous push injection.

J0597-J0598

J0597 Injection, C-1 esterase inhibitor (human), Berinert, 10 units

J0598 Injection, C-1 esterase inhibitor (human), Cinryze, 10 units

Lay Description

C1 esterase inhibitor is a protein found in the blood that inactivates two components of C1 protease. Human plasma is used to develop the C1 esterase inhibitor protein. A deficiency of C1 esterase inhibitor gives rise to hereditary angioedema (HAE), a rare condition that affects the immune system and is passed down in families. HAE can cause sudden, severe swelling of arms, legs, lips, eyes, tongue, throat, or the intestinal tract. Berinert is used to treat acute attacks of abdominal or facial attacks HAE. Recommended dose is 20 units per kg body weight administered by slow intravenous injection at a rate of approximately 4 mL per minute. Cinryze is used as a prevention of the angioedema attacks. The recommended dose is 1,000 units every three or four days and is administered by IV infusion.

J0600

J0600 Injection, edetate calcium disodium, up to 1,000 mg

Lay Description

Edetate calcium disodium is a chelating drug that is used as an antidote for lead poisoning and lead encephalopathy in adults and children. The mode of action of the drug is to form a stable chelate with any metal that has the ability to displace calcium, particularly lead. Edetate calcium disodium is used alone for patients with very high blood lead levels (>70 mcg/dl). When lead poisoning is present, the drug should be used in combination with dimercaprol. Therapy is administered over a five-day period, followed by an interruption of two to four days (to allow for redistribution of the lead, as well as to prevent depletion of other essential metals such as zinc), and then another treatment course is administered. Most often two courses of therapy are administered. Edetate calcium disodium is provided in injectable form only. The drug may be administered intramuscularly (preferred route for pediatric patients), as well as for all patients with lead encephalopathy. Intravenously, the drug is administered as a slow infusion over a period of eight to 12 hours.

J0610

J0610 Injection, calcium gluconate, per 10 ml

Lay Description

Calcium is a metallic element that is the most abundant element in the human body. It is found in almost all organized tissues. Calcium, in combination with phosphorus, forms calcium phosphate, the dense, hard material of the teeth and bones. It is an essential dietary element, an electrolyte essential for the maintenance of normal heartbeat and functioning of nerves and muscles. Calcium also plays a role in multiple phases of blood coagulation and in many enzymatic processes. Calcium gluconate is a form of calcium used to replace and maintain adequate levels of calcium. It is indicated as a nutritional supplement, for the prophylaxis and treatment of hypocalcemia related to hypoparathyroidism, rickets, osteomalacia, lead poisoning, and magnesium sulfate overdose. It is also indicated as treatment of hyperkalemia and as an adjunct treatment for cardiac arrest.

J0620

J0620 Injection, calcium glycerophosphate and calcium lactate, per 10 ml

Lay Description

Calcium is a metallic element that is the most abundant element in the human body. It is found in almost all organized tissues. Calcium, in combination with phosphorus, forms calcium phosphate, the dense, hard material of the teeth and bones. It is an essential dietary element, an electrolyte essential for the maintenance of normal heartbeat and functioning of nerves and muscles. Calcium also plays a role in multiple phases of blood coagulation and in many enzymatic processes. Calcium glycerophosphate and calcium lactate are electrolytes used to replace and maintain adequate levels of calcium. They are indicated for the prophylaxis and treatment of hypocalcemia. Calcium glycerophosphate and calcium lactate are administered by intramuscular or intravenous injection.

J0630

J0630 Injection, calcitonin salmon, up to 400 units

Lay Description

Calcitonin-salmon is a synthetic version of the hormone calcitonin originally obtained from salmon, but now produced by recombinant DNA technology. The salmon version has a slightly different amino acid sequence than the human form, but it produces the same effects. Calcitonin lowers plasma calcium and phosphate levels, inhibits bone resorption, and acts as an antagonist to the parathyroid hormone. Calcitonin-salmon is indicated for the treatment of symptomatic Paget's disease of bone, hypercalcemia, and postmenopausal osteoporosis. The drug is provided in injection solution for subcutaneous or intramuscular injection.

J0636

J0636 Injection, calcitriol, 0.1 mcg

Lay Description

Calcitrol is a form of cholecalciferol that is a parathyroid-like hormone. It increases the ability of the body to absorb vitamin D and to distribute calcium throughout the body. It is indicated for the treatment of hypocalcemia, hypophosphatemia, rickets, osteodystrophy associated with long-term dialysis, and such disorders as hypoparathyroidism and pseudo-hypoparathyroidism. It is available in oral and injectable forms. The injectable form is administered by intravenous injection. Dosages vary from 0.25 to 3 mcg depending upon the form and indication.

J0637

J0637   Injection, caspofungin acetate, 5 mg

Lay Description
Caspofungin acetate is an antifungal with the ability to inhibit one of the integral components of the cell wall of the fungus. It is indicated for treatment of presumed fungal infections in patients that are febrile and neutropenic, esophageal candidiasis, intra-abdominal candidiasis, pleural space candida infection, candida peritonitis, and for the treatment of invasive aspergillosis in patients who are intolerant of or refractory to other therapies. Caspofungin acetate is administered by slow intravenous infusion over one hour. It should not be mixed or infused with another drug. For the majority of indications, a 70 mg initial loading dose is administered on the first day, followed by 50 mg daily.

J0638

J0638   Injection, canakinumab, 1 mg

Lay Description
Canakinumab is a recombinant monoclonal antibody used to treat cryopyrin-associated periodic syndromes (CAPS), including familial cold autoinflammatory syndrome (FCAS) and Muckle-Wells syndrome (MWS). Canakinumab is also indicated as a treatment for systemic juvenile idiopathic arthritis (SJIA). CAPS are syndromes usually caused by a genetic mutation. The ultimate result of this mutation is increased interleukin-1 beta that stimulates inflammation. Canakinumab binds to the interleukin-1 beta, which counteracts its ability to bind with the receptors. SJIA is a severe autoinflammatory disease, driven by proinflammatory cytokines such as interleukin 1β (IL-1β). Recommended dose for CAPS or MWS is 150 mg for patients who weigh more than 40 kg every eight weeks. For patients under that weight or children, dose is based on body weight. The recommended dose for SJIA patients with a body weight greater than or equal to 7.5 kg is 4mg/kg (with a maximum of 300 mg) administered every four weeks. Canakinumab is administered by subcutaneous injection.

J0640

J0640   Injection, leucovorin calcium, per 50 mg

Lay Description
Leucovorin calcium (folinic acid, citrovorum factor) is a form of folic acid. When used with the chemotherapy drug 5-fluorouraci (Adrucil, 5-FU), it increases the ability of that drug to reduce or stop cell growth in advanced colorectal cancer. Leucovorin calcium is also indicated as a treatment for or to prevent toxicities associated with folic acid antagonists including methotrexate (MTX, Rheumatrex), trimetrexate (Neutrexin), trimethoprim (Proloprim, Trimpex), trimethoprim/sulfamethoxazole (Bactrim, Septra), pyrimethamine (Daraprim), and pyrimethamine/sulfadoxine (Fansidar). Leucovorin calcium is also used for the treatment of folate-deficient megoblastic anemias. Leucovorin calcium is available in injectable and oral forms. Doses and route of administration vary with regards to the condition being treated.

J0641

J0641   Injection, levoleucovorin calcium, 0.5 mg

Lay Description
Levoleucovorin is similar to folate and used to reduce the toxicity in high-dose methotrexate therapy in osteosarcoma. Methotrexate is a folic acid antagonist. Folate is one of the B vitamins necessary for the production of DNA and RNA. Recommended dose is 7.5 mg administered as an IV infusion. It should not be mixed with other agents in the same mixture.

J0670

J0670   Injection, mepivacaine HCl, per 10 ml

Lay Description
Mepivacaine hydrochloride is a local anesthetic available in concentrations of 1%, 1.5%, and 2% for injection. As a local anesthetic, mepivacaine hydrochloride blocks the generation and conduction of nerve impulses. It may be administered by local infiltration, as a peripheral nerve block, or for caudal and lumbar epidural blocks. Dosages and concentrations of the drug vary with regards to how it is being administered.

J0690

J0690   Injection, cefazolin sodium, 500 mg

Lay Description
Cefazolin sodium is a semi-synthetic cephalosporin that inhibits synthesis of the cell wall used to prevent and treat a wide range of bacterial infections. Susceptibility studies should be performed prior to the administration of cefazolin sodium. Susceptible bacteria include *S. pneumoniae, Klebsiella* species, *H. influenzae, S. aureus*, group A beta-hemolytic streptococci, *E. coli, P. mirabilis, S. aureus*, and some strains of *Enterobacter* and enterococci. Cefazolin sodium is available in an injectable form for intravenous and intramuscular injection or

intravenous infusion. Dosages vary from 25 mg to 1 g depending on the indication and for children, their body weight.

J0692

J0692   Injection, cefepime HCl, 500 mg

Lay Description

Cefepime hydrochloride is a semi-synthetic, broad spectrum, fourth generation cephalosporin antibiotic. It works by inhibiting synthesis of the cell wall and is used to treat a wide range of bacterial infections, as well as for empiric treatment for febrile neutropenia. Susceptibility studies should be performed prior to the administration of cefazolin sodium. Susceptible bacteria include *Streptococcus pneumoniae, Pseudomonas aeruginosa, Klebsiella pneumoniae, Enterobacter* species, *Escherichia coli, Proteus mirabilis, Staphylococcus aureus, Streptococcus pyogenes, Bacteroides fragilis,* and some strains of *Enterobacter* and streptococci. Intramuscular administration is used only for infections caused by *E. coli.* Otherwise, the intravenous route is used and the drug is administered by infusion over a period of 30 minutes. Dosages vary from 0.5 to 2 g depending on the indication and for children, their body weight.

J0694

J0694   Injection, cefoxitin sodium, 1 g

Lay Description

Cefoxitin sodium is a broad spectrum, third generation cephalosporin antibiotic. It works by inhibiting synthesis of the cell wall and is used to treat a wide range of bacterial infections. Cefoxitin sodium is administered by intravenous or intramuscular injection. Dosages vary from 80 mg to 2 g depending on the type and severity of the infection being treated and for children, their body weight.

J0696

J0696   Injection, ceftriaxone sodium, per 250 mg

Lay Description

Ceftriaxone sodium is a semisynthetic, third generation, broad-spectrum cephalosporin antibiotic for intravenous or intramuscular administration. It works by inhibiting synthesis of the cell wall and is used to treat a wide range of bacterial infections, as well as preoperative prevention. For IV use, it is mixed with 50 to 100 ml of compatible solution for infusion over a period of 30 minutes. Dosages depend on the type of infection being treated, as well as the patient's age and the weight of children. For adults, the dosage ranges from 1 to 2 g IV daily. For children age 12 or younger, 50 to 100 mg/kg IM or IV every 12 hours.

J0697

J0697   Injection, sterile cefuroxime sodium, per 750 mg

Lay Description

Cefuroxime sodium is a semisynthetic, second generation, broad-spectrum cephalosporin antibiotic for intravenous or intramuscular administration. It works by inhibiting synthesis of the cell wall and is used to treat a wide range of bacterial infections, as well as preoperative prevention. For IV use, it may be infused over a period of 15 to 60 minutes or injected directly over a period of three to five minutes. Dosages and the form of administration depend on the type and severity of the infection being treated, as well as the patient's age and the weight of children. There is also an oral form, cefuroxime axetil that is available in a suspension as well as tablets.

J0698

J0698   Injection, cefotaxime sodium, per g

Lay Description

Cefotaxime sodium is a semisynthetic, third generation, broad-spectrum cephalosporin antibiotic for intravenous or intramuscular administration. It works by inhibiting synthesis of the cell wall and is used to treat a wide range of bacterial infections, as well as preoperative prevention. For IV use, it may be infused over a period of 20 to 30 minutes or injected directly over a period of three to five minutes. Dosages and the form of administration depend on the type and severity of the infection being treated, as well as the patient's age and the weight of children.

J0702

J0702   Injection, betamethasone acetate 3 mg and betamethasone sodium phosphate 3 mg

Lay Description

Betamethasone acetate and betamethasone sodium phosphate are injectable corticosteroid suspensions with anti-inflammatory and immunosuppressive abilities. The injectable corticosteroid suspensions are used to treat a wide variety of medical problems, including endocrine disorders, rheumatic disorders, collagen diseases, allergic states, ophthalmic diseases, gastrointestinal diseases, respiratory diseases, dermatologic diseases, hematologic disorders, neoplastic disorders, edematous states, nervous system disorders, tuberculous meningitis, and trichinosis with neurologic or myocardial involvement. The route of administration depends on the condition being treated. For most conditions, betamethasone acetate and betamethasone sodium phosphate are administered by intramuscular injection. For conditions such as bursitis, tenosynovitis, peritendinitis, ganglion cysts, or bone cysts, the injection is administered directly into the bursa, tendon sheath, or cystic lesions. For rheumatoid arthritis and osteoarthritis, administration is by intra-articular injection.

J0706

J0706 Injection, caffeine citrate, 5 mg

Lay Description
Caffeine is a methylxanthine that is a central nervous system stimulant, bronchial smooth muscle relaxant, cardiac stimulant, and a diuretic. Caffeine citrate is a compound of caffeine and citric acid. It is indicated for adjunct treatment of apnea in premature neonates between 28 to 33 weeks gestational age. The exact action of caffeine citrate is not known, but it is thought to stimulate the respiratory center; increase minute ventilate; diminish diaphragm fatigue; increase metabolic rate skeletal tone, and oxygen consumption response; and decrease the threshold to and increase the response to hypercapnia. A loading dose of 1 mg per kg of body weight is administered by intravenous infusion over a period of 30 minutes using an infusion pump followed by a maintenance dose of 5 mg per kg of body weight over a 10-minute period every 24 hours.

J0710

J0710 Injection, cephapirin sodium, up to 1 g

Lay Description
Per the FDA, this drug is no longer available in the United States.

J0712

J0712 Injection, ceftaroline fosamil, 10 mg

Lay Description
Ceftaroline fosamil is a semisynthetic, fourth generation, broad-spectrum, beta-lactamase resistant cephalosporin antibiotic. It works by inhibiting synthesis of the cell wall and is used to treat a wide range of gram-positive and gram-negative microorganisms: *Staphylococcus aureus* (including methicillin-susceptible and -resistant isolates), *Streptococcus pyogenes, Streptococcus agalactiae, Escherichia coli, Klebsiella pneumoniae, Klebsiella oxytoca,* and *Streptococcus pneumoniae.* Ceftaroline fosamil is the water-soluble prodrug of the bioactive ceftaroline. The recommended dose is 600 mg every 12 hours administered by IV infusion.

J0713

J0713 Injection, ceftazidime, per 500 mg

Lay Description
Ceftazidime is a cephalosporin, a bactericidal agent that prevents cell wall production, causing osmotic imbalance in cellular pressure, and leading to cell death. This drug is used to treat serious infections of the lower respiratory and genitourinary tract, the central nervous system, and skin. It is also used in cases of bacteremia and septicemia from susceptible *Streptococci, Staphylococcus aureus, E. coli, Klebsiella, Enterobacter,* and *Pseudomonas.* Side effects include

phlebitis, thrombophlebitis, rashes, urticaria, sterile abscesses of the skin, vaginitis, candidiasis, cramps, vomiting, diarrhea, hypersensitivity reactions, and other hematologic conditions. Concomitant use with aminoglycosides produces an additive effect against some microorganisms and may increase nephrotoxicity. Chloramphenicol is antagonistic to the action of ceftazidime. This anti-infective is administered by IV or IM injection with sodium carbonate, arginine, or as a premix infusion solution.

J0715

J0715 Injection, ceftizoxime sodium, per 500 mg

Lay Description
Ceftizoxime sodium is a semisynthetic, third generation, broad-spectrum, beta-lactamase resistant cephalosporin antibiotic. It works by inhibiting synthesis of the cell wall and is used to treat a wide range of bacterial infections. Susceptibility studies should be performed prior to the administration of ceftizoxime sodium. Susceptible bacteria include *Klebsiella, Serratia, Enterobacter, Pseudomonas, Peptococcus, Peptostreptococcus, Bacteroides* species, *Proteus mirabilis, Escherichia coli, Haemophilus influenzae, Staphylococcus aureus, P. vulgaris, Providencia rettgeri, Morganella morganii, Neisseria gonorrhoeae, Streptococcus agalactiae, Staphylococcus epidermidis,* and *Streptococcus* species excluding enterococci. Ceftizoxime sodium is administered by intravenous or intramuscular injection. Dosages vary from 200 mg to 2 g depending on the type and severity of the infection and for children, their body weight.

J0716

J0716 Injection, Centruroides immune f(ab)2, up to 120 mg

Lay Description
Centruroides (scorpion) immune f(ab)2 (equine) is used to treat stings by Centruroides scorpions. Scorpion stings can cause serious reactions, such as loss of muscle control, roving or abnormal eye movements, slurred speech, respiratory distress, excessive salivation, frothing at the mouth, and vomiting. It is derived from horse plasma. The horses are immunized with the scorpion venom. The product is obtained by pepsin digestion of horse plasma and is fractionated and purified. The f(ab)2 fragments of immunoglobulin bind to the venom toxins to neutralize them. The recommended dose is three vials initially and additional doses if necessary. Centruroides (scorpion) immune f(ab)2 (equine) is administered by IV infusion over 10 minutes.

J0717

J0717   Injection, certolizumab pegol, 1 mg (code may be used for Medicare when drug administered under the direct supervision of a physician, not for use when drug is self administered)

Lay Description

Certolizumab pegol is a tumor necrosis factor (TNF) blocker used to treat rheumatoid arthritis and the symptoms of Crohn's disease in patients who have not responded to conventional treatment. It is a recombinant humanized antibody Fab fragment that is manufactured in *E. coli*. For rheumatoid arthritis, the initial recommended dose is 400 mg (given as two subcutaneous injections of 200 mg). The same dose is given at weeks two and four. It is then reduced to 200 mg every other week. For maintenance, 200 mg may be given every four weeks. For Crohn's disease, the recommended initial adult dose is 400 mg (given as two subcutaneous injections of 200 mg). The same dose is given at weeks two and four. In patients who obtain a clinical response, the recommended maintenance regimen is 400 mg every four weeks. Certolizumab pegol is given as a subcutaneous injection.

J0720

J0720   Injection, chloramphenicol sodium succinate, up to 1 g

Lay Description

Chloramphenicol sodium is a potent antibiotic that is useful for, and should be reserved for, serious infections caused by organisms susceptible to its antimicrobial effects when other therapeutic agents that are potentially less hazardous are ineffective or contraindicated. The drug is able to inhibit bacterial protein synthesis and exert a bacteriostatic effect. Chloramphenicol is injected intravenously over a period of three to five minutes. Dosages depend on the type and severity of the infection being treated, as well as the patient's age, weight, and the presence of hepatic or renal function impairment. It should be used very cautiously in children and newborns with immature metabolic function. The adult dose is 50 to 100 mg/kg IV daily, divided into doses every six hours. For children, the dose is 50 mg/kg per day divided into four doses at six hour intervals. When cerebrospinal fluid concentrations of the drug are required, such as for meningitis, a dosage of up to 100 mg/kg a day can be administered. In newborns that are less than 2 weeks of age, a total of 25 mg/kg per day is administered in four equal doses at intervals of six hours.

J0725

J0725   Injection, chorionic gonadotropin, per 1,000 USP units

Lay Description

Chorionic gonadotropin is a hormone with actions nearly the same as luteinizing hormone (LH), which is produced by the pituitary gland and is the same as the hormone produced by the placenta during pregnancy. Indications for the use of chorionic gonadotropin vary with males and females. Used in many in vitro fertilization programs, chorionic gonadotropin is used to aid conception and is usually administered in combination with other drugs, including menotropins and urofollitropin. In male patients, LH and chorionic gonadotropin stimulate the testes to produce male hormones such as testosterone to treat cryptorchidism, male infertility, and hypogonadism. Although chorionic gonadotropin may be prescribed as a weight loss drug, it should not be used for this indication. It is available in an injectable form only. The dose and the frequency with which it is administered are determined based on the indication for its use. For the treatment of male patients with low male hormone levels, 1,000 to 4,000 units are provided intramuscularly (IM) two or three times weekly. Treatment may range from several weeks to several months. For women undergoing fertility treatment, 5,000 to 10,000 units are administered IM per the physician's instructions. Children being treated for cryptorchidism receive 1,000 to 5,000 units IM two or three times weekly for up to a total of 10 doses.

J0735

J0735   Injection, clonidine HCl, 1 mg

Lay Description

Clonidine hydrochloride is used in addition to opiates to treat severe pain caused by cancer. Although the action of the drug is not known, it is thought to stimulate alpha2-adrenergic receptors and inhibit central vasomotor centers, which lowers sympathetic outflow to the kidneys, heart, and peripheral vascular system lowering vascular resistance, blood pressure, and heart rate.

J0740

J0740   Injection, cidofovir, 375 mg

Lay Description

Cidofovir is an injectable antiviral that is indicated for the treatment of cytomegalovirus (CMV) retinitis in patients with AIDS. By selective inhibition of viral DNA synthesis, Cidofovir is able to suppress the replication of CMV. Dosage is based on the weight of the patient and is 5 mg/kg. It is infused intravenously over a period of one hour given every two weeks.

J0743

J0743 Injection, cilastatin sodium; imipenem, per 250 mg

Lay Description
Cilastatin sodium imipenem is a potent, broad-spectrum antibiotic for intravenous (IV) and intramuscular (IM) administration. Its action is to inhibit bacterial cell-wall synthesis. Because of breakdown in the kidneys, it is able to provide adequate levels of drug in the urine. Dosage and the route and frequency of administration are determined by the type of infection and the body area affected, the weight of the patient, and the age of the patient (e.g., adult, child 3 months of age and older, infants, and neonates).

J0744

J0744 Injection, ciprofloxacin for intravenous infusion, 200 mg

Lay Description
Ciprofloxacin is a fluoroquinolone antibiotic that inhibits the synthesis of bacterial DNA. The broad-spectrum action of the drug makes it useful against a wide range of infections and organisms. Dosage, route, and frequency of administration depend on the type of infection, the age of patient (adult or child), and the weight of children.

J0745

J0745 Injection, codeine phosphate, per 30 mg

Lay Description
Codeine phosphate is an opioid analgesic indicated for the treatment of mild to moderate pain. Although the action is unknown, it is known to bind with opiate receptors in the central nervous system and alter the perception of and response to pain. It is provided in an injectable form for subcutaneous (SC), intramuscular (IM), and intravenous (IV) use. The dosage, route of, and frequency of administration are determined by the degree of pain (e.g., mild to moderate), as well as the age of the patient. When administered by IV, it is injected slowly into a large vein.

J0760

J0760 Injection, colchicine, per 1 mg

Lay Description
Colchicine is an antigout drug. Although the action is not known, it is thought to decrease WBC motility, phagocytosis, and the production of lactic acid, which in turn reduces the deposits of urate crystals and inflammation. The drug may be administered intravenously (IV) by slow IV push over a period of two to five minutes. It is also provided orally as tablets. The dosage and route of administration depend on whether it is being used to prevent acute attacks of gout, including preoperatively, or for the treatment of an acute attack. For prophylactic and maintenance therapy, oral doses of 0.5 to 0.6 mg are administered three to four times weekly. Patients who have more

than one attack of gout a year should take the medication daily. As much as 1 to 1.8 mg may be administered daily in severe cases. For preoperative prophylaxis, patients are given 0.5 to 0.6 mg three times daily for the three days prior to and after surgery. For acute attacks, patients receive an initial oral dose of 0.5 to 1.2 mg, repeated every one or two hours until the pain is relieved, gastrointestinal symptoms appear, or the maximum dose of 8 mg is attained. Intravenously, the patient is given 2 mg IV to start with, then 0.5 mg every six hours as needed up to a maximum of 4 mg. As an alternative, 3 mg IV may be administered.

J0770

J0770 Injection, colistimethate sodium, up to 150 mg

Lay Description
Colistimethate sodium is an antibiotic that disrupts the bacterial cell membrane causing its death. It is effective against *Enterobacter aerogenes, Escherichia coli, Klebsiella pneumoniae,* and *Pseudomonas aeruginosa.* Recommended dose is 2.5 mg/kg based on ideal body weight divided into two to four doses a day. Medication can be administered by intravenous infusion over three to five minutes every 12 hours or one half of the dose by intravenous infusion over three to five minutes and the rest by continuous intravenous infusion.

J0775

J0775 Injection, collagenase, clostridium histolyticum, 0.01 mg

Lay Description
Collagenase clostridium histolyticum is a purified form of the exotoxin collagenase produced by the bacteria *Clostridium histolyticum.* Collagenases are enzymes that break down collagen. This drug is indicated as a treatment for Dupuytren's contracture, which causes a build up of collagen in tendon sheaths in the hands. This drug is administered as an injection directly into the collagen cord of the hand.

J0780

J0780 Injection, prochlorperazine, up to 10 mg

Lay Description
Prochlorperazine/prochlorperazine maleate is an antiemetic used for severe nausea and vomiting, such as that associated with the administration of chemotherapy and prior to induction of anesthesia to control nausea and vomiting during and after surgery. The drug inhibits nausea and vomiting by acting on the chemoreceptor trigger zone and partially depresses the vomiting center. Prochlorperazine is also indicated for treating adult psychiatric illnesses including schizophrenia, non-psychotic anxiety, and mild psychotic disorders. Prochlorperazine is available in injection form for intramuscular (IM) and intravenous (IV) use, in tablets, extended release

capsules and syrup for oral administration, and in suppository form. The dosage, route of administration, and frequency of administration depends on the patient's diagnosis, the severity of symptoms, and, in the injectable form, by the patient's weight. Parenteral adult doses range from 2.5 to 10 mg at no more than 5 mg/minute IV for adults or 5 to 20 mg IM. The maximum parenteral adult dose is 40 mg a day. The drug should be injected or infused slowly. For children, 0.132 mg/kg may be administered IM. Oral doses range from 5 to 10 mg three or four times a day for tablets, or for extended-release capsules, 15 mg daily or 10 mg every 12 hours.

J0795

J0795   Injection, corticorelin ovine triflutate, 1 mcg

Lay Description
Corticorelin ovine triflutate is used to differentiate pituitary and ectopic production of adrenocorticotropic hormone (ACTH) in Cushing's syndrome. After the hypercortisolism is determined to be caused from Cushing's syndrome and autonomous adrenal hyperfunction is eliminated as the cause, the corticorelin test is used to determine the source of the excessive ACTH. Blood samples are drawn 15 minutes before and immediately before the medication is administered. A baseline is determined by averaging the two samples. The corticorelin is administered by intravenous infusion over 30 to 60 second intervals at a dose of 1 mcg/kg body weight. Additional blood samples are drawn 15, 30, and 60 minutes after the patient receives the medication.

J0800

J0800   Injection, corticotropin, up to 40 units

Lay Description
Corticotropin is a pituitary hormone released in response to corticotrophin-releasing hormone (CRH), which is released by the hypothalamus. Corticotropin is administered as a diagnostic indicator or adrenocortical function, as well as an anti-inflammatory or immunosuppressant for conditions such as multiple sclerosis. Corticotropin replaces the body's own hormones and stimulates the adrenal cortex to secrete hormones. Corticotropin may be administered intravenously (IV), intramuscularly (IM), or subcutaneously (SC). Intravenously it is administered over a period of eight hours. Dosages, frequency, and method of administration vary according to the indication for the drug, as well as the age of the patient (adult or child). IV doses range from 10 to 25 units every 12 hours for one or two days. IM and SC doses range from 20 to 120 units every 24 to 72 hours.

J0833-J0834

J0833   Injection, cosyntropin, not otherwise specified, 0.25 mg

J0834   Injection, cosyntropin (Cortrosyn), 0.25 mg

Lay Description
Cosyntropin is a synthetic version of adrenocorticotropic hormone (ACTH). It is a polypeptide that comprises the first 24 of the 39 amino acids of natural ACTH and has the same effect as natural ACTH. Cosyntropin is used as a diagnostic agent to screen patients with presumed adrenocortical insufficiency. Since it exerts a rapid effect on the adrenal cortex, it may be used to perform a 30-minute test of adrenal function (plasma cortisol response) as an office or outpatient procedure. Cosyntropin may be administered by intramuscular or intravenous injection for a rapid screening test of adrenal function. It may also be administered as an intravenous infusion over four to eight hours for greater stimulus to the adrenal glands. One of the rapid screening tests of adrenal function involves the collection of a control blood sample followed by an intramuscular injection of cosyntropin. A dose of 0.25 mg is provided to adults; for children 2 years of age or younger; a dose of 0.125 mg is adequate. A second blood sample is collected exactly 30 minutes after injection. When administered as an infusion, 0.25 mg is given over a six-hour period.

J0840

J0840   Injection, crotalidae polyvalent immune fab (ovine), up to 1 g

Lay Description
Crotalidae polyvalent immune fab is an antivenin used to treat the effects of venomous snake bites. The medication is created by immunizing sheep with one of four different venoms. The four different antivenins are extracted from the sheep serum and combined to create the final immunoglobulin product. The immunoglobulin binds to the toxins and neutralizes them. The recommended dose is based on the patient's response to treatment. Crotalidae polyvalent immune fab is administered by intravenous infusion.

J0850

J0850   Injection, cytomegalovirus immune globulin intravenous (human), per vial

Lay Description
Immune globulins are glycoproteins in the blood that function as antibodies. Immune globulins specific to a certain disease are antibodies with specific amino acid sequences that interact only with the antigen that stimulated its creation or with antigens that are closely related to the stimulating antigen. Immune globulins are usually derived from the pooled plasma of human donors who have antibodies to the specific disease. The antibodies from the exogenous immune globulin help the body to fight off a disease.

Cytomegalovirus (CMV) is a virus of the subfamily Betaherpesvirinae that produces unique large cells with intranuclear inclusions. The majority of CMV infections are very mild. Depending on the age and immune status of the person, CMV infections can cause several serious diseases. CMV infections can include mononucleosis, encephalitis, retinitis, and pneumonia. In immunocompromised patients, CMV can cause a disseminated and sometimes fatal illness. In severely infected infants, CMV may cause hepatosplenomegaly, jaundice, retinitis, purpura, microcephaly, cerebral calcifications, blindness, deafness, quadriplegia, and mental retardation. CMV can be transmitted by respiratory droplets or from the mother to infant during birth or breast-feeding. CMV immune globulin is administered intravenously for the treatment and prophylaxis of CMV disease in transplant recipients and other immunocompromised patients.

J0878

J0878   Injection, daptomycin, 1 mg

Lay Description
Daptomycin is an antibiotic of the class cyclic lipopeptide. It binds to the bacterial membrane causing a rapid depolarization that leads to bacterial cell death. Daptomycin is indicated for the treatment of complicated skin and skin-structure infections caused by susceptible gram-positive bacteria. Susceptible bacteria include *Staphylococcus aureus*, including methicillin-resistant strains (MRSA); *Streptococcus pyogenes; Streptococcus agalactiae; Streptococcus dysgalactiae subspecies equisimilis*; and vancomycin-susceptible strains of *Enterococcus faecalis*. Daptomycin may be given in combination with other antibiotics. It is administered by intravenous infusion over a 30-minute period once every 24 hours for seven to 14 days. Dosage is based upon body weight with a recommended dose of 4 mg per kg.

J0881-J0882

J0881   Injection, darbepoetin alfa, 1 mcg (non-ESRD use)

J0882   Injection, darbepoetin alfa, 1 mcg (for ESRD on dialysis)

Lay Description
Darbepoetin alfa is a drug used to stimulate red blood cell production. It is produced by recombinant DNA technology in Chinese hamster ovaries. Darbepoetin alfa contains more carbohydrate chains and sialic acid residues than epoetin alfa. This reduces the rate of clearance, extends the half-life, and allows for less frequent administration. It acts in the body similar to erythropoietin, which is produced by the kidneys. Erythropoietin is a hormone that is released into the blood system by the kidneys to prompt the production of red blood cells when low levels of oxygen are detected in the blood. Patients with chronic renal failure will not be able to produce

adequate levels of erythropoietin in the kidneys. Darbepoetin alfa is used to treat patients with anemia due to chronic renal failure or due to chemotherapy for patients with nonmyeloid cancer. Dose is based on patient condition and indication. Darbepoetin alfa can be administered by subcutaneous or intravenous injection.

J0885-J0886

J0885   Injection, epoetin alfa, (for non-ESRD use), 1000 units

J0886   Injection, epoetin alfa, 1000 units (for ESRD on dialysis)

Lay Description
Epoetin alfa is used to stimulate red blood cell production. It is produced by recombinant DNA technology in mammalian cells. It acts in the body similarly to erythropoietin, which is produced by the kidneys. Erythropoietin is a hormone the kidneys release into the blood system to prompt the production of red blood cells when low levels of oxygen are detected in the blood. Patients with chronic renal failure are not able to produce adequate levels of erythropoietin in the kidneys. Epoetin alfa is used to treat patients with anemia due to chronic renal failure due to chemotherapy for patients with non-myeloid cancer, or anemia for HIV patients being treated with zidovudine. Epoetin alfa is also indicated in the preoperative treatment of anemic patients scheduled to undergo surgery with significant, anticipated blood loss who cannot donate autologous blood. The dose is based on the patient's condition and indication. Epoetin alfa can be administered by subcutaneous or intravenous injection.

J0887-J0888

J0887   Injection, epoetin beta, 1 microgram, (for ESRD on dialysis)

J0888   Injection, epoetin beta, 1 microgram, (for non-ESRD use)

Lay Description
Epoetin beta, trade name Mircera, is used to stimulate red blood cell production. It is an erythropoietin receptor activator that acts in the body similarly to erythropoietin, which is produced by the kidneys. Erythropoietin is a hormone the kidneys release into the blood system to prompt the production of red blood cells when low levels of oxygen are detected in the blood. Patients with chronic renal failure are not able to produce adequate levels of erythropoietin in the kidneys. Epoetin beta is used to treat patients with anemia due to chronic renal failure for patients on dialysis and patients not on dialysis. Epoetin beta is not indicated for treatment of anemia due to cancer chemotherapy. The drug is formulated as a sterile, preservative free protein solution for intravenous or subcutaneous administration. The IV route is recommended for patients receiving hemodialysis because the IV route may be less immunogenic. The initial treatment is 0.6 mcg per kg body weight

administered once every two weeks. When the drug is initiated or the dose adjusted, hemoglobin should be monitored every two weeks until stabilized, and every two to four weeks thereafter. The dose should be individualized to achieve and maintain hemoglobin levels within the range of 10.6 to 12 g/dL.

J0890

J0890 Injection, peginesatide, 0.1 mg (for ESRD on dialysis)

Lay Description
Peginesatide is an erythropoiesis-stimulating agent (ESA) used to treat anemia caused by renal failure in patients who are on dialysis. It binds with a hormone produced by the kidney to stimulate the formation of blood cells in the bone marrow and increases the reticulocyte count, which are the young blood cells found in the blood. This elevation is an indicator that the red cell production is increasing quickly in the blood. The recommended starting dose of peginesatide for patients who are not currently being treated with an ESA is 0.04 mg/kg body weight administered as a single intravenous or subcutaneous injection once monthly. The dose for patients who are currently being treated with an ESA is based on a conversion table.

J0894

J0894 Injection, decitabine, 1 mg

Lay Description
Decitabine is an antineoplastic drug that is an analogue of the nucleoside 2-deoxycytidine. It incorporates itself into cellular DNA suppressing methylation. It is thought that suppression of the methylation of DNA may restore normal function to genes. Decitabine is indicated as a treatment for patients with myelodysplastic syndromes (MDS), both previously treated and untreated. The drug may be used for newly diagnosed and secondary MDS. The recommended dosage is 15 mg per m² of body surface. Decitabine is administered by intravenous infusion over three hours and is repeated every eight hours for three days. This cycle is repeated every six weeks for a recommended four cycles. Patient response may take longer than four cycles and treatments may be continued as long as the patient benefits.

J0895

J0895 Injection, deferoxamine mesylate, 500 mg

Lay Description
Deferoxamine mesylate is an iron-chelating agent that forms a stable complex with the iron and prevents it from being broken down any further in the body. It is indicated for the treatment of both acute iron intoxication and for chronic iron overload due to transfusion-dependent anemias. In acute iron intoxication, deferoxamine mesylate is administered

along with standard measures for the treatment of acute iron intoxication. In patients with chronic iron overload secondary to multiple transfusions, deferoxamine mesylate can promote the excretion of iron. With long-term use, the drug can slow the accumulation of hepatic iron and slow or stop the progression of hepatic fibrosis. The action of the drug has been found to be poor in patients younger than 3 years of age without significant iron overload and should not be used unless the mobilization of 1 mg (or more) of iron per day can be demonstrated. This drug is not indicated for treating primary hemochromatosis. The drug is provided for intramuscular, subcutaneous, and intravenous administration.

J0897

J0897 Injection, denosumab, 1 mg

Lay Description
Denosumab is a monoclonal antibody used for the treatment of osteoporosis in postmenopausal women with a high risk of bone fractures that were not successful with other osteoporosis therapies. Denosumab reduces the possibility of fractures of the hip and vertebral and non-vertebral fractures because it is a RANK Ligand inhibitor. It works by binding to the Rank Ligand inhibiting osteoclast formation, function, and survival, therefore preventing the osteoclasts from resorbing bone. The recommended dose is 60 mg every six months. Denosumab is administered by subcutaneous injection.

J0945

J0945 Injection, brompheniramine maleate, per 10 mg

Lay Description
Brompheniramine maleate is an antihistamine that blocks the effects of histamine in the body and provides relief of allergy symptoms including hives, rashes, itching, watery eyes, runny nose, and sneezing. It is also indicated for the treatment of motion sickness, anxiety or tension, and sleeplessness. Brompheniramine maleate is available in oral and injectable forms. The injectable form is administered by intramuscular injection.

J1000

J1000 Injection, depo-estradiol cypionate, up to 5 mg

Lay Description
Depo-estradiol cypionate is a long-acting estrogen in a sterile oil solution for intramuscular use. Depo-estradiol cypionate increases the synthesis of RNA, DNA and protein in tissues and inhibits the release of follicle stimulating and luteinizing hormones from the pituitary gland. Depo-estradiol cypionate is indicated for the treatment of atrophic vaginitis, the palliative treatment of inoperable breast and prostate cancer, severe vasomotor symptoms

associated with menopause, and hypoestrogenism due to hypogonadism, castration, or primary ovarian failure. Dosage is based on the condition being treated as well as the patient's response to treatment and ranges from 10 mg every four weeks to 30 mg every week.

J1020-J1040

J1020   Injection, methylprednisolone acetate, 20 mg

J1030   Injection, methylprednisolone acetate, 40 mg

J1040   Injection, methylprednisolone acetate, 80 mg

Lay Description
Methylprednisolone is a corticosteroid used to treat a variety of conditions. Indications include allergic disorders, arthritis, blood diseases, breathing problems, certain cancers, eye diseases, intestinal disorders, and collagen and skin diseases. Methylprednisolone may also be used with other medications as a replacement for certain hormones. Methylprednisolone works by decreasing the body's immune response to these diseases and reducing symptoms such as swelling and redness. Methylprednisolone may be administered orally, by intramuscular injection in the form of methylprednisolone acetate, or by intravenous infusion in the form of methylprednisolone sodium succinate.

J1050

J1050   Injection, medroxyprogesterone acetate, 1 mg

Lay Description
Medroxyprogesterone acetate is a progestin used in a variety of disorders and as a long-term injectable contraceptive. Medroxyprogesterone acetate suppresses ovulation by inhibiting the secretion of pituitary gonadotropin, which prevents maturation of follicles and causes thinning of the endometrial lining. It is indicated as antineoplastic treatment in endometrial, breast, and renal carcinoma. Medroxyprogesterone acetate is administered by subcutaneous or intramuscular injection.

J1060

Lay Description
Testosterone cypionate is an androgen. Estradiol cypionate is an estrogen. Please see the separate entries for each drug for additional information. This combination is indicated for the treatment of menopausal symptoms including hot flashes, unusual sweating, dizziness, and chills. It is administered by intramuscular injection.

J1071

J1071   Injection, testosterone cypionate, 1 mg

Lay Description
Testosterone cypionate is an anabolic steroid that stimulates the normal development of target tissues in men with androgen deficiency. It also has antiestrogen qualities that make it useful to treat estrogen dependent breast cancers. Administered intramuscularly (IM) or subcutaneously (SC), the dosages of testosterone cypionate and the frequency with which it is administered vary with regards to the condition being treated. For the treatment of male hypogonadism, the dose is 50 to 400 mg of testosterone cypionate IM every two to four weeks. For the treatment of metastatic breast cancer in women after menopause, 200 to 400 mg is administered IM every two to four weeks. In combination with estradiol cypionate, it is also indicated for the treatment of menopausal symptoms including hot flashes, unusual sweating, dizziness, and chills.

J1094-J1100

J1094   Injection, dexamethasone acetate, 1 mg

J1100   Injection, dexamethasone sodium phosphate, 1 mg

Lay Description
Dexamethasone is a synthetic corticosteroid that is similar to a natural hormone produced by the adrenal gland. It is 25 times as potent as cortisol. Dexamethasone has anti-inflammatory, antiemetic, and immunosuppressant properties. It is used to treat a wide variety of disorders. It is also used as a diagnostic aid in the detection of Cushing's syndrome in dexamethasone suppression testing.

J1110

J1110   Injection, dihydroergotamine mesylate, per 1 mg

Lay Description
Dihydroergotamine mesylate is indicated for acute treatment of migraine and cluster headaches. By stimulating alpha receptors, it causes peripheral vasoconstriction and may abort vascular headaches by direct vasoconstriction of the dilated carotid artery bed. It may be administered intravenously (IV), intramuscularly (IM), or subcutaneously (SC) with a dose of 1 mg that may be repeated every hour or two up to a maximum of 2 mg IV or 3 mg IM and SC in a 24-hour period. When administered by IV, it is given by a slow injection over three minutes. The weekly maximum is 6 mg.

J1120

J1120   Injection, acetazolamide sodium, up to 500 mg

Lay Description
Acetazolamide sodium is a carbonic anhydrase inhibitor indicated as adjunctive treatment of edema caused by congestive heart failure or drugs, and for rapid relief of ocular tension. Acetazolamide sodium is a non-bacteriostatic sulfonamide that acts to inhibit secretion of aqueous humor, reduce abnormal discharges from central nervous system neurons, and increase diuresis in the kidneys. The drug is administered by venous injection of a reconstituted powder that has been mixed with sterile water.

J1160

J1160   Injection, digoxin, up to 0.5 mg

Lay Description
Digoxin is a cardiac glycoside extracted from the leaf of the digitalis (foxglove) plant. Digoxin acts directly on cardiac muscle and indirectly on the cardiovascular system and autonomic nervous system to both strengthen heart contractions and slow the heart rate. It is a therapy for congestive heart failure, paroxysmal supraventricular tachycardia, and atrial fibrillation.

J1162

J1162   Injection, digoxin immune fab (ovine), per vial

Lay Description
Digoxin immune Fab (ovine) is an antigen binding fragment (Fab) substance raised in sheep. Sheep are immunized with human antibodies specific to digoxin to produce antibodies specific for the antigenic determinants of the digoxin molecule. The antibody is then papin digested and the digoxin specific Fab fragments of the antibody are isolated and purified by affinity chromatography. Digoxin immune Fab is used to treat life-threatening toxicity due to digoxin or digitoxin overdose. Life-threatening manifestations include severe ventricular arrhythmias, progressive bradyarrhythmias, or second- or third-degree heart block. The drug can be administered by intravenous injection if cardiac arrest seems eminent, or by intravenous infusion over 30 minutes. Improvement ordinarily is seen within a half hour after administration.

J1165

J1165   Injection, phenytoin sodium, per 50 mg

Lay Description
Phenytoin sodium is an anticonvulsant medication for the control of tonic-clonic and temporal lobe seizures. It can be taken daily as an oral medication for prophylactic treatment of seizures or be administered intravenously for treatment of acute episodes. Phenytoin sodium is somewhat related to barbiturates in chemical structure and acts upon the motor cortex to inhibit seizure activity. Therapeutic levels vary greatly among patients.

J1170

J1170   Injection, hydromorphone, up to 4 mg

Lay Description
Hydromorphone is a narcotic and opioid analgesic classified as a schedule II controlled substance. This drug binds to opiate nerve center receptors and alters the human pain response, as well as suppressing the cough reflex. It is available in oral and injectable forms. The injectable form can be administered by intramuscular, subcutaneous, and intravenous injection, or by intravenous infusion. Hydromorphone hydrochloride is indicated for the relief of moderate to severe pain.

J1180

J1180   Injection, dyphylline, up to 500 mg

Lay Description
Dyphylline is a derivative of theophylline. Theophylline is a xanthine compound that naturally occurs in tea leaves and can be made synthetically. Dyphylline acts directly on the bronchial smooth muscles as a bronchodilator. It is indicated to treat and prevent the symptoms of bronchial asthma, chronic bronchitis, and emphysema by relaxing the bronchial airways and improving the air flow through the lungs. The injectable form is administered by intramuscular injection for acute conditions. Dosage varies based on the severity of the condition and response.

J1190

J1190   Injection, dexrazoxane HCl, per 250 mg

Lay Description
Dexrazoxane hydrochloride is an intracellular chelating agent derived from ethylenediaminetetraacetic acid (EDTA). Dexrazoxane hydrochloride acts as a cardioprotective agent when used in conjunction with chemotherapeutic agents classified as anthracyclines. Anthracyclines, such as doxorubicin and daunorubicin, are known for their high rate of cardiotoxicity. The method of action is not entirely understood. However, in laboratory studies, dexrazoxane hydrochloride is converted intracellularly to a chelating agent that interferes with iron-mediated free radical generation thought to be responsible, in part, for anthracycline-induced cardiomyopathy. Dexrazoxane hydrochloride is supplied in 250 mg or 500 mg single use vials and is administered by intravenous infusion.

J1200

J1200   Injection, diphenhydramine HCl, up to 50 mg

Lay Description
Diphenhydramine hydrochloride is an antihistamine, a histamine receptor antagonist that has anticholinergic, antitussive, antiemetic, antivertigo,

antipruritic, antidyskinetic, and sedative effects. It blocks the effects of histamine on the smooth muscle of the bronchial tubes, GI tract, uterus, and blood vessels. It also acts as a local anesthetic by preventing transmission of nerve impulses. Diphenhydramine hydrochloride is indicated for the treatment of anaphylaxis, Parkinsonism when the patient cannot tolerate other medications, drug-induced extrapyramidal disorders, motion sickness, allergies, vertigo, insomnia, and to suppress nausea and prevent vomiting. Its antiemetic effects allow it to be prescribed to treat nausea and vomiting associated with chemotherapy. Diphenhydramine hydrochloride is available in self-administrable oral forms and in an injectable form. The injectable form is administered by intramuscular or intravenous injection.

J1205
J1205   Injection, chlorothiazide sodium, per 500 mg

Lay Description
Chlorothiazide sodium is a thiazide diuretic. The mechanism of action of thiazides is unknown. They affect the distal renal tubular process of electrolyte reabsorption, increasing the excretion of sodium and chloride and, to a lesser extent, potassium and bicarbonate. Chlorothiazide sodium does not usually affect normal blood pressure. It is indicated, solely or in combination, for the treatment of edema associated with congestive heart failure, hepatic cirrhosis, diabetes insipidus, and renal dysfunction. It is administered by intravenous injection or infusion. Dosages are dependent upon response and are individualized to the patient.

J1212
J1212   Injection, DMSO, dimethyl sulfoxide, 50%, 50 ml

Lay Description
Dimethyl sulfoxide, also known as DMSO, is an industrial solvent produced as a chemical byproduct of wood pulp in the production of paper. DMSO is FDA approved only as a preservative for transplant organs and for treating interstitial cystitis. It is also used as a preservative for stem cells collected from newborn umbilical cords, and has many off-label uses for medication delivery and pain control. DMSO has the ability to pass through membranes, including the skin barrier, carrying other drugs with it across those membranes. For interstitial cystitis, a 50 percent solution of DMSO is instilled in the bladder via catheter or syringe. The DMSO remains in the bladder for 15 minutes, when the patient is instructed to void.

J1230
J1230   Injection, methadone HCl, up to 10 mg

Lay Description
Methadone hydrochloride is a synthetic opioid analgesic that has effects similar to those of morphine and heroin. It is a schedule II controlled substance. Methadone hydrochloride is indicated for the treatment of severe pain and also as a substitute drug in the detoxification of heroin dependence. It is available in injectable and self-administrable oral forms. The injectable form can be administered by intrathecal, intravenous, subcutaneous, or intramuscular injection. Generally speaking, injections and tablets are administered as pain treatment and the oral solution or dissolved tablets administered as part of a detoxification program. The usual dosage for detoxification is 15 to 20 mg. Dosages for pain management vary dependent upon the severity of the pain and the response.

J1240
J1240   Injection, dimenhydrinate, up to 50 mg

Lay Description
Dimenhydrinate is a histamine receptor antagonist that has anticholinergic, antiemetic, antivertigo, and sedative effects. It is used as an antiemetic in the treatment and prevention of motion sickness or in cases of nausea and dizziness due to inner ear disturbances. It is thought that antihistamines may affect neural pathways that originate in the labyrinth, which inhibits nausea and vomiting.

J1245
J1245   Injection, dipyridamole, per 10 mg

Lay Description
Dipyridamole inhibits platelet aggregation and is a coronary vasodilator. It is indicated as a prophylaxis to prevent thromboembolisms in patients with prosthetic heart valves, and to prevent additional events in patients who have had transient ischemic attacks or an ischemic stroke due to thrombosis. An infusion of dipyridamole may also be administered during diagnostic thallium myocardial perfusion imaging as an alternative to exercise. It is available in oral and injectable forms. The injectable form is administered by intravenous injection. The recommended dosage for prophylactic use is 75 to 100 mg. The recommended dosage for diagnostic testing is 0.142 mg/kg of body weight.

J1250
J1250   Injection, Dobutamine HCl, per 250 mg

Lay Description
Dobutamine hydrochloride is a synthetic catecholamine that acts primarily on beta1 adrenergic receptors. It directly stimulates the heart muscle to increase its contractions and blood flow. Dobutamine hydrochloride is indicated for the treatment of cardiac decompensation in congestive heart failure or following cardiac surgery. It is administered by intravenous infusion through a central line or large peripheral vein. Dosage varies depending upon body weight and response.

J1260

J1260 Injection, dolasetron mesylate, 10 mg

Lay Description

Dolasetron mesylate is an antiemetic drug with a chemical compound that is a selective blocker of serotonin 5-HT3 receptors. Serotonin 5-HT3 receptors are present on the vagal nerve and at sensory nerve endings. Cytotoxic chemotherapy appears to trigger the release of serotonin in the small intestine, which may trigger the 5-HT3 receptors and initiate the vomiting reflex. It is indicated to prevent and treat nausea and vomiting associated with chemotherapy or surgery.

J1265

J1265 Injection, dopamine HCl, 40 mg

Lay Description

Dopamine hydrochloride (HCl) is a sympathomimetic amine vasopressor. This drug causes a release of norepinephrine and acts on the nerves in the central nervous system. It is a chemical naturally produced in the brain that increases heart rate and blood pressure. It is used to treat hemodynamic imbalances caused by myocardial infarction, trauma, endotoxic septicemia, open-heart surgery, renal failure, and chronic cardiac decompensation as in heart failure. Dopamine is administered via intravenous infusion.

J1267

J1267 Injection, doripenem, 10 mg

Lay Description

Doripenem is a synthetic, broad-spectrum carbapenem antibiotic structurally related to beta-lactam antibiotics. It inhibits bacterial cell wall synthesis by binding to penicillin binding proteins. It is used to treat complicated intraabdominal and urinary tract infections. The normal dose for doripenem is 500 mg administered by IV infusion over one hour.

J1270

J1270 Injection, doxercalciferol, 1 mcg

Lay Description

Doxercalciferol is a synthetic analogue of vitamin D that acts directly upon the parathyroid glands to suppress parathyroid hormone synthesis and secretion in order to control the levels of calcium and phosphate in the blood and bones. It is indicated in the treatment of secondary hyperparathyroidism in dialysis patients with chronic renal failure.

J1290

J1290 Injection, ecallantide, 1 mg

Lay Description

Ecallantide is a chemical compound that is a selective reversible inhibitor of plasma kallikrein. Kallikreins are enzymes that break peptide bonds in proteins. Ecallantide binds to the plasma kallikrein preventing the creation of bradykinin. Bradykinin is a vasodilator thought to be responsible for edema, inflammations, and pain. This medication is used to treat acute attacks of hereditary angioedema for patients who are 16 years of age or older. The recommended dosage is 30 mg administered subcutaneously in three injections.

J1300

J1300 Injection, eculizumab, 10 mg

Lay Description

Eculizumab is a monoclonal antibody produced from murine myeloma cell cultures. The antibody in the drug binds specifically to the complement protein C5, preventing the generation of a terminal complement complex that hemolyzes red blood cells. Eculizumab is indicated as a treatment for patients with paroxysmal nocturnal hemoglobinuria (PNH) to reduce hemolysis. PNH is a chronic acquired blood cell dysplasia with proliferation of a clone of stem cells producing erythrocytes, platelets, and granulocytes that are abnormally susceptible to lysis by complement. PHN patients have episodes of intravascular hemolysis causing hemolytic anemia, and venous thromboses, especially of the hepatic veins. Eculizumab is administered via intravenous infusion over 35 minutes. It should not be administered as a push or bolus. If an adverse reaction occurs during the administration, the infusion may be slowed, but total infusion time should not exceed two hours. The recommended dosage is 600 mg every seven days for the first four weeks, followed by 900 mg for the fifth dose seven days later, then 900 mg every 14 days thereafter. Since the use of this drug increases a patient's susceptibility to serious meningococcal infections (septicemia and/or meningitis), all patients without a history of prior meningococcal vaccination must receive the vaccine at least two weeks prior to receiving the first dose of eculizumab and be revaccinated according to current medical guidelines.

J1320

J1320 Injection, amitriptyline HCl, up to 20 mg

Lay Description

Amitriptyline is a tricyclic antidepressant, a dibenzocycloheptadiene derivative with additional sedative effects. It inhibits the membrane pump mechanism responsible for uptake of norepinephrine and serotonin. It is indicated for the treatment of depression, enuresis, and bulimia nervosa. The recommended dosage is 20 to 30 mg four times a day.

J1322

J1322 Injection, elosulfase alfa, 1 mg

Lay Description

Elosulfase alfa is an exogenous form of a human enzyme produced by recombinant DNA technology in a Chinese hamster ovary cell line. It is a hydrolytic lysosomal glycosaminoglycan-specific enzyme that hydrolyzes sulfate. The absence or a marked reduction in the activity of this enzyme, N-acetylgalactosamine-6-sulfatase, results in the accumulation of metabolic byproducts in the lysosomal compartment of cells throughout the body. The accumulation leads to widespread cellular, tissue, and organ dysfunction. Elosulfase alfa is intended to provide the exogenous enzyme that will be taken up into the lysosomes and help ready the cell of the protein byproducts. Elosulfase alfa is indicated for patients with Mucopolysaccharidosis type IVA (MPS IVA; Morquio A syndrome). The recommended dose is 2 mg per kg given intravenously over a minimum range of 3.5 to 4.5 hours, once every week.

J1324

J1324   Injection, enfuvirtide, 1 mg

Lay Description
Enfuvirtide is a synthetic peptide that inhibits the fusion of HIV, serotype 1 (HIV-1) into CD4+ cells. HIV-1 causes the majority of infections worldwide. Enfuvirtide, in combination with other antiretroviral agents, is indicated as a second-line therapy for the treatment of HIV-1 infections in patients who have evidence of continued HIV-1 replication despite ongoing antiretroviral therapy. The drug is administered by subcutaneous injection into the upper arm, anterior thigh, or abdomen. Recommended dosage is 90 mg twice a day. Enfuvirtide may be self-administered.

J1325

J1325   Injection, epoprostenol, 0.5 mg

Lay Description
Epoprostenol is a prostaglandin that acts as a direct vasodilator of pulmonary and systemic arteries and an inhibitor of platelet aggregation. It is usually administered parenterally through a permanent indwelling central venous catheter as a long-term medication to treat primary pulmonary hypertension and pulmonary hypertension secondary to scleroderma in NYHA Class III and IV patients. Initial administration may be through a peripheral intravenous infusion until a central venous catheter is established. It is manufactured as a powder that must be reconstituted with sterile diluent specific to the epoprostenol. Dosages vary dependent upon body weight and response. Once a regimen of epoprostenol has been established, it should never be stopped suddenly.

J1327

J1327   Injection, eptifibatide, 5 mg

Lay Description
Eptifibatide is an intravenous cyclical heptapeptide that prevents platelet aggregation and has a short half-life of 2.5 hours. It prevents the binding of fibrinogen, von Willebrand factor, and other ligands to glycoprotein IIb/IIIa stopping the platelets from joining. Eptifibatide is indicated as a treatment for acute coronary syndrome and to prevent thrombosis in patients undergoing percutaneous coronary interventions. Eptifibatide is administered by continuous intravenous infusion. Patients generally receive an infusion of eptifibatide for up to 96 hours following surgery or during medical hospitalization. Dosage is based on body weight.

J1330

J1330   Injection, ergonovine maleate, up to 0.2 mg

Lay Description
Ergonovine maleate is a natural or synthetic version of an ergot alkaloid. It is an oxytocic medication that acts to stimulate uterine and vascular smooth muscle contractions to reduce postpartum or post-abortion bleeding. It also is used to induce coronary artery spasms in diagnostic testing. Ergonovine maleate is available in oral and injectable forms. The injectable form is administered by intravenous or intramuscular injection.

J1335

J1335   Injection, ertapenem sodium, 500 mg

Lay Description
Ertapenem sodium is a synthetic parenteral antibiotic that is structurally related to penicillin and cephalosporin. It works by prohibiting the creation of bacterial cells walls, causing cellular death. Susceptibility studies should be performed prior to the administration of ertapenem sodium. Susceptible bacteria includes *E. coli, Clostridium clostridiiforme, Eubacterium lentum, Peptostreptococcus* species, *Bacteroides fragilis, Bacteroids distasonis, Bacteroids ovatus, Bacteroids thetaiotaomicron, Bacteroids uniformis, Staphylococcus aureus, Streptococcus agalactiae, Streptococcus pyogenes, Klebsiella pneumoniae, Proteus mirabilis, Porphyromonas asaccharolytica, Prevotella bivia, Streptococcus pneumoniae, Haemophilus influenzae,* and *Moraxella catarrhalis*. Ertapenem sodium is administered as a daily 30-minute intravenous infusion. The recommended dosage for a patient age 13 years or older is 1 g daily.

J1364

J1364   Injection, erythromycin lactobionate, per 500 mg

Lay Description
Erythromycin lactobionate is a macrolide antibiotic produced by the bacterium *Streptomyces erythreus*. It inhibits protein synthesis causing cellular death. Susceptibility studies should be performed prior to the administration of erythromycin lactobionate. Susceptible bacteria include *Streptococcus pyogenes, Streptococcus pneumoniae, Haemophilus influenzae, Listeria monocytogenes, Bordetella pertussis, Mycoplasma pneumoniae, Staphylococcus aureus,*

Corynebacterium diphtheriae, Corynebacterium minutissimum, Treponema pallidum, Neisseria gonorrhoeae, Chlamydia trachomatis, Ureaplasma urealyticum, and *Legionella pneumophila.* Erythromycin lactobionate is administered by intravenous injection or infusion. Dosage varies depending on the indication and the extent of the infection.

J1380

J1380   Injection, estradiol valerate, up to 10 mg

Lay Description
Estradiol valerate is an exogenous form of the natural hormone estrogen produced semisynthetically. Estradiol is produced naturally by the ovaries and placenta. It increases synthesis of DNA, RNA, and protein in responsive tissues and reduces the release of FSH from the pituitary gland. Estradiol valerate is a long-acting estrogen suspended in oil. It is indicated as a hormone replacement therapy for female hypogonadism, primary ovarian failure, absence of ovaries, postmenopausal osteoporosis, vasomotor menopausal symptoms, atrophic vaginitis, atrophic urethritis, and vulvar squamous metaplasia. It may also be used to treat advanced prostate cancer. Estradiol valerate is administered by deep intramuscular injection.

J1410

J1410   Injection, estrogen conjugated, per 25 mg

Lay Description
Estrogen conjugates are an exogenous form of the natural hormone estrogen. They may be derived from the urine of pregnant mares or produced synthetically. It increases synthesis of RNA, DNA, and protein in responsive tissue and inhibit release of FSH and luteinizing hormones from the pituitary gland. Estrogen conjugates are indicated as a hormone replacement therapy for female hypogonadism, primary ovarian failure, absence of ovaries, dysfunctional uterine bleeding, postmenopausal osteoporosis, vasomotor menopausal symptoms, atrophic vaginitis, atrophic urethritis, and vulvar squamous metaplasia. It may also be used to treat advanced prostate cancer.

J1430

J1430   Injection, ethanolamine oleate, 100 mg

Lay Description
Ethanolamine oleate is a mild sclerosing agent consisting of ethanolamine combined with oleic acid in an aqueous solution. When injected intravenously for local use, it irritates the venous endothelium and produces an inflammatory response that results in fibrosis and potential occlusion of the vein. It is indicated as a treatment for varicose veins and esophageal varices.

J1435

J1435   Injection, estrone, per 1 mg

Lay Description
Estrone is the oxidation product of estradiol, a long-acting exogenous form of the natural hormone. Estrone may be produced synthetically or derived from human or animal urine, human ovarian fluid or placenta, or palm kernel oil. It is produced naturally by the ovaries and placenta. It is less potent than estradiol but more so than estriol and is metabolically convertible to estradiol. Estrone increases synthesis of DNA, RNA, and protein in responsive tissues and reduces the release of FSH from the pituitary gland. It is a long-acting estrogen and is given as an intramuscular injection. Estrone is indicated as a hormone replacement therapy for female hypogonadism, primary ovarian failure, absence of ovaries, dysfunctional uterine bleeding, postmenopausal osteoporosis, vasomotor menopausal symptoms, atrophic vaginitis, atrophic urethritis, and vulvar squamous metaplasia. It may also be used to treat advanced prostate cancer.

J1436

J1436   Injection, etidronate disodium, per 300 mg

Lay Description
Etidronate disodium is a diphosphate compound, also known as EHDP, that regulates bone metabolism. It inhibits formation and growth of hydroxyapatite crystals to calcium surfaces, and in so doing, slows resorption and accretion in abnormal bone turnover. Etidronate disodium is indicated as a treatment for osteitis deformans, heterotopic ossification, and hypercalcemia of malignancy. The drug is available in oral and injectable forms. The injectable form is administered by intravenous infusion over a two-hour period.

J1438

J1438   Injection, etanercept, 25 mg (code may be used for Medicare when drug administered under the direct supervision of a physician, not for use when drug is self-administered)

Lay Description
Etanercept is an antirheumatic agent that binds to tumor necrosis factor, blocking its action and thereby causing a decrease in inflammation and autoimmune response. It is indicated for the treatment of juvenile rheumatoid arthritis, rheumatoid arthritis, psoriatic arthritis, ankylosing spondylitis, and chronic plaque psoriasis. Etanercept is administered by subcutaneous injection, typically the thigh, abdomen, or upper arm, once or twice weekly. The recommended adult dosage is 50 mg per week. The recommended dosage for patients 4 to 17 years of age is 0.8 mg/kg of body weight. The drug may be self-administered by the patient.

J1439

J1439   Injection, ferric carboxymaltose, 1 mg

Lay Description

Ferric Carboxymaltose is an iron replacement for the treatment of iron deficiency anemia (IDA) in adult patients who have intolerance or poor response to oral iron products or who have nondialysis dependent chronic kidney disease. IDA etiologies may include cancer, gastrointestinal disorders, abnormal uterine bleeding, or chronic kidney disease. The drug is administered intravenously by an undiluted slow push or by infusion. When administering as a slow intravenous push, it is given at the rate of approximately 100 mg (2 mL) per minute. For patients weighing 50 kg (110 lb) or more, it is administered in two doses separated by at least seven days. A dose of 750 mg for a total cumulative dose not to exceed 1,500 mg of iron is administered per course. For patients weighing less than 50 kg (110 lb), two doses are given separated by at least seven days. The dose should be 15 mg/kg body weight for a total cumulative dose not to exceed 1,500 mg of iron per course.

J1442

J1442   Injection, filgrastim (G-CSF), 1 microgram

Lay Description

Filgrastim is a synthetic, human granulocyte colony stimulating factor (G-CSF). It is produced by recombinant DNA technology using *E. coli* bacteria. The drug binds to surface receptors on hematopoietic and stimulates neutrophil production, differentiation, maturation, and function. It is indicated as a treatment for neutropenia in patients receiving myelosuppressive therapy for nonmyeloid malignancies. Filgrastim is also used to mobilize hematopoietic progenitor cells for leukapheresis to be used for bone marrow transplants. The drug is administered by subcutaneous or intravenous injection and intravenous infusion. Recommended dosage varies from 5 to 10 mcg/kg of body weight per day depending on the indication.

J1446

J1446   Injection, TBO-filgrastim, 5 micrograms

Lay Description

TBO-filgrastim is a non-glycosylated recombinant methionyl human granulocyte colony-stimulating growth factor (G-CSF) manufactured by recombinant DNA technology using the bacterium E. coli. It is composed of 175 amino acids. The endogenous human G-CSF is glycosylated and does not have the additional methionine amino acid residue. TBO-filgrastim is produced by recombinant DNA technology. It binds to G-CSF receptors and stimulates proliferation of neutrophils. G-CSF is known to stimulate differentiation and some end-cell functional activation, which increases neutrophil counts and activity. TBO-filgrastim is indicated for treatment of severe neutropenia in patients with nonmyeloid malignancies receiving myelosuppressive anticancer drugs. The product is available in prefilled syringes that contain either 300 mcg or 480 mcg of TBO-filgrastim. The recommended dose is 5 mcg per kilogram of body weight per day administered as a subcutaneous injection.

J1450

J1450   Injection, fluconazole, 200 mg

Lay Description

Fluconazole is a synthetic triazole antifungal agent. It is indicated as a treatment for vaginal, oropharyngeal, and esophageal candidiasis and cryptococcal meningitis. Fluconazole is also used as a prophylaxis for candidiasis in patients undergoing bone marrow transplantation, radiation therapy, or cytotoxic chemotherapy. It is available in oral and injectable forms. The injectable form is administered by intravenous infusion. Recommended dosage varies from 3 to 12 mg/kg of body weight depending on the indication.

J1451

J1451   Injection, fomepizole, 15 mg

Lay Description

Fomepizole is a competitive inhibitor of alcohol dehydrogenase, the enzyme that catalyzes the initial steps in the metabolism of ethylene glycol and methanol and prevents these two substances from forming the toxic metabolites that cause metabolic acidosis and renal damage. Fomepizole is indicated for use as an antidote in confirmed or suspected ethylene glycol (antifreeze) poisoning and methanol poisoning. It may be used alone or with hemodialysis. Fomepizole is administered by intravenous infusion. The usual initial dose is 15 mg/kg of body weight administered over 30 minutes. Subsequent doses are usually reduced to 10 mg/kg of body weight given every 12 hours over 30 minutes until ethylene glycol or methanol concentration decreases to less than 20 mg per dl.

J1452

J1452   Injection, fomivirsen sodium, intraocular, 1.65 mg

Lay Description

Fomivirsen sodium intravitreal injection is indicated for the local treatment of cytomegalovirus (CMV) retinitis in patients with acquired immunodeficiency syndrome (AIDS). Fomivirsen intravitreal injection is a local treatment that does not affect CMV infections of other sites. Treatment of bilateral CMV retinal infections requires injections in both eyes. Fomivirsen inhibits human cytomegalovirus (HCMV) replication by binding to the target mRNA and inhibiting IE2 protein synthesis, which prevents virus replication. Initial intravitreal injection for treatment of CMV retinitis is 330 mcg into the affected eye every other week for two doses. After the two initial doses, maintenance doses of 330 mcg are administered every four weeks.

J1453

J1453   Injection, fosaprepitant, 1 mg

Lay Description

Fosaprepitant is a lyophilized prodrug of aprepitant. When fosaprepitant is administered intravenously, it is quickly converted to aprepitant. It is administered before chemotherapy to eliminate or reduce acute nausea and vomiting. Fosaprepitant is administered 30 minutes prior to chemotherapy by IV infusion over 15 minutes. The recommended dose is 115 mg.

J1455

J1455   Injection, foscarnet sodium, per 1,000 mg

Lay Description

Foscarnet sodium is an antiviral indicated for treatment of cytomegalovirus (CMV) retinitis in patients with acquired immune deficiency syndrome. It is also indicated for treatment of herpes simplex virus types 1 and 2 (HPV-1, HPV-2) mucocutaneous infections in immunocompromised patients. It works by inhibiting in vitro viral replication by binding to the pyrophosphate binding site on virus-specific DNA polymerases. Foscarnet sodium is administered by intravenous infusion over one to two hours. Dose is dependent on the specific viral infection being treated, as well as the patient's body weight.

J1457

J1457   Injection, gallium nitrate, 1 mg

Lay Description

Gallium is a rare metal that is liquid at room temperature. Gallium nitrate is a hydrated nitrate salt of gallium used in the treatment of symptomatic cancer-related hypercalcemia that has not responded to hydration therapy. Generally, patients should have serum calcium (corrected for albumin) equal to or greater than 12 mg/dl. The recommended usage for gallium nitrate is 200 mg per m2 of body surface daily infused over 24 hours for five consecutive days.

J1458

J1458   Injection, galsulfase, 1 mg

Lay Description

Galsulfase is a human enzyme produced by recombinant DNA technology in a Chinese hamster ovary. Galsulfase is an orphan drug used to treat the inherited metabolic disorder mucopolysaccharidosis VI (MPS VI or Maroteaux-Lamy Syndrome). Mucopolysaccharidosis VI is caused by a lack of the enzyme arylsulfatase B that normally breaks down certain carbohydrates known as glycosaminoglycans. While intelligence is not affected, MPS VI causes widespread cumulative organ and tissue damage. The drug is administered via a four-hour infusion every week.

J1459

J1459   Injection, immune globulin (Privigen), intravenous, nonlyophilized (e.g., liquid), 500 mg

Lay Description

Immune globulins are glycoproteins in the blood that function as antibodies. Immune globulins specific to a certain disease are antibodies with specific amino acid sequences that interact only with the antigen that stimulated its creation or with antigens that are closely related to the stimulating antigen. Immune globulins are usually derived from the pooled plasma of human donors who have antibodies to the specific disease. The antibodies from the exogenous immune globulin help the body to fight off a disease. The term intravenous immune globulin, IVIg, used with a qualifier generally refers to the full range of immunoglobulins contained within the blood. Immunoglobulins are divided into five classes, IgM, IgG, IgA, IgD, and IgE, on the basis of structure and biologic activity. IVIg is administered by intravenous injection or infusion. IVIg is indicated as a treatment for primary immune deficiency disorders, idiopathic thrombocytopenia purpura, autoimmune diseases, and as an adjunct treatment of Kawasaki disease. It is also indicated as a prophylaxis of infectious diseases associated with chronic lymphocytic leukemia, pediatric HIV infection, and bone marrow transplants. IVIg is available as a solution or in a lyophilized or freeze-dried form.

J1460, J1560

J1460   Injection, gamma globulin, intramuscular, 1 cc

J1560   Injection, gamma globulin, intramuscular, over 10 cc

Lay Description

Gamma globulins are serum globulins having the least rapid electrophoretic migration. Since the gamma globulin fractions are composed almost entirely of immune globulin, gamma globulin has come to be used as a synonym of immune globulin or immunoglobulin. Immune globulins are glycoproteins in the blood that function as antibodies. Immune globulins specific to a certain disease are antibodies with specific amino acid sequences that interact only with the antigen that stimulated its creation or with antigens that are closely related to the stimulating antigen. Immune globulins are usually derived from the pooled plasma of human donors who have antibodies to the specific disease. The antibodies from the exogenous immune globulin help the body to fight off a disease. The term immune globulin used with a qualifier generally refers to the full range of immunoglobulins contained within the blood. Immunoglobulins are divided into five classes, IgM, IgG, IgA, IgD, and IgE, on the basis of structure and biologic activity. Gamma globulins are administered by intramuscular injection. They are indicated as a treatment for primary immune deficiency disorders or as a prophylaxis after exposure to hepatitis A, measles, rubella, and varicella.

J1556

J1556 Injection, immune globulin (bivigam), 500 mg

Lay Description
Bivigam is an exogenous source of human immunoglobulin G (IgG) antibodies used as replacement therapy. It is a concentrated human immunoglobulin purified from human plasma that undergoes rigorous testing. The drug is administered via intravenous infusion and is indicated for the treatment of primary humoral immunodeficiency. The recommended dosage is 300 mg to 800 mg per kg of body weight, which can be adjusted to achieve desired clinical response.

J1557

J1557 Injection, immune globulin, (Gammaplex), intravenous, nonlyophilized (e.g., liquid), 500 mg

Lay Description
Immune globulin (Gammaplex), intravenous, nonlyophilized (e.g., liquid) is an immune globulin liquid used in the treatment of replacement therapy of primary humoral immunodeficiency (PI). Gammaplex may also be used for treatment of a humoral immune defect in common variable immunodeficiency, Wiskott-Aldrich syndrome, X linked agammaglobulinemia, congenital agammaglobulinemia, and severe combined immunodeficiencies. Recommended dose is 300 to 800 mg/kg every three to four weeks. The dose and schedule may vary based on individual response to treatment. Gammaplex is administered by intravenous infusion.

J1559

J1559 Injection, immune globulin (Hizentra), 100 mg

Lay Description
Immune globulins are glycoproteins in the blood that function as antibodies. Immune globulins specific to a certain disease are antibodies with specific amino acid sequences that interact only with the antigen that stimulated its creation or with antigens that are closely related to the stimulating antigen. Immune globulins are usually derived from the pooled plasma of human donors who have antibodies to the specific disease. The antibodies from the exogenous immune globulin help the body to fight off a disease. It is indicated as a treatment for primary immune deficiency disorders. This includes, but is not limited to, the humoral immune defect in congenital agammaglobulinemia, common variable immunodeficiency, X-linked agammaglobulinemia, Wiskott-Aldrich syndrome, and severe combined

immunodeficiencies. Subcutaneous injections are administered with the use of an infusion pump.

J1561-J1569, J1572

J1561 Injection, immune globulin, (Gamunex/Gamunex-C/Gammaked), nonlyophilized (e.g., liquid), 500 mg

J1562 Injection, immune globulin (Vivaglobin), 100 mg

J1566 Injection, immune globulin, intravenous, lyophilized (e.g., powder), not otherwise specified, 500 mg

J1568 Injection, immune globulin, (Octagam), intravenous, nonlyophilized (e.g., liquid), 500 mg

J1569 Injection, immune globulin, (Gammagard liquid), nonlyophilized, (e.g., liquid), 500 mg

J1572 Injection, immune globulin, (Flebogamma/Flebogamma Dif), intravenous, nonlyophilized (e.g., liquid), 500 mg

Lay Description
Immune globulins are glycoproteins in the blood that function as antibodies. Immune globulins specific to a certain disease are antibodies with specific amino acid sequences that interact only with the antigen that stimulated its creation or with antigens that are closely related to the stimulating antigen. Immune globulins are usually derived from the pooled plasma of human donors who have antibodies to the specific disease. The antibodies from the exogenous immune globulin help the body to fight off a disease. The term intravenous immune globulin, IVIg, used with a qualifier generally refers to the full range of immunoglobulins contained within the blood. Immunoglobulins are divided into five classes, IgM, IgG, IgA, IgD, and IgE, on the basis of structure and biologic activity. IVIg is administered by intravenous injection or infusion. IVIg is indicated as a treatment for primary immune deficiency disorders, idiopathic thrombocytopenia purpura, autoimmune diseases, and as an adjunct treatment of Kawasaki disease. It is also indicated as a prophylaxis of infectious diseases associated with chronic lymphocytic leukemia, pediatric HIV infection, and bone marrow transplants. IVIg is available as a solution or in a lyophilized or freeze-dried form.

J1570

J1570 Injection, ganciclovir sodium, 500 mg

Lay Description
Ganciclovir sodium is a synthetic guanine derivative active against cytomegalovirus (CMV). It is indicated for treatment and prevention of CMV in patients with acquired immunodeficiency syndrome (AIDS). It is also indicated for prevention of CMV in organ transplant patients. It works by inhibiting the replication of the virus. Ganciclovir is available as sterile lyophilized powder in 500 mg vials for

intravenous administration. It is also available in 250 mg and 500 mg capsules for oral administration. For AIDS patients with CMV infection, initial treatment is by intravenous injection infused over one hour every 12 hours for 14 to 21 days. The dose depends on body weight. Following the intravenous course of treatment, maintenance therapy is administered by intravenous infusion once per day five to seven days per week or in oral capsule form. Maintenance intravenous therapy dose depends on body weight. Usual oral dose is 1,000 mg tid. Organ transplant patients typically receive initial intravenous therapy for up to 21 days, followed by maintenance doses given orally or by intravenous infusion.

J1571, J1573

J1571 Injection, hepatitis B immune globulin (Hepagam B), intramuscular, 0.5 ml

J1573 Injection, hepatitis B immune globulin (Hepagam B), intravenous, 0.5 ml

Lay Description
Immune globulins are glycoproteins in the blood that function as antibodies. Immune globulins specific to a certain disease are antibodies with specific amino acid sequences that interact only with the antigen that stimulated its creation or with antigens that are closely related to the stimulating antigen. Immune globulins are usually derived from the pooled plasma of human donors who have antibodies to the specific disease. The antibodies from the exogenous immune globulin help the body to fight off a disease. Hepatitis B is a viral infection of the liver. The virus is shed in all body fluids from infected individuals. While it is possible to become infected via oral transmission, it is more commonly transmitted by parenteral routes, such as blood transfusion, contaminated needles, and sexual contact. Hepatitis B has an incubation period of about 90 days with a range of 40 to 180 days. It can cause fever, malaise, anorexia, nausea and vomiting, jaundice, urticaria, angioedema, arthritis, and, rarely, glomerulonephritis or a serum sickness-like syndrome. Hepatitis B can cause massive liver necrosis. It is thought that the disease may be a cause of cirrhosis and primary liver cancer. Most patients recover completely. Some may remain chronic carriers or develop chronic active or persistent hepatitis. The disease is endemic worldwide. Hepatitis B immune globulin is derived from persons with high titers of antibodies against the hepatitis B surface antigen. It is administered by intramuscular injection for the prophylaxis of persons exposed to the virus or infants of mothers who test positive for the antigen.

J1572

J1572 Injection, immune globulin, (Flebogamma/Flebogamma Dif), intravenous, nonlyophilized (e.g., liquid), 500 mg

Lay Description
Please refer to code J1561 for the description, coding, and billing information.

J1580

J1580 Injection, garamycin, gentamicin, up to 80 mg

Lay Description
Garamycin/gentamicin is an antibiotic used to treat a wide variety of bacterial infections. It is indicated for use in the treatment of primary and secondary infections caused by sensitive strains of Group A beta-hemolytic, alpha-hemolytic streptococci, S. aureus, P. aeruginosa, A. aerogenes, E. coli, P. vulgaris, and K. pneumoniae.

J1590

J1590 Injection, gatifloxacin, 10 mg

Lay Description
Gatifloxacin falls into the category of drugs known as fluoroquinolones. It is used in treating chronic bronchitis, acute sinusitis, and community-acquired pneumonia caused by streptococcus pneumoniae as well as skin infections caused by streptococcus aureus. Gatifloxacin acts by inhibiting bacterial replication. Some adverse reactions may include headache, palpitations, hematuria, dyspnea, and/or back pain. It is contraindicated in patients with untreated hypokalemia. This code reports a 10 mg injection.

J1595

J1595 Injection, glatiramer acetate, 20 mg

Lay Description
Glatiramer acetate is used in the treatment of relapsing-remitting multiple sclerosis (MS) and is indicated to reduce the frequency of relapses. The mechanism by which glatiramer acetate exerts its effects in patients with MS is not fully understood; however, it is thought that it has an effect on immune processes that are believed to be responsible for the origin and development of MS. Glatiramer acetate is available in 20 mg single dose, prefilled vials and is administered by subcutaneous injection. The recommended dose is 20 mg per day. Glatiramer acetate may be self-administered.

J1599

J1599   Injection, immune globulin, intravenous, nonlyophilized (e.g., liquid), not otherwise specified, 500 mg

Lay Description

Immune globulins are glycoproteins in the blood that function as antibodies. Immune globulins specific to a certain disease are antibodies with specific amino acid sequences that interact only with the antigen that stimulated its creation or with antigens that are closely related to the stimulating antigen. Immune globulins are usually derived from the pooled plasma of human donors who have antibodies to the specific disease. The antibodies from the exogenous immune globulin help the body to fight off a disease. Immune globulins may be administered intravenously or by subcutaneous injection. This code represents 500 mg of nonlyophilized (e.g., liquid) immunoglobulin, not otherwise specified in other HCPCS Level II codes.

J1600

J1600   Injection, gold sodium thiomalate, up to 50 mg

Lay Description

Gold sodium thiomalate is a gold salt indicated for the treatment of adult and juvenile rheumatoid arthritis. The mechanism of action in gold salts is not well understood. However, in patients with inflammatory arthritis, such as adult and juvenile rheumatoid arthritis, gold salts decrease the inflammation of the joint lining, preventing destruction of bone and cartilage. Gold salts, such as gold sodium thiomalate, are second-line drugs prescribed when anti-inflammatory drugs, such as nonsteroidal anti-inflammatory drugs (NSAID) and corticosteroids, are ineffective in preventing the progression of inflammatory arthritis. Gold sodium thiomalate is available as a 50 mg/ml injectable suspension to be administered by intramuscular injection

J1602

J1602   Injection, golimumab, 1 mg, for intravenous use

Lay Description

Golimumab is a human IgG1? monoclonal antibody specific for human tumor necrosis factor alpha. It was created using genetically engineered mice immunized with human TNF, resulting in a human-derived antibody produced by a recombinant cell line cultured by continuous perfusion and purified. Elevated TNF levels in the blood, synovium, and joints have been implicated in the pathophysiology of several chronic inflammatory diseases, such as rheumatoid arthritis, psoriatic arthritis, and ankylosing spondylitis. The specific mechanism by which golimumab treats ulcerative colitis is unknown. Golimumab is indicated for the treatment of adult patients in combination with methotrexate for moderately to severely active rheumatoid arthritis alone or in combination with methotrexate for active psoriatic arthritis, active ankylosing spondylitis, and for moderate to severe ulcerative colitis patients who have an inadequate response or intolerance to prior treatment or requiring continuous steroid therapy. Recommended dosage is 2 mg per kg administered as an intravenous infusion over 30 minutes. Each single use vial contains 50 mg of golimumab per 4 mL of solution (12.5 mg of golimumab per mL). A different formulation is available in prefilled syringes or autoinjectors of 50 and 100 mg and is administered by subcutaneous injection. It may be self-injected. There is no HCPCS code for the version that is injected subcutaneously.

J1610

J1610   Injection, glucagon HCl, per 1 mg

Lay Description

Glucagon hydrochloride is a synthetic polypeptide identical to human glucagon. It is produced by recombinant DNA technology using E. coli bacteria. An injection of glucagon stimulates the liver to release stored glycogen and convert it to glucose in order to raise blood glucose levels. It also relaxes smooth muscles of the gastrointestinal tract. Its principal use is in an emergency setting as a treatment for severe insulin reaction in which the patient is unconscious or otherwise unable to eat or drink. An emergency glucagon kit containing a vial of powdered glucagon and a syringe of sterile water is usually maintained in the homes of insulin-dependent diabetics. Glucagon is also useful as a diagnostic aid in radiological examination of the stomach and lower gastrointestinal tract when diminished motility would be advantageous, because glucagon acts as a smooth muscle relaxant. The diagnostic kit also contains a vial of powdered glucagon and a syringe of sterile water. Glucagon can be administered by subcutaneous, intravenous, or intramuscular injection. It can be administered in a nonmedical setting by nonmedical personnel.

J1620

J1620   Injection, gonadorelin HCl, per 100 mcg

Lay Description

Gonadorelin HCl is used primarily as a diagnostic agent for evaluating the functional capacity and response of the anterior pituitary gonadotropins. Side effects may include headache, abdominal discomfort, flushing, bronchospasm, and/or local swelling at the injection site. The use of gonadorelin is contraindicated in patients who are hypersensitive to gonadorelin hydrochloride or any of its components. This code reports a 100 mcg injection.

J1626

J1626   Injection, granisetron HCl, 100 mcg

Lay Description

Granisetron HCl is an antiemetic used to prevent postoperative and chemotherapy or radiation related nausea and vomiting. It is a selective antagonist of serotonin receptors located in the vagus nerve and in the central nervous system's chemoreceptor trigger zone. Granisetron hydrochloride may be administered orally in solution or tablets or by intravenous injection. It is usually given 30 minutes to one hour before chemotherapy, with a second oral dose often following 12 hours later.

J1630-J1631

J1630   Injection, haloperidol, up to 5 mg
J1631   Injection, haloperidol decanoate, per 50 mg

Lay Description

Haloperidol and haloperidol decanoate are antipsychotics that are used in treating chronic psychosis due to schizophrenia, Tourette's syndrome, and other psychotic disorders. These drugs block the postsynaptic dopamine receptors in the brain. The injectable form is available in 5 mg/ml doses and may be administered by intravenous or intramuscular injection. Haloperidol decanoate is a long-acting form of haloperidol and is administered by intramuscular injection only. Haloperidol decanoate is available in 50 mg/ml and 100 mg/ml doses. Dosing is dependent on individual patient requirements and response to treatment.

J1640

J1640   Injection, hemin, 1 mg

Lay Description

Hemin is an iron containing metalloporphyrin. It is an enzyme inhibitor derived from processed red blood cells and acts to limit the hepatic and marrow synthesis of porphyrin. Hemin is an orphan drug indicated for the treatment of acute intermittent porphyria, porphyria variegata, and hereditary coproporphyria. Hemin therapy must be administered under close supervision of a physician, and it is not curative. The drug is administered by an intravenous infusion of 10 to 15 minutes. Recommended dosage is 1 to 4 mg/kg of body weight daily. The infusions are given for three to 14 days depending on the clinical signs.

J1642-J1644

J1642   Injection, heparin sodium, (heparin lock flush), per 10 units
J1644   Injection, Heparin sodium, per 1000 units

Lay Description

Heparin is an anticoagulant indicated for the treatment and prevention of blood clots, including pulmonary embolism and deep vein thrombosis. It is also used to ensure patency of indwelling intravenous catheters. Heparin inhibits reactions that lead to the clotting of blood and the formation of fibrin clots. It works by acting as an accelerant in forming antithrombin III-thrombin complex, which deactivates thrombin. This prevents the conversion of fibrinogen to fibrin. Heparin sodium is derived from bovine or porcine pulmonary or intestinal tissue and standardized for anticoagulant activity. It is administered by subcutaneous or intravenous injection. Heparin sodium is available in doses of 1,000, 5,000, and 10,000 units/ml. Heparin lock flush is available in 10 and 100 units/ml syringes or vials.

J1645

J1645   Injection, dalteparin sodium, per 2500 IU

Lay Description

Dalteparin sodium is a low molecular weight heparin that is produced through controlled nitrous acid depolymerization of sodium heparin from porcine intestinal mucosa followed by a chromatographic purification process. It acts by enhancing the inhibition of Factor Xa and thrombin by antithrombin. Dalteparin sodium is an injected drug that is used for the prophylaxis of ischemic complications in unstable angina and non-Q-wave myocardial infarction when administered in conjunction with aspirin therapy. This drug is also indicated for the prophylaxis of deep vein thrombosis (DVT), which may lead to pulmonary embolism (PE) for patients who are undergoing hip replacement surgery or abdominal surgery and are at risk for thromboembolic complications or a patient who is at risk for thromboembolic complications due to severely restricted mobility during acute illness. The dosage recommended for patients with unstable angina or non-Q-wave myocardial infarction is 120 IU per kg of body weight (but not more than 10,000 IU) subcutaneously every 12 hours with concurrent oral aspirin therapy for a duration of five to eight days. Dosage for hip replacement therapy varies as to the regime, but the first dose of 2,500 or 5,000 IU is administered prior to surgery and follow-up administration of 2,500 to 5,000 IU is administered postoperatively. In patients undergoing abdominal surgery with a risk of thromboembolic complications, the recommended dosage is 2,500 IU once daily beginning one to two hours prior to surgery and then once daily for five to 10 days. If the patient is at high risk of thromboembolic complications, dosage is increased to 5,000 IU. Dosage for patients with severely restricted mobility is 5,000 IU administered once daily. Dalteparin sodium is administered by subcutaneous injection.

J1650

J1650   Injection, enoxaparin sodium, 10 mg

Lay Description

Enoxaparin sodium is a low molecular weight heparin that has antithrombotic properties. When given at a dose of 1.5 mg/kg, enoxaparin has a higher ratio of anti-Factor Xa to anti-Factor IIa activity when compared to the ratios observed for heparin. Enoxaparin sodium is used for the prophylaxis of ischemic complications in unstable angina and non-Q-wave myocardial infarction when administered in conjunction with aspirin therapy and for the prophylaxis of deep vein thrombosis (DVT), which may lead to pulmonary embolism (PE) for patients who are undergoing hip or knee replacement surgery or abdominal surgery and are at risk for thromboembolic complications. It is also prescribed to patients who are at risk for thromboembolic complications due to severely restricted mobility during acute illness. This drug is administered via subcutaneous injection. Dosage varies depending upon the clinical indication. When administered to patients undergoing abdominal surgery, the usual dosage is 40 mg once per day beginning two hours prior to surgery for a seven to 10 day duration. When administered to patients undergoing hip or knee replacement surgery, 30 to 40 mg is injected subcutaneously 12 to 24 hours prior to surgery and then once daily for seven to 10 days. When administered to patients who are at risk for thromboembolic complications due to severely restricted mobility during an acute illness, the recommended dosage is 40 mg per day for six to 11 days. An Injection of 1 mg/kg of enoxaparin sodium subcutaneously every 12 hours in conjunction with aspirin therapy is administered for treatment of unstable angina.

J1652

J1652   Injection, fondaparinux sodium, 0.5 mg

Lay Description

Fondaparinux sodium is a synthetic inhibitor of activated factor X (Xa). It has no known effect on platelet function because it does not affect thrombin (activated factor II). Fibrinolytic activity or bleeding times are not affected. Fondaparinux sodium is a low molecular weight heparin that has antithrombotic properties. It is indicated for the prophylaxis of deep vein thrombosis, which may lead to pulmonary embolism in patients undergoing hip fracture surgery, including extended prophylaxis, hip replacement surgery, knee replacement surgery, and abdominal surgery for patients who are at risk for thromboembolic complications. Fondaparinux sodium is also indicated for the treatment of acute deep vein thrombosis when administered in conjunction with warfarin sodium, and the treatment of acute pulmonary embolism when administered in conjunction with warfarin sodium when initial therapy is administered in the hospital. The dosage depends on the condition being treated and body weight.

J1655

J1655   Injection, tinzaparin sodium, 1000 IU

Lay Description

Tinzaparin sodium is a low weight heparin that is used to treat deep vein thrombosis with or without pulmonary embolism. Tinzaparin interferes with the body's natural blood clotting mechanism by inactivating thrombin. Thrombin is an important constituent in blood clot formation. Tinzaparin is available in multiple use 2 ml vials. Each ml contains 20,000 IU of tinzaparin for a total of 40,000 IU per vial. Tinzaparin is administered by subcutaneous injection. The recommended dosage for the treatment of deep vein thrombosis is 175 IU/kg of body weight once daily for at least six days.

J1670

J1670   Injection, tetanus immune globulin, human, up to 250 units

Lay Description

Immune globulins are glycoproteins in the blood that function as antibodies. Immune globulins specific to a certain disease are antibodies with specific amino acid sequences that interact only with the antigen that stimulated its creation or with antigens that are closely related to the stimulating antigen. Immune globulins are usually derived from the pooled plasma of human donors who have antibodies to the specific disease. The antibodies from the exogenous immune globulin help the body fight off a disease. Tetanus is an acute, often fatal, infectious disease caused by the bacterium Clostridium tetani. This bacterium produces a neurotoxin called tetanospasmin. Generalized tetanus is characterized by muscular contractions and hyperreflexia, resulting in trismus (lockjaw), glottal spasm, generalized muscle spasm, opisthotonos, respiratory spasm, seizures, and paralysis. Localized tetanus may be mild, with localized muscular twitching and spasm of muscle groups near the site of injury. Localized tetanus may progress to the generalized form. Tetanus usually enters the body through a puncture wound, such as a splinter or bite. It may also enter through a burn, surgical wound, skin ulcer, injection site of drug abusers, umbilical stump, or postpartum uterus. Tetanus immune globulin is administered by intramuscular injection. It is administered for the prophylaxis or treatment of tetanus.

J1675

J1675   Injection, histrelin acetate, 10 mcg

Lay Description

Histrelin acetate is the acetate salt of a synthetic nonapeptide that corresponds to a component of naturally occurring human growth hormone. Initially the drug stimulates release of human growth hormone-releasing hormone. However, chronic use desensitizes responsiveness of the pituitary gonadotropin, causing a reduction in ovarian and testicular steroidogenesis. Decreases in LH, FSH, and sex steroid levels are observed within three months of initiation of therapy. It is an orphan drug indicated for the treatment of children with central precocious puberty (idiopathic or neurogenic) occurring before 8 years of age in girls or 9.5 years of age in boys.

J1700–J1720

J1700   **Injection, hydrocortisone acetate, up to 25 mg**

J1710   **Injection, hydrocortisone sodium phosphate, up to 50 mg**

J1720   **Injection, hydrocortisone sodium succinate, up to 100 mg**

Lay Description

Hydrocortisone is a steroid hormone produced by the adrenal cortex. A preparation of this hormone may be obtained from natural sources or produced synthetically. It is a corticosteroid that decreases inflammation and suppresses the immune system. Hydrocortisone acetate, sodium phosphate, and sodium succinate are used to treat severe inflammation, shock reactions, adrenal insufficiency, ulcerative colitis, and other inflammatory processes.

J1725

J1725   **Injection, hydroxyprogesterone caproate, 1 mg**

Lay Description

Hydroxyprogesterone caproate is a progestin medication used to treat women who have a history of delivering a single premature baby. It is not used to treat multiple gestation premature delivery. Recommended dose is 250 mg once a week beginning between 16 weeks, 0 days and 20 weeks, 6 days of gestation and continuing through delivery or 37 weeks, whichever occurs first. Hydroxyprogesterone caproate is administered by IM injection.

J1730

J1730   **Injection, diazoxide, up to 300 mg**

Lay Description

Diazoxide is a vasodilator when administered intra-venously and a drug used to treat hypoglycemia when administered orally. Intravenous administration is indicated in the emergency reduction of blood pressure in severe nonmalignant and malignant hypertension. It is also used to reduce extremely high blood pressure caused by kidney disease where other medicines have not been effective. Diazoxide works by causing the muscle in the walls of the blood vessels to relax. This allows the arteries to widen rapidly and reduces blood pressure. Intravenous dose is dependent on body weight.

J1740

J1740   **Injection, ibandronate sodium, 1 mg**

Lay Description

Ibandronate sodium is a chemical compound that inhibits bone resorption. It binds to hydroxyapatite, which is part of the mineral matrix of bone. Ibandronate inhibits osteoclast activity reducing bone resorption and turnover. The drug is indicated for the prophylaxis and treatment of osteoporosis in postmenopausal women where it reduces the elevated rate of bone turnover, leading to a net gain in bone mass density.

J1741

J1741   **Injection, ibuprofen, 100 mg**

Lay Description

Injectable ibuprofen is a nonopioid, nonsteroidal anti-inflammatory drug (NSAID). This code represents the intravenous formulation of ibuprofen. This drug is indicated for the management of mild to moderate pain, the management of moderate to severe pain with adjunctive opioid analgesics, and for fever reduction. It is administered intravenously over 30 minutes. The recommended adult dosage varies from 100 to 800 mg depending on the indication and patient response. This code represents 1 mg of intravenous ibuprofen.

J1742

J1742   **Injection, ibutilide fumarate, 1 mg**

Lay Description

Ibutilide fumarate is an antiarrhythmic drug. Ibutilide fumarate is indicated for the rapid conversion of atrial fibrillation or atrial flutter of recent onset. It prolongs action potential duration in isolated adult cardiac myocytes and increases both atrial and ventricular refractoriness. This allows prolongation of atrial and ventricular action potential duration and refractoriness, aiding in a normal cardiac rhythm. It is supplied in single dose 10 ml vials containing 1 mg of ibutilide fumarate for intravenous injection. Usual adult dose is 1 mg administered by intravenous push over a 10-minute period.

J1743

J1743   **Injection, idursulfase, 1 mg**

Lay Description

Idursulfase is an exogenous, purified form of a human enzyme produced by recombinant DNA technology in a human cell line. Idursulfase is an orphan drug used to treat the inherited metabolic disorder mucopolysaccharidosis II (MPS II or Hunter's syndrome). MPS II is caused by a lack of the enzyme iduronate-2-sulfase that normally breaks down certain carbohydrates known as glycosaminoglycans. MPS II causes widespread cumulative organ and tissue damage. The recommended dosage is 0.5 mg per kg of body weight. The drug is administered as an intravenous infusion every week over one to three hours.

J1744

J1744   Injection, icatibant, 1 mg

Lay Description
Icatibant is a synthetic chain of 10 amino acids that is a bradykinin B2 receptor antagonist indicated as a treatment for acute attacks of hereditary angioedema. Hereditary angioedema is caused by the absence or dysfunction of C1-esterase-inhibitor, which regulates a chain of reactions that lead to bradykinin production. Bradykinin is a vasodilator that is thought to cause hereditary angioedema. The drug may be self-administered. It is injected subcutaneously into the abdomen. The recommended dose is 30 mg, which can be repeated every six hours, up to three doses in a 24-hour period.

J1745

J1745   Injection infliximab, 10 mg

Lay Description
Infliximab is an injectable antibody that blocks the effects of tumor necrosis factor alpha (TNF alpha), a substance made by cells of the body that has an important role in promoting inflammation. Specifically, infliximab is used for treating the inflammation of Crohn's disease, rheumatoid arthritis, and psoriatic arthritis. Infliximab is administered by intravenous infusion, and dosage varies depending on the condition being treated. Dosage may range from 3 mg/kg of body weight (rheumatoid arthritis) to 5 mg/kg of body weight for moderate to severe Crohn's disease.

J1750

J1750   Injection, iron dextran, 50 mg

Lay Description
Iron dextran is used to treat iron deficiency anemia. It is a complex of ferric hydroxide and dextran. It is absorbed from the injection site into the capillaries and the lymphatic system. The iron is bound to the protein and forms iron. This iron is used to resupply the body with iron. Recommended dose of iron dextran varies based on the patient's hemoglobin level. It is administered by IV or intramuscular injection.

J1756

J1756   Injection, iron sucrose, 1 mg

Lay Description
Iron sucrose is a form of iron that is safe for the treatment of iron deficiency anemias in patients with kidney disease. It is used primarily in patients receiving ongoing hemodialysis and patients who are taking the hormone erythropoietin to help balance the iron deficiency caused by hemodialysis. Iron sucrose provides elemental iron, which is essential in the formation of hemoglobin. Iron sucrose is

administered by intravenous injection over a 15-minute period. The dosage varies dependent on the degree of iron deficiency and type of renal disease the patient suffers.

J1786

J1786   Injection, imiglucerase, 10 units

Lay Description
Imiglucerase is an enzyme used to treat and alleviate the symptoms of Gaucher's disease, a lysosomal storage disorder caused by a genetic lack of the enzyme glucocerebrosidase. Gaucher cells accumulate in the liver, spleen, and bone marrow, resulting in severe abdominal swelling, causing the spleen to break down red blood cells more rapidly than they are produced. Imiglucerase is a synthetic form of protein beta-glucocerebrosidase that works by catalyzing the hydrolysis of glucocerebrosidase to glucose and ceramide. Imiglucerase is used for the treatment of Type 1 Gaucher's disease that results in one or more of the following: anemia, thrombocytopenia, bone disease, hepatomegaly, or splenomegaly. Dosage is determined by body weight. The usual dose is 15 to 60 units/kg of body weight administered by intravenous injection over one to two hours.

J1790

J1790   Injection, droperidol, up to 5 mg

Lay Description
Droperidol is used as an adjunct to general or regional anesthesia or as a general anesthetic in diagnostic procedures. It also has an antiemetic effect and may be used prior to surgery or postoperatively to prevent nausea and vomiting. It is administered by intramuscular or intravenous injection. Dosage is dependent upon patient's age and weight.

J1800

J1800   Injection, propranolol HCl, up to 1 mg

Lay Description
Propranolol is a nonselective beta-blocker used to treat tremors, angina, heart rhythm disorders, hypertension, and other cardiac conditions. It has also been found to prevent myocardial infarction and lessen the severity of migraine headaches. It works by blocking catecholamine-induced increases in heart rate, blood pressure, and force of myocardial contraction, thereby reducing cardiac oxygen demand. It also depresses renin secretion and prevents vasodilation of the cerebral arteries. It may be administered orally by capsule, tablet, or oral suspension, or by intravenous injection or infusion. Intravenous administration is only used in life-threatening arrhythmias or those occurring under anesthesia. The usual dose ranges from 1 to 3 mg.

J1810

J1810   Injection, droperidol and fentanyl citrate, up to 2 ml ampule

Lay Description
Per the FDA, this drug is no longer available in the United States.

J1815-J1817

J1815   Injection, insulin, per 5 units

J1817   Insulin for administration through DME (i.e., insulin pump) per 50 units

Lay Description
Insulin is a hormone secreted by the beta cells of the pancreas that controls the metabolism and cellular uptake of sugars, proteins, and fats. As a drug, it is used principally to control Type I diabetes mellitus. Different forms of insulin may also be used to control blood sugar levels in patients with gestational diabetes to prevent fetal complications caused by maternal hyperglycemia. The use of insulin in Type II diabetes mellitus is typically only for patients who have failed to control their blood sugars with diet, exercise, and oral drugs. In the past, insulin for injection was obtained from beef or porcine pancreas. Most insulin now in use is made by recombinant DNA technology and is equivalent to human insulin from an immunological perspective. Dosage varies by the level of control of blood sugar needed. Insulin is administered by subcutaneous injection or by insulin pump.

J1826

J1826   Injection, interferon beta-1a, 30 mcg

Lay Description
Interferon beta-1a is a synthetic version of natural interferon beta-1a produced by recombinant DNA technology from Chinese hamster ovaries. Interferons are small, naturally occurring proteins that bind to specific cell membranes and initiate a series of events that include the inhibition of virus replication and the enhancement of macrophage and lymphocyte destruction of foreign cells. There are several types of interferons. Interferon beta-1a has been shown to control symptoms of muscular sclerosis, but its exact mechanism of action is unknown. Interferon beta-1a is indicated for the treatment of patients with relapsing forms of multiple sclerosis to decrease the frequency of clinical exacerbations and delay the onset of the physical disabilities associated with the disease. The drug may be self-administered as a subcutaneous injection. Interferon beta-1a is also available as an intramuscular injection.

J1830

J1830   Injection interferon beta-1b, 0.25 mg (code may be used for Medicare when drug administered under the direct supervision of a physician, not for use when drug is self-administered)

Lay Description
Interferon beta-1b is a biologic response modifier possessing both antiviral and immunoregulatory activities. Interferon beta-1b is indicated for the treatment of relapsing-remitting multiple sclerosis in ambulatory patients. The mechanisms by which interferon beta-1b exerts its actions in multiple sclerosis are not clearly understood. However, the biologic response-modifying properties are known to be mediated through its interactions with specific cell receptors found on the cell membrane, which cause cellular changes, including increased protein synthesis of human cells. The usual dosage is 0.25 mg self-injected subcutaneously every other day.

J1835

J1835   Injection, itraconazole, 50 mg

Lay Description
Itraconazole is an antifungal used for the treatment of patients with aspergillosis, blastomycosis, histoplasmosis, esophageal and oropharyngeal candidiasis, and onychomycosis. It is also used to prevent fungal infections in patients with human immunodeficiency virus (HIV) or acquired immunodeficiency syndrome (AIDS). Itraconazole is in a class of antifungals called triazoles. It works by slowing the growth of fungi that cause infection. It may be administered orally as a capsule or oral solution or by intravenous infusion. Itraconazole administered by intravenous infusion is used primarily for immunocompromised patients with severe lung or systemic fungal infections. Usual intravenous dosage is 200 mg infused over one hour.

J1840-J1850

J1840   Injection, kanamycin sulfate, up to 500 mg

J1850   Injection, kanamycin sulfate, up to 75 mg

Lay Description
Kanamycin sulfate is a bacterial antibiotic used to treat E. coli, Proteus species (both indole-positive and indole-negative), Enterobacter aerogenes, Klebsiella pneumoniae, Serratia marcescens, and Acinetobacter species. It inhibits the synthesis of protein in susceptible microorganisms. The recommended dose is 15 mg per kg per day divided equally for intramuscular injection and should not exceed 15 mg per kg per day for intravenous infusion. Kanamycin can be administered intramuscularly or intravenously over 30 to 60 minutes.

J1885

J1885   Injection, ketorolac tromethamine, per 15 mg

Lay Description
Ketorolac tromethamine is a nonsteroidal anti-inflammatory drug (NSAID) that is indicated for short-term (up to five days in adults) management of moderately severe acute pain that requires analgesia at the opioid level. Ketorolac tromethamine is available for intravenous (IV) or intramuscular (IM) administration as 15 mg in 1 mL (1.5%) and 30 mg in 1 mL (3%) in sterile solution; 60 mg in 2 mL (3%) of ketorolac tromethamine in sterile solution is available for IM administration only.

J1890

J1890   Injection, cephalothin sodium, up to 1 g

Lay Description
Cephalosporins are used in the treatment of infections caused by bacteria. They work by killing bacteria or preventing their growth. Cephalosporins are used to treat infections in many different parts of the body. They are sometimes given with other antibiotics. Some cephalosporins given by injection are also used to prevent infections before, during, and after surgery. Cephalothin will not work against infections caused by viruses such as colds or the flu. Per the FDA, this drug is no longer available for human use in the United States.

J1930

J1930   Injection, lanreotide, 1 mg

Lay Description
Lanreotide is an orphan drug used to treat acromegaly, often due to a benign pituitary gland tumor. It is a rare and potentially life-threatening disease in which abnormal growth hormone is secreted by the pituitary gland. This abnormal growth hormone can cause enlargement of the hands, feet, facial bones, and internal organs such as the heart and liver. Patients who are untreated may have a shortened life span from heart and respiratory diseases, diabetes mellitus, and colon cancer. Lanreotide is used to treat patients who are not able to undergo surgery or radiotherapy. The recommended dose is 90 milligrams. This medication is administered by deep subcutaneous injection every four weeks for three months.

J1931

J1931   Injection, laronidase, 0.1 mg

Lay Description
Laronidase is a polymorphic variant of the human enzyme L-iduronidase that is produced by recombinant DNA technology in a Chinese hamster ovary cell line. It is used to treat Hurler and Hurler-Scheie forms of mucopolysaccharidosis in patients who have moderate to severe symptoms. Laronidase has been shown to improve pulmonary function and walking capacity. Laronidase has not been evaluated for effects on the central nervous system manifestations of the disorder. The recommended dosage is 0.58 mg/kg of body weight administered once weekly as an intravenous infusion.

J1940

J1940   Injection, furosemide, up to 20 mg

Lay Description
Furosemide is a diuretic that is an anthranilic acid derivative. It is used to treat edema, hypertension, and pulmonary edema. Dosage recommendations vary by the type of condition being treated, route of administration (oral, IV, or IM), and age and size of patient.

J1945

J1945   Injection, lepirudin, 50 mg

Lay Description
Lepirudin is a bivalent direct thrombin inhibitor derived from yeast cells that reduces the risk of serious consequences of heparin-induced thrombocytopenia (HIT). It is indicated for anticoagulation in patients with HIT and associated thromboembolic diseases. The usual dosage is 0.4 mg/kg body weight (up to 110 kg) administered slowly intravenously (e.g., over 15 to 20 seconds) as a bolus dose, followed by 0.15 mg/kg body weight (up to 110kg/hour) as a continuous intravenous infusion for two to 10 days or longer if clinically needed.

J1950

J1950   Injection, leuprolide acetate (for depot suspension), per 3.75 mg

Lay Description
Leuprolide acetate is a synthetic analogue of the luteinizing hormone-releasing hormone (LHRH) that is used as an antineoplastic drug and a treatment for central precocious puberty, endometriosis, and uterine fibroids. It first stimulates and then suppresses follicle stimulating and luteinizing hormone release, resulting in suppression of testosterone and estrogen. A depot suspension is a drug that remains in the body long-term in storage and is slowly released into the blood. The leuprolide acetate depot suspension in dosages of 3.75 mg monthly and the 12.25 mg every three months are injected intramuscularly to treat endometriosis and uterine fibroids. When used to treat central precocious puberty, the dosage is individualized to the child and can range from 7.5 to 15 mg. Leuprolide acetate in doses of 7.5 mg and greater is injected subcutaneously and is used as a palliative treatment for advanced prostate cancer.

J1953

J1953　Injection, levetiracetam, 10 mg

Lay Description
Levetiracetam is an anticonvulsant indicated as an adjunctive therapy to help control partial onset seizures or myoclonic seizures in adults with juvenile myoclonic epilepsy. This injection is used when oral administration is not feasible. The precise mechanism by which levetiracetam controls seizure activity is unknown. The recommended dose is 500 milligrams twice a day. The dose can be increased every two weeks up to 3,000 milligrams. Levetiracetam is administered by IV injection over 15 minutes.

J1955

J1955　Injection, levocarnitine, per 1 g

Lay Description
Levocarnitine is a naturally occurring substance required for energy metabolism. It has been shown to facilitate long-chain, fatty acid entry into cellular mitochondria, therefore delivering substrate for oxidation and subsequent energy production. With the exception of the brain, all tissues use fatty acids as an energy substrate and serve as a major fuel source in skeletal tissue and cardiac muscle. Levocarnitine is prescribed for the treatment of patients with an inherent error of metabolism that results in secondary carnitine deficiency. It is also used to prevent and treat carnitine deficiency in patients with end-stage renal disease who are on hemodialysis. The recommended dosage is a loading dose of 50 mg/kg given as a bolus injection over two to three minutes followed by 50 mg/kg daily by intravenous infusion.

J1956

J1956　Injection, levofloxacin, 250 mg

Lay Description
Levofloxacin is a quinolone antibiotic. It inhibits DNA synthesis causing cell death. Susceptibility studies should be performed prior to the administration of levofloxacin. Susceptible bacteria include *Streptococcus pneumoniae, Haemophilus influenzae, Moraxella catarrhalis, Staphylococcus aureus, Haemophilus parainfluenzae, Pseudomonas aeruginosa, Serratia marcescens, E. coli, Klebsiella pneumoniae, Chlamydia pneumoniae, Legionella pneumophila, Mycoplasma pneumoniae, Enterococcus faecalis, Streptococcus pyogenes, Proteus mirabilis, Staphylococcus epidermidis, Enterobacter cloacae, Staphylococcus saprophyticus*, and *Bacillus anthracis*.

J1960

J1960　Injection, levorphanol tartrate, up to 2 mg

Lay Description
Levorphanol tartrate is a potent synthetic opioid analgesic used to manage moderate to severe pain or as a pre- or postoperative medication where an opioid analgesic is appropriate. It may be administered by injection, intravenous infusion, or orally. The usual recommended starting dose for intravenous administration is up to 1 mg, given in divided doses, by slow push technique. This may be repeated every three to six hours as needed. The usual recommended starting dose administration by injection is 1 to 2 mg subcutaneously or intramuscularly repeated every six to eight hours as needed.

J1980

J1980　Injection, hyoscyamine sulfate, up to 0.25 mg

Lay Description
Hyoscyamine sulfate is a component of belladonna alkaloid and is used as an anticholinergic and antispasmodic. Hyoscyamine sulfate inhibits gastrointestinal propulsive motility and decreases gastric acid secretion. This drug also decreases pharyngeal, tracheal, and bronchial secretions. Hyoscyamine sulfate is used as an adjunct therapy for the treatment of peptic ulcer disease, to control gastric secretion or excessive saliva production, and to decrease visceral spasm and hypermotility in such conditions as spastic colitis, spastic bladder, cystitis, and pylorospasm. It may also be used to prevent drug induced bradycardia during surgery. Hyoscyamine sulfate may be administered by several forms including sublingual, oral, injection, or intravenously. Dosage varies depending upon the condition being treated, patient age, and the size and weight of the patient. It can range from 0.25 mg to 0.5 mg for adults.

J1990

J1990　Injection, chlordiazepoxide HCl, up to 100 mg

Lay Description
Chlordiazepoxide is a member of the benzodiazepine class of drugs. It acts on the gamma amino butyric acid (GABA) receptors in the brain resulting in the release of GABA and reducing the function of certain areas of the brain. GABA is a major inhibitory chemical in the brain that assists with inducing sleepiness and helps to control anxiety. Chlordiazepoxide is most commonly used to treat insomnia; however, it can also be used to relieve anxiety, particularly preoperative anxiety, and help alleviate alcohol withdrawal symptoms. It can be habit forming and is only used on a short-term basis. Dosage is dependent upon the condition being treated and the response of the individual patient.

J2001

J2001　Injection, lidocaine HCl for intravenous infusion, 10 mg

Lay Description
Lidocaine hydrochloride stabilizes the neuronal membrane by inhibiting the conduction of pain impulses, thereby providing local anesthesia. It also stabilizes heart rhythms when administered

intravenously. Lidocaine hydrochloride is indicated for local or regional anesthesia by infiltration techniques, such as percutaneous injection and intravenous regional peripheral nerve block techniques, and for treatment of cardiac arrhythmias. The drug is available in topical and injectable forms. The injectable form can be administered by intravenous infusion, caudal, epidural, retrobulbar, peripheral nerve block, and sympathetic nerve block.

J2010

J2010   Injection, lincomycin HCl, up to 300 mg

Lay Description
Lincomycin hydrochloride (HCl) is an antibiotic used to treat serious, susceptible strains of streptococci, pneumococci, and staphylococci infections. It is specifically effective against the following organisms: *Streptococcus pyogenes, Viridans* group, *streptococci, Corynebacterium diphtheriae, Propionibacterium acnes, Clostridium tetani, and Clostridium perfringens.* It is used for patients who are allergic to penicillin or for whom penicillin treatment is inappropriate. Recommended dose is 600 mg intramuscularly every 24 hours and 600 mg to 1 gram via intravenous infusion every eight to 12 hours. Intravenous lincomycin should be infused over one hour or more.

J2020

J2020   Injection, linezolid, 200 mg

Lay Description
Linezolid is a synthetic antibacterial of the oxazolidinone class. This drug inhibits bacterial protein synthesis by binding to a specific site on RNA and preventing the translation process. This method of action is different from other antibacterials; cross-resistance between linezolid and other antibiotics is unlikely. Susceptibility studies should be performed prior to the administration of cefazolin sodium. Susceptible bacteria include vancomycin-resistant *Enterococcus faecium,* methicillin-susceptible and resistant *Staphylococcus aureus, Streptococcus pneumoniae, Streptococcus pyogenes,* and *Streptococcus agalactiae.* Linezolid is available in injectable and oral forms. The injectable form is administered by intravenous infusion over a period of 30 to 120 minutes. The dosage varies by the route of administration, and by type and severity of the infection.

J2060

J2060   Injection, lorazepam, 2 mg

Lay Description
Lorazepam is a psychotropic drug with potent hypnotic and sedative effects. Lorazepam injection may be prescribed as a preanesthetic medication. Lorazepam is also indicated for the management of anxiety disorders or for the short-term relief of symptoms of anxiety or anxiety associated with depressive symptoms. When administered by

intramuscular injection, usual dosage is 0.05 mg/kg of body weight up to a maximum of 4 mg. For intravenous injection for the purposes of sedation or relief of anxiety, the usual dose is 0.02 mg/kg of body weight to a maximum of 2 mg.

J2150

J2150   Injection, mannitol, 25% in 50 ml

Lay Description
Mannitol is an osmotic diuretic that is readily diffused through the kidney. It is used to induce diuresis in the treatment and/or prevention of the oliguric phase of acute renal failure before irreversible damage is established. Mannitol is also used to reduce intracranial pressure and cerebral edema by reducing brain mass, to reduce elevated intraocular pressure, and to promote urinary excretion of toxic substances. Mannitol is administered by intravenous infusion. Dosage is dependent upon the condition being treated, with usual adult dosage ranging from 20 to 100 g in a 24-hour period.

J2170

J2170   Injection, mecasermin, 1 mg

Lay Description
Mecasermin is a synthesized version of human insulin-like growth factor-1 (IGF-1). It is produced by recombinant DNA technology using strains of *E. coli* bacteria. IGF-1 (formerly called somatomedin C) is a serum peptide formed within the liver and other tissues. IGF-1 in the human body is stimulated by human growth hormone and in turn stimulates cell growth and replication by increasing the metabolic uptake of glucose, fatty acids, and amino acids. Mecasermin is indicated for the long-term treatment of growth failure in children with severe primary IGF-1 deficiency or with genetic growth gene deletion that has developed neutralizing antibodies to growth hormone. The drug is not indicated for treatment of secondary forms of IGF-1 deficiency. Mecasermin should not be used in patients with closed epiphyses. Dosage is individualized for each patient and varies from an initial dose of 0.5 mg to 2 mg per kg of patient body weight. Mecasermin is administered subcutaneously and can be self-administered.

J2175

J2175   Injection, meperidine HCl, per 100 mg

Lay Description
Meperidine hydrochloride is a narcotic analgesic with similar effects as morphine. Meperidine hydrochloride is used for analgesia and sedation. It is primarily used to treat moderate to severe pain, as a preoperative medicate, and as a form of anesthesia.

J2180

J2180   Injection, meperidine and promethazine HCl, up to 50 mg

Lay Description

Meperidine and promethazine hydrochloride is a compound of a narcotic analgesic with similar effects as morphine (meperidine hydrochloride) and a phenothiazine derivative that provides antiemetic, sedative, and antihistaminic actions. It is primarily used to treat moderate to severe pain, as a preoperative medicate, and as a form of anesthesia. This drug is usually administered intramuscularly but the intravenous route may be employed. When used intravenously, it is preferable to use a push technique. Usual adult dosage is 50 mg every three to four hours; children's dosage is 0.5 mg/kg.

J2185

J2185   Injection, meropenem, 100 mg

Lay Description

Meropenem is a broad spectrum carbapenem antibiotic for intravenous administration. It is indicated for the treatment of infections of the skin, intra-abdominal infections such as peritonitis, and bacterial meningitis when caused by susceptible bacterial agents. Dosage varies depending upon the severity of the condition and the age and weight of the patient. In adults, the recommended dosage is 500 mg every eight hours for skin infections and 1 g given every eight hours for intra-abdominal infections. Pediatric patients receive doses of 10, 20, or 40 mg/kg every eight hours depending on the type of infection. The usual technique is intravenous infusion over 15 to 30 minutes; however, a bolus dose over three to five minutes may be prescribed.

J2210

J2210   Injection, methylergonovine maleate, up to 0.2 mg

Lay Description

Methylergonovine maleate is a blood-vessel constrictor that is used to prevent or control postpartum hemorrhage caused by subinvolution or uterine atony. It works by causing the uterine muscles to contract, thereby reducing blood loss. Methylergonovine maleate is available in tablet and injectable forms. The injectable form can be administered by intramuscular or intravenous injection; however, intravenous injection is administered only for life-threatening postpartum hemorrhage.

J2212

J2212   Injection, methylnaltrexone, 0.1 mg

Lay Description

Methylnaltrexone bromide is a peripheral acting mu-opioid receptor antagonist. The drug targets tissues such as those in the gastrointestinal tract and blocks the effects of opioids. Opioids slow gastrointestinal motility and transit, which creates constipation. Methylnaltrexone bromide is indicated for the treatment of constipation in patients receiving palliative care when constipation is not relieved by laxatives. The recommended dosage is 8 mg for patients weighing 38 to 62 kg or 12 mg for patients weighing 62 to 114 kg. The drug is given as a subcutaneous injection every other day. It should not be administered more than once every 24-hour period.

J2248

J2248   Injection, micafungin sodium, 1 mg

Lay Description

Micafungin sodium is a semisynthetic lipopeptide produced from Coleophoma empetri, a plant fungus. It is used as an antifungal drug. Micafungin sodium disrupts the synthesis of a component of the fungal cellular membrane. This component is not present in mammalian cells. Micafungin sodium is indicated for the treatment of esophageal candidiasis and as a prophylactic therapy to prevent candida infections in patients undergoing hematopoietic stem cell transplants. The drug may cause allergic reactions including anaphylaxis. Micafungin sodium must be administered via an intravenous infusion over one hour. It should not be mixed with or infused with any other medication.

J2250

J2250   Injection, midazolam HCl, per 1 mg

Lay Description

Midazolam hydrochloride is a benzodiazepine, a group of chemically similar psychotropic drugs. Because midazolam hydrochloride is associated with a high incidence of partial or complete recall impairment, it is used as preoperative sedation, sedation during diagnostic or therapeutic procedures, or for induction of general anesthesia. Dosage varies depending on the reason for administration and the age and weight of the patient.

J2260

J2260   Injection, milrinone lactate, 5 mg

Lay Description

Milrinone lactate is a member of a class of bipyridine inotropic/vasodilator agents with phosphodiesterase inhibitor activity that is distinct from digitalis or catecholamines. Milrinone lactate is indicated for the short-term intravenous treatment of acute heart failure. It is administered intravenously with a loading dose of 50 mcg/kg followed by a maintenance dose of no more than 1.13 mg/kg/day.

J2265

J2265   Injection, minocycline HCl, 1 mg

Lay Description

Minocycline HCl is an antibiotic used to treat a wide variety of gram negative and gram positive infections.

It is thought to inhibit the protein synthesis. The recommended adult dose of minocycline HCl is initially 200 mg and then 100 mg every 12 hours. For children, an initial dose of 4 mg/kg, then 2 mg/kg every 12 hours. It is administered by IV infusion.

J2270–J2275

J2270   Injection, morphine sulfate, up to 10 mg

Lay Description
Morphine sulfate is an opioid analgesic that principally affects the central nervous system and gastrointestinal tract. The drug increases the patient's tolerance for pain and decreases patient discomfort. The patient, however, may still recognize the presence of pain. Sedation also occurs. Dosage varies by route of administration, patient's age, weight, severity of illness, and comorbidities.

J2274

J2274   Injection, morphine sulfate, preservative-free for epidural or intrathecal use, 10 mg

Lay Description
Preservative-free morphine sulfate injection is a systemic narcotic analgesic for administration by epidural or intrathecal routes. It is used for the management of chronic, intractable pain not responsive to nonnarcotic analgesics. Morphine sulfate, administered epidurally or intrathecally, provides pain relief for extended periods without attendant loss of motor, sensory, or sympathetic function. The solution contains no antioxidant, bacteriostat, or antimicrobial agent and is intended as a single-dose injection to provide analgesia via the intravenous, epidural, or intrathecal routes. When the epidural route of administration is used, more time is required for the morphine to cross the dura and reach the dorsal horn in the spinal cord. In contrast, intrathecal morphine binds with opiate receptors in the spinal cord without having to cross the dura. Therefore, intrathecal delivery results in faster analgesic. Each ampul and vial is intended for single use only. Epidural adult dosage: Initial injection of 5 mg in the lumbar region may provide satisfactory pain relief for up to 24 hours. If adequate pain relief is not achieved within one hour, careful administration of incremental doses of 1 to 2 mg at intervals sufficient to assess effectiveness may be given. No more than 10 mg/24 hours should be administered. Intrathecal adult dosage: A single injection of 0.2 to 1 mg may provide satisfactory pain relief for up to 24 hours. Repeated intrathecal injections of preservative-free morphine sulfate injection are not recommended. A constant intravenous infusion of naloxone hydrochloride, 0.6 mg/hr, for 24 hours after intrathecal injection may be used to reduce the incidence of potential side effects. For aged or debilitated patients, administer with extreme caution. A lower dosage is usually satisfactory. Repeat dosage: If pain recurs, alternative routes of administration should be considered, since experience with repeated doses of morphine by the intrathecal route is limited. Pediatric use: No information on the use in pediatric patients is available.

J2278

J2278   Injection, ziconotide, 1 mcg

Lay Description
Ziconotide is a synthetic equivalent conopeptide produced from piscivorous marine snails. It binds to N-type calcium channels in the afferent nerves of the dorsal horn in the spinal column preventing the transmission of pain sensation. This drug must be administered intrathecally via an implanted variable-rate microinfusion device or an external microinfusion device and catheter. Ziconotide is indicated for the management of severe chronic pain in patients who are intolerant or refractory to other treatments. The effective dose of ziconotide is variable and the dose should be adjusted according to the patient's severity of pain, response to therapy, and the occurrence of adverse events.

J2280

J2280   Injection, moxifloxacin, 100 mg

Lay Description
Moxifloxacin hydrochloride is a synthetic, broad spectrum antibacterial agent. It is used to treat adult patient with acute bacterial sinusitis, acute bacterial exacerbation of chronic bronchitis, community acquired pneumonia, skin infections, and complicated intra-abdominal infections when caused by susceptible bacterial organism such as *Streptococcus pneumoniae, Haemophilus influenzae, Haemophilus parainfluenzae, Klebsiella pneumoniae,* methicillin-susceptible *Staphylococcus aureus,* or *Moraxella catarrhalis.* The usual dosage is 400 mg daily.

J2300

J2300   Injection, nalbuphine HCl, per 10 mg

Lay Description
Nalbuphine hydrochloride is a synthetic opioid analgesic that is chemically related to naloxone and oxymorphone. Nalbuphine hydrochloride is prescribed for the relief of moderate to severe pain or as a supplement to balanced anesthesia. It is also used for pre- and postoperative pain relief or obstetrical analgesia during labor and delivery. It may be administered by subcutaneous, intramuscular, or intravenous injection. The usual adult dose is 10 mg for every 70 kg every three to six hours as needed, adjusted according to the pain severity, condition of the patient, and other medications.

J2310

J2310   Injection, naloxone HCl, per 1 mg

Lay Description

Naloxone hydrochloride injection is indicated for the complete or partial reversal of narcotic depression induced by opioids, including natural and synthetic narcotics. Naloxone hydrochloride injection is also indicated for the diagnosis of suspected acute opioid overdosage. It may be administered intravenously, intramuscularly, or subcutaneously. The most rapid onset of action is achieved by intravenous administration, and this route is recommended in emergency situations. The usual intravenous dosage is 2 mg of naloxone hydrochloride in 500 mL of IV solution. Intramuscular or subcutaneous injection dosage varies depending upon patient's response.

J2315

J2315   Injection, naltrexone, depot form, 1 mg

Lay Description

Naltrexone depot is an opioid antagonist. The drug binds to specific opioid receptors blocking the effects stimulated by alcohol ingestion. A depot suspension is a drug that remains in the body long term in storage and is slowly released into the blood. The depot form is indicated as a treatment of alcohol dependence in patients who are unable to abstain from alcohol consumption during outpatient therapy treatments. The drug should be a part of a comprehensive treatment management program. Patients should not actively consume alcohol during the initiation of naltrexone depot treatment. Naltrexone depot is administered by intramuscular injection into the gluteus once a month. The recommended dosage is 380 mg once a month. The depot form is not self-administrable.

J2320

J2320   Injection, nandrolone decanoate, up to 50 mg

Lay Description

Nandrolone decanoate is a long-acting synthetic version of testosterone that has strong anabolic properties and weak androgenic or masculinizing properties. Anabolic properties are any constructive metabolic process by which organisms convert substances into other components of the organism's chemical architecture. Nandrolone decanoate stimulates erythropoiesis, promotes tissue growth and building processes, and reverses tissue destruction. It is indicated as a treatment for chronic wasting diseases and anemia associated with renal insufficiency. Nandrolone decanoate is administered by intramuscular injection.

J2323

J2323   Injection, natalizumab, 1 mg

Lay Description

Natalizumab is a monoclonal antibody produced with recombinant DNA technology in murine myeloma cells. Natalizumab binds to the surface of leukocyte cells (except neutrophils) preventing their migration to the site of inflamed tissue. It is indicated as a monotherapy for the treatment of relapsing forms of multiple sclerosis in patients who cannot tolerate or have not adequately responded to other treatments. The recommended dose is 300 mg administered via intravenous infusion every four weeks. Note that this drug can only be prescribed, distributed and infused by providers, infusion centers and pharmacies registered with the manufacturer's TOUCH program. Patients must also be enrolled with the program.

J2325

J2325   Injection, nesiritide, 0.1 mg

Lay Description

Nesiritide is a human, B-type natriuretic peptide produced by recombinant DNA technology from E. coli. It has the same amino acid sequence as the endogenous peptide produced by the ventricular myocardium. Nesiritide binds to receptors of vascular smooth muscle and endothelial cells and increases intracellular concentrations of guanosine cyclic monophosphate (cGMP), which creates smooth muscle cell relaxation. Use of this drug should be strictly limited to patients with acutely decompensated heart failure with a clinical presentation severe enough to warrant hospitalization. The drug should be administered in a clinical setting where blood pressure can be closely monitored. Nesiritide is currently in a clinical trial to asses its use in intermittent and scheduled infusions to treat severely ill congestive heart failure patients in an outpatient setting. However, this setting and indication are not recommended and have not yet been approved. Nesiritide is not intended for use as a diuretic. The drug is administered by intravenous infusion, and the recommended dose is an initial intravenous bolus of 2 mcg/kg of body weight followed by a continuous infusion of 0.01 mcg/kg of body weight per minute.

J2353-J2354

J2353   Injection, octreotide, depot form for intramuscular injection, 1 mg

J2354   Injection, octreotide, nondepot form for subcutaneous or intravenous injection, 25 mcg

Lay Description

Octreotide is a synthetic analogue of the natural hormone somatostatin. It causes the same effects as somatostatin but has a prolonged duration. Somatostatin is a peptide produced by the hypothalamus gland and by pancreatic islet cells that inhibit the release of growth hormone, thyrotropin, corticotropin, insulin, glucagon, gastrin, renin, and secretin. The depot version is octreotide encased in biodegradable microspheres. The microspheres control the rate of drug release and allow it to be dispensed over longer periods of time. Both depot and non-depot formulations of octreotide are indicated as a treatment for acromegaly, as a symptomatic treatment for diarrhea, and flushing associated with metastatic carcinoid and vasoactive intestinal peptide tumors. Non-depot octreotide is administered by subcutaneous or intravenous injection. Dosages for the non-depot version vary from 50 to 600 mcg depending on the disease and response to treatment. Octreotide depot is administered by deep intramuscular injection into the buttocks every four weeks. The dosage for the depot version is usually 20 mg for patients who have been receiving the non-depot version.

J2355

J2355   Injection, oprelvekin, 5 mg

Lay Description

Oprelvekin is a synthetic interleukin-11 produced by recombinant DNA technology using *E. coli* bacteria. Interleukin-11 is a growth factor produced by bone marrow stromal cells that stimulates the production of hematopoietic stem cells and megakaryocyte progenitor cells and B cell differentiation. Oprelvekin is indicated for prevention of thrombocytopenia following myelosuppressive chemotherapy in patients with non-myeloid malignancies. It is administered by subcutaneous injection. The recommended dosage is 50 mg/kg of body weight.

J2357

J2357   Injection, omalizumab, 5 mg

Lay Description

Omalizumab is a monoclonal antibody produced by recombinant DNA technology using Chinese hamster ovaries. It binds specifically to human immunoglobulin E (IgE) and inhibits the binding of IgE to mast cells and basophils. The reduction in IgE binding limits the allergic response. Omalizumab is indicated for patients age 12 years or older with moderate to severe persistent asthma who are reactive to air-borne allergens and whose symptoms are not adequately controlled by inhaled corticosteroids. It is administered by subcutaneous injection. Dosages vary from 150 to 375 mg every two to four weeks. Dosage depends on the patient's body weight and the serum level of IgE. HCPCS Level II code J2357 represents 5 mg of omalizumab.

J2358

J2358   Injection, olanzapine, long-acting, 1 mg

Lay Description

Olanzapine is a psychotropic agent that belongs to the thienobenzodiazepine class. It is used to treat schizophrenia, acute mixed or manic episodes associated with bipolar disorder, agitation associated with schizophrenia, and bipolar disorder. Olanzapine is administered by deep intramuscular injection into the gluteal muscle.

J2360

J2360   Injection, orphenadrine citrate, up to 60 mg

Lay Description

Orphenadrine citrate is a synthetic analogue of diphenhydramine having analgesic, antihistaminic, anti-cholinergic, and antispasmodic properties. The drug acts on the brain stem selectively blocking facilitatory functions of the reticular formation. This produces a blocking of the pain transmission signals. Its therapeutic effects are not completely understood, but appear to be related to its analgesic properties. Orphenadrine is indicated for symptomatic relief of pain associated with acute musculoskeletal disorders. It can be used as an adjunct to rest, physical therapy, and other analgesic measures. Orphenadrine is available in an oral, self-administrable form and in an injectable form. The oral form is usually combined with aspirin and caffeine. Dosages of the oral form vary from 25 to 200 mg per day. Recommended dosage of the injectable form is 60 mg twice a day. The Injectable form is administered by intravenous or intramuscular injection.

J2370

J2370   Injection, phenylephrine HCl, up to 1 ml

Lay Description

Phenylephrine hydrochloride is an amine that is related to epinephrine and ephedrine. The drug is longer-acting than epinephrine or ephedrine. It affects the sympathetic nervous system by stimulating alpha adrenergic receptors. It functions predominately as a vasoconstrictor. Injectable phenylephrine hydrochloride is indicated for the treatment of hypotension, vascular failure in shock, and paroxysmal supraventricular tachycardia. The drug is also used to maintain adequate blood pressure during inhalation and spinal anesthesia and as a vasoconstrictor in regional analgesia. Injectable phenylephrine hydrochloride may be administered by intramuscular, subcutaneous, or intravenous injection and by intravenous infusion.

J2400

J2400   Injection, chloroprocaine HCl, per 30 ml

Lay Description

Chloroprocaine hydrochloride (HCl) is a local anesthetic that blocks the feeling of pain by inhibiting the conduction of nerve impulses. The order of loss of nerve function is pain, temperature, touch, proprioception, and skeletal muscle tone. This anesthetic is often used for dental procedures and during labor and delivery. Chloroprocaine can be administered by infiltration, caudal, epidural, or peripheral block.

J2405

J2405   Injection, ondansetron HCl, per 1 mg

Lay Description

Ondansetron hydrochloride is a chemical compound that is a selective blocker of serotonin 5-HT3 receptors. It is an antiemetic drug available in oral and injectable forms. Serotonin 5-HT3 receptors are present on the vagal nerve and at sensory nerve endings. Cytotoxic chemotherapy appears to trigger the release of serotonin in the small intestine, which may trigger the 5-HT3 receptors and initiate the vomiting reflex. Ondansetron hydrochloride is indicated for the prevention of nausea and vomiting associated with surgery and antineoplastic drugs. The oral version is also indicated for the prevention of nausea and vomiting associated with radiation therapy. The drug is available in oral and injectable versions. The injectable version is administered by intravenous injection. When administered in conjunction with antineoplastic drugs, ondansetron hydrochloride should be diluted. The recommended dosage for this indication is a single 32 mg or three doses at 0.15 mg/kg of body weight infused over 15 minutes. Subsequent dosages may be infused at four and eight hours after the initial dose. When used to suppress postoperative vomiting, the drug does not need to be diluted. The recommended dose is 4 mg or 0.1 mg/kg of body weight administered by intravenous or intramuscular injection. Dosages for the oral version vary from 8 to 24 mg depending on the indication and patient.

J2410

J2410   Injection, oxymorphone HCl, up to 1 mg

Lay Description

Oxymorphone hydrochloride is a semi-synthetic opioid substitute for morphine that is a potent analgesic and sedative. Oxymorphone hydrochloride exerts its effect on the central nervous system (CNS) and gastrointestinal tract. It binds to specific opiate receptors in the CNS providing an analgesic effect. The exact mechanism of action for its analgesic effect is unknown. Oxymorphone hydrochloride also produces respiratory depression; decreases gastric, biliary, and pancreatic secretions; and increases smooth muscle tone in the urinary tract. It is a schedule II controlled substance. Oxymorphone hydrochloride is indicated for the relief of moderate to severe pain, as an anesthetic premedication, and for the relief of anxiety related to dyspnea associated with pulmonary edema in patients with acute left ventricular dysfunction.

J2425

J2425   Injection, palifermin, 50 mcg

Lay Description

Palifermin is a human keratinocyte growth factor (KGF) produced by recombinant DNA technology in *Escherichia coli* (*E. coli*). It is different from endogenous human growth factor (EGF) in that the first 23 N-terminal amino acids have been deleted to improve protein stability. It stimulates the epithelial cells that line and protect the oral mucosa. It is used to treat severe oral mucositis that is often found as a side effect of high dose chemotherapy and/or radiation therapy in patients with hematologic malignancies. The recommended dose of palifermin is 60 mcg per kg per day. The medication is administered for three consecutive days prior to the myelotoxic therapy and three consecutive days after. Palifermin is administered by intravenous bolus injection.

J2426

J2426   Injection, paliperidone palmitate extended release, 1 mg

Lay Description

Paliperidone palmitate is a psychotropic agent used to treat schizophrenia in adults. The recommended dose is 234 mg on the first day of treatment and 156 mg one week later administered as an IM injection into the deltoid muscle. The recommended maintenance dose is 117 mg monthly administered as in IM injection in the deltoid or gluteal muscle. The maintenance dose may vary based on individual response to the treatment.

J2430

J2430   Injection, pamidronate disodium, per 30 mg

Lay Description

Pamidronate disodium is used to treat hypercalcemia from cancer, Paget's disease, osteolytic bone metastases of breast cancer, and osteolytic bone lesions of multiple myeloma. Pamidronate disodium acts as an antihypercalcemic, inhibiting the resorption of bone and blocking the formation of mature osteoclasts. Cardiovascular side effects of atrial fibrillation and tachycardia may occur, with hypertension a common side-effect as well as fatigue, abdominal pain, nausea, constipation, anorexia, and anemia.

J2440

J2440   Injection, papaverine HCl, up to 60 mg

Lay Description

Papaverine hydrochloride is an alkaloid extracted from opium or synthetically produced. The drug relaxes smooth muscles, especially when is has been contracted in spasm. The drug directly relaxes the cardiac and vascular systems, bronchial muscles, and gastrointestinal, biliary, and urinary tracts. Its effect on the vascular system includes coronary, cerebral, peripheral, and pulmonary arteries. It has minimal effect on the central nervous system, though large doses can cause some sedation. Papaverine hydrochloride is indicated in erectile dysfunction and various conditions where spasms occur, such as vascular spasm associated with acute myocardial infarction, angina pectoris, peripheral embolism, pulmonary embolism, and visceral spasms such as gastrointestinal colic and ureteral or biliary spasms. It may also be useful in peripheral vascular disease with vasospastic elements and certain cerebral angiospasms.

J2460

J2460   Injection, oxytetracycline HCl, up to 50 mg

Lay Description
Oxytetracycline hydrochloride is a broad-spectrum antibiotic of the tetracycline group produced by the bacterium Streptomyces rimosus. Its mechanism of action is not known, but it is thought to inhibit protein synthesis. Oxytetracycline is effective against a wide range of both gram-positive and gram-negative organisms. Susceptibility studies should be performed prior to the administration of this drug. Cross resistance among drugs in the tetracycline family is common. Susceptible organisms include rickettsiae, *Mycoplasma pneumoniae, Borrelia recurrentis, Escherichia coli, Enterobacter aerogenes, Pseudomonas aeruginosa, Haemophilus aegyptius, Shigella* species, *Mima* species, *Herellea* species, *Haemophilus influenzae, Klebsiella* species, *Diplococcus pneumoniae, Staphylococcus aureus, Neisseria gonorrhoeae, Treponema pallidum, Treponema pertenue, Listeria monocytogenes, Clostridium* species, *Bacillus anthracis, Fusobacterium fusiforme*, and *Actinomyces* species. It may also be used in combination with amebicides to treat acute intestinal amebiasis.

J2469

J2469   Injection, palonosetron HCl, 25 mcg

Lay Description
Palonosetron hydrochloride is a chemical compound that is a selective blocker of serotonin 5-HT3 receptors. Serotonin 5-HT3 receptors are present on the vagal nerve and at sensory nerve endings. Cytotoxic chemotherapy appears to trigger the release of serotonin in the small intestine, which may trigger the 5-HT3 receptors and initiate the vomiting reflex. It is indicated to prevent and treat nausea and vomiting associated with chemotherapy. Palonosetron hydrochloride is administered by intravenous injection. The recommended dosage of the injectable form is 25 mcg.

J2501

J2501   Injection, paricalcitol, 1 mcg

Lay Description
Paricalcitol is a synthetic analogue of calcitriol, vitamin D. Vitamins are organic compounds necessary to the metabolic functioning of the body. Vitamin D is a fat-soluble vitamin that is a group of related compounds commonly called calciferol. Two common forms are cholecalciferol and ergocalciferol. Vitamin D is a steroid hormone precursor and helps to maintain calcium and phosphorus levels throughout the body. Human skin can produce vitamin D when exposed to sunlight, specifically UVB. Secondary hyperparathyroidism is characterized by an increase in parathyroid hormone to compensate for inadequate levels of active vitamin D hormone. Paricalcitol is indicated for the prevention and treatment of hyperparathyroidism secondary to chronic renal failure. The injectable form is administered by intravenous injection and is primarily used when the patient has stage 5 chronic renal disease.

J2503

J2503   Injection, pegaptanib sodium, 0.3 mg

Lay Description
Pegaptanib sodium is a pegylated oligonucleotide for intravitreous injection. Pegylating is the addition of a polyethylene glycol (PEG) molecule, which allows a slow release of the carried substance. Pegaptanib sodium is a selective vascular endothelial growth factor antagonist that inhibits the growth of additional blood vessels. Pegaptanib sodium is indicated for the treatment of neovascular or wet age-related macular degeneration. The recommended dose is 0.3 mg administered by intravitreous injection to the affected eye once every six weeks.

J2504

J2504   Injection, pegademase bovine, 25 IU

Lay Description
Pegademase bovine is an orphan drug that provides an exogenous source for the enzyme adenosine deaminase. It is derived from bovine intestines. A deficiency of adenosine deaminase allows adenosine and some of its derivatives to accumulate in cells. This accumulation is toxic to lymphocytes, which are a main component of the immune system. Pegademase is indicated as a replacement enzyme in patients with severe combined immunodeficiency disease in whom the disease is due to the lack of adenosine deaminase. Pegademase is administered by intramuscular injection. Dosage needs to be individualized to the patient and varies from 10 to 30 IU/kg of body weight.

J2505

J2505   Injection, pegfilgrastim, 6 mg

Lay Description

Pegfilgrastim is a pegylated form of filgrastim. Pegylated means that polyethylene glycol, a dispensing agent, has been added to the drug. Filgrastim is a synthetic human granulocyte colony-stimulating factor (G-CSF). Pegfilgrastim is produced by recombinant DNA technology using E. coli bacteria. The drug binds to surface receptors on hematopoietic and stimulates neutrophil production, differentiation, maturation, and function. Pegfilgrastim is longer acting than filgrastim. It is indicated as a treatment for neutropenia in patients receiving myelosuppressive therapy for nonmyeloid malignancies. The drug is administered by subcutaneous injection. Recommended dosage is 6 mg once each chemotherapy cycle.

J2507

J2507   Injection, pegloticase, 1 mg

Lay Description

Pegloticase is an exogenous source of the human enzyme uricase, which is recreated by recombinant DNA technology in *E. coli* bacteria. The enzyme is pegylated, attached to a polyethylene glycol molecule. Pegylation increases the molecular weight and stability of the enzyme and masks it from the patient's immune system. This uric acid specific enzyme is indicated as a treatment for chronic gout in patients who have not responded to other treatment. The medication stimulates the oxidation of uric acid to allantoin, which lowers the uric acid levels. The recommended dose of pegloticase is 8 mg every two weeks administered by IV infusion.

J2510

J2510   Injection, penicillin G procaine, aqueous, up to 600,000 units

Lay Description

Penicillin G procaine is a version of penicillin that contains procaine, a local anesthetic agent. Penicillins block the actions of transpeptidase, an enzyme needed to create the cell wall. This weakens the bacterial cell wall causing cellular death. The procaine provides a local anesthetic action and contributes to a slower release of the penicillin G from the injection site. Penicillin G procaine is not as long acting as penicillin G benzathine. Once in the body, penicillin G procaine is hydrolyzed to penicillin G. The hydrolysis and slow absorption provide sustained, but lower blood levels of penicillin. Susceptibility studies should be performed prior to the administration of penicillin G procaine. This formulation is administered by deep intramuscular injection. Dosage depends upon the bacterial infection being treated.

J2513

J2513   Injection, pentastarch, 10% solution, 100 ml

Lay Description

Pentastarch is a derivative of starch composed of 90 percent amylopectin. It is used in plasma volume expander. Intravenous infusion of pentastarch results in expansion of the plasma volume in excess of the volume infused. This expansion persists for approximately 18 to 24 hours and is expected to improve the hemodynamic status for 12 to 18 hours. It is indicated for plasma volume expansion when needed to manage shock due to hemorrhage, surgery, sepsis, burns, or other trauma. It is not a substitute for red blood cells or coagulation factors in plasma. Pentastarch is administered by intravenous infusion only. Total dosage and rate of infusion depend upon the amount of blood or plasma lost.

J2515

J2515   Injection, pentobarbital sodium, per 50 mg

Lay Description

Pentobarbital sodium is a short- to intermediate-acting barbiturate. Barbiturates are derivatives of barbituric acid that act as central nervous system depressants producing a wide variety of effects, from mild sedation to anesthesia. They enhance the neurotransmitter gamma aminobutyric acid (GABA), which inhibits the excitation of nerves. Pentobarbital sodium is indicated as a sedative, presurgical adjunct to anesthesia, as a short-term treatment for insomnia, and as an anticonvulsant.

J2540

J2540   Injection, penicillin G potassium, up to 600,000 units

Lay Description

Penicillin G potassium is a version of penicillin that contains potassium. Penicillins block the actions of transpeptidase, an enzyme needed to create the cell wall. This weakens the bacterial cell wall causing cellular death. Susceptibility studies should be performed prior to the administration of penicillin G potassium. The drug is available in oral and injectable forms. The injectable form can be administered by intramuscular, subcutaneous, intracavity, and intrathecal injection or continuous intravenous infusion. Dosage depends upon the bacterial infection being treated, as well as the form of the penicillin.

J2543

J2543   Injection, piperacillin sodium/tazobactam sodium, 1 g/0.125 g (1.125 g)

Lay Description

Piperacillin is a semisynthetic broad-spectrum penicillin. Penicillins block the actions of transpeptidase, an enzyme needed to create the cell wall. This weakens the bacterial cell wall causing cellular death. Many bacteria have developed a resistance to penicillin. Resistant bacteria produce an enzyme, penicillinase or beta-lactamase that protects it from the effects of penicillin. Tazobactam inhibits the penicillinase so the piperacillin is effective against a greater number of bacteria. Susceptibility studies should be performed prior to the administration of piperacillin. Susceptible bacteria include *E. coli*, *Pseudomonas aeruginosa, enterococci, Clostridium* spp., *Bacteroides* spp., *Klebsiella* spp., *Proteus* spp., *Neisseria gonorrhoeae, Enterobacter* spp., *Serratia* spp., *Streptococcus pneumoniae, Haemophilus influenzae, Acinetobacter* spp., *Morganella morganii*, and *Providencia rettgeri*. Piperacillin/tazobactam is administered by intramuscular injection or intravenous injection and infusion. Dosage varies from 2 to 6 g depending on the organism and extent of the infection.

J2545

J2545   Pentamidine isethionate, inhalation solution, FDA-approved final product, noncompounded, administered through DME, unit dose form, per 300 mg

Lay Description
Pentamidine isethionate is an aromatic diamidine that is an antimicrobial. Its mechanism of action is not completely known. It is thought the drug interferes with the synthesis of DNA, RNA, and protein causing cell death. Pentamidine isethionate is indicated as a treatment for *Pneumocystis Jiroveci* (previously classified as *P. carinii*), trypanosomiasis, and leishmaniasis. The drug may be administered by intramuscular injection, inhalation, or intravenous infusion over one hour. Dosage is usually 300 mg.

J2550

J2550   Injection, promethazine HCl, up to 50 mg

Lay Description
Promethazine hydrochloride is a phenothiazine derivative with antihistamine, sedative, antiemetic, and anticholinergic properties. The drug binds to histamine receptors preventing the histamine from dilating capillaries, constricting the bronchial smooth muscles, and increasing gastric secretions. Promethazine hydrochloride is indicated as an antiemetic, a sedative in anesthesia, as a treatment for motion sickness, and for allergic reactions, including rhinitis and pruritic skin reactions. The drug may be combined with other drugs in cough and cold preparations. Promethazine hydrochloride is available in injectable, oral, and rectal suppository forms. The injectable form is administered by intramuscular or intravenous injection although the preferred method is by IM injection. Dosage varies from 25 to 50 mg.

J2560

J2560   Injection, phenobarbital sodium, up to 120 mg

Lay Description
Phenobarbital sodium is a long-acting barbiturate. Barbiturates are derivatives of barbituric acid that act as central nervous system depressants that produce a wide variety of effects, from mild sedation to anesthesia. They enhance the neurotransmitter gamma aminobutyric acid (GABA), which inhibits the excitation of nerves. Phenobarbital sodium is indicated as a sedative, presurgical adjunct to anesthesia, as a short-term treatment for insomnia, and as an anticonvulsant. It is a schedule IV narcotic.

J2562

J2562   Injection, plerixafor, 1 mg

Lay Description
Plerixafor is a hematopoietic stem cell mobilizer that helps move hematopoietic stem cells to the peripheral blood for collection prior to autologous transplant in patients with non-Hodgkin's lymphoma and multiple myeloma (MM). It inhibits the CXCR4 chemokine receptor and blocks binding the stromal cell-derived factors. Those factors direct the hematopoietic stem cells to the bone marrow. Once the stem cells are circulating in the peripheral blood, they can be extracted and prepared for transplant. The recommended dose is 0.24 mg/kg body weight about 11 hours before starting the apheresis for up to four consecutive days. Plerixafor is given by subcutaneous injection.

J2590

J2590   Injection, oxytocin, up to 10 units

Lay Description
Oxytocin is an animal-derived or synthetic form of the hormone secreted by the hypothalamus and stored in the pituitary gland. Oxytocin promotes uterine contractions and stimulates milk secretion. It is indicated to induce labor, to promote uterine contractions after delivery of the placenta or abortion, and to control postpartum hemorrhage. Dosage depends upon uterine response.

J2597

J2597   Injection, desmopressin acetate, per 1 mcg

Lay Description
Desmopressin acetate, also known as DDAVP, is a potent synthetic analogue of the natural hormone vasopressin. Vasopressin is a hormone produced by the posterior pituitary gland. Vasopressin has an antidiuretic effect causing the renal tubules to reabsorb water. Desmopressin acetate is indicated for the treatment of diabetes insipidus, primary nocturnal enuresis, treatment of temporary polyuria and polydipsia secondary to trauma to or surgery in the pituitary region, and to increase coagulation factor VIII

activity before surgical procedures in patients with hemophilia A and von Willebrand's disease.

J2650

J2650   Injection, prednisolone acetate, up to 1 ml

Lay Description
Prednisolone is a synthetic adrenal corticosteroid. Corticosteroids are natural substances produced by the adrenal glands located adjacent to the kidneys. Corticosteroids are widely used to treat allergies, inflammation, and many disease processes. Prednisolone is used to treat a wide variety of conditions. Oral and injectable prednisolone is used to suppress inflammation in many inflammatory and allergic conditions. Examples include rheumatoid arthritis, systemic lupus, acute gouty arthritis, psoriatic arthritis, ulcerative colitis, and Crohn's disease. Severe allergic conditions that fail conventional treatment may also be treated with prednisolone. Examples include bronchial asthma, allergic rhinitis, drug-induced dermatitis, and contact and atopic dermatitis. Prednisolone is also used in the treatment of leukemia and lymphomas, idiopathic thrombocytopenia purpura, and autoimmune hemolytic anemia. Other miscellaneous conditions treated with this medication include thyroiditis and sarcoidosis. Prednisolone is used as a hormone replacement in patients whose adrenal glands are unable to produce sufficient amounts of corticosteroids. Prednisolone injection or sterile suspension can be injected into a muscle, joint, lesion, or soft tissue. When used as an intra-articular injection, prednisolone is indicated as a treatment for joint pain and inflammation, epicondylitis, bursitis, and synovitis.

J2670

J2670   Injection, tolazoline HCl, up to 25 mg

Lay Description
Tolazoline hydrochloride is a chemical compound that is an adrenergic blocking agent and peripheral vasodilator. Per the FDA, this drug is no longer available in the United States for human use. It is still available for veterinary use.

J2675

J2675   Injection, progesterone, per 50 mg

Lay Description
Progesterone is an animal-derived or synthetic form of the natural human hormone produced by the adrenal cortex, ovaries, and placenta. The hormone prepares the uterus for the reception and development of the fertilized ovum and maintains an optimal intrauterine environment for pregnancy. Exogenous progesterone is used as a treatment for dysfunctional uterine bleeding, secondary amenorrhea, infertility, and as part of postmenopausal hormone replacement therapy.

J2680

J2680   Injection, fluphenazine decanoate, up to 25 mg

Lay Description
Fluphenazine decanoate is a phenothiazine derivative that blocks dopamine receptors in hypothalamus and pituitary glands. Fluphenazine decanoate has a slower release from the injection site than the fluphenazine hydrochloride, which results in a prolonged duration of action. The precise mechanism of action is not known, but it is believed to depress the reticular activating system. Fluphenazine decanoate is indicated in the management of manifestations of schizophrenia. Adult dosage varies from 1 to 10 mg daily depending on the severity and duration of symptoms. Fluphenazine decanoate is administered by intramuscular or subcutaneous injection.

J2690

J2690   Injection, procainamide HCl, up to 1 g

Lay Description
Procainamide hydrochloride is a benzoic acid derivative that depresses heart function. The drug increases the refractory period of the cardiac atria and ventricles. Procainamide hydrochloride is indicated as a treatment for documented life-threatening ventricular arrhythmias, such as sustained ventricular tachycardia. The drug is available in injectable and oral forms. The injectable form is administered by intramuscular or intravenous injection or intravenous infusion. Dosage varies from 100 to 1,000 mg depending upon response.

J2700

J2700   Injection, oxacillin sodium, up to 250 mg

Lay Description
Oxacillin sodium is a semi-synthetic penicillin that is penicillinase resistant. Penicillins block the actions of transpeptidase, an enzyme needed to create the cell wall. This weakens the bacterial cell wall causing cellular death. Many bacteria have developed a resistance to penicillin. Resistant bacteria produce an enzyme, penicillinase or beta-lactamase, that protects it from the effects of penicillin. Susceptibility studies should be performed prior to the administration of oxacillin sodium. Oxacillin sodium is indicated in the treatment of infections caused by penicillinase-producing staphylococci.

J2704

J2704   Injection, propofol, 10 mg

Lay Description
Propofol is a short-acting intravenous anesthetic agent suitable for induction and maintenance of general anesthesia and monitored anesthesia care sedation in adults, induction anesthesia in children at least 3 years of age, and maintenance anesthesia in children at least 2 months of age. It may also be used for sedation of ventilated patients receiving intensive

care for up to three days. Induction of anesthesia with propofol is rapid and maintenance can be achieved with continuous infusion or intermittent bolus injections.

J2710

J2710   Injection, neostigmine methylsulfate, up to 0.5 mg

Lay Description
Neostigmine methylsulfate is a chemical that blocks the passage of nerve signals in the parasympathetic system. It competes with acetylcholine by attaching itself to the same receptors on a cell. Neostigmine methylsulfate is indicated for treatment of myasthenia gravis, prevention and postoperative treatment of distention and urinary retention, and reversal of the effects of nondepolarizing neuromuscular blocking agents, such as tubocuranne, metocurine, gallamine, or pancuronium following surgery. The recommended dose is dependent on the condition being treated. For myasthenia gravis, the recommended dose is 1:2000 solution (0.5 mg) administered by subcutaneous or intramuscular injection. For prevention and postoperative treatment of distention and urinary retention, the recommended dose is 1:4000 solution (0.25 mg) administered by subcutaneous or intramuscular injection. For reversal of the effects of nondepolarizing neuromuscular blocking agents, the recommended dose is 1:2000 solution (0.5 mg) administered by subcutaneous or intramuscular injection.

J2720

J2720   Injection, protamine sulfate, per 10 mg

Lay Description
Protamine sulfate is a simple protein with a low molecular weight. It occurs naturally in the sperm of salmon and certain other species of fish. When given alone, it has a weak anticoagulant effect. However, when given in the presence of heparin, a stable salt is formed and both drugs lose their anticoagulant effect. Protamine sulfate is indicated for the treatment of heparin overdose. Protamine sulfate is administered intravenously and has a rapid onset of action. Neutralization of heparin occurs within five minutes following intravenous administration. Each mg of protamine will neutralize approximately 90 USP units of heparin activity derived from beef lung tissue or about 115 USP units of heparin activity derived from porcine intestinal mucosa. Protamine sulfate is given by very slow intravenous injection in doses 50 mg or less over a 10-minute period.

J2724

J2724   Injection, protein C concentrate, intravenous, human, 10 IU

Lay Description
Protein C concentrate is used to replace congenitally deficient protein C. Protein C is a vitamin K-dependent plasma protein. When activated by thrombin, protein C inhibits the clotting mechanism by enzymatically breaking up the activated forms of clotting factors V and VIII. It also enhances fibrinolysis. Protein C concentrate is derived from pooled human plasma and uses a column of mouse monoclonal antibodies. It is indicated for the treatment of severe congenital protein C deficiency for the prevention and treatment of venous thrombosis and purpura fulminans. Protein C concentrate may be used for an acute episode, short-term prophylaxis, and long-term prophylaxis. The dosage, frequency, and duration of treatment depends on the severity of the patient's deficiency and the patient's age, clinical condition, and the plasma levels of protein C. Protein C concentrate is administered by intravenous infusion.

J2725

J2725   Injection, protirelin, per 250 mcg

Lay Description
Protirelin is a synthetic peptide similar to the endogenous thyrotropin releasing hormone produced by the hypothalamus. Thyrotropin releasing hormone stimulates the anterior pituitary gland to release thyroid stimulating hormone (TSH). Protirelin is indicated for diagnosis of mild hyperthyroidism, Graves' disease, and for differentiating between primary, secondary, and tertiary hypothyroidism. The drug is administered via an intravenous bolus with a recommended dosage of 500 mcg. TSH serum levels are then measured at different intervals.

J2730

J2730   Injection, pralidoxime chloride, up to 1 g

Lay Description
Pralidoxime chloride, also known as p2-PAM chloride, is a chemical that reactivates the parasympathetic nervous system. Pralidoxime chloride is indicated as an antidote in the treatment of poisoning due to pesticides and chemicals of the organophosphate class that block nerve signal transmission in the parasympathetic nervous system. Pralidoxime chloride is also indicated in the control of overdosage by some drugs used in the treatment of myasthenia gravis. The principal indications for the use of pralidoxime chloride are muscle weakness and respiratory depression. The principal action of pralidoxime chloride is to reactivate cholinesterase that has been inactivated by an organophosphate pesticide or related compound. This facilitates destruction of accumulated acetylcholine, which allows nerve signals to function normally. The most critical effect of pralidoxime chloride is in relieving paralysis of the respiratory muscles. Because pralidoxime chloride is less effective in relieving depression of the respiratory center, atropine is always administered concomitantly to block the effect of accumulated acetylcholine of the respiratory center. Pralidoxime chloride is administered by intravenous, intramuscular, or subcutaneous injection or infusion.

J2760

J2760   Injection, phentolamine mesylate, up to 5 mg

Lay Description
Phentolamine mesylate is a chemical compound that produces a short-term block of the adrenal hormones epinephrine and norepinephrine. It is indicated for the diagnosis of pheochromocytoma, the prophylaxis and treatment of hypertensive episodes in patients with pheochromocytoma, and the prophylaxis and treatment of dermal necrosis following intravenous administration or extravasation of norepinephrine. Pheochromocytoma is a neoplasm, usually benign, of the adrenal medulla or sympathetic paraganglia that results in increased secretion of epinephrine and norepinephrine. The drug is administered by intramuscular or intravenous injection. Dosage ranges from 5 to 10 mg.

J2765

J2765   Injection, metoclopramide HCl, up to 10 mg

Lay Description
Metoclopramide hydrochloride is a chemical compound that acts as a dopamine receptor antagonist. Dopamine produces nausea and vomiting by stimulating the chemoreceptor trigger zones. Metoclopramide hydrochloride blocks the stimulation of these zones. It stimulates upper gastrointestinal tract motility without stimulating the gastric, biliary, or pancreatic secretions. Metoclopramide hydrochloride is indicated for use as an antiemetic and in the treatment of gastroesophageal reflux and gastroparesis.

J2770

J2770   Injection, quinupristin/dalfopristin, 500 mg (150/350)

Lay Description
Quinupristin-dalfopristin is an antibiotic in the class known as streptogramins. The streptogramins are macromolecular antibiotics produced by Streptomyces pristinaepiralis.
Quinupristin-dalfopristin is indicated for treatment of susceptible bacterial infections caused by antibiotic-resistant, gram-positive organisms, including severe infections caused by vancomycin-resistant E. faecium, nosocomial pneumonia, infections due to the use of intravascular catheters, and complicated skin and skin structure infections caused by methicillin-susceptible Staphylococcus aureus and Streptococcus pyogenes (group A streptococcus). The mechanism of action of quinupristin-dalfopristin is primarily inhibition of protein synthesis. Dalfopristin acts to block an early step in protein synthesis forming a bond with a ribosome and preventing elongation of the peptide chain. Quinupristin acts to block a later step preventing the extension of peptide chains and causing incomplete chains to be released. Quinupristin-dalfopristin is administered by intravenous injection or infusion.

J2778

J2778   Injection, ranibizumab, 0.1 mg

Lay Description
Ranibizumab is a monoclonal antibody produced by recombinant DNA technology using a strain of E. coli bacteria. The drug binds to receptor sites of human vascular endothelial growth factor A (VEGF-A) and inhibits its activity. VEGF-A has been shown to cause new vascularization and leakage of blood vessels in the eye and contributes to the progression of age-related macular degeneration. Ranibizumab is indicated as a treatment for neovascular or wet, age-related macular degeneration. The drug is administered by intravitreal injection only. Recommended dosage is 0.5 mg once a month.

J2780

J2780   Injection, ranitidine HCl, 25 mg

Lay Description
Ranitidine hydrochloride is a chemical compound that binds to histamine receptors preventing the histamine from increasing gastric acid secretions. Ranitidine hydrochloride, singularly or in combination, is indicated as a treatment and as maintenance therapy for gastric ulcers, duodenal ulcers, gastroesophageal reflux disease, pathological gastric hypersecretory conditions, and erosive esophagitis. Oral forms of ranitidine hydrochloride are available in smaller dosages over-the-counter. Larger dosages are prescription only and available in oral and injectable forms. The injectable form is administered by intramuscular or intravenous injection.

J2783

J2783   Injection, rasburicase, 0.5 mg

Lay Description
Rasburicase is a synthetic enzyme produced by recombinant DNA technology in Saccharomyces cerevisiae yeast. It catalyzes the oxidation of uric acid into an inactive and soluble metabolite. Rasburicase is indicated for the initial management of plasma uric acid levels in pediatric patients with leukemia, lymphoma, and solid tumor malignancies who are receiving antineoplastic therapy expected to result in tumor lysis and subsequent elevation of plasma uric acid. The drug is administered by intravenous infusion over 30 minutes. Recommended dosage is 0.15 or 0.20 mg/kg of body weight daily for five days.

J2785

J2785   Injection, regadenoson, 0.1 mg

Lay Description
Regadenoson is a vasodilator medication used as a cardiac stressing agent prior to myocardial perfusion imaging. This is an alternate to exercise stress when

the patient is not a candidate for exercise stress. It is administered as a rapid IV push. The recommended dose is 0.4 mg of regadenoson.

J2788-J2792

J2788 Injection, Rho D immune globulin, human, minidose, 50 mcg (250 i.u.)

J2790 Injection, Rho D immune globulin, human, full dose, 300 mcg (1500 i.u.)

J2791 Injection, Rho(D) immune globulin (human), (Rhophylac), intramuscular or intravenous, 100 IU

J2792 Injection, Rho D immune globulin, intravenous, human, solvent detergent, 100 IU

Lay Description
Rh factors are a group of antigens present on the membrane of erythrocytes. When a person who is Rh-negative receives an Rh-positive transfusion or becomes pregnant with an Rh-positive fetus, the person develops antibodies against Rh-positive blood. These antibodies will in future exposures attack and kill any Rh-positive erythrocytes. Rho (D) immune globulin suppresses the immune response of the Rh-negative person preventing antibody formation against the Rh-positive blood. Recommendations for administration during a pregnancy include a full dose of 300 mcg antepartum at 28 weeks and another full dose within 72 hours of delivery when there is known incompatibility between the mother and fetus. In cases of abortion, spontaneous or induced, of a fetus of less than 12 weeks, a mini-dose of 50 mcg is recommended. The mini-dose should be administered within three hours of the event. Dosages administered when an Rh incompatible blood transfusion occurs depend upon the volume of incompatible blood transfused and should be administered within 72 hours of the transfusion. Rho (D) immune globulin may be treated in several different ways to ensure that the pooled donor plasma has no pathogens. The immune globulin may be ultrafiltered, solvent washed, or detergent washed. It can be administered by intramuscular or intravenous injection.

J2793

J2793 Injection, rilonacept, 1 mg

Lay Description
Rilonacept is an interleukin 1 blocker used in the treatment and prevention of genetic conditions; cryopyrin associated periodic syndromes (CAPS), including Muckle Wells Syndrome (MWS); and familial cold auto inflammatory syndrome (FCAS) in adults and children age 12 or older. Although, used to treat and prevent these conditions, Rilonacept cannot cure these inherited conditions. Rilonacept is expressed in recombinant Chinese hamster ovary cells and comes in a sterile single use glass vial containing lyophilized powder for reconstitution. Recommended dose for adults is a loading dose of 320 mg administered by two separate subcutaneous injections. A maintenance dose of 160 mg is administered once a week by subcutaneous injection. Patients 12 to 17 years of age should receive a loading dose of 4.4 mg/kg with a maximum of 320 mg administered as one or two subcutaneous injections. Following that, the patient should receive 2.2 mg/kg with a maximum of 160 mg, once a week.

J2794

J2794 Injection, risperidone, long acting, 0.5 mg

Lay Description
Risperidone is an antipsychotic drug of the class of benzisoxazole derivatives. The drug's mechanism of action is unknown. It is thought that the drug acts by mediating dopamine and serotonin levels. Long-acting risperidone is encased within microspheres so that the drug is slowly released over a two-week period. Risperidone is indicated for the treatment of schizophrenia. Long-acting risperidone is injected via deep muscular gluteal injection every two weeks with a recommended initial dosage of 25 mg. This drug should not be administered intravenously. If patients do not respond to the 25 mg injections, 37.5 mg or 50 mg injections may be administered every two weeks. Different strengths should not be combined within a single administration.

J2795

J2795 Injection, ropivacaine HCl, 1 mg

Lay Description
Ropivacaine hydrochloride is a chemical compound that is an amino amide local anesthetic agent. It locally blocks the generation and conduction of nerve transmissions. Ropivacaine hydrochloride is used as a peripheral nerve block, for percutaneous infiltration anesthesia, and as an epidural block. It may also be administered by continuous epidural infusion for acute postoperative pain management. Dosage varies by indication and extent of the anesthesia required.

J2796

J2796 Injection, romiplostim, 10 mcg

Lay Description
Romiplostim increases platelet production and is used to treat patients with idiopathic thrombocytopenic purpura (ITP) for whom other treatments have not been successful. It should be used for patients who have bleeding problems and not only for normalizing a patient's platelet count. Romiplostim is derived using DNA segments in Escherichia coli (E. coli). Recommended dose is 1 mcg/kg based on the patient's weight. The dose is adjusted depending on the patient's platelet count. Romiplostim is administered by subcutaneous injection.

J2800

J2800　Injection, methocarbamol, up to 10 ml

Lay Description
Methocarbamol is a skeletal muscle relaxant,
indicated for the treatment of muscle spasms and
muscle pain and stiffness. Methocarbamol acts on the
central nervous system to produce its muscle relaxant
effects.

J2805

J2805　Injection, sincalide, 5 mcg

Lay Description
Sincalide is a gastrointestinal hormone peptide
injected intravenously. It is used to stimulate
gallbladder contractions for assessment via a
cholecystogram or ultrasound; to stimulate pancreatic
secretin prior to the obtaining of a duodenal aspirate;
or to accelerate the transit of barium through the
small bowel for fluoroscopic or x-ray examination of
the intestinal tract.

J2810

J2810　Injection, theophylline, per 40 mg

Lay Description
Theophylline is a methylxanthine drug with structural
and pharmacological similarity to caffeine. It is
naturally found in black and green tea. Theophylline's
exact mechanism of action is unknown. It is
suggested that it is a nonspecific inhibitor of
phosphodiesterase enzymes, which are enzymes that
control the tissue concentration of various hormones
and other enzymes. Inhibiting the phosphodiesterase
enzymes would allow for increases in intracellular
cyclic AMP. Cyclic AMP is a nucleotide involved in the
activities of many hormones and cellular functions.
Theophylline relaxes the smooth bronchial muscles
and allows for easier breathing. It also increases the
force of contraction of the diaphragmatic muscles. It is
indicated for the prophylaxis and treatment of chronic
asthma and COPD. Theophylline is also indicated as an
emergency treatment in an acute severe asthma
episode. Theophylline carries a high incidence of
side-effects when used at its upper therapeutic range.
The drug is also affected by many other drugs,
including antibiotics, cimetidine, and phenytoin
among others.

J2820

**J2820　Injection, sargramostim (GM-CSF), 50
mcg**

Lay Description
Sargramostim is a synthetic granulocyte-macrophage
colony-stimulating factor (GM-CSF) produced by
recombinant DNA technology in S. cerevisiae yeast.
GM-CSF binds to receptor sites on stem cells and
supports the survival, expansion, and differentiation
of hematopoietic progenitor cells into granulocytes
and macrophages. Sargramostim is indicated to
stimulate hematopoiesis and decrease neutropenia as
an adjunct to myelosuppressive cancer chemotherapy
in patients with acute myelogenous leukemia and
non-Hodgkin's lymphoma, to promote myeloid
engraftment in bone marrow transplantation or
hematopoietic stem cell transplantation, and to
enhance peripheral progenitor cell yield in
autologous hematopoietic stem cell transplantation.
The drug is administered by intravenous infusion.
Dosage varies from 250 mcg per m^2 of body surface
per day.

J2850

**J2850　Injection, secretin, synthetic, human, 1
mcg**

Lay Description
Secretin is a synthetic version of the natural hormone
secretin secreted by the mucosa of the duodenum
and upper jejunum. Secretin stimulates the release of
pancreatic juice by the pancreas and bile by the liver.
Both bile and the pancreatic juices contain
bicarbonate and change the pH of the duodenum
from acid to alkaline which facilitates the action of
intestinal digestive enzymes. Secretin is used in
diagnostic tests for gastrinoma and pancreatic
exocrine function, and to facilitate the identification
of the ampulla of Vater and accessory papilla during
endoscopic retrograde cholangiopancreatography
(ERCP). Dosage is 0.2-0.4 mcg per kg of body weight
depending on the indication. The drug is
administered by intravenous injection.

J2910

J2910　Injection, aurothioglucose, up to 50 mg

Lay Description
Aurothioglucose is a gold salt used in treating
inflammatory arthritis. The mechanism of action in
gold salts is not well understood. However, in patients
with inflammatory arthritis, such as adult and juvenile
rheumatoid arthritis, gold salts decrease the
inflammation of the joint lining, preventing
destruction of bone and cartilage. Gold salts, such as
aurothioglucose, are second-line drugs prescribed
when anti-inflammatory drugs, such as nonsteroidal
anti-inflammatory drugs (NSAID) and corticosteroids,
are ineffective in preventing the progression of
inflammatory arthritis. Aurothioglucose is available as
a 50 mg/ml injectable suspension to be administered
by intramuscular injection.

J2916

**J2916　Injection, sodium ferric gluconate
complex in sucrose injection, 12.5 mg**

Lay Description
Sodium ferric gluconate is an iron oxide hydrate
directly bound to sucrose and chelated with
gluconate. The drug replenishes iron, which is critical
for normal hemoglobulin synthesis to maintain
oxygen transport. Iron is also required for the
metabolism and synthesis of DNA and various

enzymes. Sodium ferric gluconate is indicated for the treatment of iron deficiency in ESRD patients undergoing hemodialysis who are also receiving erythropoietin therapy. It is administered by intravenous infusion over one hour. The recommended dosage is 125 mg.

J2920-J2930

J2920   Injection, methylprednisolone sodium succinate, up to 40 mg

J2930   Injection, methylprednisolone sodium succinate, up to 125 mg

Lay Description
Methylprednisolone is a corticosteroid used to treat a variety of conditions. Indications include allergic disorders, arthritis, blood diseases, breathing problems, certain cancers, eye diseases, intestinal disorders, and collagen and skin diseases. Methylprednisolone may also be used with other medications as a replacement for certain hormones. Methylprednisolone works by decreasing the body's immune response to these diseases and reducing symptoms such as swelling and redness. Methylprednisolone may be administered orally, by intramuscular injection in the form of methylprednisolone acetate, or by intravenous infusion in the form of methylprednisolone sodium succinate.

J2940

J2940   Injection, somatrem, 1 mg

Lay Description
Somatrem is a version of human growth hormone (HGH) produced by recombinant DNA technology from a strain of E. coli bacteria. It contains the identical sequence of the 191 amino acids that compromise endogenous HGH. HGH has a direct effect on the metabolism of protein, carbohydrates, and fat and controls skeletal and visceral growth. Somatrem is indicated for the treatment of idiopathic HGH deficiency in children with growth failure. Treatment with somatrem should be discontinued when the epiphyses are fused. The drug is administered subcutaneously or intramuscularly at a dosage of 0.30 mg per body weight and may be self-administered.

J2941

J2941   Injection, somatropin, 1 mg

Lay Description
Somatropin is another name for human growth hormone (HGH). Most versions are produced by recombinant DNA technology from a strain of E. coli bacteria. It contains the identical sequence of the 191 amino acids that compromise endogenous HGH. HGH has a direct effect on the metabolism of protein, carbohydrates, and fat and controls skeletal and visceral growth. Somatrem is indicated for the treatment of growth failure in children born small for their gestational age, children with growth failure due to HGH deficiency, chronic renal insufficiency, Turner's syndrome, or Prader-Willi syndrome. Another indication is the treatment of adult patients with HGH deficiency, either primary or secondary to pituitary or hypothalamic diseases, radiation therapy, surgery, or trauma. The drug is administered subcutaneously or intramuscularly at a dosage of 0.30 mg per body weight and may be self-administered.

J2950

J2950   Injection, promazine HCl, up to 25 mg

Lay Description
Promazine hydrochloride belongs to a group of medications known as the phenothiazine antipsychotics. Promazine hydrochloride is indicated for the treatment of agitation alone and agitation and restlessness in the elderly. The mechanism of action involves blocking a variety of receptors in the brain, particularly dopamine receptors. Dopamine is a chemical that aids in transmission of signals between brain cells. An excess of dopamine in the brain can cause over-stimulation of dopamine receptors. Because dopamine receptors normally act to modify behavior, over-stimulation can result in psychotic illness. Promazine hydrochloride prevents over-stimulation by blocking these receptors, which then helps to control psychotic illness.

J2993

J2993   Injection, reteplase, 18.1 mg

Lay Description
Reteplase is a longer-acting derivative of alteplase, a synthetic tissue plasminogen activator. Reteplase is produced by recombinant DNA technology in E. coli bacteria. Tissue plasminogen activators are enzymes produced by endothelial cells that catalyze the breakdown of thrombi or blood clots. The drug is indicated as a treatment of acute myocardial infarction. Treatment should begin as soon as possible after the onset of symptoms. The drug is administered by two intravenous bolus injections. Each bolus should be 18.1 mg.

J2995

J2995   Injection, streptokinase, per 250,000 IU

Lay Description
Streptokinase is a protein produced by beta hemolytic streptococci bacteria that binds to plasminogen and breaks down thrombi or blood clots. Streptokinase is indicated as a treatment of acute myocardial infarction, acute pulmonary embolism, deep venous thrombosis, acute arterial thrombi or emboli, and occlusion of an arteriovenous shunt. Treatment of the acute myocardial infarction should begin within four hours of the onset of symptoms. Treatment of acute pulmonary embolism, deep venous thrombosis, and acute arterial thrombi or emboli should begin as soon as possible from onset of the event, preferably within

seven days. The drug is administered by intravenous infusion. Recommended dosage varies from 1,000,000 to 1,500,000 units depending upon the indication.

J2997

J2997   Injection, alteplase recombinant, 1 mg

Lay Description
Alteplase is a synthetic tissue plasminogen activator produced by recombinant DNA technology in Chinese hamster ovaries. Tissue plasminogen activators are enzymes produced by endothelial cells that catalyze the breakdown of thrombi or blood clots. Alteplase is indicated as a treatment of acute myocardial infarction, acute ischemic stroke, acute massive pulmonary embolism, or to restore the function of a thrombosed central venous access device. Treatment of the acute myocardial infarction should begin as soon as possible after the onset of symptoms. Treatment of acute ischemic stroke should begin within three hours of the onset of symptoms and after it has been determined that no intracranial hemorrhage has occurred. Treatment of acute massive pulmonary embolism should begin after objective confirmation of the diagnosis has been obtained. The drug is administered by intravenous injection and infusion. Recommended total dosage is based upon body weight, but should not exceed 100 mg.

J3000

J3000   Injection, streptomycin, up to 1 g

Lay Description
Streptomycin was the first of the aminoglycoside antibiotics. Aminoglycoside antibiotics are derived from various species of Streptomyces bacteria or produced synthetically. Aminoglycosides inhibit bacterial protein synthesis by binding with the 30S ribosomal subunit and are bactericidal. Streptomycin is derived from *Streptomyces griseus*. It inhibits protein synthesis, causing cell death. Streptomycin is now in limited use due to the emergence of resistant bacterial strains. Susceptibility studies should be performed prior to the administration of streptomycin. It is indicated in the treatment of tuberculosis in combination with other drugs. Streptomycin is indicated in the treatment of infections caused by gram-negative bacillary bacteria, *Pasteurella pestis, Francisella tularensis, Brucella, Calymmatobacterium granulomatis, H. ducreyi, H. influenzae, K. pneumoniae, E. coli, Proteus, A. aerogenes, K. pneumoniae, Enterococcus faecalis, Streptococcus viridans,* and *Enterococcus faecalis*. Streptomycin is available only in an injectable form. It is administered by intramuscular injection to the buttocks or thigh. Dosages vary from 15 to 40 mg/kg of body weight depending on the frequency of administration, patient age, and indication.

J3010

J3010   Injection, fentanyl citrate, 0.1 mg

Lay Description
Fentanyl is a schedule II, controlled substance pain medication in the narcotic and opioid analgesic class. Fentanyl is used as an adjunct to anesthesia, to manage chronic pain, and breakthrough persistent pain in cancer patients who have an increased physical tolerance to current opioid therapy. Fentanyl interacts primarily with the opioid mu-receptor. These mu-binding sites are distributed throughout the human brain, spinal cord, and other tissues. In clinical settings, fentanyl exerts its principal pharmacologic effects on the central nervous system. It is administered via intravenous push injection, intramuscular injection, transdermal patch, or transmucosal lozenges.

J3030

J3030   Injection, sumatriptan succinate, 6 mg (code may be used for Medicare when drug administered under the direct supervision of a physician, not for use when drug is self-administered)

Lay Description
Sumatriptan succinate is given to treat migraines and acute treatment of cluster headaches. It is thought to act by stimulating the specific serotonin receptors of the cranial arteries and the dura mater to cause vasoconstriction of the cerebral arteries, without affecting systemic vessels or blood pressure. Recommended injection dose is 6 mg. It can be administered by subcutaneous injection, through tablets, or nasal inhalation. The injection can be self-administered.

J3060

J3060   Injection, taliglucerace alfa, 10 units

Lay Description
Taliglucerase alfa is a recombinant active form of the lysosomal enzyme beta-glucocerebrosidase, which is produced in a culture of genetically modified carrot plant root cells. It is an orphan drug used to treat Type 1 Gaucher's disease caused by a lack of the enzyme glucocerebrosidase, which is crucial to the metabolism of fats. Taliglucerase alfa assists in the breakdown of glucocerebroside to glucose and ceramide. The recommended dose is 60 units per kg of body weight administered once every two weeks as a 60 to 120 minute intravenous infusion. However, dosages can range from 11 units/kg to 73 units/kg every other week depending on disease severity and individual patient response to treatment.

J3070

J3070   Injection, pentazocine, 30 mg

Lay Description
Pentazocine is an opioid analgesic used for moderate to severe pain and during labor. It is thought that

pentazocine HCl binds with opiate receptors in the central nervous system (CNS), which then alters both the emotional response to and perception of pain.

J3095

J3095 Injection, telavancin, 10 mg

Lay Description
Telavancin is a lipoglycopeptide antibacterial that is a synthetic derivative of vancomycin. It is indicated for the treatment of adults with complicated skin and skin structure infections caused by susceptible gram-positive bacteria, including *Staphylococcus aureus, Streptococcus pyogenes, Streptococcus agalactiae,* the *Streptococcus anginosus* group, or vancomycin susceptible *Enterococcus faecalis.* Telavancin is supplied in single use vials that contain 250 mg or 750 mg of a sterile and lyophilized powder. It should be administered as an infusion over 60 minutes.

J3101

J3101 Injection, tenecteplase, 1 mg

Lay Description
Tenecteplase is a thrombolytic enzyme used in treating the effects of a myocardial infarction. It is a tissue plasminogen activator (TPA) produced by recombinant DNA technology using Chinese hamster ovary cells. It binds with fibrin and converts plasminogen to plasmin. Tenecteplase is used to treat acute myocardial infarction and should be administered as soon as possible after the onset of symptoms. This medication is administered intravenously.

J3105

J3105 Injection, terbutaline sulfate, up to 1 mg

Lay Description
Terbutaline sulfate is a bronchodilator that relaxes both bronchial and uterine smooth muscle by stimulating beta2 receptors and is used primarily to treat bronchospasm in patients with reversible obstructive airway disease. It is available as tablets, aerosol inhaler, or subcutaneous injection. Side effects may include nervousness, palpitations, tachycardia, and/or diaphoresis.

J3110

J3110 Injection, teriparatide, 10 mcg

Lay Description
Teriparatide is a recombinant human parathyroid hormone (1-34) that has an identical structure to the naturally occurring hormone. Teriparatide is manufactured from a strain of *Escherichia coli,* and modified by recombinant DNA technology. Teriparatide is indicated for the treatment of postmenopausal women with osteoporosis who are at high risk for fracture. This includes women with a history of osteoporotic fracture, who have multiple risk factors for fracture, or who have failed or are

intolerant of previous osteoporosis therapy. Teriparatide is also indicated to increase bone mass in men with primary or hypogonadal osteoporosis who are at high risk for fracture. This includes men with a history of osteoporotic fracture, who have multiple risk factors for fracture, or who have failed or are intolerant to previous osteoporosis therapy. Recommended dose is 20 mcg of teriparatide each day for up to 28 days. Teriparatide should be administered as a subcutaneous injection into the thigh or abdominal wall and can be self-administered.

J3121

J3121 Injection, testosterone enanthate, 1 mg

Lay Description
Testosterone enanthate is a hormonal drug in the androgens grouping for injection. Testosterone is used in treating male hypogonadism and delayed puberty, as it stimulates the targeted gonadal tissue to develop normally. It is also used in treating some estrogen-dependent breast cancers as it has some counter-estrogenic action in women. Testosterone enanthate is absorbed more slowly so it can be given less often than free testosterone. Doses vary from 50 to 400 mg every two to four weeks. Testosterone enanthate is administered by intramuscular injection.

J3140

Lay Description
Testosterone is an anabolic steroid used primarily to treat male hypogonadism. It stimulates targeted tissues to develop normally in androgen-deficient men. Testosterone may also have some anti-estrogen properties, making it useful in treating certain estrogen-dependent breast cancers. This drug is used to treat male hypogonadism, unusually late sexual maturity, myotonia congenita, inflammation and rotation of the testes, undescended testicle, absence of testicles, Klinefelter syndrome, anemia, and in the prevention of breast pain and engorgement in postpartum women.

J3145

J3145 Injection, testosterone undecanoate, 1 mg

Lay Description
Testosterone undecanoate is a Schedule II controlled substance. It is an androgen used for replacement therapy in adult males for conditions associated with a deficiency or absence of natural testosterone in primary, congenital or acquired, hypogonadism; or congenital or acquired, hypogonadotropic hypogonadism. The hormone is for IM use only into the buttocks. Recommended dosage is 750 mg (3 ml) at initiation, at four weeks, and then every 10 weeks. Testosterone undecanoate is an ester of testosterone and mixed with refined castor oil. These facts lead to a warning about the risks of pulmonary oil microembolism reactions (POME). The drug is

available only under a risk evaluation and mitigation strategy (REMS).

J3150

Lay Description
Testosterone propionate is a hormonal drug in the androgens grouping for injection. Testosterone is used in treating male hypogonadism and delayed puberty, as it stimulates the targeted gonadal tissue to develop normally. Testosterone propionate is absorbed more slowly so it can be given less often than free testosterone. Testosterone propionate is administered via intramuscular injection.

J3230

J3230   Injection, chlorpromazine HCl, up to 50 mg

Lay Description
Chlorpromazine hydrochloride (HCl) is used in the treatment of manic psychosis, preoperative sedation, acute intermittent porphyria, an adjunct treatment for tetanus, intractable hiccups, some behavior problems in children, and nausea and vomiting. The main pharmacological actions are psychotropic. The mechanism of action is not known. It has a sedative and antiemetic effect.

J3240

J3240   Injection, thyrotropin alpha, 0.9 mg, provided in 1.1 mg vial

Lay Description
Thyrotropin alpha is indicated for use as an adjunctive diagnostic tool for serum thyroglobulin (Tg) testing in the follow-up of patients with well-differentiated thyroid cancer. This may be done with or without radioiodine imaging. It contains a highly purified recombinant form of human thyroid stimulating hormone (TSH), a glycoprotein that is produced by recombinant DNA technology in Chinese hamster ovaries. A dose of 0.9 mg can be administered every day for three days. Thyrotropin alpha is administered via intramuscular injection.

J3243

J3243   Injection, tigecycline, 1 mg

Lay Description
Tigecycline is an antibiotic of the class glycylcycline. The drug disrupts RNA protein synthesis in bacteria causing cellular death. Tigecycline has proven effective in drug-resistant strains of many anaerobic and aerobic, gram-negative, and positive microorganisms. It is indicated in the treatment of complicated skin and skin-structure infections, and complicated intra-abdominal infections caused by susceptible strains of bacteria in patients 18 years of age or older. Susceptible bacteria include *Escherichia coli; Staphylococcus aureus*, including methicillin-resistant strains (MRSA); *Streptococcus pyogenes; Streptococcus agalactiae;* the *Streptococcus*

anginosis group; vancomycin-susceptible strains of *Enterococcus faecalis; Bacteroides fragilis; Citrobacter freundii; Enterobacter cloacae; Klebsiella oxytoca; Klebsiella pneumoniae; Bacteroides thetaiotaomicron; Bacteroides uniformis; Bacteroides vulgatus; Clostridium perfringens;* and *Peptostreptococcus micros.* Tigecycline should be administered via an intravenous infusion over 30 to 60 minutes every 12 hours.

J3246

J3246   Injection, tirofiban HCl, 0.25 mg

Lay Description
Tirofiban hydrochloride is an antiplatelet drug used to treat or prevent blood clots. It is used to treat certain types of angina, such as acute coronary syndrome, and may also be used prophylactically prior to angiography and angioplasty procedures. Tirofiban hydrochloride is a reversible antagonist of fibrinogen binding to the GP IIb/IIIa receptor, the major platelet surface receptor involved in platelet aggregation, thereby inhibiting ex vivo platelet aggregation. Tirofiban hydrochloride is administered by intravenous infusion at a recommended infusion rate of 0.4 mcg/kg/min initially for 30 minutes and then continuing at 0.1 mcg/kg/min for the duration of the infusion.

J3250

J3250   Injection, trimethobenzamide HCl, up to 200 mg

Lay Description
Trimethobenzamide hydrochloride (HCl) is an antiemetic used to alleviate nausea and vomiting. The mechanism of action is not known but it appears to act on the chemoreceptor trigger zone (CTZ) in the brain where vomiting impulses are transmitted. It can be administered via intramuscular injection. Trimethobenzamide HCl also comes in capsule and suppository forms.

J3260

J3260   Injection, tobramycin sulfate, up to 80 mg

Lay Description
Tobramycin is an aminoglycoside antibiotic. Aminoglycoside antibiotics are those derived from various species of Streptomyces bacteria or produced synthetically. Aminoglycosides inhibit bacterial protein synthesis by binding with the 30S ribosomal subunit and are bactericidal. Streptomycin is derived from *Streptomyces tenebrarius.* It inhibits protein synthesis causing cell death. Susceptibility studies should be performed prior to the administration of tobramycin. It is indicated in the treatment of infections caused by gram-negative bacillary bacteria including *Pseudomonas aeruginosa, Staphylococcus aureus, Escherichia coli, Klebsiella* species, *Enterobacter* species, *Serretia* species, *Proteus* species, *Providencia* species, and *Citrobacter* species. The injectable form is administered by intramuscular injection and

intravenous infusion. Dosages vary depending on the form of administration, frequency of administration, and indication.

J3262

J3262 Injection, tocilizumab, 1 mg

Lay Description
Tocilizumab is a chemical compound that is an interleukin-6 receptor inhibitor. Interleukin-6 is a protein secreted by a variety of cells to stimulate immune response to trauma or other tissue damage leading to inflammation. Tocilizumab is indicated for adult patients with moderate to severe active rheumatoid arthritis who have had an inadequate response to one or more tumor necrosis factor inhibitors. This medication may be used as monotherapy or with methotrexate or other disease modifying antirheumatic drugs. The recommended dose is 4 mg to 8 mg per kg of patient weight. The drug is administered as a 60 minute IV infusion.

J3265

J3265 Injection, torsemide, 10 mg/ml

Lay Description
Torsemide is a diuretic that is used to treat patients with heart or liver failure, hypertension, or for those with hepatic cirrhosis. Torsemide acts on the loop of Henle by enhancing excretion of sodium, water, and chloride.

J3280

J3280 Injection, thiethylperazine maleate, up to 10 mg

Lay Description
Thiethylperazine maleate is indicated for the relief of nausea and vomiting. The exact mechanism of action is not known. However, it appears to have an effect on the vomiting center and the chemoreceptor trigger zone (CTZ) of the brain. Recommended oral dose is 10 to 30 mg a day. Thiethylperazine maleate can be administered orally or by intramuscular injection. Recommended intramuscular injection dose is 10 mg one to three times a day.

J3285

J3285 Injection, treprostinil, 1 mg

Lay Description
Treprostinil is a prostacyclin, an analogue of prostaglandin that is a vasodilator. The drug directly dilates pulmonary and systemic arterial beds and inhibits platelet aggregation. Treprostinil is indicated for the treatment of pulmonary arterial hypertension patients who have New York Heart Association Class II-IV symptoms. The drug may be administered via a continuous subcutaneous infusion. If the patient cannot tolerate subcutaneous infusion, the drug may be administered via continuous intravenous infusion by a central venous line. Treprostinil may be self-administered using an infusion pump. Dosage is dependent upon the patient's body weight and the relief of symptoms.

J3300-J3303

J3300 Injection, triamcinolone acetonide, preservative free, 1 mg

J3301 Injection, triamcinolone acetonide, not otherwise specified, 10 mg

J3302 Injection, triamcinolone diacetate, per 5 mg

J3303 Injection, triamcinolone hexacetonide, per 5 mg

Lay Description
Triamcinolone is a synthetic corticosteroid, which is analogous to corticosteroids produced by the adrenal cortex. The drug is one to two times more potent than prednisone. Its mechanism of action is not clearly defined. Triamcinolone does decrease inflammation by stabilizing leukocytes, suppress the chemicals normally released in immune response, and stimulate bone marrow. Triamcinolone acetonide is a more potent derivative of triamcinolone, approximately eight times more potent than prednisone. Triamcinolone acetonide is the version most commonly used in preparations. Diacetate and hexacetonide are different formulations of triamcinolone with hexacetonide having the longest acting effect. The drug has a number of uses, including hormone replacement when the adrenal gland does not produce adequate supplies. The injectable version may be administered intramuscularly, intra-articularly, intravitreally, or intralesionally. The injectable version is indicated for the treatment of a large number of symptoms and diseases, which are far too numerous to list.

J3305

J3305 Injection, trimetrexate glucuronate, per 25 mg

Lay Description
Trimetrexate glucoronate is a nonclassical folate antagonist. It is a synthetic inhibitor of the enzyme dihydrofolate reductase (DHFR) and is used as an alternative therapy for the treatment of moderate-to-severe *Pneumocystis Jiroveci* pneumonia in immunocompromised patients. It interferes with the RNA, DNA, and protein synthesis, which results in cell death. Leucovorin calcium should be given with this medication to protect the patient from life-threatening toxicities. Trimetrexate glucuronate is administered by intravenous infusion over 60 minutes.

J3310

J3310 Injection, perphenazine, up to 5 mg

Lay Description
Perphenazine is used in treating psychosis and severe nausea and vomiting. The mechanism of action is not known. However, it does have an effect on the entire

central nervous system particularly the hypothalamus. Dose is based on the condition and response of the patient. Perphenazine is administered orally. Per the FDA, the injectable form is no longer available in the United States.

J3315

J3315   Injection, triptorelin pamoate, 3.75 mg

Lay Description

Triptorelin pamoate is a synthetic decapeptide agonist analog of luteinizing hormone releasing hormone (LHRH or GnRH) with greater potency than the naturally occurring LHRH. It is used in the palliative treatment of advanced prostate cancer. This medication prevents gonadotropin secretion when given continuously in therapeutic doses. After the first dose there is an increase in the luteinizing hormone (LH), follicle-stimulating hormone (FSH), testosterone, and estradiol levels. Following continuous administration, there is a persistent decrease in LH and FSH secretion. There is also a significant decrease of testicular and ovarian steroidogenesis. The reduction of serum testosterone is that usually found in surgically castrated men. Recommended dose is 3.75 mg monthly. Triptorelin pamoate is administered by intramuscular injection.

J3320

J3320   Injection, spectinomycin dihydrochloride, up to 2 g

Lay Description

Spectinomycin dihydrochloride is an aminocyclitol antibiotic produced by the *Streptomyces spectabilis* species of soil microorganism. Spectinomycin dihydrochloride is indicated for treatment of susceptible, drug-resistant strains of acute *N. gonorrhea*. Spectinomycin dihydrochloride works by inhibiting protein synthesis in the bacterial cell. Spectinomycin dihydrochloride is administered by intramuscular injection.

J3350

J3350   Injection, urea, up to 40 g

Lay Description

Urea is an organic compound of carbon, nitrogen, oxygen, and hydrogen. It is the chief nitrogenous end-product from the metabolism of proteins. Intravenous infusions of urea are used as a diuretic and to lower intracranial pressure. Intravenous urea is indicated as a treatment for fluid accumulation in the brain, high intraocular pressure, or glaucoma.

J3355

J3355   Injection, urofollitropin, 75 IU

Lay Description

Urofollitropin is a highly purified, follicle-stimulating hormone extracted from the urine of post-menopausal women. Follicle stimulating hormone is a gonadotropic hormone produced in the anterior pituitary gland. It stimulates the growth and maturation of follicles in the ovary. Urofollitropin is used to induce ovulation in polycystic ovary disease. It is administered by subcutaneous or intramuscular injection.

J3357

J3357   Injection, ustekinumab, 1 mg

Lay Description

Ustekinumab is a human monoclonal antibody that is a human interleuken-12 and 23 antagonist. This drug is indicated as a treatment for adult patients diagnosed with moderate to severe plaque psoriasis. The recommended dose is based on the patient's body weight. After initial administration, the second dose is given four weeks later and then every 12 weeks thereafter. Ustekinumab is administered by subcutaneous administration.

J3360

J3360   Injection, diazepam, up to 5 mg

Lay Description

Diazepam is an antianxiety drug that acts on the central nervous system (CNS). This benzodiazepine produces anxiolytic effects by aiding the action of a specific inhibitory neurotransmitter in the brain, depressing the CNS in the limbic and subcortical areas, as well as seizure activity focused in the cortex and thalamus. Diazepam is used for anxiety, acute alcohol withdrawal, muscle spasm, and before endoscopic procedures. Dosages range from 2 to 20 mg based on patient condition. Diazepam can be administered via intramuscular injection or intravenous push.

J3364-J3365

J3364   Injection, urokinase, 5,000 IU vial

J3365   Injection, IV, urokinase, 250,000 IU vial

Lay Description

Urokinase is urokinase-type plasminogen activator (uPA) and is a serine protease. It is a thrombolytic agent obtained from human neonatal kidney cells grown in tissue culture. Urokinase is a thrombolytic enzyme used for treatment of acute pulmonary embolism, acute coronary arterial thrombosis, and to clear thrombi from intravenous catheters. Urokinase binds to fibrin, converts plasminogen into plasmin, and breaks down the thrombus into smaller components. Urokinase is administered via intravenous infusion.

J3370

J3370   Injection, vancomycin HCl, 500 mg

Lay Description

Vancomycin is used to treat serious infections, including septicemia, bone infections, endocarditis, lower respiratory tract infections, and skin and skin structure infections. It is effective against

Diphtheroids, Enterococci (e.g., Enterococcus faecalis), Staphylococci including Staphylococcus aureus and Staphylococcus epidermidis (including heterogeneous methicillin-resistant strains), Streptococcus bovis, Viridans group streptococci, Listeria monocytogenes, Streptococcus pyogenes, Streptococcus pneumoniae (including penicillin-resistant strains), Streptococcus agalactiae, Actinomyces species, and Lactobacillus species. Oral vancomycin HCl is used in treating antibiotic-associated pseudomembranous colitis caused by C. difficile and staphylococcal enterocolitis. Vancomycin HCl is not effective by the oral route for other types of infections. Vancomycin interferes with RNA synthesis and damages the bacterial cell's plasma membrane, making it susceptible to the forces of osmotic pressure.

J3385

J3385   Injection, velaglucerase alfa, 100 units

Lay Description
Velaglucerase alfa is a hydrolytic lysosomal glucocerebroside specific enzyme used in the treatment of long-term enzyme replacement therapy (ERT) for adults or pediatric patients who are diagnosed with Type 1 Gaucher disease. Gaucher disease occurs in patients who do not produce an adequate amount of an enzyme called glucocerebrosidase, which can result in harmful amounts of lipid buildup in the spleen, bones, liver, nervous system, and bone marrow and may also prevent organs and cells from functioning properly. Velaglucerase alfa is used as a replacement for another enzyme replacement therapy, imiglucerase. Velaglucerase alfa comes in the form of a lyophilized powder to be reconstituted with diluted water and is administered by intravenous infusion.

J3396

J3396   Injection, verteporfin, 0.1 mg

Lay Description
Verteporfin is a benzoporphyrin derivative that is a photosensitizer or light-activated drug. Verteporfin is used together with a nonthermal red laser light to treat abnormal blood vessel formation in a part of the eye that, if left untreated, can lead to a loss of eyesight. Treatment with verteporfin and laser light occurs in two steps. First, the verteporfin is injected into the body. Second, 15 minutes later, a laser light is directed at the affected eye. Photodynamic therapy with verteporfin is approved to treat age-related macular degeneration (AMD) with neovascular changes, known as choroidal neovascularization (CNV). CNV can be described as classic or occult, based on appearance on fluorescein angiography. CNV can also be described by its location: extrafoveal, juxtafoveal, and subfoveal. Verteporfin is indicated for patients with predominately classic subfoveal CNV due to AMD, pathologic myopia, or presumed ocular histoplasmosis. Laser light treatment must follow verteporfin injection 15 minutes after the start of the injection. Once activated, the drug probably creates free radical formation, which causes cellular damage and eventually results in thrombosis of the vessels and slowing of the progression of CNV. The drug is injected intravenously into the patient's arm.

J3400

J3400   Injection, triflupromazine HCl, up to 20 mg

Lay Description
Per the FDA, this drug is no longer available in the United States.

J3410

J3410   Injection, hydroxyzine HCl, up to 25 mg

Lay Description
Hydroxyzine is a piperazine derivative that has central nervous system depressant, antispasmodic, antihistamine, and antifibrillatory properties. It is used to treat a variety of conditions such as anxiety, pruritus from allergies, psychiatric and emotional emergencies, and nausea and vomiting. Hydroxyzine may be used as a complete therapeutic substitute for intravenous antiemetic therapy at the time of a chemotherapy treatment. It is often used as a preoperative medication. It tends to increase the effect of meperidine and barbiturates. It can be administered via intravenous push, intramuscular injection, or orally. Hydroxyzine hydrochloride is used to treat anxiety, manifestations of allergic dermatoses, as an antiemetic, and as a preoperative medication. It is administered by intramuscular injection or orally. Hydroxyzine pamoate has uses similar to the hydrochloride version.

J3411

J3411   Injection, thiamine HCl, 100 mg

Lay Description
Vitamins are organic compounds that are necessary for the metabolic functioning of the body. Thiamine, also known as vitamin B1, is a water-soluble vitamin that acts by binding with adenosine triphosphate to form a coenzyme needed for carbohydrate metabolism. It is found particularly in pork, organ meats, legumes, nuts, and whole grain or enriched cereals and breads. Thiamine hydrochloride is used to treat deficiency states including beriberi, alcoholic neuritis, and Wernicke-Korsakoff syndrome. It is available in injectable and oral forms. Oral forms are sold over-the-counter in singular or combined products and are self-administered. The injectable form can be administered by intramuscular or intravenous injection.

J3415

J3415 Injection, pyridoxine HCl, 100 mg

Lay Description
Pyridoxine is one of the forms of vitamin B6. Vitamins are organic compounds that are necessary for the metabolic functioning of the body. Vitamin B6 is a water-soluble vitamin used by the body in the metabolism of amino acids, in the degradation of tryptophan, and in the breakdown of glycogen to glucose-1-phosphate. Pyridoxine hydrochloride is used for patients with vitamin B6 deficiency, to prevent seizures during cycloserine therapy, and as an antidote for isoniazid and cycloserine poisoning.

J3420

J3420 Injection, vitamin B-12 cyanocobalamin, up to 1,000 mcg

Lay Description
Vitamin B12 cyanocobalamin is a coenzyme that stimulates metabolic cell function. It is required for cell replication, hematopoiesis, and nucleoprotein and myelin production. This medication is indicated for treatment of pernicious anemia, vitamin B12 malabsorption, and/or methylmalonicaciduria. Malabsorption can be caused by many conditions including neoplasms, AIDS, Crohn's Disease, parasites, and tapeworms.

J3430

J3430 Injection, phytonadione (vitamin K), per 1 mg

Lay Description
Phytonadione (vitamin K injection) is given to prevent hemorrhagic conditions and promote liver formation of prothrombin. Hypoprothrombinemia occurs when the body lacks vitamin K, sometimes occurring secondary to malabsorption, oral anticoagulants, drug therapy, or too much vitamin A. Phytonadione is often used for pregnant women, those who are breast-feeding, and neonates who have hemorrhagic disease or vitamin K deficiency through breast milk. Phytonadione is administered by subcutaneous injection, intramuscular injection, intravenous infusion over two or three hours, or orally.

J3465

J3465 Injection, voriconazole, 10 mg

Lay Description
Voriconazole is an antifungal used to treat infections of the skin, abdomen, bladder wall, kidney, and esophageal candidiasis. It inhibits an essential protein found in the mitochondria of the cell that is needed for biosynthesis. This medication is effective against species of *Aspergillus* other than *A. fumigatus*, *Scedosporium apiospermum* (asexual form of *Pseudallescheria boydii*), and *Fusarium* species, including *Fusarium solani*, in patients intolerant of, or refractory to, other therapy. Voriconazole is

administered via intravenous infusion over one to two hours or orally.

J3470

J3470 Injection, hyaluronidase, up to 150 units

Lay Description
Hyaluronidase is a protein enzyme produced from purified bovine testicular tissue. Hyaluronidase is a diffusing substance that modifies the permeability of connective tissue through the hydrolysis of hyaluronic acid, a polysaccharide. Hyaluronidase hydrolyzes hyaluronic acid by splitting the glucosaminidic bond between C1 of the glucosamine moiety and C4 of glucuronic acid. This temporarily decreases the viscosity of the cellular cement and promotes diffusion of injected fluids or of localized transudates or exudates facilitating their absorption. Hyaluronidase is indicated as an adjunct to increase the absorption and dispersion of other injected drugs, for hypodermoclysis, and as an adjunct in subcutaneous urography for improving resorption of radiopaque agents.

J3471-J3472

J3471 Injection, hyaluronidase, ovine, preservative free, per 1 USP unit (up to 999 USP units)

J3472 Injection, hyaluronidase, ovine, preservative free, per 1,000 USP units

Lay Description
Hyaluronidase is a protein enzyme. The ovine version is manufactured from purified testicular tissue and is preservative-free. Hyaluronidase is a diffusing substance that modifies the permeability of connective tissue through the hydrolysis of hyaluronic acid, a polysaccharide. Hyaluronidase hydrolyzes hyaluronic acid by splitting the glucosaminidic bond between C1 of the glucosamine moiety and C4 of glucuronic acid. This temporarily decreases the viscosity of the cellular cement and promotes diffusion of injected fluids or of localized transudates or exudates facilitating their absorption. Hyaluronidase is indicated as an adjunct to increase the absorption and dispersion of other injected drugs, for hypodermoclysis, and as an adjunct in subcutaneous urography for improving resorption of radiopaque agents.

J3473

J3473 Injection, hyaluronidase, recombinant, 1 USP unit

Lay Description
Hyaluronidase is a protein enzyme. The ovine version is manufactured from purified testicular tissue and is preservative free. The recombinant version is a purified protein produced by recombinant DNA technology in Chinese hamster ovaries. Hyaluronidase is a diffusing substance that modifies the permeability of connective tissue through the hydrolysis of

hyaluronic acid, a polysaccharide. Hyaluronidase hydrolyzes hyaluronic acid by splitting the glucosaminidase bond between C1 of the glucosamine moiety and C4 of glucuronic acid. This temporarily decreases the viscosity of the cellular cement and promotes diffusion of injected fluids or of localized transudates or exudates facilitating their absorption. Hyaluronidase is indicated as an adjunct to increase the absorption and dispersion of other injected drugs, for hypodermoclysis, and as an adjunct in subcutaneous urography for improving resorption of radiopaque agents.

J3475

J3475   Injection, magnesium sulfate, per 500 mg

Lay Description
Magnesium sulfate is used to prevent or control seizures occurring in eclampsia or pre-eclampsia, for hypomagnesemia, acute nephritis in children, uterine tetany management of paroxysmal atrial tachycardia, and for constipation. Magnesium sulfate functions as an anticonvulsant and as a fluid and electrolyte replacement. Its anticonvulsant properties are thought to come by inhibiting the release of acetylcholine at the myoneural junction and thus reducing muscle contractions.

J3480

J3480   Injection, potassium chloride, per 2 mEq

Lay Description
Potassium chloride is an electrolyte that is used to prevent hypokalemia, digitalis intoxication, hypokalemic familial periodic paralysis, and to treat an acute myocardial infarction. Dose is based on age, weight, and clinical condition of the patient. Potassium ions are necessary for many essential physiological functions, including the maintenance of intracellular tonicity; the transmission of nerve impulses; the contraction of cardiac, skeletal, and smooth muscle; and the maintenance of normal renal function.

J3485

J3485   Injection, zidovudine, 10 mg

Lay Description
Zidovudine (formerly called azidothymidine or AZT) is a synthetic nucleoside analogue used as an antiviral for the treatment of human immunodeficiency virus (HIV) infection and to prevent maternal-fetal transmission of HIV. Zidovudine incorporates itself into the DNA chain preventing elongation and stopping DNA growth. Zidovudine can be administered via intravenous infusion over one hour or orally. Recommended dose is 1mg/kg given five to six times a day by IV infusion over one hour.

J3486

J3486   Injection, ziprasidone mesylate, 10 mg

Lay Description
Ziprasidone mesylate is used in the treatment of schizophrenia by inhibiting both the dopamine and serotonin-2 receptors, reducing schizophrenic symptoms. Some adverse reactions may include orthostatic hypotension, dry mouth, dysmenorrhea, rash, flu-like syndrome, and/or dyspepsia. Ziprasidone is contraindicated in patients who have experienced a recent myocardial infarction (MI) or have a history of long QT (time between the beginning of the QRS [ventricular depolarization] complex and the end of the T-wave) syndrome.

J3489

J3489   Injection, zoledronic acid, 1 mg

Lay Description
Zoledronic acid is a bisphosphate used to slow bone breakdown, decrease the amount of calcium released from the bones into the blood, and to treat hypercalcemia of malignancy. It is indicated as a treatment and prevention for postmenopausal osteoporosis and glucosteroid-induced osteoporosis, as a treatment of Paget's disease in men and women, and to increase bone mass in men with osteoporosis. It also appears to counteract the bone mineral density loss seen in patients with multiple myeloma and bone metastases from solid tumor cancers. Hypercalcemia is an abnormally high concentration of calcium in the bloodstream and results in malignancy cases from secretions by the cancer cells that promote the release of calcium stored in the bones into the bloodstream. Zoledronic acid is administered by intravenous infusion over no less than 15 minutes.

J3490

J3490   Unclassified drugs

Lay Description
Use this code to represent a drug that has been administered and that does not have any other specified level I or level II HCPCS code to represent it.

J3520

J3520   Edetate disodium, per 150 mg

Lay Description
Edetate disodium is indicated for the treatment of severe acute hypercalcemia and digitalis toxicity. It forms chelates, which displace calcium from molecules. A stable chelate will form with any metal that has the ability to displace calcium from the molecule, a feature shared by lead, zinc, cadmium, manganese, iron, and mercury. Edetate disodium is not well absorbed in the gastrointestinal tract. It does not seem to penetrate cells and is found mainly in the extracellular fluid. Edetate disodium is administered by intravenous infusion over three or more hours.

J3530

J3530   Nasal vaccine inhalation

Lay Description
Use this code to represent a drug that has been administered, when the route of administration is nasal, and it does not have any other specified level I or level II HCPCS code to represent it.

J3535

J3535   Drug administered through a metered dose inhaler

Lay Description
Use this HCPCS code to represent a drug that has been administered through a meter does inhaler and the drug does not have any other specified level I or level II HCPCS code to represent it.

J3570

J3570   Laetrile, amygdalin, vitamin B-17

Lay Description
Laetrile is a compound that contains a chemical called amygdalin. Amygdalin is found in the pits of many fruits, raw nuts, and plants. It is believed that the active anticancer ingredient in laetrile is cyanide. Laetrile has shown little anticancer effects in laboratory studies, animal studies, and human studies. The side effects of laetrile are like the symptoms of cyanide poisoning. Laetrile is not approved by the Food and Drug Administration (FDA). Laetrile is given by intravenous injection.

J3590

J3590   Unclassified biologics

Lay Description
Use this code to represent a biologic that as been administered and does not have any other specified level I or level II HCPCS code to represent it.

J7030-J7040, J7050

J7030   Infusion, normal saline solution, 1,000 cc
J7040   Infusion, normal saline solution, sterile (500 ml=1 unit)
J7050   Infusion, normal saline solution, 250 cc

Lay Description
The infusion of normal saline solution replaces electrolytes and fluid loss in hyponatremia and/or severe salt depletion. Oral tablet form is also available. Normal saline solution may cause edema or pulmonary edema if administered too rapidly. Lab values may show electrolyte imbalance.

J7042

J7042   5% dextrose/normal saline (500 ml = 1 unit)

Lay Description
Dextrose/normal saline is a water-soluble sugar that minimizes glyconeogenesis and promotes anabolism in patients whose oral caloric intake is limited. It is used to provide fluid replacement and caloric supplementation for patients with cirrhosis, hepatitis, high metabolic stress, and for nutritional support for patients with renal failure. Some side effects may include fever, nausea, glycosuria, weight gain, and/or osteoporosis.

J7050

J7050   Infusion, normal saline solution, 250 cc

Lay Description
Please refer to codes J7030-J7040 for the description, coding, and billing information.

J7060

J7060   5% dextrose/water (500 ml = 1 unit)

Lay Description
A 5 percent dextrose/water solution is used to replace fluid and calories in patients that are not able to maintain adequate oral intake or are restricted from doing so. Side effects may include fever, confusion, hypertension, and/or pulmonary edema. Dextrose/water is contraindicated in patients with a known allergy to corn or corn related products.

J7070

J7070   Infusion, D-5-W, 1,000 cc

Lay Description
D5W is 5 percent dextrose in water. A 5 percent dextrose/water solution is used to replace fluid and calories in patients that are not able to maintain adequate oral intake or are restricted from doing so. This is also known as glucose, which is the main source of energy for all cells. D5W is administered via intravenous infusion.

J7100-J7110

J7100   Infusion, dextran 40, 500 ml
J7110   Infusion, dextran 75, 500 ml

Lay Description
Dextran is used as a hemodiluent in extracorporeal circulation, for plasma volume expansion, and in the prevention of venous thrombosis. It is made from glucose molecules and binds to platelets, red blood cells, and the lining of the vessel walls. This decreases their capability of binding together and forming clots. Dextran is administered by intravenous infusion.

J7120

J7120   Ringers lactate infusion, up to 1,000 cc

Lay Description
Ringer's lactate solution, or infusion, is a replacement solution for treating fluid and electrolyte imbalance. It contains sodium, potassium, calcium, chloride, and lactate in amounts that approximate the levels found in blood plasma. Ringer's lactate is administered by intravenous infusion.

J7131

J7131   Hypertonic saline solution, 1 ml

Lay Description
Hypertonic saline solution is a high concentration of sodium chloride and is approximately eight times saltier than physiologic saline used in most hospital IVs.

J7178

J7178   Injection, human fibrinogen concentrate, 1 mg

Lay Description
Fibrinogen (factor I) is a component in the blood that helps with clotting and is used to treat patients with congenital fibrinogen deficiency, including afibrinogenemia and hypofibrinogenemia. It is a physiological substrate of three enzymes—thrombin, factor XIIIa, and plasmin—and is manufactured from pooled human plasma that has been purified and concentrated. During the coagulation process, its molecules are used by the thrombin, factor XIIIa, and plasmin to produce a fibrin monomer. This monomer, along with calcium ions and factor XIII, makes the clot stronger and more elastic. The dose is dependent on the patient's body weight, condition, and blood levels. The solution is administered by intravenous injection.

J7180

J7180   Injection, factor XIII (antihemophilic factor, human), 1 IU

Lay Description
Antihemophilic factor XIII injection is used to treat a rare genetic bleeding disorder. Factor XIII is usually found in the blood platelets, monocytes, and macrophages. It helps stabilize the blood clot, give it strength, and make it more pliable and resistant to fibrinolysis. It is made from heat treated pooled human plasma and the factor XIII is concentrated. It is then sterilized and purified. Recommended dose is 40 units per kg body weight administered by IV injection every 28 days.

J7181

J7181   Injection, factor XIII A-subunit, (recombinant), per IU

Lay Description
Factor XIII A-subunit (antihemophilic factor, recombinant), trade name Tretten, is a recombinant human factor XIII-A2, composed of two factor XIIIA-subunits. It is manufactured as a soluble protein in yeast, extracted and purified. No human or animal products are used in its manufacture. Factor XIII is the final enzyme in the blood coagulation process. When activated by thrombin at the site of a vessel injury, it crosslinks fibrin and other proteins in the fibrin clot. Factor XIII A-subunit is indicated for routine prophylaxis for bleeding in patients with congenital factor XIII A-subunit deficiency. The dose for routine

prophylaxis is 35 IU per kilogram of body weight administered once a month.

J7183

J7183   Injection, von Willebrand factor complex (human), Wilate, 1 IU vWF:RCo

Lay Description
Von Willebrand's factor complex is a concentrated blood-clotting factor extracted from human blood, pasteurized and used to treat hemophilia A. It contains highly concentrated levels of antihemophiliac/von Willebrand factors and ristocetin cofactor (vWF:RCo). It is indicated for use in adult and pediatric patients for treatment of spontaneous and trauma-induced bleeding episodes in severe von Willebrand's disease and in mild to moderate von Willebrand's disease where use of desmopressin is known or suspected to be inadequate. Other indications include the treatment of adult patients with hemophilia A (classic hemophilia). Von Willebrand's factor complex is administered by intravenous injection and can be self administered.

J7185

J7185   Injection, factor VIII (antihemophilic factor, recombinant) (XYNTHA), per IU

Lay Description
Antihemophilic factor recombinant is used as a preventive measure before a surgical procedure for patients with hemophilia A (congenital factor VIII deficiency). XYNTHA does not contain plasma or albumin. The antihemophilic factor is secreted by Chinese hamster ovary cells and is grown in a culture medium that contains recombinant insulin. It does not contain von Willebrand factor and is not appropriate for patients with von Willebrand's disease. It is used as a short-term, routine prophylaxis to reduce bleeding incidences during surgery. Dose and length of treatment is based on the patient's body weight, condition, the procedure being performed, and the extent of bleeding. Antihemophilic factor recombinant is administered by IV infusion. The medication can be self-administered.

J7186

J7186   Injection, antihemophilic factor VIII/von Willebrand factor complex (human), per factor VIII i.u.

Lay Description
Von Willebrand's factor complex is a concentrated blood-clotting factor extracted from human blood and pasteurized. It contains highly concentrated levels of antihemophiliac/von Willebrand factors. It is indicated for use in adult and pediatric patients for treatment of spontaneous and trauma-induced bleeding episodes in severe von Willebrand's disease and in mild to moderate von Willebrand's disease where use of desmopressin is known or suspected to be inadequate. Other indications include the

treatment of adult patients with hemophilia A (classic hemophilia).Von Willebrand's factor complex is administered by intravenous injection and can be self-administered.

J7187

J7187 Injection, von Willebrand factor complex (Humate-P), per IU VWF:RCO

Lay Description
Von Willebrand's factor complex is a concentrated blood-clotting factor extracted from human blood and pasteurized used to treat hemophilia A. It contains highly concentrated levels of antihemophiliac/von Willebrand factors and ristocetin cofactor (VWF:RCo). It is indicated for use in adult and pediatric patients for treatment of spontaneous and trauma-induced bleeding episodes in severe von Willebrand's disease and in mild to moderate von Willebrand's disease where use of desmopressin is known or suspected to be inadequate. Other indications include the treatment of adult patients with hemophilia A (classic hemophilia). Von Willebrand's factor complex is administered by intravenous injection and can be self-administered.

J7189

J7189 Factor VIIa (antihemophilic factor, recombinant), per 1 mcg

Lay Description
Factor VIIa recombinant is an antihemophilia drug that is a purified protein produced by recombinant DNA technology in baby hamster kidney cells. It is a vitamin K-dependent glycoprotein that is involved in the extrinsic pathway of blood coagulation. In conjunction with tissue factor, it activates coagulation Factor X and Factor IX to Factor IXa. These factors then assist in the conversion of prothrombin to thrombin and fibrinogen to fibrin inducing local hemostasis. Factor VIIa recombinant is indicated for the treatment of bleeding episodes in hemophilia A or B patients with inhibitors to Factor VIII or Factor IX. The drug is available only in an injectable form. It should be administered as an intravenous bolus only under the direct supervision of a physician experienced in the treatment of hemophilia. The recommended dosage for hemophilia A or B patients with inhibitors varies from 35 to 120 µg/kg of body weight every two hours until hemostasis is achieved, or until the treatment has been judged to be inadequate. Dosage and administration intervals are dependent upon the severity of the bleeding and patient response.

J7190-J7192

J7190 Factor VIII (antihemophilic factor, human) per IU

J7191 Factor VIII (antihemophilic factor (porcine)), per IU

J7192 Factor VIII (antihemophilic factor, recombinant) per IU, not otherwise specified

Lay Description
Factor VIII, antihemophilic factor is used to replace deficient clotting factor and treat bleeding in patients with hemophilia A or to prevent bleeding when surgery is needed. The desired level of factor VIII to be given is calculated from a formula multiplying body weight in kilograms by the level of desired factor VIII increase (or the percent of normal) by 0.5. The percent of normal used depends on the purpose of administration: to prevent spontaneous hemorrhage, 5 percent of normal is used; for moderate hemorrhage and minor surgery, 30 to 50 percent of normal is used. Severe hemorrhage requires 80 to 100 percent of normal antihemophilic factor. Factor VIII is administered by intravenous injection and can be self-administered.

J7193

J7193 Factor IX (antihemophilic factor, purified, nonrecombinant) per IU

Lay Description
Factor IX nonrecombinant is an antihemophilia drug. Factor IX nonrecombinant is a sterile, stable, lyophilized concentrate of factor IX prepared from pooled human plasma and is indicated for treatment of factor IX deficiency, also known as hemophilia B or Christmas disease. Factor IX is isolated from the source material by use of a murine monoclonal antibody, and extraneous plasma-driven proteins, including factors II, VII, and X, are removed by use of immunoaffinity chromatography. Once factor IX has been isolated and other proteins removed, the factor IX is dissociated from the monoclonal antibody and further purified, resulting in a highly purified form of factor IX. Each vial of factor IX nonrecombinant, which is administered by intravenous infusion, contains the labeled amount of factor IX activity expressed in international units (IU). One IU represents the activity of factor IX present in 1 ml of normal, pooled plasma.

J7194

J7194 Factor IX complex, per IU

Lay Description
Factor IX complex is an antihemophilia drug that is a sterile, dried, plasma fraction containing coagulation factors II, IX, X, and low levels of factor VII. Factors II, VII, IX, and X are the vitamin K dependent coagulation factors synthesized in the liver. Factor IX complex is indicated for treatment of factor IX deficiency, also known as hemophilia B or Christmas disease, in patients with current or impending bleeding

episodes. It is also indicated for treatment of bleeding episodes in patients with hemophilia A (factor VIII deficiency) who have inhibitors to factor VIII. Factor IX complex is also used in emergency situations, usually as a secondary measure following the administration of fresh frozen plasma, to treat patients with Coumadin-induced hemorrhage when prompt reversal is required. Factor IX complex administered for these indications raises the plasma level of factor IX and restores hemostasis in patients with the listed conditions. Each vial of factor IX complex, which is administered by intravenous infusion, contains the labeled amount of factor IX activity expressed in international units (IU). One IU represents the activity of factor IX present in 1 ml of normal, pooled plasma.

J7195

J7195   Injection, factor IX (antihemophilic factor, recombinant) per IU, not otherwise specified

Lay Description
Factor IX recombinant is an antihemophilia drug. Factor IX recombinant is a purified protein produced by recombinant DNA technology and indicated in the treatment of factor IX deficiency, also known as hemophilia B or Christmas disease. Indications also include control or prevention of bleeding during surgery in factor IX deficient individuals. Recombinant DNA technology involves the use of a genetically engineered animal cell line that secretes recombinant factor IX into a cell culture medium. It uses a genetically engineered Chinese hamster ovary (CHO) cell line shown to be free of infectious agents. The stored cell banks are also free of blood or plasma products. The CHO cell line secretes recombinant factor IX into a defined cell culture medium that does not contain any proteins derived from animal or human sources. The recombinant factor IX is then purified by a chromatography purification process without the use of a monoclonal antibody yielding a high-purity, active product. The potency is verified by use of in vitro clotting assay. Factor IX recombinant is administered by intravenous infusion. Each vial of factor IX recombinant contains the labeled amount of factor IX activity expressed in international units (IU).One IU represents the activity of factor IX present in 1 ml of normal, pooled plasma.

J7196

J7196   Injection, antithrombin recombinant, 50 IU

Lay Description
Antithrombin III is a sterile, nonpyrogenic, stable, lyophilized preparation of purified recombinant human antithrombin. Antithrombin III is normally present in human plasma and is the major plasma inhibitor of thrombin. It is produced by introducing the DNA coding sequence for human antithrombin and mammary gland DNA sequence into a genetically engineered goat and is expressed in the goat's milk.

Antithrombin III is indicated for the treatment of patients with hereditary antithrombin III deficiency in connection with surgical or obstetrical procedures or when they suffer from thromboembolism. Antithrombin III is prepared from pooled units of human plasma from normal donors. Antithrombin III is administered by intravenous infusion. Each vial of antithrombin III contains the labeled amount of antithrombin III activity expressed in international units (IU).

J7197

J7197   Antithrombin III (human), per IU

Lay Description
Antithrombin III is a sterile, nonpyrogenic, stable, lyophilized preparation of purified human antithrombin III. Antithrombin III is normally present in human plasma and is the major plasma inhibitor of thrombin. Antithrombin III is indicated for the treatment of patients with hereditary antithrombin III deficiency in connection with surgical or obstetrical procedures or when they suffer from thromboembolism. Antithrombin III is prepared from pooled units of human plasma from normal donors. Antithrombin III is administered by intravenous infusion. Each vial of antithrombin III contains the labeled amount of antithrombin III activity expressed in international units (IU).

J7198

J7198   Antiinhibitor, per IU

Lay Description
Anti-inhibitor is a sterile product prepared from pooled human plasma. Anti-inhibitor contains, in concentrated form, variable amounts of activated and precursor vitamin K-dependent clotting factors. Factors of the kinin generating system are also present. The product is standardized by its ability to correct the clotting time of Factor VIII deficient plasma or Factor VIII deficient plasma that contains inhibitors to Factor VIII. Anti-inhibitor is indicated for use in patients with Factor VIII or Factor IX inhibitors who are bleeding or are to undergo surgery. Anti-inhibitor is intended to control bleeding episodes in such patients. Anti-inhibitor is administered by intravenous infusion. Anti-inhibitor is labeled with the number of Hyland Factor VIII Correctional Units that it contains. One Hyland Factor VIII Correctional Unit is that quantity of activated prothrombin complex that, upon addition to an equal volume of Factor VIII deficient or inhibitor plasma, will correct the clotting time to a normal time of 35 seconds. The recommended dosage depends on the severity of hemorrhage and ranges from 25 to 100 Hyland Factor VIII Correctional Units per kg of body weight. The dose may be repeated if no improvement is observed approximately six hours following the initial administration.

J7199

J7199   Hemophilia clotting factor, not otherwise classified

Lay Description
Use this code to represent a hemophilia clotting factor that has been administered and does not have any other specified level I or level II HCPCS code to represent it.

J7200

J7200   Injection, factor IX, (antihemophilic factor, recombinant), Rixubis, per IU

Lay Description
Factor IX recombinant is produced from a genetically engineered Chinese hamster ovary (CHO) cell line with no human or animal proteins. The CHO cell line secretes the factor IX protein, which is then purified by chromatography. Deficiencies of factor IX, called hemophilia B or Christmas disease, is an inherited blood clotting disorder mainly affecting males. It is caused by mutations in the factor IX gene and leads to deficiency of factor IX. Factor IX recombinant, trade name Rixubis, is indicated for use in people with hemophilia B who are 16 years of age and older. It is indicated for the control and prevention of bleeding episodes, perioperative (period extending from the time of hospitalization for surgery to the time of discharge) management, and routine prophylactic use to prevent or reduce the frequency of bleeding episodes. Factor IX recombinant is administered by intravenous injection after reconstitution with sterile water. When used for the routine prevention of bleeding episodes, it is administered twice weekly.

J7201

J7201   Injection, factor IX, FC fusion protein (recombinant), per IU

Lay Description
Factor IX (antihemophilic factor, recombinant), trade name Alprolix, is a recombinant coagulation factor IX protein that has a primary amino acid sequence identical to the human plasma derived factor IX. It is produced from a human embryonic kidney cell line that contains no animal or human protein. The drug has no human blood or preservatives. Factor IX is indicated for adults and children with hemophilia B for the control of bleeding episodes, perioperative management, or routine prophylaxis. Dosage and the duration of treatment depend upon the severity of the Factor IX deficiency, the patient's clinical condition, and the location and extent of bleeding. Recombinant antihemophilic factor IX is administered intravenously.

J7300

J7300   Intrauterine copper contraceptive

Lay Description
An intrauterine copper contraceptive, also called the copper IUD, is a long-term, reversible, method of birth control that is comparable to oral contraceptives and tubal ligation in efficacy. This is an alternative choice for women who do not use hormonal contraceptives due to smoking or other conditions that contraindicate their use. The contraceptive device is about the size of a quarter in a T-shape, made of soft, flexible plastic with copper, and is designed to fit in the uterus. The physician inserts in the device, which requires no further attention outside of monthly chain checks and may be left in for continuous use up to 10 years. The copper IUD may be removed at any time. Use of this device is contraindicating in women with pelvic inflammatory disease (PID) or any history of PID.

J7301

J7301   Levonorgestrel-releasing intrauterine contraceptive system, 13.5 mg

Lay Description
A levonorgestrel-releasing intrauterine contraceptive system contains 13.5 mg of levonorgestrel (LNG), a progestin, in a T-shaped polyethylene frame, or T-body, with a steroid reservoir that provides an initial release rate of about 14 mcg/day of LNG after 24 days. The rate decreases to 5 mcg/day after three years, its expected life. Use this code for SKYLA.

J7302

J7302   Levonorgestrel-releasing intrauterine contraceptive system, 52 mg

Lay Description
Levonorgestrel-releasing intrauterine contraceptive system (LNG-IUS) consists of a Nova T-device and a Silastic rod impregnated with 52 mg of levonorgestrel. The silastic rod is attached to the vertical arm of the device and is covered with a rate limiting silastic membrane that allows release of progestin levonorgestrel at a constant rate of 20 mcg per day directly to the lining of the uterus. The LNG-IUS is a combination hormonal and intrauterine method of birth control. The LNG-IUS appears to work by suppressing the production of human chorionic gonadotropin, thereby preventing fertilization. A physician must fit the LNG-IUS into the uterus. The LNG-IUS is an effective, long-acting, reversible contraceptive, with an effective life span of at least five years. After five years, it must be removed and replaced.

J7303

J7303   Contraceptive supply, hormone containing vaginal ring, each

Lay Description
This code reports the contraceptive supply of a hormone containing vaginal ring. Unlike the daily contraceptive pill, hormone containing vaginal rings are used on a monthly basis. The ring is inserted once a month in the vaginal wall and stays in place for about three weeks depending on the product used.

During this time the contraceptive medication releases a dose of hormones needed to prevent pregnancy. The patient usually takes a week break before inserting a new ring. The two hormones released include estrogen and progestin, which prevent the ovaries from producing mature eggs. The hormones are absorbed by the vaginal walls and distributed in the bloodstream.

J7304

J7304   Contraceptive supply, hormone containing patch, each

Lay Description
A birth control patch is applied to the skin and releases hormones through the skin into the bloodstream to prevent pregnancy. The progesterone and estrogen prevents ovulation (mature eggs are not produced). The patch will also thicken the mucus produced in the cervix making it difficult for sperm to enter and reach an egg that may have been released. The hormones may also affect the lining of the uterus so that if an egg is fertilized it may have a hard time attaching itself to the wall of the uterus. The patch must be placed on the skin on the first day of the menstrual cycle (there may be differences with difference suppliers of birth control patches). The patch should only be applied to one of four areas: abdomen, buttocks, upper arm, or upper torso, except for the breasts. The patch is worn for three weeks and no patch for the fourth week. Follow all manufacturers' instructions.

J7306

J7306   Levonorgestrel (contraceptive) implant system, including implants and supplies

Lay Description
Levonorgestrel is a synthetic hormone used as contraception in females. A long-term administration is available as an implant system. Typically, the contraceptive is available as a kit of soft plastic capsules, which are imbedded under the skin of the upper arm. Depending on the kit selected, one, two, or up to six rods may be inserted. A small subdermal incision is made and a trocar is used to deliver each matchstick-sized capsule. The six capsules are arranged in a fanlike manner to facilitate drug dispersion and later removal of the capsules. The drug diffuses gradually through the walls of the capsule into the bloodstream. Protection can last up to five years with the six-capsule system. Fertility is restored within weeks upon removal of the implants.

J7307

J7307   Etonogestrel (contraceptive) implant system, including implant and supplies

Lay Description
An etonogestrel implant system is a progestin-only female contraceptive that is implanted under the skin. Once the rod is implanted under the skin, it slowly

releases the hormone that can prevent pregnancy for a period of up to 3 years. This is a completely reversible method of contraception. The implant system works in three ways: first, it suppresses ovulation; second, the hormone increases the thickness of the cervical mucus in order to prevent the egg from implanting itself into the uterine wall; third, the hormone alters that inner lining of the uterus also in an effort to prevent the egg from implanting itself.

J7308

J7308   Aminolevulinic acid HCl for topical administration, 20%, single unit dosage form (354 mg)

Lay Description
Aminolevulinic acid hydrochloride is a topical solution that photosensitizes the skin to which it is applied. It is applied topically, directly on the individual lesions. Aminolevulinic acid hydrochloride is used in conjunction with blue light photodynamic therapy applied 14 to 18 hours later. This photodynamic therapy is indicated as a treatment for nonhyperkeratotic actinic keratoses of the face or scalp. This drug should not be applied to the eyes or mucous membranes. Actinic keratoses are precancerous skin lesions, appearing as scaly red or brown patches of skin, which if left untreated may become malignant.

J7309

J7309   Methyl aminolevulinate (MAL) for topical administration, 16.8%, 1 g

Lay Description
Methyl aminolevulinate (MAL) is a topical cream that is used in addition to red light photodynamic therapy. Photodynamic therapy is used to treat nonhyperkeratotic, nonpigmented actinic keratoses of the face and scalp. The treatment sessions are provided once a week for two weeks. Recommended dose of MAL is not more than 1 gram per treatment session. The lesion is prepped by removing scales and crust with a dermal curette and the cream is applied about 1 mm thick to the lesion and surrounding normal tissue. The lesion is covered with an occlusive dressing for three hours prior to the light treatment. The photodynamic illumination is targeted at the treated lesion for about seven to 10 minutes. Nitrile gloves should be worn when handling the cream.

J7310

J7310   Ganciclovir, 4.5 mg, long-acting implant

Lay Description
Ganciclovir implant is an antiviral indicated for the treatment of cytomegalovirus (CMV) retinitis in individuals with acquired immune deficiency syndrome (AIDS). The ganciclovir implant does not cure the CMV retinitis; however, it does keep the infection under control and can help to prevent the CMV retinitis from worsening. The implant is surgically

inserted. The ganciclovir is released into the eye over a five to eight month period after which it is surgically removed. At the time of removal, another ganciclovir implant may be inserted to provide ongoing treatment for the CMV retinitis. The implants contain a minimum of 4.5 mg of ganciclovir.

J7311

J7311   Fluocinolone acetonide, intravitreal implant

Lay Description
The fluocinolone acetonide intravitreal implant is a tablet designed to slowly release the synthetic corticosteroid fluocinolone to the posterior segment of the eye. It must be placed via a surgical incision into the ciliary disk or pars plana. Each tablet contains 0.59 mg of fluocinolone acetonide. The implant is indicated for the treatment of chronic noninfectious uveitis affecting the posterior segment of the eye. It is contraindicated in most viral diseases, vaccina, varicella, mycobacterial and fungal eye infections. The fluocinolone acetonide implant has a life of approximately 30 months. If uveitis recurs, the implant may be replaced.

J7312

J7312   Injection, dexamethasone, intravitreal implant, 0.1 mg

Lay Description
Dexamethasone intravitreal implant is a corticosteroid indicated for the treatment of macular edema following branch retinal vein occlusion or central retinal vein occlusion, and for the treatment of noninfectious uveitis affecting the posterior segment of the eye. Each intravitreal implant contains 0.7 mg of dexamethasone.

J7315

J7315   Mitomycin, opthalmic, 0.2 mg

Lay Description
Mitomycin is an antibiotic isolated from the bacterium *Streptomyces verticillus Yingtanensis*. It selectively inhibits DNA synthesis. Ophthalmic mitomycin is an antimetabolite indicated for use as an adjunct to glaucoma surgery. It is not intended for intraocular administration, which can severely damage the eye. The ophthalmic mitomycin is intended for topical application at the site of glaucoma filtration surgery.

J7316

J7316   Injection, ocriplasmin, 0.125 mg

Lay Description
Ocriplasmin is a proteolytic enzyme (or proteinase) that breaks down the long chain proteins into peptides and eventually into amino acids. Its activity is directed against the protein components of the vitreous body and the vitreoretinal interface where it dissolves the vitreomacular adhesions. Ocriplasmin is a truncated version of human plasmin produced by recombinant DNA technology created in yeast *Pichia pastoris*. Ocriplasmin is indicated for the treatment of symptomatic vitreomacular adhesion, which is a progressive sight-threatening condition. It is for intravitreal injection only. Recommended dosage is 0.125 mg as a single dose to the affected eye.

J7321-J7325

J7321   Hyaluronan or derivative, Hyalgan or Supartz, for intra-articular injection, per dose

J7323   Hyaluronan or derivative, Euflexxa, for intra-articular injection, per dose

J7324   Hyaluronan or derivative, Orthovisc, for intra-articular injection, per dose

J7325   Hyaluronan or derivative, Synvisc or Synvisc-One, for intra-articular injection, 1 mg

Lay Description
Hyaluronan, also known as hyaluronic acid or hyaluronate, is a glycosaminoglycan, which is a high-molecular-mass polysaccharide found in the extracellular matrix that is widely distributed throughout connective, epithelial, and neural tissues. Hyaluronan has various physiological functions in the intercellular matrix, providing a significant contribution to cell proliferation and migration. Hyaluronan is anchored firmly in the plasma membrane or bound via hyaluronan-specific binding proteins (receptors). These receptors have been identified on many different cells. Hyaluronan is a major component of synovial fluid and articular cartilage. In the cartilage, it coats each chondrocyte cell providing resilience. Hyaluronan described in J7321 is a polymer that is derived from avian hyaluronan. Hyaluronan described by J7323 and J7324 is derived from purified bacterial cells. Hyaluronan described by J7325 is derived from avian hyaluronan. Hyaluronan is injected directly into the knee joint to supplement the knee joint's natural synovial fluid, relieving pain and improving use of the knee. This treatment is also called visco supplementation. Hyaluronan is used to treat osteoarthritis of the knee that has not improved with other treatment, such as analgesics and physical therapy. Treatment includes three or five shots into the knee joint over three to five weeks. Some study results have indicated improved symptoms of osteoarthritis and joint function, while other studies have been inconclusive about the effectiveness of hyaluronan injections.

J7326

J7326   Hyaluronan or derivative, Gel-One, for intra-articular injection, per dose

Lay Description
Hyaluronan, also known as hyaluronic acid or hyaluronate, is a glycosaminoglycan, which is a high-molecular-mass polysaccharide found in the extracellular matrix that is widely distributed

throughout connective, epithelial, and neural tissues. Hyaluronan has various physiological functions in the intercellular matrix providing a significant contribution to cell proliferation and migration. Hyaluronan is anchored firmly in the plasma membrane or bound via hyaluronan-specific binding proteins (receptors). These receptors have been identified on many different cells. Hyaluronan is a major component of synovial fluid and articular cartilage. In the cartilage, it coats each chondrocyte cell providing resilience. This code describes a derivative from avian hyaluronan. In this product, strands of hyaluronan are cross-linked or bound to each other with cinnamic acid, which increases its viscoelasticity. Hyaluronan is injected directly into the knee joint to supplement the knee joint's natural synovial fluid, relieving pain and improving use of the knee. This treatment is also called visco supplementation. Hyaluronan is used to treat osteoarthritis of the knee that has not improved with other treatment, such as analgesics and physical therapy. Treatment is one injection into the knee joint. Some study results have indicated improved symptoms of osteoarthritis and joint function, while other studies have been inconclusive about the effectiveness of hyaluronan injections.

J7327

J7327   Hyaluronan or derivative, Monovisc, for intra-articular injection, per dose

Lay Description

Monovisc is a high molecular weight hyaluronic acid. It is intended to deliver a single injection to supplement the synovial fluid of an osteoarthritic knee joint. This injection treats the pain and improves joint stability. The hyaluronic acid is derived from bacterial fermentation in *Streptococcus equi* cells and is ultra-purified. The drug is supplied in prefilled 5 ml syringes containing 4 ml of Monovisc. Recommended dosage is one syringe.

J7330

J7330   Autologous cultured chondrocytes, implant

Lay Description

Autologous cultured chondrocytes, also known as Carticel, are a type of cartilage tissue graft indicated for the repair of cartilage defects of the knee, including meniscal knee injuries, osteochondritis dissecans, chondromalacia, and other disorders of cartilage of the knee. Autologous cultured chondrocytes are derived from healthy cartilage tissue cells that are harvested from the patient. The harvested cells are sent to a laboratory and grown in a tissue culture. The cultured chondrocytes are then implanted into the patient's knee at the site of the injury or defect by periosteal injection. The amount of autologous cultured chondrocytes needed to repair damaged knee cartilage varies and is dependent on the size of the damaged area. Most patients receive

between 0.64 million and 3.3 million cells for each square centimeter of damaged area.

J7336

J7336   Capsaicin 8% patch, per sq cm

Lay Description

A capsaicin patch is a localized dermal delivery system. It is a synthetic version of the natural occurring substance found in chili peppers. Capsaicin is an irritant that causes sensation of heat and pain. The capsaicin selectively binds to a protein known as TRPV1 (i.e., capsaicin receptor) that resides on pain and heat sensing neurons. When capsaicin binds to TRPV1, it overwhelms the neuron and depletes one of the neurotransmitters for pain and heat. Neurons that do not contain TRPV1 are unaffected. The capsaicin patch is indicated to relieve the pain of postherpetic neuralgia caused by shingles.

J7500-J7501

J7500   Azathioprine, oral, 50 mg

J7501   Azathioprine, parenteral, 100 mg

Lay Description

Azathioprine is an immunosuppressant used to prevent rejection of kidney transplants. It is also indicated to treat severe rheumatoid arthritis when other medications and treatments have not helped. Less frequently, azathioprine is used to treat ulcerative colitis. Azathioprine is available in oral and injectable forms. Its mechanism of action is not known. The drug suppresses hypersensitivities of the cell-mediated type and causes variable alterations in antibody production.

J7502

J7502   Cyclosporine, oral, 100 mg

Lay Description

Cyclosporine is used to prevent rejection of skin, pancreas, kidney, liver, heart, small intestine, and bone marrow transplants. When a patient receives an allogenic tissue or organ transplant, lymphocytes in the allograft recipient recognize the foreign tissue and attack the transplanted tissue or organ. Cyclosporine can also be used to treat rheumatoid arthritis that is not responding to methotrexate and severe psoriasis. The exact mechanism of action is not known. T-lymphocytes are preferentially inhibited. The 1-helper cell is the primary target, but the 1-suppressor cell may also be suppressed. Cyclosporine also inhibits lymphokine production and release, including interleukin-2 or 1-cell growth factor (TCGF). It should be administered with adrenal corticosteroids but not with other immunosuppressive agents.

J7504

J7504 Lymphocyte immune globulin, antithymocyte globulin, equine, parenteral, 250 mg

Lay Description

Lymphocyte immune globulin, antithymocyte globulin helps to prevent organ rejection in renal allograft transplant patients. It is given at the time of rejection or as an adjunct with other immunosuppressants to delay onset of the first rejection episode. It reduces the number of thymus-dependent lymphocytes and changes the T lymphocyte immunity, which is partially responsible for cell-mediated immunity. Other medications may be prescribed to help prevent rejection of the transplanted kidney (e.g., corticosteroids, azathioprine) and/or prevent infection (e.g., antibiotics, antifungals, antivirals). Lymphocyte immune globulin, antithymocyte globulin is also used for the treatment of moderate to severe aplastic anemia in patients who cannot undergo bone marrow transplantation. It is administered via intravenous infusion over at least four hours.

J7505

J7505 Muromonab-CD3, parenteral, 5 mg

Lay Description

Muromonab-CD3 is a murine monoclonal antibody specific to the CD3 antigen of human T cells. It inhibits the functioning of T cells, which play a major role in acute allograft rejection. It is an immunosuppressant. Muromonab is a monoclonal antibody used to prevent organ transplant rejection in patients who have received kidney, heart, and liver transplants. It blocks the function of the T cells, which play a major role in organ transplant rejection. Recommended adult dose is 5 mg per day in an intravenous injection.

J7506

J7506 Prednisone, oral, per 5 mg

Lay Description

Prednisone is a corticosteroid. Corticosteroids are widely used in medicine to control allergies, inflammation, and many disease processes. Prednisone is similar to a natural hormone produced by the adrenal glands. It is often used to replace this chemical when the body does not make enough. It relieves inflammation and is used to treat certain forms of arthritis; skin, blood, kidney, eye, thyroid, and intestinal disorders; severe allergies; and asthma. Prednisone also is used with other drugs to prevent rejection of transplanted organs and to treat certain types of cancer.

J7507-J7508

J7507 Tacrolimus, immediate release, oral, 1 mg
J7508 Tacrolimus, extended release, oral, 0.1 mg

Lay Description

Tacrolimus is used to reduce the risk of rejection by the body of liver and kidney allogeneic transplants and of bone marrow transplants, usually used with corticosteroids. Recent trials show it to be effective in managing heart, pancreas, pancreatic island cell transplants, and small bowel disease patients. Tacrolimus prevents rejection by impeding T lymphocyte cells, cells that are in the immune system. A lower dose can be used than with cyclosporine because of its potency. Tacrolimus should not be used at the same time as cyclosporine. The current drug should be stopped at least 24 hours before beginning the other one. Tacrolimus can be administered orally, topically, or via intravenous infusion.

J7509

J7509 Methylprednisolone, oral, per 4 mg

Lay Description

Methylprednisolone is a corticosteroid used to treat a variety of conditions. Indications include allergic disorders, arthritis, blood diseases, breathing problems, certain cancers, eye diseases, intestinal disorders, and collagen and skin diseases. Methylprednisolone may also be used with other medications as a replacement for certain hormones. Methylprednisolone works by decreasing the body's immune response to these diseases and reducing symptoms such as swelling and redness. Methylprednisolone may be administered orally, by intramuscular injection in the form of methylprednisolone acetate, or by intravenous infusion in the form of methylprednisolone sodium succinate.

J7510

J7510 Prednisolone, oral, per 5 mg

Lay Description

Prednisolone is a synthetic adrenal corticosteroid. Corticosteroids are natural substances produced by the adrenal glands located adjacent to the kidneys. Corticosteroids are widely used to treat allergies, inflammation, and many disease processes. Prednisolone is used to treat a wide variety of conditions. Oral and injectable prednisolone is used to suppress inflammation in many inflammatory and allergic conditions. Examples include rheumatoid arthritis, systemic lupus, acute gouty arthritis, psoriatic arthritis, ulcerative colitis, and Crohn's disease. Severe allergic conditions that fail conventional treatment may also be treated with prednisolone. Examples include bronchial asthma, allergic rhinitis, drug-induced dermatitis, and contact and atopic dermatitis. Prednisolone is also used in the treatment of leukemia and lymphomas, idiopathic thrombocytopenia purpura, and autoimmune hemolytic anemia. Other miscellaneous conditions treated with this medication include thyroiditis and sarcoidosis. Prednisolone is used as a hormone replacement in patients whose adrenal glands are unable to produce sufficient amounts of corticosteroids. Prednisolone injection or sterile suspension can be injected into a muscle, joint, lesion, or soft tissue.

J7511

J7511   Lymphocyte immune globulin, antithymocyte globulin, rabbit, parenteral, 25 mg

Lay Description
Lymphocyte immune globulin, antithymocyte globulin helps prevent organ rejection in renal allograft transplant patients. It is given at the time of rejection or as an adjunct with other immunosuppressants to delay onset of the first rejection episode. It reduces the number of thymus-dependent lymphocytes and changes the T lymphocyte immunity, which is partially responsible for cell-mediated immunity. Other medications may be prescribed to help prevent rejection of the transplanted kidney (e.g., corticosteroids, azathioprine) and/or prevent infection (e.g., antibiotics, antifungals, antivirals). Lymphocyte immune globulin, antithymocyte globulin is also used for the treatment of moderate to severe aplastic anemia in patients who cannot undergo bone marrow transplantation. It is administered via intravenous infusion over at least four hours.

J7513

J7513   Daclizumab, parenteral, 25 mg

Lay Description
Daclizumab is an immunosuppressive agent indicated to prevent organ rejection in kidney transplant patients. Immunosuppressive agents work to lower the body's natural immunity in patients who receive tissue and organ transplants. When a patient receives a kidney transplant, lymphocytes in the allograft recipient recognize the foreign tissue and attack the transplanted kidney. Daclizumab works by preventing lymphocytes from rejecting the allograft. More specifically, daclizumab works by inhibiting IL2 mediated activation of lymphocytes, a critical pathway in the cellular immune response involved in allograft rejection. The dose of daclizumab varies, but the recommended dose is 1 mg per kg (0.45 mg per pound) of body weight. Daclizumab is administered by intravenous infusion.

J7515-J7516

J7515   Cyclosporine, oral, 25 mg
J7516   Cyclosporine, parenteral, 250 mg

Lay Description
Cyclosporine is used to prevent rejection of skin, pancreas, kidney, liver, heart, small intestine, and bone marrow transplants. When a patient receives an allogenic tissue or organ transplant, lymphocytes in the allograft recipient recognize the foreign tissue and attack the transplanted tissue or organ. Cyclosporine can also be used to treat rheumatoid arthritis that is not responding to methotrexate and severe psoriasis. The exact mechanism of action is not known. T-lymphocytes are preferentially inhibited. The 1-helper cell is the primary target, but the 1-suppressor cell may also be suppressed. Cyclosporine also inhibits lymphokine production and release including interleukin-2 or 1-cell growth factor (TCGF). It should be administered with adrenal corticosteroids but not with other immunosuppressive agents.

J7517

J7517   Mycophenolate mofetil, oral, 250 mg

Lay Description
Mycophenolate mofetil is an immunosuppressive agent indicated to prevent organ rejection in kidney, heart, and liver transplant patients. Immunosuppressive agents work to lower the body's natural immunity in patients who receive tissue and organ transplants. When a patient receives an allogenic tissue or organ transplant, lymphocytes in the allograft recipient recognize the foreign tissue and attack the transplanted tissue or organ. Mycophenolate mofetil works in two ways to prevent rejection. First, it inhibits rejection by preventing the production of T-cells, lymphocytes, and development of antibodies from B-cells that stimulate rejection. Second, mycophenolate mofetil inhibits mobilization of leukocytes to inflammatory sites. It is generally used in conjunction with cyclosporin and corticosteroids to prevent rejection. Mycophenolate mofetil may be administered orally by tablet (available in 250 mg or 500 mg doses) or in a liquid suspension (available in a dose of 200 mg/ml). This agent may also be administered by intravenous infusion in the form of mycophenolate mofetil hydrochloride (available in 500 mg vials) at a suggested rate not to exceed 500 mg over a two-hour period.

J7518

J7518   Mycophenolic acid, oral, 180 mg

Lay Description
Mycophenolic acid is a formulation of mycophenolate sodium. It acts by inhibiting lymphocyte proliferation and antibody production and is an immunosuppressive agent indicated to prevent organ rejection in kidney transplant patients. Mycophenolic

acid is generally used in conjunction with cyclosporine and corticosteroids to prevent rejection. The recommended dose of mycophenolic acid is 720 mg orally twice a day on an empty stomach.

J7520

J7520   Sirolimus, oral, 1 mg

Lay Description
Sirolimus is an immunosuppressive agent formerly known as rapamycin. It is a macrocyclic lactone found in the soil of Easter Island. Sirolimus resembles tacrolimus and binds to the same intracellular binding protein or immunophilins known as FKBP-12. Sirolimus, in combination with cyclosporine or tacrolimus and steroids, is used for the prevention of acute kidney allograft rejection. Sirolimus is administered orally.

J7525

J7525   Tacrolimus, parenteral, 5 mg

Lay Description
Tacrolimus is used to reduce the risk of rejection by the body of liver and kidney allogeneic transplants and of bone marrow transplants, usually used with corticosteroids. Recent trials show it to be effective in managing heart, pancreas, pancreatic island cell transplants, and small bowel disease patients. Tacrolimus prevents rejection by impeding T lymphocyte cells, cells that are in the immune system. A lower dose can be used than with cyclosporine because of its potency. Tacrolimus should not be used at the same time as cyclosporine. The current drug should be stopped at least 24 hours before beginning the other one. Tacrolimus can be administered orally, topically, or via intravenous infusion.

J7527

J7527   Everolimus, oral, 0.25 mg

Lay Description
Everolimus inhibits a serine-threonine kinase protein pathway that does not function appropriately in certain human cancers. Everolimus binds to a protein site within the cell preventing the completion of the kinase pathway. It ultimately reduces the expression of vascular endothelial growth factor, which retards cell growth. Everolimus is indicated as a treatment for pancreatic progressive neuroendocrine tumors in patients who cannot be treated with surgery or who have advanced metastatic disease, advanced renal cell carcinoma after failed treatment with sunitinib or sorafenib, and subependymal giant cell astrocytoma (SEGA) associated with tuberous sclerosis who are not candidates for surgical resection. Recommended dose is 2.5 to 10 mg daily based on patient condition and disease process.

J7599

J7599   Immunosuppressive drug, not otherwise classified

Lay Description
Immunosuppressive drugs are chemical compounds that inhibit or prevent the activity of the immune system. These drugs are indicated for the prevention of rejection of a transplanted organ or tissue, to treat autoimmune diseases (e.g., rheumatoid arthritis, ulcerative colitis), and to treat inflammatory diseases not of autoimmune origin (e.g., long-term asthma). This code should be used only for immunosuppressive drugs that are not otherwise classified among the other HCPCS Level II codes.

J7604, J7608

J7604   Acetylcysteine, inhalation solution, compounded product, administered through DME, unit dose form, per g

J7608   Acetylcysteine, inhalation solution, FDA-approved final product, noncompounded, administered through DME, unit dose form, per g

Lay Description
Acetylcysteine is a derivative of the naturally occurring amino acid L-cysteine. The drug is available in inhalation solution, oral, and injectable forms. It is a mucolytic agent when inhaled, used to lower the viscosity (i.e., thin) mucous secretions to allow easier expulsion or easier breathing. The oral and injectable forms are used as an antidote for acetaminophen overdose to prevent life-threatening liver damage. Acetylcysteine reacts with the acetaminophen, rendering some of the acetaminophen harmless. The inhaled form is indicated as an adjunct treatment for patients with acute and chronic bronchopulmonary diseases, cystic fibrosis, tracheostomies, pulmonary complications associated with surgery, post-traumatic chest conditions, and atelectasis due to mucous obstruction. It is also used during anesthesia and in diagnostic bronchial studies. As an antidote for acetaminophen poisoning, acetylcysteine should be administered as soon as possible, but within 24 hours after the overdose. The inhaled form is administered by nebulizer, tent, or as a compressed gas. The injectable form is administered by intravenous infusion over 60 minutes. The oral form should be administered after gastric lavage or emesis. The dosage depends on the indication and drug form.

J7605

J7605   Arformoterol, inhalation solution, FDA approved final product, noncompounded, administered through DME, unit dose form, 15 mcg

Lay Description
Arformoterol tartrate is a mirror image of the drug formoterol that exhibits slightly different properties. The drug, similar to formoterol, is a long-acting,

selective, beta$_2$-adrenergic receptor agonist. Arformoterol has twice as much potency as formoterol. Inhaled arformoterol acts locally in the lung as a bronchodilator. Arformoterol tartrate inhalation solution is indicated for the long-term maintenance treatment of patients with chronic obstructive pulmonary disease (COPD), including chronic bronchitis and emphysema. The recommended dosage is 15 mcg administered twice a day (morning and evening) by nebulization. The drug is inhaled and should be administered by a standard nebulizer connected to an air compressor.

J7606

J7606   Formoterol fumarate, inhalation solution, FDA approved final product, noncompounded, administered through DME, unit dose form, 20 mcg

Lay Description
Formoterol fumarate is a long-acting selective beta$_2$-adrenergic receptor agonist 33 (beta$_2$-agonist). Inhaled formoterol acts locally in the lung as a bronchodilator. This is a long-term medication used to treat chronic obstructive pulmonary disease (COPD), including bronchitis and emphysema. The recommended dose is 20 micrograms twice a day through a nebulizer.

J7607, J7609-J7615

J7607   Levalbuterol, inhalation solution, compounded product, administered through DME, concentrated form, 0.5 mg

J7609   Albuterol, inhalation solution, compounded product, administered through DME, unit dose, 1 mg

J7610   Albuterol, inhalation solution, compounded product, administered through DME, concentrated form, 1 mg

J7611   Albuterol, inhalation solution, FDA-approved final product, noncompounded, administered through DME, concentrated form, 1 mg

J7612   Levalbuterol, inhalation solution, FDA-approved final product, noncompounded, administered through DME, concentrated form, 0.5 mg

J7613   Albuterol, inhalation solution, FDA-approved final product, noncompounded, administered through DME, unit dose, 1 mg

J7614   Levalbuterol, inhalation solution, FDA-approved final product, noncompounded, administered through DME, unit dose, 0.5 mg

J7615   Levalbuterol, inhalation solution, compounded product, administered through DME, unit dose, 0.5 mg

Lay Description
Albuterol and levalbuterol are selective beta2-adrenergic receptor agonists that function as bronchodilators. The drugs block the actions of enzymes that cause the smooth muscles within the respiratory tract to contract. This relaxation of smooth muscles allows easier breathing. Albuterol and levalbuterol are indicated for the prevention and relief of bronchospasm in patients with reversible obstructive pulmonary disease and for the prevention of exercise-induced bronchospasm. Effects of the drug may last up to six hours after administration.

J7608

J7608   Acetylcysteine, inhalation solution, FDA-approved final product, noncompounded, administered through DME, unit dose form, per g

Lay Description
Please refer to code J7604 for the description.

J7609-J7610

J7609   Albuterol, inhalation solution, compounded product, administered through DME, unit dose, 1 mg

J7610   Albuterol, inhalation solution, compounded product, administered through DME, concentrated form, 1 mg

Lay Description
Please refer to code J7607 for the description.

J7615

J7615   Levalbuterol, inhalation solution, compounded product, administered through DME, unit dose, 0.5 mg

Lay Description
Please refer to code J7607 for the description.

J7620

J7620   Albuterol, up to 2.5 mg and ipratropium bromide, up to 0.5 mg, FDA-approved final product, noncompounded, administered through DME

Lay Description
Albuterol and ipratropium bromide is a combination bronchodilator used in inhalation solutions. Albuterol is a selective beta2 -adrenergic receptor agonist that blocks the actions of enzymes that cause the smooth muscles within the respiratory tract to contract. This relaxation of smooth muscles allows easier breathing. Ipratropium bromide is an anticholinergic agent that binds to receptors of vascular smooth muscle and endothelial cells and increases intracellular concentrations of guanosine cyclic monophosphate (cGMP), which creates smooth muscle cell relaxation. Albuterol and ipratropium bromide is indicated as a treatment for bronchospasms associated with chronic obstructive pulmonary disease (COPD). One vial

usually contains 2.5 mg or albuterol combined with 0.5 mg of ipratropium bromide. The drug is available as a metered dose inhaler or in a solution for administration via a reusable nebulizer. Recommended dosage for inhalation is one vial four times a day administered administration via a reusable nebulizer.

J7622

J7622   Beclomethasone, inhalation solution, compounded product, administered through DME, unit dose form, per mg

Lay Description
Beclomethasone is a corticosteroid. Beclomethasone is indicated for the treatment of bronchial asthma when administered as an oral inhalant. Beclomethasone controls symptoms of asthma and other lung diseases but does not cure them.

J7624

J7624   Betamethasone, inhalation solution, compounded product, administered through DME, unit dose form, per mg

Lay Description
Betamethasone valerate is a corticosteroid with anti-inflammatory and immunosuppressive abilities. The inhalation solution is used to prevent moderate to severe asthma.

J7626-J7627

J7626   Budesonide, inhalation solution, FDA-approved final product, noncompounded, administered through DME, unit dose form, up to 0.5 mg

J7627   Budesonide, inhalation solution, compounded product, administered through DME, unit dose form, up to 0.5 mg

Lay Description
Budesonide is a corticosteroid with anti-inflammatory and immunosuppressive abilities. It is available as an inhalation solution in several formulations including a non-compounded unit dose form, a powder compounded for inhalation, and a concentrated form. The inhalation solution is used to prevent wheezing, shortness of breath, and difficulty breathing caused by severe asthma and other lung diseases. Budesonide controls symptoms of asthma and other lung diseases but does not cure them. Budesonide is usually inhaled once or twice a day.

J7628-J7629

J7628   Bitolterol mesylate, inhalation solution, compounded product, administered through DME, concentrated form, per mg

J7629   Bitolterol mesylate, inhalation solution, compounded product, administered through DME, unit dose form, per mg

Lay Description
Bitolterol mesylate is a bronchodilator used in the treatment of bronchospasm associated with asthma. It may also be helpful in the treatment of emphysema and chronic bronchitis. Asthma is a condition that causes narrowing of the bronchial tubes due to muscle spasm and inflammation within the bronchial tubes. Bitolterol mesylate relaxes the smooth muscles surrounding these airway tubes, thereby increasing the diameter and ease of air flow through the tubes. Bitolterol mesylate is unique in that it is a "prodrug" because the body must first metabolize it before it becomes active. Bitolterol is administered in an aerosol inhaled by mouth. It usually is taken as needed to relieve symptoms or every eight hours to prevent symptoms.

J7631-J7632

J7631   Cromolyn sodium, inhalation solution, FDA-approved final product, noncompounded, administered through DME, unit dose form, per 10 mg

J7632   Cromolyn sodium, inhalation solution, compounded product, administered through DME, unit dose form, per 10 mg

Lay Description
Cromolyn sodium is a nonsteroidal anti-inflammatory that works by preventing the release of substances in the body that cause inflammation. More specifically, cromolyn sodium acts indirectly by blocking calcium ions from entering the mast cell, thereby preventing mediator release. This prevents the release of substances that cause inflammation in the air passages of the lungs. Cromolyn sodium is used to prevent wheezing, shortness of breath, and difficulty breathing caused by asthma. It is also used to prevent breathing difficulties (bronchospasm) during exercise. Cromolyn comes as powder-filled capsules and solution to take by mouth and an aerosol to inhale by mouth. The inhalant form is used to prevent asthma attacks and other conditions involving inflammation of the lung tissues. It is usually inhaled three or four times a day to prevent asthma attacks or within an hour before activities to prevent breathing difficulties caused by exercise.

J7633-J7634

J7633 Budesonide, inhalation solution, FDA-approved final product, noncompounded, administered through DME, concentrated form, per 0.25 mg

J7634 Budesonide, inhalation solution, compounded product, administered through DME, concentrated form, per 0.25 mg

Lay Description
Budesonide is a corticosteroid with anti-inflammatory and immunosuppressive abilities. It is available as an inhalation solution in several formulations, including a non-compounded unit dose form, a powder compounded for inhalation, and a concentrated form. The inhalation solution is used to prevent wheezing, shortness of breath, and difficulty breathing caused by severe asthma and other lung diseases. Budesonide controls symptoms of asthma and other lung diseases but does not cure them. Budesonide is usually inhaled once or twice a day.

J7635-J7636

J7635 Atropine, inhalation solution, compounded product, administered through DME, concentrated form, per mg

J7636 Atropine, inhalation solution, compounded product, administered through DME, unit dose form, per mg

Lay Description
Atropine is an extract of an alkaloid from the plants belladonna, hyoscyamus, or stramonium. It is also made synthetically. Atropine sulfate is a highly toxic compound of atropine and sulfuric acid that has the same uses and effects as atropine. It blocks the neurotransmitter acetylcholine in muscarinic receptors of the parasympathetic system. Muscarinic receptors occur throughout the nervous system including in the heart, smooth muscles of the blood vessels, lungs, salivary glands, gastrointestinal tract, and eye. Atropine sulfate in clinical doses counteracts the peripheral vessel dilatation and abrupt decrease in blood pressure produced by other drugs or biologicals. Atropine is used to reduce secretions in the respiratory tract.

J7637-J7638

J7637 Dexamethasone, inhalation solution, compounded product, administered through DME, concentrated form, per mg

J7638 Dexamethasone, inhalation solution, compounded product, administered through DME, unit dose form, per mg

Lay Description
Dexamethasone is a synthetic corticosteroid that is similar to a natural hormone produced by the adrenal gland. It is 25 times as potent as cortisol. Dexamethasone has anti-inflammatory, antiemetic

and immunosuppressant properties. It is used to treat a wide variety of disorders.

J7639

J7639 Dornase alfa, inhalation solution, FDA-approved final product, noncompounded, administered through DME, unit dose form, per mg

Lay Description
Dornase alpha is an inhaled drug indicated for the treatment of cystic fibrosis. Healthy lungs continually secrete fluid into the airways to keep them moist. However, in cystic fibrosis, a reduced amount of water is present in the secretions making them thick and difficult to cough up or spit out. These thickened secretions block the airways, causing labored breathing and promoting the growth of bacteria and infection. These thickened secretions contain high concentrations of deoxyribonucleic acid (DNA) and dornase alpha, a genetically engineered form of the human enzyme deoxyribonuclease or DNAse. Dornase alpha works by breaking down the DNA, thereby reducing the thickness of the fluids. Dornase alpha is supplied in single-use ampules that contain 2.5 ml of a sterile, clear, colorless solution containing 1 mg/ml of dornase alpha.

J7640

J7640 Formoterol, inhalation solution, compounded product, administered through DME, unit dose form, 12 mcg

Lay Description
Formoterol is a long-acting selective beta2 adrenergic receptor agonist 33 (beta2 agonist). Inhaled formoterol acts locally in the lung as a bronchodilator. This is a long-term medication used to treat asthma and to prevent exercise-induced bronchospasm in adults and children older than 12. It can also be used long term to treat chronic obstructive pulmonary disease (COPD), including bronchitis and emphysema. The usual dose is 12 micrograms every 12 hours through an inhaler.

J7641

J7641 Flunisolide, inhalation solution, compounded product, administered through DME, unit dose, per mg

Lay Description
Flunisolide is a corticosteroid used as maintenance treatment for asthma. It is shown to be several hundred times stronger in animal anti-inflammatory assays than the cortisol standard. This may reduce or eliminate the need for oral corticosteroids. Corticosteroids reduce or eliminate inflammation in the lining of the airways. They may also reduce the reaction to inhaled allergen and can be used for the management of the nasal symptoms of seasonal or perennial rhinitis. The recommended dose varies depending on the treatment.

J7642-J7643

J7642   Glycopyrrolate, inhalation solution, compounded product, administered through DME, concentrated form, per mg

J7643   Glycopyrrolate, inhalation solution, compounded product, administered through DME, unit dose form, per mg

Lay Description

Glycopyrrolate is an anticholinergic drug that inhibits the action of acetylcholine on structures innervated by postganglionic cholinergic nerves and on smooth muscles that respond to acetylcholine but lack cholinergic innervation. It reduces the amount of free acidity of gastric secretions and controls excessive pharyngeal, tracheal, and bronchial secretions. Glycopyrrolate inhalation solution is used for maintenance treatment for asthma and chronic obstructive pulmonary disease (COPD). It has been shown to be an effective bronchodilator when used once a day.

J7644-J7645

J7644   Ipratropium bromide, inhalation solution, FDA-approved final product, noncompounded, administered through DME, unit dose form, per mg

J7645   Ipratropium bromide, inhalation solution, compounded product, administered through DME, unit dose form, per mg

Lay Description

Ipratropium bromide is an anticholinergic agent that functions as a bronchodilator when inhaled. The drug binds to receptors of vascular smooth muscle and endothelial cells and increases intracellular concentrations of guanosine cyclic monophosphate (cGMP), which creates smooth muscle cell relaxation. Inhaled ipratropium bromide, singularly or in combination with other bronchodilators, is for the treatment of bronchospasms associated with chronic obstructive pulmonary disease (COPD) including chronic bronchitis and emphysema. Recommended dosage for inhalation is 36 mcg four times a day.

J7647, J7650

J7647   Isoetharine HCl, inhalation solution, compounded product, administered through DME, concentrated form, per mg

J7650   Isoetharine HCl, inhalation solution, compounded product, administered through DME, unit dose form, per mg

Lay Description

Isoetharine hydrochloride is a bronchodilator that relaxes the smooth muscles of the lungs that constrict due to inflammation or disease. It is used to treat asthma, emphysema, bronchitis, and chronic obstructive pulmonary disease (COPD). The medication comes in a solution that is used with a nebulizer and in a hand-held aerosol form.

J7648-J7649

J7648   Isoetharine HCl, inhalation solution, FDA-approved final product, noncompounded, administered through DME, concentrated form, per mg

J7649   Isoetharine HCl, inhalation solution, FDA-approved final product, noncompounded, administered through DME, unit dose form, per mg

Lay Description

Isoetharine hydrochloride (HCl) is a bronchodilator that relaxes the smooth muscles of the lungs that constrict due to inflammation or disease. It is used to treat asthma, emphysema, bronchitis, and chronic obstructive pulmonary disease (COPD).

J7650

J7650   Isoetharine HCl, inhalation solution, compounded product, administered through DME, unit dose form, per mg

Lay Description

Please refer to code J7647 for the description.

J7657-J7660

J7657   Isoproterenol HCl, inhalation solution, compounded product, administered through DME, concentrated form, per mg

J7658   Isoproterenol HCl, inhalation solution, FDA-approved final product, noncompounded, administered through DME, concentrated form, per mg

J7659   Isoproterenol HCl, inhalation solution, FDA-approved final product, noncompounded, administered through DME, unit dose form, per mg

J7660   Isoproterenol HCl, inhalation solution, compounded product, administered through DME, unit dose form, per mg

Lay Description

Isoproterenol hydrochloride (HCl) is a synthetic sympathometic amine that is similar to epinephrine but acts almost entirely on beta-receptors. It lowers peripheral vascular resistance in skeletal muscle, renal, and mesenteric vascular beds. Cardiac output is increased due to the lowered peripheral resistance. The inhalation form is used to treat bronchospasms. Commercial inhalation forms of isoproterenol have been discontinued.

J7665

J7665   Mannitol, administered through an inhaler, 5 mg

Lay Description

Mannitol inhalation substance is used in bronchial challenge tests to help diagnose patients with symptoms of asthma. It is a sugar alcohol substance that constricts the bronchial constriction. Respiratory measurements are taken prior to and after the administration of the mannitol inhaler. The mannitol is administered to the patient in graduated doses until the patient has a positive response or 635 mg of mannitol has been administered.

J7667-J7670

J7667 **Metaproterenol sulfate, inhalation solution, compounded product, concentrated form, per 10 mg**

J7668 **Metaproterenol sulfate, inhalation solution, FDA-approved final product, noncompounded, administered through DME, concentrated form, per 10 mg**

J7669 **Metaproterenol sulfate, inhalation solution, FDA-approved final product, noncompounded, administered through DME, unit dose form, per 10 mg**

J7670 **Metaproterenol sulfate, inhalation solution, compounded product, administered through DME, unit dose form, per 10 mg**

Lay Description
Metaproterenol sulfate is a bronchodilator used to treat asthma, bronchitis, and emphysema. It acts on the beta receptors in the bronchial smooth muscles to relax bronchospasms that cause difficulty breathing. The medication comes in powder form and in a solution that is used with a nebulizer and in a hand-held aerosol.

J7674

J7674 **Methacholine chloride administered as inhalation solution through a nebulizer, per 1 mg**

Lay Description
Methacholine chloride is a synthetic choline ester that acts to induce bronchoconstriction. This medication is used in a bronchospasm provocation test to diagnose asthma. This is often done when spirometry alone does not provide a definitive diagnosis. Two different dilution schedules are used in North America to perform the test. Both use 100 mg of methacholine. One is based on a two minute tidal breathing dosing protocol and the other is a five breath dosimeter protocol. Both methods utilize a nebulizer to administer the medication.

J7676

J7676 **Pentamidine isethionate, inhalation solution, compounded product, administered through DME, unit dose form, per 300 mg**

Lay Description
Pentamidine isethionate is an aromatic diamidine that is an anti-protozoal. Its mechanism of action is not completely known. It is thought the drug interferes with the synthesis of DNA, RNA, and protein causing cell death. Pentamidine isethionate is indicated as a treatment for *Pneumocystis Jiroveci*, trypanosomiasis,

and leishmaniasis. The drug may be administered by intramuscular injection, inhalation, or intravenous infusion over one hour. The inhalation solution is inhaled through a special breathing unit that ensures the drug reaches deep into the lungs. The recommended dosage for the inhalation solution is 300 mg once a month and administered via a nebulizer. Treatment usually takes 30-45 minutes.

J7680-J7681

J7680 **Terbutaline sulfate, inhalation solution, compounded product, administered through DME, concentrated form, per mg**

J7681 **Terbutaline sulfate, inhalation solution, compounded product, administered through DME, unit dose form, per mg**

Lay Description
Terbutaline sulfate is a beta$_2$-adrenergic agonist that functions as a bronchodilator. It works, in part, by stimulating the conversion of adenosine triphosphate (ATP) to cyclic 3',5'-adenosine monophosphate, which relaxes bronchial muscles. Terbutaline sulfate is indicated for the prevention and reversal of bronchospasm in asthma, bronchitis, and emphysema.

J7682

J7682 **Tobramycin, inhalation solution, FDA-approved final product, noncompounded, unit dose form, administered through DME, per 300 mg**

Lay Description
Tobramycin is an aminoglycoside antibiotic, which is derived from various species of *Streptomyces* bacteria or produced synthetically. Aminoglycosides inhibit bacterial protein synthesis by binding with the 30S ribosomal subunit and are bactericidal. Streptomycin is derived from *Streptomyces tenebrarius* and inhibits protein synthesis, causing cell death. Susceptibility studies should be performed prior to the administration of tobramycin. It is indicated in the treatment of infections caused by gram-negative bacillary bacteria, including *Pseudomonas aeruginosa*, *Staphylococcus aureus*, *Escherichia coli*, *Klebsiella* species, *Enterobacter* species, *Serretia* species, *Proteus* species, *Providencia* species, and *Citrobacter* species. The inhalation form is indicated in the treatment of *Pseudomonas aeruginosa* in patients with cystic fibrosis.

J7683-J7684

J7683 Triamcinolone, inhalation solution, compounded product, administered through DME, concentrated form, per mg

J7684 Triamcinolone, inhalation solution, compounded product, administered through DME, unit dose form, per mg

Lay Description
Triamcinolone is a synthetic corticosteroid, which is analogous to corticosteroids produced by the adrenal cortex. The drug is one to two times more potent than prednisone. Its mechanism of actions is not clearly defined. Triamcinolone does decrease inflammation by stabilizing leukocytes, suppress the chemicals normally released in immune response, and stimulate bone marrow. Inhaled triamcinolone is a local anti-inflammatory delivering the drug directly to the lungs. The drug has no effect on acute bronchospasms, but is indicated for prophylactic and maintenance therapy of asthma.

J7685

J7685 Tobramycin, inhalation solution, compounded product, administered through DME, unit dose form, per 300 mg

Lay Description
Tobramycin is an aminoglycoside antibiotic, which is derived from various species of Streptomyces bacteria or produced synthetically. Aminoglycosides inhibit bacterial protein synthesis by binding with the 30S ribosomal subunit and are bactericidal. Streptomycin is derived from *Streptomyces tenebrarius* and inhibits protein synthesis, causing cell death. Susceptibility studies should be performed prior to the administration of tobramycin. It is indicated in the treatment of infections caused by gram-negative bacillary bacteria, including *Pseudomonas aeruginosa*, *Staphylococcus aureus*, *Escherichia coli*, *Klebsiella* species, *Enterobacter* species, *Serretia* species, *Proteus* species, *Providencia* species, and *Citrobacter* species. The inhalation form is indicated in the treatment of *Pseudomonas aeruginosa* in patients with cystic fibrosis.

J7686

J7686 Treprostinil, inhalation solution, FDA-approved final product, noncompounded, administered through DME, unit dose form, 1.74 mg

Lay Description
Treprostinil inhalation solution is used for the treatment of pulmonary arterial hypertension to improve exercise activities. Treprostinil is a prostacyclin analogue and provides direct vasodilation of pulmonary and systemic arterial vascular beds and inhibition of platelet aggregation. Recommended dose is an initial treatment of three breaths per treatment session, four times daily. The dose is increased by an additional three breaths at approximately one to two week intervals, if tolerated, until nine breaths are reached per treatment session, four times daily. The medication is administered through an ultrasonic, pulsed-delivery nebulizer.

J7699

J7699 NOC drugs, inhalation solution administered through DME

Lay Description
Use this code to represent an inhalation drug that has been administered through DME and is not represented by any other level I or level II HCPCS code.

J7799

J7799 NOC drugs, other than inhalation drugs, administered through DME

Lay Description
Use this code to represent a drug that has been administered through DME, but is not an inhalation drug. Be sure the drug does not have any other specified level I or level II HCPCS code to represent it.

J8498

J8498 Antiemetic drug, rectal/suppository, not otherwise specified

Lay Description
Antiemetic medication may be used in conjunction with anti-cancer drugs such as chemotherapeutic agents and acts to prevent or relieve nausea and vomiting. Antiemetics are antagonists for a specific serotonin subtype receptor located on the nerve terminals of the vagus in the small intestine.

J8499

J8499 Prescription drug, oral, nonchemotherapeutic, NOS

Lay Description
Use this code to represent an oral prescription drug that is not a form of chemotherapy and is not represented by any other Level I or Level II HCPCS code.

J8501

J8501 Aprepitant, oral, 5 mg

Lay Description
Aprepitant is a chemical complex used as an oral antiemetic drug. It seeks cell receptors of human substance P/neurokinin 1 (NK1). NK1s are peptides found in the central and peripheral nervous systems involved in the transmission of a signal from outside the cell wall into the cell. Aprepitant blocks those transmissions. It is used in combination with a corticosteroid and a 5-HT3 antagonist to prevent acute and delayed nausea and vomiting associated with initial and repeat courses of certain chemotherapies, including high-dose cisplatin.

J8510

J8510   Busulfan, oral, 2 mg

Lay Description

Busulfan is an alkylating agent that is used to reduce tumor growth. It causes breaks in the DNA, which prevent replication, thus interfering with tumor cell reproduction. It is used in the treatment of chronic myelogenous leukemia, and disorders such as severe thrombocytosis and polycythemia vera. Side effects commonly reported from busulfan are brittle or thinned hair, dry skin, diarrhea, weight loss, fatigue, and blistering of the mouth. This code is for the oral administration per 2 mg.

J8515

J8515   Cabergoline, oral, 0.25 mg

Lay Description

Cabergoline is a chemical complex that binds to a dopamine receptor on cells and inhibits the secretion of prolactin. Prolactin is a hormone produced by the anterior pituitary gland that stimulates and sustains lactation. Cabergoline is indicated for the treatment of hyperprolactinemia, whether idiopathic or caused by a pituitary adenoma. The recommended initial dosage is 0.25 mg twice weekly increasing to 1 mg twice weekly depending upon the prolactin levels in the patient's blood. Cabergoline is available only as a self-administrable oral tablet.

J8520-J8521

J8520   Capecitabine, oral, 150 mg
J8521   Capecitabine, oral, 500 mg

Lay Description

Capecitabine is an antineoplastic drug that is broken down in the liver into fluorouracil, also known as 5 FU. Fluorouracil is a fluorinated analogue of uracil. Uracil is a chemical compound found in nucleic acids that interferes with the synthesis of DNA and RNA causing cell death. Capecitabine, singularly or in combination with other chemotherapeutic drugs, is indicated as a treatment for colorectal cancer and metastatic breast cancer. The drug is self-administered orally.

J8530

J8530   Cyclophosphamide, oral, 25 mg

Lay Description

Cyclophosphamide is a synthetic antineoplastic drug chemically related to the nitrogen mustards. The drug itself is inert and functions only after transformation in the liver to active alkylating metabolites. These metabolites interfere with the growth of susceptible rapidly proliferating malignant cells. The mechanism of action is thought to be its interference with the DNA of the tumor cell causing cell death. Cyclophosphamide is indicated singularly or in combination with other chemotherapeutic drugs, to treat a wide variety of cancers including Hodgkin's disease, lymphosarcoma, acute lymphocytic leukemia, Burkitt's lymphoma, carcinoma of the breast, multiple myeloma, chronic lymphocytic leukemia, bronchogenic carcinoma, neuroblastoma, ovarian carcinoma, and carcinoma of the uterine cervix. It is also used as an immunosuppressant to prevent transplant rejection and in the treatment of certain diseases with abnormal immune function, including severe lupus manifestations and vasculitis. Cyclophosphamide may be administered via intravenous injection or infusion, or may be injected intramuscularly, intraperitoneally, or intrapleurally. An oral version is also available. Dosage depends upon body weight and the disease being treated. The lyophilized version of cyclophosphamide is a freeze-dried version of the drug.

J8540

J8540   Dexamethasone, oral, 0.25 mg

Lay Description

Dexamethasone is a synthetic corticosteroid that is similar to a natural hormone produced by the adrenal gland. It is 25 times as potent as cortisol. Dexamethasone has anti-inflammatory, antiemetic and immunosuppressant properties. It is used to treat a wide variety of disorders.

J8560

J8560   Etoposide, oral, 50 mg

Lay Description

Etoposide is a semisynthetic derivative of podophyllotoxin, a toxic compound found in the rhizomes and roots of the mandrake plant. It is believed to inhibit the repair of DNA, causing cell death. Etoposide is an antineoplastic drug used in combination with other chemotherapeutic agents. It is available in injectable or oral versions. Injectable etoposide is indicated for the treatment of small-cell lung cancer and refractory testicular cancer that has been treated previously with surgery, radiation, or other chemotherapy. The oral version is indicated for the treatment of small-cell lung cancer. The recommended dosage of the injectable version ranges from 35 to 100 mg per m^2 of body surface depending on which disease is being treated. The injectable version is administered by intravenous infusion over 30 to 60 minutes. The recommended dosage for the oral version is two times the intravenous version.

J8562

J8562   Fludarabine phosphate, oral, 10 mg

Lay Description

Fludarabine phosphate is an antineoplastic drug that is a fluorinated nucleotide analogue of the antiviral agent vidarabine. It is rapidly broken down into 2-fluoro-ara-A, which inhibits DNA synthesis and causes cell death. Fludarabine phosphate is indicated for the treatment of beta-cell chronic lymphocytic leukemia for patients who have not responded to an alkylating drug treatment. This drug is available in liquid form for IV infusions or in tablet form for oral administration. The recommended dose for oral administration is 40 mg per meter squared of body surface area.

J8565

J8565   Gefitinib, oral, 250 mg

Lay Description
Gefitinib is a chemical complex used as an antineoplastic drug. It inhibits forms of the amino acid tyrosine from binding to epidermal growth factor receptor (EGFR) sites. EGFR is expressed on the cell surface of many normal and cancer cells. Gefitinib is indicated for the treatment of patients with locally advanced or metastatic non-small-cell lung cancer after failure of both platinum-based and docetaxel chemotherapies. It is available only as an oral self-administrable drug. The recommended dosage is 250 mg daily. Gefitinib has limited distribution under a risk management plan called the IRESSATM Access Program, to the following patient populations: patients currently receiving and benefiting from gefitinib; patients who have previously received and benefited from gefitinib; and previously enrolled patients or new patients in non-investigational new drug (IND) clinical trials approved by an institutional review board prior to June 17, 2005. New patients may also be able to obtain gefitinib if the manufacturer decides to make it available under IND and the patients meet the criteria for enrollment under the IND.

J8597

J8597   Antiemetic drug, oral, not otherwise specified

Lay Description
This code is used to report the supply of oral antiemetic drugs that do not have another specific HCPCS Level II code. An antiemetic drug is given to prevent or relieve nausea and vomiting. An oral antiemetic may be indicated at the time of chemotherapy treatment to help allay the side effect of nausea and vomiting that often accompanies chemotherapy.

J8600

J8600   Melphalan, oral, 2 mg

Lay Description
Melphalan hydrochloride is a derivative of nitrogen mustard used as an antineoplastic drug. It interferes with RNA synthesis causing cell death. Melphalan is indicated for the treatment of multiple myeloma and advanced epithelial ovarian cancer. The injectable form is used for the treatment of multiple myeloma when the oral form is inappropriate. The recommended oral dosage for ovarian cancer is 0.2 mg pr kg of body weight for five days. The recommended oral dosage for multiple myeloma is 6

mg per day for two to three weeks. Each course can be repeated after four weeks.

J8610

J8610   Methotrexate, oral, 2.5 mg

Lay Description
Methotrexate sodium is a chemical complex that blocks cell metabolism. It works by hindering the production of an enzyme needed for the metabolism of dividing cells, like those involved in inflammation and the immune response. Methotrexate has been found useful in treating diseases linked with abnormally rapid cell growth. It is indicated singularly or in combination as a treatment for gestational choriocarcinoma, chorioadenoma destruens, hydatidiform mole, breast cancer, epidermoid cancers of the head and neck, advanced mycosis fungoides, squamous and small cell lung cancer, advanced non-Hodgkin's lymphoma, acute lymphocytic leukemia, Burkitt's lymphoma, and lymphosarcoma. It is also used to treat rheumatoid and psoriatic arthritis and severe psoriasis that is unresponsive to other treatments.

J8650

J8650   Nabilone, oral, 1 mg

Lay Description
Nabilone is a Schedule II, synthetic cannabinoid that is similar to the active ingredient found in the marijuana plant. Nabilone, like its natural counterpart, produces complex effects on the central nervous system, including alterations in mental status. It is suggested that the antiemetic effect of nabilone is caused by the cannabinoid receptor system in neural tissues. Nabilone is indicated for the treatment of nausea and vomiting associated with cancer chemotherapy in patients who have not adequately responded to conventional antiemetics. Patients should use this drug only when they are under the close supervision of another person. These restrictions are required as many of the patients treated with nabilone experience altered mental states not observed with other antiemetic drugs. Nabilone has the potential for abuse and misuse. This is an oral drug with a recommended dosage of one to two mg twice a day during each cycle of chemotherapy. Maximum recommended dosage is six mg per day. If needed, administration of the drug may continue for 48 hours after the last dose of each chemotherapy cycle.

J8700

J8700   Temozolomide, oral, 5 mg

Lay Description
Temozolomide is a chemical complex that is broken down in the liver into monomethyltriazene, also known as MTIC. MTIC causes breaks in the DNA, which prevents replication, thus interfering with tumor cell reproduction. Temozolomide is indicated for the treatment of adult patients with newly diagnosed

glioblastoma multiforme, and for the treatment of adult patients with refractory anaplastic astrocytoma. Temozolomide is available only as a self-administrable oral drug. The recommended dosage is 75 mg per m2 of body surface.

J8705

J8705   Topotecan, oral, 0.25 mg

Lay Description
Topotecan hydrochloride is an antineoplastic drug that is a semisynthetic derivative of camptothecin, an alkaloid extract from plants such as Camptotheca acuminata. The drug works by causing breaks in DNA that the cell cannot repair leading to cell death. Topotecan hydrochloride is indicated as a treatment for metastatic carcinoma of the ovaries after failure of prior chemotherapy. It is also indicated as a treatment for small cell lung cancer that responded to chemotherapy, but subsequently progressed. The recommended dose is 2.3 mg per m2 of body surface once daily for five consecutive days.

J8999

J8999   Prescription drug, oral, chemotherapeutic, NOS

Lay Description
Use this code to represent an oral prescription drug that has been taken as a form of chemotherapy, and is not represented by any other level I or level II HCPCS code.

J9000

J9000   Injection, doxorubicin HCl, 10 mg

Lay Description
Doxorubicin hydrochloride is an anthracycline antibiotic antineoplastic drug isolated from the bacterium *Streptomyces peucetius* var. *caesius*. It binds to DNA and inhibits RNA synthesis, causing cell death. It is utilized to treat many forms of cancer, such as bladder, breast, lung, stomach, and thyroid cancer, as well as Hodgkin's and non-Hodgkin's disease, acute lymphoblastic (ALL) and myeloblastic (AML) leukemia, and Wilms' tumor. The liposome version is the doxorubicin hydrochloride enclosed in a spherical lipid bilayer membrane. Doxorubicin hydrochloride liposome is indicated as a treatment for patients with ovarian cancer whose disease has recurred or progressed after platinum-based chemotherapy, and for patients with AIDS-related Kaposi's sarcoma whose disease has progressed on prior combination chemotherapy or who cannot tolerate such therapy. Both versions are administered via intravenous injection.

J9010

J9010   Injection, alemtuzumab, 10 mg

Lay Description
Alemtuzumab is a monoclonal antibody produced by recombinant DNA technology in Chinese hamster ovaries. This monoclonal antibody is directed against the CD52 antigen, which is found on the surface of normal and malignant B and T lymphocytes, NK cells, monocytes, macrophages, and tissues of the male reproductive system. Alemtuzumab is indicated for the treatment of chronic B cell lymphocytic leukemia in patients who have been treated with alkylating agents and who have failed fludarabine therapy. The recommended initial dose is 3 mg rising to 30 mg as a maintenance dose. The drug is administered as a two-hour intravenous infusion.

J9015

J9015   Injection, aldesleukin, per single use vial

Lay Description
Aldesleukin is an interleukin-2 product produced by recombinant DNA technology using a strain of *Escherichia coli* bacterium. Interleukin-2 is a non-antibody protein produced by T cells in response to an antigen or mitogenic stimulation. It stimulates the production of other T cells, the growth and cytolytic function of NK cells to produce lymphokine-activated killer cells, and is a growth factor for and stimulates antibody synthesis in B cells. It is also thought to promote cell death in antigen-activated T cells. Aldesleukin is indicated for the treatment of adults with metastatic renal cell carcinoma and for the treatment of adults with metastatic melanoma. The recommended dosage is 600,000 IU per kg of body weight administered every eight hours by a 15-minute IV infusion for a maximum of 14 doses. Following nine days of rest, the schedule is repeated for another 14 doses, for a maximum of 28 doses per course.

J9017

J9017   Injection, arsenic trioxide, 1 mg

Lay Description
Arsenic trioxide is a toxic element used as an antineoplastic agent. The actions of the drug are not completely understood. It is known to cause structural cell changes and DNA fragmentation leading to cellular death. Arsenic trioxide is indicated for the induction of remission and consolidation in patients with relapsing or refractory acute promyelocytic leukemia who have undergone retinoid or anthracycline chemotherapy and whose disease has a specific gene expression. The drug must be diluted and administered via an intravenous infusion over one to two hours. The infusion may be extended up to four hours if the patient develops acute vasomotor reactions. Recommended dosage for induction of remission is 0.15 mg per kg of body weight daily until bone marrow remission. The total induction dose should not exceed 60 doses. Recommended dosage for consolidation treatment is 0.15 mg per kg daily for 25 doses over a period up to five weeks. Consolidation treatment should begin three to six weeks after completion of induction therapy.

J9019

J9019   Injection, asparaginase (Erwinaze), 1,000 IU

Lay Description

Asparaginase Erwinia chrysanthemi is an asparaginase derived from the gram negative enterobacterium *Erwinia chrysanthemi*. This is a plant pathogen closely related to *E. coli*. Asparaginase is an enzyme that breaks down the amino acid asparagine into aspartic acid and ammonium. Leukemia cells cannot synthesize their own asparagine and rely on circulating sources to maintain protein survival. This drug deprives the leukemia cells of asparagine and ultimately causes cell death. Asparaginase Erwinia chrysanthemi is indicated as a component of a multi-drug treatment for acute lymphoblastic leukemia in patients who have developed a hypersensitivity to *E. coli* derived asparaginase.

J9020

J9020   Injection, asparaginase, not otherwise specified, 10,000 units

Lay Description

Asparaginase is a synthetic version of the enzyme L-asparaginase produced by recombinant DNA technology using a strain of Escherichia coli bacterium. The enzyme catalyzes the breakdown of asparagine, an amino acid. Leukemia cells cannot synthesize asparagine and depend upon exogenous sources. Asparaginase deletes asparagine throughout the body. This depletion kills the leukemia cells. Normal cells can synthesize the asparagine and are unaffected. Asparaginase is indicated in the treatment of acute lymphocytic leukemia for pediatric and adult patients. The dosage depends upon body weight and whether the use is for induction or maintenance therapy. The drug may be administered as an intravenous infusion via an existing IV over 30 minutes. Asparaginase can also be injected intramuscularly with the volume administered at each injection site limited to 2 ml. When used to induce remission, the drug is usually given in combination with other chemotherapeutic agents.

J9025

J9025   Injection, azacitidine, 1 mg

Lay Description

Azacitidine is a pyrimidine nucleoside used as an antineoplastic agent. The drug disrupts the chemistry of DNA and causes cellular death in rapidly dividing cells, including cancer cells that no longer respond to normal growth control mechanism. Azacitidine is indicated for the treatment of myelodysplastic syndrome subtypes: refractory anemia or refractory anemia with sideroblasts (if accompanied by neutropenia, thrombocytopenia, or requiring transfusions), refractory anemia with excess blasts, refractory anemia with excess blasts in transformation, and chronic myelomonocytic

leukemia. The recommended initial treatment therapy is 75 mg per m^2 of body surface subcutaneously injected daily for seven days, every four weeks. The dosage may be increased to 100 mg per m^2 if no beneficial effect is seen after two treatment cycles and if no side effects other than nausea and vomiting occur. A minimum of four treatment cycles is recommended. However, treatment can continue as long as beneficial effects are evident.

J9027

J9027   Injection, clofarabine, 1 mg

Lay Description

Clofarabine is a purine nucleoside that is an antineoplastic agent. The drug inhibits DNA synthesis and cellular repair leading to cell death. Clofarabine is attracted to rapidly proliferating cells and quiescent cancer cell types. It is indicated for the treatment of pediatric patients, ages 1 to 21 years, with relapsed or refractory acute lymphoblastic leukemia who have undergone at least two prior treatment regimens. Recommended dosage is 52 mg per m^2 of body surface infused intravenously over two hours for five consecutive days. This regimen may be repeated every two to six weeks.

J9031

J9031   BCG (intravesical) per instillation

Lay Description

BCG live, intravesical is a freeze-dried preparation of Bacillus Calmette and Guerin, which is a weakened version of Mycobacterium bovis. Mycobacterium bovis is a form of tuberculous originally isolated from cattle. It is used as an antineoplastic agent. The BCG is reconstituted and administered intravesically into the urinary bladder. One dose is usually 81 mg of BCG reconstituted by a diluent and further diluted by 50 ml of sterile water. It causes a local acute inflammation with macrophage and lymphocyte infiltration of the bladder. The exact anti-tumor mechanism is unknown, but it is thought to be created by the lymphocyte reaction. BCG live, intravesical is indicated for the treatment and prophylaxis of carcinoma in situ of the urinary bladder, and for the prophylaxis of primary or recurrent stage Ta and/or stage T1 papillary tumors following transurethral resection.

J9033

J9033   Injection, bendamustine HCl, 1 mg

Lay Description

Bendamustine HCl is an antineoplastic alkylating drug. It is indicated as a treatment for chronic lymphocytic leukemia and indolent B-cell non-Hodgkin's lymphoma when the disease has progressed after being treated with rituximab. The recommended dose is 100 mg per m^2 administered by IV administration on days one and two of a 28-day cycle, for up to six cycles.

J9035

J9035   Injection, bevacizumab, 10 mg

Lay Description
Bevacizumab is a monoclonal antibody produced by recombinant DNA technology in Chinese hamster ovaries. This monoclonal antibody binds to and inhibits the biologic activity of human vascular endothelial growth factor preventing the formation of new blood vessels. Bevacizumab, used in combination with intravenous 5-fluorouracil, is indicated for first-line treatment of patients with metastatic carcinoma of the colon or rectum. The recommended dose is 5 mg per kg of body weight administered once every 14 days disease progression is detected. Bevacizumab is administered by intravenous infusion. The initial dose infusion should be delivered over 90 minutes. If the first infusion is well tolerated, the second infusion may be administered over 60 minutes. If the 60-minute infusion is well tolerated, all subsequent infusions may be administered over 30 minutes.

J9040

J9040   Injection, bleomycin sulfate, 15 units

Lay Description
Bleomycin sulfate is an antibiotic antineoplastic drug produced from a strain of Streptomyces verticillus. It is thought to cause cell death by the inhibition of DNA synthesis with some inhibition of RNA and protein synthesis. Bleomycin sulfate is indicated as a single agent or in combination with other therapeutic agents for squamous cell carcinoma, Hodgkin's disease, non-Hodgkin's lymphoma, testicular carcinoma, and for treatment of malignant pleural effusion. It can be administered as an intravenous, intramuscular, or subcutaneous injection. Bleomycin sulfate may also be administered into the pleural cavity. The recommended dosage for pleural cavity administration is 60 units. The recommended dosage for other administration is 0.25 to 0.50 units per kg of body weight administered once or twice a week.

J9041

J9041   Injection, bortezomib, 0.1 mg

Lay Description
Bortezomib is a modified form of boronic acid used as an antineoplastic agent. Boron is a nonmetallic element and boric acid is a form of boron. The drug inhibits the activity of a protein complex that regulates the intracellular concentration of specific proteins within a cell. This disruption of cell stability can lead to cell death. Bortezomib is indicated for the treatment of multiple myeloma in patients who have received at least two prior therapies and who have demonstrated disease progression on the last therapy. The recommended therapy is 1.3 mg per m^2 of body surface injected intravenously twice weekly for two weeks with a subsequent 10-day rest period. This three-week period is considered one treatment cycle.

Bortezomib may be administered for a maximum of eight treatment cycles.

J9042

J9042   Injection, brentuximab vedotin, 1 mg

Lay Description
Brentuximab vedotin is an antibody-drug conjugate (ADC) used to treat patients with Hodgkin lymphoma (HL) after at least two multi-agent chemotherapy treatment courses have failed. It is also used to treat patients with systemic anaplastic large cell lymphoma (sALCL) after at least one prior multi-agent chemotherapy treatment course has been unsuccessful. The antibody binds to CD30-expressing cells and ultimately causes the cell destruction. The ecommended dose of brentuximab vedotin is 1.8 mg/kg administered only as an intravenous infusion over 30 minutes every three weeks. The dose for patients weighing greater than 100 kg should be calculated based on a weight of 100 kg.

J9043

J9043   Injection, cabazitaxel, 1 mg

Lay Description
Cabazitaxel is an antineoplastic taxane class agent extracted from yew needles. It is indicated as a treatment for hormone-refractory metastatic prostate cancer previously treated with a docetaxel-containing treatment regimen. The medication binds with the tubulin and disrupts the function and reproduction of the cell. Recommended dose is based on body surface area and is administered by IV infusion over the course of one hour.

J9045

J9045   Injection, carboplatin, 50 mg

Lay Description
Carboplatin is a chemical complex containing the metal platinum used as an antineoplastic drug. It binds to DNA disrupting synthesis and causing cell death. Carboplatin is similar to, but more stable than cisplatin. It is indicated as an initial treatment for advanced ovarian cancer in combination with other chemotherapeutic agents. Carboplatin is also indicated as a secondary treatment of recurrent ovarian carcinoma after prior chemotherapy, including patients who have been previously treated with cisplatin. Dosage depends upon patient body surface, patient reactions to the drug, and whether it is used as a single agent or in combination. Carboplatin is administered by an intravenous infusion lasting 15 minutes or longer. Aluminum reacts with carboplatin causing a loss of potency, therefore, needles or intravenous sets containing aluminum parts that may come in contact with the drug must not be used for its preparation or administration.

J9047

J9047   Injection, carfilzomib, 1 mg

Lay Description

Carfilzomib is a proteasome inhibitor. Proteasomes are protein complexes that assist in the breakdown and elimination of other damaged or unneeded cellular proteins. Proteasome inhibitors block the action of proteasomes allowing debris to build and ultimately causing cellular death. This drug is indicated for the treatment of patients with multiple myeloma who have received at least two prior therapies, including bortezomib and an immunomodulatory agent, and have demonstrated disease progression on or within 60 days of completion of the last therapy. Carfilzomib is administered intravenously over two to 10 minutes, on two consecutive days each week for three weeks (days one, two, eight, nine, 15, and 16), followed by a 12-day rest period (days 17 to 28). The recommended cycle 1 dose is 20 mg/m2/day. If the initial cycle is tolerated, then subsequent cycles can be increased to 27 mg/m2/day.

J9050

J9050   Injection, carmustine, 100 mg

Lay Description

Carmustine is one of the nitrosoureas, alkylating agents used as antineoplastic drugs. Nitrosoureas are a group of similar drugs that are highly lipid-soluble and cross the blood-brain barrier. Carmustine inhibits DNA repair causing cell death. It is indicated as a single agent or in combination therapy for the treatment of brain tumors, multiple myeloma, colorectal cancer, Hodgkin's disease, and non-Hodgkin's lymphoma. Dosage depends upon patient body surface, patient reactions to the drug, and whether it is used as a single agent or in combination. Carmustine is administered as an intravenous injection.

J9055

J9055   Injection, cetuximab, 10 mg

Lay Description

Cetuximab is monoclonal antibody produced by recombinant DNA technology in a murine cell culture. This antibody binds specifically to the epidermal growth factor receptor (EGFR, HER1, c-ErbB-1) on both normal and tumor cells resulting in inhibition of cell growth and causing cell death. Cetuximab, used in combination with irinotecan, is indicated for the treatment of EGFR-expressing, metastatic colorectal carcinoma in patients who are refractory to irinotecan-based chemotherapy. Cetuximab, administered as a single agent, is also indicated for the treatment of EGFR-expressing, metastatic colorectal carcinoma in patients who are intolerant to irinotecan-based chemotherapy. The recommended initial dosage for combination or as a single agent is 400 mg per m2 of body surface administered as a 120-minute intravenous infusion. The recommended weekly maintenance dose is 250 mg per m2 of body surface infused intravenously over 60 minutes.

J9060

J9060   Injection, cisplatin, powder or solution, 10 mg

Lay Description

Cisplatin is a chemical complex containing the metal platinum used as an antineoplastic drug. It binds to DNA disrupting synthesis and causing cell death. Cisplatin is indicated in combination therapy for treatment of metastatic testicular and ovarian cancer after surgical and radiation therapy. Cisplatin is indicated as a single agent treatment for advanced transitional cell bladder cancer that can no longer be treated locally, such as with surgery or radiation therapy. As a single agent, it may also be used as a secondary treatment for metastatic ovarian cancer that is refractory to standard chemotherapy where cisplatin has not been previously administered. Cisplatin is administered as an intravenous infusion. Dosage depends upon patient body surface, patient reactions to the drug, and whether it is used as a single agent or in combination. Aluminum reacts with cisplatin causing a loss of potency; therefore, needles or intravenous sets containing aluminum parts that may come in contact with the drug must not be used for its preparation or administration.

J9065

J9065   Injection, cladribine, per 1 mg

Lay Description

Cladribine is a synthetic version of adenosine used as an antineoplastic drug. Cladribine interferes with DNA repair and causes cell death. Cladribine is indicated as a treatment for active hairy cell leukemia. The recommended initial dosage is 0.9 mg per kg of body weight. It is administered by a continuous intravenous infusion over 24 hours. This continuous infusion is repeated daily for seven consecutive days.

J9070

J9070   Cyclophosphamide, 100 mg

Lay Description

Cyclophosphamide is a synthetic antineoplastic drug chemically related to the nitrogen mustards. The drug itself is inert and functions only after transformation in the liver to active alkylating metabolites. These metabolites interfere with the growth of susceptible rapidly proliferating malignant cells. The mechanism of action is thought to be its interference with the DNA of the tumor cell causing cell death. Cyclophosphamide is indicated singularly or in combination with other chemotherapeutic drugs, to treat a wide variety of cancers including Hodgkin's disease, lymphosarcoma, acute lymphocytic leukemia, Burkitt's lymphoma, carcinoma of the breast, multiple myeloma, chronic lymphocytic leukemia, bronchogenic carcinoma, neuroblastoma, ovarian carcinoma, and carcinoma of the uterine cervix. It is also used as an immunosuppressant to prevent transplant rejection and in the treatment of certain diseases with abnormal immune function, including severe lupus manifestations and vasculitis. Cyclophosphamide may be administered via intravenous injection or infusion, or may be injected intramuscularly, intraperitoneally, or intrapleurally. An oral version is also available. Dosage depends upon body weight and the disease being treated. The lyophilized version of cyclophosphamide is a freeze-dried version of the drug.

J9098-J9100

J9098 Injection, cytarabine liposome, 10 mg
J9100 Injection, cytarabine, 100 mg

Lay Description
Cytarabine is a synthetic nucleoside used as an antineoplastic drug. The drug interferes with DNA synthesis causing cell death. Cytarabine is indicated singularly or in combination with other chemotherapeutic drugs to induce remission in acute nonlymphocytic leukemia in adults and children and to treat acute lymphocytic leukemia and the blast phase of chronic myelocytic leukemia. Intrathecal cytarabine is indicated in the prophylaxis and treatment of meningeal leukemia. Cytarabine may be administered via intravenous injection or infusion, or may be injected intramuscularly, intraperitoneally, intrapleurally, or intrathecally. Dosage depends upon body weight and the disease being treated. The liposome version of cytarabine is a suspension of cytarabine encapsulated with liposomes. The liposome version is administered intrathecally to treat meningitis associated with lymphoma.

J9120

J9120 Injection, dactinomycin, 0.5 mg

Lay Description
Dactinomycin, also known as actinomycin D, is an antibiotic produced by a strain of *Streptomyces parvulus* bacterium that is used as an antineoplastic agent. The drug inhibits RNA synthesis, leading to cellular death. Dactinomycin is indicated in combination therapy for the treatment of Wilms' tumor, childhood rhabdomyosarcoma, Ewing's sarcoma, and metastatic nonseminomatous testicular cancer. The drug may be used as a single agent or in combination as a treatment for gestational trophoblastic neoplasia. Dactinomycin is also indicated as a part of a regional perfusion for the palliative and/or adjunctive treatment of locally recurrent or locoregional sarcoma, carcinoma, and adenocarcinoma. Recommended dosages vary by the type of neoplasm being treated and the patient's body surface or weight. The drug is highly toxic even in powdered form and is extremely corrosive to soft tissue. Dactinomycin is administered intravenously.

J9130

J9130 Dacarbazine, 100 mg

Lay Description
Dacarbazine, also known as DTIC, is a chemical complex that is an antineoplastic agent. The drug interferes with DNA synthesis causing cell death. Dacarbazine is indicated in the treatment of metastatic malignant melanoma. It is also used in combination with other chemotherapeutic agents as a treatment for Hodgkin's disease. The drug is administered by intravenous injection or infusion. The recommended dosage depends upon body surface, the disease being treated, and the treatment plan.

J9150-J9151

J9150 Injection, daunorubicin, 10 mg
J9151 Injection, daunorubicin citrate, liposomal formulation, 10 mg

Lay Description
Daunorubicin hydrochloride is an anthracycline antibiotic, produced by a strain of Streptomyces coeruleorubidus bacterium, that is used as an antineoplastic agent. The drug interrupts DNA synthesis creating breaks within the DNA strands leading to cellular death. Daunorubicin hydrochloride is indicated in combination with other chemotherapeutic agents for the remission induction of acute nonlymphocytic leukemia (myelogenous, monocytic, and erythroid) in adults and for acute lymphocytic leukemia in both children and adults. Recommended dosages are 25 to 30 mg per m2 of body surface infused intravenously. In children younger than 2 years of age, it is recommended that the dose be based on body weight rather than body surface. The drug should never be given by intramuscular or subcutaneous injection. The length of a regimen and the subsequent courses of therapy depend upon the patient and type of leukemia being treated. Daunorubicin citrate liposome is indicted for the treatment of HIV-related advanced Kaposi's sarcoma.

J9155

J9155 Injection, degarelix, 1 mg

Lay Description
Degarelix is a gonadotropin releasing hormone (GnRH) receptor inhibitor used to treat patients with advanced prostate cancer. It inhibits the testosterone, which retards the growth of cancer in the prostate. It's a synthetic mixture that contains seven amino acids. The recommended dose is 240 mg initially administered by two subcutaneous injections of 120 mg each. The recommended maintenance dose is 80 mg given as a single subcutaneous injection every 28 days.

J9160

J9160 Injection, denileukin diftitox, 300 mcg

Lay Description

Denileukin diftitox is a modified form of the diphtheria toxin produced from E. coli bacterium using recombinant DNA technology. This biological is used as an antineoplastic agent. It binds to IL-2 receptor sites on certain cells delivering the diphtheria toxin, which inhibits cellular protein synthesis causing the death of the cell. This receptor is usually highly active in activated B and T lymphocytes and macrophages. Denileukin diftitox is indicated for the treatment of persistent or recurrent cutaneous T cell lymphoma where the cells express the CD25 component of the IL-2 receptor. The biological is administered via an intravenous infusion of at least 15 minutes, daily for five consecutive days. This regimen should be administered every 21 days. The recommended dose is 9 or 18 mcg per kg of body weight.

J9165

J9165 Injection, diethylstilbestrol diphosphate, 250 mg

Lay Description

Diethylstilbestrol (DES) diphosphate is a synthetic estrogen used as a hormone treatment for advanced prostate cancer. Estrogen is a hormone produced by the ovaries, adrenal gland, testis, and placenta. While small amounts are present in males, it is generally referred to as the female sex hormone. The high levels of estrogen within the body cause a decrease in testosterone production that can slow the growth of prostatic cancer cells.

J9171

J9171 Injection, docetaxel, 1 mg

Lay Description

Docetaxel is a semisynthetic antineoplastic drug created from the needles of the yew tree. The drug inhibits cell division, which stops the cancer cells from reproducing. Docetaxel is indicated as a single agent for the treatment of locally advanced or metastatic breast cancer after failure of prior chemotherapy and for locally advanced or metastatic non-small-cell lung cancer after failure of prior platinum-based chemotherapy. In combination with other chemotherapeutic agents, it is indicated as induction treatment for patients with inoperable locally advanced squamous cell carcinoma of the head and neck and adjuvant treatment of patients with operable node-positive breast cancer and hormone refractory metastatic prostate cancer; patients with unresectable, locally advanced or metastatic non-small-cell lung cancer who have not previously received chemotherapy for this condition; and those with advanced gastric adenocarcinoma who have not received prior chemotherapy for advanced disease. Docetaxel is infused intravenously over one hour.

Dosage depends upon m2 of patient body surface and the disease being treated.

J9175

J9175 Injection, Elliotts' B solution, 1 ml

Lay Description

Elliotts' B solution is a diluent of buffered electrolytes and dextrose that is comparable in pH, composition, and osmolarity to cerebrospinal fluid. Elliotts' B solution is indicated as a diluent for the intrathecal administration of methotrexate sodium and cytarabine for the prevention or treatment of meningeal leukemia or lymphocytic lymphoma.

J9178

J9178 Injection, epirubicin HCl, 2 mg

Lay Description

Epirubicin hydrochloride (HCl) is an anthracycline, antibiotic, antineoplastic drug that is chemically similar to doxorubicin hydrochloride, but has a lower toxicity. It binds to DNA inhibiting RNA and protein synthesis creating cell death. Epirubicin hydrochloride is used as an adjunctive therapy for patients with primary breast cancer who have evidence of axillary node involvement following surgical resection. It is also indicated in the treatment of cancers of the lung, stomach, ovary, colon, and rectum, and for treatment of leukemia, lymphoma, and multiple myeloma. The initial recommended dosage is 100 to 120 mg per m2 of body surface administered as an intravenous infusion over 15 to 20 minutes. Dosages administered after the initial dose depend upon the patient's reaction and the infusion time for subsequent doses may be significantly decreased.

J9179

J9179 Injection, eribulin mesylate, 0.1 mg

Lay Description

Eribulin mesylate is used to treat patients with metastatic breast cancer who have received at least two other forms of treatment, including taxane-based and anthracycline-based therapy. The drug inhibits the growth phase of microtubules. Recommended dose of eribulin mesylate is 1.4 mg/m2 administered intravenously over two to five minutes on days one and eight of a 21-day cycle. The dose may vary based on renal and hepatic function.

J9181

J9181 Injection, etoposide, 10 mg

Lay Description

Etoposide is a semisynthetic derivative of podophyllotoxin, a toxic compound found in the rhizomes and roots of the mandrake plant. It is believed to inhibit the repair of DNA causing cell death. Etoposide is an antineoplastic drug used in combination with other chemotherapeutic agents. It is available in injectable or oral versions. Injectable etoposide is indicated for the treatment of small cell lung cancer and refractory testicular cancer that has been previously treated with surgery, radiation, or other chemotherapy. The oral version is indicated for the treatment of small cell lung cancer. The recommended dosage of the injectable version ranges from 35 to 100 mg per m2 of body surface depending on which disease is being treated. The injectable version is administered by intravenous infusion over 30 to 60 minutes. The recommended dosage for the oral version is two times the intravenous version.

J9185

J9185   Injection, fludarabine phosphate, 50 mg

Lay Description
Fludarabine phosphate is an antineoplastic drug that is a fluorinated nucleotide analogue of the antiviral agent vidarabine. It is rapidly broken down into 2-fluoro-ara-A which inhibits DNA synthesis and causes cell death. Fludarabine phosphate is indicated for the treatment of beta-cell chronic lymphocytic leukemia for patients who have not responded to an alkylating drug treatment. It is administered through intravenous infusion over 30 minutes for five consecutive days. The recommended dosage is 25 mg per m2 of body surface.

J9190

J9190   Injection, fluorouracil, 500 mg

Lay Description
Fluorouracil, also known as 5 FU, is an antineoplastic drug that is a fluorinated analogue of uracil. Uracil is a chemical compound found in nucleic acids. Once broken down, it interferes with the synthesis of DNA and RNA causing cell death. Fluorouracil is available in injectable and topical versions. The injectable version is indicated for the treatment of many different cancers, among them cancer of the breast, stomach, pancreas, and colon. The topical version is used to treat actinic or solar keratoses and superficial basal cell carcinomas. Dosage for the injectable version depends upon body weight and is administered by intravenous injection.

J9200

J9200   Injection, floxuridine, 500 mg

Lay Description
Floxuridine, also known as FUDR, is an antineoplastic drug that is broken down into the same substance as fluorouracil. It interferes with the synthesis of DNA and RNA causing cell death. Floxuridine is administered by continuous intra-arterial infusion using a pump. It is indicated as a palliative treatment of gastrointestinal adenocarcinoma that has metastasized to the liver in patients who are considered incurable by surgery or other means. The recommended dosage is 0.1 to 0.6 mg per kg of body weight per day.

J9201

J9201   Injection, gemcitabine HCl, 200 mg

Lay Description
Gemcitabine hydrochloride is a nucleoside analogue used as an antineoplastic drug. It interferes with the synthesis of DNA and RNA causing cell death. Gemcitabine hydrochloride in combination with paclitaxel is indicated as a treatment for metastatic breast cancer after the failure of prior chemotherapy. It is indicated in combination with cisplatin in the treatment of inoperable locally advanced or metastatic non-small cell lung cancer. As a sole agent, gemcitabine hydrochloride is indicated as a treatment for inoperable locally advanced or metastatic pancreatic cancer previously treated with fluorouracil. The recommended initial dosage is from 1,000 to 1,250 mg per m2 of body surface administered by intravenous infusion over 30 minutes.

J9202

J9202   Goserelin acetate implant, per 3.6 mg

Lay Description
Goserelin acetate is a synthetic analogue of the luteinizing hormone-releasing hormone (LHRH) used as an antineoplastic drug. The implant is a biodegradable tube containing 3.6 mg of goserelin acetate that is slowly released over 28 days. This continued administration leads to suppression of pituitary gonadotropins and subsequently to lower levels of estrogen and testosterone. The goserelin acetate implant is indicated as a palliative treatment for advanced breast and prostatic cancer. In combination with flutamide, it is indicated for treatment of locally confined prostate cancer stage T2b-T4 (Stage B2-C). It may also be indicated as a treatment for endometriosis and as an endometrial-thinning agent prior to ablation. The goserelin acetate implant is injected subcutaneously into the upper abdominal wall every 28 days.

J9206

J9206   Injection, irinotecan, 20 mg

Lay Description
Irinotecan hydrochloride (HCL) is an antineoplastic drug that is a semisynthetic derivative of camptothecin, an alkaloid extract from plants such as Camptotheca acuminata. The drug works by causing strand breaks in DNA that the cell cannot repair leading to cell death. Irinotecan is indicated as a first line treatment in combination with fluorouracil and leucovorin for metastatic carcinoma of the colon or rectum. Irinotecan is also indicated for patients with metastatic carcinoma of the colon or rectum whose disease has recurred or progressed following initial fluorouracil-based therapy. The recommended dosage varies from 125 to 300 mg depending on the regimen. Irinotecan hydrochloride is administered by intravenous infusion over 90 minutes.

J9207

J9207   Injection, ixabepilone, 1 mg

Lay Description

Ixabepilone is an antineoplastic drug used to treat metastatic or locally advanced breast cancer that is resistant to anthracycline and taxane or if those treatments are contraindicated. It inhibits cell division, which leads to cell death. The recommended dose is 40 mg/m^2 by intravenous infusion over three hours. The treatment is administered every three weeks.

J9208

J9208   Injection, ifosfamide, 1 g

Lay Description

Ifosfamide is an antineoplastic that is a synthetic analogue of cyclophosphamide and is related to the nitrogen mustards. The drug functions only after transformation in the liver to active alkylating metabolites. These metabolites interfere with the DNA causing cell death. Ifosfamide is indicated as a third-line treatment for germ cell testicular cancer. The recommended dosage is 1.2 g per m^2 of body surface administered by slow intravenous infusion over 30 minutes, through five consecutive days. Mesna is often given with ifosfamide as a prophylactic agent against hemorrhagic cystitis.

J9209

J9209   Injection, mesna, 200 mg

Lay Description

Mesna is a synthetic sulfur-hydrogen compound that is used as a detoxifying agent to inhibit the hemorrhagic cystitis caused by ifosfamide. Once broken down in the body, the drug combines with the urotoxic byproducts of ifosfamide rendering them harmless. Mesna is available in injectable and oral versions. The dosage is dependent upon the amount of ifosfamide given calculated at 20 percent the amount of ifosfamide. Mesna is administered as an intravenous injection at the time of ifosfamide administration, and then repeated at four and eight hours following the administration. Alternately, the first does may be by intravenous injection and the subsequent doses may be oral.

J9211

J9211   Injection, idarubicin HCl, 5 mg

Lay Description

Idarubicin hydrochloride is an antineoplastic drug that is a semisynthetic analogue of daunorubicin. It interferes with DNA synthesis causing cell death. Idarubicin hydrochloride is indicated in combination with other chemotherapeutic drugs for the treatment of acute myeloid leukemia. The recommended dosage is 12 mg per m^2 of body surface. Idarubicin hydrochloride is administered by intravenous infusion over 10 to 15 minutes.

J9212

J9212   Injection, interferon alfacon-1, recombinant, 1 mcg

Lay Description

Interferon alfacon-1 is a non-natural form of human interferon alpha proteins that are produced by recombinant DNA technology. Interferons are small, naturally occurring proteins that bind to specific cell membranes and initial a series of events that include the inhibition of virus replication and the enhancement of macrophage and lymphocyte destruction of foreign cells. Interferon alfacon-1 is indicated for the treatment of chronic hepatitis C. The recommended dosage is 9 to 15 mcg administered as a subcutaneous injection every 48 hours for 24 weeks.

J9213

J9213   Injection, interferon, alfa-2a, recombinant, 3 million units

Lay Description

Interferon alfa-2a is a purified form of human interferon alpha proteins that are produced by recombinant DNA technology using Escherichia coli bacteria. Interferons are small, naturally occurring proteins that bind to specific cell membranes and initial a series of events that include the inhibition of virus replication and the enhancement of macrophage and lymphocyte destruction of foreign cells. Interferon alfa-2a is indicated for the treatment of AIDS-related Kaposi's sarcoma, hairy cell leukemia, chronic hepatitis C, and in Philadelphia chromosome-positive chronic myelogenous leukemia. The recommended dosage is 3 to 9 million IU depending upon the disease being treated. Interferon alfa-2a is administered as an intramuscular or subcutaneous injection daily. Prefilled syringes are intended for subcutaneous injection only.

J9214

J9214   Injection, interferon, alfa-2b, recombinant, 1 million units

Lay Description

Interferon alfa-2b is a purified form of human interferon alpha proteins that are produced by recombinant DNA technology using Escherichia coli bacteria. Interferons are small, naturally occurring proteins that bind to specific cell membranes and initial a series of events that include the inhibition of virus replication and the enhancement of macrophage and lymphocyte destruction of foreign cells. Interferon alfa-2b is indicated for the treatment of hairy cell leukemia, malignant melanoma, genital or venereal warts, Kaposi's sarcoma, and chronic hepatitis B and C. It is also indicated in combination with other chemotherapeutic agents as an initial treatment of clinically aggressive follicular non-Hodgkin's lymphoma. The recommended dosage varies from 5 to 25 million IU depending upon the disease being treated. Interferon alfa-2b can be administered as an intramuscular, subcutaneous, or intravenous infusion over 20 minutes or intralesional injection.

J9215

J9215   Injection, interferon, alfa-N3, (human leukocyte derived), 250,000 IU

Lay Description
Interferon alfa-N3 is a purified form of human interferon alpha proteins that is derived from human leukocytes. The human leukocytes are induced by inoculation with a murine virus to produce the interferon alfa proteins. Interferons are small naturally occurring proteins that bind to specific cell membranes and initiate a series of events that include the inhibition of virus replication and the enhancement of macrophage and lymphocyte destruction of foreign cells. Interferon alfa-N3 is indicated for the treatment of condylomata acuminata (genital warts) where it is injected intralesionally. Interferon alfa-N3 has also been used off-label to treat multiple sclerosis, hepatitis C, and some cancers.

J9216

J9216   Injection, interferon, gamma 1-b, 3 million units

Lay Description
Interferon gamma-1b is a purified form of human interferon gamma proteins that are produced by recombinant DNA technology using Escherichia coli bacteria. Interferons are small, naturally occurring proteins that bind to specific cell membranes and initial a series of events that include the inhibition of virus replication and the enhancement of macrophage and lymphocyte destruction of foreign cells. Interferon gamma-1b is indicated for the treatment of chronic granulomatous disease and severe malignant osteopetrosis. The recommended dosage varies from 1 to 1.5 million units per m2 of body surface. Interferon gamma-1b is administered as a subcutaneous injection.

J9217-J9219

J9217   Leuprolide acetate (for depot suspension), 7.5 mg
J9218   Leuprolide acetate, per 1 mg
J9219   Leuprolide acetate implant, 65 mg

Lay Description
Leuprolide acetate is a synthetic analogue of the luteinizing hormone-releasing hormone (LHRH) that is used as an antineoplastic drug and a treatment for central precocious puberty, endometriosis, and uterine fibroids. It first stimulates and then suppresses follicle stimulating and luteinizing hormone release, resulting in suppression of testosterone and estrogen. A depot suspension is a drug that remains in the body long-term in storage and is slowly released into the blood. The leuprolide acetate depot suspension in dosages of 3.75 mg monthly and the 12.25 mg every three months are injected intramuscularly to treat endometriosis and uterine fibroids. When used to treat central precocious puberty, the dosage is individualized to the child and can range from 7.5 to 15 mg. Leuprolide acetate in doses of 7.5 mg and greater is injected subcutaneously and is used as a palliative treatment for advanced prostate cancer. The leuprolide acetate implant is a non-biodegradable tube containing 72 mg. The implant delivers the drug over a 12-month period. The implant is inserted subcutaneously in the inner portion of the upper arm. It must be removed or replaced when the drug is depleted. The leuprolide acetate implant is used as a palliative treatment of advanced prostate cancer.

J9225-J9226

J9225   Histrelin implant (Vantas), 50 mg
J9226   Histrelin implant (Supprelin LA), 50 mg

Lay Description
A histrelin implant is a thin, flexible tube inserted subcutaneously that contains 50 mg of histrelin acetate, a synthetic version of luteinizing hormone-releasing hormone or gonadotropin-releasing hormone. Luteinizing hormone-releasing hormone is produced by the pituitary gland that stimulates the ovaries (to release an ovum), the release of estrogen, and certain cells in the testis. A histrelin implant is indicated as a palliative treatment for advanced prostate cancer. Histrelin decreases testosterone levels to castrate levels. A histrelin implant is also indicated for the treatment of children with central precocious puberty, who have an early onset of secondary sexual characteristics (earlier than 8 years of age in females and 9 years of age in males). They also show a significantly advanced bone age that can result in diminished adult height attainment. The implant contains 50 mg of histrelin, administered continuously over a 12-month period. When depleted, the implant must be removed and can be replaced with another implant.

J9228

J9228   Injection, ipilimumab, 1 mg

Lay Description
Ipilimumab is a recombinant, human monoclonal antibody used as an antineoplastic agent. The drug is an IgG1 kappa immunoglobulin produced in Chinese hamster ovary cell cultures. Ipilimumab binds and blocks the cytotoxic T-lymphocyte antigen-4 (CTLA-4). This augments T-cell activation and proliferation, which indirectly enhances the T-cell mediated anti-tumor immune response. Ipilimumab is indicated for the treatment of unresectable or metastatic melanoma. The recommended dosage is 3 mg/kg administered every three weeks for a total of four doses. Ipilimumab is administered as an IV infusion over 90 minutes and should not be administered as IV push or bolus injection.

J9230

J9230   Injection, mechlorethamine HCl, (nitrogen mustard), 10 mg

Lay Description
Mechlorethamine hydrochloride, also known as nitrogen mustard, is a highly toxic chemical complex used as an antineoplastic drug. In water or body fluids, it is rapidly transformed and acts by interfering with RNA synthesis causing an imbalance of growth, which then leads to cell death. Administered as an intravenous injection, mechlorethamine hydrochloride is indicated for the treatment of Hodgkin's disease, lymphosarcoma, polycythemia vera, chronic lymphocytic and myelocytic leukemias, mycosis fungoides, and bronchogenic cancers. When administered intrapleurally, intraperitoneally, or intrapericardially, it is used to treat malignant effusions. The recommended dosage is 0.4 mg per kg of body weight per day. The dosage may be divided into smaller doses.

J9245

J9245   Injection, melphalan HCl, 50 mg

Lay Description
Melphalan hydrochloride is a derivative of nitrogen mustard used as an antineoplastic drug. It interferes with RNA synthesis causing cell death. Melphalan is indicated for the treatment of multiple myeloma and advanced epithelial ovarian cancer. The drug is available in oral and injectable form. The injectable form is used for the treatment of multiple myeloma when the oral form is inappropriate. The recommended oral dosage for ovarian cancer is 0.2 mg per kg of body weight for five days. The recommended intravenous dosage is 16 mg per m^2 of body surface administered as a single infusion over 15 to 20 minutes. The intravenous dosage is administered at two-week intervals for four doses, then at four-week intervals.

J9250-J9260

J9250   Methotrexate sodium, 5 mg
J9260   Methotrexate sodium, 50 mg

Lay Description
Methotrexate sodium is a chemical complex that blocks cell metabolism. It works by hindering the production of an enzyme needed for the metabolism of dividing cells, like those involved in inflammation and the immune response. Methotrexate has been found useful in treating diseases linked with abnormally rapid cell growth. It is indicated singularly or in combination as a treatment for gestational choriocarcinoma, chorioadenoma destruens, hydatidiform mole, breast cancer, epidermoid cancers of the head and neck, advanced mycosis fungoides, squamous and small cell lung cancer, advanced non-Hodgkin's lymphoma, acute lymphocytic leukemia, Burkitt's lymphoma, and lymphosarcoma. It is also used to treat rheumatoid and psoriatic arthritis

and severe psoriasis that is unresponsive to other treatments.

J9261

J9261   Injection, nelarabine, 50 mg

Lay Description
Nelarabine is an antineoplastic prodrug that is converted in the body into arabinofuranosylguanine (ara-G). Ara-G accumulates in leukemic blast cells and is incorporated into cellular DNA. The ara-G inhibits synthesis and causes cell death. Nelarabine is indicated for the treatment of T-cell acute lymphoblastic leukemia and T-cell lymphoblastic lymphoma in patients who have not responded or relapsed following treatment with at least two chemotherapeutic regimens. The drug is administered by intravenous infusion. Recommended adult dosage is 1,500 mg per mc2 of body surface administered over two hours on days one, three, and five. Recommended pediatric dosage is 650 mg per mc2 of body surface administered over one hour daily for five consecutive days. This chemotherapy cycle is repeated every 21 days until induction of complete response.

J9262

J9262   Injection, omacetaxine mepesuccinate, 0.01 mg

Lay Description
Omacetaxine mepesuccinate is derived from the leaves of the *Cephalotaxus harringtonia* plant (Cowtail Pine or Japanese Plum Yew). The drug functions as a protein synthesis inhibitor. The mechanism of action of omacetaxine mepesuccinate is not fully understood. It binds to the center of a large ribosomal unit and reduces protein levels in cells harboring the BCR-ABL T3151I mutation. Omacetaxine mepesuccinate is indicated for the treatment of chronic or accelerated phase chronic myeloid leukemia that is resistant to tyrosine kinase inhibitors. Omacetaxine mepesuccinate is administered by subcutaneous injection. Recommended induction and maintenance dose is 1.25 mg per m^2 administered twice daily for 14 consecutive days in a 28-day period.

J9263

J9263   Injection, oxaliplatin, 0.5 mg

Lay Description
Oxaliplatin is a chemical complex containing the metal platinum used as an antineoplastic drug. It binds to DNA disrupting synthesis and causing cell death. It is thought to have a greater cytotoxicity than cisplatin and carboplatin, which are other antineoplastic drugs containing platinum. The exact mechanism of action of oxaliplatin is not known. Oxaliplatin forms reactive platinum. Oxaliplatin is indicated with fluorouracil and leucovorin as a treatment for metastatic colon or rectum cancer that

has recurred or progressed following irinotecan, fluorouracil, and leucovorin therapy. The recommended dosage is 85 mg per m² of body surface. Oxaliplatin is administered by intravenous infusion over two hours. It is administered in a separate bag, but simultaneously with leucovorin.

J9264

J9264   Injection, paclitaxel protein-bound particles, 1 mg

Lay Description
Paclitaxel protein-bound particles are an albumin-bound form of paclitaxel, an antineoplastic agent. Paclitaxel protein-bound particles are indicated for the treatment of breast cancer after the failure of combination chemotherapy for metastatic disease, or relapse within six months of chemotherapy. The recommended therapy is 260 mg per m² of body surface infused intravenously over 30 minutes every three weeks. Paclitaxel protein-bound particles are contraindicated in patients with baseline neutrophil counts of less than 1,500.

J9266

J9266   Injection, pegaspargase, per single dose vial

Lay Description
Pegaspargase is a modified version of the enzyme L-asparaginase produced from *E. coli* bacterium and used as an antineoplastic agent. The enzyme catalyzes the breakdown of asparagine, an amino acid. Leukemia cells cannot synthesize asparagine and depend upon exogenous sources. Pegaspargase depletes asparagine throughout the body. This depletion kills the leukemia cells. Normal cells can synthesize the asparagine and are unaffected. Pegaspargase is indicated as a treatment for acute lymphoblastic leukemia in patients who have developed hypersensitivity to native forms of L-asparaginase. The drug is usually administered in combination with other chemotherapeutic agents and should only be administered as a single therapy when multi-agent therapy is inappropriate. The recommended dose is 2,500 IU per m² of body surface via intravenous or intramuscular injection every 14 days. Lower doses of 82.5 IU per kg are recommended for children with a body surface of less than 0.6 m².

J9267

J9267   Injection, paclitaxel, 1 mg

Lay Description
Paclitaxel is a chemical compound isolated from the Pacific yew tree used as an antineoplastic drug. It disrupts intercellular functions causing cell death. Paclitaxel, singularly or in combination with other chemotherapeutic drugs, is indicated as a treatment for Kaposi's sarcoma, advanced breast cancer, advanced ovarian cancer, and non-small cell lung cancer. Recommended dosage varies from 100 to 175 mg per m² of body surface depending on the disease and treatment regimen. It is administered via intravenous infusion over three hours or over 24 hours depending on the treatment regimen.

J9268

J9268   Injection, pentostatin, 10 mg

Lay Description
Pentostatin is an antibiotic isolated from the soil bacterium Streptomyces antibioticus used as antineoplastic drug. It interferes with enzyme activity preventing cellular reproduction. Pentostatin is indicated as a treatment for hairy cell leukemia refractory to alpha interferon. Pentostatin is given by intravenous injection or diluted in normal saline and infused over approximately 30 minutes. The recommended dosage is 4 mg per m² of body surface.

J9270

J9270   Injection, plicamycin, 2.5 mg

Lay Description
Plicamycin, also known as mithramycin, is an antibiotic with antineoplastic effects. The drug is derived from *Streptomyces plicatus*. It binds to DNA inhibiting RNA synthesis. Plicamycin is indicated for the treatment of testicular cancer in patients for whom surgery or radiotherapy is not an option. Plicamycin may also be considered in the treatment of symptomatic patients with hypercalcemia caused by chemotherapy for whom conventional therapy has failed. The drug may lower serum calcium by blocking the actions of vitamin D and inhibiting the effects of parathyroid hormone. The recommended antineoplastic dose is 25 to 30 mcg per kg of ideal body weight for a period of eight to 10 days. The recommended dose for hypercalcemia treatment is 25 mcg per kg of body weight for a period of three or four days. Plicamycin is administered via an intravenous infusion over four to six hours. The drug may cause severe thrombocytopenia and hemorrhagic syndrome.

J9280

J9280   Injection, mitomycin, 5 mg

Lay Description
Mitomycin is an antibiotic with antineoplastic effects. The drug is derived from Streptomyces caespitosus plicatus. It selectively inhibits DNA synthesis. Mitomycin is not recommended as a single agent primary therapy. Mitomycin is indicated for the treatment of disseminated adenocarcinoma of the stomach or pancreas in combination with other approved chemotherapeutic agents, or as a palliative treatment when other modalities have failed. The drug is not recommended as a replacement for surgery or radiotherapy. Mitomycin is administered intravenously via a catheter with a recommended dosage of 20 mg per m² of body surface in six to eight week cycles. The patient must have a full

hematological recovery from any previous therapy prior to the administration of mitomycin. The drug has a cumulative effect on bone marrow causing suppression and may cause hemolytic uremic syndrome at doses higher than 60 mg.

J9293

J9293   Injection, mitoxantrone HCl, per 5 mg

Lay Description

Mitoxantrone hydrochloride is a synthetic antineoplastic anthracenedione drug that disrupts the DNA of cells causing cell death. The drug is used in combination with corticosteroids as an initial treatment for pain related to advanced hormone-refractory prostate cancer. Mitoxantrone hydrochloride is also indicated in combination with other approved drugs as the initial treatment for acute nonlymphocytic leukemia, including myelogenous, promyelocytic, monocytic, and erythroid leukemias. Mitoxantrone is also indicated for the treatment of secondary progressive, progressive relapsing, or worsening relapsing-remitting multiple sclerosis. The drug must be diluted and administered via an intravenous infusion.

J9300

J9300   Injection, gemtuzumab ozogamicin, 5 mg

Lay Description

Gemtuzumab ozogamicin is a monoclonal antibody produced by recombinant DNA coupled with an antineoplastic antibiotic, calicheamicin. Calicheamicin is derived from the bacterium Micromonospora echinospora subsp. calichensis. The antibody portion of the drug binds specifically to the CD33 antigen, a protein found on the surface of leukemic blasts and immature normal cells of myelomonocytic lineage, but not on normal hematopoietic stem cells. Once bound with the CD33 antigen, the calicheamicin interferes with DNA replication and causes cell death. Gemtuzumab ozogamicin is indicated for the treatment of patients with CD33 positive acute myeloid leukemia in first relapse who are 60 years of age or older and who are not considered candidates for other chemotherapy. The recommended dosage is 9 mg per m2 of body surface administered by intravenous infusion over two hours.

J9301

J9301   Injection, obinutuzumab, 10 mg

Lay Description

Obinutuzumab is a humanized monoclonal antibody that is produced using Chinese hamster ovaries. It targets the CD20 antigen found on the surface of pre and mature B-lymphocytes. After binding to these sites, obinutuzumab activates intracellular pathways that lead to the death of the cell. Obinutuzumab, in combination with chlorambucil, is indicated as a treatment for patients with chronic lymphocytic leukemia that have not been previously treated. It is

administered as an intravenous infusion. Six cycles are recommended with a dosage of 1,000 mg except for day one and day two of cycle one. Recommended dosage for day one of cycle one is 100 mg with 900 mg recommended for day two of cycle one.

J9302

J9302   Injection, ofatumumab, 10 mg

Lay Description

Ofatumumab is a human monoclonal antibody produced in murine cells. The drug binds specifically to the CD20 molecule contained in B lymphocytes, causing the breakdown of the cell. This drug is indicated for the treatment of patients who have chronic lymphocytic leukemia refractory to fludarabine and alemtuzumab. The drug is administered as a prolonged IV infusion. The recommended dosage is 2,000 mg after an initial 300 mg dose.

J9303

J9303   Injection, panitumumab, 10 mg

Lay Description

Panitumumab is a monoclonal antibody produced by recombinant DNA technology using Chinese hamster ovaries. The drug binds to human epidermal growth factor receptor (EGFR) sites inhibiting its effects. EGFR is a glycoprotein expressed in many normal epithelial cells including skin and hair follicles. Over-expression of EGFR usually accompanies many human epithelial cells including those of the colon and rectum. Panitumumab is indicated for the treatment of EGFR-expressing metastatic colorectal cancer in patients whose disease has progressed after treatment with fluoropyrimidine, oxaliplatin and irinotecan chemotherapy regimens. The drug is administered via an intravenous infusion over 60 minutes. Recommended dosage is 6 mg per kg of patient body weight every 14 days. Total dosages greater than 1000 mg should be administered over 90 minutes.

J9305

J9305   Injection, pemetrexed, 10 mg

Lay Description

Pemetrexed is a chemical complex used as an antineoplastic drug. It disrupts folate-dependent metabolic processes essential for cell reproduction. Pemetrexed in combination with cisplatin is indicated for the treatment of patients with malignant pleural mesothelioma whose disease is unresectable or who are otherwise not candidates for curative surgery metastatic lung cancer. As a singular agent, pemetrexed is indicated as a treatment for locally advanced or metastatic non-small cell lung cancer after prior chemotherapy. The recommended dosage is 500 mg per m2 of body surface administered by intravenous injection.

J9306

J9306   Injection, pertuzumab, 1 mg

Lay Description
Pertuzumab is a monoclonal antibody produced in Chinese hamster ovaries using recombinant DNA technology. The drug targets the human epidermal growth factor 2 protein (HER2) inhibiting two intracellular signal pathways, which can halt cellular growth and cause cell destruction. Pertuzumab is indicated for use in combination with trastuzumab and docetaxel for the treatment of patients with HER2-positive metastatic breast cancer who have not received prior anti-HER2 therapy or chemotherapy. The initial dose of pertuzumab is 840 mg administered as a 60-minute intravenous infusion. Subsequent recommended dose is 420 mg in an intravenous infusion over 30 to 60 minutes, administered every three weeks.

J9307

J9307   Injection, pralatrexate, 1 mg

Lay Description
Pralatrexate is a folate analogue that is a metabolic inhibitor that prevents the synthesis of thymidine. Thymidine is one of the nucleosides in DNA. This drug is used to treat patients with relapsed or refractory peripheral T-cell lymphoma. The drug is administered via an IV push over three to five minutes. The recommended dose is 30 mg per meter squared of body surface area.

J9310

J9310   Injection, rituximab, 100 mg

Lay Description
Rituximab is a monoclonal antibody produced by recombinant DNA in Chinese hamster ovaries used as an antineoplastic drug. It binds to the CD20 antigen on the surface of normal and malignant B-lymphocytes and causes cell death. This drug is used to treat the relapsed or refractory, low-grade, or follicular, CD20-positive, B-cell non-Hodgkin's lymphoma. In combination with other chemotherapeutic drugs, it is indicated as a treatment for diffuse large B-cell, CD20-positive non-Hodgkin's lymphoma, chronic lymphocystic leukemia, and moderate to severe active rheumatoid arthritis that has displayed inadequate response to other therapies. Rituximab is also approved for use in Wegener's granulomatosis and microscopic polyangiitis. The recommended dosage is 375 mg per m^2 of body surface administered by intravenous infusion.

J9315

J9315   Injection, romidepsin, 1 mg

Lay Description
Romidepsin is a chemical compound that functions as a histone deacetylase inhibitor. Histone deacetylases are a class of enzymes that remove acetyl groups from an amino acid on a histone. Histones are strong alkaline proteins found in cell nuclei, which package and order the DNA into structural units. The accumulation of acetylated histones interrupts the cell cycle and induces death. Romidepsin is indicated in the treatment of cutaneous T-cell lymphoma in patients who have received at least one prior systemic therapy. The recommended dose is 14 mg per meter squared of body surface area administered as an IV infusion over a four-hour period.

J9320

J9320   Injection, streptozocin, 1 g

Lay Description
Streptozocin is a synthetic antineoplastic drug chemically related to other nitro ureas that inhibits DNA synthesis causing cell death. Streptozocin is indicated for the treatment of metastatic islet cell carcinoma of the pancreas for both functioning and nonfunctioning carcinomas. Due to its renal toxicity, streptozocin should be limited to patients with symptomatic or progressive metastatic disease. The drug is administered intravenously by injection or via infusion.

J9328

J9328   Injection, temozolomide, 1 mg

Lay Description
Temozolomide is a chemical complex that is broken down in the liver into monomethyl triazine, also known as MTIC. MTIC causes breaks in the DNA, which prevents replication, thus interfering with tumor cell reproduction. Temozolomide is indicated for the treatment of adult patients with newly diagnosed glioblastoma multiforme and for the treatment of adult patients with refractory anaplastic astrocytoma. Dosage is calculated based on the patient's body surface area. Temozolomide is administered by IV infusion.

J9330

J9330   Injection, temsirolimus, 1 mg

Lay Description
Temsirolimus is an antineoplastic drug used to treat advanced renal cancer. It inhibits mammalian target of rapamycin (mTOR) and binds to the protein that controls cell division. The recommended dose of temsirolimus is 25 mg administered by IV infusion over 30 to 60 minutes. The drug is usually administered once a week.

J9340

J9340   Injection, thiotepa, 15 mg

Lay Description
Thiotepa is a synthetic antineoplastic compound drug related chemically and pharmacologically to nitrogen mustard. The drug disrupts cell DNA producing cell death. Thiotepa may be administered intravenously, intracavitary, or intravesically. The drug has been tried in the treatment of a wide variety of neoplastic

diseases with varying results. It has shown success in treating adenocarcinoma of the breast and ovary, superficial papillary carcinoma of the urinary bladder, and in controlling intracavity effusions secondary to diffuse or localized neoplastic diseases of various serosal cavities. While usually superseded by other treatments, thiotepa has been effective in the treatment of other lymphomas such as lymphosarcoma and Hodgkin's disease.

J9351

J9351   Injection, topotecan, 0.1 mg

Lay Description

Topotecan hydrochloride is an antineoplastic drug that is a semisynthetic derivative of camptothecin, an alkaloid extract from plants such as Camptotheca acuminata. The drug works by causing breaks in DNA that the cell cannot repair leading to cell death. Topotecan hydrochloride is indicated as a treatment for metastatic carcinoma of the ovaries after failure of prior chemotherapy. It is also indicated as a treatment for small cell lung cancer that responded to chemotherapy, but subsequently progressed. The recommended dosage is 1.5 mg per m^2 of body surface administered by intravenous infusion over 30 minutes for five consecutive days.

J9354

J9354   Injection, ado-trastuzumab emtansine, 1 mg

Lay Description

Ado-trastuzumab emtansine is an HER-2 targeted therapy. It consists of an antibody linked to a drug, called an ADC or antibody-drug conjugate. The antibody links to the target cell. The ADC is then internalized by the cell and the drug is released to perform its function. The trastuzumab is a humanized anti-HER2 IgG1 that is linked to a microtubule inhibitory drug, DM1 with a chemical link called MCC. The emtansine refers to the MCC-DM1 links. Trastuzumab is a monoclonal antibody produced by recombinant technology in Chinese hamster ovaries. After internalization, the DM1 disrupts the microtubule networks of the cell causing cellular death. Ado-trastuzumab emtansine is indicated as a treatment for HER2-positive, metastatic breast cancer in patients who have previously received trastuzumab and a taxane. Ado-trastuzumab emtansine is administered via an IV infusion every three weeks. The recommended dosage is 3.6 mg per kg of patient weight.

J9355

J9355   Injection, trastuzumab, 10 mg

Lay Description

Trastuzumab is a monoclonal antibody produced using recombinant DNA technology from Chinese hamster ovaries. The drug is an antineoplastic agent indicated for treatment of metastatic breast cancer

that over expresses the human epidermal growth factor receptor 2 (HER2) protein. Trastuzumab selectively binds to the HER2 protein site and inhibits the production of cells that over express HER2. Trastuzumab is indicated as a treatment for HER2 over expressing breast cancer in patients who do not have heart failure or cardiomyopathy in the following circumstances: as a single therapy for patients who have undergone one or more chemotherapy regimens for metastatic breast cancer; in combination therapy with doxorubicin, cyclophosphamide, and paclitaxel for node-positive breast cancer that has been surgically treated; and in combination with paclitaxel for patients who have not received chemotherapy for metastatic breast cancer. The drug is administered via an intravenous infusion and should not be given as an IV push or bolus. Recommended dosage for the initial infusion is 4 mg per kg of patient body weight infused over 90 minutes. Subsequent recommended dosage is 2 mg per kg of patient body weight infused over 30 minutes. The infusions are administered every seven days.

J9357

J9357   Injection, valrubicin, intravesical, 200 mg

Lay Description

Valrubicin intravesical is a synthetic version of anthracycline doxorubicin that is an antineoplastic agent instilled into the urinary bladder. The drug disrupts cell DNA causing chromosomal damage. Valrubicin is indicated for the intravesical treatment of BCG-refractory carcinoma in situ of the urinary bladder for those patients who cannot undergo an immediate cystectomy.

J9360

J9360   Injection, vinblastine sulfate, 1 mg

Lay Description

Vinblastine sulfate is an antineoplastic drug that is an alkaloid extract from the herb known as Madagascar periwinkle or Vinca rosea Linn. It interferes with the cell metabolism of amino acids and nucleic acid synthesis causing cell death. Vinblastine sulfate, singularly or in combination, is indicated for the treatment of Hodgkin's disease, lymphocytic lymphoma, histiocytic lymphoma, mycosis fungoides, Kaposi's sarcoma, Letterer-Siwe disease, advanced carcinoma of the testis, choriocarcinoma resistant to other chemotherapeutic agents, and breast cancer that is unresponsive to surgery and hormonal therapy. The recommended dosage varies from 2.5 mg to 18.5 mg per m^2 of body surface depending upon the patient's age and response. Vinblastine sulfate is administered by intravenous injection.

J9370-J9371

J9370 Vincristine sulfate, 1 mg

J9371 Injection, vincristine sulfate liposome, 1 mg

Lay Description
Vincristine sulfate is an antineoplastic drug that is an alkaloid extract from the herb known as Madagascar periwinkle or Vinca rosea Linn. It interferes with the cell metabolism of amino acids and nucleic acid synthesis causing cell death. Vincristine sulfate, singularly or in combination, is indicated for the treatment of acute leukemia, non-Hodgkin's lymphoma, Hodgkin's disease, neuroblastoma, rhabdomyosarcoma, and Wilms' tumor. A liposome is an artificially prepared vesicle composed of a lipid bilayer. It is used to deliver nutrients and drugs . The recommended dosage varies from 0.5 to 1.4 mg per m^2 of body surface depending upon the patient's age and response. Vincristine sulfate is administered by intravenous injection.

J9390

J9390 Injection, vinorelbine tartrate, 10 mg

Lay Description
Vinorelbine tartrate is an antineoplastic drug that is a semisynthetic derivative of vinblastine. Vinblastine is an alkaloid extract from the herb known as Madagascar periwinkle or Vinca rosea Linn. It interferes with the cell metabolism of amino acids and nucleic acid synthesis causing cell death. Vinorelbine tartrate, singularly or in combination with cisplatinum, is indicated for the treatment of unresectable, advanced nonsmall cell lung cancer. The recommended dosage is from 25 to 30 mg per m^2 of body surface depending upon the regimen. It is administered by intravenous injection over six to 10 minutes.

J9395

J9395 Injection, fulvestrant, 25 mg

Lay Description
Fulvestrant is an antineoplastic estrogen receptor antagonist. Many breast cancers have estrogen receptors and their growth can be stimulated by estrogen. Fulvestrant binds to the estrogen receptor preventing the estrogen from reaching the cells. It is indicated for the treatment of estrogen receptor, positive metastatic breast cancer in postmenopausal women who have not responded to other antiestrogen therapy. The recommended dosage is 250 mg. Fulvestrant is administered as a slow intramuscular injection into the buttocks. It may be administered as a single 5 ml injection or as two 2.5 ml injections.

J9400

J9400 Injection, ziv-aflibercept, 1 mg

Lay Description
Ziv-aflibercept is a recombinant fusion protein composed of vascular endothelial growth factor (VEGF)-binding portions from the domains of human VEGF Receptors 1 and 2 then fused to a portion of the human Immunoglobulin G (IgG1). When the drug binds to these receptors, it blocks their activation and can result in the decreased growth of new blood vessels and decreased vascular permeability. Ziv-aflibercept is produced by recombinant DNA technology in a Chinese hamster ovary. Ziv-aflibercept is indicated for patients with metastatic colorectal cancer that is resistant to or has progressed following an oxaliplatin-containing regimen. It is to be used in combination with 5-fluorouracil (5-FU), leucovorin, and irinotecan. The recommended dosage is 4 mg/kg as an intravenous infusion over one hour every two weeks.

J9600

J9600 Injection, porfimer sodium, 75 mg

Lay Description
Porfimer sodium is a mixture of porphyrins that sensitizes cells to light. The drug is injected into neoplastic cells as step one of a two-step photodynamic treatment. Two to three days following injection, the neoplasm is irradiated with a laser light producing a cytotoxic reaction that destroys the cells. As the penetration of the light is limited, the photodynamic therapy is primarily used to treat small thin lesions on accessible surfaces. This type of photodynamic therapy is indicated for the palliative care of patients with completely obstructing esophageal cancer, patients with have partially obstructing esophageal cancer who cannot be satisfactorily treated with laser therapy alone, patients with partially or completely obstructive endobrachial nonsmall cell lung cancer, or patients who have microinvasive endobrachial nonsmall cell lung cancer for whom surgery and radiotherapy are not indicated.

J9999

J9999 Not otherwise classified, antineoplastic drugs

Lay Description
Use this code to represent an antineoplastic drug that has been administered and is not represented by any other HCPCS Level I or Level II code.

K

K0001

K0001   Standard wheelchair

Lay Description

A standard wheelchair has a seat width of 16 (narrow) or 18 inches (adult), a seat depth of 16 inches, and 21 inches from seat to floor. It comes with a nonadjustable back height of 16 to 21 inches, a chrome plated frame, 24 inch molded rear wheels, 8 inch molded casters, nylon or vinyl upholstery, and fixed or swing away detachable footrests. The footplate extension is between 16 and 21 inches. The standard wheelchair weighs more than 36 pounds.

K0002

K0002   Standard hemi (low seat) wheelchair

Lay Description

This code reports a standard hemi (low seat) wheelchair. A hemi wheelchair has a seat height of 16 to 18 inches and is made for patients with a short stature or for patients who have an inability to place feet directly on the ground for propulsion. The hemi wheelchair has a weight capacity of 250 pounds and weighs 36 pounds or less. It comes with a chrome plated frame, 24-inch molded rear wheels, 8-inch molded casters, nylon or vinyl upholstery, and fixed or swing away detachable footrests.

K0003

K0003   Lightweight wheelchair

Lay Description

A lightweight wheelchair is indicated for patients requiring a chair for self-propulsion, and when the seat measurements required cannot be accommodated by a standard or hemi standard wheelchair. This device weighs less than 36 pounds, is fully reclining, and has swing away detachable legrests. The seat width is 14, 16, or 18 inches, has a seat depth of 16 inches, and seat height between 17 and 21 inches. It has a nonadjustable back height of 16 to 17 inches, 24 inch molded rear wheels; 8 inch molded casters, nylon or vinyl upholstery, fixed-height detachable arms, and fixed or swing away detachable footrests. The footplate extension is between 14 and 17 inches.

K0004

K0004   High strength, lightweight wheelchair

Lay Description

A high strength, lightweight wheelchair is indicated for patients requiring a chair for self propulsion that is extra strong in frame construction, and when the seat measurements required cannot be accommodated by a standard or hemi standard wheelchair. This device weighs less than 34 pounds, with cross braces. The seat width is 14, 16, or 18 inches, has a seat depth of 14 (child) or 16 inches (adult), and a seat height

between 17 and 21 inches. It has a sectional or adjustable back height of 15 to 19 inches. It has 24 inch molded rear wheels, 8 inch molded casters, nylon upholstery, fixed-height detachable arms, and fixed or swing away detachable footrests. The footplate extension is 16 to 21 inches.

K0005

K0005   Ultralightweight wheelchair

Lay Description

An ultra-lightweight wheelchair weighs less than 30 pounds, with cross braces, has a seat width of 14, 16, or 18 inches, a seat depth of 14 (child) or 16 inches (adult), and a seat height between 17 and 21 inches. It has an adjustable rear axle position, nylon upholstery, fixed or detachable arms, and fixed or swing away detachable footrests. The footplate extension is 16 to 21 inches.

K0006-K0007

K0006   Heavy-duty wheelchair
K0007   Extra heavy-duty wheelchair

Lay Description

Wide, heavy-duty, and extra heavy-duty wheelchairs are indicated for obese patients when the seat measurements required cannot be accommodated by a standard wheelchair. The seat width is 18 inches, has a seat depth of 16 to 17 inches, and a seat height between 19 and 21 inches. It has a nonadjustable back height of 16 to 17 inches. It has reinforced back and seat upholstery, fixed-height detachable arms, and fixed or swing away detachable footrests. The footplate extension is 16 to 21 inches.

K0008

K0008   Custom manual wheelchair/base

Lay Description

A custom manual wheelchair or base is a uniquely constructed or substantially modified wheelchair or base adapted to a specific patient according to the physician's description and orders. Customized items are rarely necessary and are rarely furnished. It is expected to be a one-of-a-kind item fabricated to meet specific needs.

K0009

K0009   Other manual wheelchair/base

Lay Description

Use this code to report manual wheelchair bases that are not described by any other HCPCS Level II code.

K0010-K0014

K0010 Standard-weight frame motorized/power wheelchair

K0011 Standard-weight frame motorized/power wheelchair with programmable control parameters for speed adjustment, tremor dampening, acceleration control and braking

K0012 Lightweight portable motorized/power wheelchair

K0013 Custom motorized/power wheelchair base

K0014 Other motorized/power wheelchair base

Lay Description

Motorized (powered) wheelchairs are those not included in the manual wheelchair categories. They can be standard, lightweight, and customized, and can be fitted with a variety of accessories. These wheelchairs are generally slow-speed and fairly good at maneuvering and negotiating corners and certain inclines. They usually work from a battery power source. Motorized wheelchairs are not suited to patients who cannot operate the controls, such as stroke patients. Wheelchairs, in general, assist the patient in the activities of daily living (ADL), both in and out of the home. They enable the patient to move about in confined and open spaces. While some patients and/or their caretakers may prefer motorized wheelchairs, depending on the patient's clinical needs and ADL restrictions, payers' policies can differ widely in coverage. The patient's medical condition may dictate whether or not the patient can operate (maneuver and control) a motorized wheelchair alone or with limited assistance and/or observation. A custom manual wheelchair or base is a uniquely constructed or substantially modified wheelchair or base adapted to a specific patient according to the physician's description and orders. It is expected to be a one-of-a-kind item fabricated to meet specific needs.

K0015-K0020

K0015 Detachable, nonadjustable height armrest, each

K0017 Detachable, adjustable height armrest, base, each

K0018 Detachable, adjustable height armrest, upper portion, each

K0019 Arm pad, each

K0020 Fixed, adjustable height armrest, pair

Lay Description

Armrests are used with wheelchairs to provide comfort to the patient. They help with the patient position, allowing for better posture. There are several different types of armrests. Fixed armrests are bolted to the chair and cannot be removed. Detachable armrests can be removed to make moving the patient easier and to allow the patient better access to tables and desks. The armrests may also be adjustable to different heights for comfort and function. Armrest pads are attached to the armrest; they may be upholstered, hard plastic, or covered with soft material.

K0037

K0037 High mount flip-up footrest, each

Lay Description

The flip up footrest forms the support surface on which the patient's foot is supported and may be flipped up out of the way when the patient is transferred in or out of the wheelchair. Use this code to report a flip up footrest that is mounted high up on the wheelchair.

K0038-K0039

K0038 Leg strap, each

K0039 Leg strap, H style, each

Lay Description

Use these codes to report the fabric strap that is placed over the legs to secure the lower leg to the legrest. The H-style leg strap covers more of the leg and provides greater stability for the patient with severely impaired legs. Typically, the H-strap is used for quadriplegics, hemiplegics, paraplegics, and patients with palsy.

K0040-K0042

K0040 Adjustable angle footplate, each

K0041 Large size footplate, each

K0042 Standard size footplate, each

Lay Description

Footplates are flat surfaces designed to support the feet while in a wheelchair. They may be aluminum (usually found in heavy duty wheelchairs) or made of a plastic composite material, which is lightweight and easy to keep clean. Footplates come in various sizes but usually support the individual's foot from the back of his/her heel to around the ball of the foot. An adjustable angle footplate is usually aluminum and has two or three adjustment features, depending on the model of the wheelchair. Adjustable angle footplates are generally longer since they support more of the foot than the standard footplates and may be adjusted with the toes pointing down or up. Use these codes to report each wheelchair footplate.

K0043-K0045

K0043 Footrest, lower extension tube, each

K0044 Footrest, upper hanger bracket, each

K0045 Footrest, complete assembly

Lay Description

Footrests are available in two or three angles, depending on the individual's needs, and may be removed. The lower extension tube attaches to the footplate. The upper hanger bracket attaches the footrest to the wheelchair. The complete assembly includes all three components.

K

K0046-K0047

K0046 Elevating legrest, lower extension tube, each

K0047 Elevating legrest, upper hanger bracket, each

Lay Description
Elevating legrests attach to the lower front of the chair and are used to support the legs. The elevating legrest can be positioned to maintain the leg in an extended position or at varying angles. These codes represent pieces of a footrest.

K0050

K0050 Ratchet assembly

Lay Description
A wheelchair ratchet assembly is a device that allows continuous linear or rotary movement in one direction while preventing motion in the opposite direction. A ratchet may allow the wheels to roll forward, but prevent any backward motion.

K0051

K0051 Cam release assembly, footrest or legrest, each

Lay Description
A cam release assembly device allows quick and easy release and removal of the legrest or footrest of a wheelchair. The legrest or footrest can be removed for access to the patient and transporting the wheelchair.

K0052

K0052 Swingaway, detachable footrests, each

Lay Description
Swing away footrests form a platform on which the foot is supported. The hinged connection enables the footrest to rotate out of the way when the patient is transferred into or out of the wheelchair. Use this code to report removable swing away footrests.

K0053

K0053 Elevating footrests, articulating (telescoping), each

Lay Description
Elevating footrests can be raised up to elevate and support the patient's legs. The telescopic feature allows the legrest to be lengthened as a support for patients with longer limbs. Use this code to report each elevating, articulating footrest.

K0056

K0056 Seat height less than 17 in or equal to or greater than 21 in for a high-strength, lightweight, or ultralightweight wheelchair

Lay Description
A standard wheelchair has a nonadjustable back height of 16 to 21 inches. The standard wheelchair weighs more than 36 pounds. This code is used to report a seat height less than 17 inches or equal to or greater than 21 inches that is designed for use in a high-strength, lightweight, or ultra lightweight wheelchair.

K0065

K0065 Spoke protectors, each

Lay Description
Wheelchair spoke protectors, or spoke guards, are lightweight discs designed to cover the back wheels of wheelchairs. These protectors prevent fingers from going into the spokes of the wheelchairs.

K0069-K0070

K0069 Rear wheel assembly, complete, with solid tire, spokes or molded, each

K0070 Rear wheel assembly, complete, with pneumatic tire, spokes or molded, each

Lay Description
The rear wheels are the large wheels on the back of a wheelchair often used for propulsion. The wheel assembly is comprised of the rear wheel, spokes, and hub. The wheels may come with solid or pneumatic tires. Use these codes to report the rear wheel assembly (based on type of tire).

K0071-K0077

K0071 Front caster assembly, complete, with pneumatic tire, each

K0072 Front caster assembly, complete, with semipneumatic tire, each

K0073 Caster pin lock, each

K0077 Front caster assembly, complete, with solid tire, each

Lay Description
Casters are the front wheels of a wheelchair and are designed to pivot and allow the patient to steer the chair. The caster assembly is composed of the front wheel and the castor fork assembly. Casters may come with pneumatic, semi pneumatic, or solid tires. Use these codes to report the complete front caster assembly (based on type of tire) or to report the pin that locks the caster in place.

K0098

K0098 Drive belt for power wheelchair

Lay Description
A drive belt is used with the belt-drive power wheelchair to connect the motor to the drive wheels.

K0105

K0105 IV hanger, each

Lay Description
The IV hanger is a pole that attaches to a wheelchair to allow the patient to receive an infusion.

K0108

K0108 Wheelchair component or accessory, not otherwise specified

Lay Description
A wheelchair component or accessory is an addition or a part of a wheelchair. Report this code for a wheelchair component or accessory that is not identified by a more specific HCPCS Level II code.

K0195

K0195 Elevating legrests, pair (for use with capped rental wheelchair base)

Lay Description
An elevating legrest is a wheelchair accessory required by patients who have musculoskeletal conditions, casts, or braces that prevent 90-degree flexion at the knee. It may also be required for patients with significant edema of the lower extremities requiring elevation of the legs and for patients who require a reclining back on the wheelchair. This code reports a single elevating legrest and all hardware required for complete assembly. Report this code twice for patients who require elevating legrests for both legs.

K0455

K0455 Infusion pump used for uninterrupted parenteral administration of medication, (e.g., epoprostenol or treprostinol)

Lay Description
Epoprostenol (Flolan) is a medication used primarily to treat pulmonary hypertension. Its brief half life typically requires continuous parenteral infusion. The infusion pump is usually delivered through the subclavian or jugular veins, sometimes through a tunneled catheter that exits in an area maintainable by the patient. The pump is typically portable, worn on a harness or belt, and powered by 9-volt or AA alkaline batteries. Often a second unit is worn, or immediately available, and alternated every 24 hours to ensure uninterrupted delivery.

K0462

K0462 Temporary replacement for patient-owned equipment being repaired, any type

Lay Description
This code is used to report temporary replacement of patient equipment that is being repaired.

K0552

K0552 Supplies for external drug infusion pump, syringe type cartridge, sterile, each

Lay Description
These codes are used to report the sterile supplies required for the syringe type cartridge external drug infusion pump. The pump runs on electrical current.

K0601-K0605

K0601 Replacement battery for external infusion pump owned by patient, silver oxide, 1.5 volt, each

K0602 Replacement battery for external infusion pump owned by patient, silver oxide, 3 volt, each

K0603 Replacement battery for external infusion pump owned by patient, alkaline, 1.5 volt, each

K0604 Replacement battery for external infusion pump owned by patient, lithium, 3.6 volt, each

K0605 Replacement battery for external infusion pump owned by patient, lithium, 4.5 volt, each

Lay Description
The external infusion pump (EIP) is a small portable device that provides a continuous infusion therapy over an extended time period. The EIP requires batteries for operation. Use these codes to report the batteries required by an EIP that is owned by the patient.

K0606-K0609

K0606 Automatic external defibrillator, with integrated electrocardiogram analysis, garment type

K0607 Replacement battery for automated external defibrillator, garment type only, each

K0608 Replacement garment for use with automated external defibrillator, each

K0609 Replacement electrodes for use with automated external defibrillator, garment type only, each

Lay Description
Automatic external defibrillators are compact and portable devices that deliver an electrical shock to a person who has a sudden cardiac arrest. Automatic external defibrillator units use a microprocessor inside of a portable defibrillator to interpret a person's heart rhythm through electrodes. The computer recognizes ventricular fibrillation or ventricular tachycardia. Once recognized, the computer advises the operator/user that electrical defibrillation is needed or it will automatically deliver a countershock. The patient wears the external defibrillator in a vest.

K0669

K0669 Wheelchair accessory, wheelchair seat or back cushion, does not meet specific code criteria or no written coding verification from DME PDAC

Lay Description
Wheelchair seat cushions can provide leg positioning, pelvic stability, and pressure management for patients with postural asymmetry. A cushion may provide support and pressure relief for individuals

K

sitting in a wheelchair. The cushions can be made out of various material and filling. The Pricing, Data Analysis and Coding (PDAC) contractor maintains the Durable Medical Equipment Coding System.

K0672

K0672 Addition to lower extremity orthotic, removable soft interface, all components, replacement only, each

Lay Description
A soft interface is worn under an orthosis to provide skin cushioning and protection. It also lessens the pressure and irritation that the orthosis can cause. The interface can be made of different kinds of fibers and are usually seam free.

K0730

K0730 Controlled dose inhalation drug delivery system

Lay Description
A controlled dose inhalation drug delivery system provides a precise, monitored dose of inhaled medication. The dose provided in nebulizers may vary somewhat from patient to patient based on breathing patterns. The medications through a nebulizer are administered in a continuous flow. Some medications require precise dosing that cannot be obtained with other nebulizers. The controlled dose inhaler monitors the patient's breathing pattern and adjusts the drug delivery. Medication is only administered during inhalation and not during exhalation.

K0733

K0733 Power wheelchair accessory, 12 to 24 amp hour sealed lead acid battery, each (e.g., gel cell, absorbed glassmat)

Lay Description
A 12 to 24 amp hour lead-acid battery is a valve-regulated type that may be referred to as sealed or maintenance-free. This type of battery fixes the acid electrolyte in a gel or in an absorptive fiberglass mat. A gel cell suspends the electrolyte in a silica-based gel producing a thick pasty material. An absorbed glassmat (AGM) suspends the electrolyte in fiberglass matt separators that act as absorbent sponges. The battery needs no added water and can be safely operated in any position.

K0738

K0738 Portable gaseous oxygen system, rental; home compressor used to fill portable oxygen cylinders; includes portable containers, regulator, flowmeter, humidifier, cannula or mask, and tubing

Lay Description
A rented portable gaseous oxygen system is equipment that includes a home compressor used to fill portable oxygen cylinders. This type of system allows individuals to fill their own oxygen cylinders in their homes. This is accomplished by attaching the home compressor to an oxygen concentrator that provides the oxygen for the cylinders. The home compressor takes the oxygen and compresses it into the portable cylinders, which the patient uses when away from home. The home compressor can be used simultaneously to receive stationary oxygen while at the same time filling portable cylinders. This code includes all delivery hardware associated with use of the portable gaseous oxygen system, including portable containers, regulator, flowmeter, humidifier, cannula/mask, and tubing.

K0739-K0740

K0739 Repair or nonroutine service for durable medical equipment other than oxygen equipment requiring the skill of a technician, labor component, per 15 minutes

K0740 Repair or nonroutine service for oxygen equipment requiring the skill of a technician, labor component, per 15 minutes

Lay Description
These codes report the repair or non-routine service of durable medical equipment, such as wheelchair repair or oxygen equipment, that requires the skill of a technician. The labor involved in the repair or service is reported in 15-minute increments.

K0743

K0743 Suction pump, home model, portable, for use on wounds

Lay Description
Home wound suction is achieved with a system of components. The wound suction pump provides a controlled atmospheric pressure without the use of a collection canister. The pump is used with separately reportable special dressings that absorb the drainage. Use this code to report use of a home suction pump.

K0744-K0746

K0744 Absorptive wound dressing for use with suction pump, home model, portable, pad size 16 sq in or less

K0745 Absorptive wound dressing for use with suction pump, home model, portable, pad size more than 16 sq in but less than or equal to 48 sq in

K0746 Absorptive wound dressing for use with suction pump, home model, portable, pad size greater than 48 sq in

Lay Description
These codes are used to report the dressing sets used with the portable suction pump that does not require a collection canister. These codes include all of the necessary components of a complete dressing change, such as the drainage tubing, the porous

K

non-adherent dressing, and an occlusive dressing that creates the seal around the wound site.

K0800-K0812

K0800 Power operated vehicle, group 1 standard, patient weight capacity up to and including 300 pounds

K0801 Power operated vehicle, group 1 heavy-duty, patient weight capacity 301 to 450 pounds

K0802 Power operated vehicle, group 1 very heavy-duty, patient weight capacity 451 to 600 pounds

K0806 Power operated vehicle, group 2 standard, patient weight capacity up to and including 300 pounds

K0807 Power operated vehicle, group 2 heavy-duty, patient weight capacity 301 to 450 pounds

K0808 Power operated vehicle, group 2 very heavy-duty, patient weight capacity 451 to 600 pounds

K0812 Power operated vehicle, not otherwise classified

Lay Description
A power operated vehicle (POV) is a battery powered mobility device with tiller operated steering and three or four wheels. POVs may also be referred to as scooters. POVs are designed for a combination of indoor use with moderate outdoor capabilities on flat terrain and hard surfaces with minimal to moderate surface irregularity. A POV assists patients for whom a wheelchair is unsuitable in the activities of daily living, but POVs are not suited to all types of patients such as stroke victims or some quadriplegic and/or hemiplegic patients who cannot operate the controls nor be left alone while the vehicle is in operation. POVs are divided into two groups. Group 1 POVs have the following specifications: length 48 inches, width 28 inches, obstacle height 20 mm, minimum top end speed-flat 3 MPH, range 5 miles, and dynamic stability incline 6 degrees. Group 2 POVs have the following specifications: length 48 inches, width 28 inches, obstacle height 50 mm, minimum top end speed-flat 4 MPH, range 10 miles, and dynamic stability incline 7.5 degrees. POVs are further classified by weight capacity. Standard refers to a weight capacity up to and including 300 pounds. Heavy duty refers to a weight capacity of between 301 and 450 pounds. Very heavy duty refers to a weight capacity of between 451 and 600 pounds.

K0813-K0816

K0813 Power wheelchair, group 1 standard, portable, sling/solid seat and back, patient weight capacity up to and including 300 pounds

K0814 Power wheelchair, group 1 standard, portable, captain's chair, patient weight capacity up to and including 300 pounds

K0815 Power wheelchair, group 1 standard, sling/solid seat and back, patient weight capacity up to and including 300 pounds

K0816 Power wheelchair, group 1 standard, captain's chair, patient weight capacity up to and including 300 pounds

Lay Description
These codes describe Group 1 standard power wheelchairs. Group 1 power wheelchairs have the following specifications: length 40 inches, width 24 inches, obstacle height 20 mm, minimum top end speed-flat 3 MPH, range 5 miles, dynamic stability incline 6 degrees, fatigue test on a level 200,000 cycles with 0.5 inch slats under all wheels, and 6,666 drop cycles. Standard wheelchairs have a maximum weight capacity of 300 pounds. Chairs represented by these four codes have been further subdivided by portability. Portable chairs are defined as being easily disassembled without the use of tools for transport in a vehicle whereas nonportable chairs cannot be easily disassembled. Each of these subcategories has been further defined by the type of chair.

K0820-K0823

K0820 Power wheelchair, group 2 standard, portable, sling/solid seat/back, patient weight capacity up to and including 300 pounds

K0821 Power wheelchair, group 2 standard, portable, captain's chair, patient weight capacity up to and including 300 pounds

K0822 Power wheelchair, group 2 standard, sling/solid seat/back, patient weight capacity up to and including 300 pounds

K0823 Power wheelchair, group 2 standard, captain's chair, patient weight capacity up to and including 300 pounds

Lay Description
These codes describe Group 2 standard power wheelchairs. Group 2 power wheelchairs have the following specifications: length 48 inches, width 34 inches, obstacle height 40 mm, minimum top speed-flat 3 MPH, range 7 miles, dynamic stability incline 6 degrees, fatigue test on a level 200,000 cycles with 0.5 inch slats under all wheels, and 6,666 drop cycles. Standard wheelchairs have a maximum weight capacity of 300 pounds. Chairs represented by these four codes have been further subdivided by portability. Portable chairs are defined as being easily disassembled without use of tools for transport in a vehicle whereas nonportable chairs cannot be easily

K

disassembled. Each of these subcategories has been further defined by the type of chair.

K0824-K0825

K0824 Power wheelchair, group 2 heavy-duty, sling/solid seat/back, patient weight capacity 301 to 450 pounds

K0825 Power wheelchair, group 2 heavy-duty, captain's chair, patient weight capacity 301 to 450 pounds

Lay Description
These codes describe Group 2 heavy duty power wheelchairs. Group 2 power wheelchairs have the following specifications: length 48 inches, width 34 inches, obstacle height 40 mm, minimum top speed-flat 3 MPH, range 7 miles, dynamic stability incline 6 degrees, fatigue test on a level 200,000 cycles with 0.5 inch slats under all wheels, and 6,666 drop cycles. Heavy duty wheelchairs have a weight capacity of between 301 to 450 pounds. Chairs represented by these two codes have been further subdivided by type of chair.

K0826-K0827

K0826 Power wheelchair, group 2 very heavy-duty, sling/solid seat/back, patient weight capacity 451 to 600 pounds

K0827 Power wheelchair, group 2 very heavy-duty, captain's chair, patient weight capacity 451 to 600 pounds

Lay Description
These codes describe Group 2 very heavy duty power wheelchairs. Group 2 power wheelchairs have the following specifications: length 48 inches, width 34 inches, obstacle height 40 mm, minimum top speed-flat 3 MPH, range 7 miles, dynamic stability incline 6 degrees, fatigue test on a level 200,000 cycles with 0.5 inch slats under all wheels, and 6,666 drop cycles. Very heavy duty wheelchairs have a weight capacity of 451 to 600 pounds. Chairs represented by these two codes have been further subdivided by type of chair.

K0828-K0829

K0828 Power wheelchair, group 2 extra heavy-duty, sling/solid seat/back, patient weight capacity 601 pounds or more

K0829 Power wheelchair, group 2 extra heavy-duty, captain's chair, patient weight 601 pounds or more

Lay Description
These codes describe Group 2 extra heavy duty power wheelchairs. Group 2 power wheelchairs have the following specifications: length 48 inches, width 34 inches, obstacle height 40 mm, minimum top speed-flat 3 MPH, range 7 miles, dynamic stability incline 6 degrees, fatigue test on a level 200,000 cycles with 0.5 inch slats under all wheels, and 6,666 drop cycles. Extra heavy duty wheelchairs have a weight

capacity of 601 pounds or more. Chairs represented by these two codes have been further subdivided by type of chair: sling/solid seat/back and a captain's chair.

K0830-K0831

K0830 Power wheelchair, group 2 standard, seat elevator, sling/solid seat/back, patient weight capacity up to and including 300 pounds

K0831 Power wheelchair, group 2 standard, seat elevator, captain's chair, patient weight capacity up to and including 300 pounds

Lay Description
These codes describe Group 2 standard power wheelchairs with the added feature of a seat elevator. Seat elevators are used to assist with transfers and to reach items that would be out of reach from a standard wheelchair height. Group 2 power wheelchairs have the following specifications: length 48 inches, width 34 inches, obstacle height 40 mm, minimum top speed-flat 3 MPH, range 7 miles, dynamic stability incline 6 degrees, fatigue test on a level 200,000 cycles with 0.5 inch slats under all wheels, and 6,666 drop cycles. Standard wheelchairs have a maximum weight capacity of 300 pounds. Chairs represented by these two codes have been further subdivided by type of chair.

K0835-K0840

K0835 Power wheelchair, group 2 standard, single power option, sling/solid seat/back, patient weight capacity up to and including 300 pounds

K0836 Power wheelchair, group 2 standard, single power option, captain's chair, patient weight capacity up to and including 300 pounds

K0837 Power wheelchair, group 2 heavy-duty, single power option, sling/solid seat/back, patient weight capacity 301 to 450 pounds

K0838 Power wheelchair, group 2 heavy-duty, single power option, captain's chair, patient weight capacity 301 to 450 pounds

K0839 Power wheelchair, group 2 very heavy-duty, single power option sling/solid seat/back, patient weight capacity 451 to 600 pounds

K0840 Power wheelchair, group 2 extra heavy-duty, single power option, sling/solid seat/back, patient weight capacity 601 pounds or more

Lay Description
These codes describe Group 2 power wheelchairs with the added feature of a single power option. Group 2 power wheelchairs have the following specifications: length 48 inches, width 34 inches, obstacle height 40

mm, minimum top speed-flat 3 MPH, range 7 miles, dynamic stability incline 6 degrees, fatigue test on a level 200,000 cycles with 0.5 inch slats under all wheels, and 6,666 drop cycles. The single power option is available in all weight capacities, including standard (weight capacity up to and including 300 pounds), heavy duty (weight capacity 301 to 450 pounds), very heavy duty (weight capacity 451 to 600 pounds), and extra heavy duty (weight capacity 601 pounds or more). Standard and heavy duty weight capacity chairs with single power option are further classified by type of chair.

K0841-K0843

K0841 **Power wheelchair, group 2 standard, multiple power option, sling/solid seat/back, patient weight capacity up to and including 300 pounds**

K0842 **Power wheelchair, group 2 standard, multiple power option, captain's chair, patient weight capacity up to and including 300 pounds**

K0843 **Power wheelchair, group 2 heavy-duty, multiple power option, sling/solid seat/back, patient weight capacity 301 to 450 pounds**

Lay Description
These codes describe Group 2 power wheelchairs with the added feature of a multiple power option. Group 2 power wheelchairs have the following specifications: length 48 inches, width 34 inches, obstacle height 40 mm, minimum top speed-flat 3 MPH, range 7 miles, dynamic stability incline 6 degrees, fatigue test on a level 200,000 cycles with 0.5 inch slats under all wheels, and 6,666 drop cycles. The multiple power option is available in only standard and heavy duty weight capacities. Standard weight capacity is defined as up to and including 300 pounds and heavy duty weight capacity is 301 to 450 pounds. Standard weight capacity chairs with single power option are further classified by type of chair.

K0848-K0851

K0848 **Power wheelchair, group 3 standard, sling/solid seat/back, patient weight capacity up to and including 300 pounds**

K0849 **Power wheelchair, group 3 standard, captain's chair, patient weight capacity up to and including 300 pounds**

K0850 **Power wheelchair, group 3 heavy-duty, sling/solid seat/back, patient weight capacity 301 to 450 pounds**

K0851 **Power wheelchair, group 3 heavy-duty, captain's chair, patient weight capacity 301 to 450 pounds**

Lay Description
These codes describe standard and heavy duty Group 3 power wheelchairs. Group 3 power wheelchairs have the following specifications: length 48 inches, width 34 inches, obstacle height 60 mm, minimum

top speed-flat 4.5 MPH, range 12 miles, dynamic stability incline 7.5 degrees, fatigue test on a level 200,000 cycles with 0.5 inch slats under all wheels, and 6,666 drop cycles. Standard weight capacity is defined as up to and including 300 pounds and heavy duty weight capacity is 301 to 450 pounds. Standard and heavy duty weight capacity chairs are further classified by type of chair.

K0852-K0855

K0852 **Power wheelchair, group 3 very heavy-duty, sling/solid seat/back, patient weight capacity 451 to 600 pounds**

K0853 **Power wheelchair, group 3 very heavy-duty, captain's chair, patient weight capacity 451 to 600 pounds**

K0854 **Power wheelchair, group 3 extra heavy-duty, sling/solid seat/back, patient weight capacity 601 pounds or more**

K0855 **Power wheelchair, group 3 extra heavy-duty, captain's chair, patient weight capacity 601 pounds or more**

Lay Description
These codes describe very heavy duty and extra heavy duty Group 3 power wheelchairs. Group 3 power wheelchairs have the following specifications: length 48 inches, width 34 inches, obstacle height 60 mm, minimum top speed-flat 4.5 MPH, range 12 miles, dynamic stability incline 7.5 degrees, fatigue test on a level 200,000 cycles with 0.5 inch slats under all wheels, and 6,666 drop cycles. Very heavy duty weight capacity is 451 to 600 pounds and extra heavy duty is 601 pounds or more. Very heavy duty and extra heavy duty weight capacity chairs are further classified by type of chair.

K0856-K0860

K0856 **Power wheelchair, group 3 standard, single power option, sling/solid seat/back, patient weight capacity up to and including 300 pounds**

K0857 **Power wheelchair, group 3 standard, single power option, captain's chair, patient weight capacity up to and including 300 pounds**

K0858 **Power wheelchair, group 3 heavy-duty, single power option, sling/solid seat/back, patient weight 301 to 450 pounds**

K0859 **Power wheelchair, group 3 heavy-duty, single power option, captain's chair, patient weight capacity 301 to 450 pounds**

K0860 **Power wheelchair, group 3 very heavy-duty, single power option, sling/solid seat/back, patient weight capacity 451 to 600 pounds**

K

Lay Description

These codes describe Group 3 power wheelchairs with the added feature of a single power option. Group 3 power wheelchairs have the following specifications: length 48 inches, width 34 inches, obstacle height 60 mm, minimum top speed-flat 4.5 MPH, range 12 miles, dynamic stability incline 7.5 degrees, fatigue test on a level 200,000 cycles with 0.5 inch slats under all wheels, and 6,666 drop cycles. The single power option is available in standard (weight capacity up to and including 300 pounds), heavy duty (weight capacity 301 to 450 pounds), and very heavy duty (weight capacity 451 to 600 pounds). Standard and heavy duty weight capacity chairs are further classified by type of chair.

K0861-K0864

K0861   **Power wheelchair, group 3 standard, multiple power option, sling/solid seat/back, patient weight capacity up to and including 300 pounds**

K0862   **Power wheelchair, group 3 heavy-duty, multiple power option, sling/solid seat/back, patient weight capacity 301 to 450 pounds**

K0863   **Power wheelchair, group 3 very heavy-duty, multiple power option, sling/solid seat/back, patient weight capacity 451 to 600 pounds**

K0864   **Power wheelchair, group 3 extra heavy-duty, multiple power option, sling/solid seat/back, patient weight capacity 601 pounds or more**

Lay Description

These codes describe Group 3 power wheelchairs with the added feature of a multiple power option. Group 3 power wheelchairs have the following specifications: length 48 inches, width 34 inches, obstacle height 60 mm, minimum top speed-flat 4.5 MPH, range 12 miles, dynamic stability incline 7.5 degrees, fatigue test on a level 200,000 cycles with 0.5 inch slats under all wheels, and 6,666 drop cycles. The multiple power option is available with sling/solid seat/back in all weight capacities.

K0868-K0871

K0868   **Power wheelchair, group 4 standard, sling/solid seat/back, patient weight capacity up to and including 300 pounds**

K0869   **Power wheelchair, group 4 standard, captain's chair, patient weight capacity up to and including 300 pounds**

K0870   **Power wheelchair, group 4 heavy-duty, sling/solid seat/back, patient weight capacity 301 to 450 pounds**

K0871   **Power wheelchair, group 4 very heavy-duty, sling/solid seat/back, patient weight capacity 451 to 600 pounds**

Lay Description

These codes describe Group 4 power wheelchairs. Group 4 power wheelchairs have the following specifications: length 48 inches, width 34 inches, obstacle height 75 mm, minimum top speed-flat 6 MPH, range 16 miles, dynamic stability incline 9 degrees, fatigue test on a level 200,000 cycles with 0.5 inch slats under all wheels, and 6,666 drop cycles. Group 4 power wheelchairs are available in three weight capacities, including standard (up to and including 300 pounds), heavy duty (301 to 450 pounds), and very heavy duty (450 to 600 pounds). Standard weight capacity chairs are further classified by type of chair. Heavy duty and very heavy duty chairs are available only as sling/solid seat/back.

K0877-K0880

K0877   **Power wheelchair, group 4 standard, single power option, sling/solid seat/back, patient weight capacity up to and including 300 pounds**

K0878   **Power wheelchair, group 4 standard, single power option, captain's chair, patient weight capacity up to and including 300 pounds**

K0879   **Power wheelchair, group 4 heavy-duty, single power option, sling/solid seat/back, patient weight capacity 301 to 450 pounds**

K0880   **Power wheelchair, group 4 very heavy-duty, single power option, sling/solid seat/back, patient weight 451 to 600 pounds**

Lay Description

These codes describe Group 4 power wheelchairs with the added feature of a single power option. Group 4 power wheelchairs have the following specifications: length 48 inches, width 34 inches, obstacle height 75 mm, minimum top speed-flat 6 MPH, range 16 miles, dynamic stability incline 9 degrees, fatigue test on a level 200,000 cycles with 0.5 inch slats under all wheels, and 6,666 drop cycles. The single power option is available in three weight capacities, including standard (up to and including 300 pounds), heavy duty (301 to 450 pounds), and very heavy duty (450 to 600 pounds). Standard weight capacity chairs with a single power option are further classified by type of chair. Heavy duty and very heavy duty chairs are available only as sling/solid seat/back.

K0884-K0886

K0884   **Power wheelchair, group 4 standard, multiple power option, sling/solid seat/back, patient weight capacity up to and including 300 pounds**

K0885   **Power wheelchair, group 4 standard, multiple power option, captain's chair, patient weight capacity up to and including 300 pounds**

K0886 Power wheelchair, group 4 heavy-duty, multiple power option, sling/solid seat/back, patient weight capacity 301 to 450 pounds

Lay Description
These codes describe Group 4 power wheelchairs with the added feature of a multiple power option. Group 4 power wheelchairs have the following specifications: length 48 inches, width 34 inches, obstacle height 75 mm, minimum top speed-flat 6 MPH, range 16 miles, dynamic stability incline 9 degrees, fatigue test on a level 200,000 cycles with 0.5 inch slats under all wheels, and 6,666 drop cycles. Group 4 power wheelchairs with a multiple power option are available in standard (up to and including 300 pounds) and heavy duty (301 to 450 pounds) weight capacities. Standard weight capacity chairs are further classified by type of chair. Heavy duty chairs are available only as sling/solid seat/back.

K0890-K0891

K0890 Power wheelchair, group 5 pediatric, single power option, sling/solid seat/back, patient weight capacity up to and including 125 pounds

K0891 Power wheelchair, group 5 pediatric, multiple power option, sling/solid seat/back, patient weight capacity up to and including 125 pounds

Lay Description
These codes describe Group 5 power wheelchairs, which are pediatric wheelchairs with a patient weight capacity up to and including 125 pounds. Group 5 power wheelchairs have the following specifications: length 48 inches, width 28 inches, obstacle height 60 mm, minimum top speed-flat 4.5 MPH, range 12 miles, dynamic stability incline 7.5 degrees, fatigue test on a level 200,000 cycles with 0.5 inch slats under all wheels, and 6,666 drop cycles. Group 5 power wheelchairs are available with single and multiple power options in a sling/solid seat/back chair.

K0898-K0899

K0898 Power wheelchair, not otherwise classified

K0899 Power mobility device, not coded by DME PDAC or does not meet criteria

Lay Description
Power wheelchairs and power mobility device codes are assigned based on specific criteria related to length, width, obstacle height, minimum top end speed on a flat surface, range, dynamic stability on incline, fatigue tests on a level with 0.5-inch slats, and drop cycles. Criteria were defined by the Pricing, Data Analysis and Coding (PDAC) contractor, a national entity that provides services under contract to CMS related to DMEPOS HCPCS coding and pricing.

K0900

K0900 Customized durable medical equipment, other than wheelchair

Lay Description
Customized durable medical equipment is uniquely constructed or substantially modified wheelchair or base adapted to a specific patient according to the physician's description and orders. Customized items are rarely necessary and are rarely furnished. It is expected to be a one-of-a-kind item fabricated to meet specific needs. Use this code for durable medical equipment, other than wheelchairs, that meet the customized requirements explained above.

K0901-K0902

K0901 Knee orthosis (KO), single upright, thigh and calf, with adjustable flexion and extension joint (unicentric or polycentric), medial-lateral and rotation control, with or without varus/valgus adjustment, prefabricated, off-the-shelf

K0902 Knee orthosis (KO), double upright, thigh and calf, with adjustable flexion and extension joint (unicentric or polycentric), medial-lateral and rotation control, with or without varus/valgus adjustment, prefabricated, off-the-shelf

Lay Description
Prefabricated knee orthoses (KO) are ready-made (prefabricated) knee braces that are purchased off-the-shelf with no custom fitting or adjustment. Report K0901 for a single upright hinge and K0902 for a double upright hinge. Both are secured to the leg at the thigh and calf, have adjustable flexion and extension joint (unicentric or polycentric), and medial-lateral and rotation control, with or without varus/valgus adjustment.

L

L0112

L0112 Cranial cervical orthotic, congenital torticollis type, with or without soft interface material, adjustable range of motion joint, custom fabricated

Lay Description
A custom fabricated cranial cervical orthosis for congenital muscular torticollis (CMT) is used to treat infants with CMT complicated by plagiocephaly. CMT is a postural deformity that results primarily from unilateral shortening and fibrosis of the sternocleidomastoid muscle. This causes the head to tilt to one side. Plagiocephaly, manifested as deformities of the skull base, cranium, or face, may occur in infants with CMT. These deformities may be the result of intrauterine compression or may occur after birth due to consistent positioning of the head to one side during sleep. A cranial cervical orthosis is

designed to treat both the torticollis and any resulting plagiocephaly. The cranial orthosis consists of a custom fabricated helmet that may be lined with a soft interface material. The helmet remolds the skull to a more normal shape. The helmet is attached to an adjustable cervical orthosis that supports the neck and relieves the tilting of the head. The cervical component can be adjusted as the sternocleidomastoid muscle lengthens and the head tilt becomes less severe.

L0113

L0113   Cranial cervical orthotic, torticollis type, with or without joint, with or without soft interface material, prefabricated, includes fitting and adjustment

Lay Description
A prefabricated cranial cervical orthosis for muscular torticollis is used to treat patients with torticollis. Torticollis is a postural deformity that results primarily from unilateral shortening and fibrosis of the sternocleidomastoid muscle. This causes the head to tilt to one side. The cranial orthosis consists of a prefabricated helmet that may be lined with a soft interface material. The helmet is attached to an adjustable cervical orthosis that supports the neck and relieves the tilting of the head. The cervical component can be adjusted as the sternocleidomastoid muscle lengthens and the head tilt becomes less severe.

L0120-L0130

L0120   Cervical, flexible, nonadjustable, prefabricated, off-the-shelf (foam collar)

L0130   Cervical, flexible, thermoplastic collar, molded to patient

Lay Description
Cervical collars are used to limit the range of motion in the head and neck. By having the jaws and chin supported, the angle between the chin and the chest is maintained, which alleviates stress on the posterior neck/nuchal and suboccipital areas. This reduces the potential for cervical root irritation and adds an extra measure of head/neck immobilization. There is still a minute degree of mobilization capability while the patient is in the cervical collar. These codes report flexible cervical collars. Cervical foam collars are nonadjustable in terms of collar width but can be easily adjusted to the circumference of the patient's neck by simply pulling the collar closed and securing it in an overlapping fashion using the Velcro anchor at the back of the collar. Some collars can be obtained in low, medium, or high contour styles, depending on the collar width and degree of head and/or neck immobilization desired.

L0140-L0160

L0140   Cervical, semi-rigid, adjustable (plastic collar)

L0150   Cervical, semi-rigid, adjustable molded chin cup (plastic collar with mandibular/occipital piece)

L0160   Cervical, semi-rigid, wire frame occipital/mandibular support, prefabricated, off-the-shelf

Lay Description
Cervical collars are used to limit the range of motion in the head and neck. By having the jaws and chin supported, the angle between the chin and the chest is maintained, which alleviates stress on the posterior neck/nuchal and suboccipital areas. This reduces the potential for cervical root irritation and adds an extra measure of head/neck immobilization. There is still a minute degree of mobilization capability while the patient is in the cervical collar. These codes report semi-rigid cervical collars. Semi-rigid collars are typically constructed from plastic or like materials, with padded inner surfaces and may have an added jaw/chin support.

L0170

L0170   Cervical, collar, molded to patient model

Lay Description
Cervical collars are used to limit the range of motion in the head and neck. By having the jaws and chin supported, the angle between the chin and the chest is maintained, which alleviates stress on the posterior neck/nuchal and suboccipital areas. This reduces the potential for cervical root irritation and adds an extra measure of head/neck immobilization. There is still a minute degree of mobilization capability while the patient is in the cervical collar.

L0172

L0172   Cervical, collar, semi-rigid thermoplastic foam, two-piece, prefabricated, off-the-shelf

Lay Description
Cervical collars are used to limit the range of motion in the head and neck. By having the jaws and chin supported, the angle between the chin and the chest is maintained, which alleviates stress on the posterior neck/nuchal and suboccipital areas. This reduces the potential for cervical root irritation and adds an extra measure of head/neck immobilization. There is still a minute degree of mobilization capability while the patient is in the cervical collar. This collar has two pieces, is semi-rigid, usually light in weight though constructed from sturdy plastics, and also has padded or lined surfaces so as not to chafe the patient's skin. Sizes vary according to source.

L0174

L0174 Cervical, collar, semi-rigid, thermoplastic foam, two piece with thoracic extension, prefabricated, off-the-shelf

Lay Description

This code reports the supply of a specific type of two-piece cervical collar. Cervical orthoses are used to restrict motion to prevent pain, to protect spinal instability before or after surgery, and as emergency protection from the effects of trauma. The cervical spine (neck) offers the ability for a wide range of motion. The head normally rotates almost 180 degrees; about 145 degrees of flexion and extension is considered a clinical base as is about 90 degrees of lateral flexion. This type of orthosis restricts these movements by immobilizing the head. The design reported by this code has two semi-rigid pieces. One piece may be a chin support component that drops into the support collar. Other models may feature front and back components. Velcro closures are used to close and adjust the two pieces. The design reported by this code also features an extension to the thoracic region to further stabilize the cervical spine. This may be an upper waistband connected by rigid bars (front and back) to the cervical collar. The thoracic component essentially converts the device to a cervical thoracic orthosis.

L0180-L0200

L0180 Cervical, multiple post collar, occipital/mandibular supports, adjustable

L0190 Cervical, multiple post collar, occipital/mandibular supports, adjustable cervical bars (SOMI, Guilford, Taylor types)

L0200 Cervical, multiple post collar, occipital/mandibular supports, adjustable cervical bars, and thoracic extension

Lay Description

These codes report the supply of multiple post cervical collars. Cervical orthoses are used to restrict motion to prevent pain or to address spinal instability before or after surgery. The healthy cervical spine (neck) offers a wide range of motion. The head normally rotates almost 180 degrees; about 145 degrees of flexion and extension is considered a clinical base as is about 90 degrees of lateral flexion. These types of orthoses restrict these movements by immobilizing the head. All collars will have more than one bar or post to support and immobilize the cervical spine. The Somi brace is named as an acronym for sternal occipital mandibular immobilizer. The Somi brace features three adjustable vertical bars on the front of the device that connects a rigid upper sternal band to the cervical and head support. The head and neck component supports against the mandible (lower jaw) and occiput (back of head). The Guilford brace is an eponym for the designer and features two

adjustable posts (front and back) that extend from a shoulder harness to a ring that supports the head. Some designs may also feature an extension to the thoracic region to further stabilize the cervical spine. This may be a rigid extension to the thoracic region. The thoracic component essentially converts the device to a cervical thoracic orthosis.

L0220

L0220 Thoracic, rib belt, custom fabricated

Lay Description

A thoracic rib belt is an elastic belt used to support the thoracic area and rib cage. This code represents a belt crafted specifically for the patient.

L0450-L0490

L0450 TLSO, flexible, provides trunk support, upper thoracic region, produces intracavitary pressure to reduce load on the intervertebral disks with rigid stays or panel(s), includes shoulder straps and closures, prefabricated, off-the-shelf

L0452 Thoracic-lumbar-sacral orthotic (TLSO), flexible, provides trunk support, upper thoracic region, produces intracavitary pressure to reduce load on the intervertebral disks with rigid stays or panel(s), includes shoulder straps and closures, custom fabricated

L0454 TLSO flexible, provides trunk support, extends from sacrococcygeal junction to above T-9 vertebra, restricts gross trunk motion in the sagittal plane, produces intracavitary pressure to reduce load on the intervertebral disks with rigid stays or panel(s), includes shoulder straps and closures, prefabricated item that has been trimmed, bent, molded, assembled, or otherwise customized to fit a specific patient by an individual with expertise

L0455 TLSO, flexible, provides trunk support, extends from sacrococcygeal junction to above T-9 vertebra, restricts gross trunk motion in the sagittal plane, produces intracavitary pressure to reduce load on the intervertebral disks with rigid stays or panel(s), includes shoulder straps and closures, prefabricated, off-the-shelf

L0456 TLSO, flexible, provides trunk support, thoracic region, rigid posterior panel and soft anterior apron, extends from the sacrococcygeal junction and terminates just inferior to the scapular spine, restricts gross trunk motion in the sagittal plane, produces intracavitary pressure to reduce load on the intervertebral disks, includes straps and closures, prefabricated item that has been trimmed, bent, molded, assembled, or otherwise customized to fit a specific patient by an individual with expertise

L0457 TLSO, flexible, provides trunk support, thoracic region, rigid posterior panel and soft anterior apron, extends from the sacrococcygeal junction and terminates just inferior to the scapular spine, restricts gross trunk motion in the sagittal plane, produces intracavitary pressure to reduce load on the intervertebral disks, includes straps and closures, prefabricated, off-the-shelf

L0458 Thoracic-lumbar-sacral orthotic (TLSO), triplanar control, modular segmented spinal system, 2 rigid plastic shells, posterior extends from the sacrococcygeal junction and terminates just inferior to the scapular spine, anterior extends from the symphysis pubis to the xiphoid, soft liner, restricts gross trunk motion in the sagittal, coronal, and transverse planes, lateral strength is provided by overlapping plastic and stabilizing closures, includes straps and closures, prefabricated, includes fitting and adjustment

L0460 TLSO, triplanar control, modular segmented spinal system, two rigid plastic shells, posterior extends from the sacrococcygeal junction and terminates just inferior to the scapular spine, anterior extends from the symphysis pubis to the sternal notch, soft liner, restricts gross trunk motion in the sagittal, coronal, and transverse planes, lateral strength is provided by overlapping plastic and stabilizing closures, includes straps and closures, prefabricated item that has been trimmed, bent, molded, or otherwise customized to fit a specific patient by an individual with expertise

L0462 Thoracic-lumbar-sacral orthotic (TLSO), triplanar control, modular segmented spinal system, 3 rigid plastic shells, posterior extends from the sacrococcygeal junction and terminates just inferior to the scapular spine, anterior extends from the symphysis pubis to the sternal notch, soft liner, restricts gross trunk motion in the sagittal, coronal, and transverse planes, lateral strength is provided by overlapping plastic and stabilizing closures, includes straps and closures, prefabricated, includes fitting and adjustment

L0464 Thoracic-lumbar-sacral orthotic (TLSO), triplanar control, modular segmented spinal system, 4 rigid plastic shells, posterior extends from sacrococcygeal junction and terminates just inferior to scapular spine, anterior extends from symphysis pubis to the sternal notch, soft liner, restricts gross trunk motion in sagittal, coronal, and transverse planes, lateral strength is provided by overlapping plastic and stabilizing closures, includes straps and closures, prefabricated, includes fitting and adjustment

L0466 TLSO, sagittal control, rigid posterior frame and flexible soft anterior apron with straps, closures and padding, restricts gross trunk motion in sagittal plane, produces intracavitary pressure to reduce load on intervertebral disks, prefabricated item that has been trimmed, bent, molded, assembled, or otherwise customized to fit a specific patient by an individual with expertise

L0467 TLSO, sagittal control, rigid posterior frame and flexible soft anterior apron with straps, closures and padding, restricts gross trunk motion in sagittal plane, produces intracavitary pressure to reduce load on intervertebral disks, prefabricated, off-the-shelf

L0468 TLSO, sagittal-coronal control, rigid posterior frame and flexible soft anterior apron with straps, closures and padding, extends from sacrococcygeal junction over scapulae, lateral strength provided by pelvic, thoracic, and lateral frame pieces, restricts gross trunk motion in sagittal, and coronal planes, produces intracavitary pressure to reduce load on intervertebral disks, prefabricated item that has been trimmed, bent, molded, assembled, or otherwise customized to fit a specific patient by an individual with expertise

L0469 TLSO, sagittal-coronal control, rigid posterior frame and flexible soft anterior apron with straps, closures and padding, extends from sacrococcygeal junction over scapulae, lateral strength provided by pelvic, thoracic, and lateral frame pieces, restricts gross trunk motion in sagittal and coronal planes, produces intracavitary pressure to reduce load on intervertebral disks, prefabricated, off-the-shelf

L0470 Thoracic-lumbar-sacral orthotic (TLSO), triplanar control, rigid posterior frame and flexible soft anterior apron with straps, closures and padding extends from sacrococcygeal junction to scapula, lateral strength provided by pelvic, thoracic, and lateral frame pieces, rotational strength provided by subclavicular extensions, restricts gross trunk motion in sagittal, coronal, and transverse planes, provides intracavitary pressure to reduce load on the intervertebral disks, includes fitting and shaping the frame, prefabricated, includes fitting and adjustment

L0472 Thoracic-lumbar-sacral orthotic (TLSO), triplanar control, hyperextension, rigid anterior and lateral frame extends from symphysis pubis to sternal notch with 2 anterior components (one pubic and one sternal), posterior and lateral pads with straps and closures, limits spinal flexion, restricts gross trunk motion in sagittal, coronal, and transverse planes, includes fitting and shaping the frame, prefabricated, includes fitting and adjustment

L0480 Thoracic-lumbar-sacral orthotic (TLSO), triplanar control, 1 piece rigid plastic shell without interface liner, with multiple straps and closures, posterior extends from sacrococcygeal junction and terminates just inferior to scapular spine, anterior extends from symphysis pubis to sternal notch, anterior or posterior opening, restricts gross trunk motion in sagittal, coronal, and transverse planes, includes a carved plaster or CAD-CAM model, custom fabricated

L0482 Thoracic-lumbar-sacral orthotic (TLSO), triplanar control, 1 piece rigid plastic shell with interface liner, multiple straps and closures, posterior extends from sacrococcygeal junction and terminates just inferior to scapular spine, anterior extends from symphysis pubis to sternal notch, anterior or posterior opening, restricts gross trunk motion in sagittal, coronal, and transverse planes, includes a carved plaster or CAD-CAM model, custom fabricated

L0484 Thoracic-lumbar-sacral orthotic (TLSO), triplanar control, 2 piece rigid plastic shell without interface liner, with multiple straps and closures, posterior extends from sacrococcygeal junction and terminates just inferior to scapular spine, anterior extends from symphysis pubis to sternal notch, lateral strength is enhanced by overlapping plastic, restricts gross trunk motion in the sagittal, coronal, and transverse planes, includes a carved plaster or CAD-CAM model, custom fabricated

L0486 Thoracic-lumbar-sacral orthotic (TLSO), triplanar control, 2 piece rigid plastic shell with interface liner, multiple straps and closures, posterior extends from sacrococcygeal junction and terminates just inferior to scapular spine, anterior extends from symphysis pubis to sternal notch, lateral strength is enhanced by overlapping plastic, restricts gross trunk motion in the sagittal, coronal, and transverse planes, includes a carved plaster or CAD-CAM model, custom fabricated

L0488 Thoracic-lumbar-sacral orthotic (TLSO), triplanar control, 1 piece rigid plastic shell with interface liner, multiple straps and closures, posterior extends from sacrococcygeal junction and terminates just inferior to scapular spine, anterior extends from symphysis pubis to sternal notch, anterior or posterior opening, restricts gross trunk motion in sagittal, coronal, and transverse planes, prefabricated, includes fitting and adjustment

L0490 Thoracic-lumbar-sacral orthotic (TLSO), sagittal-coronal control, 1 piece rigid plastic shell, with overlapping reinforced anterior, with multiple straps and closures, posterior extends from sacrococcygeal junction and terminates at or before the T-9 vertebra, anterior extends from symphysis pubis to xiphoid, anterior opening, restricts gross trunk motion in sagittal and coronal planes, prefabricated, includes fitting and adjustment

Lay Description

A thoracic-lumbar-sacral orthosis (TLSO) is a rigid or semirigid brace used to support weak or deformed areas of the spine or to restrict or eliminate motion (immobilization) in diseased or injured areas of the spine. An orthosis can be either prefabricated (custom fitted) or custom fabricated. These particular orthoses can have various features and can be constructed or have component parts of different types of materials. The benefits from orthotics use, specifically during convalescence from an injury or illness (useful to the weak or deformed body area) or as a postoperative treatment measure, can include the following: restricted range of motion of the affected area (immobilization); support of the affected area; and/or protection from injury, reinjury, suture tearing, and/or wound dehiscence. A prefabricated or custom-fitted orthosis is one that the manufacturer has produced in quantity, without a specific patient in mind. A prefabricated orthosis may be trimmed, bent, molded (with or without heat), or otherwise modified for use by a specific patient (i.e., custom fitted). An orthosis that is assembled from prefabricated components is considered prefabricated. Any orthosis that does not meet the definition of a custom-fabricated orthosis is considered prefabricated. A custom-fabricated orthosis is individually made for a specific patient, starting with basic materials, including but not limited to plastic, metal, leather, or cloth in the form of sheets, bars, and so forth. This type of orthosis must involve substantial work, such as cutting, bending, molding, sewing, and so forth. Although it may involve the incorporation of some prefabricated components, the device involves more than trimming, bending, or making other modifications to a substantially prefabricated item. A molded-to-patient-model orthosis is a particular type of custom-fabricated orthosis in which an impression of the specific body part is made (by means of a plaster cast, CAD-CAM technology, etc.). This impression is then used to make a positive model (of plaster or other material) of the body part to be braced. The orthosis is then molded on this positive model to be fit exactly to the patient's body part.

L0491-L0492

L0491 Thoracic-lumbar-sacral orthotic (TLSO), sagittal-coronal control, modular segmented spinal system, 2 rigid plastic shells, posterior extends from the sacrococcygeal junction and terminates just inferior to the scapular spine, anterior extends from the symphysis pubis to the xiphoid, soft liner, restricts gross trunk motion in the sagittal and coronal planes, lateral strength is provided by overlapping plastic and stabilizing closures, includes straps and closures, prefabricated, includes fitting and adjustment

L0492 Thoracic-lumbar-sacral orthotic (TLSO), sagittal-coronal control, modular segmented spinal system, 3 rigid plastic shells, posterior extends from the sacrococcygeal junction and terminates just inferior to the scapular spine, anterior extends from the symphysis pubis to the xiphoid, soft liner, restricts gross trunk motion in the sagittal and coronal planes, lateral strength is provided by overlapping plastic and stabilizing closures, includes straps and closures, prefabricated, includes fitting and adjustment

Lay Description

A thoracic-lumbar-sacral orthosis (TLSO) is a brace that is a rigid or semirigid device used for the purpose of supporting weak or deformed areas of the spine, or for restricting or eliminating motion (immobilization) in diseased or injured areas of the spine. An orthosis can be prefabricated (custom fitted) or custom fabricated. These particular orthoses can have various features and can be constructed or have component parts of different types of materials. The benefits from orthotics use, specifically during convalescence from an injury or illness or as a postoperative treatment measure, can include the following: restricted range of motion of the affected area (immobilization), support of the affected area (useful to the weak or deformed body area), and/or protection from injury, reinjury, suture tearing, and/or wound dehiscence. A prefabricated (also known as custom-fitted) orthosis is one that the manufacturer has produced in quantity, without a specific patient in mind. A prefabricated orthosis may be trimmed, bent, molded (with or without heat), or otherwise modified for use by a specific patient (i.e., custom fitted). An orthosis that is assembled from prefabricated components is considered prefabricated. Any orthosis that does not meet the definition of a custom-fabricated orthosis is considered prefabricated. In contrast to a prefabricated orthosis, a custom-fabricated orthosis is individually made for a specific patient, starting with basic materials including, but not limited to, plastic, metal, leather, or cloth in the form of sheets, bars, and so forth. It involves substantial work, such as cutting, bending, molding, sewing, and so forth. Although it may involve the incorporation of some prefabricated components, it involves more than trimming, bending, or making other modifications to a prefabricated item. A molded-to-patient-model orthosis is a particular type of custom-fabricated orthosis in which an impression of the specific body part is made (by means of a plaster cast, CAD-CAM technology, etc.). This impression is then used to make a positive model (of plaster or other material) of the body part to be braced. The orthosis is then molded on this positive model to be fit exactly to the patient's body part.

L0621-L0624

L0621 Sacroiliac orthosis, flexible, provides pelvic-sacral support, reduces motion about the sacroiliac joint, includes straps, closures, may include pendulous abdomen design, prefabricated, off-the-shelf

L0622 Sacroiliac orthotic, flexible, provides pelvic-sacral support, reduces motion about the sacroiliac joint, includes straps, closures, may include pendulous abdomen design, custom fabricated

L0623 Sacroiliac orthosis, provides pelvic-sacral support, with rigid or semi-rigid panels over the sacrum and abdomen, reduces motion about the sacroiliac joint, includes straps, closures, may include pendulous abdomen design, prefabricated, off-the-shelf

L0624 Sacroiliac orthotic, provides pelvic-sacral support, with rigid or semi-rigid panels placed over the sacrum and abdomen, reduces motion about the sacroiliac joint, includes straps, closures, may include pendulous abdomen design, custom fabricated

Lay Description
Sacroiliac orthoses may be flexible, rigid, or semi-rigid. These orthoses provide support for the lower portion of the torso, including the pelvic region, and reduce motion about the sacroiliac joint. Because of the narrow width of theses types of orthoses, they are commonly referred to as belts or corsets. An orthosis can be prefabricated or custom fabricated. A prefabricated (also known as custom fitted) orthosis is one that the manufacturer has produced in quantity, without a specific patient in mind. A prefabricated orthosis may be trimmed, bent, molded (with or without heat), or otherwise modified for use by a specific patient (i.e., custom fitted). An orthosis that is assembled from prefabricated components is considered prefabricated. In contrast, a custom-fabricated orthosis is one that is individually made for a specific patient, starting with basic materials, including plastic, metal, leather, or cloth in the form of sheets, bars, and so forth. It involves substantial work, such as cutting, bending, molding,

sewing, and so forth. It may involve the incorporation of some prefabricated components. It involves more than trimming, bending, or making other modifications to a prefabricated item. Sacroiliac orthoses are usually prescribed to reduce sacroiliac diastasis or to reduce pelvic symphysis separation, and can even be given on a prophylactic basis to workers whose day-to-day tasks involve heavy lifting.

L0625-L0627

L0625 Lumbar orthosis, flexible, provides lumbar support, posterior extends from L-1 to below L-5 vertebra, produces intracavitary pressure to reduce load on the intervertebral discs, includes straps, closures, may include pendulous abdomen design, shoulder straps, stays, prefabricated, off-the-shelf

L0626 Lumbar orthosis, sagittal control, with rigid posterior panel(s), posterior extends from L-1 to below L-5 vertebra, produces intracavitary pressure to reduce load on the intervertebral discs, includes straps, closures, may include padding, stays, shoulder straps, pendulous abdomen design, prefabricated item that has been trimmed, bent, molded, assembled, or otherwise customized to fit a specific patient by an individual with expertise

L0627 Lumbar orthosis, sagittal control, with rigid anterior and posterior panels, posterior extends from L-1 to below L-5 vertebra, produces intracavitary pressure to reduce load on the intervertebral discs, includes straps, closures, may include padding, shoulder straps, pendulous abdomen design, prefabricated item that has been trimmed, bent, molded, assembled, or otherwise customized to fit a specific patient by an individual with expertise

Lay Description
Lumbar orthoses may be flexible, rigid, or semi-rigid. These orthoses provide support to the lumbar (L1-L5) spinal area. They function by producing pressure within the abdominal and body cavities, creating space between the vertebrae, and allowing the intervertebral disk enough space to comfortably fit between the vertebrae. An orthosis can be prefabricated (custom fitted) or custom fabricated. A prefabricated (also known as custom fitted) orthosis is one that the manufacturer has produced in quantity, without a specific patient in mind. A prefabricated orthosis may be trimmed, bent, molded (with or without heat), or otherwise modified for use by a specific patient (i.e., custom fitted). An orthosis that is assembled from prefabricated components is considered prefabricated. In contrast to a prefabricated orthosis, a custom fabricated orthosis is one that is individually made for a specific patient, starting with basic materials including, but not limited

to, plastic, metal, leather, or cloth in the form of sheets, bars, and so forth. It involves substantial work, such as cutting, bending, molding, sewing, and so forth. It may involve the incorporation of some prefabricated components. Flexible lumbar orthoses are used to treat mild spinal instability, painful arthritis, vertebral fractures of the lumbar and lower thoracic spine, and may be used immediately after lumbar surgery (e.g., discectomy, fusion) to provide back support. The rigid lumbar orthoses are used postfracture to reduce risk of further injury, or postoperatively for complex spinal surgeries when increased support is required. Rigid devices are also recommended for the treatment of scoliosis.

L0628-L0651

L0628 Lumbar-sacral orthosis, flexible, provides lumbo-sacral support, posterior extends from sacrococcygeal junction to T-9 vertebra, produces intracavitary pressure to reduce load on the intervertebral discs, includes straps, closures, may include stays, shoulder straps, pendulous abdomen design, prefabricated, off-the-shelf

L0629 Lumbar-sacral orthotic, flexible, provides lumbo-sacral support, posterior extends from sacrococcygeal junction to T-9 vertebra, produces intracavitary pressure to reduce load on the intervertebral discs, includes straps, closures, may include stays, shoulder straps, pendulous abdomen design, custom fabricated

L0630 Lumbar-sacral orthosis, sagittal control, with rigid posterior panel(s), posterior extends from sacrococcygeal junction to T-9 vertebra, produces intracavitary pressure to reduce load on the intervertebral discs, includes straps, closures, may include padding, stays, shoulder straps, pendulous abdomen design, prefabricated item that has been trimmed, bent, molded, assembled, or otherwise customized to fit a specific patient by an individual with expertise

L0631 Lumbar-sacral orthosis, sagittal control, with rigid anterior and posterior panels, posterior extends from sacrococcygeal junction to T-9 vertebra, produces intracavitary pressure to reduce load on the intervertebral discs, includes straps, closures, may include padding, shoulder straps, pendulous abdomen design, prefabricated item that has been trimmed, bent, molded, assembled, or otherwise customized to fit a specific patient by an individual with expertise

L0632 Lumbar-sacral orthotic (LSO), sagittal control, with rigid anterior and posterior panels, posterior extends from sacrococcygeal junction to T-9 vertebra, produces intracavitary pressure to reduce load on the intervertebral discs, includes straps, closures, may include padding, shoulder straps, pendulous abdomen design, custom fabricated

L0633 Lumbar-sacral orthosis, sagittal-coronal control, with rigid posterior frame/panel(s), posterior extends from sacrococcygeal junction to T-9 vertebra, lateral strength provided by rigid lateral frame/panels, produces intracavitary pressure to reduce load on intervertebral discs, includes straps, closures, may include padding, stays, shoulder straps, pendulous abdomen design, prefabricated item that has been trimmed, bent, molded, assembled, or otherwise customized to fit a specific patient by an individual with expertise

L0634 Lumbar-sacral orthotic (LSO), sagittal-coronal control, with rigid posterior frame/panel(s), posterior extends from sacrococcygeal junction to T-9 vertebra, lateral strength provided by rigid lateral frame/panel(s), produces intracavitary pressure to reduce load on intervertebral discs, includes straps, closures, may include padding, stays, shoulder straps, pendulous abdomen design, custom fabricated

L0635 Lumbar-sacral orthotic (LSO), sagittal-coronal control, lumbar flexion, rigid posterior frame/panel(s), lateral articulating design to flex the lumbar spine, posterior extends from sacrococcygeal junction to T-9 vertebra, lateral strength provided by rigid lateral frame/panel(s), produces intracavitary pressure to reduce load on intervertebral discs, includes straps, closures, may include padding, anterior panel, pendulous abdomen design, prefabricated, includes fitting and adjustment

L0636 Lumbar-sacral orthotic (LSO), sagittal-coronal control, lumbar flexion, rigid posterior frame/panels, lateral articulating design to flex the lumbar spine, posterior extends from sacrococcygeal junction to T-9 vertebra, lateral strength provided by rigid lateral frame/panels, produces intracavitary pressure to reduce load on intervertebral discs, includes straps, closures, may include padding, anterior panel, pendulous abdomen design, custom fabricated

L0637 Lumbar-sacral orthosis, sagittal-coronal control, with rigid anterior and posterior frame/panels, posterior extends from sacrococcygeal junction to T-9 vertebra, lateral strength provided by rigid lateral frame/panels, produces intracavitary pressure to reduce load on intervertebral discs, includes straps, closures, may include padding, shoulder straps, pendulous abdomen design, prefabricated item that has been trimmed, bent, molded, assembled, or otherwise customized to fit a specific patient by an individual with expertise

L0638 Lumbar-sacral orthotic (LSO), sagittal-coronal control, with rigid anterior and posterior frame/panels, posterior extends from sacrococcygeal junction to T-9 vertebra, lateral strength provided by rigid lateral frame/panels, produces intracavitary pressure to reduce load on intervertebral discs, includes straps, closures, may include padding, shoulder straps, pendulous abdomen design, custom fabricated

L0639 Lumbar-sacral orthosis, sagittal-coronal control, rigid shell(s)/panel(s), posterior extends from sacrococcygeal junction to T-9 vertebra, anterior extends from symphysis pubis to xyphoid, produces intracavitary pressure to reduce load on the intervertebral discs, overall strength is provided by overlapping rigid material and stabilizing closures, includes straps, closures, may include soft interface, pendulous abdomen design, prefabricated item that has been trimmed, bent, molded, assembled, or otherwise customized to fit a specific patient by an individual with expertise

L0640 Lumbar-sacral orthotic (LSO), sagittal-coronal control, rigid shell(s)/panel(s), posterior extends from sacrococcygeal junction to T-9 vertebra, anterior extends from symphysis pubis to xyphoid, produces intracavitary pressure to reduce load on the intervertebral discs, overall strength is provided by overlapping rigid material and stabilizing closures, includes straps, closures, may include soft interface, pendulous abdomen design, custom fabricated

L0641 Lumbar orthosis, sagittal control, with rigid posterior panel(s), posterior extends from L-1 to below L-5 vertebra, produces intracavitary pressure to reduce load on the intervertebral discs, includes straps, closures, may include padding, stays, shoulder straps, pendulous abdomen design, prefabricated, off-the-shelf

L0642 Lumbar orthosis, sagittal control, with rigid anterior and posterior panels, posterior extends from L-1 to below L-5 vertebra, produces intracavitary pressure to reduce load on the intervertebral discs, includes straps, closures, may include padding, shoulder straps, pendulous abdomen design, prefabricated, off-the-shelf

L0643 Lumbar-sacral orthosis, sagittal control, with rigid posterior panel(s), posterior extends from sacrococcygeal junction to T-9 vertebra, produces intracavitary pressure to reduce load on the intervertebral discs, includes straps, closures, may include padding, stays, shoulder straps, pendulous abdomen design, prefabricated, off-the-shelf

L0648 Lumbar-sacral orthosis, sagittal control, with rigid anterior and posterior panels, posterior extends from sacrococcygeal junction to T-9 vertebra, produces intracavitary pressure to reduce load on the intervertebral discs, includes straps, closures, may include padding, shoulder straps, pendulous abdomen design, prefabricated, off-the-shelf

L0649 Lumbar-sacral orthosis, sagittal-coronal control, with rigid posterior frame/panel(s), posterior extends from sacrococcygeal junction to T-9 vertebra, lateral strength provided by rigid lateral frame/panels, produces intracavitary pressure to reduce load on intervertebral discs, includes straps, closures, may include padding, stays, shoulder straps, pendulous abdomen design, prefabricated, off-the-shelf

L0650 Lumbar-sacral orthosis, sagittal-coronal control, with rigid anterior and posterior frame/panel(s), posterior extends from sacrococcygeal junction to T-9 vertebra, lateral strength provided by rigid lateral frame/panel(s), produces intracavitary pressure to reduce load on intervertebral discs, includes straps, closures, may include padding, shoulder straps, pendulous abdomen design, prefabricated, off-the-shelf

L0651 Lumbar-sacral orthosis, sagittal-coronal control, rigid shell(s)/panel(s), posterior extends from sacrococcygeal junction to T-9 vertebra, anterior extends from symphysis pubis to xyphoid, produces intracavitary pressure to reduce load on the intervertebral discs, overall strength is provided by overlapping rigid material and stabilizing closures, includes straps, closures, may include soft interface, pendulous abdomen design, prefabricated, off-the-shelf

Lay Description

A lumbosacral orthotic (LSO) can be flexible, rigid, or semi-rigid. An LSO provides lumbosacral support from the sacrococcygeal junction to the T-9 vertebrae. It is a device that is used for the purpose of supporting weak or deformed areas of the spine, or for restricting or eliminating motion (immobilization) in diseased or injured areas of the spine. An orthosis can be prefabricated or custom fabricated. A prefabricated (also known as custom fitted) orthosis is one that the manufacturer has produced in quantity, without a specific patient in mind. A prefabricated orthosis may be trimmed, bent, molded (with or without heat), or otherwise modified for use by a specific patient (i.e., custom fitted). An orthosis that is assembled from prefabricated components is considered prefabricated. In contrast, a custom-fabricated orthosis is one that is individually made for a specific patient, starting with basic materials including plastic, metal, leather, or cloth in the form of sheets, bars, and so forth. It involves substantial work, such as cutting, bending, molding, sewing, and so forth. It may involve the incorporation of some prefabricated components. It involves more than trimming, bending, or making other modifications to a prefabricated item. The benefits of orthotics use, specifically during convalescence from an injury or illness (useful to the weak or deformed body area) or as a postoperative treatment measure, can include the following: restricted range of motion of the affected area (immobilization); support of the affected area; and/or protection from injury, reinjury, suture tearing, and/or wound dehiscence. An LSO can be designed to control movement of both the trunk and between the segments of the vertebrae in one or more planes of motion. The most common planes are coronal/frontal, sagittal, and transverse.

L0700-L0710

L0700   Cervical-thoracic-lumbar-sacral orthotic (CTLSO), anterior-posterior-lateral control, molded to patient model, (Minerva type)

L0710   Cervical-thoracic-lumbar-sacral orthotic (CTLSO), anterior-posterior-lateral-control, molded to patient model, with interface material, (Minerva type)

Lay Description

These codes report a specific type of cervical thoracic lumbar sacral orthosis (CTLSO). These orthoses control all spinal movement, lateral as well as anterior and posterior. Since the unit has a cervical component, the patient's head and neck are also immobilized. In addition to immobilization, the orthosis reduces compression load on the affected area of the spine. These devices are usually prepared ahead of a planned surgery. Measurements, scans, and moldings are taken by an orthotist. The orthosis is fashioned out of plastic polymers based on the patient data. The orthosis is bivalved, or cut into front and back pieces

for donning and adjustment. Ventilation holes may be cut into the body of the orthosis, since they are typically worn over the course of the day. The Minerva component is an extension from the body of the orthosis that supports the mandible and occiput and stabilizes the cervical spine.

L0810-L0861

L0810   Halo procedure, cervical halo incorporated into jacket vest

L0820   Halo procedure, cervical halo incorporated into plaster body jacket

L0830   Halo procedure, cervical halo incorporated into Milwaukee type orthotic

L0859   Addition to halo procedure, magnetic resonance image compatible systems, rings and pins, any material

L0861   Addition to halo procedure, replacement liner/interface material

Lay Description

This system represents the non-conductive halo traction ring and skull pins. These component parts represent pieces of what is commonly called the halo system. The halo system consists of a metal ring that is secured to the upper part of the skull (mid-forehead area) with pins. A cervical halo is used to immobilize the cervical spine usually due to an odontoid fracture (fracture of the second cervical vertebrae). Two metal rods extend from the halo along the sides of the head to the shoulder area and are attached to a well-fitted plastic vest, jacket, or other type of orthotic. While the patient is wearing the halo system, the patient may be required to have diagnostic imaging such as MRI or CT procedures. These additions to the halo system ensure patient safety by eliminating the risk of scalp burns, while also allowing for a clearer, higher-quality image.

L0970-L0976

L0970   Thoracic-lumbar-sacral orthotic (TLSO), corset front

L0972   Lumbar-sacral orthotic (LSO), corset front

L0974   Thoracic-lumbar-sacral orthotic (TLSO), full corset

L0976   Lumbar-sacral orthotic (LSO), full corset

Lay Description

This range of codes reports specific corset additions to spinal orthoses. Some spinal orthoses, such as the "chair back" designs, require a closure addition for the anterior of the device. The corset front is attached to this type of posterior orthosis and provides a means to close and adjust tension of the device. The corset closure is a lace-and-eyelet configuration. Some designs feature a full corset design. These devices will have a stiff fabric body, sometimes with semi-rigid ribbing, and a corset closure, usually on the front.

L0978

L0978 Axillary crutch extension

Lay Description
This code reports the supply of an axillary crutch extension. The axillary crutch is the most common type of crutch in use today. A pad under the armpit, or axilla, bears most of the user's weight over the length of double uprights that extend to the floor. An extra upright piece makes the crutch adjustable (extension crutch). A handle bridges the double uprights about one-third the length down the crutch.

L0980

L0980 Peroneal straps, prefabricated, off-the-shelf, pair

Lay Description
This code reports the supply of each pair of perineal straps. These straps, or belts, are used occasionally with spinal orthoses that tend to migrate upward as the wearer engages in activities. The belt connects to the lower aspect of the orthosis, front to rear, by passing in a criss-cross fashion under the groin, or perineum. Certain ankle straps used to provide traction during endoscopic surgery may be referred to as peroneal straps, but are not reported by this spinal orthosis code.

L0982

L0982 Stocking supporter grips, prefabricated, off-the-shelf, set of four (4)

Lay Description
Compression and support stocking are frequently singular stockings not permanently attached to a panty or other support garment. Stocking supporter grips are devices that attach to the top of the stocking and the bottom of the support garment, such as a garter belt. The grips help to hold the stockings in place.

L0984

L0984 Protective body sock, prefabricated, off-the-shelf, each

Lay Description
A protective body sock is a garment made up of soft, cushiony fabric that is used under spinal orthotics and body jackets. This item does not meet the definition of a brace and is considered more as a convenience item for the patient.

L0999

L0999 Addition to spinal orthotic, not otherwise specified

Lay Description
A spinal orthotic is a flexible, rigid, or semi-rigid device that provides support to the spinal area. It functions by producing pressure within the abdominal and body cavities, creating space between the vertebrae, and allowing the intervertebral disk enough space to comfortably fit between the vertebrae. Use this code to report an addition to a spinal orthotic that is not identified by a more specific code.

L1000

L1000 Cervical-thoracic-lumbar-sacral orthotic (CTLSO) (Milwaukee), inclusive of furnishing initial orthotic, including model

Lay Description
This code reports the supply of a Milwaukee-style cervical thoracic lumbar sacral orthosis (CTLSO). This is among the oldest designs of spinal braces still in use today, most commonly as treatment for idiopathic scoliosis, a lateral curvature of the spine that usually presents around puberty. A variety of brace configurations is seen, but all reported by this code will have a component that supports the head, limiting movement of the cervical spine (neck). Traditional braces were made of rigid leather, although most modern versions are constructed of thermoplastic and natural and artificial padding. The classic model features rigid waist and upper torso components. Metal rods, front and back, connect these components and the cervical support. Various padding may be placed to further manipulate the spine. Computer models based on detailed patient measurements and radiographs are used to calculate spinal geometries and loading. Several initial orthoses may be generated before a long-term brace is fabricated.

L1001

L1001 Cervical-thoracic-lumbar-sacral orthotic (CTLSO), immobilizer, infant size, prefabricated, includes fitting and adjustment

Lay Description
This is a cervical thoracic lumbar sacral orthosis (CTLSO) that is intended for use on infants with suspected or diagnosed spinal injury resulting from trauma or delivery complications or a tumor impinging on the spine, or it can be used for temporary immobilization for IV placement. This orthotic stabilizes the child's head and spine, and its unique shape keeps the child's spine aligned with the airway to promote an optimal healing process.

L1005

L1005 Tension based scoliosis orthotic and accessory pads, includes fitting and adjustment

Lay Description
This code reports the supply of a tension based scoliosis orthosis. Idiopathic scoliosis is a lateral curvature of the spine that usually presents by adolescence. Girls are affected at a ratio of five to one over boys. The classic nonsurgical approach is to

stabilize the spine and manipulate development toward normal anatomy through the use of cervical thoracic lumbar sacral orthoses (CTLSO) or TLSOs. Tension based orthoses address scoliosis by exerting correctional forces on the spine through use of elastic fabrics and bands. Fabrics with elastic properties, pads, and elastic bands are fitted on the patient, often in configurations that change as development occurs. The orthosis is worn over the trunk, without a cervical component.

L1010

L1010   Addition to cervical-thoracic-lumbar-sacral orthotic (CTLSO) or scoliosis orthotic, axilla sling

Lay Description
This code reports the addition of an axilla sling to a scoliosis orthosis. Idiopathic scoliosis is a lateral curvature of the spine that usually presents by adolescence. Girls are affected at a ratio of five to one over boys. The classic nonsurgical approach is to stabilize the spine and manipulate development toward normal anatomy through the use of cervical thoracic lumbar sacral orthoses (CTLSO) or TLSOs. An axilla sling may be added to an orthosis to provide corrective leverage on the upper spine, usually in combination with fabric pads elsewhere on the apparatus. As the name implies, the sling runs under the armpit and connects the anterior and posterior components of the orthosis. It may be added to either a CTLSO or TLSO.

L1020-L1025

L1020   Addition to cervical-thoracic-lumbar-sacral orthotic (CTLSO) or scoliosis orthotic, kyphosis pad

L1025   Addition to cervical-thoracic-lumbar-sacral orthotic (CTLSO) or scoliosis orthotic, kyphosis pad, floating

Lay Description
These codes report the addition of pads to a scoliosis orthosis. Idiopathic scoliosis is a lateral curvature of the spine that usually presents by adolescence. Girls are affected at a ratio of five to one over boys. The classic non-surgical approach is to stabilize the spine and manipulate development toward normal anatomy through the use of cervical thoracic lumbar sacral orthoses (CTLSO) or TLSOs. Fabric pads are often added to an orthosis, often at the area of greatest thoracic curve (kyphosis) and usually in combination with a thoracic strap or axilla sling. When a pad is suspended from the apparatus on a movable strap, it is known as a "floating" pad, as opposed to one that is mounted onto the rigid shell. Maximum pad adjustment is ideal to adjust the amount of pressure and angle of applied force.

L1030-L1040

L1030   Addition to cervical-thoracic-lumbar-sacral orthotic (CTLSO) or scoliosis orthotic, lumbar bolster pad

L1040   Addition to cervical-thoracic-lumbar-sacral orthotic (CTLSO) or scoliosis orthotic, lumbar or lumbar rib pad

Lay Description
These codes report addition of specific types of pads to a scoliosis orthosis. Idiopathic scoliosis is a lateral curvature of the spine that usually presents by adolescence. Girls are affected at a ratio of five to one over boys. The classic non-surgical approach is to stabilize the spine and manipulate development toward normal anatomy through the use of cervical thoracic lumbar sacral orthoses (CTLSO). Fabric or foam pads are often added to an orthosis, often at the area of lumbar curve. The pads are considered accessories to flexible corset-style orthoses and occasionally to rigid models. The pads are typically rectangular shaped and may be referred to informally as a "shingle." The actual pad may be fabric-based, urethane, closed cell foam, or other material. Lumbar pads may be available as inflatable units. The addition may be made to a CTLSO or other type of scoliosis orthosis.

L1050

L1050   Addition to cervical-thoracic-lumbar-sacral orthotic (CTLSO) or scoliosis orthotic, sternal pad

Lay Description
This code reports the addition of a sternal pad to a scoliosis orthosis. Idiopathic scoliosis is a lateral curvature of the spine that usually presents by adolescence. Girls are affected at a ratio of five to one over boys. The classic non-surgical approach is to stabilize the spine and manipulate development toward normal anatomy through the use of cervical thoracic lumbar sacral orthoses (CTLSO). Other forms of scoliosis may be treated with orthoses as well. The padded sternal component reported by this code may be added to a scoliosis orthosis to provide a pressure point against the sternal bone. Some may be applied and held in place by straps. But most models feature an integrated pad and rigid outer shell, sometimes including a tension hinge on an armature to adjust pressure on the sternum. The actual pad may be fabric-based, urethane, closed cell foam, or other material. The addition may be made to a CTLSO or other type of scoliosis orthosis.

L1060

L1060 Addition to cervical-thoracic-lumbar-sacral orthotic (CTLSO) or scoliosis orthotic, thoracic pad

Lay Description
This code reports the addition of a thoracic pad to a scoliosis orthosis. Idiopathic scoliosis is a lateral curvature of the spine that usually presents by adolescence. Girls are affected at a ratio of five to one over boys. The classic non-surgical approach is to stabilize the spine and manipulate development toward normal anatomy through the use of cervical thoracic lumbar sacral orthoses (CTLSO). These devices rely on pressure points to manipulate spinal development and strategically placed padding provides this pressure. Other forms of scoliosis may be treated with orthoses as well. Thoracic pads may be applied and held in place by straps. Others are integrated into the rigid shell that comprises the thoracic component of the orthosis.

L1070

L1070 Addition to cervical-thoracic-lumbar-sacral orthotic (CTLSO) or scoliosis orthotic, trapezius sling

Lay Description
This code reports the addition of a trapezius sling to a scoliosis orthosis. Idiopathic scoliosis is a lateral curvature of the spine that usually presents by adolescence. Girls are affected at a ratio of five to one over boys. The classic non-surgical approach is to stabilize the spine and manipulate development toward normal anatomy through the use of cervical thoracic lumbar sacral orthoses (CTLSO). These devices rely on pressure points to manipulate spinal development and strategically placed padding provides this pressure. Other forms of scoliosis may be treated with orthoses as well. The trapezius muscle is on the upper back and works to move the shoulder blade. A trapezius sling is an addition to the anterior and posterior thoracic components that cross high on the shoulder near the neck. Padding on the sling provides a pressure point, usually to address the upper thoracic and lower cervical vertebra.

L1080-L1085

L1080 Addition to cervical-thoracic-lumbar-sacral orthotic (CTLSO) or scoliosis orthotic, outrigger

L1085 Addition to cervical-thoracic-lumbar-sacral orthotic (CTLSO) or scoliosis orthotic, outrigger, bilateral with vertical extensions

Lay Description
These codes report outrigger additions to scoliosis orthoses. Idiopathic scoliosis is a lateral curvature of the spine that usually presents by adolescence. Girls are affected at a ratio of five to one over boys. The classic non-surgical approach is to stabilize the spine and manipulate development toward normal anatomy through the use of cervical thoracic lumbar sacral orthoses (CTLSO). These devices rely on pressure points to manipulate spinal development. Other forms of scoliosis may be treated with orthoses as well. Outriggers are components added to the rigid portion of the orthosis. They are most often associated with Milwaukee-style orthoses. Outriggers themselves are often stainless steel bars and attachment may be to a vertical bar of the orthosis. The outrigger usually contributes leverage for pressure points.

L1090

L1090 Addition to cervical-thoracic-lumbar-sacral orthotic (CTLSO) or scoliosis orthotic, lumbar sling

Lay Description
A lumbar sling is an addition to a scoliosis orthotic device. Scoliosis is an abnormal curvature of the spine from side to side, giving the spine an "S" shape. The sling addition is a padded strap or sling used to hold or put pressure on the lumbar spine.

L1100-L1110

L1100 Addition to cervical-thoracic-lumbar-sacral orthotic (CTLSO) or scoliosis orthotic, ring flange, plastic or leather

L1110 Addition to cervical-thoracic-lumbar-sacral orthotic (CTLSO) or scoliosis orthotic, ring flange, plastic or leather, molded to patient model

Lay Description
These codes report the addition of a custom molded ring flange to a scoliosis orthosis. This device supports the mandible and occiput of a cervical thoracic lumbar sacral orthoses (CTLSO). Idiopathic scoliosis is a lateral curvature of the spine that usually presents by adolescence. Girls are affected at a ratio of five to one over boys. The classic nonsurgical approach is to stabilize the spine and manipulate development toward normal anatomy through the use of CTLSO. Certain CTLSO models employ a plastic ring to immobilize the cervical spine and head, which is less visible than the larger supports seen on some models.

L1120

L1120 Addition to cervical-thoracic-lumbar-sacral orthotic (CTLSO), scoliosis orthotic, cover for upright, each

Lay Description
A CTLSO is an orthosis used for the treatment of scoliosis and/or kyphosis, and consists of pelvic interface molded to the patient. Metal anterior and posterior uprights attach to the pelvic interface and

terminate in the occipital mandibular area. The cover for the uprights protects the skin and prevents skin breakdown.

L1200

L1200 Thoracic-lumbar-sacral orthotic (TLSO), inclusive of furnishing initial orthotic only

Lay Description
This code reports the supply of a thoracic lumbar sacral orthosis (TLSO). These devices are sometimes referred to as "low profile" because they lack the "high profile" of a cervical component and many designs fit unobtrusively under clothing. These braces are not specifically limited to correction of scoliosis. Some may be prescribed following certain surgeries or to treat symptoms of trauma. Numerous fittings may be required, as idiopathic scoliosis requires adjustments as the patient's spine develops. Report this code for an initial TLSO only.

L1210

L1210 Addition to thoracic-lumbar-sacral orthotic (TLSO), (low profile), lateral thoracic extension

Lay Description
A TLSO is an orthotic designed for scoliosis and/or kyphosis. It is a heat moldable plastic insert for rigid support of the lower areas of the spine. This orthotic is used on the lateral aspect of a patient.

L1220

L1220 Addition to thoracic-lumbar-sacral orthotic (TLSO), (low profile), anterior thoracic extension

Lay Description
A TLSO is an orthotic designed for scoliosis and/or kyphosis. It is a heat moldable plastic insert for rigid support of the lower areas of the spine. This orthotic is used on the anterior aspect of a patient in a low profile scoliosis TLSO.

L1230

L1230 Addition to thoracic-lumbar-sacral orthotic (TLSO), (low profile), Milwaukee type superstructure

Lay Description
This code reports the addition of a Milwaukee type superstructure to a thoracic lumbar sacral orthosis (TLSO). The Milwaukee brace is among the oldest designs of spinal braces still in use today, most commonly as treatment for idiopathic scoliosis, a lateral curvature of the spine that usually presents around puberty. A variety of Milwaukee brace configurations are seen, but the classic model features rigid waist and upper torso components. Vertical metal rods, front and back, connect these components. Various padding arrangements and slings may be placed to further manipulate the spine.

L1240

L1240 Addition to thoracic-lumbar-sacral orthotic (TLSO), (low profile), lumbar derotation pad

Lay Description
A TLSO is an orthotic made from molded plastic designed for scoliosis and/or kyphosis in the lower areas of the spine. TLSOs have built-in pads (derotation) in the lumbar area that exert pressure on the spinal column at three points to apply the corrective force to improve the malposition of the spinal column. These three point corsets are fitted with derotation pressure pads along the lumbar spine, around the outer pelvis, and along the rib cage. Correction of the existing spinal malposition is achieved through derotation pad pressure in a low profile scoliosis TLSO.

L1250

L1250 Addition to thoracic-lumbar-sacral orthotic (TLSO), (low profile), anterior ASIS pad

Lay Description
This code reports the addition of an anterior ASIS pad to a thoracic lumbar sacral orthosis (TLSO). The acronym ASIS stands for anterior sacroiliac spine, which is the prominence of the hipbone at the front of the waist. This type of pad typically is used to provide a pressure point across the lower abdomen. Pressure here raises intraabdominal pressure, which in turn supports the lumbosacral spine.

L1260

L1260 Addition to thoracic-lumbar-sacral orthotic (TLSO), (low profile), anterior thoracic derotation pad

Lay Description
A TLSO is a molded plastic orthotic designed for scoliosis and/or kyphosis in the lower areas of the spine. TLSOs have built-in pads (derotation) in the anterior thoracic area that exert pressure on the spinal column at three points to apply the corrective force to improve the malposition of the spinal column. These three point corsets are fitted with derotation pressure pads along the anterior thoracic spine, around the outer pelvis, and along the rib cage. Correction of the existing spinal malposition is achieved through derotation pad pressure in a low profile scoliosis TLSO.

L1270

L1270 Addition to thoracic-lumbar-sacral orthotic (TLSO), (low profile), abdominal pad

Lay Description
A pad is attached to or incorporated into the abdominal area of a low profile scoliosis TLSO to counteract rotation of the thoracic spine.

L1280

L1280 Addition to thoracic-lumbar-sacral orthotic (TLSO), (low profile), rib gusset (elastic), each

Lay Description
A rib gusset is an addition to a spinal orthotic. It is an elastic support used to provide structural integrity and to lower the pressure on the ribs.

L1290

L1290 Addition to thoracic-lumbar-sacral orthotic (TLSO), (low profile), lateral trochanteric pad

Lay Description
A pad is installed in the trochanter area to control the lumbar curve.

L1300-L1310

L1300 Other scoliosis procedure, body jacket molded to patient model

L1310 Other scoliosis procedure, postoperative body jacket

Lay Description
These codes report the supply of a body jacket to treat scoliosis. Idiopathic scoliosis is a lateral curvature of the spine that usually presents by adolescence. Girls are affected at a ratio of five to one over boys. The non-surgical approach to idiopathic scoliosis is to stabilize the spine and manipulate development toward normal anatomy, and may include use of a body jacket. Body jackets may also be used for other cases of scoliosis. Preparation of a body jacket entails taking a plaster mold of the patient's body. Radiography, body scans, and computer modeling may also be employed. A plastic shell is prepared from the modeling and manipulated for optional therapy. The jacket may be bi-valved, or split into front and back halves for entry. The shell is vented and lined with cushion material. In some instances, a body jacket is required for recovery from surgery. In these cases, the casting and measurements are usually, but not always, taken prior to surgery.

L1499

L1499 Spinal orthotic, not otherwise specified

Lay Description
A spinal orthotic is an external apparatus that is applied to the body to limit the motion of, correct a deformity in, reduce the axial load on, or improve the function of a particular segment of the spine. Report this code for any spinal orthotic device not described in more specific HCPCS Level II codes.

L1600-L1650

L1600 Hip orthosis, abduction control of hip joints, flexible, Frejka type with cover, prefabricated item that has been trimmed, bent, molded, assembled, or otherwise customized to fit a specific patient by an inidividual with expertise

L1610 Hip orthosis, abduction control of hip joints, flexible, (Frejka cover only), prefabricated item that has been trimmed, bent, molded, assembled, or otherwise customized to fit a specific patient by an individual with expertise

L1620 Hip orthosis, abduction control of hip joints, flexible, (Pavlik harness), prefabricated item that has been trimmed, bent, molded, assembled, or otherwise customized to fit a specific patient by an individual with expertise

L1630 Hip orthotic (HO), abduction control of hip joints, semi-flexible (Von Rosen type), custom fabricated

L1640 Hip orthotic (HO), abduction control of hip joints, static, pelvic band or spreader bar, thigh cuffs, custom fabricated

L1650 Hip orthotic (HO), abduction control of hip joints, static, adjustable, (Ilfled type), prefabricated, includes fitting and adjustment

Lay Description
This range of codes reports the supply of flexible hip orthoses designed to control hip abduction (spreading the legs). Many of these designs address congenital anomalies, such as hip dysplasia in infants and pre-toddlers. The Frejka orthosis is a pillow-like device that separates and immobilizes the legs. The Pavlik harness features cuffs that fit to the femurs; front and back harness arrangement fits over the shoulders and chest and may be adjusted to maintain the desired leg position. Like the Frejka device, this design also immobilizes the upper legs in a flexed and abducted position. The Von Rosen orthosis is a cross-shaped, semi-rigid pad that is custom fitted to the baby and then fixed into the desired position. The Ilfeld-style device uses a spreader bar fitted to cuffs on the baby's thighs and is prefabricated or custom fabricated. Either is adjustable and the degree of abduction is controlled by adjusting the length of the cross bar. A waistband is generally used to hold the splint in place more securely. None of the above devices completely immobilize the legs and hips. All prefabricated devices include fitting and adjustment.

L1652-L1686

L1652 Hip orthotic, bilateral thigh cuffs with adjustable abductor spreader bar, adult size, prefabricated, includes fitting and adjustment, any type

L1660 Hip orthotic (HO), abduction control of hip joints, static, plastic, prefabricated, includes fitting and adjustment

L1680 Hip orthosis (HO), abduction control of hip joints, dynamic, pelvic control, adjustable hip motion control, thigh cuffs (Rancho hip action type), custom fabricated

L1685 Hip orthosis (HO), abduction control of hip joint, postoperative hip abduction type, custom fabricated

L1686 Hip orthotic (HO), abduction control of hip joint, postoperative hip abduction type, prefabricated, includes fitting and adjustment

Lay Description

These codes report supply of prefabricated hip orthoses designed to control hip abduction (spreading the legs) in adults. Such devices may be for any number of disorders, following certain surgeries, or to treat symptoms of trauma.

L1690

L1690 Combination, bilateral, lumbo-sacral, hip, femur orthotic providing adduction and internal rotation control, prefabricated, includes fitting and adjustment

Lay Description

This code represents a type of assistive technology often referred to as SWASH (standing, walking, and sitting hip orthosis). A SWASH is most commonly used on children with cerebral palsy, who often have difficulties with dystonia, hip migration, and a scissoring gait that interferes with ambulation and limits independent sitting. When properly fitted, the SWASH stabilizes the hip and prevents excessive adduction and internal rotation. This ultimately helps the child with stability while standing and gait during walking. When the child sits, the orthosis dictates continuous abduction, resulting in a wider base. This allows for a balanced posture and keeps the child from having to use their hands for support. Because of the technical nature of the SWASH orthosis, providers interested in using the device are required to attend a specialized training course.

L1700-L1755

L1700 Legg Perthes orthotic, (Toronto type), custom fabricated

L1710 Legg Perthes orthotic, (Newington type), custom fabricated

L1720 Legg Perthes orthotic, trilateral, (Tachdijan type), custom fabricated

L1730 Legg Perthes orthotic, (Scottish Rite type), custom fabricated

L1755 Legg Perthes orthotic, (Patten bottom type), custom fabricated

Lay Description

These codes report supply of a specific type of custom fabricated orthosis used to treat Legg Calve Perthes disease (LCPD or, more commonly, Legg Perthes). Legg Perthes disease is an osteonecrosis of the femoral head and hip socket found only in children, usually boys between the ages of 2 and 12. Bone death occurs in the ball of the hip due to interruption in blood flow. The disease is of unknown etiology. The Toronto type orthosis addresses the disorder with an unusual splint design. Each leg is secured by cuffs high on the thigh. A single vertical tube is connected to these thigh cuffs near the crotch. The lower end is connected to horizontal spreader bars fixed to special shoes. A ball joint between the vertical tube and the spreader bar allows knee flexibility. Shoe blocks are attached to the shoes to maintain alignment.

L1810-L1833

L1810 Knee orthosis, elastic with joints, prefabricated item that has been trimmed, bent, molded, assembled, or otherwise customized to fit a specific patient by an individual with expertise

L1812 Knee orthosis, elastic with joints, prefabricated, off-the-shelf

L1820 Knee orthotic, elastic with condylar pads and joints, with or without patellar control, prefabricated, includes fitting and adjustment

L1830 Knee orthosis, immobilizer, canvas longitudinal, prefabricated, off-the-shelf

L1831 Knee orthotic, locking knee joint(s), positional orthotic, prefabricated, includes fitting and adjustment

L1832 Knee orthosis, adjustable knee joints (unicentric or polycentric), positional orthosis, rigid support, prefabricated item that has been trimmed, bent, molded, assembled, or otherwise customized to fit a specific patient by an individual with expertise

L1833 Knee orthosis, adjustable knee joints (unicentric or polycentric), positional orthosis, rigid support, prefabricated, off-the shelf

Lay Description

Knee orthotics (braces) come in a variety of sizes and shapes, and are made differently depending on their intended use. A prophylactic brace is used to prevent or reduce the severity of knee ligament injuries. A rehabilitative brace allows protected movement of the injured knee, and usually has hinges that allow the knee to be locked into certain positions. A functional brace is used to support an unsteady knee during daily activities or is used during a sporting activity. A derotation brace is used after an injury to a ligament and typically has bars, straps, and hinges; it is used during sporting activities and is most often made up of lightweight materials so that it allows significant motion and speed. An unloader brace is specifically designed for patients suffering from pain and disability due to osteoarthritis. This brace works by keeping the knee in the valgus position, which allows unloading of the compressive forces on the medial compartment.

L1834

L1834   Knee orthotic (KO), without knee joint, rigid, custom fabricated

Lay Description

This code reports the supply of a rigid knee orthotic, without knee joint, custom fabricated. Certain knee orthoses are designed to immobilize the knee completely and therefore do not feature a joint system. These devices may be applied to a knee injury to facilitate healing or to protect the joint following surgery.

L1836

L1836   Knee orthosis, rigid, without joint(s), includes soft interface material, prefabricated, off-the-shelf

Lay Description

This code reports the supply of a prefabricated rigid knee orthosis. Certain knee orthoses (KO) are designed to immobilize the knee completely and therefore do not feature a joint system. Such devices may be applied to a knee injury to facilitate healing, or to protect the joint following surgery. The orthosis holds the knee in a fixed position, usually slightly flexed. Cushion material to interface between the rigid orthosis and the patient's skin is included in the code description as are fitting sessions.

L1840

L1840   Knee orthotic (KO), derotation, medial-lateral, anterior cruciate ligament, custom fabricated

Lay Description

This code reports supply of a custom made knee orthosis that limits medial and lateral rotation of the knee for patients with compromised anterior cruciate ligament function. This is a dynamic rigid body orthosis, meaning that muscle actions against the orthosis work to stabilize the joint. The anterior cruciate ligament (ACL) is the most often injured ligament in the knee, often without external contact. The ACL limits forward motion and rotation of the tibia. Patients with compromised ACL exhibit muscle movement abnormalities in activities as simple as walking on level surfaces. Stopping, landing from a jump, running downhill, or making rapid lateral maneuvers causes a sense of instability. Most knee orthoses that address ACL instability exert pressures to prevent the knee from coming into full extension. Devices such as the Lenox-Hill orthosis also work to control torque, or twisting, actions of the tibia.

L1843-L1846

L1843   Knee orthosis, single upright, thigh and calf, with adjustable flexion and extension joint (unicentric or polycentric), medial-lateral and rotation control, with or without varus/valgus adjustment, prefabricated item that has been trimmed, bent, molded, assembled, or otherwise customized to fit a specific patient by an individual with expertise

L1844   Knee orthotic (KO), single upright, thigh and calf, with adjustable flexion and extension joint (unicentric or polycentric), medial-lateral and rotation control, with or without varus/valgus adjustment, custom fabricated

L1845   Knee orthosis, double upright, thigh and calf, with adjustable flexion and extension joint (unicentric or polycentric), medial-lateral and rotation control, with or without varus/valgus adjustment, prefabricated item that has been trimmed, bent, molded, assembled, or otherwise customized to fit a specific patient by an individual with expertise

L1846   Knee orthotic, double upright, thigh and calf, with adjustable flexion and extension joint (unicentric or polycentric), medial-lateral and rotation control, with or without varus/valgus adjustment, custom fabricated

Lay Description

Knee orthotic devices (braces) come in a variety of sizes and shapes, and are made differently depending on their intended use. A prophylactic brace is use to prevent or reduce the severity of knee ligament injuries. A rehabilitative brace allows protected movement of the injured knee, and usually has hinges that allow the knee to be locked into certain positions. A functional brace is used to support an unsteady knee during daily activities or is used during a sporting activity. A derotation brace is used after an injury to a ligament and typically has bars, straps, and hinges; it is used during sporting activities and is most often made up of lightweight materials so that it allows significant motion and speed. An unloader brace is specifically designed for patients suffering from pain and disability due to osteoarthritis. This brace works by keeping the knee in the valgus position, which allows unloading of the compressive forces on the medial compartment.

L1847-L1848

L1847   Knee orthosis, double upright with adjustable joint, with inflatable air support chamber(s), prefabricated item that has been trimmed, bent, molded, assembled, or otherwise customized to fit a specific patient by an individual with expertise

L1848   Knee orthosis, double upright with adjustable joint, with inflatable air support chamber(s), prefabricated, off-the-shelf

Lay Description
This code reports the supply of a specific type of prefabricated knee orthosis that uses air-support chambers. Many varieties of knee brace orthoses are available, and many feature a lateral and medial upright and an adjustable joint. The type reported by this code, however, also supports the knee with air-filled chambers rather than cushion material alone. This type of orthosis may be used to initially stabilize the joint following trauma.

L1850

L1850   Knee orthosis, swedish type, prefabricated, off-the-shelf

Lay Description
This code reports the supply of a particular design of knee orthosis (KO) known as the Swedish cage, or Swedish type. Great varieties of knee brace orthoses are available, and many feature a lateral and medial upright and an adjustable joint. The Swedish cage design also features a posterior support piece to further stabilize the joint and prevent hyperextension. The Swedish style brace is further distinguished by its longer length. The thigh and calf cuffs are generally positioned at a further extreme than similar hinged KOs. This type of orthosis is "off-the-shelf," or prefabricated.

L1860

L1860   Knee orthotic (KO), modification of supracondylar prosthetic socket, custom fabricated (SK)

Lay Description
This code reports a custom fabricated modification to a knee orthosis (KO) that is fitted in combination with a specific type of prosthetic socket. A prosthetic socket is the device that secures to the residual limb. The prosthetic leg attaches to the socket. In this instance, the socket is a variety that fits above the bony protuberance, or condyles, that constitute the distal end of the femur and the proximal end of the tibia (supracondylar). A KO may be required in

patients with lower limb prosthetics to stabilize the joint, particularly during training in the use of an artificial limb.

L1900

L1900   Ankle-foot orthotic (AFO), spring wire, dorsiflexion assist calf band, custom fabricated

Lay Description
This code reports the supply of a custom made, specialty ankle foot orthosis (AFO). Most AFOs employ medial and lateral upright bars attached from a calf band to an orthotic shoe or footplate. This device uses heavy gauge stainless steel spring wire rather than upright bars. The coiled spring action is at the attachment to the shoe or footplate and assists in dorsiflexion of the ankle joint (raising the foot at the ankle). These devices hold an advantage in being lightweight while offering good dorsiflexion assistance.

L1902-L1906

L1902   Ankle foot orthosis, ankle gauntlet, prefabricated, off-the-shelf

L1904   Ankle orthosis, ankle gauntlet, custom-fabricated

L1906   Ankle foot orthosis, multiligamentus ankle support, prefabricated, off-the-shelf

Lay Description
Ankle orthotics, gauntlets, and supports are generalized under the heading ankle-foot orthosis (AFO). (An exception within this range is the simple, prefabricated neoprene sock-type device.) AFOs within this range are prescribed for a variety of conditions for ambulatory patients, including congenital anomalies, pronation of the ankle, tendon problems, arthritis, and amputation. These devices generally extend well above the ankle, often to the upper calf, and may accommodate multiple planes of ankle movement. Some devices also limit ankle movement. The units may be built from standardized molds or custom fabricated from a plaster impression taken of the patient's foot and ankle. The units themselves may be made of metal, plastic polymers, or leather, sometimes in combination, and usually with various fabrics, cushions, and closure systems. A custom-fabricated orthosis involves substantial work, such as cutting, bending, molding, or sewing. It may involve the incorporation of some prefabricated components. It involves more than trimming, bending, or making other modifications to a substantially prefabricated item. Polypropylene models are close fitting and are often worn inside the shoe. Gauntlets usually feature lateral and medial stabilizers to address eversion and inversion, arch support, heel lock, padded tongue to facilitate application, and side panels for additional reinforcement. Fitting and adjustment is included in the supply of the product. Some gauntlets use natural

heat therapy to gently warm troubled areas on the ankle and foot. They consist of stabilizers (usually plastic) on either side to help resist inversion and eversion. Other features usually offered are arch support and complete heel lock, elastic back section to eliminate blistering, padded tongue to facilitate application, and side panels for more reinforcement. A molded-to-patient-model orthosis is a particular type of custom fabricated orthosis in which an impression of the foot is taken, by means of a plaster cast, CAD-CAM technology, etc. This impression is then used to make a positive model (of plaster or other material) of the body part to be braced. The orthosis is then molded on this positive model to be fit exactly to the patient's foot. It may require several castings and fittings by an orthotist/MD.

L1907

L1907 Ankle orthosis, supramalleolar with straps, with or without interface/pads, custom fabricated

Lay Description

Ankle foot orthotics (AFO) are orthoses or braces made of plastic or other material encompassing the ankle joint and all (or part) of the foot. AFOs are externally applied and intended to control position and motion of the ankle, compensate for weakness, or correct deformities. A variety of straps are available, including standard Velcro turn-back straps or custom designed leather and Dacron straps with padding.

L1910

L1910 Ankle-foot orthotic (AFO), posterior, single bar, clasp attachment to shoe counter, prefabricated, includes fitting and adjustment

Lay Description

This code reports the supply of a prefabricated single bar ankle foot orthosis (AFO). This type of AFO involves a single upright bar that attaches to a cuff near the top of the back of the calf and spans to an attachment that fits at the heel of the foot with a clasp attachment. The bar is shaped to the curve of the back of the calf and ankle. The AFO is available "off-the-shelf," and fitting and adjustment to a specific patient is required.

L1920

L1920 Ankle-foot orthotic (AFO), single upright with static or adjustable stop (Phelps or Perlstein type), custom fabricated

Lay Description

The type of ankle-foot orthosis (AFO) represented by this code involves a single upright bar that attaches to a band near the top of the calf and spans to an attachment that fits at the ankle-foot. The bar is usually on the lateral side of the orthotic and its length may be adjustable. The AFO is custom

fabricated to address a specific disorder and to fit a specific patient.

L1930-L1940

L1930 Ankle-foot orthotic (AFO), plastic or other material, prefabricated, includes fitting and adjustment

L1932 Ankle-foot orthotic (AFO), rigid anterior tibial section, total carbon fiber or equal material, prefabricated, includes fitting and adjustment

L1940 Ankle-foot orthotic (AFO), plastic or other material, custom fabricated

Lay Description

Ankle-foot orthoses extend well above the ankle (usually to near the top of the calf) and are fastened around the lower leg above the ankle. A prefabricated ankle-foot orthosis (AFO) involves producing many generic AFOs from a single mold. This device is constructed for many patients and is generic in design, made of plastic or other material. A custom fabricated (molded to patient model) AFO involves taking a mold of the patient first and fabricating an AFO from that mold. This device is constructed for only one patient and is not generic in design. It is made of plastic or other material.

L1945

L1945 Ankle-foot orthotic (AFO), plastic, rigid anterior tibial section (floor reaction), custom fabricated

Lay Description

This code reports the supply of a specific type of custom-made ankle foot orthosis (AFO). Typically a plaster mold is made of the patient's calf, ankle, and foot, although scans and computer modeling may also be used. A thermoplastic orthosis is created based on the patient's image. The device reported by this code features an anterior plastic upright piece, known as floor reaction. This upright is integrated into a solid footplate. A floor reaction AFO is often used for patients with lower limb weaknesses, since it prevents dorsiflexion collapse at the ankle. It is ordinarily prescribed bilaterally. The orthosis is rear-entry with Velcro or strap closures.

L1950

L1950 Ankle-foot orthotic (AFO), spiral, (Institute of Rehabilitative Medicine type), plastic, custom fabricated

Lay Description

This code reports supply of a specific type of custom-made ankle foot orthosis (AFO). The IRM is typically a single-piece AFO. The calf cuff is integrated into a single upright that spirals around the lower calf to join a footplate. Some designs are hemi-spiral others make a full spiral. This thermoplastic component is based on patient specific measurements or moldings.

L1951

L1951 Ankle-foot orthotic (AFO), spiral, (Institute of rehabilitative Medicine type), plastic or other material, prefabricated, includes fitting and adjustment

Lay Description

Ankle foot orthotics (AFO) are orthoses or braces made of plastic or other material encompassing the ankle joint and all (or part) of the foot. AFOs are externally applied and intended to control position and motion of the ankle, compensate for weakness, or correct deformities. The spiral AFO helps patients control medial-lateral movement. This code includes the fitting and adjustment of the AFO.

L1960

L1960 Ankle-foot orthotic (AFO), posterior solid ankle, plastic, custom fabricated

Lay Description

A custom fabricated (molded to patient model) ankle-foot orthosis (AFO) involves taking a mold of a patient first and fabricating an AFO from that mold. This device is constructed of plastic for only one patient and has a posterior solid ankle.

L1970

L1970 Ankle-foot orthotic (AFO), plastic with ankle joint, custom fabricated

Lay Description

A custom-fabricated orthosis is one that is individually made for a specific patient starting with basic materials including, but not limited to, plastic, metal, leather, or cloth in the form of sheets, bars, and so forth. It involves substantial work, such as cutting, bending, molding, sewing, and so forth. It may involve the incorporation of some prefabricated components. It involves more than trimming, bending, or making other modifications to a substantially prefabricated item. A molded-to-patient-model orthosis is a particular type of custom fabricated orthosis in which an impression of the ankle joint is made by means of a plaster cast, CAD-CAM technology, etc. This impression is then used to make a model of plastic of the ankle joint to be braced. The orthosis is then molded on this model to be fit exactly to the ankle. This provides for free limited motion or assists in dorsiflexion and plantar flexion while limiting inversion and eversion of the ankle. The plastic design is lightweight and allows the patient to interchange shoes. It may provide critical foot and arch support. Neutral arch position promotes healing of injured ligaments. Side supports help position the brace correctly and tightly to move in harmony with the foot and ankle and assure full time protection and support.

L1971

L1971 Ankle-foot orthotic (AFO), plastic or other material with ankle joint, prefabricated, includes fitting and adjustment

Lay Description

Ankle foot orthotics (AFO) are orthoses or braces made of plastic or other material encompassing the ankle joint and all (or part) of the foot. AFOs are externally applied and intended to control position and motion of the ankle, compensate for weakness, or correct deformities.

L1980-L1990

L1980 Ankle-foot orthotic (AFO), single upright free plantar dorsiflexion, solid stirrup, calf band/cuff (single bar 'BK' orthotic), custom fabricated

L1990 Ankle-foot orthotic (AFO), double upright free plantar dorsiflexion, solid stirrup, calf band/cuff (double bar 'BK' orthotic), custom fabricated

Lay Description

This type of ankle-foot orthosis (AFO) involves use of upright bars that attach to a band near the top of the calf and spans to a stirrup attachment that fits at the ankle-foot. A single bar is usually on the lateral side of the orthotic. The double bar model has upright supports on the medial and lateral sides of the AFO. Both models allow for free plantarflexion and dorsiflexion (movement to raise and lower the foot) at the hinged stirrup. The AFO is custom fabricated to address a specific disorder and to fit a specific patient.

L2000-L2034

L2000 Knee-ankle-foot orthotic (KAFO), single upright, free knee, free ankle, solid stirrup, thigh and calf bands/cuffs (single bar 'AK' orthotic), custom fabricated

L2005 Knee-ankle-foot orthotic (KAFO), any material, single or double upright, stance control, automatic lock and swing phase release, any type activation, includes ankle joint, any type, custom fabricated

L2010 Knee-ankle-foot orthotic (KAFO), single upright, free ankle, solid stirrup, thigh and calf bands/cuffs (single bar 'AK' orthotic), without knee joint, custom fabricated

L2020 Knee-ankle-foot orthotic (KAFO), double upright, free ankle, solid stirrup, thigh and calf bands/cuffs (double bar 'AK' orthotic), custom fabricated

L2030 Knee-ankle-foot orthotic (KAFO), double upright, free ankle, solid stirrup, thigh and calf bands/cuffs, (double bar 'AK' orthotic), without knee joint, custom fabricated

L2034 Knee-ankle-foot orthotic (KAFO), full plastic, single upright, with or without free motion knee, medial-lateral rotation control, with or without free motion ankle, custom fabricated

Lay Description
These codes report the supply of specific custom fabricated knee-ankle-foot orthotics (KAFO). Designs for KAFO devices are similar to ankle-foot devices. Similar materials are employed. Some units may be built from standardized molds, but most are custom fabricated for a specific patient based on plaster molds and measurements. In addition to the solid stirrup ankle-foot features reported by this range of codes, a KAFO has an upper thigh band or plastic shell and a hinged apparatus to eliminate (static) or limit knee movement.

L2035

L2035 Knee-ankle-foot orthotic (KAFO), full plastic, static (pediatric size), without free motion ankle, prefabricated, includes fitting and adjustment

Lay Description
A knee-ankle-foot orthotic (KAFO) is a device that extends from the thigh to the foot and is generally used to control instabilities in the lower limb by maintaining alignment and controlling motion. In L2035, a prefabricated plastic KAFO is designed to hold a child's ankle and knee in a fixed position. It is non-adjustable and is sometimes used to treat infantile club foot disorders. Fitting and adjustment is included in this code.

L2036-L2038

L2036 Knee-ankle-foot orthotic (KAFO), full plastic, double upright, with or without free motion knee, with or without free motion ankle, custom fabricated

L2037 Knee-ankle-foot orthotic (KAFO), full plastic, single upright, with or without free motion knee, with or without free motion ankle, custom fabricated

L2038 Knee-ankle-foot orthotic (KAFO), full plastic, with or without free motion knee, multi-axis ankle, custom fabricated

Lay Description
A knee-ankle-foot orthotic (KAFO) is a device that extends from the thigh to the foot and is generally used to control instabilities in the lower limb by maintaining alignment and controlling motion. These codes describe a custom-fabricated KAFO that is used to control the knee and ankle, with free motion joints or rigid control at the ankle, with or without bilateral unicentric free motion joints at the knee, and molded plastic thigh and calf/ankle/foot sections. A single or double upright metal KAFO is an AFO with one or two metal uprights extending proximally to the thigh to control knee motion and alignment. This orthosis

consists of a mechanical knee joint and two thigh bands between one or two uprights. Free motion knee joint refers to a joint that has unrestricted knee flexion and extension with a stop to prevent hyperextension. The free motion knee joint is used for patients with recurvatum but good strength of the quadriceps to control knee motion. A multi-axis ankle allows movement along multiple planes.

L2040

L2040 Hip-knee-ankle-foot orthotic (HKAFO), torsion control, bilateral rotation straps, pelvic band/belt, custom fabricated

Lay Description
This custom fabricated hip-knee-ankle-foot orthotic (HKAFO) is used to assist in controlling rotation at the hips. It consists of a pelvic band and belt with elastic or webbing straps that twist around the legs and attach to shoes.

L2050

L2050 Hip-knee-ankle-foot orthotic (HKAFO), torsion control, bilateral torsion cables, hip joint, pelvic band/belt, custom fabricated

Lay Description
This custom fabricated hip-knee-ankle-foot orthotic (HKAFO) is used to control the internal or external rotation of the hips and consists of a pelvic band and belt, unicentric free motion hip joints, bilateral torsion cables, and calf straps attached to shoes.

L2060

L2060 Hip-knee-ankle-foot orthotic (HKAFO), torsion control, bilateral torsion cables, ball bearing hip joint, pelvic band/ belt, custom fabricated

Lay Description
This custom fabricated hip-knee-ankle-foot orthotic (HKAFO) is used to control the internal or external rotation of the hips and consists of a pelvic band and belt, unicentric free motion ball bearing hip joints, bilateral torsion cables, and calf straps attached to shoes.

L2070-L2090

L2070 Hip-knee-ankle-foot orthotic (HKAFO), torsion control, unilateral rotation straps, pelvic band/belt, custom fabricated

L2080 Hip-knee-ankle-foot orthotic (HKAFO), torsion control, unilateral torsion cable, hip joint, pelvic band/belt, custom fabricated

L2090 Hip-knee-ankle-foot orthotic (HKAFO), torsion control, unilateral torsion cable, ball bearing hip joint, pelvic band/ belt, custom fabricated

Lay Description

These custom fabricated hip-knee-ankle-foot orthotics (HKAFO) are used to assist in controlling rotation of one hip. In L2070, the orthotic includes a pelvic band and belt with an elastic or a webbing rotation strap that twists around the leg and attaches to a shoe. In L2080 and L2090, the orthotic includes a unicentric free motion hip joint (L2080) or a unicentric ball bearing free motion hip joint (L2090) in conjunction with a unilateral torsion cable, calf strap, pelvic band, and belt to control the internal or external rotation of one hip. The orthosis attaches to a shoe and is custom fabricated.

L2106–L2116

L2106 Ankle-foot orthotic (AFO), fracture orthotic, tibial fracture cast orthotic, thermoplastic type casting material, custom fabricated

L2108 Ankle-foot orthotic (AFO), fracture orthotic, tibial fracture cast orthotic, custom fabricated

L2112 Ankle-foot orthotic (AFO), fracture orthotic, tibial fracture orthotic, soft, prefabricated, includes fitting and adjustment

L2114 Ankle-foot orthotic (AFO), fracture orthotic, tibial fracture orthotic, semi-rigid, prefabricated, includes fitting and adjustment

L2116 Ankle-foot orthotic (AFO), fracture orthotic, tibial fracture orthotic, rigid, prefabricated, includes fitting and adjustment

Lay Description

Certain tibial fractures may be treated with ankle-foot orthoses (AFO). These devices generally extend well above the ankle, often to the upper calf. Ankle movement may be locked or limited, or multiple planes of ankle movement allowed. The units may be built from standardized prefabricated molds or custom fabricated from a plaster impression taken of the patient's foot, ankle, and lower leg. The units themselves may be made of metal, plastic polymers, or leather, sometimes in combination, and usually with various fabrics, cushions, and closure systems. Some models are "thermoplastic," which means shape can be adjusted by application of heat. Fracture AFOs may also be custom built from rigid materials such as plaster or synthetic polymers, as well as from prefabricated and easily manipulated semi-rigid (polypropylene) and soft materials (rubber, plastic foam). Fitting and adjustment is included in the supply of the product.

L2126–L2136

L2126 Knee-ankle-foot orthotic (KAFO), fracture orthotic, femoral fracture cast orthotic, thermoplastic type casting material, custom fabricated

L2128 Knee-ankle-foot orthotic (KAFO), fracture orthotic, femoral fracture cast orthotic, custom fabricated

L2132 Knee-ankle-foot orthotic (KAFO), fracture orthotic, femoral fracture cast orthotic, soft, prefabricated, includes fitting and adjustment

L2134 Knee-ankle-foot orthotic (KAFO), fracture orthotic, femoral fracture cast orthotic, semi-rigid, prefabricated, includes fitting and adjustment

L2136 Knee-ankle-foot orthotic (KAFO), fracture orthotic, femoral fracture cast orthotic, rigid, prefabricated, includes fitting and adjustment

Lay Description

These codes report the supply of specific femoral fracture cast orthoses. Codes are differentiated by casting material and rigidity and whether the device is custom made or prefabricated. Custom fabricated orthoses are generally manufactured for a specific patient based on measurements, castings, and sometimes computer modeling. Prefabricated orthoses are generally produced in volume, with variations only for size, and are intended for use by any patient in need of such a device. Prefabricated devices require fitting and adjustment sessions. Knee ankle foot orthotics (KAFO) typically extend well above the knee and in these instances address fractures of the femur. Thermoplastic is shaped and contoured by heat application.

L2180–L2192

L2180 Addition to lower extremity fracture orthotic, plastic shoe insert with ankle joints

L2182 Addition to lower extremity fracture orthotic, drop lock knee joint

L2184 Addition to lower extremity fracture orthotic, limited motion knee joint

L2186 Addition to lower extremity fracture orthotic, adjustable motion knee joint, Lerman type

L2188 Addition to lower extremity fracture orthotic, quadrilateral brim

L2190 Addition to lower extremity fracture orthotic, waist belt

L2192 Addition to lower extremity fracture orthotic, hip joint, pelvic band, thigh flange, and pelvic belt

Lay Description

Fracture orthoses stabilize the fracture site and promote callus formation, while allowing weight bearing and joint movement after initial subsiding pain and edema. The bony motion at the fracture site is prevented through circumferential compression of the soft tissue. Fracture orthoses include the tibial fracture orthosis and femoral fracture orthosis. Fracture orthoses are commonly referred to as "removable casts." These codes report additions to lower extremity fracture orthotics.

L2200

L2200 Addition to lower extremity, limited ankle motion, each joint

Lay Description
This code reports an addition to a previously provided orthosis. This code represents the supply of a device or service to limit ankle motion on an ankle-foot orthosis. The ankle joint moves the foot in flexion (plantarflexion is the dropping of the foot downward and dorsiflexion moves the foot upward), as well as inversion and eversion. A previously supplied orthosis is adjusted to limit ankle motion. This may entail molding a block to the interface of the ankle/foot parts of the orthosis, or otherwise manipulating the orthosis to limit movement.

L2210-L2265

L2210 Addition to lower extremity, dorsiflexion assist (plantar flexion resist), each joint

L2220 Addition to lower extremity, dorsiflexion and plantar flexion assist/resist, each joint

L2230 Addition to lower extremity, split flat caliper stirrups and plate attachment

L2232 Addition to lower extremity orthotic, rocker bottom for total contact ankle-foot orthotic (AFO), for custom fabricated orthotic only

L2240 Addition to lower extremity, round caliper and plate attachment

L2250 Addition to lower extremity, foot plate, molded to patient model, stirrup attachment

L2260 Addition to lower extremity, reinforced solid stirrup (Scott-Craig type)

L2265 Addition to lower extremity, long tongue stirrup

Lay Description
This range of codes reports additions to previously provided orthoses. Dorsiflexion assist (as well as plantarflexion assist/resist) devices involve the application of a small spring-loaded cylinder on the ankle portion of the orthosis that works against a piston rod on the foot section. The spring tension assists or resists the flexing action of the foot as prescribed. (Plantarflexion is the dropping of the foot downward; dorsiflexion moves the foot upward.) Certain devices, such as caliper plates, stirrup plates, and stirrups can be mounted to an existing orthosis. Others may be molded directly to a plastic polymer

orthosis. These additions are used to manipulate the flexion mobility of the ankle joint.

L2270-L2275

L2270 Addition to lower extremity, varus/valgus correction (T) strap, padded/lined or malleolus pad

L2275 Addition to lower extremity, varus/valgus correction, plastic modification, padded/lined

Lay Description
Varus/valgus is usually a congenital condition (or pathological condition, such as in poliomyelitis). Varus is the condition where the joint is bent outward; valgus is the condition where the joint is bent inward, or medially. Treatment may entail an ankle-foot orthosis (AFO). Valgus of the ankle, or inversion, might be treated by an AFO with a bar on the medial side and a t-strap on the lateral side. Varus, or eversion, might be treated by an AFO with a bar on the lateral side and a t-strap on the medial side.

L2280

L2280 Addition to lower extremity, molded inner boot

Lay Description
A molded inner boot is a rigid protective covering for the ankle and foot. It is usually composed of polypropylene or a similar material and is vacuum formed to a plaster mold of the patient's foot and ankle.

L2300-L2310

L2300 Addition to lower extremity, abduction bar (bilateral hip involvement), jointed, adjustable

L2310 Addition to lower extremity, abduction bar, straight

Lay Description
These codes report the supply of abduction bars added to a fracture orthosis. The fracture bar added to the orthosis maintains abduction (legs spread) during healing. The bar is jointed and adjustable.

L2320-L2340

L2320 Addition to lower extremity, nonmolded lacer, for custom fabricated orthotic only

L2330 Addition to lower extremity, lacer molded to patient model, for custom fabricated orthotic only

L2335 Addition to lower extremity, anterior swing band

L2340 Addition to lower extremity, pretibial shell, molded to patient model

Lay Description
A leather, or similar material, lacer is a cuff-like support that fits around the calf area. It may be custom to measurement or molded from a model of

the patient. An anterior swing band is a rigid anterior (front) articulating metal band for attachment to a lower extremity orthosis. An anterior (front) pretibial shell is a lower limb orthoses that is custom molded to a model of the patient's leg.

L2350

L2350 Addition to lower extremity, prosthetic type, (BK) socket, molded to patient model, (used for PTB, AFO orthoses)

Lay Description
This code is used to report a custom fabricated plastic prosthetic type socket, molded from a model of the patient's knee section, used on ankle-foot orthotics (AFO). It includes casting and cast preparation.

L2360

L2360 Addition to lower extremity, extended steel shank

Lay Description
This orthotic is a steel shank inserted between the inner and outer sole of a shoe to provide more rigidity to the shoe.

L2370

L2370 Addition to lower extremity, Patten bottom

Lay Description
This code reports the addition to a lower extremity orthosis of a Patten bottom. A Patten bottom is a type of strike boot added to the bottom of a knee ankle foot orthosis (KAFO). The Patten bottom is connected to the rigid outer shell of the orthotic so that with the limb slightly flexed, weight is transferred to the orthosis and upper leg rather than on the foot and ankle.

L2375

L2375 Addition to lower extremity, torsion control, ankle joint and half solid stirrup

Lay Description
This orthosis is a half stirrup attached to a shoe and a free motion ankle joint for torsion control.

L2380

L2380 Addition to lower extremity, torsion control, straight knee joint, each joint

Lay Description
This code is used to report a lower extremity addition and refers to a free motion knee joint used only for torsion control.

L2385

L2385 Addition to lower extremity, straight knee joint, heavy-duty, each joint

Lay Description
This code is used to report a free motion knee joint used only for torsion control. It is a heavy duty, 180-degree stop unicentric knee joint for a knee orthotic (KO) or a knee-ankle-foot orthotic (KAFO).

L2387

L2387 Addition to lower extremity, polycentric knee joint, for custom fabricated knee-ankle-foot orthotic (KAFO), each joint

Lay Description
This code is used to report a polycentric knee joint for a custom knee-ankle-foot orthotic (KAFO) only. It provides stability at full extension and easy movement during swing phase.

L2390-L2395

L2390 Addition to lower extremity, offset knee joint, each joint

L2395 Addition to lower extremity, offset knee joint, heavy-duty, each joint

Lay Description
These codes refer to an orthosis that has a design of a 180-degree stop unicentric knee joint or heavy-duty knee joint for a knee orthotic (KO) or knee-ankle-foot orthotic (KAFO). This addition puts the joint center posterior to the weight line providing more knee stability.

L2397

L2397 Addition to lower extremity orthotic, suspension sleeve

Lay Description
Orthoses of the lower extremities are sometimes attached by a suspension sleeve. These interface devices often feature a soft silicone or neoprene liner that makes a non-slip suction-type contact to the skin.

L2405-L2492

L2405 Addition to knee joint, drop lock, each

L2415 Addition to knee lock with integrated release mechanism (bail, cable, or equal), any material, each joint

L2425 Addition to knee joint, disc or dial lock for adjustable knee flexion, each joint

L2430 Addition to knee joint, ratchet lock for active and progressive knee extension, each joint

L2492 Addition to knee joint, lift loop for drop lock ring

Lay Description
This range of codes addresses additions to external knee joint orthoses used to treat knee dysfunctions.

The codes report additions or adaptations to the joint mechanism of a base orthosis. Many of these types of orthoses minimally feature a manual adjustment that locks the joint for walking and another to release the knee for comfortable sitting. The traditional manual drop lock system requires the patient to lift a locking mechanism to release the fixed walking position. More advanced adaptations automatically lock and unlock the joint as the patient goes through gait motions (swing-phase or pendulum lock systems). Some adaptations add a release mechanism, such as a bail or cable, or a dial lock. A polycentric joint works like a cam, offering more rigidity as the joint is extended and less during flexion. A ratchet joint features a series of locking positions that can be selected or skipped over by the wearer, either for active use or as a means to progressively increase range of motion. A lift loop is a gripping device for the wearer to raise the locking ring of a drop lock mechanism.

L2500

L2500   Addition to lower extremity, thigh/weight bearing, gluteal/ischial weight bearing, ring

Lay Description
This code is used to report an addition to the upper part of a knee-ankle-foot orthotic (KAFO) designed to assist with weight bearing at the ischium during walking and standing.

L2510

L2510   Addition to lower extremity, thigh/weight bearing, quadri-lateral brim, molded to patient model

Lay Description
A molded plastic model of a patient's thigh is constructed. It is then used at the upper portion of a knee-ankle-foot orthotic (KAFO) to reduce the weight off the extremity during walking and standing. This custom fabricated quadrilateral socket design includes casting and cast preparation.

L2520

L2520   Addition to lower extremity, thigh/weight bearing, quadri-lateral brim, custom fitted

Lay Description
This code is used to report a prefabricated, adjustable plastic brim that is used at the upper portion of a knee-ankle-foot orthotic (KAFO). It is designed to reduce the weight off the extremity during walking and standing. It is custom fitted.

L2525-L2526

L2525   Addition to lower extremity, thigh/weight bearing, ischial containment/narrow M-L brim molded to patient model

L2526   Addition to lower extremity, thigh/weight bearing, ischial containment/narrow M-L brim, custom fitted

Lay Description
These codes are used to report a thigh/weight bearing orthosis that has a foam cast brim that may be custom fitted or custom molded. These models have a tighter medial-lateral (M-L) design and greater weight bearing ability from the standard quadrilateral model.

L2530-L2540

L2530   Addition to lower extremity, thigh/weight bearing, lacer, nonmolded

L2540   Addition to lower extremity, thigh/weight bearing, lacer, molded to patient model

Lay Description
These codes are used to report a thigh/weight bearing lacer, which is a corset-like device wrapped around a thigh, and used at the top portion of a knee-ankle-foot orthotic (KAFO) to reduce the weight off the extremity during walking and standing. It may be molded to a patient model or nonmolded.

L2550

L2550   Addition to lower extremity, thigh/weight bearing, high roll cuff

Lay Description
This code is used to report a high roll cuff used for thigh/weight bearing. A high roll cuff is a padded and rolled special top edge of a lacer, which is a corset-like device wrapped around a thigh to give greater support and comfort.

L2570

L2570   Addition to lower extremity, pelvic control, hip joint, Clevis type 2 position joint, each

Lay Description
This code is used to report a specially designed hip joint that can be locked in 90- and 180-degree positions.

L2580

L2580   Addition to lower extremity, pelvic control, pelvic sling

Lay Description
This code is used to report a narrow band of leather or some flexible material that is attached to an orthotic hip joint to apply pressure to the gluteal area to stabilize the pelvic area.

L2600

L2600 Addition to lower extremity, pelvic control, hip joint, Clevis type, or thrust bearing, free, each

Lay Description
This code is used to report a free motion unicentric hip joint for a knee-ankle-foot orthotic (KAFO). This device controls motion at the hip, knee, and ankle.

L2610

L2610 Addition to lower extremity, pelvic control, hip joint, Clevis or thrust bearing, lock, each

Lay Description
This refers to a free motion unicentric hip joint. This KAFO device controls motion at hip, knee, and ankle and has a drop lock.

L2620

L2620 Addition to lower extremity, pelvic control, hip joint, heavy-duty, each

Lay Description
This is a free motion, unicentric hip joint KAFO that is heavy duty. This device controls motion at hip, knee, and ankle.

L2622

L2622 Addition to lower extremity, pelvic control, hip joint, adjustable flexion, each

Lay Description
This is an adjustable flexion, free motion unicentric hip joint for a KAFO. This device controls motion at hip, knee, and ankle. The adjustable flexion control range of motion of the affected limb.

L2624

L2624 Addition to lower extremity, pelvic control, hip joint, adjustable flexion, extension, abduction control, each

Lay Description
This code is used to report an adjustable extension, flexion, and abduction free, motion unicentric hip joint on a knee-ankle-foot orthotic (KAFO). These hip joints control flexion/extension and abduction/adduction and control range of motion of the affected area.

L2627

L2627 Addition to lower extremity, pelvic control, plastic, molded to patient model, reciprocating hip joint and cables

Lay Description
This refers to a hip/pelvic control system that provides a reciprocating gait action. The way RGA works is with every step a patient takes, as one leg flexes, the other leg must extend and thereby stretch out the hip contracting structures. This orthoses is custom fabricated, a molded plastic pelvic section, molded from a model of the patient, special hip joints, vertical lateral uprights, and a thoracic belt.

L2628

L2628 Addition to lower extremity, pelvic control, metal frame, reciprocating hip joint and cables

Lay Description
This refers to a hip/pelvic control system that provides a reciprocating gait action. The way RGA works is with every step a patient takes, as one leg flexes, the other leg must extend and thereby stretch out the hip contracting structures. This KAFO orthoses includes a metal pelvic band, special hip joints, vertical lateral uprights, and a thoracic belt. It is custom fabricated.

L2630

L2630 Addition to lower extremity, pelvic control, band and belt, unilateral

Lay Description
This refers to a pelvic band and belt for use with a unilateral KAFO that is secured to the hip joint for control and is custom fabricated

L2640

L2640 Addition to lower extremity, pelvic control, band and belt, bilateral

Lay Description
This refers to a pelvic band and belt for use with bilateral orthosis and is secured to both hip joints for control and is custom fabricated.

L2650

L2650 Addition to lower extremity, pelvic and thoracic control, gluteal pad, each

Lay Description
This code is used to report a specially designed pad that provides gluteal pressure. This aids in support and balance and is custom fabricated.

L2660

L2660 Addition to lower extremity, thoracic control, thoracic band

Lay Description
This code is used to report a thoracic band that is added to a bilateral hip-knee-ankle-foot orthotic (HKAFO). A pelvic band and paraspinal uprights are also used to provide greater torso control and spinal alignment.

L2670-L2680

L2670 Addition to lower extremity, thoracic control, paraspinal uprights

L2680 Addition to lower extremity, thoracic control, lateral support uprights

Lay Description
These codes are used to report thoracic bands that are added to a bilateral hip-knee-ankle-foot orthotic (HKAFO). One has paraspinal uprights (L2670) between the pelvic and thoracic bands to provide greater control of the torso and spinal alignment. The other has lateral uprights (L2680) between the pelvic and thoracic bands to provide greater control of the torso and spinal alignment.

L2750

L2750 Addition to lower extremity orthotic, plating chrome or nickel, per bar

Lay Description
This refers to a process of adding a durable, protective finish to steel components on any orthoses.

L2755

L2755 Addition to lower extremity orthotic, high strength, lightweight material, all hybrid lamination/prepreg composite, per segment, for custom fabricated orthotic only

Lay Description
This code reports supply of a segmental addition to a lower extremity orthosis of high strength, lightweight material, such as carbon graphite laminates. These high-end materials are extremely lightweight yet posses good torsional and structural properties. This additional segment is for custom fabricated orthosis only.

L2760-L2780

L2760 Addition to lower extremity orthotic, extension, per extension, per bar (for lineal adjustment for growth)

L2768 Orthotic side bar disconnect device, per bar

L2780 Addition to lower extremity orthotic, noncorrosive finish, per bar

Lay Description
This range of codes reports supply of additions to lower extremity orthoses support bars and associated devices. These bars are usually paired medially and laterally on the orthosis, although single-bar units are also used. Growth in children necessitates regular changing of bars and disconnect devices may be added to facilitate bar change and adjustment.

L2785

L2785 Addition to lower extremity orthotic, drop lock retainer, each

Lay Description
This refers to a clip or a spring and a steel ball inserted into a metal upright on an orthoses. It is designed to hold a drop lock in a locked or unlocked position.

L2795-L2810

L2795 Addition to lower extremity orthotic, knee control, full kneecap

L2800 Addition to lower extremity orthotic, knee control, knee cap, medial or lateral pull, for use with custom fabricated orthotic only

L2810 Addition to lower extremity orthotic, knee control, condylar pad

Lay Description
This range of codes reports supply of additions to lower extremity orthoses designed to improve knee stability and control through manipulative padding and coverings. These additions may allow for greater loading or unloading of a side of the joint, possibly relieving pressure on an arthritic or injured site.

L2820-L2830

L2820 Addition to lower extremity orthotic, soft interface for molded plastic, below knee section

L2830 Addition to lower extremity orthotic, soft interface for molded plastic, above knee section

Lay Description
These codes report supply of soft interface additions to lower extremity orthoses. This is padding against the skin for molded plastic pieces. A great deal of orthosis design engineering focuses on above-the-joint and below-the-joint supports. These supports must work through the skin surface to stabilize skeletal bone as well as softer-tissue structures such as ligaments, cartilage, and musculature.

L2840-L2850

L2840 Addition to lower extremity orthotic, tibial length sock, fracture or equal, each

L2850 Addition to lower extremity orthotic, femoral length sock, fracture or equal, each

Lay Description
These codes report supply of fracture socks, or the equivalent. These are highly elastic stockings, often with a natural fabric liner on the skin contact side. The stockings are often made of a closed mesh that can be trimmed for length. Fracture socks may be applied for certain types of closed fractures of the lower extremity, usually in combination with a rigid orthosis. The sock/orthosis combination holds certain

advantages over traditional plaster casting in that patients often experience less muscle shrinkage.

L2861

L2861 Addition to lower extremity joint, knee or ankle, concentric adjustable torsion style mechanism for custom fabricated orthotics only, each

Lay Description

This code describes concentric adjustable torsion style mechanisms used for the lower extremity joint, knee or ankle, for custom fabricated orthotics only. These components incorporate adjustable and removable dynamic power assist. The power assist add-on component is mounted to a conventionally functioning knee or ankle component within a custom orthotic and adds the prescribed function to dynamic assist/resist as required. These additions are used to improve stability and walking functions.

L2999

L2999 Lower extremity orthotic, not otherwise specified

Lay Description

This code reports the supply of an orthosis of the lower extremity that is not defined elsewhere in the HCPCS listing. Certain wraps, splints, shoes, or other supplies may be reported by the code. Generally speaking, a Medicare claim for L2999 must include "a narrative description of the item, the brand name and model name/number of the item, and a statement defining the medical necessity of the item for the particular patient."

L3000-L3030

L3000 Foot insert, removable, molded to patient model, UCB type, Berkeley shell, each

L3001 Foot, insert, removable, molded to patient model, Spenco, each

L3002 Foot insert, removable, molded to patient model, Plastazote or equal, each

L3003 Foot insert, removable, molded to patient model, silicone gel, each

L3010 Foot insert, removable, molded to patient model, longitudinal arch support, each

L3020 Foot insert, removable, molded to patient model, longitudinal/metatarsal support, each

L3030 Foot insert, removable, formed to patient foot, each

Lay Description

This range of codes reports supply of a variety of prescription orthosis shoe inserts, differentiated largely by product type, construction material, and method of preparation and fitting. These devices fit inside the shoe. Most are molded to a plaster or foam replica of the patient's foot, but some are modeled to electronic images of the foot. Inserts molded to the patient's foot directly are often made of thermo-formable materials that can be heat softened, custom applied, and trimmed in a single session. The UCB (also known as UCBL or "Berkeley shell") is named for the University of California Biomechanics Laboratories, the developer of several types of rigid inserts. Materials for this range of codes include high and low heat plastic, leather, and various synthetics. Plastazote is a type of closed cell polyethylene foam and Spenco is manufactured from closed cell neoprene. Most inserts address a variety of foot corrections.

L3031

L3031 Foot, insert/plate, removable, addition to lower extremity orthotic, high strength, lightweight material, all hybrid lamination/prepreg composite, each

Lay Description

This code refers to a lower extremity orthosis of high strength, lightweight material, such as carbon graphite laminates. These high-end materials are extremely lightweight and have good structural properties. This device fits inside the shoe.

L3040-L3060

L3040 Foot, arch support, removable, premolded, longitudinal, each

L3050 Foot, arch support, removable, premolded, metatarsal, each

L3060 Foot, arch support, removable, premolded, longitudinal/metatarsal, each

Lay Description

This range of codes reports the supply of arch support products that are available premolded and not modeled to a replica of the patient's foot. These prefabricated "stock" devices may still require a custom fitting, however. Materials are usually various synthetics.

L3070-L3090

L3070 Foot, arch support, nonremovable, attached to shoe, longitudinal, each

L3080 Foot, arch support, nonremovable, attached to shoe, metatarsal, each

L3090 Foot, arch support, nonremovable, attached to shoe, longitudinal/metatarsal, each

Lay Description

These codes report the supply of nonremovable arch support products that are attached to the patient's shoe. Materials are usually various synthetics.

L3100

L3100 Hallus-valgus night dynamic splint, prefabricated, off-the-shelf

Lay Description
This type of night splint addresses poor alignment of the base joint of the great toe (hallux-valgus) through strapping, padding, and rigid splinting. A slip-on type splint is applied to the great toe and straps are applied to correctly align the toe while the patient sleeps.

L3140-L3150

L3140 Foot, abduction rotation bar, including shoes

L3150 Foot, abduction rotation bar, without shoes

Lay Description
These codes report the supply of abduction rotation bars. Abduction is the movement away from the median plane, in this case of the foot outward. These bars maintain the position of the feet and, consequently, the femoral head in a fixed position. The abduction bar is often prescribed to treat cases of talipes (clubfoot) and genu varus (pigeon toe-in) and certain types of hip dysplasia in toddlers. The prototypical orthosis is the Denis-Browne splint, which is an abduction rotation bar that attaches to the footplate of a baby shoe or is wrapped to the foot. The variety that attaches to a shoe may be adjusted with a special wrench.

L3160

L3160 Foot, adjustable shoe-styled positioning device

Lay Description
This is a pediatric two piece shoe that enables the forefoot and hind foot can be positioned independently for the forefoot adduction or abduction. The two pieces have separate closures for control.

L3170

L3170 Foot, plastic, silicone or equal, heel stabilizer, prafabricated, off-the-shelf, each

Lay Description
Report this code for supply of prefabricated plastic silicone or equivalent heel stabilizer bars to control abduction and rotation. Ordinarily, this is an insert or modification to a shoe that is part of a lower extremity orthosis system.

L3201-L3203

L3201 Orthopedic shoe, Oxford with supinator or pronator, infant

L3202 Orthopedic shoe, Oxford with supinator or pronator, child

L3203 Orthopedic shoe, Oxford with supinator or pronator, junior

Lay Description
These codes report supply of specific orthopedic footwear. The codes are differentiated by whether the footwear is modeled for infants, children, or juniors. The shoes reported by this range of codes are oxford style. The shoes are fitted with adjustment for supination or pronation. Supination is bowing out of the foot and adjustment is usually to raise the lateral edge of the shoe or to lower the medial edge. Pronation is a "flat foot" or bowing in of the foot. Adjustment is usually to raise the medial edge or lower the lateral edge of the shoe.

L3204-L3207

L3204 Orthopedic shoe, hightop with supinator or pronator, infant

L3206 Orthopedic shoe, hightop with supinator or pronator, child

L3207 Orthopedic shoe, hightop with supinator or pronator, junior

Lay Description
These codes report supply of specific orthopedic footwear. The codes are differentiated by whether the footwear is modeled for infants, children, or juniors. The shoes reported by this range of codes are high-top style. The shoes are fitted with adjustment for supination or pronation. Supination is bowing out of the foot and adjustment is usually to raise the lateral edge of the shoe or to lower the medial edge. Pronation is a "flat foot" or bowing in of the foot. Adjustment is usually to raise the medial edge or lower the lateral edge of the shoe.

L3208-L3211

L3208 Surgical boot, each, infant

L3209 Surgical boot, each, child

L3211 Surgical boot, each, junior

Lay Description
A surgical boot or shoe is a special type of footwear, usually high-top style, designed to accommodate post-surgical wrappings and dressings and to allow the patient a degree of mobility. Ordinarily these boots are manufactured without left-foot or right-foot design considerations and are sold as single units.

L3212-L3214

L3212   Benesch boot, pair, infant
L3213   Benesch boot, pair, child
L3214   Benesch boot, pair, junior

Lay Description
Benesch boots are shoes that have a clear plastic window in the back that permit a view of the heel while in the shoe. It is used to ensure that the heel is held in the correct position within the shoe.

L3215-L3230

L3215   Orthopedic footwear, ladies shoe, oxford, each
L3216   Orthopedic footwear, ladies shoe, depth inlay, each
L3217   Orthopedic footwear, ladies shoe, hightop, depth inlay, each
L3219   Orthopedic footwear, mens shoe, oxford, each
L3221   Orthopedic footwear, mens shoe, depth inlay, each
L3222   Orthopedic footwear, mens shoe, hightop, depth inlay, each
L3224   Orthopedic footwear, woman's shoe, oxford, used as an integral part of a brace (orthotic)
L3225   Orthopedic footwear, man's shoe, oxford, used as an integral part of a brace (orthotic)
L3230   Orthopedic footwear, custom shoe, depth inlay, each

Lay Description
This range of codes reports supply of orthopaedic footwear. The codes are differentiated by whether the footwear is modeled for men or women, whether the shoe is an integral part of a lower-extremity orthosis, and the style of the shoe. Depth inlay is a design feature to accommodate an in-the-shoe component of a lower-extremity orthosis. The inlay may be removable for use of the shoe with or without the brace component. Shoes that are an integral part of a lower-extremity orthosis generally feature a stirrup or caliper and plate attachment system to an external brace. Custom shoes are made for a specific patient. Generally, a code reports supply of a single shoe when sold as a single unit.

L3250

L3250   Orthopedic footwear, custom molded shoe, removable inner mold, prosthetic shoe, each

Lay Description
Report this code for each prosthetic shoe that is custom molded for a patient and has a removable inner mold and a custom fabricated insert designed for toe or distal partial foot amputation.

L3251

L3251   Foot, shoe molded to patient model, silicone shoe, each

Lay Description
This code is used to report a custom-fabricated shoe molded from a model of the patient that is lined with a silicone material. It is designed for sensitive feet and accommodates pressure areas. Casting and cast preparation is included.

L3252

L3252   Foot, shoe molded to patient model, Plastazote (or similar), custom fabricated, each

Lay Description
This is a custom fabricated shoe. It is molded from a model of the patient. The upper portion of the shoe is made of foam plastic or a similar material. It is designed to accommodate pressure areas. This code includes the casting and cast preparation.

L3253

L3253   Foot, molded shoe, Plastazote (or similar), custom fitted, each

Lay Description
This code is used to report a molded foam plastic (or like material) shoe, designed for temporary use. It is custom fitted and designed for sensitive feet and pressure areas.

L3254-L3255

L3254   Nonstandard size or width
L3255   Nonstandard size or length

Lay Description
These codes are used to report a shoe or shoes that are not a normal size or width or a shoe or shoes that are not a normal size or length.

L3257

L3257   Orthopedic footwear, additional charge for split size

Lay Description
This code is used to report an additional charge when the two orthopedic shoes for a patient are of different sizes (split shoes).

L3260

L3260   Surgical boot/shoe, each

Lay Description
A surgical boot or shoe is a special type of footwear, usually high-top style, designed to accommodate post-surgical wrappings and dressings and to allow the patient a degree of mobility. Ordinarily these boots are manufactured without left-foot or right-foot design considerations and are sold as single units.

L3265

L3265   Plastazote sandal, each

Lay Description
Plastazote is a type of closed cell polyethylene foam and this code reports supply of each Plastazote sandal. This type of footwear is often prescribed for patients who have undergone surgery of the toes or metatarsal area or who have problems in the forefoot zone. The sole of the sandal is manufactured from polyethylene foam to protect and cushion the plantar surface. Closures are usually Velcro strapping.

L3300-L3334

L3300   Lift, elevation, heel, tapered to metatarsals, per in

L3310   Lift, elevation, heel and sole, neoprene, per in

L3320   Lift, elevation, heel and sole, cork, per in

L3330   Lift, elevation, metal extension (skate)

L3332   Lift, elevation, inside shoe, tapered, up to one-half in

L3334   Lift, elevation, heel, per in

Lay Description
This range of codes reports lift modification to shoes. The codes are differentiated largely by type of material, style, and application in the shoe.

L3340-L3350

L3340   Heel wedge, SACH

L3350   Heel wedge

Lay Description
Heel wedges are modifications to shoes to lift medial or lateral aspects of the foot (pronation or supination) or otherwise address foot or posture problems. SACH is an acronym for solid ankle, cushioned heel.

L3360-L3370

L3360   Sole wedge, outside sole

L3370   Sole wedge, between sole

Lay Description
Heel wedges are modifications to shoes to lift medial or lateral aspects of the foot (pronation or supination) or otherwise address foot or posture problems.

L3380

L3380   Clubfoot wedge

Lay Description
This code reports a shoe modification wedge to address clubfoot. Talipes equinovarus is the Latin-based medical term for clubfoot. Equino is a reference to horse and varus means to "toe-in." Babies born with clubfoot exhibit extreme plantarflexion, which, as in horses, means weight is born on the extreme forefoot and toes. The feet are also characteristically turned inward. Talipes refers to the talus bone of the foot, which is not fully developed in clubfoot. Optimally, cases of clubfoot are aggressively addressed early in life. Shoe wedges may be of some benefit to those patients who still exhibit characteristics as children, teens, and adults. The wedge is usually fitted to fill the extreme arch of the foot seen in these patients.

L3390

L3390   Outflare wedge

Lay Description
An outflare wedge refers to a heel or sole that is extended and flared out from the shoe to provide greater efficiency in controlling pronation and supination of the ankle.

L3400

L3400   Metatarsal bar wedge, rocker

Lay Description
Bar wedges and rockers are used to transfer and alleviate pressure and improve the gait. Rocker soles assist in the burring of energy that forces the body forward after the center of gravity goes over the peak of the rocker. The rockers also assist in cases of limited range of motion with regards to the ankle or metatarsophalangeal joints. Rockers are created by adding extra crepe to the midsole portion of the shoe and then beveling it away just proximal to the point of pressure. There are different types of rockers, but they should all have a stable flat area at mid-stance. There are also many styles of rockers. There are also metatarsophalangeal bars that refer to specific shoe modifications. All metatarsophalangeal bars are to help metatarsalgia and relieve plantar pressure by adding a wedge of firm material across the sole of the shoe. By placing the bar to the metatarsophalangeal heads it unloads the pressure from the metatarsophalangeal heads, which allows transfer from the shafts of the metatarsals to the distal end of the toes.

L3410

L3410   Metatarsal bar wedge, between sole

Lay Description
This code is used to report a style of metatarsal bar that is placed between the sole layers.

L3420

L3420   Full sole and heel wedge, between sole

Lay Description
This refers to a wedge that is placed between sole layers over the full length of the shoe.

L3430-L3440

L3430   Heel, counter, plastic reinforced

L3440   Heel, counter, leather reinforced

Lay Description
These codes are used to report a firm plastic liner or a firm leather liner that reinforces the heel section of a shoe. These are permanently attached to a shoe.

L3450

L3450   Heel, SACH cushion type

Lay Description

This code is used to report a solid ankle cushion heel, also known as a SACH cushion heel. It is made of a softer durometer material that replaces a portion of the posterior heel base. SACH heels reduce shock at heel strike and compensate for the absence of ankle motion.

L3455-L3460

L3455   Heel, new leather, standard
L3460   Heel, new rubber, standard

Lay Description

These codes are used to report a conventional leather heel or a conventional rubber heel for shoes.

L3465-L3470

L3465   Heel, Thomas with wedge
L3470   Heel, Thomas extended to ball

Lay Description

These codes report modifications to a shoe heel known as the Thomas wedge. This is a bar applied to the exterior of the sole of the shoe posterior to the metatarsal heads. The bar is shaved at either end. The wedge provides pressure relief off the metatarsal heads, or ball of the foot.

L3480-L3485

L3480   Heel, pad and depression for spur
L3485   Heel, pad, removable for spur

Lay Description

Bone spurs often form on the bones of the feet, particularly on the calcaneus or heel bone. These spurs can be extremely painful, particularly as pressure is placed against them.

L3500

L3500   Orthopedic shoe addition, insole, leather

Lay Description

This code is used to report a full leather insole to an orthopedic shoe.

L3510

L3510   Orthopedic shoe addition, insole, rubber

Lay Description

This code is used to report a full rubber or similar material insole for an orthopedic shoe.

L3520

L3520   Orthopedic shoe addition, insole, felt covered with leather

Lay Description

This code is used to report a full-length lining made of felt and leather that is placed inside of an orthopedic shoe.

L3530-L3540

L3530   Orthopedic shoe addition, sole, half
L3540   Orthopedic shoe addition, sole, full

Lay Description

These codes are used to report an addition, repair, and/or modification to half of the sole or the complete sole of an orthopedic shoe.

L3550-L3560

L3550   Orthopedic shoe addition, toe tap, standard
L3560   Orthopedic shoe addition, toe tap, horseshoe

Lay Description

These codes are used to report a small metal insert, sometimes shaped like a horseshoe (L3560), secured to the sole (near the toe) of an orthopedic shoe to reduce wear.

L3570

L3570   Orthopedic shoe addition, special extension to instep (leather with eyelets)

Lay Description

This code is used to report an extension piece added to an existing lace area of an orthopedic shoe that allows a patient with an extremely high instep or deformity to tie his or her own shoes.

L3580

L3580   Orthopedic shoe addition, convert instep to Velcro closure

Lay Description

This code is used to report an addition to an orthopedic shoe that converts an instep of a shoe that has laces to an instep that has straps with Velcro, which is a hook/loop tape fastener. This is easier for donning and removing shoes.

L3590

L3590   Orthopedic shoe addition, convert firm shoe counter to soft counter

Lay Description

This code is used to report when a firm counter (the cup your heel fits into) of an orthopedic shoe is converted to a soft counter.

L3595

L3595   Orthopedic shoe addition, March bar

Lay Description

This code is used to report an external sole buildup to an orthopedic shoe that has an elevation placed behind the metatarsal heads to relieve pressure.

L3600-L3610

L3600 Transfer of an orthotic from one shoe to another, caliper plate, existing

L3610 Transfer of an orthotic from one shoe to another, caliper plate, new

Lay Description

These codes report the transfer or replacement of caliper plates from one shoe to another. The caliper plate is the footplate of an ankle foot orthosis (AFO) or knee ankle foot orthosis (KAFO). The plate features short, integrated medial and lateral uprights that connect to the upper portion of the AFO. The caliper plate is usually incorporated into a shoe, typically by cutting or splitting the sole. These plates are subject to some wear and occasionally need to be replaced. More commonly, though, the shoe becomes worn and the caliper plate is switched to a new shoe.

L3620-L3630

L3620 Transfer of an orthotic from one shoe to another, solid stirrup, existing

L3630 Transfer of an orthotic from one shoe to another, solid stirrup, new

Lay Description

These codes report the transfer or replacement of solid stirrups from one shoe to another. The solid stirrup is a particular design component of many ankle foot orthoses (AFO) or knee ankle foot orthoses (KAFO). Stirrups usually are attached directly to the shoe between the sole and heel, although the footplate inside the shoe occasionally is used. A solid stirrup reported by these codes integrates the upright with the footplate portion. A medial and lateral upright connects to the upper portion of the AFO. The stirrup may be subject to some wear and occasionally needs to be replaced. More commonly, though, the shoe becomes worn and the stirrup is switched to a new shoe.

L3640

L3640 Transfer of an orthotic from one shoe to another, Dennis Browne splint (Riveton), both shoes

Lay Description

This code reports the transfer of a specific type of orthosis from one shoe to another. The Denis Browne splint is named for the British pediatric surgeon who invented the device early in the last century. It is a static orthotic device used to treat babies and young children with congenital disorders such as hip dysplasia and congenital genu varus (toe-in). An abduction bar is attached to a special footplate of the patient's baby shoes. The bar and footplates fix the patient's feet and, therefore, the femoral heads into a therapeutic position. Adjustment on the footplate allows for positioning of the feet. In infancy, the splint may be left on for long periods. In toddlers, the splint may be used only at night and during nap times. As the patient grows, new shoes must be fitted. The

Denis Browne splint can be detached from the old pair of shoes and mounted to the new pair.

L3649

L3649 Orthopedic shoe, modification, addition or transfer, not otherwise specified

Lay Description

This code is used to report any orthopedic shoe modification or addition that has not been individually listed in previous HCPCS Level II codes.

L3650-L3660

L3650 Shoulder orthosis, figure of eight design abduction restrainer, prefabricated, off-the-shelf

L3660 Shoulder orthosis, figure of eight design abduction restrainer, canvas and webbing, prefabricated, off-the-shelf

Lay Description

A shoulder orthosis (SO) or shoulder immobilizer is a support device (usually not rigid or semirigid) used for sustaining injured, postsurgical, and/or weak or deformed areas of the shoulder girdle and for restricting or eliminating motion (immobilization). The benefits from orthotic and immobilizer use, specifically during convalescence from an injury (strain, chip fracture with strain, fracture) or illness or as a postoperative treatment measure can include the following: restricted range of motion of the affected area (immobilization), support of the affected area, and/or protection from injury, reinjury, suture tearing, and/or wound dehiscence. Some of the devices support the shoulder while limiting most ranges of motion, particularly abduction, which is the movement that raises the arm. All of these items usually require the assistance of a person other than the patient for appropriate application. Most of these items can be adjusted to fit the patient and come in a variety of sizes.

L3670-L3678

L3670 Shoulder orthosis, acromio/clavicular (canvas and webbing type), prefabricated, off-the-shelf

L3671 Shoulder orthotic (SO), shoulder joint design, without joints, may include soft interface, straps, custom fabricated, includes fitting and adjustment

L3674 Shoulder orthotic, abduction positioning (airplane design), thoracic component and support bar, with or without nontorsion joint/turnbuckle, may include soft interface, straps, custom fabricated, includes fitting and adjustment

L3675 Shoulder orthosis, vest type abduction restrainer, canvas webbing type or equal, prefabricated, off-the-shelf

L3677 Shoulder orthosis, shoulder joint design, without joints, may include soft interface, straps, prefabricated item that has been trimmed, bent, molded, assembled, or otherwise customized to fit a specific patient by an individual with expertise

L3678 Shoulder orthosis, shoulder joint design, without joints, may include soft interface, straps, prefabricated, off-the-shelf

Lay Description

A shoulder orthosis (SO) or shoulder immobilizer is a support device (usually not rigid or semirigid) used for sustaining injured, postsurgical, and/or weak or deformed areas of the shoulder girdle and for restricting or eliminating motion (immobilization). The benefits from orthotic and immobilizer use, specifically during convalescence from an injury (strain, chip fracture with strain, fracture) or illness or as a postoperative treatment measure, can include the following: restriction of the range of motion of the affected area (immobilization); support of the affected area; and/or protection from injury, reinjury, suture tearing, and/or wound dehiscence. Some of the devices support the shoulder while limiting most ranges of motion, particularly abduction, which is the movement that raises the arm. All of these items usually require the assistance of a person other than the patient for appropriate application. Most of these items can be adjusted to fit the patient and come in a variety of sizes.

L3702

L3702 Elbow orthotic (EO), without joints, may include soft interface, straps, custom fabricated, includes fitting and adjustment

Lay Description

This code is used to report a static/rigid elbow orthotic that is custom fabricated and may have a soft interface. It is used particularly for elbow immobilization in patients who have had recent elbow surgery and/or inflammation.

L3710

L3710 Elbow orthosis, elastic with metal joints, prefabricated, off-the-shelf

Lay Description

This code reports supply of a simple, prefabricated elastic elbow orthotic with metal joints. The device is prefabricated, which means the orthotist selects from mass produced products based on the size of the patient and fits the device accordingly. These devices may be neoprene or Lycra sleeves pulled over the elbow or wrapped around the elbow and closed with Velcro straps. Incorporated into the fabric of the orthosis are rigid, jointed bars, typically on the medial and lateral sides.

L3720

L3720 Elbow orthotic (EO), double upright with forearm/arm cuffs, free motion, custom fabricated

Lay Description

This code is used to report a custom fitted elbow orthotic designed to provide control of the elbow joint. It consists of upper and lower arm sections made of plastic or leather and bilateral unicentric free motion joints.

L3730

L3730 Elbow orthotic (EO), double upright with forearm/arm cuffs, extension/ flexion assist, custom fabricated

Lay Description

This code is used to report a custom fabricated elbow orthotic that provides control of the elbow and flexion or extension support. It consists of upper and lower arm sections made of plastic or leather, bilateral unicentric free motion joints, and a unilateral spring device at a joint.

L3740

L3740 Elbow orthotic (EO), double upright with forearm/arm cuffs, adjustable position lock with active control, custom fabricated

Lay Description

This code is used to report a custom fabricated elbow orthotic designed to provide control and function to a weak elbow. It consists of upper and lower arm sections made of plastic or leather, bilateral unicentric joints (one of which is lockable at various levels of flexion), and a shoulder harness assembly with a cable used to operate the elbow lock.

L3760

L3760 Elbow orthotic (EO), with adjustable position locking joint(s), prefabricated, includes fitting and adjustments, any type

Lay Description

This code is used to report a custom fitted elbow orthosis that is designed to control the elbow. It consists of upper and lower arm sections and has adjustable locking joints.

L3762

L3762 Elbow orthosis, rigid, without joints, includes soft interface material, prefabricated, off-the-shelf

Lay Description

This code reports the supply of a prefabricated, rigid elbow orthosis. In certain instances the elbow must be immobilized as completely as possible, such as following trauma or during recovery from a surgery of the joint capsule. This type of orthosis acts much like a cast in that the joint is locked in position, usually in several degrees of flexion. The brace is rigid and includes cushion material between the hard structure and the patient's skin. The device is prefabricated, which means the orthotist selects from mass produced products based on the size of the patient and fits the device accordingly.

L3763-L3766

L3763 Elbow-wrist-hand orthotic (EWHO), rigid, without joints, may include soft interface, straps, custom fabricated, includes fitting and adjustment

L3764 Elbow-wrist-hand orthotic (EWHO), includes one or more nontorsion joints, elastic bands, turnbuckles, may include soft interface, straps, custom fabricated, includes fitting and adjustment

L3765 Elbow-wrist-hand-finger orthotic (EWHFO), rigid, without joints, may include soft interface, straps, custom fabricated, includes fitting and adjustment

L3766 Elbow-wrist-hand-finger orthotic (EWHFO), includes one or more nontorsion joints, elastic bands, turnbuckles, may include soft interface, straps, custom fabricated, includes fitting and adjustment

Lay Description
Fracture orthoses may be similar in design, depending on the manufacturer and the intended application. These are bracing devices, typically containing hardware such as aluminum or other lightweight arm supports for the desired degree of abduction, as well as plastic, polyethylene, or foam. These devices may use the patient torso or neck as an anchor, as well as the phalanges. There may be hinges at certain points in the device to allow for a certain degree of elbow or wrist motion. The treating provider must initially apply these items, but a person other than the patient can be instructed in the proper application when/if the patient removes the device during specified intervals. Sizes can vary according to the manufacturer (there may be pediatric sizes as well). The items are generally manufactured in right and left models. Shoulder braces with arm, elbow, and wrist immobilization support and control the range of motion of the upper extremity, including the upper arm, scapula, clavicle, elbow, forearm, and/or wrist. They also support most muscles and ligamentous tissues related to the movement of the upper extremity. They maintain a degree of abduction between the patient's torso and the affected upper limb, at the degree desired (usually 45-90 degrees). Each of these devices typically leaves the fingers free, but grasping heavy items is usually unable to be accomplished and is not advised. They are used posttraumatically for severe fractures.

L3806-L3809, L3900-L3935

L3806 Wrist-hand-finger orthotic (WHFO), includes one or more nontorsion joint(s), turnbuckles, elastic bands/springs, may include soft interface material, straps, custom fabricated, includes fitting and adjustment

L3807 Wrist hand finger orthosis, without joint(s), prefabricated item that has been trimmed, bent, molded, assembled, or otherwise customized to fit a specific patient by an individual with expertise

L3808 Wrist-hand-finger orthotic (WHFO), rigid without joints, may include soft interface material; straps, custom fabricated, includes fitting and adjustment

L3809 Wrist hand finger orthosis, without joint(s), prefabricated, off-the-shelf, any type

L3900 Wrist-hand-finger orthotic (WHFO), dynamic flexor hinge, reciprocal wrist extension/ flexion, finger flexion/extension, wrist or finger driven, custom fabricated

L3901 Wrist-hand-finger orthotic (WHFO), dynamic flexor hinge, reciprocal wrist extension/ flexion, finger flexion/extension, cable driven, custom fabricated

L3904 Wrist-hand-finger orthotic (WHFO), external powered, electric, custom fabricated

L3905 Wrist-hand orthotic (WHO), includes one or more nontorsion joints, elastic bands, turnbuckles, may include soft interface, straps, custom fabricated, includes fitting and adjustment

L3906 Wrist-hand orthosis (WHO), without joints, may include soft interface, straps, custom fabricated, includes fitting and adjustment

L3908 Wrist hand orthosis, wrist extension control cock-up, non molded, prefabricated, off-the-shelf

L3912 Hand finger orthosis (HFO), flexion glove with elastic finger control, prefabricated, off-the-shelf

L3913 Hand finger orthotic (HFO), without joints, may include soft interface, straps, custom fabricated, includes fitting and adjustment

L3915 Wrist hand orthosis, includes one or more nontorsion joint(s), elastic bands, turnbuckles, may include soft interface, straps, prefabricated item that has been trimmed, bent, molded, assembled, or otherwise customized to fit a specific patient by an individual with expertise

L3916 Wrist hand orthosis, includes one or more nontorsion joint(s), elastic bands, turnbuckles, may include soft interface, straps, prefabricated, off-the-shelf

L3917 Hand orthosis, metacarpal fracture orthosis, prefabricated item that has been trimmed, bent, molded, assembled, or otherwise customized to fit a specific patient by an individual with expertise

L3918 Hand orthosis, metacarpal fracture orthosis, prefabricated, off-the-shelf

L3919 Hand orthotic (HO), without joints, may include soft interface, straps, custom fabricated, includes fitting and adjustment

L3921 Hand finger orthotic (HFO), includes one or more nontorsion joints, elastic bands, turnbuckles, may include soft interface, straps, custom fabricated, includes fitting and adjustment

L3923 Hand finger orthosis, without joints, may include soft interface, straps, prefabricated item that has been trimmed, bent, molded, assembled, or otherwise customized to fit a specific patient by an individual with expertise

L3924 Hand finger orthosis, without joints, may include soft interface, straps, prefabricated, off-the-shelf

L3925 Finger orthosis, proximal interphalangeal (PIP)/distal interphalangeal (DIP), non-torsion joint/spring, extension/flexion, may include soft interface material, prefabricated, off-the-shelf

L3927 Finger orthosis, proximal interphalangeal (PIP)/distal interphalangeal (DIP), without joint/spring, extension/flexion (e.g., static or ring type), may include soft interface material, prefabricated, off-the-shelf

L3929 Hand finger orthosis, includes one or more nontorsion joint(s), turnbuckles, elastic bands/springs, may include soft interface material, straps, prefabricated item that has been trimmed, bent, molded, assembled, or otherwise customized to fit a specific patient by an individual with expertise

L3930 Hand finger orthosis, includes one or more nontorsion joint(s), turnbuckles, elastic bands/springs, may include soft interface material, straps, prefabricated, off-the-shelf

L3931 Wrist-hand-finger orthotic (WHFO), includes one or more nontorsion joint(s), turnbuckles, elastic bands/springs, may include soft interface material, straps, prefabricated, includes fitting and adjustment

L3933 Finger orthotic (FO), without joints, may include soft interface, custom fabricated, includes fitting and adjustment

L3935 Finger orthotic, nontorsion joint, may include soft interface, custom fabricated, includes fitting and adjustment

Lay Description
A wrist-hand-finger orthosis (WHFO) is typically a rigid or semirigid device used for the purpose of supporting injured, post-surgical, and/or weak or deformed areas of the wrist, hand, and metacarpal regions (phalanges are usually freely mobile with these types of devices) and for restricting or eliminating motion (immobilization) of the affected structure. While orthoses are usually prefabricated (custom fitted) or custom fabricated, these types of orthoses are generally not customized. Many of these items appear as sleeves or stockinette types of items. The benefits from WHFO use, specifically during convalescence from an injury or illness or as a postoperative treatment measure, can include the following: restricted range of motion of the affected area (immobilization); support of the affected area; and/or protection from injury, reinjury, suture tearing, and/or wound dehiscence.

L3891

L3891 Addition to upper extremity joint, wrist or elbow, concentric adjustable torsion style mechanism for custom fabricated orthotics only, each

Lay Description
This code describes concentric adjustable torsion style mechanisms used for the upper extremity joint, wrist or elbow, for custom fabricated orthotics only. Each component is used to describe the removable components used with custom orthotics. These components incorporate adjustable and removable dynamic power assist. The power assist add-on component is mounted to a conventionally functioning wrist or elbow within a custom orthotic and they add the prescribed function to dynamic assist/resist as required. These additions are used to improve reach, grasp, and pinching functions.

L3956

L3956 Addition of joint to upper extremity orthotic, any material; per joint

Lay Description
This code is used to report the incorporation of a joint into an upper extremity orthosis where the base code does not include an articulation.

L3960-L3962

L3960 Shoulder-elbow-wrist-hand orthotic (SEWHO), abduction positioning, airplane design, prefabricated, includes fitting and adjustment

L3961 Shoulder elbow wrist hand orthotic (SEWHO), shoulder cap design, without joints, may include soft interface, straps, custom fabricated, includes fitting and adjustment

L3962 Shoulder-elbow-wrist-hand orthotic (SEWHO), abduction positioning, Erb's palsy design, prefabricated, includes fitting and adjustment

Lay Description

A shoulder-elbow-wrist-hand orthosis (SEWHO) is used for the purpose of supporting injured, post-surgical, and/or weak or deformed areas of the shoulder, elbow, wrist, or hand. These codes may be similar in design, depending on the manufacturer and the intended application. These are bracing devices used on wheelchairs, typically containing hardware such as aluminum or other lightweight arm supports for the desired degree of abduction, as well as plastic, polyethylene, or foam. These devices may use the patient torso or neck as an anchor as well as the phalanges. There may be hinges at certain points in the device to allow for a certain degree of elbow or wrist motion. The treating provider must initially apply these items, but a person other than the patient can be instructed in the proper application when/if the patient removes the device during specified intervals. Sizes can vary according to the manufacturer (there may be pediatric sizes as well). The items are generally manufactured in right and left models. Shoulder braces, with arm, elbow, and wrist immobilization, support and control the range of motion of the upper extremity, including the upper arm, scapula, clavicle, elbow, forearm, and/or wrist. They also support most muscles and ligamentous tissues related to the movement of the upper extremity. They maintain a degree of abduction between the patient's torso and the affected upper limb, at the degree desired (usually 45-90 degrees). Each of these devices will typically leave the fingers free, but grasping heavy items is usually unable to be accomplished and is not advised. They are used post-traumatically for severe fractures and for certain types of surgical procedures, such as partial or total shoulder replacement. A prefabricated or custom fitted orthosis is one that the manufacturer has produced in quantity, without a specific patient in mind. A prefabricated orthosis may be trimmed, bent, molded (with or without heat), or otherwise modified for use by a specific patient (i.e., custom fitted). An orthosis that is assembled from prefabricated components is considered prefabricated. Any orthosis that does not meet the definition of a custom fabricated orthosis is considered prefabricated. A custom fabricated orthosis is one that is individually made for a specific patient, starting with basic materials including, but not limited to, plastic, metal, leather, or cloth in the form of sheets, bars, and so forth. It involves substantial work, such as cutting, bending, molding, sewing, and so forth. It may involve the incorporation of some prefabricated components. It involves more than trimming, bending, or making other modifications to a substantially prefabricated item. A molded-to-patient-model orthosis is a particular type of custom fabricated orthosis in which an impression of the specific body part is made (by means of a plaster cast, CAD-CAM technology, etc.).

L3967-L3978

L3967 Shoulder-elbow-wrist-hand orthotic (SEWHO), abduction positioning (airplane design), thoracic component and support bar, without joints, may include soft interface, straps, custom fabricated, includes fitting and adjustment

L3971 Shoulder-elbow-wrist-hand orthotic (SEWHO), shoulder cap design, includes one or more nontorsion joints, elastic bands, turnbuckles, may include soft interface, straps, custom fabricated, includes fitting and adjustment

L3973 Shoulder-elbow-wrist-hand orthotic (SEWHO), abduction positioning (airplane design), thoracic component and support bar, includes one or more nontorsion joints, elastic bands, turnbuckles, may include soft interface, straps, custom fabricated, includes fitting and adjustment

L3975 Shoulder-elbow-wrist-hand-finger orthotic (SEWHO), shoulder cap design, without joints, may include soft interface, straps, custom fabricated, includes fitting and adjustment

L3976 Shoulder-elbow-wrist-hand-finger orthotic (SEWHO), abduction positioning (airplane design), thoracic component and support bar, without joints, may include soft interface, straps, custom fabricated, includes fitting and adjustment

L3977 Shoulder-elbow-wrist-hand-finger orthotic (SEWHO), shoulder cap design, includes one or more nontorsion joints, elastic bands, turnbuckles, may include soft interface, straps, custom fabricated, includes fitting and adjustment

L3978 Shoulder-elbow-wrist-hand-finger orthotic (SEWHO), abduction positioning (airplane design), thoracic component and support bar, includes one or more nontorsion joints, elastic bands, turnbuckles, may include soft interface, straps, custom fabricated, includes fitting and adjustment

Lay Description

A shoulder-elbow-wrist-hand orthosis (SEWHO) is used for the purpose of supporting injured, post-surgical, and/or weak or deformed areas of the shoulder, elbow, wrist, or hand. These codes may be similar in design, depending on the manufacturer and the intended application. These are bracing devices attached to wheelchairs, typically containing hardware such as aluminum or other lightweight arm supports for the desired degree of abduction, as well as plastic, polyethylene, or foam. These devices may use the patient torso or neck as an anchor, as well as the phalanges. There may be hinges at certain points in the device to allow for a certain degree of elbow or wrist motion. The treating provider must initially apply these items, but a person other than the patient can be instructed in the proper application when/if the patient removes the device during specified intervals. Sizes can vary according to the manufacturer (there may be pediatric sizes as well). The items are generally manufactured in right and left models. Shoulder braces with arm, elbow, and wrist immobilization support and control the range of motion of the upper extremity, including the upper arm, scapula, clavicle, elbow, forearm, and/or wrist. They also support most muscles and ligamentous tissues related to the movement of the upper extremity. They maintain a degree of abduction between the patient's torso and the affected upper limb, at the degree desired (usually 45-90 degrees). Each of these devices typically leaves the fingers free, but grasping heavy items is usually unable to be accomplished and is not advised. They are used posttraumatically for severe fractures and for certain types of surgical procedures, such as partial or total shoulder replacement. A prefabricated or custom fitted orthosis is one that the manufacturer has produced in quantity, without a specific patient in mind. A prefabricated orthosis may be trimmed, bent, molded (with or without heat), or otherwise modified for use by a specific patient (i.e., custom fitted). An orthosis that is assembled from prefabricated components is considered prefabricated. Any orthosis that does not meet the definition of a custom fabricated orthosis is considered prefabricated. A custom fabricated orthosis is one that is individually made for a specific patient, starting with basic materials including, but not limited to, plastic, metal, leather, or cloth in the form of sheets, bars, and so forth. It involves substantial work, such as cutting, bending, molding, sewing, and so forth. It may involve the incorporation of some prefabricated components. It involves more than trimming, bending, or making other modifications to a substantially prefabricated item. A molded-to-patient-model orthosis is a particular type of custom fabricated orthosis in which an impression of the specific body part is made (by means of a plaster cast, CAD-CAM technology, etc.). These codes describe shoulder-elbow-wrist-hand orthoses that are supports attached to a wheelchair.

L3980-L3984

L3980 Upper extremity fracture orthotic, humeral, prefabricated, includes fitting and adjustment

L3982 Upper extremity fracture orthotic, radius/ulnar, prefabricated, includes fitting and adjustment

L3984 Upper extremity fracture orthotic, wrist, prefabricated, includes fitting and adjustment

Lay Description

Fracture orthoses may be similar in design, depending on the manufacturer and the intended application. These are bracing devices, typically containing hardware such as aluminum or other lightweight arm supports for the desired degree of abduction, as well as plastic, polyethylene, or foam. These devices may use the patient torso or neck as an anchor as well as the phalanges. There may be hinges at certain points in the device to allow for a certain degree of elbow or wrist motion. The treating provider must initially apply these items, but a person other than the patient can be instructed in the proper application when/if the patient removes the device during specified intervals. Sizes can vary according to the manufacturer (there may be pediatric sizes as well). The items are generally manufactured in right and left models. Shoulder braces, with arm, elbow, and wrist immobilization, support and control the range of motion of the upper extremity, including the upper arm, scapula, clavicle, elbow, forearm, and/or wrist. They also support most muscles and ligamentous tissues related to the movement of the upper extremity. They maintain a degree of abduction between the patient's torso and the affected upper limb, at the degree desired (usually 45-90 degrees). Each of these devices will typically leave the fingers free, but grasping heavy items is usually unable to be accomplished and is not advised. They are used post-traumatically for severe fractures. A prefabricated or custom fitted orthosis is one that the manufacturer has produced in quantity, without a specific patient in mind. A prefabricated orthosis may be trimmed, bent, molded (with or without heat), or otherwise modified for use by a specific patient (i.e., custom fitted). An orthosis that is assembled from prefabricated components is considered prefabricated. Any orthosis that does not meet the definition of a custom fabricated orthosis is considered prefabricated. A custom fabricated orthosis is one that is individually made for a specific patient, starting with basic materials including, but not limited to, plastic, metal, leather, or cloth in the form of sheets, bars, and so forth. It involves substantial work, such as cutting, bending, molding, sewing, and so forth. It may involve the incorporation of some prefabricated components. It involves more than trimming, bending, or making other modifications to a substantially prefabricated item. A molded-to-patient-model orthosis is a particular type of custom fabricated orthosis in which an impression of the specific body part is made (by means of a plaster cast, CAD-CAM technology, etc.).

L3995

L3995 **Addition to upper extremity orthotic, sock, fracture or equal, each**

Lay Description
This code is used to report an addition to an upper extremity fracture orthosis. It consists of a special sock that is used as an interface between the arm and the orthosis.

L3999

L3999 **Upper limb orthotic, not otherwise specified**

Lay Description
This code is used to report an upper limb orthosis not specified in previous HCPCS Level II codes. Upper extremity orthoses are devices applied externally to restore or improve functional and structural characteristics of the musculoskeletal and nervous systems.

L4000

L4000 **Replace girdle for spinal orthotic (cervical-thoracic-lumbar-sacral orthotic (CTLSO) or spinal orthotic SO)**

Lay Description
This code is used to report replacement of a molded plastic or leather pelvic girdle for a spinal orthosis. It is custom fabricated from a model of the patient and includes casting and cast preparation.

L4002

L4002 **Replacement strap, any orthotic, includes all components, any length, any type**

Lay Description
This code is used to report replacement of a dysfunctional strap on an orthosis and includes all attachment components.

L4010-L4030

L4010 **Replace trilateral socket brim**

L4020 **Replace quadrilateral socket brim, molded to patient model**

L4030 **Replace quadrilateral socket brim, custom fitted**

Lay Description
These codes are used to report replacement of a molded plastic ischial weight bearing socket of trilateral (L4010) or quadrilateral design for a knee-ankle-foot orthotic (KAFO). The quadrilateral design can be custom fabricated from a model of a patient (L4020) and/or custom fitted (L4030). Casting and cast preparation are included.

L4040-L4055

L4040 **Replace molded thigh lacer, for custom fabricated orthotic only**

L4045 **Replace nonmolded thigh lacer, for custom fabricated orthotic only**

L4050 **Replace molded calf lacer, for custom fabricated orthotic only**

L4055 **Replace nonmolded calf lacer, for custom fabricated orthotic only**

Lay Description
These codes report the replacement of molded lacers. Lacers are cuff-like devices that fit around a portion of a limb. They have a slit opening on one side to don the device and a lace-string corset-style closure of gussets and eyelets. Often they are of thermoplastic material with cushion liners built from patient molds, but many are still manufactured of leather, or have leather incorporated into the design. An orthotic device may attach to this device. Many are used for suspension of a prosthetic attachment.

L4060-L4130

L4060 **Replace high roll cuff**

L4070 **Replace proximal and distal upright for KAFO**

L4080 **Replace metal bands KAFO, proximal thigh**

L4090 **Replace metal bands KAFO-AFO, calf or distal thigh**

L4100 **Replace leather cuff KAFO, proximal thigh**

L4110 **Replace leather cuff KAFO-AFO, calf or distal thigh**

L4130 **Replace pretibial shell**

Lay Description
These codes are used to report replacements/repairs of any dysfunctional pieces to various parts of a knee-ankle-foot orthotic (KAFO) and/or ankle-foot orthotic (AFO).

L4205

L4205 **Repair of orthotic device, labor component, per 15 minutes**

Lay Description
This code is used for the labor component of repair of a previously provided orthosis except for any labor involved in the replacement of an orthotic component that has a specific L code. Report the time in 15-minute increments.

L4210

L4210 **Repair of orthotic device, repair or replace minor parts**

Lay Description
This code is used to report the replacement or repair of any minor parts on any type of orthosis.

L4350

L4350 Ankle control orthosis, stirrup style, rigid, includes any type interface (e.g., pneumatic, gel), prefabricated, off-the-shelf

Lay Description
This code is used to report a prefabricated ankle brace support comprised of a stirrup that goes under the foot with pads on both sides, which are wrapped around the ankle. Rigid brace shells fit the ankle comfortably and provide the needed medial/lateral stabilization.

L4360-L4361

L4360 Walking boot, pneumatic and/or vacuum, with or without joints, with or without interface material, prefabricated item that has been trimmed, bent, molded, assembled, or otherwise customized to fit a specific patient by an individual with expertise

L4361 Walking boot, pneumatic and/or vacuum, with or without joints, with or without interface material, prefabricated, off-the-shelf

Lay Description
This code is used to report a boot-shaped brace for an injured foot. It is a lightweight, rigid knee-length boot with a reinforced sole and other supporting devices embedded in the plaster to facilitate walking. This device has compressing air in chambers between the rigid outer shell and the patient's leg.

L4370

L4370 Pneumatic full leg splint, prefabricated, off-the-shelf

Lay Description
This code reports the supply of pneumatic splints or air splints. These devices immobilize the limb by compressing air in chambers between the rigid outer shell and the patient's leg. These orthoses are used commonly in first response situations to trauma. But some models may be prescribed for more extended use to support the knee joint. The devices reported by these codes are prefabricated and may require fitting and adjustment sessions to suit individual patient needs. Typically, the chambers are inflated by a hand pump or electric pump until the desired level of pressure against the limb is attained.

L4386-L4387

L4386 Walking boot, non-pneumatic, with or without joints, with or without interface material, prefabricated item that has been trimmed, bent, molded, assembled, or otherwise customized to fit a specific patient by an individual with expertise

L4387 Walking boot, non-pneumatic, with or without joints, with or without interface material, prefabricated, off-the-shelf

Lay Description
This code is used to report a boot-shaped brace for an injured foot. It is a lightweight, rigid knee-length boot with a reinforced sole and other supporting devices embedded in the plaster to facilitate walking. It is prefabricated and includes fitting and adjustment.

L4392-L4394

L4392 Replacement, soft interface material, static AFO

L4394 Replace soft interface material, foot drop splint

Lay Description
These codes represent replacements of softer interface materials for static ankle foot orthotics and foot drop splints. Ankle flexion contracture is a condition in which there is shortening of the muscles and/or tendons that plantarflex the ankle with the resulting inability to bring the ankle to 0 degrees by passive range of motion (0 degrees ankle position is when the foot is perpendicular to the lower leg). "Foot drop" is a condition in which there is weakness and/or lack of use of the muscles that dorsiflex the ankle, but there is the ability to bring the ankle to 0 degrees by passive range of motion. A foot drop splint/recumbent positioning device is a prefabricated ankle-foot orthosis, with a soft interface, that has all of the following characteristics: designed to maintain the foot at a fixed position of 0 degrees (i.e., perpendicular to the lower leg), not designed to accommodate an ankle with a plantar flexion contracture, and used by a patient who is nonambulatory.

L4396-L4397

L4396 Static or dynamic ankle foot orthosis, including soft interface material, adjustable for fit, for positioning, may be used for minimal ambulation, prefabricated item that has been trimmed, bent, molded, assembled, or otherwise customized to fit a specific patient by an individual with expertise

L4397 Static or dynamic ankle foot orthosis, including soft interface material, adjustable for fit, for positioning, may be used for minimal ambulation, prefabricated, off-the-shelf

Lay Description
A static ankle foot orthosis (AFO) is a prefabricated AFO that may be adjustable for fit and positioning and is designed to accommodate an ankle with a plantar flexion contracture up to 45 degrees. It applies a dorsiflexion force to the ankle, allows pressure reduction, is used by a patient who is minimally ambulatory or nonambulatory, and has a soft

interface. AFOs extend well above the ankle (usually to near the top of the calf) and are fastened around the lower leg above the ankle. A dynamic AFO allows a more gradual stretch, and allows the patient to progress as tolerance is increased. The low-load stretching also allows the patient to maintain gains in range of motion. The dynamic AFO has an adjustable cord and articulating dorsal shell that assists in controlling the degree of stretch, while at the same time allowing for an adjustment of the cord's tension. This code includes the fitting, adjustment, and supply of a static or dynamic ankle foot orthosis.

L4398

L4398   Foot drop splint, recumbent positioning device, prefabricated, off-the-shelf

Lay Description
A foot drop splint/recumbent positioning device is a prefabricated ankle-foot orthosis that is designed to maintain the foot at a fixed position of 0 degrees (i.e., perpendicular to the lower leg), but not designed to accommodate an ankle with a plantar flexion contracture. The foot drop splint is used by a patient who is nonambulatory and has a soft interface. This code includes the fitting and adjustment as well as the supply of the static ankle foot orthosis.

L4631

L4631   Ankle-foot orthotic, walking boot type, varus/valgus correction, rocker bottom, anterior tibial shell, soft interface, custom arch support, plastic or other material, includes straps and closures, custom fabricated

Lay Description
This code is used to report an ankle-foot orthotic (AFO) intended to protect the affected ankle/foot from further damage by replacing the shoe with a device suitable for ambulation. This AFO includes a metal "rocker" to the sole of the plastic form to reduce plantar pressures during gait and a varus/valgus correction wedging lift. It is custom fabricated and includes straps and closures.

L5000-L5020

L5000   Partial foot, shoe insert with longitudinal arch, toe filler
L5010   Partial foot, molded socket, ankle height, with toe filler
L5020   Partial foot, molded socket, tibial tubercle height, with toe filler

Lay Description
These codes report the supply of partial foot orthoses. Partial amputations of the foot often entail disarticulation of the forefoot (phalanges and metatarsals), leaving the heel (calcaneus) intact. Prosthesis preparation for partial foot amputations is complicated by several factors, including socket fitting to the foot remnant and filler material for the

amputation. Typically, a toe filler is prepared from artificial materials to resemble the size and shape of the missing toes and metatarsal pad. This is designed to fit into a conventional shoe. Based on moldings or castings taken before amputation, a flexible sleeve is custom fabricated from rubber or other material with elastic properties. The fore end is designed to attach to the toe filler. The proximal end may be fitted with a zipper that closes up the back of the ankle in the general area over the Achilles tendon. This design is usually fitted up to the tibial tubercle, the bony prominence at the ankle. Other designs simply fit over the residual foot/ankle by elastic compression. A molded socket is the interface between the residual foot/ankle and the toe filler. The prosthesis is designed to fit into a conventional or orthotic shoe.

L5050-L5060

L5050   Ankle, Symes, molded socket, SACH foot
L5060   Ankle, Symes, metal frame, molded leather socket, articulated ankle/foot

Lay Description
These codes report the supply of specific prostheses for Symes-type amputations. The Symes amputation is a disarticulation at the ankle joint with preservation of the fatty heel pad, which is rotated over the distal closure. The heel pad becomes the most distal part of the residual limb and an interface for a prosthesis. Based on moldings or castings taken before or after amputation, a flexible sleeve is custom fabricated from rubber or other material with elastic properties. This constitutes the molded socket that interfaces between the residual ankle and the prosthetic foot. A solid ankle, cushioned heel (SACH) foot prosthesis is a basic passive device.

L5100-L5105

L5100   Below knee, molded socket, shin, SACH foot
L5105   Below knee, plastic socket, joints and thigh lacer, SACH foot

Lay Description
These codes report the supply of specific prostheses for below-the-knee amputations. Based on moldings or castings taken before or after amputation, a flexible sleeve is custom fabricated from rubber or other material with elastic properties. This constitutes the molded socket that interfaces between the residual limb and the prosthesis that attaches to it. Plastic sockets are typically custom fabricated, sometimes from thermoplastic materials that are molded and shaped as heat is applied. A thigh lacer is a cuff-like device that fits around that portion of the residual limb. It has a slit opening on the front side to don the device and a lace-string corset-style closure of gussets and eyelets. Often lacers are of thermoplastic material with cushion liners built from patient molds, but many are still manufactured of leather, or have leather incorporated into the design. The thigh lacer supports and suspends the below-the-knee prosthesis from

above. A solid ankle, cushioned heel (SACH) foot prosthesis is a basic passive device.

L5150-L5160

L5150 Knee disarticulation (or through knee), molded socket, external knee joints, shin, SACH foot

L5160 Knee disarticulation (or through knee), molded socket, bent knee configuration, external knee joints, shin, SACH foot

Lay Description
These codes report the supply of specific prostheses for knee disarticulation (or through knee) amputations. A flexible sleeve is custom fabricated from rubber or other material with elastic properties based on moldings or castings taken before or after amputation. This constitutes the molded socket that interfaces between the residual limb and the prosthesis that attaches to it. Plastic sockets are typically custom fabricated, sometimes from thermoplastic materials that are molded and shaped as heat is applied. Knee disarticulation results in an excellent weight-bearing stump.

L5200-L5230

L5200 Above knee, molded socket, single axis constant friction knee, shin, SACH foot

L5210 Above knee, short prosthesis, no knee joint (stubbies), with foot blocks, no ankle joints, each

L5220 Above knee, short prosthesis, no knee joint (stubbies), with articulated ankle/foot, dynamically aligned, each

L5230 Above knee, for proximal femoral focal deficiency, constant friction knee, shin, SACH foot

Lay Description
These codes are used to report the supply of a specific above-the-knee prosthetic system. Based on moldings or castings taken before or after amputation, a flexible sleeve is custom fabricated from rubber or other material with elastic properties. This constitutes the molded socket that interfaces between the residual limb and the prosthetic system that attaches to it. Plastic sockets may be custom fabricated from moldings as well, sometimes from thermoplastic materials that are molded and shaped as heat is applied. A single-axis friction knee is a prosthetic component to replace the knee joint. This type of joint is among the oldest designs and consists of a simple axle connecting the thigh and shank segments. The joint is capable of flexion and extension, but cannot bear the user's weight unless locked in an extended position. Constant friction is applied to the joint hinge to keep it from swinging too freely, particularly in gait. A solid ankle, cushioned heel (SACH) foot prosthesis is a basic passive device. These prostheses are considered inexpensive and simple to manufacture.

L5250-L5270

L5250 Hip disarticulation, Canadian type; molded socket, hip joint, single axis constant friction knee, shin, SACH foot

L5270 Hip disarticulation, tilt table type; molded socket, locking hip joint, single axis constant friction knee, shin, SACH foot

Lay Description
These codes report the supply of prostheses for patients who have had hip disarticulation amputations (removal of the entire leg at the juncture of the hip socket and femoral head). The Canadian type prosthesis consists of a plastic waistband at the trunk line of the iliac crests. Any residual stump may also be utilized for prosthesis attachment and a molded plastic socket encloses the ischial tuberosity to bear weight. The artificial hip joint is toward the anterior of the prosthesis and is unlocked, as is the knee joint. The "tilt table" type prosthesis refers to a specific device that takes the patient's weight off the fresh incisions during early rehabilitation following disarticulation. Based on moldings or castings taken before or after amputation, a flexible sleeve is custom fabricated from rubber or other material with elastic properties. This constitutes the molded socket that interfaces between the residual limb and the prosthetic system that attaches to it. Plastic sockets may be custom fabricated from moldings as well, sometimes from thermoplastic materials that are molded and shaped as heat is applied. A single-axis friction knee is a prosthetic component to replace the knee joint. This type of joint is among the oldest designs and consists of a simple axle connecting the thigh and shank segments. The joint is capable of flexion and extension, but cannot bear the user's weight unless locked in an extended position. Constant friction is applied to the joint hinge to keep it from swinging too freely, particularly in gait. A solid ankle, cushioned heel (SACH) foot prosthesis is a basic passive device. The knee and foot components are considered inexpensive and simple to manufacture.

L5280

L5280 Hemipelvectomy, Canadian type; molded socket, hip joint, single axis constant friction knee, shin, SACH foot

Lay Description
This code is used to report a Canadian type prosthesis that consists of a plastic waistband at the trunk line of the iliac crests. Any residual stump may also be utilized for prosthesis attachment and a molded plastic socket encloses the ischial tuberosity to bear weight. The artificial hip joint is toward the anterior of the prosthesis and is unlocked, as is the knee joint. A single-axis friction knee is a prosthetic component to replace the knee joint and consists of a simple axle connecting the thigh and shank segments. The joint is capable of flexion and extension, but cannot bear the user's weight unless locked in an extended position.

Constant friction is applied to the joint hinge to keep it from swinging too freely, particularly in gait. A solid ankle, cushioned heel (SACH) foot prosthesis is a basic passive device.

L5301

L5301   Below knee, molded socket, shin, SACH foot, endoskeletal system

Lay Description
The code is used to report a below knee prosthesis. Based on moldings or castings taken before or after amputation, a flexible sleeve is custom fabricated from rubber or other material with elastic properties. This constitutes the molded socket that interfaces between the residual limb and the prosthetic system that attaches to it. Plastic sockets may be custom fabricated from moldings as well, sometimes from thermoplastic materials that are molded and shaped as heat is applied. A solid ankle, cushioned heel (SACH) foot prosthesis is a basic passive device.

L5312

L5312   Knee disarticulation (or through knee), molded socket, single axis knee, pylon, SACH foot, endoskeletal system

Lay Description
This code is used to report a through the knee prosthesis. Based on moldings or castings taken before or after amputation, a flexible sleeve is custom fabricated from rubber or other material with elastic properties. This constitutes the molded socket that interfaces between the residual limb and the prosthetic system that attaches to it. Plastic sockets may be custom fabricated from moldings as well, sometimes from thermoplastic materials that are molded and shaped as heat is applied. A pylon is a post-like structure fitted to the plaster socket on one end and the prosthetic foot component on the other. It is a feature of many lower limb prosthetic designs. The pylon may be a tube made of aluminum, titanium, steel, or carbon fiber reinforced plastic and in early fittings is usually adjustable for length. The artificial knee component is a single axis, which means the joint is capable of simple flexion and extension actions only. A solid ankle, cushioned heel (SACH) foot prosthesis is a basic passive device.

L5321

L5321   Above knee, molded socket, open end, SACH foot, endoskeletal system, single axis knee

Lay Description
This code is used to report an above-the-knee prosthesis. Based on moldings or castings taken before or after amputation, a flexible sleeve is custom fabricated from rubber or other material with elastic properties. This constitutes the molded socket that interfaces between the residual limb and the prosthetic system that attaches to it. Plastic sockets

may be custom fabricated from moldings as well, sometimes from thermoplastic materials that are molded and shaped as heat is applied. The artificial knee component is single axis, which means the joint is capable of simple flexion and extension actions only. Rather than internal rigid supports, this type of prosthesis uses the external hard shell to transfer the patient's weight from the thigh and knee to the foot component. A solid ankle, cushioned heel (SACH) foot prosthesis is a basic passive device.

L5331-L5341

L5331   Hip disarticulation, Canadian type, molded socket, endoskeletal system, hip joint, single axis knee, SACH foot

L5341   Hemipelvectomy, Canadian type, molded socket, endoskeletal system, hip joint, single axis knee, SACH foot

Lay Description
These codes report a prosthetic system for patients who have undergone a hemipelvectomy (removal of half of the pelvic girdle and an entire leg). This type of amputation presents numerous problems for the prosthetist, since there is no residual limb with which to anchor a device. The socket is based on moldings and castings taken before or after amputation and may extend well up the torso. The Canadian type prosthesis features a molded plastic socket to enclose the remaining ischial tuberosity to bear weight. An artificial hip joint is toward the anterior of the prosthesis and is unlocked, as is the knee joint, which is single axis. This means the joint is capable of simple flexion and extension actions only. Rather than internal rigid supports, this type of leg prosthesis uses the external hard shell to transfer the patient's weight from the thigh and knee to the foot component (endoskeletal). A solid ankle, cushioned heel (SACH) foot prosthesis is a basic passive device.

L5400-L5430

L5400   Immediate postsurgical or early fitting, application of initial rigid dressing, including fitting, alignment, suspension, and one cast change, below knee

L5410   Immediate postsurgical or early fitting, application of initial rigid dressing, including fitting, alignment and suspension, below knee, each additional cast change and realignment

L5420   Immediate postsurgical or early fitting, application of initial rigid dressing, including fitting, alignment and suspension and one cast change AK or knee disarticulation

L5430   Immediate postsurgical or early fitting, application of initial rigid dressing, including fitting, alignment and suspension, AK or knee disarticulation, each additional cast change and realignment

Lay Description

These codes report supply of early fittings and dressings following below-the-knee amputation or disarticulation at the knee joint. A major consideration for prosthetists is the constantly changing size and shape of the residual limb, or stump, which is the attachment site for a prosthesis. Following amputation of the limb, post-surgical or "early" dressings are applied to the surgical stump, sometimes during the same operative session. These early applications are designed to compress and prepare the distal tissues in anticipation of fitting a test socket and later a permanent socket. Early applications may be known as immediate post-surgical fittings (IPSF). The accepted plan for most lower limb amputations is to transition the patient as quickly as possible to use of a prosthesis. This minimizes muscle atrophy and limb weakness seen in longer convalescences. In some instances, a plaster cast or other rigid dressing is hand molded to the residual limb as the amputation session is completed. In other instances, the initial dressing is applied up to several days following surgery. As swelling diminishes and also to access the surgical closure, the dressing must be periodically changed out. These early dressings may be fitted to interface with test prosthetic devices.

L5450-L5460

L5450   **Immediate postsurgical or early fitting, application of nonweight bearing rigid dressing, below knee**

L5460   **Immediate postsurgical or early fitting, application of nonweight bearing rigid dressing, above knee**

Lay Description

These codes report supply of early non-weight bearing fittings and dressings following amputation of a lower limb. Following amputation of the limb, post-surgical or "early" dressings are applied to the surgical stump, sometimes during the same operative session. These early applications are designed to compress and prepare the distal tissues in anticipation of fitting a test socket and later a permanent socket. In some instances, a plaster cast or other rigid dressing is hand molded to the residual limb as the amputation session is completed. In other instances, the initial dressing is applied up to several days following surgery. As swelling diminishes and also to access the surgical closure, the dressing must be periodically changed out. For plaster and rigid dressings, this entails cutting off the cast and reapplying the dressing. In some cases, removable casts or caps are devised. These devices may be removed and reapplied several times. The dressings reported by these codes are never fitted to interface with test prostheses.

L5500-L5505

L5500   **Initial, below knee PTB type socket, nonalignable system, pylon, no cover, SACH foot, plaster socket, direct formed**

L5505   **Initial, above knee, knee disarticulation, ischial level socket, nonalignable system, pylon, no cover, SACH foot, plaster socket, direct formed**

Lay Description

These codes report the supply of initial hand molded plaster socket systems for amputation of a lower limb. These are initial sockets that are the transition between the initial rigid dressings applied post-surgery and the test socket systems that prepare the patient for a long-term prosthesis. A patella tendon bearing (PTB) type socket generally features an adjustable cuff worn just above the knee joint. This cuff suspends the lower components, comprised in this instance of the direct-formed plaster socket over the stump, the pylon, and foot components. Plaster sockets may be directly formed from bandages saturated with plaster of paris. Once fitted, the plaster socket cannot be aligned. A pylon is a post-like structure fitted to the plaster socket on one end and the prosthetic foot component on the other. It is a feature of most lower limb prosthetic designs. The pylon may be a tube made of aluminum, titanium, steel, or carbon fiber reinforced plastic and in early fittings is usually adjustable for length. Unlike many long-term prostheses, this unit does not feature a cosmetic covering. A solid ankle, cushioned heel (SACH) foot prosthesis is a basic passive device. A high, above-the-knee amputation or disarticulation at the femoral head presents numerous challenges for the prosthetist, since there is very little residual limb to attach the prosthesis. An ischial level socket in this instance is a direct-formed plaster encasement of the ischial tuberosity, to bear the patient's weight. Once fitted, it cannot be aligned. A pylon is fitted to the plaster socket on one end and the prosthetic foot component on the other.

L5510-L5540

L5510   **Preparatory, below knee PTB type socket, nonalignable system, pylon, no cover, SACH foot, plaster socket, molded to model**

L5520   **Preparatory, below knee PTB type socket, nonalignable system, pylon, no cover, SACH foot, thermoplastic or equal, direct formed**

L5530   **Preparatory, below knee PTB type socket, nonalignable system, pylon, no cover, SACH foot, thermoplastic or equal, molded to model**

L5535   **Preparatory, below knee PTB type socket, nonalignable system, no cover, SACH foot, prefabricated, adjustable open end socket**

L5540 Preparatory, below knee PTB type socket, nonalignable system, pylon, no cover, SACH foot, laminated socket, molded to model

Lay Description

These codes report a variety of non-alignable preparatory prostheses for below-the-knee amputations. Preparatory prostheses are transition devices between the initial rigid dressings and pylons applied post-surgery and the finished long-term prosthetic system. The codes are differentiated by the style of socket and the material used in its fabrication. As is typical with preparatory sockets, none can be aligned once fitted. A patella tendon bearing (PTB) type socket generally features an adjustable cuff worn just above the knee joint. This cuff suspends the socket, which can be made of any of a variety of materials. A plaster socket, in this instance, is formed from bandages saturated with plaster of paris applied over a previously cast model of the stump. A thermoplastic socket may be formed by applying heat to the rough-formed socket and modeling it to the patient's stump directly or to a previously cast model of the stump. Another style of preparatory socket involves laminating together two or more resin-saturated materials over a previously cast model of the stump. Other preparatory sockets are prefabricated or selected from mass produced components based only on patient size. This type of preparatory socket is adjustable. A pylon is a post-like structure fitted to the plaster socket on one end and the prosthetic foot component on the other. It is a feature of most lower limb prosthetic designs. The pylon may be a tube made of aluminum, titanium, steel, or carbon fiber reinforced plastic and in early fittings is usually adjustable for length. Unlike many long-term prostheses, none of these units feature cosmetic coverings. A solid ankle, cushioned heel (SACH) foot prosthesis is a basic passive device.

L5560-L5590

L5560 Preparatory, above knee, knee disarticulation, ischial level socket, nonalignable system, pylon, no cover, SACH foot, plaster socket, molded to model

L5570 Preparatory, above knee - knee disarticulation, ischial level socket, nonalignable system, pylon, no cover, SACH foot, thermoplastic or equal, direct formed

L5580 Preparatory, above knee, knee disarticulation, ischial level socket, nonalignable system, pylon, no cover, SACH foot, thermoplastic or equal, molded to model

L5585 Preparatory, above knee - knee disarticulation, ischial level socket, nonalignable system, pylon, no cover, SACH foot, prefabricated adjustable open end socket

L5590 Preparatory, above knee, knee disarticulation, ischial level socket, nonalignable system, pylon, no cover, SACH foot, laminated socket, molded to model

Lay Description

These codes report preparatory prostheses for knee disarticulations with ischial level sockets. Preparatory prostheses are transition devices between the initial rigid dressings and pylons applied post-surgery and the finished long-term prosthetic system. The codes are differentiated by the style of socket and the material used in its fabrication. Ischial level sockets embrace the thigh to the level of the ischial tuberosity, or so-called "sit bones." Preparatory sockets extending to this level are for transition and are unsuitable for aggressive ambulation. Permanent sockets for knee disarticulations are usually three-quarter-thigh length. As is typical with preparatory sockets, none can be aligned once fitted. A plaster socket, in this instance, is formed from bandages saturated with plaster of Paris applied over a previous cast model of the stump and ischium. A thermoplastic socket may be formed by applying heat to the rough-formed socket and modeling it to either the patient's stump and ischium directly or to a previously cast model of the stump. Another style of preparatory socket involves laminating together two or more resin-saturated materials over a previously cast model of the stump. Other preparatory sockets are prefabricated selected from mass-produced components based only on patient size and are adjustable. A pylon is a post-like structure fitted to the socket on one end and the prosthetic foot component on the other. It is a feature of most lower limb prosthetic designs. The pylon may be a tube made of aluminum, titanium, steel, or carbon fiber reinforced plastic and in early fittings is usually adjustable for length. Unlike many long-term prostheses, none of these units features cosmetic coverings, and none of the units reported by this range of codes features knee joints. A solid ankle, cushioned heel (SACH) foot prosthesis is a basic passive device.

L5595-L5600

L5595 Preparatory, hip disarticulation/hemipelvectomy, pylon, no cover, SACH foot, thermoplastic or equal, molded to patient model

L5600 Preparatory, hip disarticulation/hemipelvectomy, pylon, no cover, SACH foot, laminated socket, molded to patient model

Lay Description

These codes report preparatory prostheses for hip disarticulation/hemipelvectomy. Preparatory prostheses are a cosmetically unfinished functional replacement for an amputated extremity, fitted and aligned in accordance with sound biomechanical principles, which is worn for a limited period of time to expedite prosthetic wear and use and to aid in the evaluation of amputee adjustment. This transition device is used between the initial rigid dressings and pylons applied postsurgery and the finished long-term prosthetic system. Preparatory sockets extending to this level are for transition and are unsuitable for aggressive ambulation. As is typical with preparatory sockets, none can be aligned once fitted. A thermoplastic socket may be formed by applying heat to the rough-formed socket and modeling it to the patient's stump directly or to a previously cast model of the stump. Another style of preparatory socket involves laminating together two or more resin-saturated materials over a previously cast model of the stump. A pylon is a post-like structure fitted to the socket on one end and the prosthetic foot component on the other. It is a feature of most lower limb prosthetic designs. The pylon may be a tube made of aluminum, titanium, steel, or carbon fiber reinforced plastic and in early fittings is usually adjustable for length. Unlike many long-term prostheses, none of these units feature cosmetic coverings. None of the units reported by this range of codes feature knee joints. A solid ankle, cushioned heel (SACH) foot prosthesis is a basic passive device.

L5610

L5610 Addition to lower extremity, endoskeletal system, above knee, hydracadence system

Lay Description

This code is used to report the addition of above knee devices to knee joints fitted to patients who have undergone above-the-knee amputation or disarticulation at the knee joint. This code reports the hydracadence system. Hydracadence knee is a single axis hydraulic knee whose specific feature is a unique functional coupling between the knee and the ankle joint during flexion and extension movements. It incorporates some ankle control, as well as swing-phase control. This system is available only in a metal frame, with a specially designed foot-ankle assembly. The swing-phase unit is a relatively simple piston type. In addition to control of the shank during swing phase, resistance to plantar flexion is controlled hydraulically, and motion between the ankle and knee are coordinated so that dorsiflexion of the ankle takes place after the knee has been flexed 20 degrees.

L5611-L5614

L5611 Addition to lower extremity, endoskeletal system, above knee, knee disarticulation, 4-bar linkage, with friction swing phase control

L5613 Addition to lower extremity, endoskeletal system, above knee, knee disarticulation, 4-bar linkage, with hydraulic swing phase control

L5614 Addition to lower extremity, exoskeletal system, above knee-knee disarticulation, 4 bar linkage, with pneumatic swing phase control

Lay Description

These codes report the addition of specific types of swing control devices to knee joints fitted to patients who have undergone above-the-knee amputation or disarticulation at the knee joint. The codes report supply of polycentric-type knee joints. Single-axis knee joints are capable of simple flexion and extension only. The polycentric joint offers greater range of motion. The center of rotation for a polycentric knee joint varies as the flexion angle changes. This feature offers the patient better toe clearance during the swing phase of gait. A common type of polycentric knee is known as the four-bar linkage. This device has four axes of rotation connected by four rigid linkages, and all codes in this range describe this type of knee component. Friction control over the knee joint means that the joint adjustments are tightened down to prevent unwanted movement during gait. Hydraulic swing phase control means the joint is fitted with a fluid-filled piston to dampen unwanted movement during gait, whereas pneumatic swing phase control involves an air-filled piston. All codes in the range report an endoskeletal prosthesis. In this type of design, a pylon, or pole, bears most of the weight load from the thigh to the prosthetic foot, rather than the exterior prosthetic shell in exoskeletal systems.

L5616

L5616 Addition to lower extremity, endoskeletal system, above knee, universal multiplex system, friction swing phase control

Lay Description

This code reports an addition to an endoskeletal above-the-knee prosthesis of a specific design of knee joint. There are two major design differences for the shank component of a leg prosthesis. Endoskeletal shank designs transfer most of the weight from the residual limb to the prosthetic foot through a pylon, a post-like structure fitted to the socket on one end and the prosthetic foot component on the other. The pylon may be a tube made of aluminum, titanium, steel, or carbon fiber reinforced plastic. The pylon may be adjustable and may feature shock absorption characteristics. Most endoskeletal systems are modular and components can be fairly easily upgraded. The endoskeletal pylon system may be covered with an entirely cosmetic outer shell that resembles an actual leg. Exoskeletal designs feature a rigid and structural outer shell that transfers most of the weight from the residual limb to the prosthetic foot. Exoskeletal designs also usually have a pylon, but most of the weight is distributed by the shell. Exoskeletal systems are usually covered and painted to resemble an actual leg. In general, exoskeletal systems are considered durable and easy to maintain.

Both systems offer special versions for active and athletic amputees. The universal multiplex is a particular design suited for moderately active use. This code reports friction swing phase control, which means the joint may be adjusted more tightly to control unwanted movement during gait. Report L5616 for addition of a universal multiplex system with friction swing phase control to an existing endoskeletal above-the-knee prosthesis.

L5617

L5617   Addition to lower extremity, quick change self-aligning unit, above knee or below knee, each

Lay Description
This code is used to report a device that allows the distal section of the prosthetic to be quickly disconnected and reconnected whenever desired without loss of alignment.

L5618-L5628

L5618   Addition to lower extremity, test socket, Symes

L5620   Addition to lower extremity, test socket, below knee

L5622   Addition to lower extremity, test socket, knee disarticulation

L5624   Addition to lower extremity, test socket, above knee

L5626   Addition to lower extremity, test socket, hip disarticulation

L5628   Addition to lower extremity, test socket, hemipelvectomy

Lay Description
A socket is the portion of a prosthesis that fits around the residual limb (or stump) and to which prosthetic components are attached. Test sockets are typically soft and often have transparent fittings that allow the prosthetist to visualize the fit. A test socket tests the interface between the prosthesis and the residual limb. The use of a test/temporary socket allows a refinement in the fit and allows repeated modifications for increased comfort.

L5629

L5629   Addition to lower extremity, below knee, acrylic socket

Lay Description
This code is used to report an acrylic resin used to laminate the socket.

L5630

L5630   Addition to lower extremity, Symes type, expandable wall socket

Lay Description
This code reports the addition of a Symes-type expandable wall socket to a test socket. A socket is the portion of a prosthesis that fits around the residual

limb (or stump) and to which prosthetic components are attached. Test sockets are typically soft and often have transparent fittings that allow the prosthetist to visualize the fit. A test socket tests the interface between the prosthesis and the residual limb. The eponym Symes derives from the Scottish surgeon James Syme, who introduced many orthopaedic procedures in the early 19th century. The Symes disarticulation at the ankle joint remains in common use.

L5631

L5631   Addition to lower extremity, above knee or knee disarticulation, acrylic socket

Lay Description
This code reports the addition of a specific variation to a test socket for knee disarticulations or above-the-knee amputations. A socket is the portion of a prosthesis that fits around the residual limb (or stump) and to which prosthetic components are attached. A test socket, also known as a "check" socket, tests the interface between the prosthesis and the residual limb. The type of socket reported by this code is of acrylic material that is often clear. A clear socket allows the prosthetist to visualize the fit and see points of contact and potential problem areas.

L5632-L5636

L5632   Addition to lower extremity, Symes type, PTB brim design socket

L5634   Addition to lower extremity, Symes type, posterior opening (Canadian) socket

L5636   Addition to lower extremity, Symes type, medial opening socket

Lay Description
These codes report the addition of specific alterations to test sockets. A socket is the portion of a prosthesis that fits around the residual limb (or stump) and to which prosthetic components are attached. Test sockets are typically soft and often have transparent fittings that allow the prosthetist to visualize the fit. A test socket tests the interface between the prosthesis and the residual limb. The eponym Symes derives from the Scottish surgeon James Syme, who introduced many orthopaedic procedures in the early 19th century. The Symes disarticulation at the ankle joint remains in common use. Among prostheses, however, Symes refers to a particular design in which a door is cut into the prosthetic device or, in this instance, the test socket. A patella tendon bearing (PTB) brim design is a socket that extends up to the area above the knee joint; the stump is held in place by the brim shape of the socket.

L5637-L5639

L5637 Addition to lower extremity, below knee, total contact

L5638 Addition to lower extremity, below knee, leather socket

L5639 Addition to lower extremity, below knee, wood socket

Lay Description

These codes address socket variations for below-the-knee prostheses. A socket is the portion of a prosthesis that fits around the residual limb and to which prosthetic components are attached. Several test sockets may be required as the dimensions of the residual limb stabilize following amputation and as the musculature changes over time. A total contact socket, also known as a total surface bearing, is one that fully interfaces with the entire residual limb (or stump). Traditionally, there is a bit of space between the stump and the contact area of the test socket. This space is accessed and injected with a substance that dries to a gel-like consistency, conforming exactly to the shape of the stump and the socket. A total contact interface allows more surface area to bear weight against the prosthesis.

L5640

L5640 Addition to lower extremity, knee disarticulation, leather socket

Lay Description

A knee-disarticulation prosthesis is very similar to an above-knee prosthesis, except for the lower part of the socket and the knee mechanism. Before the introduction of the present day polycentric knee units, sockets for the prosthesis were usually made of leather and metal hinges were used to attach the socket to the shin. Leather sockets are held on by a lacing.

L5642

L5642 Addition to lower extremity, above knee, leather socket

Lay Description

This code is used to report an above knee leather socket. A leather socket has several advantages, including it is available almost everywhere, is more comfortable in hot weather, and can easily be adjusted to the stump as it becomes smaller. Also, leather is soft and easily takes the shape of the stump, and therefore self-corrects molding mistakes.

L5643

L5643 Addition to lower extremity, hip disarticulation, flexible inner socket, external frame

Lay Description

This code is used to report a hip disarticulation socket that utilizes a semi flexible, molded plastic inner socket that is supported by a rigid structural frame.

Plastic sockets usually have a foam liner in the lower part for the bulbous end of the stump to slip by so as to keep the socket in place.

L5644

L5644 Addition to lower extremity, above knee, wood socket

Lay Description

The oldest, traditional way of making artificial limbs is to make the socket out of wood. Wood always has a preponderant place in the fabrication of above knee sockets. Wood is easier to work on the actual object (the socket) rather than on its negative image (positive plaster). In the first fitting, corrections of depth, volume, and form are easy to make while maintaining an acceptable aspect for a definitive socket. When it comes to performing the final adjustments to a finished socket, the thickness of the medial border enables modifications to be effected that are difficult to make on a plastic socket, just as are modifications of volume.

L5645-L5653

L5645 Addition to lower extremity, below knee, flexible inner socket, external frame

L5646 Addition to lower extremity, below knee, air, fluid, gel or equal, cushion socket

L5647 Addition to lower extremity, below knee, suction socket

L5648 Addition to lower extremity, above knee, air, fluid, gel or equal, cushion socket

L5649 Addition to lower extremity, ischial containment/narrow M-L socket

L5650 Additions to lower extremity, total contact, above knee or knee disarticulation socket

L5651 Addition to lower extremity, above knee, flexible inner socket, external frame

L5652 Addition to lower extremity, suction suspension, above knee or knee disarticulation socket

L5653 Addition to lower extremity, knee disarticulation, expandable wall socket

Lay Description

This range of codes addresses additions to lower extremity prostheses of test sockets. Above and below the knee amputations are addressed. A socket is the portion of a prosthesis that fits around the residual limb and to which prosthetic components are attached. Amputees consistently report that the comfort and fit of the socket is crucial to the success of the prosthesis. Test sockets are used to determine optimal interface between the patient's skin at the residual limb and the artificial material of the prosthesis. Several test sockets may be required as the dimensions of the residual limb stabilize following amputation and as the musculature changes over time. Some socket designs feature a flexible inner socket combined with an external frame and/or strapping. Air cushion sockets were developed for aggressive ambulation and running. Suction sockets usually employ a silicone interface. The vacuum is created by the natural properties of the silicone as the socket is donned and weight placed against the interface. Some systems feature a release button to aid in removal. An ischial containment socket is a traditional above-the-knee design by which the ischial tuberosity is contained within the walls of the socket (also known as "plug fit" or anatomical fit). The M-L socket is another variety of anatomical fit, above-the-knee designs. The M-L (medial-lateral) socket is tight fitting with most of the squeezing taking place on the lateral side followed by the medial side.

L5654-L5658

L5654 Addition to lower extremity, socket insert, Symes, (Kemblo, Pelite, Aliplast, Plastazote or equal)

L5655 Addition to lower extremity, socket insert, below knee (Kemblo, Pelite, Aliplast, Plastazote or equal)

L5656 Addition to lower extremity, socket insert, knee disarticulation (Kemblo, Pelite, Aliplast, Plastazote or equal)

L5658 Addition to lower extremity, socket insert, above knee (Kemblo, Pelite, Aliplast, Plastazote or equal)

Lay Description
Socket inserts help to protect the fragile skin of the residual limb while compensating for daily changes in limb volume. Some manufacturers of prostheses require socket inserts. Other designs can be comfortably fit without use of an insert. Irregular or bony residual limbs present complications that can be addressed by inserts. The codes in this range are differentiated by type of amputation and length of residual limb. Symes-type disarticulation occurs at the ankle joint with the fat pad of the heel preserved and rotated over the closure. The specific insert materials mentioned in the code descriptions are trade names for foams or other synthetic materials that are generally lightweight and can be molded and shaped when heat is applied.

L5661-L5665

L5661 Addition to lower extremity, socket insert, multidurometer Symes

L5665 Addition to lower extremity, socket insert, multidurometer, below knee

Lay Description
These codes report the supply of multidurometer socket inserts for either a Symes-type disarticulation at the ankle or a below-the-knee amputation. Some manufacturers of prostheses require socket inserts. Other designs can be comfortably fit without use of an insert. A durometer is a device to measure surface resiliency of material, and a firmness scale is used by fabricators of prosthetic devices. Multidurometer, in

this context, is used to define an insert material made up of three or more materials, each with a different firmness rating. Combinations may include laminates of Plastazote, Poron, or other materials.

L5666

L5666 Addition to lower extremity, below knee, cuff suspension

Lay Description
This code reports supply of a specific type of suspension socket for patients who have had below-the-knee amputation. A cuff is a gripping device that fits, in this instance, around the residual limb below the knee. A cuff is smaller than a corset or "lacer" but works similarly. It is made of rigid or semi-rigid material lined on the inside with cushioning material. The cuff may be closed snugly around the limb by straps, Velcro, or eyelet and gusset lacing. The socket and prosthesis may make full contact with the residual limb, particularly when weight is brought to bear, but the attachment integrity of the system is the suspension from the cuff.

L5668

L5668 Addition to lower extremity, below knee, molded distal cushion

Lay Description
This code reports supply of a molded distal cushion addition to a prosthesis liner. These types of cushions are now made of viscoelastic materials; gel-like substances that may be molded or provided off-the-shelf. In this instance, the cushion is molded to a positive image of the residual distal stump for precise fit.

L5670-L5672

L5670 Addition to lower extremity, below knee, molded supracondylar suspension (PTS or similar)

L5671 Addition to lower extremity, below knee/above knee suspension locking mechanism (shuttle, lanyard, or equal), excludes socket insert

L5672 Addition to lower extremity, below knee, removable medial brim suspension

Lay Description
These codes report suspension style additions to lower extremity prostheses. A patella tendon bearing (PTB) type of prosthesis may have already been fitted to a below-the-knee amputation. Above-the-knee amputations may require the addition of a suspension-locking device to hold the prosthesis. The supracondylar suspension (PTS) is a prosthesis that suspends from the prominence of the condyles of the tibial plateau just distal to the knee joint. The prosthesis is allowed to hang from just below the knee joint until weight is placed upon it. A shuttle system incorporates a pin and lock at the bottom of

the socket to suspend the prosthesis and may be used for amputations above or below the knee.

L5673

L5673 Addition to lower extremity, below knee/above knee, custom fabricated from existing mold or prefabricated, socket insert, silicone gel, elastomeric or equal, for use with locking mechanism

Lay Description
This socket insert has an interface that surrounds the residual limb in a layer of skin-friendly, mineral-oil based gel. Made from thermoplastic elastomer, the gel gently adheres to the skin to protect against abrasion and breakdown. The gel is covered in a layer of durable fabric that helps to extend the life of the liners and allows the amputees to easily slide into the sockets. These locking liners are designed for use with a shuttle lock and 10mm pin.

L5676

L5676 Additions to lower extremity, below knee, knee joints, single axis, pair

Lay Description
This basic lower-extremity prosthesis includes a single-axis, constant friction knee. This device is a basic knee that acts as a door-and-hinge device, is free swinging and does not allow stance control. It allows one-speed ambulation and is often used in children.

L5677

L5677 Additions to lower extremity, below knee, knee joints, polycentric, pair

Lay Description
The polycentric knee is a device that has multiple rotational axes and is sometimes referred to as the "four bar" knee. It has four points of rotation connected by a linkage bar. The device is very stable in early stance and easy to flex in swing phase.

L5678

L5678 Additions to lower extremity, below knee, joint covers, pair

Lay Description
This is an accessory that aids in the effective use of a lower-limb prosthetic.

L5679

L5679 Addition to lower extremity, below knee/above knee, custom fabricated from existing mold or prefabricated, socket insert, silicone gel, elastomeric or equal, not for use with locking mechanism

Lay Description
This socket insert has an interface that surrounds the residual limb in a layer of skin-friendly, mineral-oil based gel. Made from thermoplastic elastomer, the gel gently adheres to the skin to protect against

abrasion and breakdown. The gel is covered in a layer of durable fabric that helps to extend the life of the liners and allows the amputees to easily slide into the sockets.

L5680, L5682

L5680 Addition to lower extremity, below knee, thigh lacer, nonmolded

L5682 Addition to lower extremity, below knee, thigh lacer, gluteal/ischial, molded

Lay Description
These codes report supply of so-called thigh lacers, or corsets, for patients who have undergone below-the-knee amputations. These corset-like cuffs are often made of leather or composites and may be custom manufactured or off-the-shelf. Custom-made devices are usually molded to a positive image of the leg. These devices are closed usually using lacing through eyelets and gussets along the anterior face. A lower leg prosthesis is attached to the corset, usually by two vertical metal sidebars, thus forming a type of suspension system. At one time thigh lacers were a common form of suspension for transtibial prostheses. With the rise of total contact sockets, however, thigh lacer suspension has seen diminishing use. Thigh lacers still offer an advantage in that much of the weight is distributed from the thigh to the lower leg over the vertical sidebars and may be prescribed for patients who do not tolerate full contact pressure on the residual limb.

L5681, L5683

L5681 Addition to lower extremity, below knee/above knee, custom fabricated socket insert for congenital or atypical traumatic amputee, silicone gel, elastomeric or equal, for use with or without locking mechanism, initial only (for other than initial, use code L5673 or L5679)

L5683 Addition to lower extremity, below knee/above knee, custom fabricated socket insert for other than congenital or atypical traumatic amputee, silicone gel, elastomeric or equal, for use with or without locking mechanism, initial only (for other than initial, use code L5673 or L5679)

Lay Description
This is a polyurethane liner that sits directly against the skin. The suspension sleeve creates a seal between the prosthesis and the residual limb. One code is for an initial liner for a congenital or atypical traumatic amputee and the other for other than a congenital or atypical traumatic amputee.

L5684

L5684 Addition to lower extremity, below knee, fork strap

Lay Description
This type of suspension incorporates a fork strap, with or without a waist belt. A fork strap has two diagonal straps attached to a third strap. The advantages of straps are that they are patient adjustable and provide auxiliary suspension for participation in activities such as sports, hunting, or hiking.

L5685

L5685 Addition to lower extremity prosthesis, below knee, suspension/sealing sleeve, with or without valve, any material, each

Lay Description
This is a suspension component consisting of a sleeve that fits over the socket and onto the thigh of the wearer. A valve may or may not be incorporated into the sleeve.

L5686

L5686 Addition to lower extremity, below knee, back check (extension control)

Lay Description
This code reports the supply of a device that, when added to a lower prosthesis, prevents the knee joint from hyperextension, or bending backward. This device may be a strap, blocking, or locking mechanism that prevents the artificial knee from moving beyond the position needed for normal standing.

L5688-L5690

L5688 Addition to lower extremity, below knee, waist belt, webbing

L5690 Addition to lower extremity, below knee, waist belt, padded and lined

Lay Description
Waist belt suspension is designed to work with transtibial prostheses. This belt is made of leather, cotton webbing, or nylon webbing and is worn around the patient's waist. Padding and/or a leather liner may be included to minimize the discomfort caused by the edges of the belt digging into the skin of the waist. An elastic strap extends from the belt to a leather strap attached to the medial and lateral (side) surfaces of the prosthetic socket. The design helps with extension of the residual limb and is indicated for patients with weak musculature. Waist belt suspension is primarily used for patients who have experienced difficulty with, or cannot tolerate, other forms of suspension.

L5692-L5695

L5692 Addition to lower extremity, above knee, pelvic control belt, light

L5694 Addition to lower extremity, above knee, pelvic control belt, padded and lined

L5695 Addition to lower extremity, above knee, pelvic control, sleeve suspension, neoprene or equal, each

Lay Description
These codes report additions of pelvic control systems to above-the-knee amputation prosthetics. These are often belt systems worn around the lower waist. A light belt is a simple fabric belt worn around the lower waist. The Silesian belt consists of a broad and often padded belt that fits around the lower back and halfway around the hips. A thinner cinch belt fits over the broad portion and closes and adjusts the system. The belt systems partially suspend the prosthesis, usually from a single location on the lateral side. A sleeve suspension is pulled over the residual limb and in this instance extends over the ischium and pelvis. Neoprene is specifically cited in the code description, but gel-like materials made from silicon are probably used most often today.

L5696

L5696 Addition to lower extremity, above knee or knee disarticulation, pelvic joint

Lay Description
This code reports the addition of a pelvic joint to an above-the-knee amputation or pelvic joint disarticulation. The pelvic joint may be single or multiple axes and typically is mounted at the anterior of the prosthesis. Various designs and features are available. The joint allows for flexibility at the hip and may allow ambulation.

L5697-L5698

L5697 Addition to lower extremity, above knee or knee disarticulation, pelvic band

L5698 Addition to lower extremity, above knee or knee disarticulation, Silesian bandage

Lay Description
These codes report the supply of additional supports to an above-the-knee amputation or pelvic joint disarticulation prosthetic system. Most modern femoral amputation prostheses are designed to attach and hold firmly to the residual limb without use of hip belts or additional supports. In some instances, however, patients may require additional support or suspension in the form of pelvic bands or bandages. These are typically broad, padded bands or wrappings worn around the lower waist and from which the prosthesis can be attached. The site of attachment is usually at a lateral and/or anterior location on the prosthesis.

L5699

L5699 All lower extremity prostheses, shoulder harness

Lay Description
This code reports the supply of a shoulder harness support to an above-the-knee amputation or a pelvic joint disarticulation prosthetic system. Most modern femoral amputation prostheses are designed to attach and hold firmly to the residual limb without use of hip belts or additional supports at the shoulder. In some instances, however, patients may require additional support or suspension in the form of a shoulder harness. This type of device may involve both shoulders or be a simpler single-shoulder harness sling. The site of attachment is usually at a lateral and/or anterior location on the prosthesis.

L5700-L5703

L5700 Replacement, socket, below knee, molded to patient model

L5701 Replacement, socket, above knee/knee disarticulation, including attachment plate, molded to patient model

L5702 Replacement, socket, hip disarticulation, including hip joint, molded to patient model

L5703 Ankle, Symes, molded to patient model, socket without solid ankle cushion heel (SACH) foot, replacement only

Lay Description
These codes report replacement for molded sockets for lower limb prosthetic systems. The codes are differentiated by the level of amputation. Amputation patients routinely see significant daily changes in the volume and physical dimensions of the residual limb, or stump. This challenge is addressed as best as possible by fitting test or "check" sockets during the early phase of adjustment to a prosthetic limb. Liners and stockings of varying thickness also compensate for volume changes in the stump. Terminal sockets designed for extended use have limited life spans and must be changed out for various reasons, including changes in stump volume. These codes report supply of a replacement socket molded to a plaster positive model taken of the residual limb. Changes in the limb may require that a new model be prepared, or an earlier model may still be workable. Increasingly, computer models and scans are used. The socket material may be heat molded or otherwise shaped to conform precisely to the patient model.

L5704-L5707

L5704 Custom shaped protective cover, below knee

L5705 Custom shaped protective cover, above knee

L5706 Custom shaped protective cover, knee disarticulation

L5707 Custom shaped protective cover, hip disarticulation

Lay Description
A custom-shaped protective covering for a prosthesis is one of two general varieties. Prostheses with internal supports (endoskeletal) usually feature an outer protective cover made of closed cell foam and a skin-color finish. Externally supported prostheses (exoskeletal) usually feature a hard, synthetic shell, also usually finished to resemble human skin. Both varieties may start out from an off-the-shelf blank but are carefully customized to match the size and length, thickness, and coloring of an opposing or lost limb. This range of codes reports the replacement of these protective outer surface cover systems (POSCS).

L5710

L5710 Addition, exoskeletal knee-shin system, single axis, manual lock

Lay Description
This code refers to an addition of a manual lock to a single-axis knee/shin system. A manual locking knee incorporates an automatic lock that can be unlocked voluntarily. The manual locking knee is appropriate for weak or unstable patients as well as more active individuals who frequently walk on unstable terrain.

L5711

L5711 Additions exoskeletal knee-shin system, single axis, manual lock, ultra-light material

Lay Description
This code refers to an addition of a manual lock to a single-axis knee/shin system made of ultra-light material. A manual locking knee incorporates an automatic lock that can be unlocked voluntarily. The manual locking knee is appropriate for weak or unstable patients as well as more active individuals who frequently walk on unstable terrain.

L5712

L5712 Addition, exoskeletal knee-shin system, single axis, friction swing and stance phase control (safety knee)

Lay Description
This is a transfemoral or hip disarticulation knee/shin unit that is unicentric and locks when weight is placed on it (otherwise known as stance locking).

L5714

L5714 Addition, exoskeletal knee-shin system, single axis, variable friction swing phase control

Lay Description
This code refers to a mechanical variable friction knee unit that utilizes two brakes to terminate the flexion and extension portions of swing phase, simulating the functions of the quadriceps and hamstring muscles. The deceleration and braking function is performed by two bumpers attached to a tubular knee bolt, which provide continuous friction throughout the gait cycle.

L5716

L5716 Addition, exoskeletal knee-shin system, polycentric, mechanical stance phase lock

Lay Description
The geometric lock feature, also referred to as a mechanical stance phase lock, locks the knee on full extension (initial contact) and does not release it until the weight line passes over the forefoot and the knee unit is hyperextended. Mechanical-knee users must exert muscular and mechanical control to alter speed and step length. This provides stability in the weight-bearing phase of gait.

L5718

L5718 Addition, exoskeletal knee-shin system, polycentric, friction swing and stance phase control

Lay Description
Friction is used in the knee to control the knee joint during walking. Friction controls how far and how fast the knee bends and straightens during gait. A manual locking knee incorporates an automatic lock that can be unlocked voluntarily. The manual locking knee is appropriate for weak or unstable patients as well as more active individuals who frequently walk on unstable terrain.

L5722

L5722 Addition, exoskeletal knee-shin system, single axis, pneumatic swing, friction stance phase control

Lay Description
This code refers to a hydraulic unit that includes piston cylinders and contains air (pneumatic) added to the knee device to allow swing control as the amputee speeds up or slows down. Swing control may allow the amputee to walk at variable speeds. The limitation of the lack of stance control can be addressed by locking knee or safety knee features.

L5724

L5724 Addition, exoskeletal knee-shin system, single axis, fluid swing phase control

Lay Description
This is a hydraulic knee control unit that includes a knee/shin set-up that is unicentric and controls swing phase only.

L5726

L5726 Addition, exoskeletal knee-shin system, single axis, external joints, fluid swing phase control

Lay Description
This is a hydraulic knee control unit that consists of a knee/shin set-up that is unicentric with external uprights above the knee center and that controls swing phase only.

L5728

L5728 Addition, exoskeletal knee-shin system, single axis, fluid swing and stance phase control

Lay Description
This is a hydraulic knee control unit that includes the knee/shin set-up that is unicentric and controls both swing and stance.

L5780

L5780 Addition, exoskeletal knee-shin system, single axis, pneumatic/hydra pneumatic swing phase control

Lay Description
This is a hydra-pneumatic knee unit that is unicentric and is for swing phase control and provides smooth, coordinated hip and knee motion.

L5781-L5782

L5781 Addition to lower limb prosthesis, vacuum pump, residual limb volume management and moisture evacuation system

L5782 Addition to lower limb prosthesis, vacuum pump, residual limb volume management and moisture evacuation system, heavy-duty

Lay Description
These codes report a specialized vacuum system for the socket. Amputation patients routinely see significant daily changes in the volume and physical dimensions of the residual limb, or stump. This volume can change significantly in the course of a day and some suction socket systems are believed to exacerbate short-term volume loss. The vacuum system reported by these codes is designed to create a greater vacuum between the liner and the wall of the socket than is found in standard suction socket systems. Moisture trapped between the liner and

socket is also removed. The system purportedly stabilizes volume fluctuation in the residual limb.

L5785-L5795

L5785 Addition, exoskeletal system, below knee, ultra-light material (titanium, carbon fiber or equal)

L5790 Addition, exoskeletal system, above knee, ultra-light material (titanium, carbon fiber or equal)

L5795 Addition, exoskeletal system, hip disarticulation, ultra-light material (titanium, carbon fiber or equal)

Lay Description

These codes report the addition of ultra-light weight material components to an exoskeletal lower limb prosthesis. The codes are differentiated by level of amputation. Two major types of lower limb prostheses are currently offered. Endoskeletal shank designs transfer most of the weight from the residual limb to the prosthetic foot through a pylon, a post-like structure fitted to the socket on one end and the prosthetic foot component on the other. The pylon may be a tube made of aluminum, titanium, steel, or carbon fiber-reinforced plastic. Most endoskeletal systems are modular and components can be fairly easily upgraded. The endoskeletal pylon system may be covered with an entirely cosmetic outer shell that resembles an actual leg. Exoskeletal designs feature a rigid and structural outer shell that transfers most of the weight from the residual limb to the prosthetic foot. Exoskeletal designs also often have a pylon, but most of the weight is distributed by the shell. Exoskeletal systems are usually covered and painted to resemble an actual leg. In general, exoskeletal systems are considered durable and easy to maintain. Both systems offer special versions for active and athletic amputees. These codes report modification to an exoskeletal system by the addition of carbon fiber, titanium, or other lightweight materials, either to the pylon component, the exoskeletal shell, or both.

L5810-L5812

L5810 Addition, endoskeletal knee-shin system, single axis, manual lock

L5811 Addition, endoskeletal knee-shin system, single axis, manual lock, ultra-light material

L5812 Addition, endoskeletal knee-shin system, single axis, friction swing and stance phase control (safety knee)

Lay Description

These codes report additions to endoskeletal prosthetic systems of single axis knees. Endoskeletal shank designs transfer most of the weight from the residual limb to the prosthetic foot through a pylon, a post-like structure fitted to the socket on one end and the prosthetic foot component on the other. The pylon may be a tube made of aluminum, titanium, steel, or carbon fiber-reinforced plastic. Most

endoskeletal systems are modular and components can be easily upgraded. The endoskeletal pylon system may be covered with a cosmetic outer shell that resembles an actual leg. Addition of a single axis knee joint to an endoskeletal system entails proper interface with the upper component and the pylon (shin) component. A single axis joint is capable of straight-on flexion and extension only. The type reported by L5810 features a locking pin that maintains the standing position. The device must be manually released for the patient to flex the joint and to sit down. Friction control over the knee joint means that the adjustments can be tightened down to prevent unwanted joint movement, especially during gait. The joint also features a braking or locking mechanism to maintain proper standing position and to prevent overextension of the joint.

L5814-L5818

L5814 Addition, endoskeletal knee-shin system, polycentric, hydraulic swing phase control, mechanical stance phase lock

L5816 Addition, endoskeletal knee-shin system, polycentric, mechanical stance phase lock

L5818 Addition, endoskeletal knee-shin system, polycentric, friction swing and stance phase control

Lay Description

These codes report additions to endoskeletal prosthetic systems of multiple axis, or polycentric knee joints. These knees flex and extend like single axis joints, but also offer limited lateral movement and twisting action. Endoskeletal shank designs transfer most of the weight from the residual limb to the prosthetic foot through a pylon, a post-like structure fitted to the socket on one end and the prosthetic foot component on the other. The pylon may be a tube made of aluminum, titanium, steel, or carbon fiber-reinforced plastic. Most endoskeletal systems are modular and components can be easily upgraded. The endoskeletal pylon system may be covered with a cosmetic outer shell that resembles an actual leg. Addition of a single axis knee joint to an endoskeletal system entails proper interface with the upper component and the pylon (shin) component. A hydraulic cylinder may be used to assist joint movement, especially during the swing phase of gait. A locking mechanism or a friction brake may be added to support the system as the patient stands.

L5822-L5830

L5822 Addition, endoskeletal knee-shin system, single axis, pneumatic swing, friction stance phase control

L5824 Addition, endoskeletal knee-shin system, single axis, fluid swing phase control

L5826 Addition, endoskeletal knee-shin system, single axis, hydraulic swing phase control, with miniature high activity frame

L5828 Addition, endoskeletal knee-shin system, single axis, fluid swing and stance phase control

L5830 Addition, endoskeletal knee-shin system, single axis, pneumatic/swing phase control

Lay Description

These codes report additions to endoskeletal prosthetic systems of single axis knee joints. Specific devices are added to the joints to assist the swing phase of gait and sometimes to control stance, or standing. Single axis knee joints are capable of simple flexion and extension only. Endoskeletal shank designs transfer most of the weight from the residual limb to the prosthetic foot through a pylon, a post-like structure fitted to the socket on one end and the prosthetic foot component on the other. The pylon may be a tube made of aluminum, titanium, steel, or carbon fiber-reinforced plastic. Most endoskeletal systems are modular and components can be easily upgraded. The endoskeletal pylon system may be covered with a cosmetic outer shell that resembles an actual leg. Friction control over the knee joint means that adjustments can be tightened down to slow down joint movement, especially during gait. Consequently, friction control joints may be fitted with assistance devices to help extend the joint during the swing phase of gait. These devices may employ a cylinder filled with air or gas (pneumatic) or fluids such as oil (hydraulic). Pressure in the cylinder forces a piston to assist movement of the joint while dampening impact during heel strike. The pressure may also be employed to act as a brake to control joint movement while standing. A high activity frame is a supportive structure around the knee joint and is designed for high levels of activity and uneven terrain. The framework may assist in special functions such as shortening the shin component for better heel and toe clearance over uneven terrain.

L5840

L5840 Addition, endoskeletal knee-shin system, 4-bar linkage or multiaxial, pneumatic swing phase control

Lay Description

This code refers to an addition of a specific endoskeletal knee-shin system known for its multiaxial features. Endoskeletal shank designs transfer most of the weight from the residual limb to the prosthetic foot through a pylon, a post-like structure fitted to the socket on one end with the prosthetic foot component on the other. The pylon may be a tube made of aluminum, titanium, steel, or carbon fiber-reinforced plastic. Most endoskeletal systems are modular, and components can be easily upgraded. The endoskeletal pylon system may be covered with a cosmetic outer shell that resembles an actual leg. As the name denotes, a four-bar joint system features four vertical bars paired anteriorly and posteriorly, and superior and inferior hinges are

linked together to pivot the joint. The additional bars affect the center of gravity and provide for a stable joint. Other multiaxial joints may feature bearings or other innovations to provide additional movement. Certain joints may be fitted with assistance devices to help extend and/or flex the joint during the swing phase of gait. These devices may employ a cylinder filled with air or gas (pneumatic). Pressure in the cylinder forces a piston to assist movement of the joint while dampening impact during heel strike.

L5845

L5845 Addition, endoskeletal knee-shin system, stance flexion feature, adjustable

Lay Description

This code refers to an addition to an endoskeletal knee-shin system of an adjustable stance flexion feature. Endoskeletal shank designs transfer most of the weight from the residual limb to the prosthetic foot through a pylon, a post-like structure fitted to the socket on one end and the prosthetic foot component on the other. The pylon may be a tube made of aluminum, titanium, steel, or carbon fiber-reinforced plastic. Most endoskeletal systems are modular, and components can be easily upgraded. The endoskeletal pylon system may be covered with a cosmetic outer shell that resembles an actual leg. This code reports the addition of an adjustable device that limits movement of the knee joint while standing, while still assisting the bending, or flexion, of the joint during gait. This type of device may be piston-driven, either pneumatic or hydraulic. Some models activate stance control as the patient "bounces" weight on the knee, which locks and unlocks the device for prolonged standing.

L5848

L5848 Addition to endoskeletal knee-shin system, fluid stance extension, dampening feature, with or without adjustability

Lay Description

This code reports the addition to a knee-shin endoskeletal system of an adjustable fluid stance extension with dampening feature, with or without adjustability addition. Endoskeletal shank designs transfer most of the weight from the residual limb to the prosthetic foot through a pylon, a post-like structure fitted to the socket on one end and the prosthetic foot component on the other. The pylon may be a tube made of aluminum, titanium, steel, or carbon fiber-reinforced plastic. Most endoskeletal systems are modular and components can be easily upgraded. The endoskeletal pylon system may be covered with a cosmetic outer shell that resembles an actual leg. This type of addition is to a knee joint prosthesis and involves the use of a hydraulic driven device. Fluid such as oil is compressed in a chamber. As the joint moves, the oil is further compressed or relaxed, which governs the stance phase of the prosthesis. The compression chamber further works to dampen shock as weight is placed on the fully extended joint to engage the stance phase. Most of these designs are integrated into the joint interior. Adjustments allow the patient to open and close valves to control fluid movement through the chambers.

L5850-L5855

L5850   Addition, endoskeletal system, above knee or hip disarticulation, knee extension assist

L5855   Addition, endoskeletal system, hip disarticulation, mechanical hip extension assist

Lay Description

These codes refer to the addition of mechanical joint assists to prosthetic joints of the knee or hip. Various prosthetic joint designs are available, particularly for endoskeletal systems with knee components. Almost all feature some type of control to temper joint movement when not needed. Constant friction control involves adjusting tension against the joint pivot, essentially making it more difficult to move throughout its range. Other designs may involve external brakes that slow or stop joint action, particularly in the full extension stance phase. Mechanical assist devices are often added to prosthetic joints to make them move more easily in one direction, particularly during the swing phase of gait. These devices may feature an air-filled or fluid-filled cylinder and piston design that helps to push the knee joint into extension. Others may entail spring action to operate the mechanical assistance. Prosthetic hip joints are usually on the anterior side near the top of the femoral pylon somewhat removed from the natural anatomic location. Disarticulation of the hip constitutes only about 2 percent of lower-limb amputations. Several types of mechanical assistance designs are used for hip joints. Some employ cords with elastic properties to assist flexion. More modern designs entail spring-driven assistance devices with components integrated into the joint.

L5856

L5856   Addition to lower extremity prosthesis, endoskeletal knee-shin system, microprocessor control feature, swing and stance phase, includes electronic sensor(s), any type

Lay Description

This is a computerized limb prosthesis that is a nonstandard, external prosthetic device that incorporates a microprocessor for movement control. This use of a microprocessor control in both the swing and stance phases of gait improves stance control and may provide increased safety, stability, and function; for example, the sensors are designed to recognize a stumble and stiffen the knee, thus avoiding a fall. Other potential benefits of microprocessor-controlled

knee prostheses are improved ability to navigate stairs, slopes, and uneven terrain, and reduction in energy expenditure and concentration required for ambulation.

L5857

L5857   Addition to lower extremity prosthesis, endoskeletal knee-shin system, microprocessor control feature, swing phase only, includes electronic sensor(s), any type

Lay Description

This is a computerized limb prosthesis that is a nonstandard, external prosthetic device incorporating a microprocessor for movement control. These devices are equipped with a sensor that detects when the knee is in full extension and adjusts the swing phase automatically, permitting a more natural walking pattern of varying speeds.

L5858

L5858   Addition to lower extremity prosthesis, endoskeletal knee shin system, microprocessor control feature, stance phase only, includes electronic sensor(s), any type

Lay Description

This is a computerized limb prosthesis that is a nonstandard, external prosthetic device incorporating a microprocessor for movement control. This device improves stance control and may provide increased safety, stability, and function; for example, the sensors are designed to recognize a stumble and stiffen the knee, thus avoiding a fall.

L5859

L5859   Addition to lower extremity prosthesis, endoskeletal knee-shin system, powered and programmable flexion/extension assist control, includes any type motor(s)

Lay Description

A motorized prosthetic knee is provided as an addition to a lower extremity prosthetic. The knee contains an electromechanical actuator that actively initiates and controls all aspects of the user's gait. It also provides powered knee flexion and extension for the patient. The knee functions based on data collected through accelerometers, gyroscopes, a torque sensor, and a load sensor. When the patient walks, the addition samples knee position and loads at a high rate of speed. It is able to help replace hip, leg, and foot muscle function to allow a more natural gait and stance. It also provides stability and support and reduces impact to the patient. The motor in the knee is battery operated.

L5910-L5920

L5910 Addition, endoskeletal system, below knee, alignable system

L5920 Addition, endoskeletal system, above knee or hip disarticulation, alignable system

Lay Description

These codes are used to report the addition of an alignable system for lower extremity endoskeletal prostheses. Alignment of the prosthesis usually occurs during the latter phases of the manufacturing process. Endoskeletal systems feature internal supports. Preliminary alignment of an above-the-knee prosthesis may occur at a fitting session before the protective covering is applied. Ordinarily, however, alignment is performed at the time of final fitting. Below-the-knee systems sometimes feature alignment settings for the foot/ankle component that can be adjusted by the person who wears the prosthesis.

L5925

L5925 Addition, endoskeletal system, above knee, knee disarticulation or hip disarticulation, manual lock

Lay Description

This code is used to report the addition of a manual lock to a hip or knee joint of an endoskeletal system for above-the-knee amputation or hip disarticulation. A manual lock to a joint prosthesis is usually designed to be easily engaged and disengaged by the wearer. Some may feature a ring or lever that pulls a cable triggering locking mechanism. The lock itself may be a simple drop-pin design that engages the two main components of the joint, usually in full extension. This allows the patient to confidently stand without worry that the joint will collapse into flexion or hyperextend backward. The wearer must actively disengage the lock to allow the joint to flex for sitting. For some prostheses, the lock is engaged for walking as well as standing. Some manual locks can be engaged while the joint is in any variety of positions as needed by the user.

L5930

L5930 Addition, endoskeletal system, high activity knee control frame

Lay Description

This code refers to the addition of a high-activity knee control frame to an endoskeletal prosthesis. Lower-limb prosthesis users are usually classified in some manner according to their physical abilities. Those with good prospects for high activity levels and athletes may be fitted with special adaptations to accommodate additional stresses on the knee prosthesis. A knee control frame is usually employed in more advanced prostheses and is most often used to support high-end joint components to accommodate extreme use. These typically include a

polycentric knee joint with hydraulic features and possibly microprocessor controls.

L5940

L5940 Addition, endoskeletal system, below knee, ultra-light material (titanium, carbon fiber or equal)

Lay Description

This is a global code that includes ultra-light materials and encompasses all areas of a below-knee prosthesis.

L5950

L5950 Addition, endoskeletal system, above knee, ultra-light material (titanium, carbon fiber or equal)

Lay Description

This is a global code that includes ultra-light materials and encompasses all areas of an above knee prosthesis.

L5960

L5960 Addition, endoskeletal system, hip disarticulation, ultra-light material (titanium, carbon fiber or equal)

Lay Description

An endoskeletal system is an internal support composed of natural skeletal parts or artificial parts that replace missing natural parts. This system is used to replace an entire lower limb that was removed at the hip joint. Ultralight materials allow greater ease in movement.

L5961

L5961 Addition, endoskeletal system, polycentric hip joint, pneumatic or hydraulic control, rotation control, with or without flexion and/or extension control

Lay Description

An endoskeletal system is an internal support composed of natural skeletal parts or artificial parts that replace missing natural parts. A polycentric hip joint with pneumatic or hydraulic control is a three-dimensional joint system using mechanical means to mimic natural hip movement.

L5962-L5966, L5969

L5962 Addition, endoskeletal system, below knee, flexible protective outer surface covering system

L5964 Addition, endoskeletal system, above knee, flexible protective outer surface covering system

L5966 Addition, endoskeletal system, hip disarticulation, flexible protective outer surface covering system

L5969 Addition, endoskeletal ankle-foot or ankle system, power assist, includes any type motor(s)

Lay Description

These codes refer to a skin-like material that is either brushed or sprayed over the soft foam covering that is attached to the outside of a definitive prosthesis that forms a water- and tear-resistant flexible surface.

L5968

L5968 Addition to lower limb prosthesis, multiaxial ankle with swing phase active dorsiflexion feature

Lay Description

This code is used to report the addition of a specific design of multiaxial ankle to a lower limb prosthesis. A multiaxial ankle prosthesis is capable of dorsiflexion and plantarflexion (the single axis movement of the foot up and down), as well as limited twisting motion and medial and lateral movement. This offers stability and allows the user to better negotiate uneven terrain. In addition, this prosthesis automatically moves the foot into dorsiflexion (foot up) during the swing phase of gait to prepare for heel strike. This feature may be accomplished several ways. A spring-loaded cylinder acting on a piston rod is one approach. Spring tension pushes the heel down and raises the forefoot into dorsiflexion. Other designs may be activated by energy storing capabilities as weight is released from the foot.

L5970-L5972

L5970 All lower extremity prostheses, foot, external keel, SACH foot

L5971 All lower extremity prostheses, solid ankle cushion heel (SACH) foot, replacement only

L5972 All lower extremity prostheses, foot, flexible keel

Lay Description

These codes are used to report the supply of a variety of prosthetic foot types. The keel of a prosthetic foot is the rigid (or spring-like) section that generally runs from heel to toe near the footplate. It may serve merely as a structural piece, as in designs using wooden or rigid keels. In other designs, the keel absorbs impact and transfers energy as weight rolls from heel strike to "toe-off," the moment when weight is released from the forefoot. The keel may be made of wood, plastic, carbon-reinforced fibers, or metal. An external keel, as the name implies, is exposed and the prosthesis may be hollow, or exoskeletal. A solid ankle, cushion heel type foot is known by the acronym SACH and a variety of models are available. In some, the external keel is part of the shell. Flexible keels are integral components of many energy storing prosthetic feet. A stationary ankle, flexible exoskeleton type of foot is known by the acronym SAFE. These types of prosthetic feet have flexible keels, either internally or as external components of the shell. The SAFE foot is known for its ability to slightly invert and evert and to absorb shock. Some designs of SACH and SAFE feet have a pylon-type bolt that penetrates through the prosthesis and connects to the ankle component and pylon. The STEN foot is named for "STored ENergy," which is largely accomplished through use of a flexible keel and other resilient materials.

L5973

L5973 Endoskeletal ankle foot system, microprocessor controlled feature, dorsiflexion and/or plantar flexion control, includes power source

Lay Description

Endoskeletal ankle foot system, microprocessor controlled feature, dorsiflexion and/or plantar flexion control, includes power source is an electronic, microprocessor controlled prosthetic ankle-foot system. This system was designed to assist lower extremity amputees with walking on level ground or on uneven terrain, up and down inclines and declines, up and down stairs, and standing up from a sitting position. The system permits a more dynamic, real-time adjustment of the prosthetic as the patient takes a step.

L5974-L5975

L5974 All lower extremity prostheses, foot, single axis ankle/foot

L5975 All lower extremity prostheses, combination single axis ankle and flexible keel foot

Lay Description

These codes are used to report the supply of specific types of prosthetic feet. A single axis ankle is capable of dorsiflexion and plantarflexion only (the movement of the foot up and down). This is among the more fundamental designs of prosthetic feet. The keel is the component of a prosthetic foot that generally runs from heel to toe near the footplate. A flexible keel may be made of carbon reinforced fibers, metal, or resilient materials. The flexible keel absorbs impact and transfers energy as weight rolls from heel strike to "toe-off," the moment when weight is released from the forefoot. Flexible keels are integral components of many energy storing prosthetic feet.

L5976

L5976 All lower extremity prostheses, energy storing foot (Seattle Carbon Copy II or equal)

Lay Description

This code refers to the supply of a specific level of energy-storing prosthetic foot, whereby some type of material deforms with weight pressure but then resumes its original shape as pressure is removed with a consequent release of energy. The keel is the component of a prosthetic foot that generally runs from heel to toe near the footplate. A flexible keel, which may be made of carbon-reinforced fibers, metal, or resilient materials, absorbs impact and transfers energy as weight rolls from heel strike to "toe-off" the moment when weight is released from the forefoot. Flexible keels are integral components of many energy-storing prosthetic feet.

L5978-L5979

L5978 **All lower extremity prostheses, foot, multiaxial ankle/foot**

L5979 **All lower extremity prostheses, multiaxial ankle, dynamic response foot, one piece system**

Lay Description
These codes are used to report the supply of a specific type of foot prosthesis. A multi-axial ankle is capable of dorsiflexion and plantarflexion (the movement of the foot up and down), as well as limited twisting motion, medial and lateral movement, and internal and external rotation. This offers stability and allows the user to better negotiate uneven terrain. The dynamic response foot is a type of energy storing prosthetic foot. It falls well within the range of active use, but somewhat short of the high-end athletic prostheses. The keel in this type of foot is energy absorbing with good transfer upon "toe-off." Sure-Flex, Genesis II, and Seattle Lite are considered in this category.

L5980-L5981

L5980 **All lower extremity prostheses, flex-foot system**

L5981 **All lower extremity prostheses, flex-walk system or equal**

Lay Description
These codes report the supply of a specific type of foot prosthesis. The original flex-foot system was a unique design to accommodate active users. The foot was developed in the early 1980s using a single L-shaped strip of carbon fiber, which at the time was a material new to prosthesis fabrication. The lower horizontal portion was fitted to sole material, and the upper vertical part was attached to the pylon. A separate strip was attached to the rear of the footplate like a leaf spring to act as the heel. The design provides springlike compression action, as well as some torque and flexibility properties. The foot is known for high flexibility and good energy-storing capabilities and remains in widespread use. The flex-walk system is a second generation of the flex-foot design and addresses the needs of amputees with longer residual limbs with moderate activity levels, as well as pediatric applications. Both versions adapt well to both endoskeletal and exoskeletal shank designs.

L5982-L5984

L5982 **All exoskeletal lower extremity prostheses, axial rotation unit**

L5984 **All endoskeletal lower extremity prostheses, axial rotation unit, with or without adjustability**

Lay Description
When the prosthesis incorporates an axial rotation device, this net torque acting about the long axis of the socket is able to rotate the socket externally, the only resistance to such rotation being the relatively weak return spring in the axial rotation device. The axial rotation tends to relieve the contact pressures that caused the torque and thus reduces pressures in the critical anteromedial region of the brim. With an axial rotation device, the socket is free to respond to the demands of the stump and relieve the pressures and torque caused by cyclic action of the musculature.

L5985

L5985 **All endoskeletal lower extremity prostheses, dynamic prosthetic pylon**

Lay Description
This code reports the supply of a dynamic pylon for a lower-extremity prosthesis system. A pylon is a post-like structure fitted to the residual limb socket on one end and the prosthetic foot component on the other. The pylon may be a tube made of aluminum, titanium, steel, or carbon fiber-reinforced plastic. A dynamic pylon has energy-storing properties, typically provided by an internal spring or series of springs. Some models, such as the Endolite telescopic torsion pylon, also allow for some twisting movement. The energy-return feature absorbs shock and in some users provides gait efficiency with less energy outlay.

L5986

L5986 **All lower extremity prostheses, multiaxial rotation unit (MCP or equal)**

Lay Description
This code reports the supply of a multiaxial system for artificial ankles that incorporate rubber compression springs bonded to reversible adapters. This allows the adapters to be bolted to the ankle plate and function with the maximum efficiency in all the planes of motion.

L5987

L5987 **All lower extremity prostheses, shank foot system with vertical loading pylon**

Lay Description
This code refers to a pylon foot system that deflects vertically on weight bearing and reflexes to its original posture as it is unloaded.

L5988

L5988 Addition to lower limb prosthesis, vertical shock reducing pylon feature

Lay Description

This code reports the supply of a vertical shock-reducing pylon for a lower-extremity prosthesis system. A pylon is a post-like structure fitted to the residual limb socket on one end and the prosthetic foot component on the other. The pylon may be a tube made of aluminum, titanium, steel, or carbon fiber-reinforced plastic. A pylon may be fitted with a device to absorb vertical shock, as occurs during heel strike. These additions have energy-storing properties, typically provided by an internal spring or series of springs. This feature absorbs shock and in some users provides gait efficiency with less energy outlay.

L5990

L5990 Addition to lower extremity prosthesis, user adjustable heel height

Lay Description

The adjustable heel height prosthetic foot is an anatomical gliding ankle that maintains appropriate foot alignment to provide knee stability and consistent performance at all heel heights. A person can adjust the heel to accommodate wearing a sandal to wearing a two-inch heel on a dress shoe.

L5999

L5999 Lower extremity prosthesis, not otherwise specified

Lay Description

A lower extremity prosthetic is used to replace function for a patient who is missing all or part of a leg or foot. Use this code to report a lower extremity prosthetic when there is not a more specific HCPCS Level II code available.

L6000-L6020

L6000 Partial hand, thumb remaining
L6010 Partial hand, little and/or ring finger remaining
L6020 Partial hand, no finger remaining

Lay Description

This range of codes reports the supply of a traditional type of shoulder-powered hand prosthesis. They are designed for patients with partial hand amputation. The prosthesis is functional through use of a simple mechanical shoulder harness with a cable extending to the prosthesis. The length of socket depends on the amputation and the types of tasks demanded of the prosthesis. Heavy-duty use typically requires a deeper socket. A cosmetic glove-like covering may finish the prosthesis. A two-position prosthetic thumb is used when that digit is missing. Other digits may feature single or multiple joints.

L6026

L6026 Transcarpal/metacarpal or partial hand disarticulation prosthesis, external power, self-suspended, inner socket with removable forearm section, electrodes and cables, two batteries, charger, myoelectric control of terminal device, excludes terminal device(s)

Lay Description

A myoelectric prosthesis of the hand is an electronic device used as a replacement for an amputation at the transcarpal or metacarpal area. This type of prosthesis uses an external battery pack to supply power to electric motors and microprocessors that control the movement of the device in different directions. The myoelectric prosthetic has a more realistic appearance and provides the patient with increased function. Control of the device is through skin electrodes inside the socket of the prosthetic. The electrodes can detect and amplify the electrical activity of muscle groups left in the hand. These impulses are cycled through the microprocessor units and result in movement of the hand through electric motors.

L6050-L6055

L6050 Wrist disarticulation, molded socket, flexible elbow hinges, triceps pad
L6055 Wrist disarticulation, molded socket with expandable interface, flexible elbow hinges, triceps pad

Lay Description

These codes report the supply of hand prostheses for disarticulations at the wrist. As is typical of traditional below-the-elbow prostheses, an upper-arm harness assists the mechanical operation. Movement is transferred by cable from the harness to the prosthesis. A cuff or half-cuff is situated over the triceps muscle. Paired medial and lateral elbow hinges act as leverage points to assist movement. The socket is the interface between the residual limb and the prosthesis. Traditionally, a plaster mold is taken of the residual stump and a positive replica is made. The socket is then vacuum fitted to the replica. A socket may be made from any variety of materials, although modern ones are increasingly fabricated from thermoplastic resins or elastic sleeves. Many are designed for use with gel liners. Patients with wrist disarticulation amputations can retain a high level of pronation and supination movement. An expandable interface at the socket end may be fashioned to accommodate limb growth in children or for interchangeable prostheses.

L6100-L6110

L6100 Below elbow, molded socket, flexible elbow hinge, triceps pad

L6110 Below elbow, molded socket (Muenster or Northwestern suspension types)

Lay Description

These codes report two types of sockets for below-the-elbow or transradial amputations. A cuff or half-cuff is situated over the triceps muscle. Paired medial and lateral elbow hinges act as leverage points to assist movement. The socket is the interface between the residual limb and the prosthesis. Traditionally, a plaster mold is taken of the residual stump, and a positive replica is made. The socket is then vacuum fitted to the replica. A socket may be made from any variety of materials, although modern ones are increasingly fabricated from thermoplastic resins or elastic sleeves. Many are designed for use with gel liners. The Muenster and Northwestern-style sockets traditionally extend proximally to the elbow condyles. The Muenster fits snugly on the anterior and posterior aspects; the Northwestern on the medial and lateral sides. Modified versions of both are available, often with the upper posterior side cut away for movement and breathability. Both styles are suspension sockets, which hold snugly to the residual limb and suspend the prosthetic components.

L6120

L6120 Below elbow, molded double wall split socket, step-up hinges, half cuff

Lay Description

This code refers to an exoskeletal prosthesis for a short, transradial amputation. It includes a custom-fitted socket fabricated from a model of a patient, custom-fabricated forearm using step-up hinges to increase range of motion, a triceps cuff, and a friction wrist unit.

L6130

L6130 Below elbow, molded double wall split socket, stump activated locking hinge, half cuff

Lay Description

This code refers to an exoskeletal prosthesis for a short, transradial amputation. It includes a custom-fitted socket fabricated from a model of a patient, custom-fabricated forearm using stump-activated locking hinges, a triceps cuff, and a friction wrist unit.

L6200-L6205

L6200 Elbow disarticulation, molded socket, outside locking hinge, forearm

L6205 Elbow disarticulation, molded socket with expandable interface, outside locking hinges, forearm

Lay Description

These codes are used to report an exoskeletal prosthesis for an elbow disarticulation or long, transhumeral amputation. It includes a custom-fitted socket fabricated from a model of a patient and a custom-fabricated forearm using an outside locking hinge and a friction wrist unit. An expandable interface allows for differences in residual limb size.

L6250

L6250 Above elbow, molded double wall socket, internal locking elbow, forearm

Lay Description

A transhumeral prothesis is an artificial limb that replaces an arm missing above the elbow. This code refers to a transhumeral amputation that includes a custom-fitted double wall socket fabricated from a model of the patient, a custom-fabricated forearm using an internal locking elbow, and a friction wrist unit.

L6300

L6300 Shoulder disarticulation, molded socket, shoulder bulkhead, humeral section, internal locking elbow, forearm

Lay Description

This code refers to an exoskeletal prosthesis for a shoulder disarticulation amputation. It includes a custom-fitted socket fabricated from a model of a patient, a custom-fabricated humeral section, and a forearm using a shoulder bulkhead, an internal locking elbow, and friction wrist unit. Exoskeletal prostheses have a hard outer shell, which can usually withstand considerable force. Exoskeletal designs are usually preferred for prostheses designed to perform work.

L6310

L6310 Shoulder disarticulation, passive restoration (complete prosthesis)

Lay Description

This code refers to an exoskeletal passive prosthesis for a shoulder disarticulation amputation. It includes a custom-fitted socket fabricated from a model of the patient, a custom-fabricated humeral section and forearm using a passive elbow, a passive terminal device (the most distal part of a prosthesis that substitutes for the hand; it may be a prosthetic hand, a hook, or another device), and a friction wrist unit and suspension. Exoskeletal prostheses have a hard outer shell, which can usually withstand considerable force. Exoskeletal designs are usually preferred for prostheses designed to perform work. A passive functional prosthesis offers very realistic cosmetics and can perform limited function.

L6320

L6320   Shoulder disarticulation, passive restoration (shoulder cap only)

Lay Description
The code refers to an upper extremity restoration (cap) prosthesis for the shoulder of a shoulder disarticulation amputation. It includes a custom-fitted socket fabricated from a model of the patient with special modifications to restore shoulder shape and protect the amputation area. A passive system is primarily cosmetic but also functions as a stabilizer. A passive system is fabricated if the patient does not have enough strength or movement to control a prosthesis or wears a prosthesis only because of cosmetic concerns.

L6350

L6350   Interscapular thoracic, molded socket, shoulder bulkhead, humeral section, internal locking elbow, forearm

Lay Description
An interscapular-thoracic amputation is the surgical separation of the humerus (upper arm bone), scapula (shoulder blade), and a portion of the clavicle (collar bone) from the body. In this procedure the entire shoulder and arm are removed. This code refers to an exoskeletal prosthesis for an interscapular thoracic amputation. It includes a custom-fitted socket fabricated from a model of the patient, a custom-fabricated humeral section, forearm utilizing a shoulder bulkhead, an internal locking elbow, and a friction wrist unit.

L6360

L6360   Interscapular thoracic, passive restoration (complete prosthesis)

Lay Description
An interscapular-thoracic amputation is the surgical separation of the humerus (upper arm bone), scapula (shoulder blade), and a portion of the clavicle (collar bone) from the body. In this procedure, the entire shoulder and arm are removed. This code refers to the complete passive restoration. A passive system is primarily cosmetic but also functions as a stabilizer. A passive system is fabricated if the patient does not have enough strength or movement to control a prosthesis or wears a prosthesis only because of cosmetic concerns.

L6370

L6370   Interscapular thoracic, passive restoration (shoulder cap only)

Lay Description
An interscapular-thoracic amputation is the surgical separation of the humerus (upper arm bone), scapula (shoulder blade), and a portion of the clavicle (collar bone) from the body. In this procedure the entire shoulder and arm are removed. This code refers to an upper-extremity restoration (shoulder cap) prosthesis for the shoulder of an interscapular thoracic amputation. It includes a custom-fitted socket fabricated from a model of the patient with special modification to restore shoulder shape and to provide protection to the amputation area.

L6380-L6384

L6380   Immediate postsurgical or early fitting, application of initial rigid dressing, including fitting alignment and suspension of components, and one cast change, wrist disarticulation or below elbow

L6382   Immediate postsurgical or early fitting, application of initial rigid dressing including fitting alignment and suspension of components, and one cast change, elbow disarticulation or above elbow

L6384   Immediate postsurgical or early fitting, application of initial rigid dressing including fitting alignment and suspension of components, and one cast change, shoulder disarticulation or interscapular thoracic

Lay Description
These codes report supply of early fittings and dressings following an upper limb amputation or disarticulation at the shoulder joint. A major consideration for prosthetists is the constantly changing size and shape of the residual limb, or stump, which is the attachment site for the prosthesis. Following amputation of the limb, post-surgical or "early" dressings are applied to the surgical stump, sometimes during the same operative session. These early applications are designed to compress and prepare the distal tissues in anticipation of fitting a test socket and later a permanent socket. Early applications may be known as immediate post-surgical fittings (IPSF). The accepted plan for most limb amputations is to transition the patient as quickly as possible to the use of prosthesis. This minimizes muscle atrophy and limb weakness seen in longer convalescences. In some instances, a plaster cast or other rigid dressing is hand molded to the residual limb as the amputation session is completed. In other instances, the initial dressing is applied up to several days following surgery. As swelling diminishes and also to access the surgical closure, the dressing must be periodically changed out. These early dressings may be fitted to interface with test prosthetic devices.

L6386

L6386 Immediate postsurgical or early fitting, each additional cast change and realignment

Lay Description
This code refers to the removal and reapplication of the direct formed socket (codes L6380, L6382, and L6384) and includes alignment and any adjustments.

L6388

L6388 Immediate postsurgical or early fitting, application of rigid dressing only

Lay Description
This code refers to an application of a dressing immediately post-op or soon after surgery, consisting of a socket fabricated directly to the amputee's residual limb at any level.

L6400

L6400 Below elbow, molded socket, endoskeletal system, including soft prosthetic tissue shaping

Lay Description
A transradial prosthesis is an artificial limb that replaces an arm missing below the elbow. This code refers to an endoskeletal prosthesis for a transradial amputation. It includes a custom-fitted socket fabricated from a patient model, a forearm (always made of similar material as the arm section), friction wrist unit, custom-shaped cover, and a nonprotective covering. An endoskeletal system is covered with a cosmetic foam that is shaped to match the sound side limb (the noninvolved limb).

L6450

L6450 Elbow disarticulation, molded socket, endoskeletal system, including soft prosthetic tissue shaping

Lay Description
This code refers to an endoskeletal prosthesis for an elbow disarticulation or long transradial amputation. It includes a custom-fitted socket fabricated from a patient model, a nonalignable forearm, friction wrist unit, custom-shaped cover, and a nonprotective covering.

L6500

L6500 Above elbow, molded socket, endoskeletal system, including soft prosthetic tissue shaping

Lay Description
This code refers to an endoskeletal prosthesis for a transradial amputation. It includes a custom-fitted socket fabricated from a patient model, nonalignable humeral section, nonalignable forearm section, friction wrist unit, custom-shaped cover, and nonprotective covering.

L6550

L6550 Shoulder disarticulation, molded socket, endoskeletal system, including soft prosthetic tissue shaping

Lay Description
This code refers to an upper-extremity, endoskeletal prosthesis for a shoulder disarticulation amputation. It includes a custom-fitted socket fabricated from a patient model, nonalignable humeral section, non-alignable forearm section, friction wrist unit, custom-shaped cover, and nonprotective covering.

L6570

L6570 Interscapular thoracic, molded socket, endoskeletal system, including soft prosthetic tissue shaping

Lay Description
This code refers to an upper-extremity, endoskeletal prosthesis for an interscapular thoracic amputation. It includes a custom-fitted socket fabricated from a patient model, nonalignable humeral section, nonalignable forearm section, friction wrist unit, custom-shaped cover, and nonprotective covering.

L6580

L6580 Preparatory, wrist disarticulation or below elbow, single wall plastic socket, friction wrist, flexible elbow hinges, figure of eight harness, humeral cuff, Bowden cable control, USMC or equal pylon, no cover, molded to patient model

Lay Description
This code refers to an upper-extremity, preparatory prosthesis for a wrist disarticulation or transradial amputation. It includes a custom-fitted socket fabricated from a patient model, single-wall construction, nonalignable pylon, triceps cuff flexible hinges, friction wrist unit, Bowden control cable, and figure-eight harness. No cover is allowed with this code.

L6582

L6582 Preparatory, wrist disarticulation or below elbow, single wall socket, friction wrist, flexible elbow hinges, figure of eight harness, humeral cuff, Bowden cable control, USMC or equal pylon, no cover, direct formed

Lay Description
This code refers to an upper-extremity, preparatory prosthesis for a wrist disarticulation or transradial amputation. It includes a direct formed socket, single-wall construction, nonalignable pylon, triceps cuff, flexible hinges, Bowden control cable, figure-eight harness, and friction wrist unit. No cover is allowed for this code.

L6584

L6584 Preparatory, elbow disarticulation or above elbow, single wall plastic socket, friction wrist, locking elbow, figure of eight harness, fair lead cable control, USMC or equal pylon, no cover, molded to patient model

Lay Description
This code refers to an upper-extremity, preparatory prosthesis for a wrist disarticulation or transradial amputation. It includes a custom-fitted socket fabricated from a patient, single-wall construction, locking elbow, nonalignable pylon, fair lead control cable, figure-eight harness, and friction wrist unit. No cover is allowed for this code.

L6586

L6586 Preparatory, elbow disarticulation or above elbow, single wall socket, friction wrist, locking elbow, figure of eight harness, fair lead cable control, USMC or equal pylon, no cover, direct formed

Lay Description
This code refers to an upper-extremity, preparatory prosthesis for a wrist disarticulation or transradial amputation. It includes a direct formed socket, single-wall construction, locking elbow, nonalignable pylon, fair lead control cable, figure-eight harness, and friction wrist unit. No cover is allowed for this code.

L6588

L6588 Preparatory, shoulder disarticulation or interscapular thoracic, single wall plastic socket, shoulder joint, locking elbow, friction wrist, chest strap, fair lead cable control, USMC or equal pylon, no cover, molded to patient model

Lay Description
This code refers to an upper-extremity, preparatory prosthesis for a shoulder disarticulation or an interscapular thoracic amputation. It includes a custom-fitted socket fabricated from a patient model, single-wall fabrication using a plastic shoulder joint, locking elbow, friction wrist joint, nonalignable pylon, fair lead control cable, and chest harness. No cover is allowed for this code.

L6590

L6590 Preparatory, shoulder disarticulation or interscapular thoracic, single wall socket, shoulder joint, locking elbow, friction wrist, chest strap, fair lead cable control, USMC or equal pylon, no cover, direct formed

Lay Description
This code refers to an upper-extremity, preparatory prosthesis for a shoulder disarticulation or an interscapular thoracic amputation. It includes a direct

formed socket, single-wall fabrication using a plastic shoulder joint, locking elbow, friction wrist unit, nonalignable pylon, fair lead control cable, and chest harness. No cover is allowed for this code.

L6600-L6611

L6600 Upper extremity additions, polycentric hinge, pair

L6605 Upper extremity additions, single pivot hinge, pair

L6610 Upper extremity additions, flexible metal hinge, pair

L6611 Addition to upper extremity prosthesis, external powered, additional switch, any type

Lay Description
In the prosthetics armamentarium (all of the equipment necessary for prosthetic fitting or use), a patient or doctor needs a complete range of components to be available to provide a proper fitting prosthesis for all sites of amputations. These codes refer to the array of components necessary for the prescription fitting of prostheses in relation to the site of upper-extremity amputation.

L6615-L6616

L6615 Upper extremity addition, disconnect locking wrist unit

L6616 Upper extremity addition, additional disconnect insert for locking wrist unit, each

Lay Description
The disconnect locking wrist unit refers to a quick disconnect wrist unit that allows interchanging of terminal device (supination and pronation of a device) in locked positions. The disconnect locking wrist unit includes one wrist unit insert. An additional insert to be utilized with the quick disconnect wrist unit is also available.

L6620

L6620 Upper extremity addition, flexion/extension wrist unit, with or without friction

Lay Description
This code refers to a wrist unit that allows flexion of the terminal device into a locked position. The wrist unit flexes in only one plane.

L6621

L6621 Upper extremity prosthesis addition, flexion/extension wrist with or without friction, for use with external powered terminal device

Lay Description
This code refers to a wrist unit that allows flexion of the terminal device into locked positions. The wrist

unit flexes in only one plane. This is for use with external powered devices.

L6623

L6623   Upper extremity addition, spring assisted rotational wrist unit with latch release

Lay Description
This code refers to a wrist unit that utilizes a spring to assist supination and pronation. A locking mechanism locks the terminal in a fixed position.

L6624

L6624   Upper extremity addition, flexion/extension and rotation wrist unit

Lay Description
Flexion and extension, along with rotation, give the prosthesis two additional degrees of freedom, and rotational wrist units are cable-controlled, positive-locking mechanisms. Flexion and extension in a prosthetic wrist make it easier for users to grip and see objects.

L6625

L6625   Upper extremity addition, rotation wrist unit with cable lock

Lay Description
This code refers to a wrist unit that utilizes a cable to unlock the terminal device to allow supination and pronation.

L6628

L6628   Upper extremity addition, quick disconnect hook adapter, Otto Bock or equal

Lay Description
The code refers to a wrist unit for an external powered prosthesis that allows for the interchange of an external powered or body powered terminal device. This device allows supination or pronation and allows the wearer to release the hand quickly in an emergency or reposition objects without having to go through the open/close cycle.

L6629

L6629   Upper extremity addition, quick disconnect lamination collar with coupling piece, Otto Bock or equal

Lay Description
This code refers to a lamination collar and a coupling piece to accept a terminal device for an external powered prosthesis. It is used in the fabrication of the forearm.

L6630

L6630   Upper extremity addition, stainless steel, any wrist

Lay Description
This code refers to any wrist unit made of stainless steel.

L6632

L6632   Upper extremity addition, latex suspension sleeve, each

Lay Description
This code refers to a suspension sleeve (which suspends the prosthesis) made of latex. These sleeves provide optimal distribution of weight between the upper arm and forearm. It is also formulated with a medical grade mineral oil that soothes and protects the skin from shearing, abrasion, and friction between the residual limb and the prosthesis.

L6635

L6635   Upper extremity addition, lift assist for elbow

Lay Description
Lift assists are used to counterbalance the weight of the forearm, making elbow flexion easier. It is a spring mechanism that somewhat compensates for gravity forces.

L6637

L6637   Upper extremity addition, nudge control elbow lock

Lay Description
This code refers to a device used by high-level amputees to lock and unlock the prosthetic elbow when shoulder excursion (linear displacement) is limited.

L6638

L6638   Upper extremity addition to prosthesis, electric locking feature, only for use with manually powered elbow

Lay Description
An electric locking feature is attached to a prosthetic elbow to allow locking in various positions. The locking mechanism is activated electronically rather than manually using a myoelectrode, touch pad, or switch.

L6640

L6640   Upper extremity additions, shoulder abduction joint, pair

Lay Description
This code is used to report shoulder joints that provide passive abduction for the humeral section of a high-level prosthesis.

L6641-L6642

L6641   Upper extremity addition, excursion amplifier, pulley type

L6642   Upper extremity addition, excursion amplifier, lever type

Lay Description
A cable-operated prosthesis uses body movements to supply power for its operation. An excursion amplifier is used to amplify the patient's motion that is necessary to operate the cables in upper extremity prosthesis. It consists of a small pulley attached near the posterior end of the chest strap of the harness or an actuation lever that can be moved to different places on the device. The pulley amplifier reduces the required body motion in half (and doubles the required body force). The lever amplifier can be varied by placement of the control strap cable on the lever.

L6645

L6645   Upper extremity addition, shoulder flexion-abduction joint, each

Lay Description
A shoulder flexion-abduction joint is a two-way joint that is attached to residual limb of the shoulder. This addition allows the patient to flex and abduct the prosthetic arm.

L6646

L6646   Upper extremity addition, shoulder joint, multipositional locking, flexion, adjustable abduction friction control, for use with body powered or external powered system

Lay Description
This code is used to report an addition to an upper extremity prosthesis. It is a shoulder joint that can swing in a natural arc and can also be locked in 36 positions, every 10 degrees. The user can free the joint manually or by using a nudge control. Abduction (pushing away) and adduction (pulling in) is achieved through a second hinge with adjustable friction. This joint can be used with body powered or external powered systems.

L6647-L6648

L6647   Upper extremity addition, shoulder lock mechanism, body powered actuator

L6648   Upper extremity addition, shoulder lock mechanism, external powered actuator

Lay Description
A locking feature is attached to a prosthetic shoulder to allow locking in various positions. The mechanism can be powered by cables that use body movements for control or it can be an externally powered locking device that is powered by electric motors and an external battery pack.

L6650

L6650   Upper extremity addition, shoulder universal joint, each

Lay Description
This code is used to report a universal shoulder joint that provides passive abduction, flexion, rotation, and circumduction.

L6655-L6660

L6655   Upper extremity addition, standard control cable, extra

L6660   Upper extremity addition, heavy-duty control cable

Lay Description
These codes are used to report a standard or heavy duty control cable and housing for a body powered prosthesis.

L6665

L6665   Upper extremity addition, Teflon, or equal, cable lining

Lay Description
Control cables are attached to the prosthesis and are used to link the patient's movements to control movement of the prosthesis. These cables run through lined housings. The housing can be lined to reduce the friction generated as the cable moves.

L6670

L6670   Upper extremity addition, hook to hand, cable adapter

Lay Description
This code is used to report a cable adapter utilized to allow a hook and hand to be interchanged on a body powered prosthesis.

L6672-L6677

L6672   Upper extremity addition, harness, chest or shoulder, saddle type

L6675   Upper extremity addition, harness, (e.g., figure of eight type), single cable design

L6676   Upper extremity addition, harness, (e.g., figure of eight type), dual cable design

L6677   Upper extremity addition, harness, triple control, simultaneous operation of terminal device and elbow

Lay Description
A harness system holds the prosthetic device securely to the residual limb, distributes the weight and lifting load, and positions the prosthesis for greatest ease of use. For the figure-8 strap, a harness wraps around the axilla on the intact side of the body. This holds the harness and provides the counterforce for suspension and control-cable forces. On the residual limb side, the front strap provides the most of the suspending forces to the prosthesis by attaching directly to the socket in transhumeral prosthesis or indirectly to a transradial

socket through an intermediate Y-strap and triceps cuff. The back strap on the side with the prosthesis attaches to the control cable. A saddle type harness provides the ability for the patient to lift heavier loads and is an alternative to the figure-8 harness. A shoulder saddle is a fairly wide leather piece that rests on the shoulder of the amputated arm. Straps are attached to the saddle and the prosthesis and the saddle is secured with a strap around the chest. This provides less pressure on the axilla than the figure-8 harness.

L6680-L6684

L6680 Upper extremity addition, test socket, wrist disarticulation or below elbow

L6682 Upper extremity addition, test socket, elbow disarticulation or above elbow

L6684 Upper extremity addition, test socket, shoulder disarticulation or interscapular thoracic

Lay Description
A socket is the portion of a prosthesis that fits around the residual limb (or stump) and to which prosthetic components are attached. Test sockets are typically soft and often have transparent fittings that allow the prosthetist to visualize the fit. A test socket tests the interface between the prosthesis and the residual limb. The use of a test/temporary socket allows a refinement in the fit and allows repeated modifications for increased comfort.

L6686

L6686 Upper extremity addition, suction socket

Lay Description
A suction socket uses a vacuum action to attach the prosthesis to the socket. The residual limb is put into the socket. It is fit with a one-way air valve to remove air and create the suction force to keep the socket in place until air is reintroduced to remove the socket. Suction sockets require total contact with the residual limb to maintain the vacuum.

L6687-L6690

L6687 Upper extremity addition, frame type socket, below elbow or wrist disarticulation

L6688 Upper extremity addition, frame type socket, above elbow or elbow disarticulation

L6689 Upper extremity addition, frame type socket, shoulder disarticulation

L6690 Upper extremity addition, frame type socket, interscapular-thoracic

Lay Description
A socket is the piece of the prosthetic that fits the residual limb of a patient who has experienced an amputation. A frame type of socket has a flexible plastic inner piece for contact and fit. This is surrounded by a flexible liner and a rigid frame for

support and to which the necessary cables and joints are attached as needed. Windows are created in the outer sock to allow movement and reduce pressure and pain over bony prominences.

L6691-L6692

L6691 Upper extremity addition, removable insert, each

L6692 Upper extremity addition, silicone gel insert or equal, each

Lay Description
A prosthetic socket insert surrounds the residual limb in a layer of skin friendly material. A gel insert gently adheres to the skin to protect against abrasion and breakdown. The gel is covered in a layer of durable fabric that helps extend the life of liners and allows amputees to easily slide into the sockets.

L6693

L6693 Upper extremity addition, locking elbow, forearm counterbalance

Lay Description
A locking elbow is an addition to an upper extremity prosthesis. It allows the elbow joint to flex and can be locked into various positions. Elbow spring-lift devices are used to counterbalance the weight of the forearm to make flexion easier for the patient.

L6694-L6697

L6694 Addition to upper extremity prosthesis, below elbow/above elbow, custom fabricated from existing mold or prefabricated, socket insert, silicone gel, elastomeric or equal, for use with locking mechanism

L6695 Addition to upper extremity prosthesis, below elbow/above elbow, custom fabricated from existing mold or prefabricated, socket insert, silicone gel, elastomeric or equal, not for use with locking mechanism

L6696 Addition to upper extremity prosthesis, below elbow/above elbow, custom fabricated socket insert for congenital or atypical traumatic amputee, silicone gel, elastomeric or equal, for use with or without locking mechanism, initial only (for other than initial, use code L6694 or L6695)

L6697 Addition to upper extremity prosthesis, below elbow/above elbow, custom fabricated socket insert for other than congenital or atypical traumatic amputee, silicone gel, elastomeric or equal, for use with or without locking mechanism, initial only (for other than initial, use code L6694 or L6695)

Lay Description

A socket insert is a soft device designed to fit around a residual limb and inside the socket to provide increased padding and comfort. This code is used to report socket inserts for prosthetic arms. The inserts may be composed of silicone gel and elastic polymers (elastomers), and can be custom-made from an existing mold or prefabricated (ready-made). Locking mechanics hold the arm or a portion thereof in a set position until the lock is released. The designation of "initial only" represents the first creation of a mold of the residual arm and the socket insert for a specific patient.

L6698

L6698 Addition to upper extremity prosthesis, below elbow/above elbow, lock mechanism, excludes socket insert

Lay Description

A prosthetic locking mechanism is a device using suction, pins, or similar means to hold the prosthesis to the residual limb.

L6703-L6704

L6703 Terminal device, passive hand/mitt, any material, any size

L6704 Terminal device, sport/recreational/work attachment, any material, any size

Lay Description

A terminal device is an addition to an upper extremity prosthesis that replaces a missing hand in function, appearance, or both. The device attaches to a base wrist unit. Terminal devices are interchangeable, and a patient may use different versions at different times. Terminal devices may be passive or active. Passive devices more cosmetically resemble a hand and are usually less functional.

L6706-L6722

L6706 Terminal device, hook, mechanical, voluntary opening, any material, any size, lined or unlined

L6707 Terminal device, hook, mechanical, voluntary closing, any material, any size, lined or unlined

L6708 Terminal device, hand, mechanical, voluntary opening, any material, any size

L6709 Terminal device, hand, mechanical, voluntary closing, any material, any size

L6711 Terminal device, hook, mechanical, voluntary opening, any material, any size, lined or unlined, pediatric

L6712 Terminal device, hook, mechanical, voluntary closing, any material, any size, lined or unlined, pediatric

L6713 Terminal device, hand, mechanical, voluntary opening, any material, any size, pediatric

L6714 Terminal device, hand, mechanical, voluntary closing, any material, any size, pediatric

L6715 Terminal device, multiple articulating digit, includes motor(s), initial issue or replacement

L6721 Terminal device, hook or hand, heavy-duty, mechanical, voluntary opening, any material, any size, lined or unlined

L6722 Terminal device, hook or hand, heavy-duty, mechanical, voluntary closing, any material, any size, lined or unlined

Lay Description

A terminal device is an addition to an upper extremity prosthesis that replaces a missing hand in function, appearance, or both. The device attaches to a base wrist unit. Terminal devices are interchangeable, and a patient may use different versions at different times. Terminal devices may be passive or active. Passive devices more cosmetically resemble a hand and are usually less functional. Active devices provide some of the normal hand functions. These active terminal devices may be in the form of a hook or a hand. A hook is a metal device with two fingers that can be opened or closed and is usually made of aluminum or steel. Hands are more esthetically pleasing and allow finger position control. Body-powered or manual prostheses use cables and gross limb movement to control the device. They are usually of moderate weight and cost. Active devices may have voluntary opening or closing mechanisms. Multiple articulating digits allow individual, multiple movements in the fingers and/or thumb. Each digit has a separate motor to control the movement. Voluntary opening mechanisms are closed at relaxation and open when the patient exerts control. Control may be mechanical or electric using patient muscle contractions. Relaxation of the muscles allows the device to close around the object. Voluntary closing mechanisms are open at rest. Residual forearm flexors control the grasp of the desired object.

L6805

L6805 Addition to terminal device, modifier wrist unit

Lay Description

A terminal device is the distal potion of an upper extremity prosthesis that replaces a missing hand in function, appearance, or both. Terminal devices are interchangeable and a patient may use different versions at different times. This device attaches to a modified wrist unit. Wrist units may be modified for use with designated sports or occupational equipment.

L6810

L6810 Addition to terminal device, precision pinch device

Lay Description
A precision grip is designed to perform more refined thumb and index finger movement. It allows the user to pinch or pick up small objects.

L6880

L6880 Electric hand, switch or myoelectric controlled, independently articulating digits, any grasp pattern or combination of grasp patterns, includes motor(s)

Lay Description
A terminal device is an addition to an upper extremity prosthesis that replaces a missing hand in function, appearance, or both. The device attaches to a base wrist unit. Terminal devices are interchangeable and a patient may use different versions at different times. Hands are more esthetic and allow finger position control. Myoelectric prostheses transmit electrical impulses from electrodes on the surface of the residual muscles to an electric motor that operates the terminal device. Myoelectric devices are heavier and more expensive than manual prostheses. Myoelectric devices use electrodes to generate muscle contraction strength controlling the function. Multi-articulating digits allow various finger and grip positions.

L6881

L6881 Automatic grasp feature, addition to upper limb electric prosthetic terminal device

Lay Description
A terminal device is an addition to an upper extremity prosthesis that replaces a missing hand in function, appearance, or both. The device attaches to a base wrist unit. Terminal devices are interchangeable and a patient may use different versions at different times. Electric prosthesis uses a small electric motor to provide movement. An automatic grasp feature in an electric hand monitors the shear force and the grip force and automatically adjusts the grip strength so that an object can be securely held within the hand even if its center of gravity changes.

L6882

L6882 Microprocessor control feature, addition to upper limb prosthetic terminal device

Lay Description
A microprocessor is a single integrated circuit that contains all the functions of a computer's central processing. In this instance, the microprocessor controls the terminal device attached to a prosthetic arm. Sensors determine the current parameters (weight load, position, etc.) of the prosthesis and send a message to the prosthesis that guides its subsequent motion. Greater control allows a more natural motion.

L6883-L6885

L6883 Replacement socket, below elbow/wrist disarticulation, molded to patient model, for use with or without external power

L6884 Replacement socket, above elbow/elbow disarticulation, molded to patient model, for use with or without external power

L6885 Replacement socket, shoulder disarticulation/interscapular thoracic, molded to patient model, for use with or without external power

Lay Description
A socket is the portion of a prosthesis that fits around the residual limb (or stump) and to which prosthetic components are attached. When the initial socket is created, a mold of the extremity is taken along with measurements and notations on cosmetic features. These codes are used to report replacement sockets created using patient models. The differentiation between these sockets is through which joint the amputation (disarticulation) occurred.

L6890-L6895

L6890 Addition to upper extremity prosthesis, glove for terminal device, any material, prefabricated, includes fitting and adjustment

L6895 Addition to upper extremity prosthesis, glove for terminal device, any material, custom fabricated

Lay Description
A terminal device is an addition to an upper extremity prosthesis that replaces a missing hand in function, appearance, or both. The device attaches to a base wrist unit. Terminal devices are interchangeable, allowing the patient to use different versions for different functions. A glove is put over the terminal device to enhance the appearance and protect the device from water and dirt. The gloves can be made from various materials, such as silicone or polyvinyl chloride (PVC). The gloves range from prefabricated gloves that may come in different skin shades to custom painted covers that closely match the patient's own skin, applying acrylic nails and even tattoos and hair to further customize the glove.

L6900-L6915

L6900 Hand restoration (casts, shading and measurements included), partial hand, with glove, thumb or one finger remaining

L6905 Hand restoration (casts, shading and measurements included), partial hand, with glove, multiple fingers remaining

L6910 Hand restoration (casts, shading and measurements included), partial hand, with glove, no fingers remaining

L6915   Hand restoration (shading and measurements included), replacement glove for above

Lay Description

Partial hand restoration replaces part of a hand. A mold is made of the affected hand and a glove is made with holes for any remaining fingers. Realistic looking custom fingers are created to replace the missing digits. The glove adheres to the hand by suction. The glove can be customized to closely match the patient's own skin, applying acrylic nails and jewelry on the prosthetic fingers to create a natural appearance.

L6920-L6925

L6920   Wrist disarticulation, external power, self-suspended inner socket, removable forearm shell, Otto Bock or equal switch, cables, 2 batteries and 1 charger, switch control of terminal device

L6925   Wrist disarticulation, external power, self-suspended inner socket, removable forearm shell, Otto Bock or equal electrodes, cables, 2 batteries and one charger, myoelectronic control of terminal device

Lay Description

These prostheses are replacement devices for an amputation at the wrist. This type of prosthesis uses a self-suspended inner socket to which a terminal device is attached. The socket and terminal device interface are covered by a removable forearm shell. The myoelectric prosthetic uses an external battery pack to supply power to electric motors and microprocessors that control the movement of the device in different directions. The myoelectric prosthetic has a more realistic appearance and provides the patient with increased function. Control of the device is through skin electrodes inside the socket of the prosthetic. They are able to detect and amplify the electrical activity of muscle groups left in the limb. These impulses are cycled though the microprocessor units and result in movement through electric motors. Switch control of the terminal device requires the user to toggle, nudge, or otherwise operate a switch to create movement in the terminal device.

L6930-L6935

L6930   Below elbow, external power, self-suspended inner socket, removable forearm shell, Otto Bock or equal switch, cables, 2 batteries and one charger, switch control of terminal device

L6935   Below elbow, external power, self-suspended inner socket, removable forearm shell, Otto Bock or equal electrodes, cables, 2 batteries and one charger, myoelectronic control of terminal device

Lay Description

These prostheses are replacement devices for a below-elbow amputation. This type of prosthesis uses a self-suspended inner socket to which a terminal device is attached. The socket and terminal device interface is covered by a removable forearm shell. A myoelectric prosthesis uses an external battery pack to supply power to electric motors and microprocessors that control the movement of the device in different directions. The myoelectric prosthetic has a more realistic appearance and provides the patient with increased function. The device is controlled through skin electrodes inside the socket of the prosthetic that can detect and amplify the electrical activity of muscle groups left in the limb. These impulses are cycled though the microprocessor units and result in movement through electric motors. Switch control of the terminal device requires the user to toggle, nudge, or otherwise operate a switch to create movement in the terminal device.

L6940-L6945

L6940   Elbow disarticulation, external power, molded inner socket, removable humeral shell, outside locking hinges, forearm, Otto Bock or equal switch, cables, 2 batteries and one charger, switch control of terminal device

L6945   Elbow disarticulation, external power, molded inner socket, removable humeral shell, outside locking hinges, forearm, Otto Bock or equal electrodes, cables, 2 batteries and one charger, myoelectronic control of terminal device

Lay Description

These prostheses are replacement devices for an amputation at the elbow. The myoelectric prosthetic uses an external battery pack to supply power to electric motors and microprocessors that control the movement of the device in different directions. The myoelectric prosthetic has a more realistic appearance and provides the patient with increased function. This type of prosthesis uses a self-suspended inner socket to which a terminal device is attached. The socket and terminal device interface are covered by a removable forearm shell. The device is controlled through skin electrodes inside the socket of the prosthetic that can detect and amplify the electrical activity of muscle groups left in the limb. These impulses are cycled though the microprocessor units and result in movement through electric motors. Switch control of the terminal device requires the user to toggle, nudge, or otherwise operate a switch to create movement in the terminal device.

L6950-L6955

L6950 Above elbow, external power, molded inner socket, removable humeral shell, internal locking elbow, forearm, Otto Bock or equal switch, cables, 2 batteries and one charger, switch control of terminal device

L6955 Above elbow, external power, molded inner socket, removable humeral shell, internal locking elbow, forearm, Otto Bock or equal electrodes, cables, 2 batteries and one charger, myoelectronic control of terminal device

Lay Description

These prostheses are replacement devices for an amputation above the elbow. The myoelectric prosthetic uses an external battery pack to supply power to electric motors and microprocessors that control the movement of the device in different directions. The myoelectric prosthetic has a more realistic appearance and provides the patient with increased function. This type of prosthesis uses a self-suspended inner socket to which a terminal device is attached. The socket and terminal device interface are covered by a removable forearm shell. The device is controlled through skin electrodes inside the socket of the prosthetic that can detect and amplify the electrical activity of muscle groups left in the limb. These impulses are cycled though the microprocessor units and result in movement through electric motors. Switch control of the terminal device requires the user to toggle, nudge, or otherwise operate a switch to create movement in the terminal device.

L6960

L6960 Shoulder disarticulation, external power, molded inner socket, removable shoulder shell, shoulder bulkhead, humeral section, mechanical elbow, forearm, Otto Bock or equal switch, cables, 2 batteries and one charger, switch control of terminal device

Lay Description

A switch controlled prosthesis device is an electronic device used as a replacement for an amputation through the shoulder joint. This type of prosthesis uses switches instead of muscle tightening to control the prosthesis. The switches are located inside the socket or harness and can be activated by pulling a harness or triggered by movement of a bony protrusion against the switch. An external battery pack is used to supply power to electric motors that control the movement of the device.

L6965

L6965 Shoulder disarticulation, external power, molded inner socket, removable shoulder shell, shoulder bulkhead, humeral section, mechanical elbow, forearm, Otto Bock or equal electrodes, cables, 2 batteries and one charger, myoelectronic control of terminal device

Lay Description

A myoelectric prosthesis is an electronic device used as a replacement for an amputation through the shoulder joint. This type of prosthesis uses an external battery pack to supply power to electric motors and microprocessors that control the movement of the device in different directions. The myoelectric prosthetic has a more realistic appearance and provides the patient with increased function. Control of the device is through skin electrodes inside the socket of the prosthetic. They are able to detect and amplify the electrical activity of muscle groups. These impulses are cycled though the microprocessor units and result in movement through electric motors.

L6970

L6970 Interscapular-thoracic, external power, molded inner socket, removable shoulder shell, shoulder bulkhead, humeral section, mechanical elbow, forearm, Otto Bock or equal switch, cables, 2 batteries and one charger, switch control of terminal device

Lay Description

A switch controlled prosthesis device is an electronic device used as a replacement for an amputation at the interscapulothoracic region, also referred to as a forequarter amputation. This type of prosthesis uses switches instead of muscle tightening to control the prosthesis. The switches are located inside the socket or harness and can be activated by pulling a harness or triggered by movement of a bony protrusion against the switch. An external battery pack is used to supply power to electric motors that control the movement of the device.

L6975

L6975 Interscapular-thoracic, external power, molded inner socket, removable shoulder shell, shoulder bulkhead, humeral section, mechanical elbow, forearm, Otto Bock or equal electrodes, cables, 2 batteries and one charger, myoelectronic control of terminal device

Lay Description

A myoelectric prosthesis is an electronic device used as a replacement for an amputation at the interscapulothoracic region, also referred to as a forequarter amputation. This type of prosthesis uses an external battery pack to supply power to electric motors and microprocessors that control the movement of the device in different directions. The myoelectric prosthetic has a more realistic appearance and provides the patient with increased function. Control of the device is through skin electrodes inside the socket of the prosthetic. They are able to detect and amplify the electrical activity of muscle groups. These impulses are cycled though the microprocessor units and result in movement through electric motors.

L7007-L7009

L7007   **Electric hand, switch or myoelectric controlled, adult**

L7008   **Electric hand, switch or myoelectric, controlled, pediatric**

L7009   **Electric hook, switch or myoelectric controlled, adult**

Lay Description

A terminal device is an addition to an upper extremity prosthesis that replaces a missing hand in function, appearance, or both. The device attaches to a base wrist unit. Terminal devices are interchangeable and a patient may use different versions at different times. Terminal devices may be passive or active. Passive devices more cosmetically resemble a hand and are usually less functional. Active devices provide some of the normal hand functions. These active terminal devices may be in the form of a hook or a hand. A hook is a metal device with two fingers that can be opened or closed and are usually made of aluminum or steel. Hands are more esthetic and allow finger position control. Body powered or manual prostheses use cables and gross limb movement to control the device. They are usually of moderate weight and cost. Electric hands may be switch activated or myoelectric. Myoelectric prostheses transmit electrical impulses from electrodes on the surface of the residual muscles to an electric motor that operates the terminal device. Myoelectric devices are heavier and more expensive than manual prostheses. Myoelectric devices can have one or two electrodes. The two electrode version has separate electrodes for flexion and extension. The one electrode version uses only one electrode for both flexion and extension with differing muscle contraction strength controlling each function.

L7040

L7040   **Prehensile actuator, switch controlled**

Lay Description

An actuator is a small mechanical device that converts energy into motion. In this case it controls the grasping action of a terminal device. It uses a switch rather than muscle signals to activate the device. The switches can be activated by movement of a residual digit or movement of a bony prominence against the switch. Another method to active the switch is by pulling on the suspension harness.

L7045

L7045   **Electric hook, switch or myoelectric controlled, pediatric**

Lay Description

A terminal device is an addition to an upper extremity prosthesis that replaces a missing hand in function, appearance, or both. The device attaches to a base wrist unit. Terminal devices are interchangeable and a patient may use different versions at different times. Terminal devices may be passive or active. Passive devices more cosmetically resemble a hand and are usually less functional. Active devices provide some of the normal hand functions. These active terminal devices may be in the form of a hook or a hand. A hook is a metal device with two fingers that can be opened or closed and are usually made of aluminum or steel. Hands are more esthetic and allow finger position control. Body powered or manual prostheses use cables and gross limb movement to control the device. They are usually of moderate weight and cost. Electric hands may be switch activated or myoelectric. Myoelectric prostheses transmit electrical impulses from electrodes on the surface of the residual muscles to an electric motor that operates the terminal device. Myoelectric devices are heavier and more expensive than manual prostheses. Myoelectric devices can have one or two electrodes. The two electrode version has separate electrodes for flexion and extension. The one electrode version uses only one electrode for both flexion and extension with differing muscle contraction strength controlling each function. This code represents the pediatric version of an electric hook, switch or myoelectric control.

L7170-L7191

L7170   **Electronic elbow, Hosmer or equal, switch controlled**

L7180   **Electronic elbow, microprocessor sequential control of elbow and terminal device**

L7181   **Electronic elbow, microprocessor simultaneous control of elbow and terminal device**

L7185   **Electronic elbow, adolescent, Variety Village or equal, switch controlled**

L7186   **Electronic elbow, child, Variety Village or equal, switch controlled**

L7190   **Electronic elbow, adolescent, Variety Village or equal, myoelectronically controlled**

L7191   **Electronic elbow, child, Variety Village or equal, myoelectronically controlled**

Lay Description

Electronic elbows are additions to arm prostheses that use an external power source, electric motor, and/or a microprocessing unit to enable the movement of the elbow in several different planes. Some allow the sequential or simultaneous movement of both the elbow and terminal device. Myoelectrically controlled devices use surface electrodes embedded in the socket to detect and amplify the electrical activity of muscle groups in the residual limb. The myoelectric impulses are then translated through microprocessors and electric motors into limb functions. Switch controlled motors allow a patient to move the prosthetic device using toggle switches or buttons. The switches can be toggled using the remaining muscles in a residual limb or by using the opposite shoulder.

L7259

L7259   Electronic wrist rotator, any type

Lay Description
Electric wrist rotator devices attach to an arm prosthesis and provide movement of the terminal device. Rotators provide pronation and supination of the terminal device and can sometimes allow for the opening and closing of the device. These devices are intended for use with the specific type of prosthetic device listed in the description.

L7360-L7368

L7360   Six volt battery, each

L7362   Battery charger, 6 volt, each

L7364   Twelve volt battery, each

L7366   Battery charger, twelve volt, each

L7367   Lithium ion battery, rechargeable, replacement

L7368   Lithium ion battery charger, replacement only

Lay Description
These codes are used to report supply of batteries and chargers for prosthetic devices. These battery systems fall into two major categories: primary or single-use batteries, which are cells containing lithium-metal anodes, and secondary or rechargeable batteries, which are systems utilizing lithium-ion chemistry. Nickel cadmium (NiCad) batteries are usually acceptable for air travel and have other advantages, but they tend to lose charge over time while not in use. All of these cells share the characteristics of high safety, reliability, energy density, and predictability of performance.

L7400-L7405

L7400   Addition to upper extremity prosthesis, below elbow/wrist disarticulation, ultralight material (titanium, carbon fiber or equal)

L7401   Addition to upper extremity prosthesis, above elbow disarticulation, ultralight material (titanium, carbon fiber or equal)

L7402   Addition to upper extremity prosthesis, shoulder disarticulation/interscapular thoracic, ultralight material (titanium, carbon fiber or equal)

L7403   Addition to upper extremity prosthesis, below elbow/wrist disarticulation, acrylic material

L7404   Addition to upper extremity prosthesis, above elbow disarticulation, acrylic material

L7405   Addition to upper extremity prosthesis, shoulder disarticulation/interscapular thoracic, acrylic material

Lay Description
These codes are used to report additions to upper arm prosthetics for amputations at various levels. Code selection is based on the material used for the addition. These codes should only be reported if a more specific HCPCS Level II code is not available.

L7499

L7499   Upper extremity prosthesis, not otherwise specified

Lay Description
An upper extremity prosthetic is used to replace function for a patient who is missing all or part of an arm or hand. This code is used to report an upper extremity prosthetic if there is not a more specific HCPCS Level II code available.

L7510

L7510   Repair of prosthetic device, repair or replace minor parts

Lay Description
Report this code for any minor materials (those without specific HCPCS codes) used as replacement parts or used to adjust and/or repair a prosthetic device.

L7520

L7520   Repair prosthetic device, labor component, per 15 minutes

Lay Description
Adjustments and repairs made to prostheses are billed as a labor charge using this code with one unit of service representing 15 minutes of labor time. The time reported must be only for laboratory repair time and associated prosthetic evaluation.

L7600

L7600   Prosthetic donning sleeve, any material, each

Lay Description
A donning sleeve is a cone-shaped sleeve that is used to help the patient place the residual limb into the prosthesis. It reduces the friction to allow the patient to more easily pull on the prosthetic liner or prosthetic. This code should be reported for a sleeve made out of any material.

L

L7900-L7902

L7900 Male vacuum erection system

L7902 Tension ring, for vacuum erection device, any type, replacement only, each

Lay Description

Vacuum erection systems are used to treat erectile dysfunction in men. In normal circumstances, sexual arousal in men causes blood to flow into the corpus cavernosum, the blood storage columns of the penis, which creates an erection for sexual activity. Erectile dysfunction occurs when blood flow is inadequate, sometimes in combination with defects in the natural blood trapping mechanism that allows an erection to be sustained. A vacuum device is usually a clear silastic cylinder that fits externally over the penis. A vacuum is created, manually or by an electronic pump, causing blood to be drawn into the penis. Typically a release valve on the device prevents too much vacuum pressure from building. A special elastic, metal, or leather ring is slipped around the base of the member, holding the blood within the erect penis. The vacuum pump is then removed. The ring is left on during intercourse and removed immediately afterward.

L8000-L8002

L8000 Breast prosthesis, mastectomy bra, without integrated breast prosthesis form, any size, any type

L8001 Breast prosthesis, mastectomy bra, with integrated breast prosthesis form, unilateral, any size, any type

L8002 Breast prosthesis, mastectomy bra, with integrated breast prosthesis form, bilateral, any size, any type

Lay Description

Mastectomy bras come in various materials and sizes to fit patients who have undergone a mastectomy. The bras provide support and shape, usually so that the patient looks the same as she did prior to the mastectomy.

L8010-L8031

L8010 Breast prosthesis, mastectomy sleeve

L8015 External breast prosthesis garment, with mastectomy form, post mastectomy

L8020 Breast prosthesis, mastectomy form

L8030 Breast prosthesis, silicone or equal, without integral adhesive

L8031 Breast prosthesis, silicone or equal, with integral adhesive

Lay Description

This range of codes reports the supply of specific breast prosthetics. A mastectomy sleeve is a full-length elastic support sleeve for the upper arm and axilla. Removal of lymph nodes during mastectomy surgery can cause lymphedema, fluid retention and swelling, in this instance in the axilla and upper arm region. Mastectomy sleeves address

this condition. Some may feature a shoulder cap and support straps around the upper torso; others just fit the arm and are held in place by the tensor properties of the fabric. Forms are external cosmetic breast devices that fit on the skin or onto garments following a patient's mastectomy surgery. Certain lightweight models may be made of silicone or other synthetics. Many designs adhere to the skin while others feature tabs to attach to bras or other garments.

L8032

L8032 Nipple prosthesis, reusable, any type, each

Lay Description

A nipple prosthesis, reusable, any type, is a washable self-sticking adhesive prosthesis formed in the shape of a human nipple. It can be used daily over several months. A nipple prosthesis allows post status nipple and breast reconstruction patients to feel whole again, by giving them natural looking breast. It is indicated for patients who undergo mastectomies and breast reconstruction, either prior to, or as an alternative to nipple reconstruction.

L8035-L8039

L8035 Custom breast prosthesis, post mastectomy, molded to patient model

L8039 Breast prosthesis, not otherwise specified

Lay Description

A custom fabricated breast prosthesis is individually made for a patient who is post-mastectomy status, starting with basic materials. This particular type of custom fabricated prosthesis involves using an initial impression of the chest wall to make a positive model of the chest wall. The breast prosthesis is molded on this positive model. Report the other code for a breast prosthesis that is not otherwise specified by other HCPCS codes.

L8040

L8040 Nasal prosthesis, provided by a nonphysician

Lay Description

A nasal prosthesis is a removable superficial prosthesis that restores all or part of the nose. It may include the nasal septum. Report this code when a nonphysician provides the prosthesis.

L8041

L8041 Midfacial prosthesis, provided by a nonphysician

Lay Description

A midfacial prosthesis is a removable superficial prosthesis that restores part or all of the nose plus significant adjacent facial tissue/structures but does not include the orbit or any intraoral maxillary component. Adjacent facial tissue or structures include one or more of the following: soft tissue of the cheek, upper lip, or forehead.

L8042

L8042 Orbital prosthesis, provided by a nonphysician

Lay Description
An orbital prosthesis is a removable superficial prosthesis that restores the eyelids and the hard and soft tissue of the orbit. It may also include the eyebrow. This code does not include the ocular prosthesis component.

L8043

L8043 Upper facial prosthesis, provided by a nonphysician

Lay Description
An upper facial prosthesis is a removable superficial prosthesis that restores the orbit plus significant adjacent facial tissue/structures but does not include the nose or any intraoral maxillary component. Adjacent facial tissue and structures include one or more of the following: soft tissue of the cheek or forehead. This code does not include the ocular prosthesis component.

L8044

L8044 Hemi-facial prosthesis, provided by a nonphysician

Lay Description
A hemifacial prosthesis is a removable superficial prosthesis that restores part or all of the nose plus the orbit and significant adjacent facial tissue/structures but does not include any intraoral maxillary component. This code does not include the ocular prosthesis component.

L8045

L8045 Auricular prosthesis, provided by a nonphysician

Lay Description
An auricular prosthesis is a removable superficial prosthesis that restores all or part of the ear.

L8046

L8046 Partial facial prosthesis, provided by a nonphysician

Lay Description
A partial facial prosthesis is a removable superficial prosthesis that restores a portion of the face but does not specifically involve the nose, orbit, or ear.

L8047

L8047 Nasal septal prosthesis, provided by a nonphysician

Lay Description
A nasal septal prosthesis is a removable prosthesis that occludes a hole in the nasal septum but does not include superficial nasal tissue.

L8048

L8048 Unspecified maxillofacial prosthesis, by report, provided by a nonphysician

Lay Description
Report this code for any materials used for repair or modification of a maxillofacial prosthesis provided by a nonphysician. This code is also used for a facial prosthesis that is not described by a specific code.

L8049

L8049 Repair or modification of maxillofacial prosthesis, labor component, 15 minute increments, provided by a nonphysician

Lay Description
Modifications or repairs of a maxillofacial prosthesis are reported using this code for the labor component by a nonphysician provider. Report the time in 15-minute increments. Time reported should be only for laboratory modification/repair time and associated prosthetic evaluation used only for services after 90 days from the date of delivery of the prosthesis.

L8300-L8330

L8300 Truss, single with standard pad
L8310 Truss, double with standard pads
L8320 Truss, addition to standard pad, water pad
L8330 Truss, addition to standard pad, scrotal pad

Lay Description
A truss is a supportive device mainly used for hernias. It can be a belt or a brief type garment that provides extra support where needed. A double truss would be used for a bilateral hernia. The pads that can add extra support and comfort can be added or replaced within the truss.

L8400-L8417

L8400 Prosthetic sheath, below knee, each
L8410 Prosthetic sheath, above knee, each
L8415 Prosthetic sheath, upper limb, each
L8417 Prosthetic sheath/sock, including a gel cushion layer, below knee or above knee, each

Lay Description
This range of codes reports supply of prosthetic sheaths. Many wearers of prostheses use nylon (or other artificial or natural fabric) sleeves over the residual limb to interface between skin and the socket

material. The sheath may be a stocking in the case of ankle/foot prostheses, although the term prosthetic sock refers to a sleeve that is closed on one end and may be used on either upper or lower extremity amputations. A special gel cushion layer may be used to improve the attachment capabilities of the socket. Sheaths and socks play an important role in adjusting for volume changes in the residual limb, and many products provide thickness padding against the socket.

L8420-L8435

L8420   **Prosthetic sock, multiple ply, below knee, each**

L8430   **Prosthetic sock, multiple ply, above knee, each**

L8435   **Prosthetic sock, multiple ply, upper limb, each**

Lay Description
The term prosthetic sock refers to a sleeve that is closed on one end and may be used on either upper or lower extremity amputations. The sock may be nylon, wool, or other artificial or natural fabric or blends. The sock plays an important role in adjusting for volume changes in the residual limb, and many products provide thickness padding against the socket. This thickness is expressed as a ply rating; generally one- to six-ply socks are most commonly available. By selecting a ply rating, usually in combination with liners, the wearer can adjust for changes in the size of the residual limb.

L8440-L8465

L8440   **Prosthetic shrinker, below knee, each**

L8460   **Prosthetic shrinker, above knee, each**

L8465   **Prosthetic shrinker, upper limb, each**

Lay Description
This range of codes reports the supply of prosthetic shrinkers, or stump shrinkers. These elastic stockings are usually applied shortly after amputation to control swelling of the residual limb and to prepare the site for a temporary prosthesis. Most shrinkers are made of elastic material, and the devices may be strapped on or simply held in place by the tensor properties of the fabric. Most devices are designed to mold and shape the site in preparation for eventual fitting of a prosthesis.

L8470-L8485

L8470   **Prosthetic sock, single ply, fitting, below knee, each**

L8480   **Prosthetic sock, single ply, fitting, above knee, each**

L8485   **Prosthetic sock, single ply, fitting, upper limb, each**

Lay Description
This range of codes reports the fitting of single ply prosthetic socks. The term prosthetic sock refers to a sleeve that is closed on one end and may be used on

either upper or lower extremity amputations. The sock may be nylon, wool, or other artificial or natural fabric or blends. The sock plays an important role in adjusting for volume changes in the residual limb, and many products provide thickness padding against the socket. This thickness is expressed as a ply rating. This range of codes reports only single-ply thickness fittings.

L8499

L8499   **Unlisted procedure for miscellaneous prosthetic services**

Lay Description
This code is used to report miscellaneous prosthetic services that are not described by more specific HCPCS Level II codes.

L8500, L8505

L8500   **Artificial larynx, any type**

L8505   **Artificial larynx replacement battery/accessory, any type**

Lay Description
An artificial larynx is a prosthetic speech device intended to assume some of the function of the natural larynx in the absence of the human organ. A natural larynx generates sound waves that become speech. It also controls the pitch and volume of the sounds. Air expelled from the lungs adds to the volume. The sound waves move from the larynx up the throat to the oral cavity where movement of the lips, teeth, palate, and tongue contribute to the final sound that emerges as speech. The artificial larynx may be electronically-controlled or pneumatically-controlled. It is held against the throat or cheek and creates sound that the user could then form into words. An electronically controlled larynx generates the sound by creating a battery driven vibration.

L8501

L8501   **Tracheostomy speaking valve**

Lay Description
A tracheostomy speaking valve is used for patients who have had a tracheostomy which is an incision in the anterior portion of the neck that opens a direct path to the trachea. A tube is usually placed in this pathway to maintain the opening. Following this procedure, patients are not able to speak normally because air is diverted through the tracheostomy tube and it doesn't pass through the vocal folds. Speaking valves can be attached to the tracheostomy tube to allow air to move through the tracheostomy tube but not out through it. This forces air around the tracheostomy tube, through the vocal cords and out the mouth upon expiration allowing the patient to speak. The vocalization may not sound like the patient's normal speech but allows a patient with a tracheostomy to be able communicate more effectively.

L8507-L8509

L8507 Tracheo-esophageal voice prosthesis, patient inserted, any type, each

L8509 Tracheo-esophageal voice prosthesis, inserted by a licensed health care provider, any type

Lay Description
A tracheo-esophageal voice prosthesis shunts air from the lungs into the esophagus and vibrates the esophageal tissue to produce speech sounds. These may be indwelling devices and are considered semi-permanent. The device is inserted into a tracheostoma and secured using flanges on the device. There is a one-way valve at the end of the prosthesis that is inserted into the esophagus that allows air to flow into the esophagus. The life span of a tracheo-esophageal voice prosthesis is three to six months after which it is replaced with a new device.

L8510

L8510 Voice amplifier

Lay Description
A voice amplifier is an external device worn or carried in a pocket, on a waistband, or in a similar manner that makes speech stronger and louder. This can be used by a person who has a weakened voice due to conditions such as vocal nodules, Parkinson's disease, Lou Gehrig's disease, multiple sclerosis, Guillain Barré, impairment of throat or chest muscles, damaged or partially paralyzed vocal cords, diminished lung capacity, artificial larynx users, and esophageal and TEP speakers. The device makes the voice louder and reduces the strain on the patient's voice.

L8511-L8515

L8511 Insert for indwelling tracheoesophageal prosthesis, with or without valve, replacement only, each

L8512 Gelatin capsules or equivalent, for use with tracheoesophageal voice prosthesis, replacement only, per 10

L8513 Cleaning device used with tracheoesophageal voice prosthesis, pipet, brush, or equal, replacement only, each

L8514 Tracheoesophageal puncture dilator, replacement only, each

L8515 Gelatin capsule, application device for use with tracheoesophageal voice prosthesis, each

Lay Description
An indwelling tracheo-esophageal voice prosthesis must be cleaned several times a day and replaced every three to six months. The tract that holds the prosthesis may need to be dilated periodically to maintain the diameter necessary for the prosthesis. Gelatin capsules aid in insertion as they dissolve within seconds and allow the prosthesis to expand and adhere to the anterior esophageal wall.

L8600

L8600 Implantable breast prosthesis, silicone or equal

Lay Description
A breast implant is a prosthesis used to modify the size, form, and feel of a woman's breast in a post-mastectomy reconstruction, improve chest wall congenital deformities, augment the breast, or perform gender transition (male to female). Breast implants are surgically placed in anatomical relation to the pectoralis major muscle.

L8603

L8603 Injectable bulking agent, collagen implant, urinary tract, 2.5 ml syringe, includes shipping and necessary supplies

Lay Description
Collagen is a protein based substance of strength and flexibility that is the major component of connective tissue, found in cartilage, bone, tendons, and skin. Collagen can be used as an implanted bulking agent to treat urinary incontinence due to intrinsic sphincter deficiency. A cystoscope is inserted into the urethra and the collagen is injected into and around the urethral sphincter to plump up the tissue and inhibit the urine leakage.

L8604

L8604 Injectable bulking agent, dextranomer/hyaluronic acid copolymer implant, urinary tract, 1 ml, includes shipping and necessary supplies

Lay Description
Dextranomer/hyaluronic acid is a bulking agent used to treat vesicoureteral reflux (VUR) in children. VUR occurs when there is a defect in the area where the ureters connect to the bladder. Dextranomer/hyaluronic acid is a biocompatible, biodegradable gel that is injected in the bladder near the opening of each ureter to prevent the flow of urine back into the ureter and kidneys. It is injected with the aid of a cystoscope.

L8605

L8605 Injectable bulking agent, dextranomer/hyaluronic acid copolymer implant, anal canal, 1 ml, includes shipping and necessary supplies

Lay Description
Dextranomer/hyaluronic acid is a bulking agent used to treat fecal incontinence in patients 18 years of age or older who have failed conservative therapy. Although the exact mechanism of action isn't known, it is theorized that it works by causing a chemical reaction within the body that may narrow the anal canal and expand the submucosal tissue, which in turn, allows better sphincter control. Using an anoscope, the physician injects 1 mL of the agent into

the submucosal layer of the anal canal in four different sites.

L8606

L8606   Injectable bulking agent, synthetic implant, urinary tract, 1 ml syringe, includes shipping and necessary supplies

Lay Description
Synthetic material such as copolymer can be used as a bulking agent to treat urinary incontinence due to intrinsic sphincter deficiency. A cystoscope is inserted into the urethra and the substance is injected into and around the urethral sphincter to plump up the tissue and inhibit the urine leakage.

L8609

L8609   Artificial cornea

Lay Description
An artificial cornea is used to treat patients who are not candidates for human donor corneas because of rejection or eye diseases that would interfere with a human cornea transplant. The cornea is made from a clear hydrogel center and surrounded by a mesh that allows the patient's tissue to secure the implant.

L8610

L8610   Ocular implant

Lay Description
An ocular implant is a spherical shaped device that can be implanted at the time of an eye removal or during a subsequent surgery. It is surgically implanted into the orbit to replace the lost volume and maintain the shape of the missing eye. It is inserted and the eye muscles are usually attached to it to allow it to move in conjunction with the other eye. This implant stays in place permanently. An artificial eye can be attached to the implant to restore a natural appearance.

L8612

L8612   Aqueous shunt

Lay Description
Aqueous shunts are small tubes used in surgery to treat glaucoma. Glaucoma is an eye disease that causes increased pressure in the eye. The increased pressure in the eye is caused by the inability of the aqueous fluid to drain normally. An aqueous shunt is surgically inserted into the anterior chamber of the eye. The shunt maintains an opening to allow drainage of the eye fluid. The fluid is absorbed into the body through the lymph nodes and blood system.

L8613

L8613   Ossicula implant

Lay Description
Ossicular implants are small surgically implanted components used to replace one or more of the ear ossicles. They can be made from various materials such as stainless steel, ceramic material, or Gelfoam.

L8614-L8629

L8614   Cochlear device, includes all internal and external components

L8615   Headset/headpiece for use with cochlear implant device, replacement

L8616   Microphone for use with cochlear implant device, replacement

L8617   Transmitting coil for use with cochlear implant device, replacement

L8618   Transmitter cable for use with cochlear implant device, replacement

L8619   Cochlear implant, external speech processor and controller, integrated system, replacement

L8621   Zinc air battery for use with cochlear implant device, replacement, each

L8622   Alkaline battery for use with cochlear implant device, any size, replacement, each

L8623   Lithium ion battery for use with cochlear implant device speech processor, other than ear level, replacement, each

L8624   Lithium ion battery for use with cochlear implant device speech processor, ear level, replacement, each

L8627   Cochlear implant, external speech processor, component, replacement

L8628   Cochlear implant, external controller component, replacement

L8629   Transmitting coil and cable, integrated, for use with cochlear implant device, replacement

Lay Description
A cochlear implant is a surgically implanted electronic device that provides a sense of sound to a person who is profoundly deaf or severely hard-of-hearing. A cochlear implant consists of one or more external microphones that pick up sound from the environment; an external speech processor that filters sound, splits it into channels, and sends the sound signals through a thin cable to a transmitter; and a transmitter, which may be a coil held in place by a magnet placed behind the external ear. The transmitter sends the power and sound to the internal receiver and stimulator that is surgically implanted in bone. The receiver and stimulator convert the signals into electric impulses and send them through an internal cable to an electrode array that winds through the cochlea. The cochlea transmits the impulses through the auditory nerve system to the brain. The external system may be worn entirely behind the ear or its parts may be worn in a pocket, belt pouch, or harness. These codes are used to report replacement pieces for the different components of a cochlear implant.

L8630-L8659

L8630 Metacarpophalangeal joint implant

L8631 Metacarpal phalangeal joint replacement, 2 or more pieces, metal (e.g., stainless steel or cobalt chrome), ceramic-like material (e.g., pyrocarbon), for surgical implantation (all sizes, includes entire system)

L8641 Metatarsal joint implant

L8642 Hallux implant

L8658 Interphalangeal joint spacer, silicone or equal, each

L8659 Interphalangeal finger joint replacement, 2 or more pieces, metal (e.g., stainless steel or cobalt chrome), ceramic-like material (e.g., pyrocarbon) for surgical implantation, any size

Lay Description

These codes are used to report implants in the hands or feet to restore function or relieve pain in those joints. Total joint replacements are usually comprised of two components that fit together to mimic joint function. They are made of various materials such a silicone or titanium or a combination of materials to best mimic joint function. A joint spacer does not replace the total joint. It is implanted into the interphalangeal joint for an interpositional arthroplasty.

L8670

L8670 Vascular graft material, synthetic, implant

Lay Description

A vascular graft consists of material used to patch a damaged, diseased, or injured area of an artery or for replacement of whole segments of vessels. Synthetic grafts are usually made from Dacron or polytetrafluoroethylene (PTFE).

L8679-L8689, L8695

L8679 Implantable neurostimulator, pulse generator, any type

L8680 Implantable neurostimulator electrode, each

L8681 Patient programmer (external) for use with implantable programmable neurostimulator pulse generator, replacement only

L8682 Implantable neurostimulator radiofrequency receiver

L8683 Radiofrequency transmitter (external) for use with implantable neurostimulator radiofrequency receiver

L8684 Radiofrequency transmitter (external) for use with implantable sacral root neurostimulator receiver for bowel and bladder management, replacement

L8685 Implantable neurostimulator pulse generator, single array, rechargeable, includes extension

L8686 Implantable neurostimulator pulse generator, single array, nonrechargeable, includes extension

L8687 Implantable neurostimulator pulse generator, dual array, rechargeable, includes extension

L8688 Implantable neurostimulator pulse generator, dual array, nonrechargeable, includes extension

L8689 External recharging system for battery (internal) for use with implantable neurostimulator, replacement only

L8695 External recharging system for battery (external) for use with implantable neurostimulator, replacement only

Lay Description

An implantable neurostimulator generator is a device that creates small electrical impulses that are transmitted to electrodes implanted near the spinal cord or a peripheral nerve. The small electrical impulses interrupt pain signals sent to the brain. The neurostimulator has either an external power source worn outside the body or batteries that can be implanted. A programmer allows signals to be sent to an internal receiver to adjust the neurostimulator impulses.

L8690-L8691, L8693

L8690 Auditory osseointegrated device, includes all internal and external components

L8691 Auditory osseointegrated device, external sound processor, replacement

L8693 Auditory osseointegrated device abutment, any length, replacement only

Lay Description

An auditory osseointegrated implant is a device that is implanted behind the patient's ear to provide hearing function for patients with a missing or diseased middle ear. It consists of an internal titanium implant that attaches to the temporal bone, an external abutment, and an external sound processor. The initial code for the osseointegrated implant includes all of the components. Occasionally, components of that implant may need to be replaced. Specific codes are used to report the replacement devices.

L8692

L8692 Auditory osseointegrated device, external sound processor, used without osseointegration, body worn, includes headband or other means of external attachment

Lay Description

This auditory osseointegrated device is an external device that produces amplified vibrational sound that is transmitted transcutaneously to the bones of the skull for transmission to the cochlea. This device is used for patients who are not candidates for implanted auditory osseointegrated systems. It consists of an adjustable headband to which the amplification disk is attached. The headband positions the device appropriately behind the ear.

L8699

L8699   Prosthetic implant, not otherwise specified

Lay Description

This code is used to report prosthetic implants that are not otherwise described in more specific HCPCS Level II codes.

L9900

L9900   Orthotic and prosthetic supply, accessory, and/or service component of another HCPCS L code

Lay Description

This code is to be used for an orthotic or prosthetic supply, accessory, and/or service that is a component of another HCPCS Level II code.

M

M0064

Lay Description

This code represents an office visit of a very short duration solely for the purpose of monitoring or changing drug prescriptions used for treating mental psychoneurotic and personality disorders. This code should be used when no other evaluation and management service is provided.

M0075

M0075   Cellular therapy

Lay Description

Cellular therapy is the practice of injecting humans with foreign proteins, such as those derived from the placenta or lungs of unborn lambs. Cellular therapy is currently without scientific or statistical evidence to document its therapeutic efficacy and, in fact, is considered a potentially dangerous practice.

M0076

M0076   Prolotherapy

Lay Description

Prolotherapy is also known as proliferative injection therapy or sclerotherapy. The practice of prolotherapy is used by physicians to treat a number of different types of chronic pain. Prolotherapy consists of a series of trigger point injections of "proliferative" solutions into ligaments and tendons near the pained area to induce the proliferation of new cells. Proponents of this treatment suggest that looseness in the

supporting ligaments and tendons around the joints causes the pain, inducing the muscles to contract against the ligament and irritate the nerve endings. Three types of solutions are used to initiate inflammation: chemical irritants (e.g., phenol), osmotic shock agents (e.g., hypertonic dextrose and glycerin), and chemotactic agents (e.g., morrhuate sodium, a fatty acid derivative of cod liver oil). These injections irritate or inflame the area where they are injected and are intended to mimic the natural healing process by causing an influx of fibroblasts that synthesize collagen at the injection site, leading to the formation of new ligament and tendon tissue. The newly produced collagen is intended to support the injured or loosened ligaments, creating a more stable and strong muscle base, in the process, alleviating pain.

M0100

M0100   Intragastric hypothermia using gastric freezing

Lay Description

Intragastric hypothermia using gastric freezing is an obsolete treatment for chronic peptic ulcer disease. The treatment is a non-surgical procedure designed to reduce or eliminate the production of gastric acid by freezing the secretory cells with a supercooled fluid introduced into a balloon positioned in the stomach. The treatment was popular about 20 years ago but now is seldom performed. Gastric freezing provided provides only temporary improvement to most patients. It has been largely abandoned due to a high complication rate and its lack of effectiveness in double-blind, controlled clinical trials.

M0300

M0300   IV chelation therapy (chemical endarterectomy)

Lay Description

Intravenous chelation therapy is infusion of a solution, traditionally a synthetic amino acid called ethylene diamine tetraacetic acid (EDTA). The EDTA binds with metals and minerals, which are then excreted from the body with the EDTA. This therapy, which removes unwanted metal ions from the body purportedly has therapeutic and preventative effects. Chelation therapy, when used as a treatment for atherosclerosis, is sometimes referred to as a chemical endarterectomy. The application of chelation therapy using EDTA for the treatment and prevention of atherosclerosis is controversial. There is no widely accepted rationale to explain the beneficial effects attributed to this therapy. Its safety is questioned and its clinical effectiveness has never been established by well-designed, controlled clinical trials.

M0301

M0301   Fabric wrapping of abdominal aneurysm

Lay Description
Fabric wrapping of an abdominal aneurysm is a treatment where the aneurysm is wrapped with cellophane or fascia lata. No other procedure is performed on the aneurysm or its surrounding tissue. The procedure has not been shown to prevent eventual rupture. In extremely rare instances, external wall reinforcement may be indicated when the current accepted treatment (excision of the aneurysm and reconstruction with synthetic materials) is not a viable alternative, but external wall reinforcement is not fabric wrapping. CMS believes that this treatment is ineffective and it is not covered by Medicare and many other payers.

P

P2028

P2028   Cephalin floculation, blood

Lay Description
Cephalin flocculation is a test performed on serum using cephalin or a cephalin-cholesterol emulation. The flocculation or dispersion of the blood into discrete visible particles may indicate the presence of liver cell disease. This test is considered obsolete.

P2029

P2029   Congo red, blood

Lay Description
Congo red is an odorless dark red or brown powder that decomposes upon exposure to acid fumes. It is used as a diagnostic aid in amyloidosis. The Congo red dye is injected intravenously. If after one hour more than 60 percent of the dye has disappeared, amyloidosis is indicated. This test is considered obsolete.

P2031

P2031   Hair analysis (excluding arsenic)

Lay Description
Laboratory analysis of hair may be used to detect the presence of drugs, chemicals, and other substances. Note that many insurance payers only cover hair analysis for the detection of arsenic. This code is used to report hair analysis, excluding arsenic.

P2033

P2033   Thymol turbidity, blood

Lay Description
Thymol turbidity is a test performed on serum using the chemical thymol. The serum precipitates into albumin and globulin, which can then be measured to look for indications of liver disease. Although popular in the past, it has been superseded by quantitative determination of specific proteins and direct

measurement of liver enzymes. This test is considered obsolete.

P2038

P2038   Mucoprotein, blood (seromucoid) (medical necessity procedure)

Lay Description
Mucoprotein is a general term for a protein-polysaccharide complex, wherein the protein component is the major part of the complex. The compound is present in all connective and supporting tissues. It is sometimes called glycoprotein, although this term usually refers to those mucoproteins that contain less than four percent carbohydrate. This code represents an assay of the mucoproteins contained in a sample of blood. Most testing performed currently are for a more specific component of the complex.

P3000-P3001

P3000   Screening Papanicolaou smear, cervical or vaginal, up to 3 smears, by technician under physician supervision
P3001   Screening Papanicolaou smear, cervical or vaginal, up to 3 smears, requiring interpretation by physician

Lay Description
A screening Papanicolaou (commonly referred to as Pap) smear, cervical or vaginal, is a microscopic examination of cells scraped from the cervix or vaginal wall. The smears are examined for any cells that appear to be abnormal. It is a screening procedure when no known disease process exists.

P7001

P7001   Culture, bacterial, urine; quantitative, sensitivity study

Lay Description
A culture is the inoculation and incubation of a growth medium. In this case, urine is inoculated onto a growth medium with the intention of determining the types and amounts of bacteria that grow. A sensitivity test follows. The bacteria that have been grown are tested against antibiotics to determine which antibiotic has the greatest efficacy against the bacteria. This code should be used only for urine cultures when both a culture and sensitivity are performed consecutively on the same specimen.

P9010-P9011

P9010   Blood (whole), for transfusion, per unit
P9011   Blood, split unit

Lay Description
Whole blood is blood without any component removed. Whole blood is the liquid medium containing the microscopic elements of erythrocytes (red blood cell), leukocytes (white blood cells), and thrombocytes (blood platelets). Whole blood is drawn from a selected donor under strict aseptic conditions.

The blood is usually mixed with a citrate ion or heparin to prevent coagulation. It may be banked and used as a replacement when blood is lost. Blood is classified into four phenotypes based upon the characteristics present: A, B, AB, and O. Additionally, an Rh factor of negative or positive is assigned, denoting the absence or presence of an Rh antigen. Before any blood, with the exception of type O negative, can be transfused into a patient, tests must be run to determine the compatibility of the donor blood with the patient's own blood. Type O negative is said to be the universal donor as this type of blood contains no factors that may adversely interact with the blood of the recipient. Due to the variety and number of incompatibilities that may exist, whole blood is used only when absolutely necessary and blood components are more routinely transfused.

P9012

P9012   Cryoprecipitate, each unit

Lay Description

Cryoprecipitate is the cold insoluble portion of plasma that precipitates (settles into solid particles) when fresh frozen plasma is thawed at 1-6 degrees C. The supernatant (or liquid plasma) is removed and the residual cryoprecipitate (approximately 15 ml) is refrozen and stored at -18 degrees C. A single unit of cryoprecipitate contains an average of 80-100 units of factor VIII and von Willebrand factor, 150-250 mg of fibrinogen and some factor XIII and fibronectin. No compatibility testing is required and typing is not necessary. When cryoprecipitate is ordered, units are thawed, suspended in sterile, normal saline (20ml/bag) and pooled. Cryoprecipitate is the only fibrinogen concentrate available for intravenous use. In the past, cryoprecipitate had been used as a treatment for von Willebrand's disease and hemophilia A. However, newer products are the treatment of choice now. Cryoprecipitate may also be used in the preparation of fibrin glue. This glue is used in neurosurgery, orthopedic, and other surgeries. Although widespread, such use is not FDA-approved. Autologous (the patient's own blood) units can be collected prior to surgery and processed into fibrin glue. This code represents one unit of cryoprecipitate.

P9016

P9016   Red blood cells, leukocytes reduced, each unit

Lay Description

Red blood cells (RBCs) are a singular component of whole blood. RBCs are prepared from whole blood by the removal of most of the plasma, or by apheresis collection. RBCs are stored in one of several saline-based anticoagulant/ preservative solutions, yielding a hematocrit (Hct) between 55-80 percent. Leukocytes (or WBCs) are reduced or removed from the unit as the leukocytes may provoke an adverse reaction or antibody formation when they interact with the patient's own blood. RBC transfusions increase the oxygen-carrying capacity of blood. Transfusions may also treat chronic anemia when pharmacologic therapy is not effective or available, active bleeding, Sickle cell disease, or other conditions. RBCs require compatibility testing. Transfusions should be completed within four hours per unit. A unit may be divided by the blood bank in advance and administered in two or more aliquots. This code represents one unit of RBCs.

P9017

P9017   Fresh frozen plasma (single donor), frozen within 8 hours of collection, each unit

Lay Description

Plasma is the liquid portion of whole blood. Plasma is prepared by separating it from whole blood using a centrifuge, or by hemapheresis using centrifugation or filtration. The volume of plasma varies and appears on the label. One unit of fresh frozen plasma contains the plasma from one unit of whole blood, approximately 250 ml, separated and frozen within eight hours of collection. While plasma may be pooled (multiple units of whole blood are separated and combined), this code represents plasma obtained from a single donor. Plasma contains all soluble clotting factors, though some may be substantially reduced, such as Factors V and VIII. Units of plasma transfused should be ABO compatible with the recipient, but crossmatching and Rh compatibility are not required. Plasma may be indicated in the treatment of thrombotic thrombocytopenic purpura and related syndromes, congenital or acquired coagulation factor deficiency when no concentrate is available, and for specific plasma protein deficiencies such as an anti-thrombin III or C-1 esterase deficiency. Plasma may also be indicated for bleeding, preoperative, or massively transfused patients with a deficiency of multiple coagulation factors, or for patients on warfarin therapy who are bleeding and/or who are facing urgent invasive procedures. This code should be used for one unit of fresh frozen plasma that was frozen within eight hours of its collection from a single donor.

P9019-P9020

P9019   Platelets, each unit
P9020   Platelet rich plasma, each unit

Lay Description

Platelets are thrombocyte cells removed from whole blood. Platelets may be separated from the whole blood of many different donors by the use of a centrifuge or may be harvested from a single donor by hemapheresis. Pooled random donor platelets are typically prepared from four to six units of random donor platelets. Platelet-rich plasma contains pooled amounts of platelets. Platelets may be suspended in donor plasma. Volume is specified on the label. Compatibility testing is not required, but units of platelets transfused should be ABO compatible when possible. Transfusion of large quantities of ABO-incompatible plasma may lead to a positive direct antiglobulin test and, rarely, clinically significant red cell destruction. Rh compatibility is important but not always possible. Platelets may be indicated for the prevention and treatment of nonsurgical bleeding due to thrombocytopenia and for patients with accelerated platelet destruction with significant bleeding (such as autoimmune or drug-induced thrombocytopenia), those with documented low-level platelet counts who are bleeding or who face major invasive procedures, and for patients with diffuse microvascular bleeding following cardiopulmonary bypass or massive transfusions.

P9021

P9021   Red blood cells, each unit

Lay Description
This code reports each unit of red blood cells. Whole blood is run through centrifugation where plasma (liquid portion of the whole blood) and red blood cells are separated. Red blood cells contain hemoglobin. Hemoglobin is a complex iron-containing protein that carries oxygen through the body and gives blood its red coloring. There are approximately 1 billion red blood cells in two to three drops of blood. Red blood cells are manufactured in the bone marrow.

P9022

P9022   Red blood cells, washed, each unit

Lay Description
Whole blood is run through centrifugation where the plasma (liquid portion of the whole blood) and the red blood cells are separated. Red blood cells contain hemoglobin. Hemoglobin is a complex iron containing protein that carries oxygen through the body and gives blood its red coloring. There are approximately one billion red blood cells in two to three drops of blood. Red blood cells are manufactured in the bone marrow. These red blood cells are washed with normal saline.

P9023

P9023   Plasma, pooled multiple donor, solvent/detergent treated, frozen, each unit

Lay Description
Plasma is the liquid portion of whole blood. Plasma is prepared by separating it from whole blood using a centrifuge, or by hemapheresis using centrifugation or filtration. The volume of plasma varies and appears on the label. One unit of fresh frozen plasma contains the plasma from one unit of whole blood, approximately 250 ml, separated and frozen within eight hours of collection. While plasma may be obtained from a single donor, this code represents plasma that has been pooled (multiple units of whole blood separated and combined). Plasma contains all

soluble clotting factors, though some may be substantially reduced, such as Factors V and VIII. Plasma may be "washed" or treated with a solvent or detergent to destroy any lipid bound viruses, including HIV1 and 2, hepatitis B and C, and HTLVI and II. The process does not destroy non-enveloped viruses or prion particles. Units of plasma transfused should be ABO compatible, but crossmatching and Rh compatibility are not required. Plasma may be indicated in the treatment of thrombotic thrombocytopenic purpura and related syndromes, congenital or acquired coagulation factor deficiency when no concentrate is available, and specific plasma protein deficiencies such as an anti-thrombin III or C-1 esterase deficiency. Plasma may also be indicated for bleeding, preoperative, or massively transfused patients with a deficiency of multiple coagulation factors, or for patients on warfarin therapy who are bleeding and/or who are facing urgent invasive procedures. This code should be used for one unit of plasma that has been pooled from multiple donors, solvent or detergent treated, and frozen.

P9031-P9037

P9031   Platelets, leukocytes reduced, each unit
P9032   Platelets, irradiated, each unit
P9033   Platelets, leukocytes reduced, irradiated, each unit
P9034   Platelets, pheresis, each unit
P9035   Platelets, pheresis, leukocytes reduced, each unit
P9036   Platelets, pheresis, irradiated, each unit
P9037   Platelets, pheresis, leukocytes reduced, irradiated, each unit

Lay Description
Platelets are the thrombocyte cells removed from whole blood. Platelets may be separated from the whole blood of many different donors by the use of a centrifuge, or may be harvested from a single donor by hemapheresis. Pooled random donor platelets are typically prepared from four to six units of random donor platelets. Platelet rich plasma contains pooled amounts of platelets. Platelets may be suspended in donor plasma. Volume is specified on the label. Compatibility testing is not required, but units of platelets transfused should be ABO compatible when possible. Rh compatibility is important but not always possible. Platelets may be leukocyte (white blood cell) reduced, which is the filtered removal of contaminating leukocytes. Platelets may be irradiated using gamma radiation to destroy the ability of lymphocytes (a type of leukocyte) to respond to foreign antigens, such as those in the recipient's blood. Leukocytes may provoke an adverse reaction or antibody formation in the patient's blood. They may also transmit certain viruses, including cytomegalovirus (CMV) and human T-cell lymphotropic virus (HTLV-I/II). Pheresis (apheresis) is a targeted removal of blood component from whole blood with the return of the remaining blood

components to the donor. Pheresis uses a centrifuge device to separate blood components. Plasma, platelet, and leukocytes are the components that may be removed using pheresis. The designated component (in this case platelets) is removed and the remaining blood components are retransfused into the donor. Platelets are indicated for the prevention and treatment of non-surgical bleeding due to thrombocytopenia, for patients with accelerated platelet destruction with significant bleeding (such as autoimmune or drug-induced thrombocytopenia), for patients with documented low level platelet counts who are bleeding or who face major invasive procedures, and for patients with diffuse microvascular bleeding following cardiopulmonary bypass or massive transfusions.

P9038-P9040

P9038   Red blood cells, irradiated, each unit
P9039   Red blood cells, deglycerolized, each unit
P9040   Red blood cells, leukocytes reduced, irradiated, each unit

Lay Description

Red blood cells (RBC) are a singular component of whole blood. RBCs are prepared from whole blood by the removal of most of the plasma, or by apheresis collection. RBCs are stored in one of several saline-based anticoagulant/ preservative solutions, yielding a hematocrit (Hct) between 55 to 80 percent. RBCs may be leukocyte (or white blood cell) reduced, which is the filter removal of contaminating leukocytes. RBCs may be irradiated using gamma radiation to destroy the ability of lymphocytes (a type of leukocyte) to respond to foreign antigens in the recipient's blood. Leukocytes may provoke an adverse reaction or antibody formation when they interact with the patient's own blood. They may also transmit certain viruses, including cytomegalovirus (CMV) and human T-cell lymphotropic virus (HTLV-I/II). Prior to freezing, glycerol may be added to the RBCs. When this glycerol is removed upon thawing, the RBCs are termed "deglycerolized." A major indication for RBC transfusions is prevention or treatment of symptoms of tissue hypoxia by increasing the oxygen-carrying capacity of blood. RBCs may also be indicated in the treatment of symptomatic chronic anemia when pharmacologic therapy is not effective or available, active bleeding with signs and symptoms of hypovolemia, preoperative anemia with impending major blood loss, Sickle cell disease, and anemia due to renal failure/hemodialysis. RBCs require compatibility testing and should be ABO and Rh compatible. The initial transfusion period may be carefully monitored with a slow transfusion rate to allow early detection of a reaction. Transfusions should be completed within four hours per unit. Alternatively, the unit may be divided by the blood bank in advance and administered in two or more aliquots.

P9041

P9041   Infusion, albumin (human), 5%, 50 ml

Lay Description

Albumin is a protein manufactured by the liver and carried throughout the body by plasma and is the most prevalent protein found in blood plasma. Plasma is collected and pooled, then fractionated to separate the albumin. Unlike other plasma proteins, albumin has several essential physiologic functions in the human body and is an important therapeutic agent. Albumin maintains the osmotic pressure that causes fluid to remain within the blood stream instead of leaking out into the tissues. It also transports thyroid hormone, drugs, and bilirubin. It increases total blood volume by drawing fluid from body tissues. Albumin may be indicated as a treatment for shock, hypovolemia, acute liver failure, burns and other thermal injuries, hypoproteinemia, adult respiratory distress syndrome, cardiopulmonary bypass, neonatal hemolytic disease, renal dialysis, acute nephrosis, erythrocyte, acute peritonitis, pancreatitis, and cellulitis. Albumin is available with varying concentrations of protein: 5 percent, 20 percent, and 25 percent. The recommended concentration and dosage depends upon the patient and reason for administration. It is administered by intravenous infusion.

P9043

P9043   Infusion, plasma protein fraction (human), 5%, 50 ml

Lay Description

Plasma protein fraction is a sterile solution of selected proteins derived from the blood plasma of adult human donors. It typically contains 4.5 to 5.5 grams of protein per 100 ml. This protein consists of 83 to 90 percent albumin, with the remainder alpha- and beta-globulins. Plasma protein fraction is the solution remaining once cryoprecipitate, fibrinogen, and immunoglobulins have been removed. Plasma protein faction is usually heat treated to destroy viruses. Indications for its use are similar to those for albumin. Administered intravenously, it increases total blood volume by drawing fluid from body tissues. Other indications include shock, hypovolemia, acute liver failure, burns and other thermal injuries, hypoproteinemia, adult respiratory distress syndrome, cardiopulmonary bypass, neonatal hemolytic disease, renal dialysis, acute nephrosis, erythrocyte resuspension, acute peritonitis, pancreatitis, mediastinitis, and cellulitis. This code represents 50 ml of a 5 percent concentration of plasma protein fraction.

P9044

P9044   Plasma, cryoprecipitate reduced, each unit

Lay Description

Cryoprecipitate reduced plasma is the solution remaining once the cold insoluble portion has been removed. Cryoprecipitate settles into solid particles when fresh frozen plasma is thawed at 1-6 degrees C. The liquid plasma removed is the cryoprecipitate-reduced plasma. Cryoprecipitate reduced plasma is deficient in Von Willebrand factor, Factor VIII, Factor XIII, fibrinogen, and fibronectin. It may be indicated for the treatment of thrombotic thrombocytopenic purpura. This code represents one unit.

P9045-P9047

P9045   Infusion, albumin (human), 5%, 250 ml
P9046   Infusion, albumin (human), 25%, 20 ml
P9047   Infusion, albumin (human), 25%, 50 ml

Lay Description

Albumin is a protein manufactured by the liver and carried throughout the body by plasma and is the most prevalent protein found in blood plasma. Plasma is collected and pooled, then fractionated to separate the albumin. Unlike other plasma proteins, albumin has several essential physiologic functions in the human body and is an important therapeutic agent. Albumin maintains the osmotic pressure that causes fluid to remain within the blood stream instead of leaking out into the tissues. It also transports thyroid hormone, drugs, and bilirubin. It increases total blood volume by drawing fluid from body tissues. Albumin may be indicated as a treatment for shock, hypovolemia, acute liver failure, burns and other thermal injuries, hypoproteinemia, adult respiratory distress syndrome, cardiopulmonary bypass, neonatal hemolytic disease, renal dialysis, acute nephrosis, erythrocyte, acute peritonitis, pancreatitis, and cellulitis. Albumin is available with varying concentrations of protein: 5 percent, 20 percent, and 25 percent. The recommended concentration and dosage depends upon the patient and reason for administration. It is administered by intravenous infusion.

P9048

P9048   Infusion, plasma protein fraction (human), 5%, 250 ml

Lay Description

Plasma protein fraction is a sterile solution of selected proteins derived from the blood plasma of adult human donors. It contains 4.5 to 5.5 grams of protein per 100 ml. This protein consists of 83 to 90 percent albumin with the remainder alpha-and beta-globulins. Plasma Protein Fraction is the solution remaining once cryoprecipitate, fibrinogen, and immunoglobulins have been removed from plasma. Plasma protein faction is usually heat treated to destroy HIV, hepatitis viruses, and CMV. Indications for its use are similar to those for albumin. Administered intravenously, it increases total blood volume by drawing fluid from body tissues. Other indications include shock, hypovolemia, acute liver failure, burns and other thermal injuries, hypoproteinemia, adult respiratory distress syndrome, cardiopulmonary bypass, neonatal hemolytic disease, renal dialysis, acute nephrosis, erythrocyte resuspension, acute peritonitis, pancreatitis, mediastinitis, and cellulitis. This code represents 250 ml of a 5 percent concentration of plasma protein fraction.

P9050

P9050   Granulocytes, pheresis, each unit

Lay Description

Granulocytes are types of leukocytes (white blood cells) consisting of neutrophils, basophils, or eosinophils. They are distinguished by the granules (insoluble nonmembranous particles) found within their cytoplasm. Granulocytes surround and destroy microorganisms. These granules within each cell are filled with chemicals, which upon their release, help to degrade the microorganism that the granulocyte surrounds. The cells are named for the way they stain in the laboratory. For example, eosinophils absorb acidic dyes such as eosin. Pheresis (apheresis) is a targeted removal of blood component from whole blood with the return of the remaining blood components to the donor. Pheresis uses a centrifuge to separate blood components. Plasma, platelet, and leukocytes are the components that may be removed using pheresis. The designated component (in this case granulocytes) is removed and the remaining blood components are retransfused into the donor. A standard adult concentrate contains approximately 20-50x109 granulocytes, 20-50 ml red blood cells, and 200-400 ml plasma. Granulocyte concentrates for neonates contain approximately 5x109 granulocytes in 30 µl plasma. Prior to the collection of granulocytes, donors are given G-CSF to stimulate their production. Granulocytes must be ABO and RH compatible with the recipient as there are large numbers of red cells in granulocyte concentrates. Granulocyte concentrates are always irradiated using gamma radiation to destroy the ability of lymphocytes to respond to foreign antigens, such as those in the recipient's blood. Granulocytes may be indicated as a treatment for infections that are unresponsive to antibiotic therapy.

P9051

P9051   Whole blood or red blood cells, leukocytes reduced, CMV-negative, each unit

Lay Description

Whole blood is blood without any component removed. Blood consists of plasma, or the liquid medium containing the microscopic elements of erythrocytes (red blood cells), leukocytes (white blood

P

cells), and thrombocytes (blood platelets). Red blood cells (RBCs) are a singular component of whole blood. RBCs are prepared from whole blood by the removal of most of the plasma, or by apheresis collection. RBCs are stored in one of several saline-based anticoagulant/ preservative solutions, yielding a hematocrit (Hct) between 55-80 percent. Both whole blood and RBCs require compatibility testing and should be ABO and Rh compatible. Leukocytes (or white blood cells) are reduced or removed from the unit as the leukocytes may provoke an adverse reaction or antibody formation when they interact with the patient's own blood. Cytomegalovirus (CMV) is a herpes type virus that is found universally throughout all geographic locations and socioeconomic groups, and infects between 50and 85percent of adults in the United States by 40 years of age. For most healthy persons who acquire CMV, there are few symptoms and no long-term health consequences. For the vast majority of people, CMV infection is not a serious problem. However, CMV infection is important to certain high-risk groups. These groups include pregnant women, people who work with children, and immunocompromised people, such as organ transplant recipients and persons infected with human immunodeficiency virus (HIV). Blood products intended for people in a high-risk group are usually tested for CMV. The major indication for RBC transfusions is prevention or treatment of symptoms of tissue hypoxia by increasing the oxygen-carrying capacity of blood. RBCs may also be indicated in the treatment of symptomatic chronic anemia when pharmacologic therapy is not effective or available, active bleeding, with signs and symptoms of hypovolemia, preoperative anemia with impending major blood loss, Sickle cell disease, and anemia due to renal failure/hemodialysis refractory to erythropoietin therapy. Due to the variety and number of incompatibilities that may exist, whole blood is used only when absolutely necessary and blood components are more routinely transfused. This code represents one unit of either whole body or RBCs that has been leukocyte reduced and has tested negative for the presence of the CMV virus.

P9052-P9053

P9052 Platelets, HLA-matched leukocytes reduced, apheresis/pheresis, each unit

P9053 Platelets, pheresis, leukocytes reduced, CMV-negative, irradiated, each unit

Lay Description

Platelets are the thrombocyte cells removed from whole blood. They may be separated from the whole blood of many different donors by the use of a centrifuge or may be harvested from a single donor by hemapheresis. Platelets may be suspended in donor plasma. Volume is specified on the label. Human leukocyte antigens (HLAs) are proteins located on the surface of white blood cells (WBCs) and certain tissues within the body. HLAs are inherited. There are three groups of HLA: HLA-A, HLA-B and HLA-DR. Each group contains many specific proteins, each labeled with a number (e.g., HLA-A1). Not every person possesses every type of protein (e.g., one person may be HLA-A1 and another HLA-A2). HLA testing determines the compatibility between the donor and recipient blood at the level of the A and B antigens. HLA-matched blood products are then crossmatched. HLA platelets are irradiated. Leukocytes (or WBCs) are reduced or removed from the unit, as the leukocytes may provoke an adverse reaction or antibody formation when they interact with the patient's own blood. Leukocytes may also transmit certain viruses, including cytomegalovirus (CMV) and human T-cell lymphotropic virus (HTLV-I/II). Pheresis (apheresis) is a targeted removal of blood component from whole blood with the return of the remaining blood components to the donor. Essentially, the blood is centrifuged to separate components, in this case the platelets. The remaining blood components are retransfused into the donor. Cytomegalovirus (CMV) is a herpes-type virus that is found universally throughout all geographic locations and socioeconomic groups, and infects between 50 and 85 percent of adults in the United States by 40 years of age. Most healthy persons who acquire CMV exhibit few symptoms and no long-term health consequences. Some persons may experience a mononucleosis-like syndrome with prolonged fever, and mild hepatitis. Once a person is infected, the virus remains alive, but usually dormant within that person's body for life. Recurrent disease rarely occurs unless the person's immune system is suppressed due to therapeutic drugs or disease. Blood products intended for people in high-risk groups are usually tested for CMV. HLA-matched platelets may be indicated for patients who have become refractory to random donor platelets. Use code P9052 for one unit of HLA-matched, leukocyte reduced platelets obtained via pheresis (apheresis).Use code P9053 for one unit of leukocyte reduced platelets that has been irradiated, has tested negative for CMV, and has been obtained via pheresis (apheresis).

P9054

P9054 Whole blood or red blood cells, leukocytes reduced, frozen, deglycerol, washed, each unit

Lay Description

Whole blood is blood without any component removed. Whole blood contains the microscopic elements of erythrocytes (red blood cells), leukocytes (white blood cells), and thrombocytes (blood platelets). Red blood cells (RBCs) are a singular component of whole blood. RBCs are prepared from whole blood by the removal of most of the plasma, or by apheresis collection. RBCs are stored in one of several saline-based anticoagulant/ preservative solutions, yielding a hematocrit (Hct) between 55-80 percent. Both whole blood and RBCs require compatibility testing. Leukocytes (or WBCs) are reduced or removed from the unit as the leukocytes may provoke an adverse reaction or antibody formation when they interact with the recipient blood. Glycerol may be added to the RBCs prior to freezing. When this glycerol is removed after thawing, the RBCs are termed "deglycerolized." Both whole blood and RBCs may be "washed" or treated with solvent to destroy any lipid bound viruses including HIV and hepatitis B and C. RBC transfusions increase the oxygen-carrying capacity of blood. Transfusions may also treat chronic anemia when pharmacologic therapy is not effective or available, active bleeding, Sickle cell disease, and other conditions. Due to the variety and number of incompatibilities that may exist, whole blood is used only when absolutely necessary and blood components are more routinely transfused. This code represents a unit of either whole body or RBCs that has been leukocyte reduced, frozen, deglycerolized, and washed.

P9055

P9055   Platelets, leukocytes reduced, CMV-negative, apheresis/pheresis, each unit

Lay Description
Platelets are the thrombocyte cells removed from whole blood. Platelets may be separated from the whole blood of many different donors by a centrifuge or may be harvested from a single donor by hemapheresis. Pooled random donor platelets are typically prepared from four to six units of random donor platelets. Platelet-rich plasma is plasma containing pooled amounts of platelets. Platelets may be suspended in donor plasma; volume is specified on the label. Compatibility type testing is not generally required. Rh compatibility is important but not always possible. Platelets may be leukocyte (or white blood cell) reduced, which is the filter removal of contaminating leukocytes. Leukocytes may provoke an adverse reaction or antibody formation when they interact with the patient's own blood. They may also transmit certain viruses, including cytomegalovirus (CMV) and human T-cell lymphotropic virus (HTLV-I/II). Blood products intended for people in a high-risk group are usually tested for CMV. Pheresis (apheresis) is a targeted removal of blood component from whole blood with the return of the remaining blood components to the donor. Essentially, the blood is centrifuged to separate components. Plasma, platelets, and leukocytes are components that may be removed by pheresis. The designated component, in this case platelets, is removed, and the remaining blood components are retransfused into the donor.

P9056

P9056   Whole blood, leukocytes reduced, irradiated, each unit

Lay Description
Whole blood is blood without any component removed. Blood consists of plasma or the liquid medium containing the microscopic elements of erythrocytes (red blood cell), leukocytes (white blood cells) and thrombocytes (blood platelets). Whole blood is drawn from a selected donor under strict aseptic conditions. The whole blood is usually mixed with a citrate ion or heparin to prevent coagulation. It is typically used as a replacement for blood loss. Blood is classified into four phenotypes based upon the characteristics present: A, B, AB, and O. Additionally, an Rh factor of negative or positive is assigned denoting the absence or presence of an Rh antigen. Tests are run to determine compatibility of the donor blood with the patient's own blood. Type O negative is said to be the universal donor, as this blood type contains no factors that may adversely affect or interact with the blood of the recipient. Whole blood may be leukocyte (white blood cell) reduced using a filter. Whole blood may be gamma irradiated to destroy the ability of lymphocytes (a type of leukocyte) to respond to foreign antigens, such as those in the recipient's blood. Leukocytes may provoke an adverse reaction or antibody formation when they interact with the patient's own blood. Due to the variety and number of incompatibilities that may exist, whole blood is used only when absolutely necessary and blood components are more routinely transfused.

P9057-P9058

P9057   Red blood cells, frozen/deglycerolized/washed, leukocytes reduced, irradiated, each unit
P9058   Red blood cells, leukocytes reduced, CMV-negative, irradiated, each unit

Lay Description
Red blood cells (RBCs) are a singular component of whole blood. RBCs are prepared from whole blood by the removal of most of the plasma, or by apheresis collection. RBCs are stored in one of several saline-based anticoagulant/preservative solutions, yielding a hematocrit (Hct) between 55 and 80 percent. RBCs require ABO and Rh compatibility testing. Leukocytes (white blood cells) are reduced or removed from the unit, as the leukocytes may provoke an adverse reaction or antibody formation when they interact with the patient's own blood. RBCs may also be gamma irradiated to destroy the ability of lymphocytes (a type of leukocyte) to respond to foreign antigens, such as those in the recipient's blood. Glycerol may be added to the RBCs prior to freezing. When this glycerol is removed after thawing, the RBCs are termed "deglycerolized." RBCs may be "washed," or treated with solvent, to destroy any lipid-bound viruses. Blood products intended for people in a high-risk group are usually tested for cytomegalovirus (CMV). RBC transfusions increase the oxygen-carrying capacity of blood. RBC transfusion may be indicated for symptomatic chronic anemia when pharmacologic therapy is not effective or available, active bleeding, preoperative anemia with impending major blood loss, and sickle cell disease,

P

among other conditions. Due to the variety and number of incompatibilities that may exist, whole blood is used only when absolutely necessary and blood components are more routinely transfused.

P9059-P9060

P9059 Fresh frozen plasma between 8-24 hours of collection, each unit
P9060 Fresh frozen plasma, donor retested, each unit

Lay Description
Plasma is the liquid portion of whole blood. Plasma is prepared by separating it from whole blood by centrifuge, or by hemapheresis using centrifugation or filtration. The volume of plasma varies and appears on the label. One unit of fresh frozen plasma contains the plasma from one unit of whole blood, approximately 250 ml, separated and frozen. Plasma may be pooled (multiple units of whole blood separated and combined). Plasma contains all soluble clotting factors, though some may be substantially reduced, such as Factors V and VIII. Units of plasma transfused should be ABO compatible with the recipient, but crossmatching and Rh compatibility are not typically required. Donors may be tested and retested for communicable diseases. Plasma may be indicated for a number of conditions and syndromes, including for preoperative or massively transfused patients with a deficiency of multiple coagulation factors.

P9603-P9604

P9603 Travel allowance, one way in connection with medically necessary laboratory specimen collection drawn from homebound or nursing homebound patient; prorated miles actually travelled
P9604 Travel allowance, one way in connection with medically necessary laboratory specimen collection drawn from homebound or nursing homebound patient; prorated trip charge

Lay Description
When a patient is unable to travel to the laboratory, some laboratories send technicians to a person's home or to a nursing home to collect the specimens necessary to perform a physician-ordered test. The laboratory may have a set travel fee that is charged for such collections, or it may charge by the number of miles traveled. HCPCS Level II code P9603 is used to report the actual number of one-way miles traveled. This mileage must be prorated or divided between all the patients that had specimen collection performed during one specific trip. Report P9604 when the laboratory has a set fee charged for each trip. This fee must also be prorated among the patients that had specimen collection performed during the trip.

P9612-P9615

P9612 Catheterization for collection of specimen, single patient, all places of service
P9615 Catheterization for collection of specimen(s) (multiple patients)

Lay Description
Patients who cannot produce a urine specimen when required for physician-ordered testing may need to be catheterized. Catheterization is the insertion of a small tube through the urethra to the bladder. Urine ordinarily flows freely through the tube, allowing for collection and testing. Catheterizations may be performed in hospitals, physician offices, nursing homes, or the patient's home.

Q

Q0035

Q0035 Cardiokymography

Lay Description
Cardiokymography involves the use of a noninvasive device to record the anterior left ventricle segmental wall motion. The device typically consists of a 5 cm diameter capacitive plate transducer as part of a high-frequency, low-power oscillator with recording probe. Changes in wall motion affect the magnetic field and thus the oscillatory frequency, which is then recorded on a multichannel analog waveform polygraph. Medicare and most payers cover this type of test only as an adjunct to electrocardiographic stress testing to evaluate coronary artery disease and only when specific clinical indications are present. For male patients there must be atypical angina pectoris or nonischemic chest pain. For female patients, there must be angina, either typical or atypical.

Q0081

Q0081 Infusion therapy, using other than chemotherapeutic drugs, per visit

Lay Description
Intravenous infusion is the administration of a liquid through the patient's veins for therapeutic or diagnostic purposes. This code should not be used for the infusion of any chemotherapeutic drug. This code should be reported only once per visit.

Q0083

Q0083 Chemotherapy administration by other than infusion technique only (e.g., subcutaneous, intramuscular, push), per visit

Lay Description
This code is used for the administration of chemotherapy by any technique other than infusion. Chemotherapy administration may include intramuscular or subcutaneous injection or a "push." A push is the direct intravenous injection of a drug

slowly over one to two minutes. Typically drugs that are pushed are not diluted with any type of intravenous solution (e.g., D5W, saline). Chemotherapy is the treatment of any disease with chemical agents, but commonly refers to the administration of anti-neoplastic drugs. This code should be reported only once per visit.

Q0084

Q0084   Chemotherapy administration by infusion technique only, per visit

Lay Description
This code is used for the administration of chemotherapy through the patient's vascular system for therapeutic purposes. Chemotherapy is the treatment of any disease with chemical agents, but commonly refers to the administration of anti-neoplastic drugs. This code should be reported only once per visit.

Q0085

Q0085   Chemotherapy administration by both infusion technique and other technique(s) (e.g. subcutaneous, intramuscular, push), per visit

Lay Description
This code is used for the administration of chemotherapy by both infusion and other techniques. Chemotherapy is the treatment of any disease with chemical agents, but commonly refers to the administration of anti-neoplastic drugs. This code should be reported only once per visit.

Q0091

Q0091   Screening Papanicolaou smear; obtaining, preparing and conveyance of cervical or vaginal smear to laboratory

Lay Description
A screening Papanicolaou (commonly referred to as Pap) smear, cervical or vaginal, is a microscopic examination of cells scraped from the cervix or vaginal wall. The smears are examined for any abnormal appearing cells. It is a screening procedure when no known disease process currently exists and the test is looking for any possible abnormalities. This code reports the collection and preparation of a screening vaginal or cervical Pap smear and includes the conveyance or transportation of the smear to the laboratory.

Q0092

Q0092   Set-up portable x-ray equipment

Lay Description
The set-up of portable x-ray equipment is the procedure of unpacking and readying portable radiologic devices for use. This code should only be used by portable x-ray suppliers when the equipment is transported and set-up in a place of residence used as the patient's home (such as a nursing home) or in a

nonparticipating institution. Portable x-ray services and their set-up must be performed under the general supervision of a physician and certain health and safety conditions must be met. Portable studies should be performed only when there is true medical necessity and when the patient cannot access or otherwise be examined on fixed conventional x-ray equipment. These studies should not be performed for "routine" purposes or for reasons of minor convenience. A set-up component can be paid for each radiological procedure (other than retakes of the same procedure) during single patient and multiple patient trips. This code should not be used when the portable x-ray supplier performs an EKG.

Q0111

Q0111   Wet mounts, including preparations of vaginal, cervical or skin specimens

Lay Description
A wet mount is the placement of a specimen on a microscope slide with the addition of a liquid. The liquid helps support the specimen and fills space between the cover slip and slide, which allows more light to pass and better visualization of the specimen. Wet mounts may be used for cervical, vaginal, and prostate smears, and examination of skin or feces specimens.

Q0112

Q0112   All potassium hydroxide (KOH) preparations

Lay Description
Potassium hydroxide (KOH) preparations are wet mounted slides where the added liquid is potassium hydroxide. The KOH dissolves cellular elements, such as skin cells, leaving only fungus and yeast visible.

Q0113

Q0113   Pinworm examinations

Lay Description
Pinworms are nematodes or round worms that live in the perianal area and migrate from the bowel to the skin to lay eggs. The eggs are very resistant to dehydration and can easily be dispersed into the air. Pinworm examinations involve the application of a special tape or swab at different times. The tape or swab is then examined for the presence of the pinworm or its eggs.

Q0114

Q0114   Fern test

Lay Description
A fern test is named for the pattern that the fluid takes when viewed under a microscope. The liquid crystallizes into a fern pattern. Cervical fluids may be analyzed in this manner to detect estrogen activity. As ovulation approaches, the pattern features more ferning. The test may also be used to detect amniotic fluid leakage in a pregnant uterus. A slide of vaginal

fluid is allowed to dry. Amniotic fluid crystallizes to form a fern-like pattern due to its concentrations of sodium chloride, proteins, and carbohydrates.

Q0115

Q0115 Postcoital direct, qualitative examinations of vaginal or cervical mucous

Lay Description
The microscopic analysis of cervical mucus may be performed within hours of timed intercourse in order to observe and evaluate the interaction of sperm, semen, and cervical mucus. A small sample is obtained and examined under a microscope to determine the quality of sperm and its interaction with the cervical mucosa.

Q0138-Q0139

Q0138 Injection, ferumoxytol, for treatment of iron deficiency anemia, 1 mg (non-ESRD use)

Q0139 Injection, ferumoxytol, for treatment of iron deficiency anemia, 1 mg (for ESRD on dialysis)

Lay Description
Ferumoxytol is an iron oxide used to treat low iron in patients with chronic kidney disease. It is coated with a carbohydrate layer that helps surround the iron from the plasma until it can be used for hemoglobin. The recommended dose starts with 510 mg with a follow-up injection three to eight days later. Ferumoxytol is administered as an IV injection.

Q0144

Q0144 Azithromycin dihydrate, oral, capsules/powder, 1 g

Lay Description
Azithromycin dehydrate is an antibiotic indicated for use in patient's with mild to moderate infections caused by susceptible strains of various microorganisms. Indications include pneumonia, pharyngitis and tonsillitis, staph and strep skin infections, cervicitis and urethritis due to gonorrhea and chlamydia, and genital ulcers. This code represents one gram of the oral tablets or powder.

Q0161

Q0161 Chlorpromazine hydrochloride, 5 mg, oral, FDA approved prescription anti-emetic, for use as a complete therapeutic substitute for an IV anti-emetic at the time of chemotherapy treatment, not to exceed a 48 hour dosage regimen

Lay Description
Chlorpromazine hydrochloride (HCl) is used in the treatment of manic psychosis, preoperative sedation, acute intermittent porphyria, an adjunct treatment for

tetanus, intractable hiccups, some behavior problems in children, and nausea and vomiting. The main pharmacological actions are psychotropic. The mechanism of action is not known. It has a sedative and antiemetic effect.

Q0162

Q0162 Ondansetron 1 mg, oral, FDA approved prescription antiemetic, for use as a complete therapeutic substitute for an IV antiemetic at the time of chemotherapy treatment, not to exceed a 48 hour dosage regimen

Lay Description
Ondansetron hydrochloride is a chemical compound that is a selective blocker of serotonin 5-HT3 receptors. It is an antiemetic drug available in oral and injectable forms. Serotonin 5-HT3 receptors are present on the vagal nerve and at sensory nerve endings. Cytotoxic chemotherapy appears to trigger the release of serotonin in the small intestine, which may trigger the 5-HT3 receptors and initiate the vomiting reflex. Ondansetron hydrochloride is indicated for the prevention of nausea and vomiting associated with surgery and antineoplastic drugs. The oral version is also indicated for the prevention of nausea and vomiting associated with radiation therapy. The drug is available in oral and injectable versions. The recommended dose is 4 mg or 0.1 mg/kg of body weight administered by intravenous or intramuscular injection. Dosages for the oral version vary from 8 to 24 mg depending on the indication and patient. This code should be used to report ondansetron hydrochloride for use as a complete therapeutic substitute for an IV antiemetic at the time of chemotherapy treatment, not to exceed a 48 hour dosage regimen.

Q0163

Q0163 Diphenhydramine HCI, 50 mg, oral, FDA approved prescription antiemetic, for use as a complete therapeutic substitute for an IV antiemetic at time of chemotherapy treatment not to exceed a 48-hour dosage regimen

Lay Description
Diphenhydramine hydrochloride is an antihistamine, a histamine receptor antagonist that has anticholinergic, antitussive, antiemetic, antivertigo, antipruritic, antidyskinetic, and sedative effects. It blocks the effects of histamine on the smooth muscle of the bronchial tubes, GI tract, uterus, and blood vessels. It also acts as a local anesthetic by preventing transmission of nerve impulses. Diphenhydramine hydrochloride is indicated for the treatment of anaphylaxis, Parkinsonism when the patient cannot tolerate other medications, drug-induced extrapyramidal disorders, motion sickness, allergies, vertigo, and insomnia, and to suppress nausea and prevent vomiting. Its antiemetic effects allow it to be

prescribed to treat nausea and vomiting associated with chemotherapy. Diphenhydramine hydrochloride is available in self-administrable oral forms and in an injectable form. The injectable form is administered by intramuscular or intravenous injection.

Q0164

Q0164 Prochlorperazine maleate, 5 mg, oral, FDA approved prescription antiemetic, for use as a complete therapeutic substitute for an IV antiemetic at the time of chemotherapy treatment, not to exceed a 48-hour dosage regimen

Lay Description
Prochlorperazine/prochlorperazine maleate is an antiemetic used for severe nausea and vomiting, such as that associated with the administration of chemotherapy and prior to induction of anesthesia to control nausea and vomiting during and after surgery. The drug inhibits nausea and vomiting by acting on the chemoreceptor trigger zone and partially depresses the vomiting center. Prochlorperazine is also indicated for treating adult psychiatric illnesses including schizophrenia, non-psychotic anxiety, and mild psychotic disorders. Prochlorperazine is available in injection form for intramuscular (IM) and intravenous (IV) use, in tablets, extended release capsules and syrup for oral administration, and in suppository form. The dosage, route of administration, and frequency of administration depends on the patient's diagnosis, the severity of symptoms, and, in the injectable form, by the patient's weight. Parenteral adult doses range from 2.5 to 10 mg at no more than 5 mg/minute IV for adults or 5 to 20 mg IM. The maximum parenteral adult dose is 40 mg a day. The drug should be injected or infused slowly. For children, 0.132 mg/kg may be administered IM. Oral doses range from 5 to 10 mg three or four times a day for tablets, or for extended-release capsules, 15 mg daily or 10 mg every 12 hours.

Q0166

Q0166 Granisetron HCl, 1 mg, oral, FDA approved prescription antiemetic, for use as a complete therapeutic substitute for an IV antiemetic at the time of chemotherapy treatment, not to exceed a 24-hour dosage regimen

Lay Description
An antiemetic is a drug given to suppress nausea and prevent vomiting. Patients receiving chemotherapy treatment have to contend with a great deal of nausea and vomiting as a side-effect and are given an antiemetic at the time of treatment. These codes all report FDA-approved prescription antiemetics to be taken orally, for use as a complete therapeutic substitute for an antiemetic given by IV injection at the time of therapy, not to exceed a 48-hour dosage regimen.

Q0167

Q0167 Dronabinol, 2.5 mg, oral, FDA approved prescription antiemetic, for use as a complete therapeutic substitute for an IV antiemetic at the time of chemotherapy treatment, not to exceed a 48-hour dosage regimen

Lay Description
Dronabinol is a cannabinoid with an active ingredient that is found in marijuana. It is used to treat anorexia associated with weight loss in patients with AIDS and nausea and vomiting for patients on chemotherapy. Dronabinol may be used as a complete therapeutic substitute for intravenous antiemetic therapy at the time of a chemotherapy treatment. When used to treat anorexia associated with AIDS or as a prolonged treatment for nausea and vomiting for patients on chemotherapy, an initial dose of 2.5 mg of dronabinol is administered before lunch and dinner. This can be gradually increased to 20 mg per day. Dronabinol is administered orally.

Q0169

Q0169 Promethazine HCl, 12.5 mg, oral, FDA approved prescription antiemetic, for use as a complete therapeutic substitute for an IV antiemetic at the time of chemotherapy treatment, not to exceed a 48-hour dosage regimen

Lay Description
Promethazine hydrochloride is a phenothiazine derivative with antihistamine, sedative, antiemetic, and anticholinergic properties. The drug binds to histamine receptors preventing the histamine from dilating capillaries, constricting the bronchial smooth muscles, and increasing gastric secretions. Promethazine hydrochloride is indicated as an antiemetic, a sedative in anesthesia, as a treatment for motion sickness, and for allergic reactions, including rhinitis and pruritic skin reactions. The drug may be combined with other drugs in cough and cold preparations. Promethazine hydrochloride is available in injectable, oral, and rectal suppository forms. The injectable form is administered by intramuscular or intravenous injection. Dosage varies from 25 to 50 mg.

Q0173

Q0173 Trimethobenzamide HCl, 250 mg, oral, FDA approved prescription antiemetic, for use as a complete therapeutic substitute for an IV antiemetic at the time of chemotherapy treatment, not to exceed a 48-hour dosage regimen

Lay Description
Trimethobenzamide hydrochloride (HCl) is an antiemetic used to alleviate nausea and vomiting. The mechanism of action is not known but it appears to act on the chemoreceptor trigger zone (CTZ) in the

brain where vomiting impulses are transmitted. It can be administered via intramuscular injection. Trimethobenzamide HCl also comes in capsule and suppository forms.

Q0174

Q0174 Thiethylperazine maleate, 10 mg, oral, FDA approved prescription antiemetic, for use as a complete therapeutic substitute for an IV antiemetic at the time of chemotherapy treatment, not to exceed a 48-hour dosage regimen

Lay Description

Thiethylperazine maleate is indicated for the relief of nausea and vomiting. The exact mechanism of action is not known. However, it appears to have an effect on the vomiting center and the chemoreceptor trigger zone (CTZ) of the brain. Recommended oral dose is 10 to 30 mg a day. Thiethylperazine maleate can be administered orally or by intramuscular injection. Recommended intramuscular injection dose is 10 mg one to three times a day.

Q0175

Q0175 Perphenazine, 4 mg, oral, FDA approved prescription antiemetic, for use as a complete therapeutic substitute for an IV antiemetic at the time of chemotherapy treatment, not to exceed a 48 hour dosage regimen

Lay Description

Perphenazine is used in treating psychosis and severe nausea and vomiting. The mechanism of action is not known. However, it does have an effect on the entire central nervous system particularly the hypothalamus. Dose is based on the condition and response of the patient. Perphenazine is administered orally.

Q0177

Q0177 Hydroxyzine pamoate, 25 mg, oral, FDA approved prescription antiemetic, for use as a complete therapeutic substitute for an IV antiemetic at the time of chemotherapy treatment, not to exceed a 48-hour dosage regimen

Lay Description

Hydroxyzine is a piperazine derivative that has central nervous system depressant, antispasmodic, antihistamine, and antifibrillatory properties. It is used to treat a variety of conditions such as anxiety, pruritus from allergies, psychiatric and emotional emergencies, and nausea and vomiting. Hydroxyzine may be used as a complete therapeutic substitute for intravenous antiemetic therapy at the time of a chemotherapy treatment. It is often used as a preoperative medication. It tends to increase the effect of meperidine and barbiturates. It can be administered via intravenous push, intramuscular

injection, or orally. Hydroxyzine hydrochloride is used to treat anxiety, manifestations of allergic dermatoses, as an antiemetic, and as a preoperative medication. It is administered by intramuscular injection or orally. Hydroxyzine pamoate has uses similar to the hydrochloride version. The pamoate version is administered orally.

Q0180

Q0180 Dolasetron mesylate, 100 mg, oral, FDA approved prescription antiemetic, for use as a complete therapeutic substitute for an IV antiemetic at the time of chemotherapy treatment, not to exceed a 24-hour dosage regimen

Lay Description

Dolasetron mesylate is an antiemetic drug with a chemical compound that is a selective blocker of serotonin 5-HT3 receptors. Serotonin 5-HT3 receptors are present on the vagal nerve and at sensory nerve endings. Cytotoxic chemotherapy appears to trigger the release of serotonin in the small intestine, which may trigger the 5-HT3 receptors and initiate the vomiting reflex. It is indicated to prevent and treat nausea and vomiting associated with chemotherapy or surgery.

Q0181

Q0181 Unspecified oral dosage form, FDA approved prescription antiemetic, for use as a complete therapeutic substitute for an IV antiemetic at the time of chemotherapy treatment, not to exceed a 48-hour dosage regimen

Lay Description

Oral antiemetic drugs are a therapeutic substitute for intravenous antiemetic drugs. Oral antiemetic drugs help patients better tolerate the effects of chemotherapy. Report this code for an unspecified oral dosage of an antiemetic drug used as a complete therapeutic substitute for an IV antiemetic at the time of chemotherapy treatment.

Q0478-Q0509

Q0478 Power adapter for use with electric or electric/pneumatic ventricular assist device, vehicle type

Q0479 Power module for use with electric or electric/pneumatic ventricular assist device, replacement only

Q0480 Driver for use with pneumatic ventricular assist device, replacement only

Q0481 Microprocessor control unit for use with electric ventricular assist device, replacement only

Q0482 Microprocessor control unit for use with electric/pneumatic combination ventricular assist device, replacement only

Q0483 Monitor/display module for use with electric ventricular assist device, replacement only

Q0484 Monitor/display module for use with electric or electric/pneumatic ventricular assist device, replacement only

Q0485 Monitor control cable for use with electric ventricular assist device, replacement only

Q0486 Monitor control cable for use with electric/pneumatic ventricular assist device, replacement only

Q0487 Leads (pneumatic/electrical) for use with any type electric/pneumatic ventricular assist device, replacement only

Q0488 Power pack base for use with electric ventricular assist device, replacement only

Q0489 Power pack base for use with electric/pneumatic ventricular assist device, replacement only

Q0490 Emergency power source for use with electric ventricular assist device, replacement only

Q0491 Emergency power source for use with electric/pneumatic ventricular assist device, replacement only

Q0492 Emergency power supply cable for use with electric ventricular assist device, replacement only

Q0493 Emergency power supply cable for use with electric/pneumatic ventricular assist device, replacement only

Q0494 Emergency hand pump for use with electric or electric/pneumatic ventricular assist device, replacement only

Q0495 Battery/power pack charger for use with electric or electric/pneumatic ventricular assist device, replacement only

Q0496 Battery, other than lithium-ion, for use with electric or electric/pneumatic ventricular assist device, replacement only

Q0497 Battery clips for use with electric or electric/pneumatic ventricular assist device, replacement only

Q0498 Holster for use with electric or electric/pneumatic ventricular assist device, replacement only

Q0499 Belt/vest/bag for use to carry external peripheral components of any type ventricular assist device, replacement only

Q0500 Filters for use with electric or electric/pneumatic ventricular assist device, replacement only

Q0501 Shower cover for use with electric or electric/pneumatic ventricular assist device, replacement only

Q0502 Mobility cart for pneumatic ventricular assist device, replacement only

Q0503 Battery for pneumatic ventricular assist device, replacement only, each

Q0504 Power adapter for pneumatic ventricular assist device, replacement only, vehicle type

Q0506 Battery, lithium-ion, for use with electric or electric/pneumatic ventricular assist device, replacement only

Q0507 Miscellaneous supply or accessory for use with an external ventricular assist device

Q0508 Miscellaneous supply or accessory for use with an implanted ventricular assist device

Q0509 Miscellaneous supply or accessory for use with any implanted ventricular assist device for which payment was not made under Medicare Part A

Lay Description
A ventricular assist device (VAD) is a mechanical device that compresses the heart to aid pumping function in patients with heart failure. The device is implanted into the chest and connects to an external controlling mechanism. The codes listed above are used to report the replacement of various components of the VAD.

Q0510-Q0512

Q0510 Pharmacy supply fee for initial immunosuppressive drug(s), first month following transplant

Q0511 Pharmacy supply fee for oral anticancer, oral antiemetic, or immunosuppressive drug(s); for the first prescription in a 30-day period

Q0512 Pharmacy supply fee for oral anticancer, oral antiemetic, or immunosuppressive drug(s); for a subsequent prescription in a 30-day period

Lay Description
Medicare pays a dispensing or supplying fee for immunosuppressive drugs, oral anti-cancer chemotherapeutic drugs, and oral anti-emetic drugs used as part of an anti-cancer chemotherapeutic regimen. These fees are payable to a pharmacy, dialysis facility in the state of Washington, or any hospital outpatient department not subject to the OPPS for each supplied prescription of the above-mentioned drugs. Medicare also pays a separately billable supplying fee of $50 for the initial supplied prescription of immunosuppressive drugs during the first month following a patient's transplant. When multiple prescriptions are supplied in a 30-day period, Medicare will pay $24 for the first prescription of the above-mentioned drugs, and $16 for each subsequent prescription. A pharmacy will be limited to one $24 fee per 30-day period even if the pharmacy supplies drugs from more than one of the above-mentioned categories to a beneficiary (e.g., an

oral-anticancer drug and an oral anti-emetic drug). Supply fees and dispensing fees must be billed on the same claim as the drug.

Q0513-Q0514

Q0513 Pharmacy dispensing fee for inhalation drug(s); per 30 days

Q0514 Pharmacy dispensing fee for inhalation drug(s); per 90 days

Lay Description
Medicare pays a dispensing or supplying fee for inhalation drugs furnished through durable medical equipment. Medicare will pay a dispensing fee of $57 to a pharmacy for the initial 30-day period of inhalation drugs furnished through DME, regardless of the number of shipments or drugs dispensed or the number of pharmacies used by a beneficiary during that time. This is a one-time fee applicable only to someone who is using inhalation drugs for the first time as a Medicare beneficiary. Subsequently, Medicare will pay a dispensing fee of $33 to a pharmacy/supplier for each 30-day supply of inhalation drugs furnished through DME, regardless of the number of shipments or drugs dispensed during the 30-day period. Medicare will pay a dispensing fee of $66 to a pharmacy/supplier for each 90-day period of inhalation drugs furnished through DME, regardless of the number of shipments or drugs dispensed during the 90 days. Only one 30-day dispensing fee will be payable per 30-day period, and only one 90-day dispensing fee will be payable per 90-day period, regardless of the number of suppliers used. A 30-day and 90-day supplying fee cannot be applied to drugs supplied for the same month. Medicare will not pay separately for compounding drugs; this cost is in the dispensing fees. Supply fees and dispensing fees must be billed on the same claim as the drug.

Q0515

Q0515 Injection, sermorelin acetate, 1 mcg

Lay Description
Sermorelin acetate is a synthetic peptide that contains a portion of the 191 amino acids that compromise natural human growth hormone (HGH). The drug stimulates the pituitary gland to produce HGH. HGH has a direct effect on the metabolism of protein, carbohydrates, and fat and controls skeletal and visceral growth. Sermorelin acetate is used in the diagnosis of HGH deficiencies and is indicated for the treatment of idiopathic HGH deficiency in children with growth failure. Treatment with sermorelin acetate should begin at a bone age of younger than 7.5 years for females and younger than 8 years for males and should be discontinued when the epiphyses are fused. The drug is administered subcutaneously daily at a dosage of 30 mcg per kg body weight and may be self-administered.

Q1004-Q1005

Q1004 New technology, intraocular lens, category 4 as defined in Federal Register notice

Q1005 New technology, intraocular lens, category 5 as defined in Federal Register notice

Lay Description
Cataracts are the clouding of the crystalline lens of the eye, which obstructs vision. An intraocular lens (IOL) is usually placed during or subsequent to cataract extraction. New-technology intraocular lenses (NTIOL) are FDA-approved prosthetic implants that demonstrate clinical advantages and superiority over existing intraocular lenses. The FDA, based upon published clinical data, determines if a lens has clinical advantages and superiority over existing IOLs with regard to reduced risk of intraoperative or postoperative complication or trauma, accelerated postoperative recovery, reduced induced astigmatism, improved postoperative visual acuity, more stable postoperative vision, or other comparable clinical advantages. Each subset or category of NTIOLs is separated into groups that meet the criteria for being treated as NTIOLs and share a common feature that distinguishes them from other IOLs. For example, all new-technology IOLs that are made of a particular bioengineered material could make up one subset, while all that rely on a particular optical innovation would encompass another. Any assignment and definition of the categories of four and five will be announced in the *Federal Register* notice prior to their use.

Q2004

Q2004 Irrigation solution for treatment of bladder calculi, for example renacidin, per 500 ml

Lay Description
Irrigation solution for treatment of bladder calculi is a liquid containing various minerals and weak acids that is used to irrigate or wash calculi from the bladder. The solution acts upon the stones by dissolving portions or all of the calculi.

Q2009

Q2009 Injection, fosphenytoin, 50 mg phenytoin equivalent

Lay Description
Fosphenytoin is a prodrug that is converted within the body to the anticonvulsant phenytoin. It is indicated for the control of status epilepticus, the prevention or control of seizures during neurosurgery, and for short-term parenteral administration when other means of phenytoin administration are unavailable, inappropriate, or less advantageous. It is thought to alter the sodium channels and block the calcium flow across the neuronal membranes, modulate the voltage-dependent calcium channels of neurons, and

enhance the sodium-potassium ATPase activity of neurons and glial cells. Fosphenytoin may be administered by intravenous injection, intravenous infusion, or intramuscular.

Q2017

Q2017   Injection, teniposide, 50 mg

Lay Description
Teniposide is a semisynthetic derivative of podophyllotoxin, a toxic compound found in the rhizomes and roots of the mandrake plant. Teniposide is closely related to etoposide. It is an antineoplastic drug used in combination with other approved antineoplastic agents for induction therapy in patients with refractory childhood acute lymphoblastic leukemia. It acts on cells by preventing them from entering mitosis. Teniposide is administered via intravenous infusion over 30 to 60 minutes.

Q2026

Q2026   Injection, Radiesse, 0.1 ml

Lay Description
Radiesse is an injectable implant placed under the skin for treatment of defects such as moderate to severe wrinkles and folds such as nasolabial folds and facial lipoatrophy in patients with human immunodeficiency virus (HIV). It is also used to treat certain dental defects, as a tissue marker, and for treatment of vocal fold insufficiency. Radiesse contains a synthetic calcium hydroxylapatite in an injectable gel. It provides temporary filling and helps stimulate the body's collagen formation. The treatment can last up to one year or more. The recommended dose varies based on location and severity of the defect.

Q2028

Q2028   Injection, sculptra, 0.5 mg

Lay Description
Sculptra is an injectable implant placed under the skin for treatment of facial lipoatrophy in patients with human immunodeficiency virus (HIV). Sculptra contains microparticles of poly-L-lactic acid, a biodegradable, biocompatible synthetic polymer from the alpha-hydroxy-acid family. It provides temporary fullness to improve the sunken appearance from the fat loss that may accompany HIV therapy. Sculptra treatments can last up to two years. The recommended dose varies based on location and size of the treatment area.

Q2034-Q2039

Q2034   Influenza virus vaccine, split virus, for intramuscular use (Agriflu)

Q2035   Influenza virus vaccine, split virus, when administered to individuals 3 years of age and older, for intramuscular use (AFLURIA)

Q2036   Influenza virus vaccine, split virus, when administered to individuals 3 years of age and older, for intramuscular use (FLULAVAL)

Q2037   Influenza virus vaccine, split virus, when administered to individuals 3 years of age and older, for intramuscular use (FLUVIRIN)

Q2038   Influenza virus vaccine, split virus, when administered to individuals 3 years of age and older, for intramuscular use (Fluzone)

Q2039   Influenza virus vaccine, split virus, when administered to individuals 3 years of age and older, for intramuscular use (not otherwise specified)

Lay Description
These codes report the supply of the vaccine only. A vaccine produces active immunization by inducing the immune system to build its own antibodies against specific microorganisms/viruses. The body retains memory of the antibody production pattern for long-term protection. A split virus suspension of the expected strains of influenza is prepared for intramuscular use. The vaccine induces active immunity to the highly contagious infection of the respiratory tract caused by a myxovirus and transmitted by airborne droplet infection. Vaccines are administered by IM injection. Report these codes with the appropriate administration code.

Q2043

Q2043   Sipuleucel-T, minimum of 50 million autologous cd54+ cells activated with PAP-GM-CSF, including leukapheresis and all other preparatory procedures, per infusion

Lay Description
Sipuleucel T is an autologous cellular immunotherapy used in the treatment of asymptomatic or minimally symptomatic metastatic castrate resistant (hormone refractory) prostate cancer. Sipuleucel T consists of autologous peripheral blood mononuclear cells (PBMC) obtained by leukapheresis and cultured or activated using a recombinant human protein (PAP GM CSF) that consists of prostatic acid phosphatase linked to granulocyte macrophage colony stimulating factor. Sipuleucel T is administered by intravenous infusion over a period of approximately 60 minutes.

Q2049

Q2049 Injection, doxorubicin hydrochloride, liposomal, imported Lipodox, 10 mg

Lay Description
Doxorubicin hydrochloride is an anthracycline antibiotic antineoplastic drug isolated from the bacterium [ital]Streptomyces peucetius var. caesius.[ital] It binds to DNA and inhibits RNA synthesis, causing cell death. It is utilized to treat many forms of cancer, such as bladder, breast, lung, stomach, and thyroid cancer, as well as Hodgkin's and non-Hodgkin's disease, acute lymphoblastic (ALL) and myeloblastic (AML) leukemia, and Wilms' tumor. The liposome version is the doxorubicin hydrochloride enclosed in a spherical lipid bilayer membrane. Doxorubicin hydrochloride liposome is indicated as a treatment for patients with ovarian cancer whose disease has recurred or progressed after platinum-based chemotherapy and for patients with AIDS-related Kaposi's sarcoma whose disease has progressed on prior combination chemotherapy or who cannot tolerate such therapy. Both versions are administered via intravenous injection.

Q2050

Q2050 Injection, doxorubicin hydrochloride, liposomal, not otherwise specified, 10 mg

Lay Description
Doxorubicin hydrochloride is an anthracycline antibiotic antineoplastic drug isolated from the bacterium *Streptomyces peucetius* var. *caesius*. It binds to DNA and inhibits RNA synthesis, causing cell death. It is utilized to treat many forms of cancer, such as bladder, breast, lung, stomach, and thyroid cancer, as well as Hodgkin's and non-Hodgkin's disease, acute lymphoblastic (ALL) and myeloblastic (AML) leukemia, and Wilms' tumor. The liposome version is the doxorubicin hydrochloride enclosed in a spherical lipid bilayer membrane. Doxorubicin hydrochloride liposome is indicated as a treatment for patients with ovarian cancer whose disease has recurred or progressed after platinum-based chemotherapy, and for patients with AIDS-related Kaposi's sarcoma whose disease has progressed on prior combination chemotherapy or who cannot tolerate such therapy. Both versions are administered via intravenous injection.

Q2052

Q2052 Services, supplies and accessories used in the home under the Medicare intravenous immune globulin (IVIG) demonstration

Lay Description
The Medicare IVIG Access and Strengthening Medicare and Repaying Taxpayers Act of 2012 established a three year demonstration to evaluate the benefits of providing payment for items and services needed for the in-home administration of intravenous immune globulin (IVIG) for the treatment of primary immune deficiency disease (PIDD). This is a not a regular or a new Medicare benefit. It is a special demonstration limited to 4,000 beneficiaries diagnosed with PIDD who voluntarily apply to participate. Medicare currently pays for IVIG medications for beneficiaries who have primary immune deficiency who wish to receive the drug at home. However, the traditional Medicare fee for service benefit does not currently cover any services to administer the drug to a beneficiary at home, such as nursing services and certain supplies. Under the demonstration, Medicare will pay a bundled payment for the administration and supplies related to the administration of IVIG for beneficiaries who are otherwise eligible to receive IVIG in the home.

Q3001

Q3001 Radioelements for brachytherapy, any type, each

Lay Description
Brachytherapy is a form of radiotherapy in which physicians place the source of irradiation close to the tumor or within a body cavity. Brachytherapy includes placing radioactive sources inside a body cavity (intracavitary brachytherapy) or putting radioactive material directly into body tissue using hollow needles (interstitial brachytherapy). Brachytherapy may be given in addition to external beam radiation or it may be used as the only form of radiotherapy. In some cases, the radioactive sources may be permanently left in place; in other cases, they are removed after a specified time. Placement of radioactive sources may be repeated several times. Use this code to report the radioelement used in brachytherapy.

Q3014

Q3014 Telehealth originating site facility fee

Lay Description
Telehealth is the delivery of health-related services via telecommunications equipment. The term encompasses technology that includes e-mail, video conferencing, and the transmission of medical images or medical data. The telecommunications most often involve a primary care practitioner with a patient at a remote site and a consulting medical specialist at an urban or referral facility. As applicable to Medicare, an originating site is the location of the patient at the time the service is being furnished via a telecommunications system. Originating sites authorized by law include the following:

- Physician or practitioner's office

- Hospital

- Critical access hospital

- Rural health clinic

- Federally qualified health center

- Community mental health center

- Skilled nursing facility

- Hospital-based or CAH-based renal dialysis center

A fee that is set annually is paid to the originating site. A separate payment is made for the professional fee(s) of the physician or practitioner at the distant site.

Q3027-Q3028

Q3027 **Injection, interferon beta-1a, 1 mcg for intramuscular use**

Q3028 **Injection, interferon beta-1a, 1 mcg for subcutaneous use**

Lay Description
Interferon beta-1a is a synthetic version of natural interferon beta-1a produced by recombinant DNA technology from Chinese hamster ovaries. Interferons are small, naturally occurring proteins that bind to specific cell membranes and initiate a series of events that include the inhibition of virus replication and the enhancement of macrophage and lymphocyte destruction of foreign cells. There are several types of interferons. Interferon beta-1a has been shown to control symptoms of muscular sclerosis, but its exact mechanism of action is unknown. Interferon beta-1a is indicated for the treatment of patients with relapsing forms of multiple sclerosis to decrease the frequency of clinical exacerbations and delay the onset of the physical disabilities associated with the disease. The drug may be self-administered as a subcutaneous injection. Interferon beta-1a is also available as an intramuscular injection.

Q3031

Q3031 **Collagen skin test**

Lay Description
This code reports the kit supplied for performing a collagen skin test. A collagen skin test is done to test for delayed hypersensitivity before any collagen procedure is carried out. The test is given as a small injection into and just under the skin, where a small lump is formed and watched for redness or irritation in the days following.

Q4001-Q4051

Q4001 **Casting supplies, body cast adult, with or without head, plaster**

Q4002 **Cast supplies, body cast adult, with or without head, fiberglass**

Q4003 **Cast supplies, shoulder cast, adult (11 years +), plaster**

Q4004 **Cast supplies, shoulder cast, adult (11 years +), fiberglass**

Q4005 **Cast supplies, long arm cast, adult (11 years +), plaster**

Q4006 **Cast supplies, long arm cast, adult (11 years +), fiberglass**

Q4007 **Cast supplies, long arm cast, pediatric (0-10 years), plaster**

Q4008 **Cast supplies, long arm cast, pediatric (0-10 years), fiberglass**

Q4009 **Cast supplies, short arm cast, adult (11 years +), plaster**

Q4010 **Cast supplies, short arm cast, adult (11 years +), fiberglass**

Q4011 **Cast supplies, short arm cast, pediatric (0-10 years), plaster**

Q4012 **Cast supplies, short arm cast, pediatric (0-10 years), fiberglass**

Q4013 **Cast supplies, gauntlet cast (includes lower forearm and hand), adult (11 years +), plaster**

Q4014 **Cast supplies, gauntlet cast (includes lower forearm and hand), adult (11 years +), fiberglass**

Q4015 **Cast supplies, gauntlet cast (includes lower forearm and hand), pediatric (0-10 years), plaster**

Q4016 **Cast supplies, gauntlet cast (includes lower forearm and hand), pediatric (0-10 years), fiberglass**

Q4017 **Cast supplies, long arm splint, adult (11 years +), plaster**

Q4018 **Cast supplies, long arm splint, adult (11 years +), fiberglass**

Q4019 **Cast supplies, long arm splint, pediatric (0-10 years), plaster**

Q4020 **Cast supplies, long arm splint, pediatric (0-10 years), fiberglass**

Q4021 **Cast supplies, short arm splint, adult (11 years +), plaster**

Q4022 **Cast supplies, short arm splint, adult (11 years +), fiberglass**

Q4023 **Cast supplies, short arm splint, pediatric (0-10 years), plaster**

Q4024 **Cast supplies, short arm splint, pediatric (0-10 years), fiberglass**

Q4025 **Cast supplies, hip spica (one or both legs), adult (11 years +), plaster**

Q4026 **Cast supplies, hip spica (one or both legs), adult (11 years +), fiberglass**

Q4027 **Cast supplies, hip spica (one or both legs), pediatric (0-10 years), plaster**

Q4028 **Cast supplies, hip spica (one or both legs), pediatric (0-10 years), fiberglass**

Q4029 **Cast supplies, long leg cast, adult (11 years +), plaster**

Q4030 **Cast supplies, long leg cast, adult (11 years +), fiberglass**

Q4031 **Cast supplies, long leg cast, pediatric (0-10 years), plaster**

Q4032 **Cast supplies, long leg cast, pediatric (0-10 years), fiberglass**

Q4033 Cast supplies, long leg cylinder cast, adult (11 years +), plaster

Q4034 Cast supplies, long leg cylinder cast, adult (11 years +), fiberglass

Q4035 Cast supplies, long leg cylinder cast, pediatric (0-10 years), plaster

Q4036 Cast supplies, long leg cylinder cast, pediatric (0-10 years), fiberglass

Q4037 Cast supplies, short leg cast, adult (11 years +), plaster

Q4038 Cast supplies, short leg cast, adult (11 years +), fiberglass

Q4039 Cast supplies, short leg cast, pediatric (0-10 years), plaster

Q4040 Cast supplies, short leg cast, pediatric (0-10 years), fiberglass

Q4041 Cast supplies, long leg splint, adult (11 years +), plaster

Q4042 Cast supplies, long leg splint, adult (11 years +), fiberglass

Q4043 Cast supplies, long leg splint, pediatric (0-10 years), plaster

Q4044 Cast supplies, long leg splint, pediatric (0-10 years), fiberglass

Q4045 Cast supplies, short leg splint, adult (11 years +), plaster

Q4046 Cast supplies, short leg splint, adult (11 years +), fiberglass

Q4047 Cast supplies, short leg splint, pediatric (0-10 years), plaster

Q4048 Cast supplies, short leg splint, pediatric (0-10 years), fiberglass

Q4049 Finger splint, static

Q4050 Cast supplies, for unlisted types and materials of casts

Q4051 Splint supplies, miscellaneous (includes thermoplastics, strapping, fasteners, padding and other supplies)

Lay Description

Casting materials are made of plaster-imbedded strips or bandages or fiberglass wraps or strips, available in varieties pertinent to the type of fracture or post-surgical state requiring the support and protection of a cast. Some of these materials are initially dry and are water-activated, while others come premoistened for immediate application. Plaster varieties can be imbedded with strength-adding chemical compounds such as polyurethane. Splints are used when a cast is not necessary but the injury or condition requires immobilization. Casts and casting materials support and protect fractured or strained extremities or other body areas. They hold manipulated (set) fractures in place or can assist other devices (pins, wires, screws) in doing so and protect against reinjury. These codes identify the different casting materials (e.g., fiberglass or plaster), the type of immobilization provided such splint or cast for adult or pediatric patients, and the length or shape of casts for the different types of

injuries or conditions (e.g., shoulder or body cast, long or short leg or arm).

Q4074

Q4074 Iloprost, inhalation solution, FDA-approved final product, noncompounded, administered through DME, unit dose form, up to 20 mcg

Lay Description

Iloprost is an inhaled form of prostacyclin, an analogue of prostaglandin. Prostaglandin is a naturally occurring, long-chain fatty acid that regulates smooth muscle contractions, is a vasodilator, lowers blood, and affects other hormones. It is an orphan drug indicated for use in pulmonary arterial hypertension (WHO group I) patients who have New York Heart Association (NYHA) Class III or IV symptoms. The NYHA classification system identifies Class II patients as those patients with marked limitation of activity, who are comfortable only at rest. NYHA Class IV patients are those patients who should be at complete rest, for whom any physical activity brings on discomfort. The drug is administered via a pulmonary drug delivery device with an initial inhaled dose of 2.5 mcg increasing to 5.0 mcg if tolerated. Iloprost should be inhaled six to nine times a day during waking hours, no more than once every two hours.

Q4081

Q4081 Injection, epoetin alfa, 100 units (for ESRD on dialysis)

Lay Description

Epoetin alfa (EPO) is a biologically engineered protein that stimulates the bone marrow to make new red blood cells. EPO is administered to treat anemia in patients with end-stage renal disease (ESRD) on a regular course of dialysis, as well as patients with other primary and secondary anemias. EPO is administered by subcutaneous or intravenous injection. This code is specific to patients with ESRD on dialysis and reports 100 units of EPO.

Q4082

Q4082 Drug or biological, not otherwise classified, Part B drug competitive acquisition program (CAP)

Lay Description

This code is used to report drugs or biologicals (not otherwise classified) that are administered as part of the Medicare Part B drug competitive acquisition program.

Q4100

Q4100 Skin substitute, not otherwise specified

Lay Description

This code represents skin substitutes that are not specifically identified by other HCPCS Level II codes. Skin substitutes may or may not contain bioactive tissue, cells, or matrices from human or animal sources. The skin substitutes are used to protect large or non-healing wounds or burns. Some products promote cellular growth and wound repair. Most substitutes are used in place of grafts.In 2014, OPPS considers this product a low cost skin substitute.

Q4101

Q4101   Apligraf, per sq cm

Lay Description

Apligraf is a skin substitute created from biological ingredients found in healthy human skin. It contains an outer layer of protective skin cells and an inner layer to aid in wound healing. It looks like a round piece of skin but does not include hair follicles, sweat glands, or blood vessels. When healthy skin cells get damaged, proteins and growth factors in the skin trigger the body to regenerate new skin. In certain conditions, such as diabetes or circulatory problems, the triggers are missing and wounds do not heal. Apligraf contains fresh cells, nutrients, and proteins that are applied directly to the wound and initiate the healing process. It is used to heal sores such as diabetic foot and venous leg ulcers that are not healing after three to four weeks, despite treatment with conventional therapies. After debriding the wound of necrotic, damaged, or infected tissue, the physician applies the Apligraf and covers it with a nonadhering dressing and an outer wrap.In 2014, OPPS considers this product a high cost skin substitute.

Q4102-Q4103

Q4102   Oasis wound matrix, per sq cm
Q4103   Oasis burn matrix, per sq cm

Lay Description

Oasis is a skin substitute created from a biomaterial found in porcine small intestine. The material is processed to remove all cells and then dehydrated. This leaves a matrix or scaffold material that the body uses to surround cells, binding it to tissue and replacing extracellular matrix (ECM). ECM is a necessary component in wound healing. Oasis is used to treat nonhealing wounds such as diabetic, venous, and pressure ulcers, as well as second-degree burns. After debriding the wound of necrotic, damaged, or infected tissue, the physician applies Oasis to the wound and a small area of surrounding tissue. The dehydrated sheet is fixed into place using Steri-strips, sutures, or staples and rehydrated with sterile saline. The wound is covered with a nonadherent dressing, an absorptive dressing for wet wounds, or a moist dressing for dry wounds, and covered with a secure dressing. Oasis is absorbed and forms a gel leaving ECM material. Oasis may be reapplied every seven days over the top of the ECM gel. In 2014, OPPS considers these products low cost skin substitutes.

Q4104

Q4104   Integra bilayer matrix wound dressing (BMWD), per sq cm

Lay Description

Integra bilayer wound matrix is a biologic matrix that provides coverage for partial and full-thickness wounds. It is used to treat chronic and traumatic wounds including pressure ulcers, venous ulcers, diabetic ulcers, chronic and vascular ulcers, surgical wounds, traumatic wound abrasions, lacerations, and draining wounds. It is a two-layer material created from three-dimensional porous material made from the fibers of a cross-linked bovine tendon collagen and a glycosaminoglycan. This provides the framework for dermal tissue and capillary growth. As the tissue is repaired, the matrix dissolves. For large wounds, an epidermal autograft may also be used. The outer layer is made of silicone and provides moisture control and a bacteria barrier. When the Integra bilayer wound matrix is applied, fluid is quickly adhered to the wound and is conforms to the shape of the wound. It can also be adhered with sutures, staples, or other materials. About 21 days after application, the outer silicone layer is removed, which allows further healing of the epidermis. The bilayer wound matrix may be used in conjunction with Integra matrix wound dressing. In 2014, OPPS considers this product a low cost skin substitute.

Q4105

Q4105   Integra dermal regeneration template (DRT), per sq cm

Lay Description

Integra dermal regeneration template is a bilayer matrix or scaffold for dermal regeneration. It is a two-layer material created from the fibers of a cross-linked bovine tendon collagen and a glycosaminoglycan. The outer layer is made of silicone and provides moisture control and bacteria barrier of the wound. The dermal layer is a collagen that provides a scaffold for dermal tissue and blood vessels. This provides a viable surface for autografting. This product is used for the immediate treatment of partial or full-thickness burns. It can also be used to treat scar contractures when there are not adequate donor sites or the patient's condition prohibits immediate grafting. As skin cells grow into the matrix, the collagen is slowly absorbed into the body and replaced with protein that the skin naturally produces. In about 14 to 21 days, new dermal skin is produced and the outer layer can be removed. The physician can then perform an autograft of the patient's epidermis. In 2014, OPPS considers this product a low cost skin substitute.

Q4106

Q4106   Dermagraft, per sq cm

Lay Description
Dermagraft is a human dermal substitute manufactured from newborn foreskin tissue. It is made of fibroblasts, extracellular matrix, and a bioabsorbable scaffold. The fibroblasts reproduce and infiltrate the scaffold and secrete human dermal collagen, matrix proteins, growth factors, and cytokines to create a three-dimensional human skin substitute. Dermagraft does not contain macrophages, lymphocytes, blood vessels, or hair follicles. Dermagraft is approved for use in the treatment of full-thickness diabetic foot ulcers lasting longer than six weeks but without exposure of the tendon, muscle, joint capsule, or bone. The physician prepares the wound bed, thaws and rinses the Dermagraft, and applies it to the site. The wound is dressed and left undisturbed for 72 hours. In 2014, OPPS considers this product a high cost skin substitute.

Q4107

Q4107   GRAFTJACKET, per sq cm

Lay Description
GRAFTJACKET is a three-dimensional, freeze dried biologic tissue matrix that forms a tissue scaffold used for diabetic foot ulcers. The material is derived from donated human skin. The epidermal and dermal cells are removed. The result is a matrix of preserved human dermal tissue, including its native protein, collagen structure, blood vessel channels, and essential biochemical composition to allow repair and revascularization. There are two distinct sides to the GRAFTJACKET. The dermal or vascular side is placed down, closest to the wound bed. The basement membrane side is exposed to the secondary dressing. The wound is prepared to receive the graft, and the graft is cut to size and rehydrated. Two or more sheets can be sewn together for larger wounds. The matrix is applied and fixed into place with sutures or staples and a moist dressing is applied. In 2014, OPPS considers this product a high cost skin substitute.

Q4108

Q4108   Integra matrix, per sq cm

Lay Description
Integra matrix is a biologic matrix that provides coverage for partial and full-thickness wounds. It is used to treat chronic and traumatic wounds including pressure ulcers, venous ulcers, diabetic ulcers, chronic and vascular ulcers, tunneled or undermined wounds, surgical wounds, traumatic wounds abrasions, lacerations, and draining wounds. It is a single layer material created of three-dimensional porous material made from the fibers of a cross-linked bovine tendon collagen. This provides the framework for tissue and capillary growth. Within seven to 14 days, the tissues and blood vessels invade the scaffold and the matrix is absorbed. For deeper wounds, Integra matrix can be used in conjunction with Integra bilayer wound dressing. An epidermal autograft can be performed 21 to 56 days later if necessary. In 2014, OPPS considers this product a low cost skin substitute.

Q4110

Q4110   PriMatrix, per sq cm

Lay Description
PriMatrix is an acellular collagen matrix that provides the framework for tissue and vascular growth. It is used to treat partial- and full-thickness wounds, pressure ulcers, diabetic ulcers, venous ulcers, second-degree burns, surgical wounds, skin tears, and tunneled or undermined wounds. It is derived from fetal bovine dermal tissue and consists of type I and type III collagen. It delivers collagen to the wound, which stimulates tissue growth and collagen production. The physician debrides the wound as appropriate. The PriMatrix is cut to size, rehydrated, and applied to the wound. It is affixed with a surgical closure and covered with a nonadherent dressing. Hydrogel is applied and the wound is dressed. In 2014, OPPS considers this product a high cost skin substitute.

Q4111

Q4111   GammaGraft, per sq cm

Lay Description
GammaGraft is a skin substitute derived from human cadaver tissue. It contains a dermal and epidermal layer of human skin that is irradiated. GammaGraft is used as a temporary covering when the patient's own skin is not available and provides a protection from bacteria and reduces fluid loss. It is used to treat burns, chronic wounds, and partial- and full-thickness wounds. The physician debrides the wound of infected or necrotic tissue. The GammaGraft is applied and affixed with sutures or other means. The wound is covered by a nonadherent dressing and covered with gauze. In 2014, OPPS considers this product a low cost skin substitute.

Q4112

Q4112   Cymetra, injectable, 1 cc

Lay Description
Cymetra is a small, particulate substance derived from donated human tissue. It contains collagens, elastin, proteins, and proteoglycans. It provides a structure for cell regrowth and helps the body produce tissue growth and vascularization. It is used as a substitute for the patient's own tissue to correct soft tissue defects and laryngoplasty.

Q4113

Q4113   GRAFTJACKET XPRESS, injectable, 1cc

Lay Description
GRAFTJACKET XPRESS is a micronized substance derived from human dermis. This substance contains

biologic components and structure of the dermal matrix. It forms a tissue scaffold and is used for damaged or inadequate integumentary tissue, such as deep dermal wounds. The freeze-dried powder is rehydrated and injected as appropriate.

Q4114

Q4114 Integra flowable wound matrix, injectable, 1 cc

Lay Description
Integra flowable wound matrix is a biologic gel that provides coverage for partial- and full-thickness wounds. It is used to treat chronic and traumatic wounds including pressure ulcers, venous ulcers, diabetic ulcers, chronic and vascular ulcers, tunneled or undermined wounds, surgical wounds, traumatic wound abrasions, lacerations, and draining wounds. This product is not used for third-degree burns. Since the wound matrix needs to be in contact with the wound bed, the flowable matrix is used for tunneled or irregular shaped defects. It is a single layer material created of three-dimensional porous material made from the fibers of a cross-linked bovine tendon collagen and mixed with sterile saline to form a gel. This provides the framework for tissue and capillary growth. The wound is debrided and probed for depth and tracking. The powdered product is mixed with sterile saline and injected into the site. A dressing is applied to ensure adherence and protect the wound.

Q4115

Q4115 AlloSkin, per sq cm

Lay Description
AlloSkin is an allograft made from donated human skin that is used for partial and full-thickness wounds. It has two layers, epidermal and dermal, and provides protection from infection by covering exposed tissue and allowing time for the wound to heal. In 2014, OPPS considers this product a low cost skin substitute.

Q4116

Q4116 AlloDerm, per sq cm

Lay Description
AlloDerm is a regenerative tissue matrix used to repair hernias and in postmastectomy reconstruction. The matrix is derived from donated human skin in which all the dermal and epidermal cells are removed. This provides a scaffold of acellular biological components that encourages revascularization, cell migration, and regeneration. In 2014, OPPS considers this product a high cost skin substitute.

Q4117

Q4117 HYALOMATRIX, per sq cm

Lay Description
Hyalomatrix is a temporary dermal substitute composed of an esterified hyaluronan (or hyaluronic acid) scaffold covered by a silicone membrane. The hyaluronan scaffold provides a biodegradable,

three-dimensional surface that promotes cellular growth. Hyalomatrix is indicated for the management of wounds or burns. In 2014, OPPS considers this product a low cost skin substitute

Q4118-Q4120

Q4118 MatriStem micromatrix, 1 mg
Q4119 MatriStem wound matrix, per sq cm
Q4120 MatriStem burn matrix, per sq cm

Lay Description
MatriStem products are extracellular matrices derived from porcine urinary bladder (also called UBM) used to promote wound healing and tissue growth. The products are non-crosslinked acellular material that is resorbable. MatriStem products contain bioactive collagens, elastins, and glycoproteins that trigger new blood vessel formation and attract numerous cell types to the wound area. They are indicated for the management of partial- and full-thickness wounds, ulcers, and burns. In 2014, OPPS considers Q4119 and Q4120 low cost skin substitutes.

Q4121

Q4121 TheraSkin, per sq cm

Lay Description
TheraSkin is a cryopreserved human skin allograft. It contains both a dermal and epidermal layer with bioactive cells including collagens, elastins, and glycoproteins that promote wound healing. TheraSkin is indicated as a wound covering for diabetic, pressure, or venous stasis ulcers; burns; dehisced surgical wounds; or any wound for which a graft is considered. In 2014, OPPS considers this product a low cost skin substitute.

Q4122

Q4122 DermACELL, per sq cm

Lay Description
DermACELL is a skin substitute used to treat second- and third-degree burns, breast reconstruction, chronic non-healing wounds, dehisced wound sites, and cosmetic reconstruction after traumatic burn injuries. DermACELL is derived from human tissue with most of the DNA removed. It provides a mechanical barrier and an allograft collagen scaffold regeneration mesh to protect the wound and promote healing. DermACELL is provided in various sizes and is sutured to the wound.

Q4123

Q4123 AlloSkin RT, per sq cm

Lay Description
AlloSkin RT is a skin replacement used to treat wounds caused by burns or trauma or chronic wounds such as venous and arterial ulcers, neuropathic diabetic ulcers, and pressure ulcers. The tissue is derived from human cadaver skin that is specially treated by low-dose, e-beam irradiation. The AlloSkin provides

protection and promotes healing of the tissue. It is applied surgically and secured into place by sutures, staples, glue, or other methods the physician deems appropriate. In 2014, OPPS considers this product a low cost skin substitute

Q4124

Q4124   OASIS ultra tri-layer wound matrix, per sq cm

Lay Description
OASIS Ultra Tri-layer Matrix is an acellular matrix derived from three layers of porcine small intestinal mucosa. It is indicated for the treatment of partial- and full-thickness wounds that are surgical or traumatic; burns; venous, vascular, diabetic, or pressure ulcers; and draining wounds. It is not for use on third-degree burns.In 2014, OPPS considers this product a low cost skin substitute.

Q4125

Q4125   Arthroflex, per sq cm

Lay Description
Arthroflex is an allograft used to treat chronic wounds such as diabetic foot ulcers and large surgical wounds. It is comprised of decellularized human skin and contains collagen, cytokines, and elastin. Collagen and elastin provide structure and growth factors to aid tissue growth and wound healing. Cytokines help with epithelizations and adjust the differentiation and growth of epithelium. Arthroflex also provides a matrix to provide a scaffold for tissue growth and stimulates cell growth. This biological also creates protection from contamination and helps decrease the rate of water, electrolyte, protein, and heat loss from the wound. It is applied to the wound and anchored using sutures, staples, or adhesive strips. In 2014, OPPS considers this product a high cost skin substitute.

Q4126

Q4126   MemoDerm, DermaSpan, TranZgraft or InteguPly, per sq cm

Lay Description
MemoDerm is a thin meshed acellular dermal matrix derived from human cadaver allograft tissue. The epidermal layer and cellular elements have been removed making the matrix acellular. MemoDerm is sterilized using gamma radiation leaving intact the collagen, proteoglycans, and elastin scaffold. The matrix assists in revascularization and in the repopulation of cells. It is indicated for use as an onlay graft for diabetic foot ulcers and other soft tissue repair. In 2014, OPPS considers this product a high cost skin substitute.

Q4127

Q4127   Talymed, per sq cm

Lay Description
Talymed is a bioactive wound matrix used to cover wounds such as diabetic ulcers, venous ulcers, pressure wounds, ulcers caused by mixed vascular etiologies, full thickness and partial thickness wounds, second-degree burns, surgical wounds, chronic vascular ulcers, and dehisced surgical wounds and bleeding surface wounds, abrasions, and lacerations. The active ingredient in Talymed is poly-N-acetylglucosamine (p-GlcNAc). It stimulates tissue growth and aids in wound closure and healing. The dressing is cut to the appropriate size and applied to the wound. It can be replaced as necessary.

Q4128

Q4128   FlexHD, AllopatchHD, or Matrix HD, per sq cm

Lay Description
FlexHD and AllopatchHD are human allograft tissue processed to remove epidermal and dermal cells. It is processed using a proprietary process that preserves and maintains the natural biochemical, biomechanical, and matrix properties of the dermal graft. It assists in revascularization and in the repopulation of cells at surgical sites. It is indicated for use as a graft to replace damaged or inadequate integumentary tissue or for the repair, reinforcement, or supplemental support of soft tissue defects. In 2014, OPPS considers this product a low cost skin substitute.

Q4129

Q4129   Unite biomatrix, per sq cm

Lay Description
Unite is a xenograft wound matrix used to treat moderate to heavy draining of partial and full thickness wounds, such as pressure ulcers, venous ulcers, chronic vascular ulcers, diabetic ulcers, and traumatic or surgical wounds. Unite is a type I collagen derived from equine pericardium. It provides a structure for cell growth and stimulates wound healing. The dressing is cut to the appropriate size and applied to the débrided wound.In 2014, OPPS considers this product a low cost skin substitute.

Q4130

Q4130   Strattice TM, per sq cm

Lay Description
Strattice TM is a surgical mesh for soft tissue repair that acts as a scaffold. It is derived from porcine skin and promotes healing and revascularization of the wound. Strattice TM is surgically implanted and used to treat partial and full thickness wounds, pressure ulcers, venous ulcers, diabetic ulcers, chronic vascular ulcers, tunneled/undermined wounds, surgical wounds, trauma wounds, draining wounds, or other bleeding surface wounds. It can also be used as

reinforcement tissue. Strattice TM comes in pliable or firm forms and in assorted sizes.

Q4131
Q4131   EpiFix, per sq cm

Lay Description
EpiFix is a biologic human tissue allograft used to treat viable, noninfected, full and partial thickness wounds, such as venous, diabetic, pressure, and chronic vascular ulcers; traumatic and surgical wounds; and burns. The amniotic tissue lines the inside layer of the placenta. The fibrous layer of the amnion contains collagen IV, V, and VII. The collagen provides an attachment for cell growth. It is a natural barrier and stimulates cell growth and wound healing. The graft is cut to the appropriate size, placed on the wound surface, and secured with sterile strips and a dressing.

Q4132
Q4132   Grafix core, per sq cm

Lay Description
Grafix Core is a skin substitute used to treat wounds that have exposed bone and tendon, such as deep diabetic foot ulcers, venous stasis ulcers, and pressure ulcers that have not responded to other wound care. It is a one layer collagen matrix that includes mesenchymal stem cells (MSC), anti-inflammatory cytokines, and regenerative growth factors. It is derived from human chorionic placental tissue. The matrix provides a scaffold that provides cellular support and growth factors that encourage cell regeneration. Grafix Core is applied to the wound every seven to 14 days as needed.

Q4133
Q4133   Grafix prime, per sq cm

Lay Description
Grafix Prime is a skin substitute used to treat acute and chronic wounds such as burns, diabetic foot ulcers, venous stasis ulcers, and pressure ulcers that have not responded to other wound care. It provides an epithelial layer and stromal layer matrix that includes mesenchymal stem cells (MSC), anti-inflammatory cytokines, and regenerative growth factors. It is derived from the amniotic membrane of human placental tissue. The matrix provides a scaffold that provides cellular support and growth factors that encourage and regulate cell regeneration and vessel growth. Grafix Prime is applied to the wound with a nonadherent dressing every seven to 14 days for up to 12 weeks until the wound has healed.

Q4134
Q4134   hMatrix, per sq cm

Lay Description
hMatrix is an acellular dermal scaffold derived from human skin. The epidermal and dermal cells are removed leaving the collagen and elastin matrix. This biological is intended to replace damaged or inadequate integumental tissue, including as a wound cover or for breast reconstruction or abdominal wall repair. In 2014, OPPS considers this product a high cost skin substitute.

Q4135
Q4135   Mediskin, per sq cm

Lay Description
Mediskin is a frozen irradiated porcine xenograft used to treat burns, abrasions, donor sites, decubitus, and chronic vascular ulcers. It provides protection from fluid loss and external contamination. It also provides a favorable environment for wound healing. Mediskin may also be used as a temporary wound cover. As the wound heals, Mediskin eventually sloughs off on its own. In 2014, OPPS considers this product a low cost skin substitute.

Q4136
Q4136   E-Z Derm, per sq cm

Lay Description
EZ-Derm is a porcine dermis xenograft that is used as temporary skin coverage for treatment of burns, abrasions, donor sites, decubitus and chronic vascular ulcers. It provides protection from fluid loss and external contamination. It also provides a favorable environment for wound healing. EZ-Derm will eventually slough off on its own and can be trimmed off to avoid shearing. In 2014, OPPS considers this product a low cost skin substitute.

Q4137
Q4137   Amnioexcel or biodexcel, per sq cm

Lay Description
BioDExCel™ (AmnioExCel) is a sterile non-crosslinked, resorbable, extracellular amniotic membrane that acts as a natural scaffold for cellular attachment creating tissue repair and regeneration. It is indicated for use in traumatic injuries, burns, surgical wounds, complex, chronic and acute wounds, and other soft tissue defects. In 2014, OPPS considers this product a low cost skin substitute.

Q4138
Q4138   Biodfence dryflex, per sq cm

Lay Description
BioDfence™ is an amniotic tissue based allograft derived from human placenta. It is composed of collagens and extracellular substrates that include growth factors, connective proteins, and cytokines. BioDfence™ provides an adhesion barrier reducing fibroblast infiltration. It is procured from live, healthy donors during childbirth and dehydrated to provide optimum handling characteristics. While this product was initially used in the acute care inpatient setting in connection with neurosurgical, orthopedic, and spine surgical procedures, it is now producing positive outcomes in individual wound care cases. The

dehydrated (and the hydrated) human amnion allografts are intended for the repair or replacement of lost or damaged dermal tissue. Indications include traumatic injuries, burns, Mohs procedures or surgical wounds; complex chronic and acute wounds, such as diabetic ulcers venous and arterial leg ulcers, pressure ulcers, or cutaneous ulcers; wounds with exposed vital structures, eg, tendon, bone, and blood vessels; and other soft tissue defects. BioDfence DryFlex™ is dehydrated, making it less sticky, and a better choice for use with instrumentation. In 2014, OPPS considers this product a low cost skin substitute.

Q4139

Q4139 Amniomatrix or biodmatrix, injectable, 1 cc

Lay Description

AmnioMatrix™ and BioDMatrix™ are viable human placental allografts composed of morselized amniotic membrane and amniotic fluid components recovered from the same human donor. The amniotic membrane is separated from the placenta and morselized into particulate form, then combined with amniotic fluid components to form the allograft. The processing method is intended to preserve the structural properties of the collagen, growth factors, cellular materials, and matrix present in the tissue to create a micro-scaffold to be used to aid in the wound healing process. AmnioMatrix™ (also to be marketed under the trade name BioDMatrix™) is intended for the treatment of wounds, including surgical wounds, burns, traumatic injury; chronic and acute wound conditions; and supportive treatment of wound-associated bone defects. The product may be mixed with normal saline for application to surgical sites and open, complex or chronic wounds or mixed with the recipient's blood to fill soft tissue defects and wound-associated bone defects. AmnoMatrix™ is cryopreserved and supplied in injectable form in sterile vials.

Q4140

Q4140 Biodfence, per sq cm

Lay Description

BioDfence™ is an amniotic tissue based allograft derived from human placenta. It is composed of collagens and extracellular substrates that include growth factors, connective proteins, and cytokines. BioDfence™ provides an adhesion barrier reducing fibroblast infiltration. It is procured from live, healthy donors during childbirth and dehydrated to provide optimum handling characteristics. While this product was initially used in the acute care inpatient setting in connection with neurosurgical, orthopedic, and spine surgical procedures, it is now producing positive outcomes in individual wound care cases. The dehydrated (and the hydrated) human amnion allografts are intended for the repair or replacement of lost or damaged dermal tissue. Indications include traumatic injuries, burns, Mohs procedures or surgical

wounds; complex chronic and acute wounds, such as diabetic ulcers venous and arterial leg ulcers, pressure ulcers, or cutaneous ulcers; wounds with exposed vital structures, eg, tendon, bone, and blood vessels; and other soft tissue defects. BioDfence™ is hydrated, which makes it a bit sticky and glue may not be needed, which may make it easier to use for procedures such as on corneal defects. In 2014, OPPS considers this product a low cost skin substitute.

Q4141

Q4141 Alloskin AC, per sq cm

Lay Description

Alloskin™ is meshed, biological cadaver dermis, which is decellularized and further processed to provide an acellular tissue allograft. Alloskin™ AC allograft is a natural skin replacement that can be used as a scaffold for regeneration of tissue through revascularization and remodeling into the host tissue to achieve wound closure of partial or full-thickness wounds due to tissue loss from burns, trauma, and chronic wounds, such as venous and arterial ulcers, diabetic foot ulcers, and pressure ulcers. After the epidermal layer is removed, the resulting dermal product is low-dose, e-beam irradiated to preserve the graft in a shelf-stable format. The tissue allograft is surgically applied and secured to the skin by the anchoring method chosen by the surgeon (sutures, staples, adhesive glue, etc.). In 2014, OPPS considers this product a low cost skin substitute.

Q4142

Q4142 XCM biologic tissue matrix, per sq cm

Lay Description

XCM Biologic Tissue Matrix™ is a sterile, non-cross-linked matrix derived from porcine dermis. It provides a support structure for cellular migration and is incorporated into the surrounding tissue. It is indicated for use in general surgical procedures for the reinforcement and repair of soft tissue where weakness exists including defect of the thoracic wall, suture line reinforcement, and muscle flap reinforcement; urogynecological surgical reinforcement, such as rectal and vaginal prolapse, reconstruction of the pelvic floor, or hernia repair; soft tissue reconstructive procedures including plastic and reconstructive surgical application; and for reinforcement of the soft tissues, which are repaired by suture or suture anchors, such as rotator cuff, patellar, Achilles, biceps, quadriceps, and other tendons. XCM Biologic Tissue Matrix™ is supplied sterile and hydrated in a foil liner pouch. It does not require refrigeration or any preparation before use. In 2014, OPPS considers this product a low cost skin substitute.

Q4143
Q4143 Repriza, per sq cm

Lay Description
Repriza® is an acellular dermal matrix. It is sterile, hydrated, ready to use upon opening, and it may be stored at ambient temperature. It has no orientation, so either side may be approximated to tissues of the wound or burn. Repriza® is indicated as a skin substitute in the treatment of various types of wounds including burns, chronic ulcers, and surgical wounds. Repriza® may also be used as an implant during plastic and reconstructive surgeries wherever an acellular dermal matrix may be used. For example, it may be used to support implants in a defined pocket such as in breast reconstruction and abdominal wall reconstruction procedures. It is available in standard sizes with custom sizes and thicknesses available upon request. In 2014, OPPS considers this product a low cost skin substitute.

Q4145
Q4145 Epifix, injectable, 1 mg

Lay Description
EpiFix® Injectable is a processed, dehydrated, sterilized cellular amniotic membrane allograft used for wound treatment when it is necessary to replace or repair lost or damaged human collagen tissue. It delivers multiple extracellular matrix proteins, growth factors, cytokines, and other specialty proteins present in amniotic tissue to help regenerate soft tissue. EpiFix® Injectable is indicated for the treatment and management of chronic wounds including neuropathic ulcers, venous stasis ulcers, post traumatic ulcers, post-surgical ulcers, and pressure ulcers. It is particularly suited to deeply creviced, irregularly shaped, or tunneling wounds. The size of the dosing used is based upon the size of the wound defect.

Q4146
Q4146 Tensix, per sq cm

Lay Description
TenSIX ™ is an acellular dermal matrix derived from aseptically processed sterile cadaver human skin. It is made from human donor skin, which undergoes a process that removes the epidermis and dermal cells, thereby creating an acellular dermis. TenSIX ™ acts as a scaffold to facilitate vessel growth and the migration of growth factors that stimulate cell migration. Once rehydrated, the allograft can be applied topically to the wound and secured by the physician in his manner of choice. It is indicated for the repair or replacement of damaged or inadequate integumental tissue, particularly for wounds resulting from chronic diabetic foot ulcers. In 2014, OPPS considers this product a low cost skin substitute.

Q4147
Q4147 Architect, architect PX, or architect FX, extracellular matrix, per sq cm

Lay Description
Architect™ ECM is type I collagen that has been stabilized and sterilized for ease of use and enhanced durability as a wound dressing. It is made from equine pericardium and utilizes a patented collagen stabilizing technology. It purportedly supports rapid healing by not promoting an inflammatory response; serves as a temporary matrix that provides a platform for cell migration; helps to optimize the wound-healing environment; and facilitates cellular activity. In 2014, OPPS considers this product a low cost skin substitute.

Q4148
Q4148 Neox 1k, per sq cm

Lay Description
NEOX™ 1k is an ultra-thick human amniotic membrane product. It is a non-implantable biological skin graft substitute comprised of human amniotic membrane retrieved from electively donated umbilical cords. NEOX™ 1k is indicated as a wound covering in chronic non-healing dermal wounds, such as diabetic ulcers. It is administered by placing the appropriately sized product to completely cover the wound bed after debridement, and is secured to the wound edges using sutures or surgical staples, at the discretion of the physician. In 2014, OPPS considers this product a low cost skin substitute.

Q4149
Q4149 Excellagen, 0.1 cc

Lay Description
Excellagen® is a highly refined fibrillar Type I bovine collagen gel for wound care management. The collagen is purified using a specialized process that removes impurities (including endotoxins), denatured molecules, and collagen fragments. Excellagen® promotes cellular adhesion, migration, and proliferation to stimulate granulation tissue formation. The flowable, ready to use gel is ideal for use in wounds of varying shapes and surface contours as well as tunneled/undermined wounds. Excellagen® is indicated for non-healing lower extremity ulcers in diabetic patients and other dermal wounds and is intended for physician use during debridement procedures. It is supplied in ready-to-use, prefilled, single-use sterile syringes.

Q4150
Q4150 Allowrap DS or dry, per sq cm

Lay Description
Allowrap DS is a biological barrier composed of human amniotic membrane that is applied to a postsurgical repaired site. The double-sided membrane has two layers of epithelial tissue with the epithelial tissue oriented outward.

Q4151

Q4151 Amnioband or guardian, per sq cm

Lay Description
Amnioband and Guardian are human tissue allografts made of donated placental membranes. The allograft is composed of native human amnion and chorion, which together create a membrane in which the amnion serves as a covering epithelium. Amnioband and Guardian are identical products. They are intended for interior and exterior wounds. They may be used as coverings for surgical sites, wounds, ulcers, and soft tissue defects.

Q4152

Q4152 Dermapure, per sq cm

Lay Description
DermaPure is derived from split thickness grafts harvested from human cadaver tissue donors. The tissue is a single layer of decellularized dermal allograft. It is indicated as a treatment for acute and chronic wounds such as diabetic foot ulcers, venous stasis ulcers, and other wounds that are refractory to more conservative care.

Q4153

Q4153 Dermavest, per sq cm

Lay Description
Dermavest is a human placental connective tissue matrix. It is intended to replace or supplement damaged or inadequate integumental tissue and to stabilize a debrided wound.

Q4154

Q4154 Biovance, per sq cm

Lay Description
Biovance is a dehydrated decellularized human amniotic membrane. It is derived from the placental amnion and includes epithelial and stromal components in a collagen-rich extracellular matrix. Biovance also contains extracellular proteins, such as elastin, glycosaminoglycans, and laminins, which are important in extracellular matrix strength, cell attraction, and migration. It is indicated for the treatment of damaged or lost soft tissue.

Q4155

Q4155 Neoxflo or clarixflo 1 mg

Lay Description
NeoxFlo and ClarixFlo are human amniotic membrane and umbilical cord products in particulate form. It is obtained from donated placentas. The particulate form is useful in treating irregularly shaped or tunneled wounds. It is indicated as a wound covering for dermal ulcers and defects, such as diabetic ulcers.

Q4156

Q4156 Neox 100, per sq cm

Lay Description
Neox 100 is a cryopreserved skin graft substitute composed of human amniotic membrane. It is indicated as a wound covering for chronic, nonhealing dermal wounds, such as diabetic ulcers and venous leg ulcers. Neox modulates inflammation and encourages healing.

Q4157

Q4157 Revitalon, per sq cm

Lay Description
Revitalon is a human allograft made from donated amniotic membrane derived from the inner lining of the placenta. It is composed of native human amnion and chorion consisting of collagen, laminin, fibronectin, nidogen, and proteoglycans. It is indicated as a covering for full-thickness wounds, damaged membranes, and as a dressing for burns.

Q4159

Q4159 Affinity, per sq cm

Lay Description
Affinity is a minimally processed amniotic fluid membrane allograft. It is comprised of the amniotic epithelial layer, the amniotic basement membrane, and the amniotic stroma. It is indicated as an on-lay graft for acute and chronic wounds, including, but not limited to, neuropathic ulcers, venous stasis ulcers, pressure ulcers, burns, posttraumatic wounds, and postsurgical wounds.

Q4160

Q4160 Nushield, per square centimeter

Lay Description
NuShield is produced from human placental membrane. It includes the amniotic epithelial layer, the amniotic basement membrane, the amniotic stroma, the chorionic basement membrane, and the chorionic stroma. It is intended as a lay-on graft for acute and chronic wounds, including, but not limited to, neuropathic ulcers, venous stasis ulcers, pressure ulcers, burns, posttraumatic wounds, and postsurgical wounds. This product comes in a meshed, expandable form.

Q5001-Q5002, Q5009

Q5001 Hospice or home health care provided in patient's home/residence
Q5002 Hospice or home health care provided in assisted living facility
Q5009 Hospice or home health care provided in place not otherwise specified (NOS)

Lay Description
These codes are used to report the location where hospice or home health care services are rendered. Hospice care services are designed to address the

physical, mental, emotional, and spiritual needs of terminally ill patients and their families. Hospice care is a palliative service that is provided when a cure is not possible. Services focus on keeping the patient comfortable by relieving pain and other symptoms and supporting the family during the terminal phase of the patient's illness. Hospice care is most often provided in a home-care setting, but may be provided in other settings if the patient's condition is such that more intensive professional services are required. Home health care is health care or supportive services provided in the patient's home by licensed health care professionals. The term home health care may also be used in reference to nonmedical care or custodial care, which is provided by persons who are not licensed medical personnel. The objective of home health care is to provide services in a non-institutional environment where the patient may be more comfortable and more relaxed.

Q5003-Q5008, Q5010

Q5003   Hospice care provided in nursing long-term care facility (LTC) or nonskilled nursing facility (NF)

Q5004   Hospice care provided in skilled nursing facility (SNF)

Q5005   Hospice care provided in inpatient hospital

Q5006   Hospice care provided in inpatient hospice facility

Q5007   Hospice care provided in long-term care facility

Q5008   Hospice care provided in inpatient psychiatric facility

Q5010   Hospice home care provided in a hospice facility

Lay Description
Hospice care services are designed to address the physical, mental, emotional, and spiritual needs of terminally ill patients and their families. Hospice care is a palliative service that is provided when a cure is not possible. Services focus on keeping the patient comfortable by relieving pain and other symptoms and supporting the family during the terminal phase of the patient's illness. Hospice services also include bereavement counseling following the patient's death. Hospice care is typically delivered by an interdisciplinary health care team of physicians, nurses, social workers, counselors, home health aides, clergy, therapists, and trained volunteers. Hospice care is most often provided in a home-care setting, but may be provided in other settings if the patient's condition is such that more intensive professional services are required. Hospitals often have inpatient hospice programs. These programs may consist of a separate hospice unit or of a hospice team that provides care to terminally ill patients throughout the hospital. There are also freestanding inpatient hospice facilities that specialize in the care of the terminally ill patient. Other facilities, such as long-term acute care facilities and inpatient psychiatric facilities, may also provide hospice services.

Q9951, Q9965-Q9967

Q9951   Low osmolar contrast material, 400 or greater mg/ml iodine concentration, per ml

Q9965   Low osmolar contrast material, 100-199 mg/ml iodine concentration, per ml

Q9966   Low osmolar contrast material, 200-299 mg/ml iodine concentration, per ml

Q9967   Low osmolar contrast material, 300-399 mg/ml iodine concentration, per ml

Lay Description
Low osmolar contrast material (LOCM) is a type of iodinated radiology contrast media that has a substantially lower concentration of particles contained in solution than high osmolar contrast material at the same iodine concentration. LOCM is supplied in radiological diagnostic procedures when the patient is known to have sensitivity to standard high osmolar contrast material or when other sensitivities or medical conditions exist that can increase the chances of a reaction in the patient. Contrast material is the dye that physicians use in diagnostic procedures to enable them to visualize the best picture possible and hence help to diagnose a patient's illness/disease, locate the point of the abnormality, or to assist in determining the extent of disease. LOCM is reported per ml based on the iodine concentration.

Q9953

Q9953   Injection, iron-based magnetic resonance contrast agent, per ml

Lay Description
Magnetic resonance imaging (MRI) is a radiation-free, noninvasive technique to produce high-quality sectional images of the inside of the body in multiple planes. MRI uses the natural magnetic properties of the hydrogen atoms in our bodies that emit radiofrequency signals when exposed to radio waves within a strong electromagnetic field. These signals are then processed and converted by the computer into high-resolution, three-dimensional, tomographic images. Iron is a common metal with strong magnetic properties. Various forms of the metal are used to enhance an MRI. The iron is administered intravenously and is taken up by reticuloendothelial cells, allowing greater detail to be captured by the MRI. The iron-based solution congregates in the spleen and liver allowing for the detection and evaluation of lesions. Dosage depends on patient body weight with a recommended dose of 0.05 ml per kg.

Q

Q9954

Q9954   Oral magnetic resonance contrast agent, per 100 ml

Lay Description
Magnetic resonance imaging (MRI) is a radiation-free, noninvasive technique to produce high-quality sectional images of the inside of the body in multiple planes. MRI uses the natural magnetic properties of the hydrogen atoms in our bodies that emit radiofrequency signals when exposed to radio waves within a strong electromagnetic field. These signals are then processed and converted by the computer into high-resolution, three-dimensional, tomographic images. Oral MRI contrast may be composed of several paramagnetic metals including magnetite, gadolinium, or iron. The contrast is administered orally and is distributed through the gastrointestinal system enhancing its delineation from other adjacent organs and tissues. Recommended dose is 600 ml.

Q9955-Q9957

Q9955   Injection, perflexane lipid microspheres, per ml

Q9956   Injection, octafluoropropane microspheres, per ml

Q9957   Injection, perflutren lipid microspheres, per ml

Lay Description
Octafluoropropane and perflutren are two names for the same substance with the chemical name of octafluoropropane. Perflutren lipid microspheres (trade name Definity) are octafluoropropane gas encapsulated in lipid shells. Optison is the trade name of an albumin microsphere that contains octafluoropropane. Perflexane lipid microspheres (trade name Imagent) is a similar product that encapsulates perfluorohexane in lipid spheres. When exposed to ultrasound waves, the spheres resonate or echo back strong signals that enhance echocardiogram imaging. They are indicated for use in suboptimal echocardiograms to opacify the left ventricular chamber and enhance delineation of the left ventricular endocardial border.

Q9958-Q9964

Q9958   High osmolar contrast material, up to 149 mg/ml iodine concentration, per ml

Q9959   High osmolar contrast material, 150-199 mg/ml iodine concentration, per ml

Q9960   High osmolar contrast material, 200-249 mg/ml iodine concentration, per ml

Q9961   High osmolar contrast material, 250-299 mg/ml iodine concentration, per ml

Q9962   High osmolar contrast material, 300-349 mg/ml iodine concentration, per ml

Q9963   High osmolar contrast material, 350-399 mg/ml iodine concentration, per ml

Q9964   High osmolar contrast material, 400 or greater mg/ml iodine concentration, per ml

Lay Description
High osmolar contrast material (HOCM) refers to a water-soluble, iodinated, monomeric, ionic radiology contrast material. Contrast material is the dye physicians use in diagnostic procedures to enable them to visualize abnormalities as clearly as possible so that they can diagnose a patient's illness/disease, locate the point of the abnormality, or determine the extent of disease. HOCM is a type of iodinated radiology contrast media that has a higher concentration of particles contained in solution than low osmolar contrast material at the same iodine concentration. HOCM is supplied in radiological diagnostic procedures when the patient does not have sensitivity to standard high osmolar contrast material or other medical conditions that would preclude the use of the higher particle concentration. HOCM is reported per ml based on the iodine concentration. High osmolar contrast is administered via intravenous push.

Q9965-Q9967

Q9965   Low osmolar contrast material, 100-199 mg/ml iodine concentration, per ml

Q9966   Low osmolar contrast material, 200-299 mg/ml iodine concentration, per ml

Q9967   Low osmolar contrast material, 300-399 mg/ml iodine concentration, per ml

Lay Description
Please refer to code Q9951 for the description, coding, and billing information.

Q9968

Q9968   Injection, nonradioactive, noncontrast, visualization adjunct (e.g., methylene blue, isosulfan blue), 1 mg

Lay Description
This code represents nonradioactive, noncontrast, visualization enhancing substances that are not represented by other specific HCPCS Level II codes. For example, methylene blue and isosulfan blue are both water-soluble chemicals to stain or mark internal structures. Both may be injected to delineate lymph nodes or to identify the sentinel node in breast cancer.

Q9969

Q9969   Tc-99m from nonhighly enriched uranium source, full cost recovery add-on, per study dose

Lay Description
Modern medical imaging frequently employs the use of radioisotopes, which are widely used in cardiac imaging predominantly for the elderly (Medicare) population. The radioisotope used in the majority of such diagnostic imaging services is Technetium-99 (Tc-99m). This radioisotope is currently produced in

legacy reactors outside of the U.S. using highly enriched uranium (HEU). Molybdenum-99 (Mo-99) may be used to manufacture technetium-99m generators. Report Molybdenum-99 for Tc-99m from non-highly enriched uranium source, full cost recovery add-on, per study dose. Any dose of Tc-99m that can be traced to a Mo-99 supply containing no more than 5 percent HEU sourced Mo-99 shall be considered to be completely derived from non-HEU sources for the purposes of payment, and any compliance practices that support it. To put it another way, a product identified as non-HEU sourced must be at least 95 percent derived from non-HEU sources.

R

R0070-R0076

R0070   **Transportation of portable x-ray equipment and personnel to home or nursing home, per trip to facility or location, one patient seen**

R0075   **Transportation of portable x-ray equipment and personnel to home or nursing home, per trip to facility or location, more than one patient seen**

R0076   **Transportation of portable EKG to facility or location, per patient**

Lay Description
These HCPCS Level II codes represent the charge for transporting portable equipment and personnel to a site to provide diagnostic imaging services or record an electrocardiogram. Payers will sometimes reimburse these additional charges. These codes should be reported conjunction with the CPT radiology codes (70000 series) and only when the x-ray equipment used was actually transported to the location where the image was taken. These codes would not apply to x-ray equipment or an electrocardiograph stored in the location where the service was performed.

S

S0012

S0012   **Butorphanol tartrate, nasal spray, 25 mg**

Lay Description
Butorphanol tartrate nasal spray is a schedule IV controlled substance. It is a synthetic opioid analgesic used for the management of moderate to severe pain. The most common indication is in the management of migraines. Although the action of the drug is not known, it binds with opiate receptors in the central nervous system and alters not only the perception of pain, but the emotional response as well.

S0014

S0014   **Tacrine HCl, 10 mg**

Lay Description
Tacrine hydrochloride is a reversible cholinesterase inhibitor. Cholinesterase is an enzyme that catalyzes the breakdown of acetylcholine, a neurotransmitter. Early changes in the brain of Alzheimer's patients result in a deficiency of acetylcholine. This deficiency is thought to account for some of the mild to moderate dementia characteristic of Alzheimer's disease. Tacrine hydrochloride inhibits the breakdown of and increases the concentration of acetylcholine in the cerebral cortex. The drug is indicated as a treatment for mild to moderate dementia of Alzheimer's disease. Tacrine hydrochloride is self-administered orally in dosages ranging from 10 to 40 mg four times a day.

S0017

S0017   **Injection, aminocaproic acid, 5 g**

Lay Description
Aminocaproic acid is an amino acid that inhibits fibrinolysis. After long-term use, this medication distributes throughout extravascular and intravascular compartments of the body, penetrating red blood cells and other tissue cells. It is used to treat fibrinolytic bleeding that may frequently be associated with surgical complications following heart surgery and portacaval shunt, hematological disorders such as aplastic anemia, abruptio placentae, hepatic cirrhosis, and neoplastic diseases such as carcinoma of the prostate, lung, stomach, and cervix. It may also be used to treat urinary fibrinolysis associated with complications following severe trauma, anoxia, shock, complications following prostatectomy, nephrectomy, or nonsurgical hematuria accompanying polycystic or neoplastic diseases of the genitourinary system. Aminocaproic acid can be administered via intravenous infusion or orally.

S0020

S0020   **Injection, bupivicaine HCl, 30 ml**

Lay Description
Bupivacaine hydrochloride (HCl) is a local anesthetic that blocks the feeling of pain by inhibiting the conduction of nerve impulses. The order of loss of nerve function is pain, temperature, touch, proprioception, and skeletal muscle tone. It is often used for dental procedures and during labor and delivery. Bupivacaine can be administered by infiltration, caudal injection, lumbar epidural injection, peripheral nerve block, retrobulbar block, or sympathetic block. Bupivacaine is not recommended for intravenous or regional anesthesia (Bier Block).

S

S0021

S0021   Injection, cefoperazone sodium, 1 g

Lay Description
Cefoperazone sodium is a broad spectrum antibiotic. It is used to treat respiratory tract infections, skin infections, and urinary tract infections. Susceptible bacteria include *S. pneumoniae, H. influenzae, S. aureus, S. pyogenes, P. aeruginosa, Klebsiella pneumoniae, E. coli, Proteus mirabilis, Enterobacter* species; anaerobic gram-negative bacilli, *Pseudomonas aeruginosa, Klebsiella, Clostridium*; anaerobic gram-positive cocci, *N. gonorrhoeae* , and *S. epidermidis*. The usual dose is two to four grams per day administered at 12-hour intervals in equally divided doses. Cefoperazone is administered via intramuscular injection or intravenous infusion.

S0023

S0023   Injection, cimetidine HCl, 300 mg

Lay Description
Cimetidine is a histamine H2 receptor antagonist that inhibits the action of histamine at the histamine H2 receptors of the parietal cells. It inhibits gastric acid secretions. It is used in treatment and maintenance therapy for duodenal ulcers, short-term treatment of gastric ulcers, gastroesophageal reflux disease (GERD), prevention of upper gastrointestinal bleeding in critically ill patients, and for the treatment of pathological hypersecretory conditions (i.e., Zollinger-Ellison syndrome, systemic mastocytosis, multiple endocrine adenomas).

S0028

S0028   Injection, famotidine, 20 mg

Lay Description
Famotidine is a histamine H2 receptor antagonist that inhibits the action of histamine at the histamine H2 receptors of the parietal cells. It inhibits gastric acid secretions. It is used for treatment and maintenance therapy for duodenal ulcers, short-term treatment of gastric ulcers, gastroesophageal reflux disease (GERD), prevention of upper gastrointestinal bleeding in critically ill patients, and for the treatment of pathological hypersecretory conditions (i.e., Zollinger-Ellison syndrome, systemic mastocytosis, multiple endocrine adenomas). Famotidine can be administered orally and via intravenous infusion.

S0030

S0030   Injection, metronidazole, 500 mg

Lay Description
Metronidazole is an antibacterial and antiprotozoal. It is thought to work in an anaerobic environment by entering the organism and being reduced by intracellular electron transport proteins. Because of this alteration to the metronidazole molecule, a concentration gradient is maintained that promotes the drug's intracellular transport. Presumably, free radicals are formed that, in turn, react with cellular components, resulting in the death of the microorganism. Metronidazole is effective against the following bacteria and protozoa: *Clostridium* species, *Eubacterium* species, *Peptococcus niger*, *Peptostreptococcus* species, *Bacteroides fragilis* group (*B. fragilis, B. distasonis, B. ovatus, B. thetaiotaomicron, B. vulgatus*), *Fusobacterium* species, *Entamoeba histolytica*, and *Trichomonas vaginalis*. Metronidazole is used to treat symptomatic trichomoniasis; asymptomatic trichomoniasis, when the organism is associated with endocervicitis, cervicitis, or cervical erosion; asymptomatic consorts; *T. vaginalis* infection; acute intestinal amebiasis (amebic dysentery) and amebic liver abscess; serious infections caused by susceptible anaerobic bacteria, peritonitis, intra-abdominal abscess, and liver abscess; skin infections; inflammatory lesions of rosacea; endometritis; endomyometritis; tubo-ovarian abscess and postsurgical vaginal cuff infection; bacterial septicemia; bone and joint infections; meningitis and brain abscess; pneumonia; empyema; lung abscess; and endocarditis. Metronidazole can be administered topically, orally, or via intravenous infusion. The loading dose is 15 mg/kg of body weight or about 1 gram infused over one hour. Following that, 500 mg is infused over one hour and administered every six hours.

S0032

S0032   Injection, nafcillin sodium, 2 g

Lay Description
Nafcillin sodium is a semisynthetic antibiotic substance derived from 6-amino-penicillanic acid. This is a penicillinase-resistant penicillin and is used to treat infections caused by penicillinase-producing staphylococci that have shown to be susceptible to the drug. The drug can be administered orally or via intramuscular injection, intravenous push, or intravenous infusion.

S0034

S0034   Injection, ofloxacin, 400 mg

Lay Description
Ofloxacin is a broad spectrum antibiotic of the quinolone class. It inhibits the DNA enzymes in bacteria that are required for the DNA to replicate. This drug is chemically different from aminoglycosides, macrolides, and beta-lactam antibiotics, including penicillins, and therefore may be used to treat bacteria resistant to these antibacterials. Ofloxacin is effective against the following bacteria: *Staphylococcus aureus* (methicillin-susceptible strains), *Staphylococcus epidermidis, Enterobacter cloacae, Streptococcus pneumoniae* (penicillin-susceptible strains), *Streptococcus pyogenes, Citrobacter (diversus) koseri, Enterobacter aerogenes, Propionibacterium acnes, Escherichia coli, Haemophilus influenzae, Serratia marcescens, Proteus mirabilis, Klebsiella pneumoniae, Neisseria gonorrhoeae, Proteus mirabilis, Chlamydia trachomatis,*

Gardnerella vaginalis, Legionella pneumophila, Mycoplasma hominis, Mycoplasma pneumonia, Ureaplasma urealyticum, and *Pseudomonas aeruginosa.* Some strains of *Pseudomonas aeruginosa* may quickly develop a resistance to ofloxacin during treatment. It is used to treat acute bacterial exacerbations of chronic bronchitis, community-acquired pneumonia, uncomplicated skin infections, conjunctivitis, corneal ulcers, acute uncomplicated urethral and cervical gonorrhea, nongonococcal urethritis and cervicitis, mixed infections of the urethra and cervix, acute pelvic inflammatory disease, uncomplicated cystitis, complicated urinary tract infections, and prostatitis. Ofloxacin can be administered orally, by ophthalmic drops, and via slow intravenous infusion over 60 minutes. It should not be administered via intramuscular injection, subcutaneous injection, or intravenous push.

S0039

S0039　Injection, sulfamethoxazole and trimethoprim, 10 ml

Lay Description
Sulfamethoxazole and trimethoprim is an antibiotic that blocks two necessary steps in the biosynthesis of nucleic acids and proteins that are critical to many bacteria. It is effective against the following bacteria: *Streptococcus pneumoniae, Haemophilus influenzae, Shigella flexneri, Shigella sonnei, Escherichia coli, Klebsiella* species, *Enterobacter* species, *Morganella morganii, Proteus mirabilis,* and *Proteus vulgaris.* Sulfamethoxazole and trimethoprim is indicated in the treatment of *Pneumocystis carinii* pneumonia, enteritis, urinary tract infections, acute otitis media, acute exacerbations of chronic bronchitis, traveler's diarrhea, and for prophylaxis against *Pneumocystis jiroveci* pneumonia in individuals who are immunosuppressed and considered to be at an increased risk of developing *Pneumocystis carinii* pneumonia. Sulfamethoxazole and trimethoprim is administered orally or via intravenous infusion over 60 to 90 minutes. This drug should not be given via rapid intravenous infusion or by intramuscular injection.

S0040

S0040　Injection, ticarcillin disodium and clavulanate potassium, 3.1 g

Lay Description
Ticarcillin disodium and clavulanate is a combination drug consisting of a semisynthetic form of penicillin and clavulanate. Penicillins block the actions of transpeptidase, an enzyme needed to create the cell wall. This weakens the bacterial cell wall causing cellular death. Many bacteria have developed a resistance to penicillin. Resistant bacteria produce an enzyme, penicillinase or beta-lactamase, that protects it from the effects of penicillin. Clavulanic acid or clavulanate binds to the penicillinase and inhibits it from blocking the actions of penicillin. Ticarcillin

disodium is indicated for the treatment of infections with susceptible anaerobic, gram-negative, and positive bacteria. Specific conditions and susceptible bacteria include septicemia/bacteremia caused by *Staphylococcus aureus, Escherichia coli, Pseudomonas aeruginosa,* and other *Pseudomonas* species; lower respiratory infections caused by *Staphylococcus aureus, haemophilus influenza, Klebsiella* species; bone and joint infections caused by *Staphylococcus aureus;* skin and skin-structure infections caused by *Staphylococcus aureus, Escherichia coli, Klebsiella* species; urinary tract infections caused by *Escherichia coli, Klebsiella* species, *Pseudomonas aeruginosa* and other *Pseudomonas* species, *Citrobacter* species, *Enterobacter cloacae, Staphylococcus aureus, Serratia marcescens;* gynecological infections caused by *Prevotella melaninogenicus, Enterobacter* species, *Escherichia coli, Klebsiella pneumoniae, Staphylococcus aureus, Staphylococcus epidermidis;* and intra-abdominal infections caused by *Escherichia coli, Klebsiella pneumoniae,* and *Bacteroides fragilis.* The drug is administered via an intravenous infusion.

S0073

S0073　Injection, aztreonam, 500 mg

Lay Description
Aztreonam is a synthetic bactericidal antibiotic originally isolated from chromobacterium violaceum. Aztreonam is effective against gram-negative organisms. Susceptibility studies should be performed prior to the administration of this drug. Susceptible organisms include *Escherichia coli, Klebsiella pneumoniae, Klebsiella oxytoca, Proteus mirabilis, Pseudomonas aeruginosa, Enterobacter* species including *E. cloacae, Citrobacter* species, including *C. freundii, Serratia* species including *S. marcescens,* and *Haemophilus influenzae.*

S0074

S0074　Injection, cefotetan disodium, 500 mg

Lay Description
Cefotetan disodium is an antibiotic that inhibits the cell wall synthesis in bacteria. It is effective against the following bacteria: *Escherichia coli, Haemophilus influenzae, Klebsiella* species, *Morganella morganii, Neisseria gonorrhoeae, Proteus mirabilis, Proteus vulgaris, Providencia rettgeri, Serratia marcescens, Staphylococcus aureus, Staphylococcus epidermidis, Streptococcus agalactiae, Streptococcus pneumoniae, Streptococcus pyogenes, Prevotella bivia, Prevotella disiens, Bacteroides fragilis, Prevotella melaninogenica, Bacteroides vulgatus, Fusobacterium* species, Gram-positive bacilli, *Peptococcus niger,* and *Peptostreptococcus* species. Cefotetan is indicated in the treatment of urinary tract infections, lower respiratory infections, skin infections, gynecological infections, intra-abdominal infections, bone and joint infections, and may be used as a preventive treatment prior to surgery. This drug can be administered via

intramuscular injection, intravenous push, or intravenous infusion, usually less than one hour.

S0077

S0077 Injection, clindamycin phosphate, 300 mg

Lay Description
Clindamycin phosphate is an antibiotic used to treat serious, susceptible strains of streptococci, pneumococci, and staphylococci infections. It is used for patients who are allergic to penicillin or for whom penicillin treatment is inappropriate. It is effective against the following bacteria: *Staphylococcus aureus*, *Staphylococcus epidermidis*, Streptococci (except *Enterococcus faecalis*), Pneumococci, *Bacteroides* species (including *Bacteroides fragilis* group and *Bacteroides melaninogenicus* group), *Fusobacterium* species, *Propionibacterium*, *Eubacterium*, *Actinomyces* species, *Peptococcus* species, *Peptostreptococcus* species, *Microaerophilic streptococci*, and *Clostridium perfringens*. The injectable form is administered by intramuscular or intravenous injection followed by an intravenous infusion over 30 minutes. The usual dose is 600 to 1,200 mg per day in two, three, or four equal doses or for more severe infections 1,200 to 2,700 mg per day in two, three, or four equal doses.

S0078

S0078 Injection, fosphenytoin sodium, 750 mg

Lay Description
Fosphenytoin is a prodrug that is converted within the body to the anticonvulsant phenytoin. It is indicated for short-term (five days or less) treatment of status epilepticus, the prevention or control of seizures during neurosurgery, and for short-term parenteral administration when other means of phenytoin administration are unavailable, inappropriate, or less advantageous. It is thought to alter the sodium channels and block the calcium flow across the neuronal membranes, modulate the voltage-dependent calcium channels of neurons, and enhance the sodium-potassium ATPase activity of neurons and glial cells. Fosphenytoin may be administered by intravenous or intramuscular injection or intravenous infusion.

S0080

S0080 Injection, pentamidine isethionate, 300 mg

Lay Description
Pentamidine isethionate is an aromatic diamidine that is an antimicrobial. Its mechanism of action is not completely known. It is thought that the drug interferes with the synthesis of DNA, RNA, and protein causing cell death. Pentamidine isethionate is indicated as a treatment for *Pneumocystis Jiroveci* (previously classified as *P. carinii*), trypanosomiasis, and leishmaniasis. The drug may be administered by intramuscular injection, inhalation, or intravenous infusion over one hour. Dosage is usually 300 mg.

S0081

S0081 Injection, piperacillin sodium, 500 mg

Lay Description
Piperacillin is a broad-spectrum antibiotic that works by inhibiting septum and cell wall synthesis in bacteria. It is effective against the following bacteria: Enterococci, including *Enterococcus faecalis*, *Streptococcus pneumoniae*, *Streptococcus pyogenes*, *Acinetobacter* species, *Enterobacter* species, *Escherichia coli*, *Haemophilus influenzae* (non-lactamase-producing strains), *Klebsiella* species, *Morganella morganii*, *Neisseria gonorrhoeae*, *Proteus mirabilis*, *Proteus vulgaris*, *Providencia rettgeri*, *Pseudomonas aeruginosa*, *Serratia* species, Anaerobic cocci, *Clostridium* species, *Bacteroides* species including *Bacteroides fragilis*, *Streptococcus agalactiae*, *Streptococcus bovis*, Viridans group streptococci, *Burkholderia cepacia*, *Citrobacter diversus*, *Citrobacter freundii*, *Pseudomonas fluorescens*, *Stenotrophomonas maltophilia*, *Yersinia enterocolitica*, *Actinomyces* species, *Eubacterium* species, *Fusobacterium necrophorum*, *Fusobacterium nucleatum*, *Porphyromonas asaccharolytica*, *Prevotella melaninogenica*, and *Veillonella* species. Piperacillin is indicated in the treatment of intraabdominal infections including hepatobiliary and surgical infections, urinary tract infections, endometritis, pelvic inflammatory disease, pelvic cellulitis, septicemia, lower respiratory tract infections, skin infections, bone and joint infections, uncomplicated gonococcal urethritis, and may be used as a preventive treatment prior to surgery. It is also effective for treatment of mixed infections and is used to treat infections prior to identification. Piperacillin can be administered via intramuscular injection, intravenous push, or intravenous infusion over 30 minutes. The maximum intramuscular dose is two grams per injection site.

S0088

S0088 Imatinib, 100 mg

Lay Description
Imatinib is an antineoplastic drug that inhibits the bcr-abl tyrosine kinase, the constitutive abnormal tyrosine kinase created by the Philadelphia chromosome abnormality in chronic myeloid leukemia (CML). It inhibits production and induces apoptosis in bcr-abl positive cell lines, as well as fresh leukemic cells from Philadelphia chromosome positive CML. It is also an inhibitor of the receptor tyrosine kinases for platelet-derived growth factor (PDGF) and stem cell factor (SCF), c-kit, and inhibits PDGF- and SCF-mediated cellular events. It is used to treat adults with newly diagnosed Philadelphia chromosome positive chronic myeloid leukemia in chronic phase. It is also indicated for the treatment of patients with Philadelphia chromosome (CML) in blast crisis, accelerated phase, or in chronic phase after failure of interferon-alpha therapy and patients with Kit (CD117) positive unresectable and/or metastatic

malignant gastrointestinal stromal tumors (GIST). Imatinib can be used for children with pH + chronic phase CML whose disease has recurred after stem cell transplant or who are resistant to interferon-alpha therapy. The adult dose is 400 to 800 mg per day.

S0090

S0090   Sildenafil citrate, 25 mg

Lay Description
Sildenafil citrate is a selective inhibitor of an enzyme that controls cyclic guanosine monophosphate. The drug is used to treat erectile dysfunction. Penile erection is a hemodynamic process that involves the release of nitric acid by the corpus cavernosum during sexual stimulation. The nitric acid activates the enzyme cyclic guanosine monophosphate, which produces smooth muscle relaxation in the corpus cavernosum and allows the inflow of blood. Another enzyme, phosphodiesterase type 5, controls the tissue concentration of the cyclic guanosine monophosphate. Sildenafil citrate inhibits the neutralizing effect of the phosphodiesterase type 5. Since the local release of nitric acid is initiated by sexual stimulation and the erectile process is catalyzed by nitric acid, this drug has no effect in the absence of sexual stimulation. The drug is self-administered orally in dosages ranging from 25 to 100 mg. The drug may be taken at anywhere from one-half hour to four hours prior to sexual activity.

S0091

S0091   Granisetron HCl, 1 mg (for circumstances falling under the Medicare statute, use Q0166)

Lay Description
Granisetron hydrochloride is a chemical compound that is a selective blocker of serotonin 5-HT3 receptors. It is an antiemetic drug available in oral and injectable forms. Serotonin 5-HT3 receptors are present on the vagal nerve and at sensory nerve endings. Cytotoxic chemotherapy appears to trigger the release of serotonin in the small intestine, which may trigger the 5-HT3 receptors and initiate the vomiting reflex.

S0092

S0092   Injection, hydromorphone HCl, 250 mg (loading dose for infusion pump)

Lay Description
Hydromorphone is a narcotic and opioid analgesic classified as a schedule II controlled substance. This drug binds to opiate nerve center receptors and alters the human pain response, as well as suppressing the cough reflex. It is available in oral and injectable forms. The injectable form can be administered by intramuscular, subcutaneous, and intravenous injection, or by intravenous infusion. Hydromorphone hydrochloride is indicated for the relief of moderate to severe pain.

S0093

S0093   Injection, morphine sulfate, 500 mg (loading dose for infusion pump)

Lay Description
Morphine is an opioid. It acts upon specific receptors in the brain and spinal cord to decrease the feeling of pain and to reduce the emotional response to pain. An implantable infusion pump is considered medically necessary when used to administer opioid drugs (e.g., morphine) and/or clonidine intrathecally or epidurally for treating severe chronic intractable pain in persons who have proven unresponsive to less invasive medical therapy as determined by the following criteria: a) previous medical history that patient has not responded adequately to noninvasive methods of pain control, such as systemic opioids (including attempts to eliminate physical and behavioral abnormalities that may cause an exaggerated reaction to pain); and b) a preliminary trial of intraspinal opioid drug administration undertaken with a temporary intrathecal/epidural catheter to substantiate adequately acceptable pain relief, the degree of side-effects (including effects on the activities of daily living), and acceptance.

S0104

S0104   Zidovudine, oral, 100 mg

Lay Description
Zidovudine (formerly called azidothymidine or AZT) is a synthetic nucleoside analogue used as an antiviral for the treatment of human immunodeficiency virus (HIV) infection and to prevent maternal-fetal transmission of HIV. Zidovudine incorporates itself into the DNA chain preventing elongation and stopping DNA growth. Zidovudine can be administered via intravenous infusion over one hour or orally.

S0106

S0106   Bupropion HCl sustained release tablet, 150 mg, per bottle of 60 tablets

Lay Description
Bupropion hydrochloride is a chemical that is used to treat major depressive disorders and as an aid to smoking cessation. The drug is a weak inhibitor of neuronal uptake of norepinephrine and dopamine. It does not inhibit monoamine oxidase or the reuptake of serotonin. The exact course of action is unknown. Bupropion hydrochloride is tablet form only.

S0108

S0108   Mercaptopurine, oral, 50 mg

Lay Description
Mercaptopurine is a potent chemotherapeutic drug belonging to a class of drugs known as antimetabolites. Antimetabolites resemble nutrients required for cancer cell growth. The cancer cells take up mercaptopurine, which interfere with cancer cell nucleic acid biosynthesis. Specifically, mercaptopurine

inhibits the first enzyme unique to the de novo pathway for purine ribonucleotide synthesis. It is not known exactly which of the biochemical effects of mercaptopurine is responsible for cell death. Mercaptopurine is used to treat acute lymphatic and acute myelogenous leukemia. It has also been shown to be effective in the treatment of some chronic myelogenous leukemias and some acute undifferentiated leukemias. Efficacy depends on the particular subclassification of the leukemia. Mercaptopurine may be used in combination with other chemotherapy drugs as an initial treatment to induce remission. It may also be used as maintenance therapy for lymphatic (lymphocytic, lymphoblastic) leukemia. The induction dose varies; however, the usual dose for both children and adults is 2.5 mg/kg of body weight. The maintenance dose is 1.5 to 2.5 mg/kg per day once the patient is in remission. This medication is administered orally.

S0109

S0109   Methadone, oral, 5 mg

Lay Description
Methadone is a synthetic opioid analgesic that has effects similar to those of morphine and heroin. It is a schedule II controlled substance. Methadone is indicated for the treatment of severe pain and also as a substitute drug in the detoxification of heroin dependence. It is available in injectable and self-administrable oral forms. Generally speaking, injections and tablets are administered as pain treatment and the oral solution or dissolved tablets administered as part of a detoxification program. Dosages for pain management vary depending upon the severity of the pain and the response.

S0117

S0117   Tretinoin, topical, 5 g

Lay Description
Tretinoin is a retinoid compound that is a metabolite of vitamin A used as an acne treatment. The exact mode of action of tretinoin is not known, but current evidence suggests that topical application decreases the cohesiveness of follicular epithelial cells, which decreases the formation of comedones and stimulates mitotic activity increasing the production of new cells.

S0119

S0119   Ondansetron, oral, 4 mg (for circumstances falling under the Medicare statute, use HCPCS Q code)

Lay Description
Ondansetron hydrochloride is a chemical compound that is a selective blocker of serotonin 5-HT3 receptors. It is an antiemetic drug available in oral and injectable forms. Serotonin 5-HT3 receptors are present on the vagal nerve and at sensory nerve endings. Cytotoxic chemotherapy appears to trigger the release of serotonin in the small intestine, which may trigger the 5-HT3 receptors and initiate the vomiting reflex. Ondansetron hydrochloride is indicated for the prevention of nausea and vomiting associated with surgery and antineoplastic drugs. The oral version is also indicated for the prevention of nausea and vomiting associated with radiation therapy. The drug is available in oral and injectable versions. The recommended dose is 4 mg or 0.1 mg/kg of body weight administered by intravenous or intramuscular injection. Dosages for the oral version vary from 8 to 24 mg depending on the indication and patient.

S0122

S0122   Injection, menotropins, 75 IU

Lay Description
Menotropins is a purified preparation of gonadotropins extracted from the urine of postmenopausal women. It contains follicle-stimulating hormone (FSH) activity and luteinizing hormone (LH) activity. Menotropins is used to treat infertility in women. The medication is administered for seven to 12 days to stimulate follicular growth in women who do not have primary ovarian failure. Menotropins treatment results in follicular growth and maturation. An additional drug has to be given to induce ovulation. Menotropins is administered by subcutaneous or intramuscular injection.

S0126

S0126   Injection, follitropin alfa, 75 IU

Lay Description
Follitropin alfa contains a human follicle stimulating hormone (FSH) preparation of recombinant DNA origin. FSH, the active component of follitropin alfa, is responsible for follicular growth, maturation, and gonadal steroid production. It is found in genetically modified Chinese hamster ovary (CHO) cells cultured in bioreactors. Follitropin alfa contains no luteinizing hormone (LH) activity. Based on available data derived from physicochemical tests and bioassays, follitropin alfa and follitropin beta are indistinguishable. Follitropin is used to treat infertility in women and to induce spermatogenesis in men with hypogonadotropic hypogonadism. Follitropin alfa stimulates ovarian follicular growth in women who do not have primary ovarian failure. In order to continue the final phase of follicle maturation, resumption of meiosis, and rupture of the follicle in the absence of an endogenous LH surge, human chorionic gonadotropin (hCG) must be given following the administration of follitropin when patient monitoring indicates that appropriate follicular development has occurred. Follitropin alfa is administered with hCG to men with hypogonadotropic hypogonadism to stimulate spermatogenesis. FSH is the primary hormone responsible for spermatogenesis. Follitropin alfa can be administered via subcutaneous injection.

S0128

S0128   Injection, follitropin beta, 75 IU

Lay Description

Follitropin beta contains a human follicle stimulating hormone (FSH) preparation of recombinant DNA origin. FSH, the active component of follitropin alfa, is responsible for follicular growth, maturation, and gonadal steroid production. It is found in genetically modified Chinese hamster ovary (CHO) cells cultured in bioreactors. Follitropin beta has a dimeric structure containing two glycoprotein subunits (alpha and beta). Follitropin beta contains no luteinizing hormone (LH) activity. Based on available data derived from physicochemical tests and bioassays, follitropin alfa and follitropin beta are indistinguishable. Follitropin is used to treat infertility in women and to induce spermatogenesis in men with hypogonadotropic hypogonadism. Follitropin alfa stimulates ovarian follicular growth in women who do not have primary ovarian failure. In order to continue the final phase of follicle maturation, resumption of meiosis, and rupture of the follicle in the absence of an endogenous LH surge, human chorionic gonadotropin (hCG) must be given following the administration of follitropin when patient monitoring indicates that appropriate follicular development has occurred. Follitropin alfa is administered with hCG to men with hypogonadotropic hypogonadism to stimulate spermatogenesis. FSH is the primary hormone responsible for spermatogenesis. Follitropin beta can be administered via subcutaneous or intramuscular injection for women and only by subcutaneous injection for men.

S0132

S0132   Injection, ganirelix acetate, 250 mcg

Lay Description

Ganirelix acetate is a synthetic decapeptide with high antagonistic activity against naturally occurring gonadotropin-releasing hormone (GnRH). The pulsatile release of GnRH stimulates the synthesis and secretion of luteinizing hormone (LH) and follicle-stimulating hormone (FSH). The large increase of GnRH at mid-cycle results in an LH surge. This results in ovulation, resumption of meiosis in the oocyte, and luteinization. Ganirelix is given to women undergoing fertility treatment to prevent the eggs from being released prematurely. The usual dose is 250 micrograms once a day. It is administered via subcutaneous injection during the mid to late portion of the follicular phase.

S0136

S0136   Clozapine, 25 mg

Lay Description

Clozapine is an atypical antipsychotic medication used to treat severely ill schizophrenic patients who do not respond effectively to standard drug treatment. It is considered an atypical antipsychotic medication because its profile of binding to dopamine receptors and its effects on various dopamine-mediated behaviors differ from those exhibited by more typical antipsychotic drug products. Specifically, although it does interfere with the binding of dopamine at D1, D2, D3, and D5 receptors and has a high affinity for the D4 receptor, it does not induce catalepsy nor inhibit apomorphine-induced stereotypy. It is a tricyclic dibenzodiazepine derivative. Doses can vary from 600 to 900 mg a day. Patients are started on small doses and the amount is gradually increased to obtain a therapeutic dose. Clozapine is administered orally.

S0137

S0137   Didanosine (ddI), 25 mg

Lay Description

Didanosine (ddI) is an antiviral used in combination with other drugs to treat human immunodeficiency virus (HIV). It is a synthetic nucleoside analogue of the naturally occurring nucleoside deoxyadenosine in which the 3-hydroxyl group is replaced by hydrogen. In the cell, didanosine is converted by cellular enzymes to, the active metabolite, dideoxyadenosine 5'- triphosphate, which inhibits the activity of HIV-1 reverse transcriptase both by competing with the natural substrate, deoxyadenosine 5'-triphosphate, and by its incorporation into viral DNA. This causes failure of viral DNA chain elongation. The usual dose is 400 mg for patients weighing > 60 kg and 250 mg for patients weighing < 60 kg. Didanosine is administered orally and should be taken on an empty stomach.

S0138

S0138   Finasteride, 5 mg

Lay Description

Finasteride is a synthetic compound that is a specific inhibitor of an intracellular steroidal enzyme that converts androgen testosterone into dihydrotestosterone (DHT). Development and enlargement of the prostate gland is dependent upon DHT. Finasteride is indicated as a treatment for symptomatic benign prostatic hypertrophy and androgenic alopecia or male pattern baldness. The drug is available in oral form only with a usual dose of 5 mg for treatment of benign prostatic hypertrophy with 1 mg doses used for treatment of hair loss.

S0139

S0139   Minoxidil, 10 mg

Lay Description

Minoxidil is a peripheral vasodilator used to treat hypertension by decreasing peripheral vascular resistance. It is usually used on patients who do not respond adequately to maximum doses of other hypertensive medications and diuretics. It is usually given in conjunction with beta-blockers and diuretics.

The recommended dose for adults older than age 12 is 5 mg a day but can be increased to a maximum of 100 mg a day. The recommended dose for children age 12 and younger is 0.2 mg per kg with a maximum dose of 50 mg per day. Minoxidil used in the treatment of hypertension is administered orally. Minoxidil is also available in topical form. The topical form is used as a hair restorer for men and women with certain types of hair loss.

S0140

S0140   Saquinavir, 200 mg

Lay Description
Saquinavir is a chemical complex that is an HIV protease inhibitor. HIV protease is an enzyme required for replication of the HIV virus. Saquinavir binds to the protease active site and inhibits the activity of the enzyme, which prevents cleavage of the virus polypeptides and results in the formation of immature noninfectious virus particles. Saquinavir in combination with ritonavir and other antiretroviral agents is indicated for the treatment of HIV infection. Saquinavir is administered orally and is available in 200 and 500 mg capsules. The recommended dose of saquinavir is 1,000 mg per day to be used in combination with ritonavir and other antiretroviral agents.

S0142

S0142   Colistimethate sodium, inhalation solution administered through DME, concentrated form, per mg

Lay Description
Colistimethate sodium is an antibiotic produced by certain strains of *Bacillus polymyxa*. Colistimethate sodium is anionic and is readily hydrolyzed to a variety of methanesulfonate derivatives. Colistimethate sodium is indicated as a treatment for *Pseudomonas aeruginosa* infections in cystic fibrosis patients, and it has come into recent use for treating multidrug-resistant *Acinetobacter* infection, but resistant forms have been reported. Colistimethate sodium powder for inhalation is administered twice daily for as long as a physician thinks beneficial. Extemporaneously prepared solutions for nebulization should be used promptly after being prepared.

S0145

S0145   Injection, pegylated interferon alfa-2a, 180 mcg per ml

Lay Description
Interferon alfa-2a pegylated is a covalent conjugate of interferon alfa-2a recombinant. It is a drug that uses a genetically engineered Escherichia coli bacterium containing DNA that codes for the human protein. In the pegylated form, a special strand (commonly called a PEG) is attached to the interferon molecule that helps to protect the interferon from being destroyed

by the immune system. Interferon alfa-2a pegylated is used to treat chronic hepatitis C with compensated liver disease and HBeAg positive and HBeAg negative chronic hepatitis B with evidence of viral replication and liver inflammation. The recommended dose is 180 micrograms once a week. Interferon alfa-2a is administered via subcutaneous injection.

S0148

S0148   Injection, pegylated interferon alfa-2B, 10 mcg

Lay Description
Interferon alfa-2b pegylated is a covalent conjugate of interferon alfa-2b recombinant. It is a drug that uses a genetically engineered *Escherichia coli* bacterium containing DNA that codes for the human protein. In the pegylated form, a special strand (commonly called a PEG) is attached to the interferon molecule that helps protect the interferon from being destroyed by the immune system. Interferon alfa-2b is used to treat chronic hepatitis C with compensated liver disease. The recommended dose is 1 microgram per kg on the same day each week for one year. Interferon alfa-2b is administered via subcutaneous injection.

S0155

S0155   Sterile dilutant for epoprostenol, 50 ml

Lay Description
Epoprostenol is a prostaglandin that acts as a direct vasodilator of pulmonary and systemic arteries and an inhibitor of platelet aggregation. It is usually administered parenterally through a permanent indwelling central venous catheter as a long-term medication to treat primary pulmonary hypertension and pulmonary hypertension secondary to scleroderma in NYHA Class III and IV patients. Initial administration may be through a peripheral intravenous infusion until a central venous catheter is established. It is manufactured as a powder that must be reconstituted with sterile diluent specific to the epoprostenol. Dosages vary dependent upon body weight and response. Once a regimen of epoprostenol has been established, it should never be stopped suddenly.

S0156

S0156   Exemestane, 25 mg

Lay Description
Exemestane is an irreversible, steroidal aromatase inactivator. It acts as a false substrate to the aromatase enzyme and binds to the active site of this enzyme in postmenopausal women to cause its inactivation. Exemestane lowers the circulating concentration in postmenopausal women. Many breast cancers have estrogen receptors, and growth of these tumors can be stimulated by estrogen. It is used in adjuvant treatment of postmenopausal women with estrogen receptor positive early breast cancer who have received two to three years of tamoxifen and are

switched to exemestane to finish a total of five consecutive years of adjuvant hormonal therapy. Exemestane has proven effective for the treatment of advanced breast cancer in postmenopausal women whose disease has progressed following tamoxifen therapy. The recommended dose is 25 mg once per day after a meal. Exemestane is administered orally.

S0157
S0157   Becaplermin gel 0.01%, 0.5 gm

Lay Description
Becaplermin gel is a human platelet-derived growth factor (PDGF), a substance naturally produced by the body, that helps to promote wound healing. Becaplermin is available as a gel that is applied to the skin, usually once per day. The amount of gel applied depends on the size of the ulcer and may be changed every one to two weeks as the ulcer heals. It is supplied in a 15 gram tube. Becaplermin gel is used to treat ulcers of the foot, ankle, or leg in patients with diabetes. When used in combination with standard ulcer care that includes cleaning, pressure relief, and infection control, it works by bringing the cells that the body uses to repair wounds to the site of the ulcer. The gel may cause localized skin rash.

S0160
S0160   Dextroamphetamine sulfate, 5 mg

Lay Description
Dextroamphetamine sulfate is an amphetamine. Amphetamines are noncatecholamine, sympathomimetic amines with central nervous system (CNS) stimulant activity. They elevate blood pressure, stimulate respirations, and are highly addictive. Dextroamphetamine is used to treat narcolepsy and as part of a treatment regimen in attention deficit disorder with hyperactivity in children ages 3 to 6. The recommended dose is 5 to 60 mg per day depending on the patient. Dextroamphetamine is administered orally.

S0164
S0164   Injection, pantoprazole sodium, 40 mg

Lay Description
Pantoprazole sodium is a compound that inhibits gastric secretions. Pantoprazole is a proton pump inhibitor (PPI) that suppresses the final step in gastric acid production by forming a covalent bond to two sites of the ATPase enzyme system at the secretory surface of the gastric parietal cell. This effect is dose-related and leads to inhibition of both basal and stimulated gastric acid secretion irrespective of the stimulus. This binding results in a period of antisecretory effect that persists longer than 24 hours for all doses tested. This drug is indicated for short-term treatment (seven to 10 days) for patients with gastroesophageal reflux disease (GERD) and a history of erosive esophagitis, and the hypersecretory conditions that may be associated with

Zollinger-Ellison syndrome or other neoplastic conditions.

S0166
S0166   Injection, olanzapine, 2.5 mg

Lay Description
Olanzapine is a psychotropic agent that belongs to the thienobenzodiazepine class. It is used to treat schizophrenia, acute mixed or manic episodes associated with bipolar disorder, agitation associated with schizophrenia, and bipolar disorder.

S0169
S0169   Calcitrol, 0.25 mcg

Lay Description
Calcitrol is a form of cholecalciferol that is a parathyroid-like hormone. It increases the ability of the body to absorb vitamin D and to distribute calcium throughout the body. It is indicated for the treatment of hypocalcemia, hypophosphatemia, rickets, osteodystrophy associated with long-term dialysis, and such disorders as hypoparathyroidism and pseudo-hypoparathyroidism. It is available in oral and injectable forms. The injectable form is administered by intravenous injection. Dosages vary from 0.25 to 3 mcg depending upon the form and indication.

S0170
S0170   Anastrozole, oral, 1 mg

Lay Description
Anastrozole is a non-steroidal aromatase inhibitor. Anastrozole is converted to estrone in adipose tissue of the breast. The estrone is further converted to estradiol, which is the primary source of estrogen in postmenopausal women. Many breast cancers have estrogen receptors and growth of these tumors can be stimulated by estrogen. Anastrozole is used to treat postmenopausal women with hormone receptor positive early breast cancer and for the first-line treatment of postmenopausal women with hormone receptor positive or hormone receptor unknown locally advanced or metastatic breast cancer. Recommended dose is 1 mg per day. Anastrozole is administered orally.

S0171
S0171   Injection, bumetanide, 0.5 mg

Lay Description
Bumetanide is a potent diuretic that is in the class of loop diuretics. It blocks fluid and sodium reabsorbsion from the kidney's tubules. This medication is used to treat mild to moderate hypertension, edema associated with heart failure, renal disease, and cirrhosis of the liver.

S0172

S0172 Chlorambucil, oral, 2 mg

Lay Description
Chlorambucil is a nitrogen mustard type of antineoplastic drug. It is used as palliative treatment for chronic lymphatic (lymphocytic) leukemia and malignant lymphomas, including lymphosarcoma, giant follicular lymphoma, and Hodgkin's disease. The usual oral dosage is 0.1 to 0.2 mg per kg body weight daily for three to six weeks. Chlorambucil is administered orally.

S0174

S0174 Dolasetron mesylate, oral 50 mg (for circumstances falling under the Medicare statute, use Q0180)

Lay Description
Dolasetron mesylate is a chemical compound that is a selective blocker of serotonin 5-HT3 receptors. It is an antiemetic drug available in oral and injectable forms. Serotonin 5-HT3 receptors are present on the vagal nerve and at sensory nerve endings. Cytotoxic chemotherapy appears to trigger the release of serotonin in the small intestine, which may trigger the 5-HT3 receptors and initiate the vomiting reflex. This code represents 50 mg of oral dolasetron mesylate.

S0175

S0175 Flutamide, oral, 125 mg

Lay Description
Flutamide is a nonsteroidal compound that actively inhibits the uptake of androgen and inhibits the nuclear binding of androgen to target cells. Prostate cancer is known to be androgen sensitive and responds to treatment that counteracts androgenic effects or removal of the androgen source. Flutamide is available only in oral form. It is indicated for use in conjunction with luteinizing hormone-releasing hormone (LHRH) agonists as a treatment for locally confined and metastatic carcinoma of the prostate.

S0176

S0176 Hydroxyurea, oral, 500 mg

Lay Description
Hydroxyurea is an antineoplastic drug used to treat melanoma, resistant chronic myelocytic leukemia, and recurrent, metastatic, or inoperable carcinoma of the ovary, and in conjunction with radiation therapy for primary squamous cell (epidermoid) carcinomas of the head and neck, excluding the lip. Hydroxyurea is administered orally.

S0177

S0177 Levamisole HCl, oral, 50 mg

Lay Description
Levamisole is an antineoplastic drug used as an adjuvant therapy in conjunction with 5-fluorouracil after surgical resection to treat patients with Dukes'

Stage C colon cancer. The initial dose is 50 mg every eight hours beginning seven to 30 days after surgery for three days. The maintenance dose is 50 mg every eight hours for three days every two weeks. Levamisole is administered orally.

S0178

S0178 Lomustine, oral, 10 mg

Lay Description
Lomustine is used to treat primary and metastatic brain tumors in patients who have already undergone surgical or radiation therapy, and as secondary therapy in Hodgkin's disease for patients who relapse while being treated with other medications or do not respond to primary therapy. Lomustine is administered orally.

S0179

S0179 Megestrol acetate, oral, 20 mg

Lay Description
Megestrol acetate is an antineoplastic medication used as palliative treatment for advanced carcinoma of the breast or endometrium. Megestrol acetate has a direct cytoxic effect on tumors in the breast. In metastatic cancer, hormone receptors may be present in some tissues but not others. The receptor mechanism is a cyclic process whereby estrogen produced by the ovaries enters the target cell, forms a complex with cytoplasmic receptor, and is transported into the cell nucleus. Inside the cell nucleus it alters the normal cell function. This medication decreases the number of hormone-dependent human breast cancer cells and can change or eliminate the way estrogen acts upon these cells. It is not known how megestrol acetate acts on endometrial cancer. Recommended dose for breast cancer is 40 mg four times a day. Recommended dose for endometrial cancer is 40 to 320 mg per day in divided doses. The usual treatment lasts two months. Megestrol acetate is administered orally.

S0182

S0182 Procarbazine HCl, oral, 50 mg

Lay Description
Procarbazine hydrochloride is used to treat stage III and stage IV Hodgkin's disease. It is used in combination with other antineoplastic drugs. The recommended dose is 50 mg per m^2 of body surface per day for the first week. After that 100 mg per m^2 of body surface per day should be given until the maximum response is obtained or until thrombocytopenia or leukopenia occurs. When the maximum response is attained, the dose may be maintained at 50 mg per m^2 of body surface per day. Procarbazine is administered orally.

S0183
S0183 Prochlorperazine maleate, oral, 5 mg (for circumstances falling under the Medicare statute, use Q0164)

Lay Description
Prochlorperazine/prochlorperazine maleate is an antiemetic used for severe nausea and vomiting, such as that associated with the administration of chemotherapy and prior to induction of anesthesia to control nausea and vomiting during and after surgery. The drug inhibits nausea and vomiting by acting on the chemoreceptor trigger zone and partially depresses the vomiting center. Prochlorperazine is also indicated for treating adult psychiatric illnesses, including schizophrenia, nonpsychotic anxiety, and mild psychotic disorders. Prochlorperazine is available in injection form for intramuscular (IM) and intravenous (IV) use, in tablets, extended release capsules and syrup for oral administration, and in suppository form. The dosage, route of administration, and frequency of administration depends on the patient's diagnosis, the severity of symptoms, and, in the injectable form, by the patient's weight.

S0187
S0187 Tamoxifen citrate, oral, 10 mg

Lay Description
Tamoxifen citrate is a nonsteroidal antiestrogen used to treat metastatic breast cancer in men and women, ductal carcinoma in situ, and women at high risk to develop breast cancer. High risk is defined as women at least 35 years of age with a five-year predicted risk of breast cancer > 1.67%, as calculated by the Gail Model. In premenopausal women with metastatic breast cancer, tamoxifen citrate is an alternative to oophorectomy or ovarian irradiation. It is believed that patients whose tumors are estrogen receptor positive are more likely to benefit from tamoxifen citrate therapy. It is recommended for postmenopausal women with node positive breast cancer who have undergone mastectomy, axillary dissection, and radiation therapy. Recommended dose is 20 to 40 mg per day. Tamoxifen citrate is administered orally.

S0189
S0189 Testosterone pellet, 75 mg

Lay Description
Testosterone is an anabolic steroid used primarily to treat male hypogonadism. It stimulates targeted tissues to develop normally in androgen-deficient men. Testosterone may also have some anti-estrogen properties, making it useful in treating certain estrogen-dependent breast cancers. This drug is used to treat male hypogonadism, unusually late sexual maturity, myotonia congenita, inflammation and rotation of the testes, undescended testicle, absence of testicles, Klinefelter syndrome, anemia, and in the prevention of breast pain and engorgement in postpartum women.

S0190
S0190 Mifepristone, oral, 200 mg

Lay Description
Mifepristone, also known as RU486, is a synthetic steroid with anti-progestational effects. The drug is used for the medical termination of an intrauterine pregnancy through the 49th day. Mifepristone binds to progesterone receptor sites blocking the effects of progesterone.

S0191
S0191 Misoprostol, oral, 200 mcg

Lay Description
Misoprostol is a synthetic prostaglandin E1 analog. It is used to reduce the risk of gastric ulcers in patients undergoing NSAID treatment who may be at high risk for complications of ulcers, including elderly patients, those with a history of gastric ulcers, and patients with a concomitant debilitating disease. Misoprostol inhibits gastric acid secretion and may have mucosal protective properties. NSAIDs reduce prostaglandin synthesis, and a lack of prostaglandins within the gastric mucosa may lead to diminishing bicarbonate and mucus secretion and may contribute to the mucosal damage caused by these agents. As a synthetic prostaglandin, misoprostol can also induce labor and dilate the cervix. Misoprostol may be used as a sole drug or in combination with mifepristone to induce a medical termination of pregnancy. The recommended dose for treatment of gastric ulcers is 200 mcg four times a day. Misoprostol is administered orally. It is sometimes administered vaginally for the induction of labor or termination of pregnancy.

S0194
S0194 Dialysis/stress vitamin supplement, oral, 100 capsules

Lay Description
Vitamins and minerals are organic compounds that are necessary for the metabolic functioning of the body. Multivitamins are combined forms of vitamins and may include minerals. Multivitamins are usually oral tablets. Pregnant patients, patients on dialysis, patients with malabsorption diseases, and those with deficient diets may need exogenous sources of multiple vitamins. Liquid forms may be added to TPN solutions. Multivitamins are sold over-the-counter and are self-administered orally.

S0195

S0195   Pneumococcal conjugate vaccine, polyvalent, intramuscular, for children from 5 years to 9 years of age who have not previously received the vaccine

Lay Description
Vaccines are suspensions of weakened, altered, or killed microorganisms of the antigen proteins derived from the microorganism administered for the prevention, improvement, or treatment of an infectious disease. The microorganism or the antigen proteins within the vaccine stimulate the immune system to produce antibodies to the specific microorganism. Pneumococcal infections are caused by the bacterium *Streptococcus pneumoniae*. There are more than 80 distinct types of polysaccharides associated with the capsule of the bacterium. Pneumococcus most commonly causes lobar pneumonia but may also cause meningitis, septicemia, empyema, and peritonitis. There are currently two different types of pneumococcal vaccines. One is a heptavalent conjugate vaccine containing purified polysaccharides of the capsular antigens of the bacterium types 4, 6B, 9V, 14, 18C, 19F, and 23F. In the conjugate vaccine, the polysaccharides are coupled with a nontoxic purified diphtheria protein. The conjugate vaccine is administered as an intramuscular injection to children younger than 23 months and children ages 24 to 59 months who are at high risk for pneumococcal infection, including those with sickle cell disease, HIV infection, those immunocompromised, and those with chronic illness, such as cardiac or pulmonary disease or diabetes mellitus. The second type of vaccine is a polyvalent, 23-valent vaccine containing the capsular polysaccharide of the bacterium, types 1-5, 8, 9, 12, 14, 17, 19, 20, 22, 23, 26, 34, 43, 51, 54, 56, 57, 68, and 70, which are responsible for about 90 percent of pneumococcal disease in the United States. The polyvalent vaccine is administered intramuscularly to individuals older than 2 years of age who are at increased risk for the disease or its complications, such as those with chronic illnesses. The polyvalent vaccine is also administered to individuals age 65 years or older and persons residing in nursing homes or other institutions.

S0197

S0197   Prenatal vitamins, 30-day supply

Lay Description
Vitamins and minerals are organic compounds that are necessary for the metabolic functioning of the body. Multivitamins are combined forms of vitamins and may include minerals. Multivitamins are usually oral tablets. Pregnant patients, patients on dialysis, patients with malabsorption diseases, and those with deficient diets may need exogenous sources of multiple vitamins. Liquid forms may be added to TPN solutions. Multivitamins are sold over-the-counter and are self-administered orally.

S0199

S0199   Medically induced abortion by oral ingestion of medication including all associated services and supplies (e.g., patient counseling, office visits, confirmation of pregnancy by HCG, ultrasound to confirm duration of pregnancy, ultrasound to confirm completion of abortion) except drugs

Lay Description
An induced abortion can be performed in several ways, including surgically or medically. In a medical abortion, certain drugs are taken to cause the abortion. It only can be done early in pregnancy. A medical abortion does not require surgery or anesthesia, but multiple visits to the doctor are needed. There are four types of medical abortion, including mifepristone and misoprostol pills, mifepristone pills and vaginal misoprostol, methotrexate and vaginal misoprostol, and vaginal misoprostol alone. This code is used for a medically induced abortion by oral ingestion of medication, including all associated services and supplies (e.g., patient counseling, office visits, confirmation of pregnancy by hCG, ultrasound to confirm duration of pregnancy, ultrasound to confirm completion of abortion) except drugs.

S0201

S0201   Partial hospitalization services, less than 24 hours, per diem

Lay Description
Partial hospitalization is a nonresidential treatment modality that includes psychiatric, psychological, social, and vocational elements under medical supervision. It is designed for patients with moderate to severe mental or emotional disorders. Partial hospitalization patients require less than 24-hour care, but more intensive and comprehensive services than are offered in outpatient treatment programs. Partial hospital (PH) programs are highly intensive, time-limited medical services intended to provide a transition from inpatient psychiatric hospitalization to community-based care or substitute for an inpatient admission.

S0207-S0208

S0207   Paramedic intercept, nonhospital-based ALS service (nonvoluntary), nontransport

S0208   Paramedic intercept, hospital-based ALS service (nonvoluntary), nontransport

Lay Description
Paramedic intercept services are advanced life support (ALS) services provided by an entity that does not provide the ambulance transport. The ambulance transport crew requests the ALS services from an independent, outside source. This additional paramedic meets the ambulance and provides

needed services, such as CPR, EKG monitoring, or IV skills.

S0207-S0208

S0207 Paramedic intercept, nonhospital-based ALS service (nonvoluntary), nontransport

S0208 Paramedic intercept, hospital-based ALS service (nonvoluntary), nontransport

Lay Description
These codes are used to report advanced life support (ALS) procedures that are done by a non-hospital-based or hospital-based ALS service. ALS procedures usually include invasive services, such as intubation, IV therapy, and drug administration. These services are rendered without providing transportation for the patient.

S0209

S0209 Wheelchair van, mileage, per mile

Lay Description
A wheelchair van is nonemergency transportation provided to patients who are wheelchair-bound. This code represents the distance traveled in miles.

S0209

S0209 Wheelchair van, mileage, per mile

Lay Description
Wheelchair vans are equipped to transport patients in wheelchairs. These vans are equipped with wide enough door openings to accommodate a wheelchair, as well as wheelchair lifts or ramps to enable to wheelchair to enter and exit the van. The wheelchair must be secured to the van while the van is in motion.

S0215

S0215 Nonemergency transportation; mileage, per mile

Lay Description
Nonemergency transportation is transportation provided to patients who are not in an emergent situation. This code represents the distance traveled in miles.

S0215

S0215 Nonemergency transportation; mileage, per mile

Lay Description
Use this code to report the mileage incurred while transporting a patient in a nonemergency setting.

S0220-S0221

S0220 Medical conference by a physician with interdisciplinary team of health professionals or representatives of community agencies to coordinate activities of patient care (patient is present); approximately 30 minutes

S0221 Medical conference by a physician with interdisciplinary team of health professionals or representatives of community agencies to coordinate activities of patient care (patient is present); approximately 60 minutes

Lay Description
A medical conference is a meeting for review, discussion, and/or care planning related to a medical illness or condition. This meeting includes the patient, the physician, and an interdisciplinary team of health professionals, and may include representatives of community agencies. The purpose of the meeting is to plan and coordinate activities of patient care.

S0250

S0250 Comprehensive geriatric assessment and treatment planning performed by assessment team

Lay Description
A comprehensive geriatric assessment involves evaluation and treatment planning designed to optimize an elderly person's ability to maintain good health, improve quality of life, reduce the need for hospital and long-term care services, and enable independent living. Because of the comprehensive scope of this exam, it must be performed by a multi-disciplinary team of experts that may include physicians, geriatric nurse practitioners, ancillary personnel, social workers, psychologists, physical/occupational therapists, dieticians, and pharmacists. The assessment begins with an examination of the elderly person's current status including physical, mental, and psycho-social health status. The ability to function independently and perform basic activities of daily living are assessed including dressing, bathing, meal preparation, and medication management. The individual's living arrangement, social network, and access to support services is evaluated. Next, current problems related to the status assessment are identified and evaluated as to their potential to cause future problems. Based on these findings a comprehensive care plan is developed that addresses all current and potential problems. Specific interventions are proposed, including recommendations regarding necessary resources and support services. Management of resources is initiated with the elderly person and family to assure that the necessary services will be provided. A plan for ongoing monitoring is provided so modifications to the care plan can be initiated as required.

S0255

S0255 Hospice referral visit (advising patient and family of care options) performed by nurse, social worker, or other designated staff

Lay Description

Hospice is a licensed program that offers an integrated set of services and supplies designed to provide comfort measures and supportive care to terminally ill patients and their families. It may include legal, financial, emotional, or spiritual counseling, in addition to meeting the patient's immediate physical needs.

S0255

S0255 Hospice referral visit (advising patient and family of care options) performed by nurse, social worker, or other designated staff

Lay Description

Hospice provides patients who have a life limiting illness with the medical care needed for relief of pain and other symptoms. During the hospice referral visit, the patient and his/her family are made aware of care options, goals are established, and a care plan is set up to try to meet these goals.

S0257

S0257 Counseling and discussion regarding advance directives or end of life care planning and decisions, with patient and/or surrogate (list separately in addition to code for appropriate evaluation and management service)

Lay Description

This code is used to report counseling and discussion regarding advance directives or end-of-life care planning and decisions. These discussions and counseling may be with the patient and/or a surrogate.

S0257

S0257 Counseling and discussion regarding advance directives or end of life care planning and decisions, with patient and/or surrogate (list separately in addition to code for appropriate evaluation and management service)

Lay Description

The advance care directive provides a clear statement of the patient's wishes about when to prolong life or withdraw care. This code reports the discussion and the counseling that is done to explain these options to the patient.

S0260

S0260 History and physical (outpatient or office) related to surgical procedure (list separately in addition to code for appropriate evaluation and management service)

Lay Description

Use this code to report the history and physical that is performed outpatient or in the physician's office that resulted in the decision for surgery.

S0265

S0265 Genetic counseling, under physician supervision, each 15 minutes

Lay Description

Individuals who have a family history of certain genetic diseases or disorders, such as cystic fibrosis, sickle cell anemia, Tay-Sachs disease, or other diseases may be referred for genetic counseling. Genetic counseling is a service that includes evaluating family history and medical records, ordering genetic tests, evaluating the test results, and helping the individuals understand the test results and reach decisions based on the results of the testing. Before meeting with a genetic counselor, information about family history, including relatives with genetic disorders, multiple miscarriages, or early or unexplained deaths, should be gathered. A personal history and medical record information related to ultrasounds, prenatal test results, past pregnancies, and medications should also be provided. The counselor reviews the family and personal history information, determines if additional tests are necessary, assists the individuals in obtaining the necessary tests, and conducts a follow-up when the results of testing are available. During the follow-up, the genetic counselor helps the patient understand options and makes any necessary referrals to other health care professionals.

S0270-S0272

S0270 Physician management of patient home care, standard monthly case rate (per 30 days)

S0271 Physician management of patient home care, hospice monthly case rate (per 30 days)

S0272 Physician management of patient home care, episodic care monthly case rate (per 30 days)

Lay Description

Use these codes to report the physician's management of standard, hospice, or episodic care in the home setting. These services are to be reported on a monthly basis and are paid as a case rate.

S0273-S0274

S0273 **Physician visit at member's home, outside of a capitation arrangement**

S0274 **Nurse practitioner visit at member's home, outside of a capitation arrangement**

Lay Description
Use these codes to report physician or nurse practitioner home care visits that are outside of the capitated case rate.

S0280-S0281

S0280 **Medical home program, comprehensive care coordination and planning, initial plan**

S0281 **Medical home program, comprehensive care coordination and planning, maintenance of plan**

Lay Description
The Multi-payer Advanced Primary Care Practice (MAPCP) Demonstration, also referred to as the patient-centered medical home, is a three-year demonstration whose purpose is to promote advanced primary care (APC) principles. Eight states are participating in this initiative. CMS has joined with Medicaid and commercial insurance payers to participate in each of these eight states' existing multi payer medical home initiatives. CMS pays a monthly care management fee for patients who are receiving primary care from APC practices. In certain circumstances, CMS may pay an additional amount to the organization that works with the APC practice by providing community-based care coordination support. CMS also pays an additional amount to the state for administering and evaluating the program. The payment is a per beneficiary monthly amount that is based on the patients under the practice's care. Use these codes to report the MAPCP services.

S0302

S0302 **Completed early periodic screening diagnosis and treatment (EPSDT) service (list in addition to code for appropriate evaluation and management service)**

Lay Description
Early periodic screening diagnosis and treatment (EPSDT) is a free service provided to children ages birth through 21 who are eligible for Medicaid. EPSDT enables children to get medical exams, check-ups, follow-up care, and any special care needed to ensure optimum health. EPSDT legislation requires states to provide Medicaid-eligible children with periodic screening, vision, dental, and hearing services. States are required to assess a child's health needs through initial and periodic examinations and evaluations to assure that health problems are diagnosed and treated early, before they become more complex. States must perform the required evaluations according to a standardized schedule, called a periodicity schedule. At a minimum, these screenings must include comprehensive health and developmental history, including assessment of both physical and mental health development; comprehensive unclothed physical exam; appropriate immunizations according to age and health history; laboratory tests, including a lead toxicity screening; health education, including anticipatory guidance; vision and hearing screens; and dental screens. In addition, EPSDT legislation requires states provide any medically necessary inter-periodic health screens and care, even if the service is not available under the state's Medicaid plan to adults. Report this code in addition to the appropriate evaluation and management service.

S0310

S0310 **Hospitalist services (list separately in addition to code for appropriate evaluation and management service)**

Lay Description
A hospitalist is a board-certified physician specializing in the care of hospitalized patients. The hospitalist is a single point person who oversees each patient's care throughout the hospital stay. The hospitalist makes daily rounds, checks on each patient as needed throughout the day, monitors the patient's in-hospital care, tracks nursing care, and works to coordinate care between the patient's primary care physician and other physician specialists. In addition, the hospitalist coordinates scheduling of tests and procedures that may be required and follows up to make sure test results are reported and reviewed by the appropriate person. Report this code in addition to the code for the appropriate evaluation and management service.

S0315-S0320

S0315 **Disease management program; initial assessment and initiation of the program**

S0316 **Disease management program, follow-up/reassessment**

S0317 **Disease management program; per diem**

S0320 **Telephone calls by a registered nurse to a disease management program member for monitoring purposes; per month**

Lay Description
Disease management is a system of coordinated health services for patients with specific disease processes, usually chronic conditions. An evolution from managed care and capitated care, disease management seeks to keep costs down and improve patient health through integrative treatments that range from patient education to life style changes and nutrition to inpatient hospitalizations. Most disease management programs are specific to one condition, such as diabetes, asthma, or heart failure.

S

S0340-S0342

S0340 Lifestyle modification program for management of coronary artery disease, including all supportive services; first quarter/stage

S0341 Lifestyle modification program for management of coronary artery disease, including all supportive services; second or third quarter/stage

S0342 Lifestyle modification program for management of coronary artery disease, including all supportive services; 4th quarter / stage

Lay Description

Lifestyle modification programs for coronary artery disease (CAD) are designed to prevent and possibly even reverse coronary artery disease. These programs may include diet modification, exercise, non-smoking, group support, stress management, and exercise. They target spiritual, psychological, and emotional healing and encourage patients to participate in their own care. The lifestyle modification program is completed over the course of a year and is conducted by a team of professionals, which may include registered dieticians, exercise physiologists, specialists in behavioral health, and nurse case managers. Use these codes to report CAD lifestyle modification program services based on the time frame the services were rendered.

S0353-S0354

S0353 Treatment planning and care coordination management for cancer initial treatment

S0354 Treatment planning and care coordination management for cancer established patient with a change of regimen

Lay Description

A treatment plan is a detailed outline of care composed of a list of problems including details on the cancer, goals, methods to achieve the goals, and estimated time necessary to achieve the goals. It may include treatment side effects and the names and addresses of individual providers. The care coordination involves the organization and monitoring of the different types of treatment or services outlined in the treatment plan.

S0390

S0390 Routine foot care; removal and/or trimming of corns, calluses and/or nails and preventive maintenance in specific medical conditions (e.g., diabetes), per visit

Lay Description

Peripheral neuropathy can be caused by many different disease or agents, such as diabetes mellitus or chemotherapeutic drugs. Decreased sensations in the feet can lead to injuries and open wounds. Periodic foot care performed on a routine basis may help to eliminate an issue before it becomes a medical problem. Routine footcare includes removal or trimming of corns, calluses, and toenails.

S0395

S0395 Impression casting of a foot performed by a practitioner other than the manufacturer of the orthotic

Lay Description

Impression casting of a foot is a cast of a foot that is to be used by a podiatrist or orthoticist to create a specialized application that can help correct painful conditions and provide assistance in ambulation. Casting materials can be plaster, wax, or a composite material. Impression casting is generally considered a part of the measurements needed to create an orthotic and is not reported separately.

S0400

S0400 Global fee for extracorporeal shock wave lithotripsy treatment of kidney stone(s)

Lay Description

The physician pulverizes a kidney stone (renal calculus) by directing shock waves through a liquid medium. Two different methods are currently available to accomplish this procedure. The physician first uses radiological guidance to determine the location and size of the renal calculus. In the first method, the patient is then immersed in a liquid medium (degassed, deionized water) with shock waves directed through the liquid to the kidney stone. In the second method, the one most often used, the patient is placed on a specially designed treatment table. A series of shock waves is directed through a water-cushion or bellow placed against the patient's body at the location of the kidney stone. Each shock wave is directed to the stone for only a fraction of a second, and the entire procedure generally takes from 30 to 50 minutes. The treatment table is equipped with video x-ray so the physician can view the pulverization process. Over several days or weeks, the tiny stone fragments pass harmlessly through the patient's urinary system and are discharged during urination.

S0500

S0500 Disposable contact lens, per lens

Lay Description

A contact lens is a corrective, therapeutic, or sometimes cosmetic lens placed on the cornea of the eye. Corrective and therapeutic lenses are intended to correct vision problems in place of glasses, or treat ophthalmological conditions such as corneal ulcers. Contact lenses may be made of hard or soft material, may be made to be worn only when awake, or can be made for continuous overnight wear. Disposable lens are intended to be worn for a specified period of time before being discarded, such a daily, two-week, or four-week disposable lens.

S0504

S0504   Single vision prescription lens (safety, athletic, or sunglass), per lens

Lay Description
A single vision lens provides one viewing surface in the lens that is concave on the back surface. This concave shape follows the shape of the eye and allows the back of the lens to stay at the same distance when the eye moves. It is used to treat refractive errors that cause the patient to have trouble seeing near or far distances. Report this code for single vision specialty prescription safety, athletic, or sunglasses, per lens.

S0506

S0506   Bifocal vision prescription lens (safety, athletic, or sunglass), per lens

Lay Description
Bifocal vision eyeglass lenses address the correction of two focal powers for distance and work, such as reading that requires a close up focus. Lenses are made from glass or plastic to the specific level of correction required to improve vision. The lens provides two viewing surfaces in the lens that is concave on the back surface. This concave shape follows the shape of the eye and allows the back of the lens to stay at the same distance when the eye moves. Use this code to report bifocal specialty prescription safety, athletic, or sunglasses, per lens.

S0508

S0508   Trifocal vision prescription lens (safety, athletic, or sunglass), per lens

Lay Description
Trifocal lenses have three visibly identifiable zones of vision divided by two segment lines of variable widths. Trifocal lenses offer three fixed fields of focus (near/intermediate/distant) for patients with higher levels of presbyopia. The lens provides a three viewing surface that is concave on the back surface. This concave shape follows the shape of the eye and allows the back of the lens to stay at the same distance when the eye moves. It is used to treat refractive errors that cause the patient to have trouble seeing near or far distances. Use this code to report trifocal specialty prescription safety, athletic, or sunglasses, per lens.

S0510

S0510   Nonprescription lens (safety, athletic, or sunglass), per lens

Lay Description
Nonprescription lenses do not correct vision but can serve as a protective covering to the eyes for work, sports participation, and as a barrier against UV rays from the sun.

S0512

S0512   Daily wear specialty contact lens, per lens

Lay Description
Daily wear specialty lenses are designed to be worn daily and removed nightly by patients after certain types of surgery and when other types of lenses are unsuitable. These may include astigmatism, patients who have undergone refractive surgery but need additional correction, and patients with penetrating keratoplasty, eye disfigurement, corneal trauma, or corneal degeneration. Report this code per specialty daily wear contact lens.

S0514

S0514   Color contact lens, per lens

Lay Description
Color contact lenses are worn directly on the cornea and may correct vision or be worn for cosmetic purposes. There are four types of colored contact lens: Light-filtering tinted lenses are intended for athletes and sports fans. These lenses enhance certain colors and mute others. For instance, contact lenses for tennis players enhance the color yellow so the tennis balls are easier to see. Visibility tinted lenses contain a mild tint to make the lenses easier to find if they are dropped. Color tinted lenses are opaque and change the color of the eyes. Enhancement tinted lenses are designed to enhance the natural color of the eyes but do not change the color. Report this code for each lens.

S0515

S0515   Scleral lens, liquid bandage device, per lens

Lay Description
Sclera lenses are a specialized type of contact lens that are larger than the regular soft contact lens and are custom made for each eye. They are designed to rest on the sclera of the eye and to vault over the cornea. The vaulted section is filled with a fluid reservoir that serves as a liquid bandage to help patients with diseased or extremely dry corneas. The fluid reservoir helps improve the patient's vision by masking irregularities of the cornea. Report this code per lens.

S0516-S0518

S0516   Safety eyeglass frames
S0518   Sunglasses frames

Lay Description
Frames are rigid or semi-rigid devices that bear lenses that are held in front of the eyes for vision correction or eye protection. Frames are made from many different materials in many different colors and shapes. Use these codes to report frames used with safety glasses or sunglasses.

S0580

S0580   Polycarbonate lens (list this code in addition to the basic code for the lens)

Lay Description
Polycarbonate lenses are developed from small pellets that are heated until melted and then rapidly injected into lens molds after which they are compressed under high pressure and cooled. These lenses are impact-resistant and often used by people participating in sports and for children and others who are apt to drop and scratch the lenses. The lenses are thin and lightweight.

S0581

S0581   Nonstandard lens (list this code in addition to the basic code for the lens)

Lay Description
A nonstandard lens is any lens that deviates from the average in curvature, size, or both. Report this code in addition to the code for the basic lens.

S0590

S0590   Integral lens service, miscellaneous services reported separately

Lay Description
Use this code to report an integral lens service that is not covered by a current HCPCS Level II code.

S0592

S0592   Comprehensive contact lens evaluation

Lay Description
The comprehensive contact lens evaluation includes the general eye examination in addition to measuring the eye's surface and curvature, possibly measuring the size of the pupils in different lighting conditions, measurement of the cornea diameter, tear film evaluation using Schirmer's test or fluorescein staining, and examining the eye's surface to determine the type of contact lens that will best meet the patient's needs.

S0595

S0595   Dispensing new spectacle lenses for patient supplied frame

Lay Description
This code is used to report the dispensing of new spectacle lenses for patients that supply their own frames. Dispensing services include following prescriptions written by ophthalmologists or optometrists and fitting the completed glasses on the patient.

S0596

S0596   Phakic intraocular lens for correction of refractive error

Lay Description
This lens is designed for people with extreme nearsightedness, from -10 to -20 diopters of myopia (nearsightedness). People with severe vision impairment may not be suitable candidates for cornea-based refractive surgery like LASIK and PRK. These lenses are not used for patients who have a cataract and have their lens replaced. This lens is a small lens implant inserted into the eye through a small incision at the edge of the cornea. The lens is placed behind the iris and in front of the natural crystalline lens without removing the natural lens. It is then adhered to the front of the iris, or colored portion of the eye, to hold it securely.

S0601

S0601   Screening proctoscopy

Lay Description
A screening proctoscopy allows visualization of the inner lining of the anus and rectum that is done through a proctoscope, a straight, rigid, hollow metal or plastic tube with a small light at the end. It is done to screen for polyps, inflammation, bleeding, and cancer and requires an enema or laxative prior to the procedure.

S0610-S0613

S0610   Annual gynecological examination, new patient

S0612   Annual gynecological examination, established patient

S0613   Annual gynecological examination; clinical breast examination without pelvic evaluation

Lay Description
The annual gynecologic (GYN) exam consists of a breast exam, a pelvic exam, and a Pap test. It is done to evaluate risk factors, monitor changes in health over time, evaluate and prescribe use of birth control methods, provide guidance in wellness, and to detect current health problems. Use these codes to report the annual GYN exam, based on whether the patient is new or established or if the GYN exam is a breast exam only.

S0618

S0618   Audiometry for hearing aid evaluation to determine the level and degree of hearing loss

Lay Description
Audiometry is a hearing test to determine the type and degree of hearing loss and to determine if the patient is a candidate for hearing aids. This exam determines if there is a need for further medical assessment or medical clearance for hearing aids.

S0620-S0621

S0620 Routine ophthalmological examination including refraction; new patient

S0621 Routine ophthalmological examination including refraction; established patient

Lay Description
The ophthalmologist or optometrist performs a routine eye (ophthalmological) examination including refraction. A complete eye examination involves a series of tests to evaluate vision and check for eye diseases. A visual exam is performed on the external eye to check the pupils' response to light, the clarity and shininess of the cornea and iris, and the position and movement of the eyes, eyelids, and eyelashes. The provider checks the eye muscles to ensure they are functioning properly. Tests on the eye muscles involve following movement of an object up and down and side to side to detect any eye muscle weakness or uncontrolled movement. A visual acuity test is performed using an eye chart. Following the visual acuity test, a refraction assessment is performed on individuals who need corrective lenses to determine the prescription required. The provider may use a computerized refractor to estimate the prescription, or alternatively a retinoscopy may be performed. A retinoscopy involves shining a light into the eye and measuring the refractive error by evaluating the movement of the light that is reflected by the retina. These results are verified and fine-tuned using a Phoroptor, which consists of a series of lenses through which the patient views an eye chart and indicates which lens provides the clearest vision. The provider checks peripheral vision by means of a visual field (perimetry) test. A slit lamp exam is performed. A slit lamp uses an intense line of light to examine the cornea, iris, lens, and anterior eye chamber. The provider performs a glaucoma test, which checks intraocular pressure. The pupils are dilated, and the retina is examined.

S0622

S0622 Physical exam for college, new or established patient (list separately in addition to appropriate evaluation and management code)

Lay Description
A physical exam is required for college admission and, depending on the college, may be an annual requirement. This code describes the college physical exam and is to be reported in addition to the evaluation and management code.

S0630

S0630 Removal of sutures; by a physician other than the physician who originally closed the wound

Lay Description
The physician removes sutures that have been placed by another physician. When a laceration or an incision

for a surgical procedure has required suturing, any non-absorbable stitches must by removed. The area is cleansed with an antiseptic cleanser to remove any dried blood and loosen any scar tissue. Sterile forceps are used to lift the suture at the knot. The suture material is then clipped as close to the skin as possible using sterile forceps and removed. When all the sutures are removed, the area is cleaned again with antiseptic. Adhesive strips and a dry dressing may be applied as needed.

S0800

S0800 Laser in situ keratomileusis (LASIK)

Lay Description
Laser in situ keratomileusis (LASIK) is a type of refractive surgery used to correct myopia, hyperopia, and astigmatism. The cornea directs or refracts light to the retina. The shape of the corneal lens can create blurry or multiple images on the retina. An ultraviolet excimer laser, which does not heat surrounding tissue, is used to ablate corneal tissue, reshaping the curvature of the lens. A flap in the cornea is created and pulled back and the laser is used to ablate the underlying corneal tissue in a pattern designed for the patient and the patient's vision problems. LASIK is intended to improve the patient's vision by improving the refraction of light and decreasing the need for glasses or contact lens.

S0810

S0810 Photorefractive keratectomy (PRK)

Lay Description
Photorefractive keratectomy (PRK) is a type of refractive surgery used to correct myopia, hyperopia, and astigmatism. The cornea directs or refracts light to the retina. The shape of the corneal lens can create blurry or multiple images on the retina. An ultraviolet excimer laser, which does not heat surrounding tissue, is used to ablate corneal tissue, reshaping the curvature of the lens. PRK reshapes the surface of the cornea rather than the underlying tissue (as in LASIK). The laser is used to ablate the corneal tissue in a pattern designed for the patient and the patient's vision problems. Photorefractive keratectomy is intended to improve the patient's vision by improving the refraction of light and decreasing the need for glasses or contact lens.

S0812

S0812 Phototherapeutic keratectomy (PTK)

Lay Description
Phototherapeutic keratectomy (PTK) is a type of eye surgery used to treat anterior corneal diseases and scars. PTK is indicated as a treatment for epithelial basement membrane dystrophy, irregular corneal surfaces, shallow corneal scars, corneal opacities, and superficial corneal dystrophies, including granular, lattice, and Reis-Buckler's. An ultraviolet excimer laser, which does not heat surrounding tissue, is used to

ablate corneal tissue to produce a smoother, clearer lens. PTK is a therapeutic procedure and is not intended to decrease the need for glasses or contact lenses.

S1001-S1002

S1001 Deluxe item, patient aware (list in addition to code for basic item)

S1002 Customized item (list in addition to code for basic item)

Lay Description
These codes can be used to report the difference between the base model of an item and the deluxe (or customized) model. For example, report the HCPCS Level II code and charge for a base model of hearing aid and on another line of the claim, list these HCPCS Level II codes to represent the deluxe (or customized) hearing aid model along with the difference in charge between the base hearing aid model and the deluxe (or customized) model.

S1015

S1015 IV tubing extension set

Lay Description
An IV tubing extension set is designed to provide longer IV tubing between the access site and the IV fluid source. This may be done to prevent the needle from dislodging and to allow greater mobility for the patient.

S1016

S1016 Non-PVC (polyvinyl chloride) intravenous administration set, for use with drugs that are not stable in PVC e.g., Paclitaxel

Lay Description
Some drugs and biologicals are unstable in a PVC environment and must be administered using IV tubing that contains no PVC. Use this code to report an IV administration that is PVC free.

S1030-S1031

S1030 Continuous noninvasive glucose monitoring device, purchase (for physician interpretation of data, use CPT code)

S1031 Continuous noninvasive glucose monitoring device, rental, including sensor, sensor replacement, and download to monitor (for physician interpretation of data, use CPT code)

Lay Description
The continuous noninvasive glucose monitoring devise is worn like a watch and has a special sensor. Without breaking the skin, this sensor measures the patient's blood sugar levels. The patient's blood sugar patterns are recorded and analyzed by the physician, who makes any necessary changes in the patient's treatment. This device is considered experimental by most payers. Use these codes to report the purchase or rental of the continuous glucose monitoring device.

S1034

S1034 Artificial pancreas device system (e.g., low glucose suspend [LGS] feature) including continuous glucose monitor, blood glucose device, insulin pump and computer algorithm that communicates with all of the devices

Lay Description
An artificial pancreas device system (APDS) links a group of devices used to detect and react to rising blood glucose levels by combining a glucose sensor, a control algorithm and an insulin infusion device. The APDS parts communicate with each other to automate the process of maintaining blood glucose concentrations at or near a specific target/range. The glucose sensor continuously detects the patient's glucose levels. The sensor then outputs the glucose level to a control system, which then computes the patient's required insulin dosage and directs the insulin pump to deliver the prescribed dosage. The system may also direct the pump to withhold delivery of insulin.

S1035-S1036

S1035 Sensor; invasive (e.g., subcutaneous), disposable, for use with artificial pancreas device system

S1036 Transmitter; external, for use with artificial pancreas device system

Lay Description
A tiny electrode called a glucose sensor is inserted under the skin to measure glucose levels in tissue fluid. The glucose sensor has a small adhesive (sticky) patch to hold it in place for a few days and then it must be replaced with a new sensor. The glucose sensor is inserted with a needle, which is removed after the glucose sensor is in place, generally in the abdominal area. The glucose sensor is easily inserted under the skin using an insertion device. The continuous glucose monitoring transmitter is a small, lightweight device that attaches to the glucose sensor, gathers glucose data, and sends it wirelessly to the glucose monitoring unit.

S1037

S1037 Receiver (monitor); external, for use with artificial pancreas device system

Lay Description
The artificial pancreas external receiver (monitor) can be a stand-alone device or built into an insulin pump. The receiver is small and can be attached to a belt, placed in a pocket, or hidden under clothing. The receiver displays the current glucose levels as well as historical trends. Notifications are issued before the patient reaches predetermined low or high glucose

limits. When built into an insulin pump, the device automatically holds or delivers insulin.

S1040

S1040 Cranial remolding orthotic, pediatric, rigid, with soft interface material, custom fabricated, includes fitting and adjustment(s)

Lay Description

This code reports the supply of a special cranial remolding orthosis used to treat plagiocephaly. Plagiocephaly refers to misshapen or flattened skull bones and a variety of causes are noted, including premature closure of cranial sutures, birth trauma, torticollis, or repetitive sleeping positions. This type of cranial remolding orthosis consists of a custom-fabricated, helmet-like device structured to address the specific cranial malformation of the infant. The orthosis has a soft interface material for comfort, as many are worn up to 23 hours per day. Some models consist of broad bands with mild elastic properties, while others are fabricated by molding to the patient's skull. The cranial remolding orthosis is designed to address plagiocephaly and manipulate skull development toward a more normal shape, or to maintain skull structure. This code reports the supply, fitting, and any required adjustments of the custom-fabricated, rigid, pediatric, cranial orthosis.

S1090

S1090 Mometasone furoate sinus implant, 370 micrograms

Lay Description

A mometasone furoate sinus implant is a self-dissolving device that delivers a sustained, localized, controlled release of the corticosteroid. The device is implanted during sinus surgery where it expands to prop open the sinus, support the bony structures inside the nose, and help prevent scar formation. The device delivers a sustained release of mometasone furoate over a 30-day period. The implant contains 370 micrograms. It is absorbed by the body within six weeks after the surgical implant. It is indicated as a treatment for chronic sinusitis in patients having ethmoid sinus surgery.

S2053-S2054

S2053 Transplantation of small intestine and liver allografts

S2054 Transplantation of multivisceral organs

Lay Description

The transplantation of organs is the removal of a healthy organ or organs from one body, usually a cadaver, and the insertion or attachment of that organ or organs into another body. Transplant types include allografts, which are transplants from the same species; autografts, which are transplants from the same patient as with skin grafts from one part of the body to another; or xenografts, which are transplants from one species to another species.

S2055

S2055 Harvesting of donor multivisceral organs, with preparation and maintenance of allografts; from cadaver donor

Lay Description

Harvesting is the process of removing living, viable organs from a cadaver for transplantation into another party. The organs of the cadaver are kept functioning with medications and machines. In a multivisceral harvest, multiple organs, such as a liver, small intestine, pancreas, and/or stomach, are removed for transplant from the cadaver. A team of physicians, nurses, and technicians remove the multiple organs that are to be transplanted. The blood supply and ducts are dissected free and isolated leaving organs that are to be transplanted together attached when possible. The organs are then perfused with a cold preservation solution and removed from the operative field. The organs remain under refrigeration, specially packed in a sealable container with some preserving solution, and kept on ice in a suitable carrier.

S2060

S2060 Lobar lung transplantation

Lay Description

The human lung is a paired organ composed of a right and left lung. The right lung represents more than one half of the total lung volume and has three lobes: superior, middle, and inferior. The left lung has a smaller volume and is composed of two lobes. In a lobar lung transplant, one of the lobes of one lung, usually a lower or inferior lobe, is transplanted into a recipient to replace the functions of the recipient's diseased lungs. Lobar lung transplants are typically from living donors. They usually replace both diseased lungs with a right lobe and a left lobe from different donors.

S2061

S2061 Donor lobectomy (lung) for transplantation, living donor

Lay Description

There are two human lungs, a right and a left lung. The right lung represents more than one half of the total lung volume and has three lobes: superior, middle, and inferior. The left lung has a smaller volume and is composed of two lobes. In a lobar lung transplant, one of the lobes of one lung, usually a lower or inferior lobe, is transplanted into a recipient to replace the functions of the recipient's diseased lungs. Report this code for the surgery performed to remove a lobe of the lung from a living donor for transplantation into another person.

S2065

S2065   Simultaneous pancreas kidney transplantation

Lay Description
Simultaneous pancreas kidney transplantation is the replacement, during the same operative session, of both a diseased or nonfunctional pancreas and kidney. This dual transplantation has become accepted therapy for patients with insulin-dependent diabetes mellitus who also have diabetic nephropathy. Both organs are removed from the same cadaver.

S2066

S2066   Breast reconstruction with gluteal artery perforator (GAP) flap, including harvesting of the flap, microvascular transfer, closure of donor site and shaping the flap into a breast, unilateral

Lay Description
Gluteal artery perforator (GAP) is breast reconstruction using the gluteal artery perforator flap, which includes harvesting the flap, the microvascular transfer, closure of the donor site, and shaping the flap into a breast. HCPCS Level II code S2066 is a unilateral procedure.

S2067

S2067   Breast reconstruction of a single breast with "stacked" deep inferior epigastric perforator (DIEP) flap(s) and/or gluteal artery perforator (GAP) flap(s), including harvesting of the flap(s), microvascular transfer, closure of donor site(s) and shaping the flap into a breast, unilateral

Lay Description
Deep inferior epigastric perforator/gluteal artery perforator (DIEP/GAP) is breast reconstruction of a single breast with a stacked deep inferior epigastric perforator or superficial inferior epigastric artery (SIEA) flap. This procedure includes harvesting of the flap, microvascular transfer, closure of the donor site, and shaping the new flap into a breast.

S2068

S2068   Breast reconstruction with deep inferior epigastric perforator (DIEP) flap or superficial inferior epigastric artery (SIEA) flap, including harvesting of the flap, microvascular transfer, closure of donor site and shaping the flap into a breast, unilateral

Lay Description
The deep inferior epigastric (DIEP) flap procedure uses tissues harvested from the patient's lower abdomen. The blood vessel that supplies blood to the abdominal muscle is the deep inferior epigastric artery. This artery also has side branches, which travel around or through the muscle to the overlying fat. These side branches or "perforators" are used as the blood supply for the DIEP procedure. As a result, the large abdominal muscle is not cut during the procedure, but the thick fascia (thick overlying tissue found over the muscle) is cut so that the perforators have enough diameter and length to supply blood to the reconstructed area. The superficial inferior epigastric artery (SIEA) flap procedure uses the same tissues as the DIEP flap. However, the blood supply for the DIEP is through the superficial inferior epigastric artery. In the SIEA procedure, neither the abdominal muscle nor its overlying fascia is touched.

S2070

S2070   Cystourethroscopy, with ureteroscopy and/or pyeloscopy; with endoscopic laser treatment of ureteral calculi (includes ureteral catheterization)

Lay Description
Cystourethroscopy is the insertion of a thin tube through the urethra to the bladder for diagnostic examination or to perform therapeutic procedures. A ureteroscopy and/or pyeloscopy is the extension of this tube through the ureter and sometimes into the kidney. A laser is passed through the tube to destroy any calcium deposits or calculi within the ureter. This code includes all components and a ureteral catheterization when performed.

S2079

S2079   Laparoscopic esophagomyotomy (Heller type)

Lay Description
A Heller type esophagomyotomy is the surgical division of the muscles surrounding the esophagus at the point where the esophagus joins the stomach, the sphincter of the esophagogastric junction. The release of the muscles allows swallowed food to pass more easily into the stomach. The procedure is most commonly performed to treat achalasia.

S2080

S2080   Laser-assisted uvulopalatoplasty (LAUP)

Lay Description
Laser-assisted uvulopalatoplasty (LAUP) is an office procedure used to treat snoring and associated obstructive sleep apnea. The uvula is the conic projection from the middle of the roof of the mouth. It is composed of connective tissue, a few glands, and muscle. The uvula contributes to the articulation of the sound of the human voice. The vibrations created by the uvula also contribute to snoring and sleep apnea. After the administration of a local anesthetic, a laser is used to vaporize the uvula and a portion of the palate. LAUP may require up to five treatments spaced four to eight weeks apart.

S2083

S2083   Adjustment of gastric band diameter via subcutaneous port by injection or aspiration of saline

Lay Description
One form of bariatric surgery uses an inflatable silicone device called a gastric band. This band is placed around the patient's stomach to reduce its size. The adjustment of the gastric band, post bariatric surgery, is accomplished by inserting a needle into the port of the band and adding or removing saline. This is done to change the width of the stomach opening.

S2095

S2095   Transcatheter occlusion or embolization for tumor destruction, percutaneous, any method, using yttrium-90 microspheres

Lay Description
Yttrium-90 microspheres are glass or plastic beads containing the radioactive element yttrium-90. These microspheres are released into the common, right, or left hepatic artery to block blood flow to a tumor and provide internal radiation. This procedure is used to treat tumors in the liver. It is a type of selective internal radiation therapy (SIRT). This code represents a percutaneous installation of yttrium-90 microspheres using a catheter.

S2102

S2102   Islet cell tissue transplant from pancreas; allogeneic

Lay Description
An islet cell tissue transplant from the pancreas is an experimental treatment for Type 1 diabetes mellitus. The pancreas is an organ that makes insulin and digestive enzymes that assist the body in the breakdown and use of food. Within the pancreas are clusters of cells called islets of Langerhans. These islets contain different types of cells, including beta cells, that make insulin. A highly purified mixture of enzymes is used to isolate islet cells from the pancreas of a deceased organ donor. The purified islet cells are then injected, under imaging guidance, into the portal vein of the liver. The islet cells attach themselves to blood vessels and begin releasing insulin. The human body treats islet cells just as it would any foreign body and immunosuppressive drugs must be taken.

S2103

S2103   Adrenal tissue transplant to brain

Lay Description
Parkinson's disease is a progressive neurodegenerative disorder caused by impaired dopamine neurons in the area of the brain that controls balance and muscle movement. Dopamine is a neurotransmitter that relays information between neurons and muscles. An adrenal tissue transplant to the brain removes adrenal gland medullary tissue

from the patient (autograft) or from another person (allograft) and places the tissue into the corpus striatum of the brain. This is an experimental procedure intended to restore dopamine activity in patients with Parkinson's disease.

S2107

S2107   Adoptive immunotherapy i.e. development of specific antitumor reactivity (e.g., tumor-infiltrating lymphocyte therapy) per course of treatment

Lay Description
Adoptive immunotherapy is a form of immunotherapy that is used for cancer treatment. It consists of removing a patient's own lymphocytes and growing them with a naturally produced growth factor (lymphokine interleukin 2 [IL-2]). These cells are then injected into the tumor site to increase local immune response.

S2112

S2112   Arthroscopy, knee, surgical for harvesting of cartilage (chondrocyte cells)

Lay Description
Normal cartilage is harvested during a knee arthroscopy with biopsy. The cells of the harvested tissue are separated from the cartilage and cultured in a medium. Over the next six weeks, these cells multiply and are stored in the frozen state. After being thawed and going through a final culture process, they are sent to the OR on the day of the implantation surgery. Under general anesthesia, an arthrotomy is done and the chondral lesion is excised and the cultured chondrocytes are injected beneath the periosteal flap.

S2115

S2115   Osteotomy, periacetabular, with internal fixation

Lay Description
A periacetabular osteotomy is performed to correct hip dysplasia. The surgeon makes an incision on the patient's hip area and divides the pelvis bone to separate the hip socket from the rest of the pelvis. The hip socket is rotated until it covers the head of the femur and is internally attached to the bone with the use of screws. Typically, no cast or other support is required by the patient after the surgery.

S2117

S2117   Arthroereisis, subtalar

Lay Description
Arthroereisis is a surgical procedure that limits the movement of a joint. The term subtalar refers to the point in the foot where the talus meets the calcaneus at the ankle. Subtalar implants are placed in the sinus tarsi to act as a spacer and prevent full flexion of the tendons. This procedure is considered an

investigational treatment for flat feet and similar foot deformities.

S2118

S2118   **Metal-on-metal total hip resurfacing, including acetabular and femoral components**

Lay Description
Total hip resurfacing is a surgical alternative to a total hip replacement. A metal cap, which is a hollow mushroom-shape, is placed over the head of the femur. A matching metal cup is used to replace the articulating surfaces of the acetabulum or pelvic socket. Synovial fluid flows between the two components as lubrication when the patient's hip moves. Total hip resurfacing is a less invasive procedure that preserves bone and provides a reduced chance of hip dislocation. This code represents the procedure, as well as the two metal components.

S2120

S2120   **Low density lipoprotein (LDL) apheresis using heparin-induced extracorporeal LDL precipitation**

Lay Description
Extracorporeal apheresis is a treatment that drains blood from the body, separates out and removes one particular blood component, and returns the blood to the body. Low density lipoprotein (LDL) is one of the five major types of lipoproteins, lipids bound with protein, that transport lipids within the bloodstream. The current theory categorizes LDL as "bad cholesterol" that contributes to cardiovascular disease and other health problems. This code represents LDL apheresis using heparin-induced LDL precipitation. The heparin binds to the LDL molecule, causing it to be removed more easily from the blood. The procedure is usually reserved for cases of severe hyperlipidemia.

S2140-S2142

S2140   **Cord blood harvesting for transplantation, allogeneic**

S2142   **Cord blood-derived stem-cell transplantation, allogeneic**

Lay Description
Cord blood harvesting is the process of collecting blood from the umbilical cord after the baby is born and the cord has been clamped. The umbilical cord contains a large amount of stem cells. After harvesting, the blood is usually screened for infectious and hereditary diseases. If there is a substantial amount of clean blood, it is cryogenically stored for future transplantation.

S2150-S2152

S2150   **Bone marrow or blood-derived stem cells (peripheral or umbilical), allogeneic or autologous, harvesting, transplantation, and related complications; including: pheresis and cell preparation/storage; marrow ablative therapy; drugs, supplies, hospitalization with outpatient follow-up; medical/surgical, diagnostic, emergency, and rehabilitative services; and the number of days of pre and post transplant care in the global definition**

S2152   **Solid organ(s), complete or segmental, single organ or combination of organs; deceased or living donor (s), procurement, transplantation, and related complications; including: drugs; supplies; hospitalization with outpatient follow-up; medical/surgical, diagnostic, emergency, and rehabilitative services, and the number of days of pre and posttransplant care in the global definition**

Lay Description
Transplants are performed to replace destroyed or damaged bone marrow or solid organs with a healthy organ or stem cells. Allogenic transplants use tissues from cadavers or living persons. Autologous transplants use the patient's own tissue. Use these codes to report all transplant-related services in the global period for stem cell and solid organ transplants.

S2202

S2202   **Echosclerotherapy**

Lay Description
Echosclerotherapy is the use of ultrasound guidance to inject a sclerosing agent into varicose veins. This office procedure is usually performed on large veins that are not visible through the skin.

S2205-S2209

S2205   **Minimally invasive direct coronary artery bypass surgery involving mini-thoracotomy or mini-sternotomy surgery, performed under direct vision; using arterial graft(s), single coronary arterial graft**

S2206   **Minimally invasive direct coronary artery bypass surgery involving mini-thoracotomy or mini-sternotomy surgery, performed under direct vision; using arterial graft(s), 2 coronary arterial grafts**

S2207 Minimally invasive direct coronary artery bypass surgery involving mini-thoracotomy or mini-sternotomy surgery, performed under direct vision; using venous graft only, single coronary venous graft

S2208 Minimally invasive direct coronary artery bypass surgery involving mini-thoracotomy or mini-sternotomy surgery, performed under direct vision; using single arterial and venous graft(s), single venous graft

S2209 Minimally invasive direct coronary artery bypass surgery involving mini-thoracotomy or mini-sternotomy surgery, performed under direct vision; using 2 arterial grafts and single venous graft

Lay Description
Unlike traditional coronary artery bypass graft (CABG) where the breast bone is divided and the patient is placed on a cardiopulmonary bypass machine to pump blood through the body, minimally invasive direct coronary artery bypass (MIDCAB) surgery is performed through a small, 2 to 5 inch incision between the ribs and does not require use of the bypass machine. A graft is connected to a diseased coronary vessel on a beating heart. MIDCAB surgery results in quicker recovery time, shorter length of stay, less infection rate, smaller incision scar, and less bleeding and blood trauma.

S2225

S2225 Myringotomy, laser-assisted

Lay Description
A laser-assisted myringotomy is performed. A myringotomy is a surgical procedure in which an incision is made in the eardrum to relieve pressure or drain fluid. A laser-assisted procedure uses a laser to create the opening in the eardrum rather than a surgical incision. The laser is less invasive and requires only topical anesthesia.

S2230

S2230 Implantation of magnetic component of semi-implantable hearing device on ossicles in middle ear

Lay Description
Semi-implantable hearing aids have been developed as another option to the external acoustic hearing aids. The semi-implantable hearing device consists of a magnetic component that is implanted in the ossicles of the middle ear, a receiver, and a sound processor. The sound vibrations are received and amplified by the sound processor. These sound pressures are transformed into electrical signals, which are received by the receiver unit. The receiver unit then converts the electrical signals into electromagnetic energy, creating an electromagnetic field with the magnetic component that is implanted on the ossicles. The electromagnetic field causes vibration of the middle ear bones, which is similar to normal vibrations. Use this code to report the implantation of the magnetic component.

S2235

S2235 Implantation of auditory brain stem implant

Lay Description
An auditory brain implant (ABI) is used for patients who have neurofibromatosis type 2, a rare disease in which cranial nerve tumors must be surgically excised. The excision of these auditory cranial nerves requires severing of the nerves and results in complete loss of hearing. In order to restore some sound, an ABI is done. This system includes a receiver/stimulator, a speech processor (pocket sized) that is worn on the body, and a microphone/headset. The receiver/stimulator is implanted behind the ear during surgery. A series of electrodes are implanted into the brainstem. A wire leads from the implanted receiver/stimulator to the implanted electrodes. The speech processor and microphone/headset pick up the sound, which is then changed to electrical impulses and sent to the receiver/stimulator. These impulses travel down the wire to the electrodes and the area that normally receives the electrical signal from the ear is stimulated.

S2260-S2267

S2260 Induced abortion, 17 to 24 weeks
S2265 Induced abortion, 25 to 28 weeks
S2266 Induced abortion, 29 to 31 weeks
S2267 Induced abortion, 32 weeks or greater

Lay Description
An induced abortion is the intentional termination of a pregnancy before the fetus is viable. The abortion may be done for therapeutic reasons or as an elective procedure, and is accomplished with the use of medication or instrumentation. The type of abortion performed can vary depending upon the age of the fetus.

S2300

S2300 Arthroscopy, shoulder, surgical; with thermally-induced capsulorrhaphy

Lay Description
Thermal capsulorrhaphy (TC), also known as thermal capsular shrinkage, is a technique developed to treat shoulder instability. Heat is used to shrink and tighten the connective tissue around the shoulder joint (shoulder capsule). TC was developed to achieve a less invasive treatment for shoulders that are frequently dislocated. TC was originally accomplished with the use of laser. Now, however, the use of radiofrequency is more commonly used in the procedure. This procedure is considered

investigational and not covered by most insurance companies.

S2325

S2325   Hip core decompression

Lay Description

The physician performs a hip core decompression of the femoral head. Hip core decompression is used in the treatment of osteonecrosis in patients with small-sized to medium-sized precollapse lesions of the femoral head. Hip core decompression relieves pressure within the rigid structure of the femoral head, thereby relieving joint pain. An incision is made over the femoral head. The soft tissues are divided. Next, one of two techniques may be used to perform the hip core decompression, which involves drilling a small hole or holes in the diseased bone. Using the more traditional technique, a hole is drilled in line with the axis of the femoral neck at the point where the lateral cortex begins to thicken. An 8 to 10 mm wide reamer is used to over-ream the drill hole. A second, newer technique utilizes a 3 mm Steinman pin to create multiple small drill holes in the diseased bone of the femoral head. Surgical instruments are then removed. The surgical area is flushed with normal saline and the incision is closed.

S2340-S2341

S2340   Chemodenervation of abductor muscle(s) of vocal cord

S2341   Chemodenervation of adductor muscle(s) of vocal cord

Lay Description

Chemodenervation is performed of the abductor muscle (S2340) of the vocal cord or the adductor muscle (S2341) of the vocal cord. Chemodenervation is the injection of a pharmacological compound into a nerve to paralyze a muscle or group of muscles. Abductor muscles open and adductor muscles close the vocal folds in the larynx. Chemodenervation of the vocal cord muscles is used to treat spasmodic dysphonia, a condition producing a variety of unusual vocal sounds. There are two main types of spasmodic dysphonia: adductor and abductor. The most common is the adductor type and it results in a strained-strangled sound, producing multiple voice breaks or pitch. Abductor spasmodic dysphonia is a "mirror image" of the adductor type. The vocal folds spasm open and create an involuntary moment of no voice, as well as a weak, breathy voice. The injection of botulinum toxin type A is used to treat both types.

S2342

S2342   Nasal endoscopy for postoperative debridement following functional endoscopic sinus surgery, nasal and/or sinus cavity(s), unilateral or bilateral

Lay Description

Postoperative debridement may be reported for the limited removal of debris, crust, or secretions from the nasal and/or sinus cavity using straight forceps, irrigation, or suction requiring topical anesthesia.

S2348

S2348   Decompression procedure, percutaneous, of nucleus pulposus of intervertebral disc, using radiofrequency energy, single or multiple levels, lumbar

Lay Description

In a typical herniated disc, the annulus fibrosis opens and the nucleus pulposus protrudes and compresses the nerves. Radiofrequency decompression is minimally invasive and was developed as a treatment for patients with low back pain due to herniated disc disease. Under fluoroscopic guidance, a small needle is inserted into the nucleus pulposus of the herniated disc. Radiofrequency is then applied to ablate the tissue and reduce the nucleus pulposus. This procedure is considered experimental and may not be reimbursed by many insurance companies.

S2350-S2351

S2350   Diskectomy, anterior, with decompression of spinal cord and/or nerve root(s), including osteophytectomy; lumbar, single interspace

S2351   Diskectomy, anterior, with decompression of spinal cord and/or nerve root(s), including osteophytectomy; lumbar, each additional interspace (list separately in addition to code for primary procedure)

Lay Description

The physician performs a lumbar discectomy to remove all or part of a herniated intervertebral disc. The patient is placed supine position. The physician makes a transverse incision in the abdominal wall overlying the intervertebral disc. Dissection and careful retraction of the abdominal contents is carried out to the disc. The physician excises the anterior anulus of the disc and uses pituitary forceps to remove as much disc material as possible. A spreader and microscope are used to enhance the evacuation. A drill is used to remove the transverse bar above and below. Graft material is obtained from the ilium and fashioned to fit into the space. The graft is placed into the disc space and traction is released. The muscles fall back into place and the incision is closed with layered sutures.

S2360-S2361

S2360 Percutaneous vertebroplasty, one vertebral body, unilateral or bilateral injection; cervical

S2361 Each additional cervical vertebral body (list separately in addition to code for primary procedure)

Lay Description
A percutaneous vertebroplasty is performed on a cervical vertebral body, unilateral or bilateral. Percutaneous vertebroplasty is used as a treatment for spinal decompression fractures commonly associated with vertebral hemangiomas, tumors, or osteoporosis. The procedure is done in the outpatient setting and lasts about 40 to 60 minutes. Local anesthetic and IV sedation are used. Under radiologic guidance, a needle is inserted into the fractured vertebra through a small incision. Bone cement is then injected into the fractured vertebra.

S2400

S2400 Repair, congenital diaphragmatic hernia in the fetus using temporary tracheal occlusion, procedure performed in utero

Lay Description
A congenital diaphragmatic hernia (CDH) is a birth defect or hole in the diaphragm that permits abdominal contents to pass into the chest cavity. Lung tissue on the affected side usually cannot develop completely. Temporary tracheal occlusion is a blocking of the trachea with the insertion of operative clips or balloons through a fetoscope. This prevents the normal outflow of fluid from the fetus' lungs, which can result in a build up of secretions. Since this build-up of secretions increases the lung size, the abdominal viscera is gradually forced out of the lung cavity and back into the abdominal cavity. During delivery, the occlusive devices are removed from the trachea. Repair of the diaphragmatic hernia is completed after birth.

S2401

S2401 Repair, urinary tract obstruction in the fetus, procedure performed in utero

Lay Description
Bilateral urinary tract obstruction can lead to distention of the bladder and is often associated with pulmonary hyperplasia. The treatment goal is to assure adequate amniotic fluid volume for the development of the lungs, and to protect the kidneys from increased pressure. A stent or shunt is placed percutaneously to achieve decompression. This procedure allows the urine from the fetus to flow into the amniotic space and bypass the urinary tract. Coverage is based on the type of obstruction among other criteria.

S2402-S2403

S2402 Repair, congenital cystic adenomatoid malformation in the fetus, procedure performed in utero

S2403 Repair, extralobar pulmonary sequestration in the fetus, procedure performed in utero

Lay Description
Congenital cystic adenomatoid malformation (CCAM) is the most common of the congenital pulmonary anomalies. The CCAM cystic lesions, which are identified as overgrowth of the terminal respiratory bronchioles, are normally found in only one part of the lung. Extralobar pulmonary sequestration (EPS) is commonly identified as masses of lung tissue that is not functioning. The extra lobar sections of lung tissue are not connected to the main tracheobronchial system, are drained by the pulmonary venous system, and are mainly supplied by anomalous artery arising from the aorta. Repair of both of these conditions is usually performed by an open in utero resection of the malformed tissue or placement of a shunt (thoracic to amniotic) in cases of large cystic lesions. Coverage of in utero repair is questionable for both conditions.

S2404

S2404 Repair, myelomeningocele in the fetus, procedure performed in utero

Lay Description
The physician repairs a myelomeningocele in a fetus. Myelomeningocele (MMC) is a developmental disorder caused by incomplete closing of the neural tube. It is the most significant, common cause of spina bifida. The spinal cord develops abnormally and is left open, resulting in the protrusion of a spinal cord sac, which is filled with cerebrospinal fluid. MMC results in disorders to the cerebrospinal fluid circulation, brain malformation, impairment to bowel and legs and bladder function, and cognitive impairment. In utero surgery to cover or repair the exposed spinal cord sac is thought to improve neurologic function but is considered experimental. Coverage is dependent on the insurance payer.

S2405

S2405 Repair of sacrococcygeal teratoma in the fetus, procedure performed in utero

Lay Description
The physician repairs a sacrococcygeal teratoma in the fetus. Sacrococcygeal teratoma (SCT) is an encapsulated neoplasm composed of germ cells that is located at the base of the coccyx. It is usually not malignant and is the most common newborn tumor. If the tumor is accompanied by fetal edema, the condition is rapidly progressive and commonly fatal.

S2409

S2409 Repair, congenital malformation of fetus, procedure performed in utero, not otherwise classified

Lay Description
The physician repairs a congenital malformation of the fetus. Most fetal malformations are handled after birth. However, there are some conditions that are considered prudent and safe to perform in utero. Report code for conditions not identified by another code.

S2411

S2411 Fetoscopic laser therapy for treatment of twin-to-twin transfusion syndrome

Lay Description
The physician performs fetoscopic laser therapy for treatment of twin-to-twin transfusion syndrome. Twin-to-twin transfusion syndrome (TTTS) is only found in identical twins that share the same placenta. Usually, the connections are balanced and the blood flows in both directions equally. However, if the connections are not balanced and one fetus (donor) is losing or donating blood to the other fetus (recipient), the donor receives insufficient nutrients and becomes dehydrated. Conversely, the recipient becomes overly large and the amniotic sac fills with excessive fluid and the recipient can develop heart failure when the extra blood volume becomes too excessive. Treatment for TTTS consists of in utero serial reductions of amniotic fluid and/or the use of fetoscopic laser photocoagulation. The laser photocoagulation is done in the OR under local, spinal, or general anesthesia. The fetoscope is placed into the uterus through a tiny incision and the laser is used to seal the blood vessels on the surface of the placenta. This restores the balance of blood and nutrients flowing to the fetuses.

S2900

S2900 Surgical techniques requiring use of robotic surgical system (list separately in addition to code for primary procedure)

Lay Description
A robotic surgical system is used, which utilizes 3-D cameras and miniature instruments to enable the surgeon to make smaller incisions and work more accurately. The surgeon is always in control but has the use of robotic tools to magnify and optimize the view, as well as guiding the surgeon's hands to achieve accurate results. The FDA has cleared two robotic systems for use in certain circumstances and for certain purposes. When using the da Vinci Surgical System, the surgeon sits at a console located several feet from the operating table. The robot has hands attached to a free standing cart. One of the hands holds the camera that has been inserted into the patient. The ZEUS Robotic Surgical System has three arms that are mounted on the operating table. Two of the arms are the extension of the surgeon's right and

left arms, and the other holds the endoscope and is voice activated and responds to the surgeon's commands. The surgeon sits at a console and wears special 3-D glasses.

S3000

S3000 Diabetic indicator; retinal eye exam, dilated, bilateral

Lay Description
A dilated retinal eye exam performed on a patient with undiagnosed diabetes may reveal bleeding of the small blood vessels of the eye. Since these vessels are highly sensitive to the toxicity of hyperglycemia, this is frequently an indicator of the presence of the diabetes. Use this code to report a bilateral exam.

S3005

S3005 Performance measurement, evaluation of patient self assessment, depression

Lay Description
A patient depression self assessment is a list of questions or symptoms to which a patient responds. The patient rates his feelings or thoughts on specific issues, including thoughts of suicide, concentration, eating, and irritability. Patient responses are evaluated by a mental health professional to determine the patient's state of mind.

S3600-S3601

S3600 STAT laboratory request (situations other than S3601)

S3601 Emergency STAT laboratory charge for patient who is homebound or residing in a nursing facility

Lay Description
A stat laboratory request indicates that all possible speed and prioritization should be used to procure, analyze, and report the results of the specimen. The results of the stat requests are necessary for an immediate critical or therapeutic decision.

S3620

S3620 Newborn metabolic screening panel, includes test kit, postage and the laboratory tests specified by the state for inclusion in this panel (e.g., galactose; hemoglobin, electrophoresis; hydroxyprogesterone, 17-d; phenylaline (PKU); and thyroxine, total)

Lay Description
Newborn screening is done on all newborns for certain metabolic, genetic, and endocrine disorders. It can identify infants who may possibly be at risk for one of the disorders that are within the screening panel. The tests included in the panel are based on state requirements. These tests are considered screening tests only. Additional testing is required to

determine if an infant truly has one of the conditions identified in the screening.

S3630

S3630 Eosinophil count, blood, direct

Lay Description
Eosinophil granulocytes are white blood cells that are part of the immune system that battle parasites and infections and regulate inflammation. The granules within their cytoplasm contain many chemical mediators that are released while the eosinophil is activated. These chemical mediators are toxic to the parasite and to the host. Eosinophil granulocytes are generally found in the GI tract, ovary, uterus, spleen, and lymph nodes. When present in the lungs, skin, or esophagus, they may signal disease.

S3645

S3645 HIV-1 antibody testing of oral mucosal transudate

Lay Description
The HIV antibody testing of oral mucosal transudate is an alternative to a standard blood test. A specially treated pad is placed in the mouth and rubbed between the lower cheek and the individual's gum. The pad collects oral mucosal transudate, which contains HIV antibodies in a person infected with HIV. It does not test for HIV in the saliva.

S3650

S3650 Saliva test, hormone level; during menopause

Lay Description
Salivary hormone test measures the biologically active component of female hormones in the bloodstream. There are some that use this test to determine the female hormone levels in women prior to initiation of hormone replacement therapy. The test was developed as a means to monitor the titration of an individual's hormone dosage.

S3652

S3652 Saliva test, hormone level; to assess preterm labor risk

Lay Description
Preterm labor is birth of an infant at less than 37 weeks gestation. One of the tests to predict preterm labor is the salivary estriol test. Estriol levels have been known to increase significantly two to four weeks prior to the onset of labor. The test is usually done with a 24-hour urine or serial blood collection. Salivary estriol has been used as a predictor of late preterm birth. Since late preterm birth has low neonatal morbidity rates, the test is rarely used and considered investigational.

S3655

S3655 Antisperm antibodies test (immunobead)

Lay Description
The presence of antibodies in the sperm may be a cause or contributing factor to infertility. Although sperm antibodies may be measured by a variety of techniques, the direct immunobead test (dIBT) is the method of choice. The test is based on the rosette formation between the viable sperm and the plastic beads coated with antiserum to human immunoglobulins. This enables the analysis of class-specific antibodies (IgM, IgA, or IgG) and their site of attachment (e.g., tail, head).

S3708

S3708 Gastrointestinal fat absorption study

Lay Description
A gastrointestinal fat absorption study is a diagnostic test for fat malabsorption. Fat is a valuable nutrient digested by enzymes in the small intestine. The simplest test involves the staining and examination under a microscope of a random fecal specimen.

S3721

S3721 Prostate cancer antigen 3 (PCA3) testing

Lay Description
Prostate cancer antigen 3 (PCA3) is a urine test that may be useful in the detection, staging, and treatment strategies of prostate cancer. The test can be used to produce more accurate predictions of benign versus malignant prostate biopsy results. The PCA3 gene is increased in certain prostate cancer cell lines and prostatic tumors. Studies are showing that the PCA3 test may provide more specific information prior to a prostate biopsy or reduce the number of biopsies necessary to detect differences in prostate disease.

S3722

S3722 Dose optimization by area under the curve (AUC) analysis, for infusional 5-fluorouracil

Lay Description
This code describes a laboratory test to determine 5-FU plasma levels for patients with colorectal cancer who are being treated with the drug. It allows more precise and accurate dosing than the body surface area methodology used to calculate doses. The information from the test allows the physician to avoid toxic levels and administered optimal levels of 5-FU to the patient to reach the target range. The assay is competitive homogenous two-reagent nanoparticle agglutination immunoassay. It is a unique service that quickly delivers quantitative 5-FU AUC results to the oncologist. This allows the physician to adjust the dose for each treatment cycle to make sure it is in the correct therapeutic range.

S

S3800

S3800   Genetic testing for amyotrophic lateral sclerosis (ALS)

Lay Description

A genetic disorder is a disease caused in whole or in part by a mutation of a gene. Genetic tests attempt to identify abnormalities in an individual's genes, which include the presence or absence of key proteins whose production is directed by specific genes. Amyotrophic lateral sclerosis (ALS) is a progressive neurodegenerative disease that affects nerve cells in the brain and spinal column. Motor neurons extend from the brain to the spinal column and from the spinal column to muscles. The progressive degeneration of these motor neurons eventually leads to their death and the loss of muscle control. It is estimated that only a very small percentage of ALS, less than 10 percent, is inherited.

S3840

S3840   DNA analysis for germline mutations of the RET proto-oncogene for susceptibility to multiple endocrine neoplasia type 2

Lay Description

DNA analysis is the study of genes or DNA and is used to detect a genetic alteration that is associated with a specific disorder. A germline mutation is a detectable and heritable variation in germ cells that can create mutations in every cell of the offspring. This code describes the DNA analysis of the RET proto-oncogene for the susceptibility of the patient to multiple endocrine neoplasia type 2 (MEN2). MEN2 is a group of medical disorders that include pheochromocytoma, medullary thyroid carcinoma, parathyroid hyperplasia, and mucocutaneous neuroma.

S3841-S3842

S3841   Genetic testing for retinoblastoma
S3842   Genetic testing for Von Hippel-Lindau disease

Lay Description

A genetic disorder is a disease caused in whole or in part by a mutation of a gene. Genetic tests attempt to identify abnormalities in an individual's genes, which include the presence or absence of key proteins whose production is directed by specific genes. Retinoblastoma is a rare type of eye cancer that develops in the retina, usually before the age of 5. Von Hippel-Lindau disease is a rare genetic disorder that arises from a mutation in the von Hippel-Lindau tumor suppressor gene. In this disorder, tumors form in different areas of the brain and body. The tumors may be benign or malignant.

S3844

S3844   DNA analysis of the connexin 26 gene (GJB2) for susceptibility to congenital, profound deafness

Lay Description

DNA analysis and the study of genes is used to detect a genetic alteration associated with a specific disorder. Connexins are gap junction proteins. Gap junctions are specialized intracellular connections between the cytoplasm of two cells that are essential for many physiologic functions. Connexin 26 is a mutation in gene GJB2 that leads to Vohwinkel syndrome as well as keratitis-ichthyosis-deafness syndrome. Vohwinkel syndrome is a mutilating keratoderma disorder with some mild to moderate hearing loss. Keratitis-ichthyosis-deafness syndrome is a disorder characterized by corneal opacification, mild generalized hyperkeratosis or erythematous plaques, and neurosensory deafness.

S3845-S3846

S3845   Genetic testing for alpha-thalassemia
S3846   Genetic testing for hemoglobin E beta-thalassemia

Lay Description

Genetic testing is used to determine mutations or variances in genes that may be responsible for certain conditions or diseases. Genetic testing for thalassemia is usually done by taking a blood sample and looking for mutations in the gene cluster causing the condition. Thalassemia is an inherited disorder that impacts the production of hemoglobin and includes a number of different types of anemia. The number of genes that are affected determines the severity and type of anemia. All types of thalassemia have three components: heme, alpha globin, and beta globin. Thalassemia results in no synthesis or a reduced rate of synthesis of one of the globin chains that make up thalassemia, which can cause abnormal hemoglobin molecules to form. Anemia is usually the only symptom of thalassemia. Alpha thalassemia includes disorders of the alpha hemoglobin chain. Beta thalassemia affects the beta hemoglobin chain.

S3849

S3849   Genetic testing for Niemann-Pick disease

Lay Description

Genetic testing for Niemann-Pick disease is performed. Genetic testing is used to determine mutations or variances in genes that may be responsible for certain conditions or diseases. Niemann-Pick disease is a group of diseases characterized by a build-up of lipids in the brain, liver, and spleen. There are four main types of this disease: A, B, C, and D. Each type can cause different symptoms and affect different organs. Types A and B are diagnosed through a blood test or bone marrow sample to measure the amount of acid sphingomyelin (found in every cell of the body) in the white blood cells. Types B and C are usually tested with a skin biopsy, which is used to study how the cells move and store cholesterol. A sphingomyelinase assay may also be done.

S3850

S3850   Genetic testing for sickle cell anemia

Lay Description
Genetic testing for sickle cell anemia is performed. Genetic testing is used to determine mutations or variances in genes that may be responsible for certain conditions or diseases. Sickle cell anemia is caused by mutations of the HBB gene. Hemoglobin is made up of four units of protein: 2 subunits called alpha-globin and 2 subunits called beta-globin. The HBB gene is responsible for providing direction for making beta-globin. Different versions of beta-globin result from different mutations of the HBB gene. At least one of the beta-globin hemoglobin subunits is replaced with hemoglobin S in sickle cell anemia. In sickle cell anemia, the normally round red blood cells are shaped like a sickle, or crescent moon. These sickle-shaped cells get stuck in the capillaries, can't carry oxygen as well and can damage muscles, bones, and organs. These sickle-shaped cells are destroyed by the body at a more rapid rate than normal blood cells, resulting in anemia. Testing is done through a blood test. It may also be performed through amniocentesis.

S3852

S3852   DNA analysis for APOE epsilon 4 allele for susceptibility to Alzheimer's disease

Lay Description
A DNA analysis for APOE epsilon 4 allele for susceptibility to Alzheimer's disease is performed. Genetic testing is used to determine mutations or variances in genes that may be responsible for certain conditions or diseases. The APOE lipoprotein is a carrier of the cholesterol that is produced in the brain cells and liver. The APOE gene has three alleles (Epsilon 2, 3, and 4). An individual carries two of the APOE alleles. When at least one of epsilons four allele is present, the risk of developing Alzheimer's disease (AD) is 1.2 to 3 times greater depending on the ethnic group. Genetic testing as a diagnostic technique for patients with AD symptoms is considered investigational and not covered by most insurance companies.

S3853

S3853   Genetic testing for myotonic muscular dystrophy

Lay Description
Genetic testing for myotonic muscular dystrophy is performed. Genetic testing is used to determine mutations or variances in genes that may be responsible for certain conditions or diseases and is the definitive test for myotonic dystrophy. Myotonic

dystrophy type 1 is caused by DMPK gene mutations. Myotonic dystrophy type 2 is caused from mutations in the CNBP gene. Mutations in each of these genes involve a small segment of DNA that is abnormally repeated many times. This abnormality forms an unstable area of the gene. The resulting changes keep cells in the muscles and other tissues from normal function. Screening for the type 1 locates the specific area on chromosome 19 and measures the size of the DNA expansion. The genetic test for type 2 was developed to measure and isolate the size of the DNA expansion on chromosome 3.

S3854

S3854   Gene expression profiling panel for use in the management of breast cancer treatment

Lay Description
Genetic testing is used to determine mutations or variances in genes that may be responsible for certain conditions or diseases. As a tool to predict the baseline risk of the recurrence of breast cancer after hormonal therapy, surgery, and radiation therapy, several panels of gene expression markers, known as "signatures" have been developed. These are used to aid in the determination of recurrence risk and can help in the decision-making process for patients who prefer to avoid chemotherapy.

S3855

Lay Description
Genetic testing for detection of mutations in the presenilin-1 gene is performed. Genetic testing is used to determine mutations or variances in genes that may be responsible for certain conditions or diseases. Early onset familial Alzheimer disease (AD) refers to multiple cases of AD in families in more than one generation, whose age at the onset is before age 60 to 65 and often before age 55. Alzheimer disease type 3 is caused by mutations in the presenilin-1 gene (PSEN 1). Presenilin 1 on chromosome 14 is the major causative gene of early onset AD. These gene mutations are sometimes responsible for such atypical presentations as prominent frontotemporal features and dementia with spastic paraplegia.

S3861

S3861   Genetic testing, sodium channel, voltage-gated, type V, alpha subunit (SCN5A) and variants for suspected Brugada Syndrome

Lay Description
Brugada syndrome is an inherited arrhythmia disorder that causes ventricular fibrillation and increases the risk of sudden cardiac death. Episodes of ventricular tachycardia exist showing a pattern of right bundle branch block and ST segment elevation. Fainting or black-outs can accompany the ventricular fibrillation. A cardiodefibrillator can be implanted to shock the

S

heart back into rhythm. The disease primarily affects males. Several mutations in the gene SCN5A, which encodes for the cardiac sodium channel, have been linked to this syndrome.

S3865-S3866

S3865   Comprehensive gene sequence analysis for hypertrophic cardiomyopathy

S3866   Genetic analysis for a specific gene mutation for hypertrophic cardiomyopathy (HCM) in an individual with a known HCM mutation in the family

Lay Description
A genetic disorder is a disease caused in whole or in part by a mutation of a gene. Genetic disorders can be passed on to family members who inherit the genetic abnormality. Genetic testing can be predictive, used to confirm a diagnosis, or used to determine if a person is a carrier for the disease. Hypertrophic cardiomyopathy (HCM) is a disorder where a portion of the myocardium becomes thickened without any obvious cause. The disorder is a leading cause of sudden cardiac death. In HCM, the sarcomeres or contractile elements replicate causing the muscle cells to increase in size and thicken the heart wall. The normal alignment of the muscle cells is disrupted creating myocardial disarray and the electrical heart functions are disrupted. HCM is most commonly due to a mutation in one of the nine sarcomeric genes resulting in mutated proteins.

S3870

S3870   Comparative genomic hybridization (CGH) microarray testing for developmental delay, autism spectrum disorder and/or intellectual disability

Lay Description
Genetic variations are often seen with developmental delay and other disorders. Standard cytogenetic analysis detects visible chromosomal alterations, such as an extra chromosome band, but smaller defects could not be reliably found. Improvements in molecular cytogenetics have enabled new more accurate and sensitive tests. Array CGH (comparative genome hybridization) is designed to detect cytogenetic imbalances that are smaller than what can be detected through routine chromosome analysis. Probes are used on glass slides as arrays to hybridize a differentially labed patient and normal DNA. The result is an identification of changes throughout the genome. They are arranged to correspond to genes that are known to affect development. The test will detect loss or duplication of chromosomes on the array.

S3890

S3890   DNA analysis, fecal, for colorectal cancer screening

Lay Description
DNA analysis is the study of genes or DNA and is used to detect a genetic alteration that is associated with a specific disorder. Since DNA is found in the stool, this test is used to detect DNA markers associated with colorectal cancer development, specifically those colorectal adenomas that are most likely to develop into cancer. Many of the markers related to this process have been found in patients' stools during the early stages of the cancer development.

S3900

S3900   Surface electromyography (EMG)

Lay Description
Surface electromyography is a non-invasive procedure in which surface electrodes, or a scanner containing electrodes, are placed on the skin to determine the overall muscle function and condition. A surface EMG is often considered not as accurate as the needle EMG.

S3902

S3902   Ballistocardiogram

Lay Description
Ballistocardiogram is a graphic recording that determines the blood volume that passes through the heart during a specific time frame, as well as the force of the contraction of the heart. It measures the body's recoil with each heartbeat as the blood is ejected from the ventricle.

S3904

S3904   Masters 2 step

Lay Description
The Masters 2 step is used to test for coronary insufficiency. It is accomplished by the patient climbing up and down two nine inch high steps while an electrocardiogram records the cardiac activity both during the exercise and at specific time intervals after the exercise is completed.

S4005

S4005   Interim labor facility global (labor occurring but not resulting in delivery)

Lay Description
This code is used by a facility to report services rendered to a patient in labor who was transferred to another facility for the delivery.

S4011

S4011 In vitro fertilization; including but not limited to identification and incubation of mature oocytes, fertilization with sperm, incubation of embryo(s), and subsequent visualization for determination of development

Lay Description
The in vitro fertilization (IVF) process is the fertilization of the egg by the sperm outside of the woman's body. After the eggs have been retrieved by the physician from the woman's ovary, the retrieved eggs are examined and the most promising ones are placed in an IVF culture medium. The father's sperm is then separated from his semen and the most mobile sperm are added to the eggs and placed in an incubator. The sperm cell penetrates an egg, usually within a very short time, and fertilizes it. The following day, fertilization is confirmed if the physician sees two pronuclei. Approximately two days after fertilization, a 2-4 cell zygote will appear, becoming an embryo when it divides. Most embryos are observed for two to four days to determine if they are developing normally and qualify to be placed in the uterus. Report this code for in vitro fertilization, including but not limited to identification and incubation of mature oocytes, fertilization with sperm, incubation of embryo(s), and subsequent visualization for determination of development.

S4013-S4014

S4013 Complete cycle, gamete intrafallopian transfer (GIFT), case rate

S4014 Complete cycle, zygote intrafallopian transfer (ZIFT), case rate

Lay Description
In gamete intrafallopian transfer (GIFT) (S4013), the physician mixes previously captured eggs with sperm and draws the mixture into a catheter. The catheter is passed through the cervix and uterus and into the tubes or passed through an abdominal incision and directly into the fimbrial end of the fallopian tube. The physician deposits the eggs and sperm in the tubes, permitting fertilization. In a zygote intrafallopian transfer (ZIFT) (S4014), a physician draws an already fertilized egg into a catheter. The catheter is passed through the cervix and uterus and into the tube where the egg is deposited. GIFT is a one-step procedure while ZIFT is a two-step process. In ZIFT, the egg is collected and fertilized and transferred to the fallopian tube at a later time. GIFT and ZIFT can be done laparoscopically or hysteroscopically.

S4015-S4021

S4015 Complete in vitro fertilization cycle, not otherwise specified, case rate

S4016 Frozen in vitro fertilization cycle, case rate

S4017 Incomplete cycle, treatment cancelled prior to stimulation, case rate

S4018 Frozen embryo transfer procedure cancelled before transfer, case rate

S4020 In vitro fertilization procedure cancelled before aspiration, case rate

S4021 In vitro fertilization procedure cancelled after aspiration, case rate

Lay Description
The in vitro fertilization (IVF) process is the fertilization of the egg by the sperm outside of the woman's body. The physician then implants the fertilized egg in the woman's uterus. An IVF cycle usually takes four to six weeks and the process may have to be done more than once to result in a pregnancy. There are five steps to IVF: (1) Ovarian stimulation: Usually done with fertility drugs, ovarian stimulation takes eight to 14 days. This usually involves the fertilization of more than one egg since not all will develop. The physician may take blood tests and use ultrasound to determine which eggs are ready for the next step. (2) Egg retrieval: The physician performs a transvaginal ultrasound aspiration once the eggs are ready for retrieval. With the use of a mild sedative or other form of anesthesia, the physician inserts a needle into the follicles in the ovary, and removes the eggs with suction. The physician may use a laparoscope if the ovaries cannot be accessed. (3) Insemination: The retrieved eggs are examined and the most promising ones are placed in an IVF culture medium. The father's sperm is then separated from his semen and the most mobile sperm are added to the eggs and placed in an incubator. (4) Fertilization and embryo culture: The sperm cell penetrates an egg, usually within a very short time, and fertilizes it. The following day, fertilization is confirmed if the physician sees two pronuclei. Approximately two days after fertilization, a two to four cell zygote appears, becoming an embryo when it divides. Most embryos are observed for two to four days to determine if they are developing normally and then placed in the uterus. (5) Embryo transfer: Approximately two to three days after fertilization, the embryo is transferred to the uterus. To do this, the physician suspends them in a drop of fluid and draws it into a catheter. The physician then guides the catheter into the uterus. The patient is usually told to rest for one to two hours to prevent any undue stress on her body. A positive pregnancy test results when the embryo attaches to the uterine wall.

S4022

S4022 Assisted oocyte fertilization, case rate

Lay Description
An oocyte is a human female germ cell involved in reproduction (an immature human egg cell). After the

S

eggs have been retrieved by the physician from the woman's ovary, the retrieved eggs are examined and the most promising ones are retrieved. Sperm is then separated from semen and the most mobile sperm are added to the eggs. An assisted fertilization typically involves the injection into the cytoplasm of the egg.

S4023

S4023   Donor egg cycle, incomplete, case rate

Lay Description
The in vitro fertilization (IVF) cycle usually takes four to six weeks. There are five steps to IVF. This code represents two of these steps. 1) Ovarian stimulation: Usually done with fertility drugs, ovarian stimulation takes eight to 14 days. This usually involves the fertilization of more than one egg since not all will develop. The physician may take blood tests and use ultrasound to determine which eggs are ready for the next step. 2) Egg retrieval: The physician performs a transvaginal ultrasound aspiration once the eggs are ready for retrieval. With the use of a mild sedative or other form of anesthesia, the physician inserts a needle into the follicles in the ovary and removes the eggs with suction. The physician may use a laparoscope if the ovaries cannot be accessed.

S4025

S4025   Donor services for in vitro fertilization (sperm or embryo), case rate

Lay Description
The in vitro fertilization (IVF) process is the fertilization of the egg by the sperm outside of the woman's body. The physician then implants the fertilized egg in the woman's uterus. This code represents the management of the services rendered to an egg or sperm donor.

S4026

S4026   Procurement of donor sperm from sperm bank

Lay Description
The in vitro fertilization (IVF) process is the fertilization of the egg by the sperm outside of the woman's body. The physician then implants the fertilized egg in the woman's uterus. This code represents charges for obtaining the sperm from a sperm bank.

S4027

S4027   Storage of previously frozen embryos

Lay Description
Women who undergo fertility treatment often produce numerous eggs that are fertilized but not all implanted. Embryos can be frozen and stored for implant at a later time. The embryos are cryogenically frozen and stored in carefully regulated tanks at a tissue bank until the woman is ready to attempt a pregnancy.

S4028

S4028   Microsurgical epididymal sperm aspiration (MESA)

Lay Description
A microsurgical epididymal sperm aspiration (MESA) is a procedure to retrieve sperm from a man who has a blockage in the reproductive system. A small incision is made in the scrotum and an operating microscope is used to identify the epididymis. The epididymis is a small tube where sperm is concentrated and stored. It is dilated and the fluid is aspirated and examined for the presence of sperm. If sperm is not present, a sample is aspirated from another tubule and examined. If sperm is identified it is processed to use immediately and can be frozen to be used later.

S4030-S4031

S4030   Sperm procurement and cryopreservation services; initial visit

S4031   Sperm procurement and cryopreservation services; subsequent visit

Lay Description
Sperm can be collected and preserved to be used later for artificial insemination. Donors can be someone known to the woman or couple or an anonymous donor. Men who are undergoing treatment that may affect fertility may also freeze sperm for later use. Anonymous sperm donors may sign a contract with a sperm bank to donate a certain number of weeks for a specified length of time. Once the specimen is obtained, it is evaluated and mixed with a substance to protect it during freezing. The sperm are placed in vials and cryopreserved with nitrogen vapor. The frozen vials are placed in liquid nitrogen and stored in cryogenic tanks at a temperature of -196°C (-321°F).

S4035

S4035   Stimulated intrauterine insemination (IUI), case rate

Lay Description
Intrauterine insemination (IUI) is a form of assisted conception. It is the placement of active washed sperm into the uterus at the time that an egg is released. Fertilization occurs within the uterus. Stimulated IUI uses hormones to cause eggs to be released. The sperm is placed in the uterus to coincide with ovulation.

S4037

S4037   Cryopreserved embryo transfer, case rate

Lay Description
This code is used to report the last stage of a complete in vitro fertilization cycle. During the IVF process, multiple embryos are frozen or cryopreserved for future use. This code represents the transfer of a thawed embryo into a uterus.

S4040

S4040 Monitoring and storage of cryopreserved embryos, per 30 days

Lay Description
Women who undergo fertility treatment often produce numerous eggs that are fertilized but not all implanted. Embryos can be frozen and stored for implant at a later time. The embryos are cryogenically frozen and stored in carefully regulated tanks at a tissue bank until the woman is ready to attempt a pregnancy.

S4042

S4042 Management of ovulation induction (interpretation of diagnostic tests and studies, nonface-to-face medical management of the patient), per cycle

Lay Description
This code is used to report the first of five in vitro fertilization (IVF) steps. Tests and studies are undertaken to determine if the woman has viable eggs that can be fertilized. Ovarian stimulation, usually done with fertility drugs, takes eight to 14 days. When the mature eggs are ready to be released, either sperm will be placed in the uterus or the eggs will be retrieved for in vitro fertilization.

S4981

S4981 Insertion of levonorgestrel-releasing intrauterine system

Lay Description
Levonorgestrel-releasing intrauterine system is a hormone-releasing system that is used to prevent pregnancy and works for up to five years. It is inserted into the uterus where it delivers a low dose of progesterone directly into the uterus lining. Use this code to report the insertion of the system.

S4989

S4989 Contraceptive intrauterine device (e.g., Progestacert IUD), including implants and supplies

Lay Description
Contraceptive intrauterine devices (IUD) prevent pregnancy by inhibiting fertilization of the egg. Although not entirely known, it is believed that the IUDs affect the way the sperm and egg move and/or affect the lining of the uterus to prevent implantation of the egg. These devices may be a loop, triangle, T-shape, or a coil. The IUD is inserted into the uterus. This code includes the implant and supplies.

S4990-S4991

S4990 Nicotine patches, legend
S4991 Nicotine patches, nonlegend

Lay Description
Nicotine patches are press-on, transdermal patches that release nicotine slowly through the skin. It is a nicotine replacement therapy. The patches help individuals to cope with withdrawal symptoms while they are trying to quit smoking by providing nicotine without the harmful effects from smoke. A legend drug is one that requires a prescription. Non-legend or over-the-counter drugs do not require a prescription.

S4993

S4993 Contraceptive pills for birth control

Lay Description
Birth control pills are oral contraceptives that are taken on a daily basis. Most of these pills contain synthetic estrogen and progestin. The hormones in the pills suppress the pituitary gland to inhibit the development and/or release of the egg, as well as help to prevent sperm from reaching the egg. The mini pill or progestin only pill works by suppressing ovulation and helps to prevent the sperm from reaching the egg.

S4995

S4995 Smoking cessation gum

Lay Description
Nicotine gum is a drug in chewing gum form to aid people in smoking cessation. Small amounts of nicotine are released from the gum, which when absorbed by the body, cuts down on the withdrawal symptoms. It is a nicotine replacement therapy. The individual is cautioned to chew very slowly until a tingling is felt in the mouth and then to hold the gum between the cheek and gum until the tingle is gone. Chew again a few more times until the tingle is felt and then move the gum to another part of the mouth. This should be repeated for 30 minutes. It is estimated that about 3 mg of nicotine is absorbed from a 4 mg piece of gum.

S5000-S5001

S5000 Prescription drug, generic
S5001 Prescription drug, brand name

Lay Description
A generic drug refers to the chemical name of the drug. Although generic drugs are chemically the same as the brand name of the drug, they are usually less expensive. The brand name drug has a trade name. It can only be produced and sold by the company that holds the patent. Brand name drugs may be available over the counter or by prescription only.

S5010

S5010 5% dextrose and 0.45% normal saline, 1000 ml

Lay Description
This code is used to report a 5% dextrose solution in half amount of normal saline. A 5% dextrose and 0.45% normal saline is a hypotonic fluid replacement that is used to replace fluid when some sodium is required in patients that are not able to maintain

adequate oral intake or are restricted from doing so. It hydrates the cells and releases fluid from the vessels. Possible side effects are hypernatremia and circulatory overload.

S5011

S5011   5% dextrose in lactated ringer's, 1000 ml

Lay Description

A 5% dextrose in ringers lactate provides potassium, electrolytes, calories, and hydration. It is used to replace fluid and calories in patients that are not able to maintain adequate oral intake or are restricted from doing so. It is a hypertonic solution that hydrates the cells and releases fluid from the vessels. Depending on the condition of the patient, it may induce diuresis.

S5012

S5012   5% dextrose with potassium chloride, 1000 ml

Lay Description

Potassium chloride in 5% dextrose solution is a sterile, nonpyrogenic solution that is used to replace fluid, electrolytes, and calories in patients that are not able to maintain adequate oral intake or are restricted from doing so. Possible side effects include hypervolemia and extravasation.

S5013-S5014

S5013   5% dextrose/0.45% normal saline with potassium chloride and magnesium sulfate, 1000 ml

S5014   5% dextrose/0.45% normal saline with potassium chloride and magnesium sulfate, 1500 ml

Lay Description

These codes are used to report a 5% dextrose solution in half amount of normal saline to which potassium chloride and magnesium sulfate have been added. It is used to replace fluid in patients that are not able to maintain adequate oral intake or are restricted from doing so. Report the code based on the volume of the IV solution.

S5035-S5036

S5035   Home infusion therapy, routine service of infusion device (e.g., pump maintenance)

S5036   Home infusion therapy, repair of infusion device (e.g., pump repair)

Lay Description

Home infusion therapy is intravenous (IV) administration of medication or fluids to patients in their own home. It is done as an alternative to receiving IV therapy in a facility or office setting. Nurses and other specially trained individuals provide the insertion and management services of the IV and IV equipment, such as the IV pump. Use these codes to report routine service and repair of the IV pump and

other equipment that is used with the home infusions.

S5100-S5105

S5100   Day care services, adult; per 15 minutes

S5101   Day care services, adult; per half day

S5102   Day care services, adult; per diem

S5105   Day care services, center-based; services not included in program fee, per diem

Lay Description

An adult day care center furnishes professional services to adults in need. These services provide social services, as well as some health care, to adults who require supervision in a safe place during the day that is outside of the home. In a community setting, the attendees are given the services by interdisciplinary professionals that are trained to meet their physical, social, and emotional needs.

S5108-S5116

S5108   Home care training to home care client, per 15 minutes

S5109   Home care training to home care client, per session

S5110   Home care training, family; per 15 minutes

S5111   Home care training, family; per session

S5115   Home care training, nonfamily; per 15 minutes

S5116   Home care training, nonfamily; per session

Lay Description

Training the home care client, family, or non-family is necessary to assure that they understand everything they need to know about the client's care. Examples of possible training topics include when and how to take medication and possible side effects, skin and wound care, monitoring IV sites and tubing, nutritional needs, fall prevention, issues related to a specific disease condition, and when to contact a health care provider.

S5120-S5121

S5120   Chore services; per 15 minutes

S5121   Chore services; per diem

Lay Description

Chore services are homemaking services provided to individuals who want to remain in their homes but are unable to do all of the necessary tasks. Companies are available to provide help with these chores, for example, shopping for groceries and supplies, planning and preparing meals, changing linens, vacuuming, making beds, housecleaning, lawn mowing, snow shoveling, trash removal, and providing transportation.

S5125-S5126

S5125   Attendant care services; per 15 minutes

S5126   Attendant care services; per diem

Lay Description
Attendant care services provide help with the activities of daily living to a patient with a physical disability, for example, help with eating, bathing, dressing, toilet and bathroom needs, and taking medications that are self administered.

S5130-S5131

S5130   Homemaker service, NOS; per 15 minutes

S5131   Homemaker service, NOS; per diem

Lay Description
These codes are used to report any homemaker services that are not explained by another HCPCS Level II code.

S5135-S5136

S5135   Companion care, adult (e.g., IADL/ADL); per 15 minutes

S5136   Companion care, adult (e.g., IADL/ADL); per diem

Lay Description
Adult companion care is the provision of nonmedical services for adults in their home. These services may include homemaking, medication reminders, personal care, and companionship. ADL refers to the activities of daily living, such as bathing, dressing, self-feeding, and walking. IADLs are instrumental activities of daily living that aren't necessary for fundamental functioning, but do assist in independent living in the community. ADLs include housework, grocery shopping, transportation, and managing money.

S5140-S5141

S5140   Foster care, adult; per diem

S5141   Foster care, adult; per month

Lay Description
Adult foster care provides a family setting for adults who are unable to live alone due to developmental, emotional, or physical impairment. These homes provide room and board and general supervision of their needs, which may include help with dressing, eating, and bathing. These codes report adult foster care on a monthly or daily basis.

S5145-S5146

S5145   Foster care, therapeutic, child; per diem

S5146   Foster care, therapeutic, child; per month

Lay Description
Therapeutic foster care services place children with foster families that have received special training in caring for children with specific medical or behavioral needs. Foster parents in these homes require greater training in order to provide more support for these children. These codes report child therapeutic foster care on a monthly or per diem basis.

S5150-S5151

S5150   Unskilled respite care, not hospice; per 15 minutes

S5151   Unskilled respite care, not hospice; per diem

Lay Description
Respite care is intended to help the patient remain living in a home environment by relieving the patient's unpaid caregiver. Typically, the "home environment" includes the home of a friend, foster home, or a licensed group home, but not a nursing home, hospital, or adult day care setting. Respite care does not refer to care provided by the patient's parent, spouse, or unpaid primary care giver. Use these codes to report respite care as a time increment or a per diem.

S5160-S5162

S5160   Emergency response system; installation and testing

S5161   Emergency response system; service fee, per month (excludes installation and testing)

S5162   Emergency response system; purchase only

Lay Description
Individuals who are at a high risk of being put in a facility are often able to remain in the home setting with the use of an emergency response system. This system is an electronic device that allows these individuals to secure help if an emergency does occur. These individuals who live alone or are alone for a large portion of the day require extensive routine supervision, and do not have a regular caregiver. These codes describe the installation and testing of the system, the monthly service fee (which includes the installation and testing), and the purchase of the system.

S5165

S5165   Home modifications; per service

Lay Description
An individual's physical condition may require physical modifications to the home setting in order to allow him or her to receive care at home and to ensure safety and welfare (e.g., the installation of hand rails).

S5170

S5170   Home delivered meals, including preparation; per meal

Lay Description
Home meal delivery usually includes two meals per day that are delivered to the patient's home or day care center.

S5175

S5175 Laundry service, external, professional; per order

Lay Description
This code is used to report laundering done by a professional service that usually includes pickup and delivery. It is to be reported on a per order basis.

S5180-S5181

S5180 Home health respiratory therapy, initial evaluation

S5181 Home health respiratory therapy, NOS, per diem

Lay Description
Home health respiratory services provide aid for patients with respiratory problems that may include COPD, emphysema, bronchitis, asthma, and sleep apnea. These services may include nebulizer and aerosol therapy, chest physical therapy, suction and tracheostomy care, monitoring of equipment, oxygen therapy, and patient education. Use these codes to report the initial evaluation and for home health respiratory therapy services that are not described by any other HCPCS Level II code.

S5185

S5185 Medication reminder service, nonface-to-face; per month

Lay Description
At specific times and dates, a medication reminder service automatically contacts the patient by phone, computer, or other personal electronic device and texts, emails, or plays a recorded message reminding the patient to take his or her medications.

S5190

S5190 Wellness assessment, performed by nonphysician

Lay Description
Wellness assessments are analyses of a person's physical and/or mental state performed in the absence of any known disease or symptom. Wellness assessments may also include evaluations of the person's social, emotional, environmental, and spiritual state. Use this code to report wellness assessments performed by a nonphysician practitioner, such as a nurse practitioner, clinical nurse specialist, or physician assistant.

S5199

S5199 Personal care item, NOS, each

Lay Description
Personal care items are used by patients to help meet their personal needs (e.g., razors, dental care products, hygiene products, and skin and hair care products). Report this code when the personal care item is not described by another existing HCPCS Level II code.

S5497-S5502

S5497 Home infusion therapy, catheter care/maintenance, not otherwise classified; includes administrative services, professional pharmacy services, care coordination, and all necessary supplies and equipment (drugs and nursing visits coded separately), per diem

S5498 Home infusion therapy, catheter care/maintenance, simple (single lumen), includes administrative services, professional pharmacy services, care coordination and all necessary supplies and equipment, (drugs and nursing visits coded separately), per diem

S5501 Home infusion therapy, catheter care/maintenance, complex (more than one lumen), includes administrative services, professional pharmacy services, care coordination, and all necessary supplies and equipment (drugs and nursing visits coded separately), per diem

S5502 Home infusion therapy, catheter care/maintenance, implanted access device, includes administrative services, professional pharmacy services, care coordination and all necessary supplies and equipment (drugs and nursing visits coded separately), per diem (use this code for interim maintenance of vascular access not currently in use)

Lay Description
Home infusion therapy is intravenous (IV) administration of medication or fluids to patients in their own home. It is done as an alternative to receiving IV therapy in a hospital setting. Nurses and other specially trained individuals provide the insertion and management services of the IV and IV equipment, such as the IV pump. These codes are used to report the catheter care, including maintaining patency of the catheter and dressing changes, as a per diem charge when it is a stand-alone therapy (not done the same day as an IV administration). Report the code based on whether the catheter care was for a single lumen, more than one lumen, or for an implanted access device that is not currently in use. Report the not otherwise specified code when there is no other HCPCS Level II code that describes the service.

S5517-S5518

S5517 Home infusion therapy, all supplies necessary for restoration of catheter patency or declotting

S5518 Home infusion therapy, all supplies necessary for catheter repair

Lay Description
Home infusion therapy is intravenous (IV) administration of medication or fluids to patients in their own home. It is done as an alternative to

receiving IV therapy in a hospital setting. Nurses and other specially trained individuals provide the insertion and management services of the IV and IV equipment, such as the IV pump. These codes are used to report the supplies used to dissolve a blockage from the catheter in order to restore patency or to repair a catheter.

S5520-S5523

S5520 **Home infusion therapy, all supplies (including catheter) necessary for a peripherally inserted central venous catheter (PICC) line insertion**

S5521 **Home infusion therapy, all supplies (including catheter) necessary for a midline catheter insertion**

S5522 **Home infusion therapy, insertion of peripherally inserted central venous catheter (PICC), nursing services only (no supplies or catheter included)**

S5523 **Home infusion therapy, insertion of midline venous catheter, nursing services only (no supplies or catheter included)**

Lay Description
Home infusion therapy is the intravenous (IV) administration of medication or fluids to patients in their own home. It is done as an alternative to receiving IV therapy in a hospital setting. Nurses and other specially trained individuals provide the insertion and management services of the IV and IV equipment, such as the IV pump. A PICC line is a catheter that is inserted into the arm and threaded through the vein to the superior vena cave, the large blood vessel that leads to the heart. A midline catheter is 6 to 8 inches long and is inserted in the arm near the elbow (basilic, cephalic, or brachial vein) and threaded to the distal axillary vein. Report the appropriate code based on site and whether supplies or catheters are included.

S5550-S5553

S5550 **Insulin, rapid onset, 5 units**

S5551 **Insulin, most rapid onset (Lispro or Aspart); 5 units**

S5552 **Insulin, intermediate acting (NPH or LENTE); 5 units**

S5553 **Insulin, long acting; 5 units**

Lay Description
Insulin is a hormone secreted by the beta cells of the pancreas that controls the metabolism and cellular uptake of sugars, proteins, and fats. As a drug, it is used principally to control Type I diabetes mellitus. Different forms of insulin may also be used to control blood sugar levels in patients with gestational diabetes to prevent fetal complications caused by maternal hyperglycemia. The use of insulin in Type II diabetes mellitus is typically only for patients who have failed to control blood sugars with diet, exercise, and oral drugs. In the past, insulin for injection was

obtained from beef or porcine pancreas. The onset of action, peak effect, and duration of the insulin effects vary with different kinds of insulin. Most insulin now in use is made by recombinant DNA technology and is equivalent to human insulin from an immunological perspective. Dosage varies by the level of control of blood sugar needed. Insulin is administered by subcutaneous injection or by insulin pump.

S5560-S5571

S5560 **Insulin delivery device, reusable pen; 1.5 ml size**

S5561 **Insulin delivery device, reusable pen; 3 ml size**

S5565 **Insulin cartridge for use in insulin delivery device other than pump; 150 units**

S5566 **Insulin cartridge for use in insulin delivery device other than pump; 300 units**

S5570 **Insulin delivery device, disposable pen (including insulin); 1.5 ml size**

S5571 **Insulin delivery device, disposable pen (including insulin); 3 ml size**

Lay Description
An insulin pen is used to inject insulin into a patient. It is comprised of an insulin cartridge and dial. Disposable needles are attached to the pen. The patient is able to use the dial on the device to adjust the dose dispense. There are two types of pens: reusable and disposable. Insulin cartridges are inserted into a reusable pen. The cartridge is replaced when it is empty but the pen is reused. A prefilled pen includes the pen and the insulin cartridge. The whole device is thrown away when it is empty. Insulin is a hormone secreted by the beta cells of the pancreas that controls the metabolism and cellular uptake of sugars, proteins, and fats. As a drug, it is used principally to control Type I diabetes mellitus. Different forms of insulin may also be used to control blood sugar levels in patients with gestational diabetes to prevent fetal complications caused by maternal hyperglycemia. The use of insulin in Type II diabetes mellitus is typically only for patients who have failed to control blood sugars with diet, exercise, and oral drugs. In the past, insulin for injection was obtained from beef or porcine pancreas. Most insulin now in use is made by recombinant DNA technology and is equivalent to human insulin from an immunological perspective. Dosage varies by the level of control of blood sugar needed.

S8030

S8030 **Scleral application of tantalum ring(s) for localization of lesions for proton beam therapy**

Lay Description
Prior to proton beam radiation therapy of a scleral tumor, the tumor must be localized. A transillumination and/or indirect ophthalmoscopy are

performed during the surgery and titanium rings are sutured to the edges of the scleral tumor.

S8032

S8032   Low-dose computed tomography for lung cancer screening

Lay Description
The U.S. preventive services task force recommends annual screening for lung cancer using low-dose computed tomography in adults aged 55 to 80 years who have a 30 pack per year smoking history and currently smoke or have quit within the past 15 years. This screening uses significantly less imaging agent to control exposure to radiation.

S8035

S8035   Magnetic source imaging

Lay Description
Magnetic source imaging is a combination of two sets of magnetic data. Brain activity is mapped using the magnetic fields generated by the natural electrical currents within the brain. The magnetic activity is gathered using arrays of superconducting quantum interference devices (SQUID). A recording of this mapping is a magnetoencephalogram or MEG. MEG provides maps of neural activity. Magnetic resonance images map blood flow and physical construction. MEG data is then superimposed on an MRI to create a magnetic source image (MSI). MSIs are used to create functional maps of the human cortex during complex cognitive tasks aiding in the targeting of lesions and epileptic foci, and can aid the identification of head trauma and vascular malformations. It has shown some promise in the classification of patients with multiple sclerosis, Alzheimer's disease, and schizophrenia.

S8037

S8037   Magnetic resonance cholangiopancreatography (MRCP)

Lay Description
Magnetic resonance cholangiopancreatography (MRCP) is magnetic resonance imaging that produces detailed images of the hepatobiliary and pancreatic systems. Multiplanar images that are parallel to the biliary tree are obtained. The MR sequence is sensitive to static fluid and does not require contrast agents. Post-processing can create multi-dimensional images of the entire area. MRCP is useful in the diagnosis and level determination of a bile duct obstruction, cystic biliary diseases, primary sclerosing cholangitis, postop complications, cholangiocarcinoma, pancreatic cancer, and chronic pancreatitis.

S8040

S8040   Topographic brain mapping

Lay Description
Topographic brain mapping, also known as brain electrical activity mapping, is an extension of conventional electroencephalography (EEG). It is the computerized analysis of EEG rhythms and evoked potential data. The analysis is used to generate maps of frequency and voltage. It is intended to identify patterns that represent progressive changes in function or deviations from normal brain activity.

S8042

S8042   Magnetic resonance imaging (MRI), low-field

Lay Description
Magnetic resonance imaging (MRI) usually requires a magnetic field of a few Tesla, which is about 10,000 to 100,000 times stronger than earth's magnetic field. Low field MRIs use approximately 30 millitesla fields, which is about 100 times weaker than the earth's magnetic field. Since the strength of the magnet is directly tied to its cost, lower field MRIs are less costly than regular MRIs. Low field MRIs are generally open and there is less danger to patients with pacemakers and metal implants.

S8055

S8055   Ultrasound guidance for multifetal pregnancy reduction(s), technical component (only to be used when the physician doing the reduction procedure does not perform the ultrasound, guidance is included in the CPT code for multifetal pregnancy reduction (59866)

Lay Description
This code is used to report the technical component of ultrasound guidance for multifetal pregnancy reduction when the physician doing the reduction procedure does not perform the ultrasound. When the physician performing the surgery is also performing the ultrasound guidance, then the guidance is included in the CPT code for multifetal pregnancy reduction. Multifetal pregnancies can result naturally or from the implantation of multiple embryos during an in vitro fertilization cycle. Fetal reductions can be done to reduce twins to a single fetus, triplets to twins, quadruplets to triplets, etc.

S8080

S8080   Scintimammography (radioimmunoscintigraphy of the breast), unilateral, including supply of radiopharmaceutical

Lay Description
A scintimammography is a nuclear medicine scan performed on women who have an abnormal or inconclusive mammogram study. It is used to help determine whether or not a patient needs a biopsy or if multiple biopsies are needed. A radioactive substance is injected into the patient's vein. The substance accumulates in the breast that has abnormal tissue. An imaging device called a gamma camera is used to detect the radioactive material. A

computer is used to analyze and measure the abnormal tissue.

S8085

S8085   Fluorine-18 fluorodeoxyglucose (F-18 FDG) imaging using dual-head coincidence detection system (nondedicated PET scan)

Lay Description
A fluorine-18 fluorodeoxyglucose (F-18 FDG) image using dual-head coincidence detection system (nondedicated positron emission tomography or PET scan) is also known as an FDG-single photon emission computed tomography (SPECT), metabolic SPECT, or PET scan using a gamma camera. F-18 FDG is a radiotracer that emits positrons as it decays. These positrons emit paired photons. Dedicated PET scanners consist of multiple detectors that simultaneously detect all high-energy photons emitted at 180 degrees from one another that produce detailed images. SPECT cameras are less expensive than PET scanners and use the photons to provide scintigraphic images reflecting the metabolic activity of the tissues. SPECT cameras can be adapted to read the higher energy photons emitted by F-18 FDG. To screen out lower energy photons, a dual head rotating SPECT camera is operated in coincidence mode, which means that the camera only counts photons that are simultaneously detected at 180 degrees from one another. However, the lower number of detectors in SPECT machines results in a loss of sensitivity and resolution.

S8092

S8092   Electron beam computed tomography (also known as ultrafast CT, cine CT)

Lay Description
Electron beam computed tomography (EBT) is also known as ultrafast CT or cine CT. In a conventional CT scanner, the x-ray source moves along a circle in space around the object to be imaged. In EBT, the x-ray tube does not move. It is large, stationary, and partially surrounds the imaging circle. The x-ray source, or electron-beam focal point, is swept electronically along a tungsten anode in the tube, tracing a large circular arc. This motion can be very fast creating an ultrafast CT. Ultrafast CT scans are needed to image the heart as its rhythm can blur images during conventional CT scans.

S8096

S8096   Portable peak flow meter

Lay Description
Portable peak flow meters are used to monitor the severity of the disease and its response to therapy in patients with asthma, chronic obstructive pulmonary disease, and other respiratory diseases. Home monitoring of peak expiratory flow is recommended by the National Heart, Lung, and Blood Institute for asthma management. The peak flow meter consists of a spring-loaded piston or vane in a drum. A forced expiration through an inlet moves the piston or vane proportional to the maximum flow. Electronic versions measure peak flow and forced expiratory volume in one second and store the measurements.

S8097

S8097   Asthma kit (including but not limited to portable peak expiratory flow meter, instructional video, brochure, and/or spacer)

Lay Description
An asthma kit includes a portable peak expiratory flow meter, instructional video and/or brochure, and/or a spacer. The kit is designed to assist asthmatics in the management of their disease. The physician should provide instructions to the patient on interpreting the peak flow levels, including normal levels, the levels that require the use of an inhaler or nebulizer, and the level requiring immediate emergency care.

S8100-S8101

S8100   Holding chamber or spacer for use with an inhaler or nebulizer; without mask

S8101   Holding chamber or spacer for use with an inhaler or nebulizer; with mask

Lay Description
A holding chamber is a valved container that holds medication that is to be administered. A spacer is a container or tube that slows the delivery of the medication from a pressurized metered dose inhaler. Spacing or controlling the dose allows the medication to more easily and effectively reach the lungs.

S8110

S8110   Peak expiratory flow rate (physician services)

Lay Description
This code is used to report physician services related to respiratory diseases and the use of peak flow meters. These services may include instructions to the patient on the use of the meter and interpretation of the peak flow levels, including normal levels, the levels that require the use of an inhaler or nebulizer, and the level requiring immediate emergency care.

S8120-S8121

S8120   Oxygen contents, gaseous, 1 unit equals 1 cubic foot

S8121   Oxygen contents, liquid, 1 unit equals 1 pound

Lay Description
Supplemental oxygen is sometimes necessary for people with respiratory illnesses. Oxygen may be contained in stationary or portable canisters or tanks and delivered in a liquid or gaseous state. These codes

are used to report the supply of oxygen used to refill the canisters or tanks.

S8130-S8131

S8130   Interferential current stimulator, 2 channel

S8131   Interferential current stimulator, 4 channel

Lay Description
Interferential current stimulator is a device that produces and delivers a high frequency (4000 HZ) carrier wave that has the same signal as a TENS device. The higher frequency penetrates more deeply than a TENS. The current generated stimulates large impulse fibers and can interfere with the transmission of pain signals at the spinal cord level. The stimulation can also be adjusted to stimulate parasympathetic nerve fibers for increased blood flow. The channels carry different frequencies, usually a high and a medium frequency electrical impulse. One channel is usually fixed and the other variable. When combined, the signals produce the desired electrical impulse. In phase electrical waves combine to deliver an amplified electrical impulse. Out of phase waves can cancel all or parts of other electrical waves, thereby decreasing or stopping the signal. Interferential therapy is used for the treatment of deep pain, to promote bone growth in delayed and nonunion fractures, to stimulate muscles to pump blood in venous insufficiency, and to depress the activity of cervical and lumbosacral sympathetic ganglia in patients with arterial constrictor tone. It has also been used to manage acute postsurgical and posttraumatic pain, edema, and inflammation.

S8185

S8185   Flutter device

Lay Description
A flutter device is used to provide positive expiratory pressure therapy for patients with respiratory conditions that produce mucus (e.g., bronchitis, bronchiectasis, asthma, atelectasis, cystic fibrosis, and COPD). The device works by vibrating the airways to loosen the mucus, helping to maintain the patency of the airway by intermittently increasing endobronchial pressure, and facilitates the movement of mucus up through the airways by increasing expiratory airflow. The device resembles a pipe with a mouthpiece at one end and a perforated cover at the opposite end. Inside the device a stainless steel ball rests on a circular cone.

S8186

S8186   Swivel adaptor

Lay Description
A swivel adaptor is used to connect ventilator circuits to endotracheal tubes. They are usually elbow shaped and allow for flexibility and help in maintaining patent airways.

S8189

S8189   Tracheostomy supply, not otherwise classified

Lay Description
Use this code to report supplies used with a tracheostomy that are not described by other HCPCS Level II codes.

S8210

S8210   Mucus trap

Lay Description
A mucus trap is a container used in respiratory section equipment to prevent sputum from going into the suction bottle so it can be sent to the lab for analysis.

S8262

S8262   Mandibular orthopedic repositioning device, each

Lay Description
The mandibular orthopedic repositioning device is typically a clear acrylic bite pad that overlays the molars and bicuspids and is connected by an oval, heavy lingual bar. It is designed to reposition the mandible with its condyle to obtain both a balanced condyle fossa relationship and optimal neuromuscular balance. The appliance is used to treat disorders of the jaw joint, grinding of the teeth, and possibly obstructive sleep apnea since the device advances the mandible and increases the upper airway size.

S8265

S8265   Haberman feeder for cleft lip/palate

Lay Description
The Haberman feeder is a bottle named after its developer that is used for babies who have impaired ability to suck due to a cleft lip/palate, congenital heart disease, a genetic disorder, or neurological disorders. The bottle has a one-way valve that helps to reduce the air that the baby takes in. It is a soft squeeze bottle that the parent can squeeze to provide an adequate amount of formula to the baby.

S8270

S8270   Enuresis alarm, using auditory buzzer and/or vibration device

Lay Description
An enuresis alarm is a device that sends out a sound or a vibration when moisture reaches the device. It is attached to the child's underwear or pajamas in the area where it would first come in contact with the drop of urine. When the child feels the vibration or hears the alarm, he or she becomes trained to get up and go to the bathroom to empty the bladder. Eventually, the child learns to respond to the sensation of a full bladder by waking up and going to the bathroom prior to the alarm going off.

S8301

S8301 Infection control supplies, not otherwise specified

Lay Description
Infection control supplies include such items as disinfectants, hand sanitizer, latex gloves, sharps containers, etc. This code is used to report infection control supplies that are not identified by another HCPCS Level II code.

S8415

S8415 Supplies for home delivery of infant

Lay Description
This code is used to report the supplies used for a home delivery of an infant. Examples include scissors, suction bulb, warm towels and receiving blankets, lubricants, cord care supplies, antiseptic, sterile gauze, OB pads, gloves, waterproof or plastic sheets, and disposable under pads.

S8420-S8429

S8420 Gradient pressure aid (sleeve and glove combination), custom made
S8421 Gradient pressure aid (sleeve and glove combination), ready made
S8422 Gradient pressure aid (sleeve), custom made, medium weight
S8423 Gradient pressure aid (sleeve), custom made, heavy weight
S8424 Gradient pressure aid (sleeve), ready made
S8425 Gradient pressure aid (glove), custom made, medium weight
S8426 Gradient pressure aid (glove), custom made, heavy weight
S8427 Gradient pressure aid (glove), ready made
S8428 Gradient pressure aid (gauntlet), ready made
S8429 Gradient pressure exterior wrap

Lay Description
When the lymphatic fluid accumulates in the interstitial tissue, especially in the subcutaneous tissue, the condition is known as lymphedema. The accumulated fluid causes gradual and progressive enlargement of the affected extremity and is accompanied by increased weight and decreased functional ability among other changes. Lymphedema may be a complication of cancer and the treatments for cancer and is usually progressive. There is no known cure for lymphedema. Gradient pressure aids are pneumatic compression devices that are used to treat lymphedema. Use these codes to report gradient pressure aids, based on the type, if they are custom or ready made, and whether they are medium or heavy weight.

S8430-S8431

S8430 Padding for compression bandage, roll
S8431 Compression bandage, roll

Lay Description
A compression bandage is an elasticized rolled bandage that provides sustained compression for treatment of venous ulcers, lymphedema, and other types of swelling or edema and related conditions. The compression bandage may also be applied as a first aid measure to control bleeding by applying pressure to stop the blood flow from an artery. Compression bandages are often used to reduce the swelling and to stabilize a limb prior to applying a cast or compression garment. Compression bandage padding may be used as an under wrap for a compression dressing or an under cast padding.

S8450-S8452

S8450 Splint, prefabricated, digit (specify digit by use of modifier)
S8451 Splint, prefabricated, wrist or ankle
S8452 Splint, prefabricated, elbow

Lay Description
A splint is a device used to support or immobilize a limb or the spine. It is commonly used right after an injury. A splint may be custom made or prefabricated. These codes represent prefabricated splints, which are usually plastic or metal and attach to the body with Velcro straps. A prefabricated splint requires very little adjustment to fit the limb or digit and does not require any expertise to trim or bend or mold the splint to fit the patient.

S8460

S8460 Camisole, postmastectomy

Lay Description
A camisole is a sleeveless undergarment for women that extends from the chest to the waist. The postmastectomy camisole has pouches and pockets sewn on the inside of the camisole and is worn with or without foam inserts. It may be used for the first six weeks post-breast surgery in place of a bra. The mastectomy camisole can hold four drains: two in the pouch and two in the underarm tabs.

S8490

S8490 Insulin syringes (100 syringes, any size)

Lay Description
A syringe is a simple pump consisting of a plunger in a tube that is used as a drug delivery device. An insulin syringe has a capacity of 1 ml or less and comes attached to a fine gauge needle (27-29 G). The syringe is marked in insulin units. This code is used to report a package of 100 insulin syringes.

S8930

S8930 Electrical stimulation of auricular acupuncture points; each 15 minutes of personal one-on-one contact with patient

Lay Description
Acupuncture was commonly used in ancient China to treat a wide variety of conditions, symptoms, and behaviors. It involves insertion of very thin needles superficially into various points in the body to produce therapy and healing in other parts of the body. The ear cartilage is thought to contain approximately 200 of these points. In western medicine, pulse electrostimulation of the needles placed in the ear cartilage provide additional stimulation of the acupuncture site.

S8940

S8940 Equestrian/hippotherapy, per session

Lay Description
Equestrian/hippotherapy, also known as therapeutic horseback riding, is the passive use of the movements of a horse to treat patients with cerebral palsy and neuromuscular disabilities. The therapist tries to facilitate normal muscle tone and discourage abnormal posture by using the horse as a treatment modality. The patient is placed in various positions on the horse (e.g., side sitting, prone across the horse, prone lengthwise on the horse, or sitting). The movement of the horse is thought to enhance balance, motor development, and coordination.

S8948

S8948 Application of a modality (requiring constant provider attendance) to one or more areas; low-level laser; each 15 minutes

Lay Description
Low-level laser therapy (LLLT) is a form of phototherapy in which low power photonic energy light is applied to lesions and injuries. It reportedly enhances wound healing, including amputation injuries, infected wounds, burns, and skin grafts. The laser infuses the body's cells with energy. LLLT is noninvasive and works quickly.

S8950

S8950 Complex lymphedema therapy, each 15 minutes

Lay Description
Complex lymphedema therapy (CLT) is a noninvasive treatment for lymphedema. Lymphedema is a result of lymphatic system failure, which causes an accumulation of lymphatic fluid or edema in the soft tissue. CLT is done to restore function of the affected limb by controlling and reducing the amount of swelling. The therapy usually consists of two phases: treatment and maintenance. CLT treatment phase includes light massage, usually for 30 to 60 minutes. The massage stimulates residual lymphatic vessels to transport the excess fluids from the edematous area. The affected limb is then wrapped in compression bandages and is subjected to range of motion movements. The treatments are usually done two to five times a week for two weeks, and then the patient moves on to the maintenance phase where the patient maintains and applies the techniques learned in the treatment phase, including continuing to wear the compressive sleeve during the day and the compression bandage wrap at night.

S8990

S8990 Physical or manipulative therapy performed for maintenance rather than restoration

Lay Description
Maintenance therapy occurs after the goals of the treatment plan have been reached, the therapy is no longer of therapeutic necessity, and it is apparent that no additional functional improvement is occurring or expected to occur. Maintenance therapy is performed to maintain the quality of life, disease prevention, and general health maintenance.

S8999

S8999 Resuscitation bag (for use by patient on artificial respiration during power failure or other catastrophic event)

Lay Description
A resuscitation bag is used to help a person breathe in a medical emergency. It is a hand-held device that consists of an air chamber (that is squeezed to force air into the patient) and a mask that is placed over the nose and mouth of the patient.

S9001

S9001 Home uterine monitor with or without associated nursing services

Lay Description
A home uterine monitor helps to detect preterm labor. The external device is worn in a belt on the abdomen of a pregnant woman twice a day for one to two hours and records contractions that may be too faint for the patient to recognize. The resulting data is transmitted via telephone modem link to nurses who analyze the data and provide assessment and counseling services to the patient on a daily basis. The uterine monitor consists of a guard ring tocodynamometer that is worn as an abdominal belt, a data transmitter, and a data recorder.

S9007

S9007 Ultrafiltration monitor

Lay Description
An ultrafiltration monitor is intended to reduce overfiltration (removal of too much fluid from tissue) and underfiltration (removal of too little fluid) during hemodialysis.

S9015
S9015   Automated EEG monitoring

Lay Description
Automated EEG monitoring is a computerized program that continuously acquires, stores, and reads electroencephalograms. It is primarily of use in neurological and neonatal intensive care units to monitor unrecognized seizures or injuries.

S9024
S9024   Paranasal sinus ultrasound

Lay Description
The paranasal sinuses are mucus lined air filled cavities and include the fontal, maxillary, ethmoid, and sphenoid sinuses. A paranasal ultrasound, which is a noninvasive procedure, may be used to help diagnose sinusitis, focal soft tissue masses, and thickening of the mucosal walls. The ultrasound applicator is placed over the sinuses on the face, including the cheekbones and nose, and high frequency sound waves are used to image the sinuses.

S9025
S9025   Omnicardiogram/cardiointegram

Lay Description
The cardiointegram or omnicardiogram may be used as a substitute for exercise tolerance testing with thallium imaging in patients for whom a resting EKG may be inadequate to identify changes compatible with coronary artery disease. The device is composed of a microcomputer that receives output from a standard 12 lead EKG. A series of integrations is used to transform the voltage versus tine format and produce a graphic representation of the heart's electrophysiologic signals.

S9034
S9034   Extracorporeal shockwave lithotripsy for gall stones (if performed with ERCP, use 43265)

Lay Description
Extracorporeal shock wave lithotripsy is a noninvasive procedure that may be done by dry method (water-filled compressible bags placed over stone area) or wet method (patient is placed in a water bath or submerged). High-intensity shock waves are electrically produced and focused sonographically on the gallstone. The procedure may be done with either epidural or general anesthesia or with the use of IV sedation.

S9055
S9055   Procuren or other growth factor preparation to promote wound healing

Lay Description
Procuren is a human platelet-derived growth factor (PDGF), a substance naturally produced by the body that helps to promote wound healing. An autologous platelet concentrate is prepared from a sample of the patient's blood, processed to separate the platelets, which are treated with a reagent to create a gel that is applied topically to the wound. Autologous platelet-derived products have also been used to treat a variety of acute surgical wounds. Please note that Procuren may no longer be available but that this code is also used to report other growth factor preparations that promote wound healing.

S9056
S9056   Coma stimulation per diem

Lay Description
A coma is a state of unconsciousness that lasts longer than six hours. Coma stimulation is done by a health care professional or a member of the patient's family (who is trained in the stimulation techniques) to increase patient responsiveness. Stimulation is applied to one or more of the patient's five senses, with the intent of facilitating awakening and enhancing the rehabilitative potential of the patient. Various stimuli can be used for each of the senses. These treatments can be given in the hospital, SNF, or patient's home and can range from hourly treatments twice a day to hourly stimulation cycles lasting 15 to 20 minutes 12 to 14 times a day six days a week. Use this code to report daily (per diem) coma stimulation.

S9061
S9061   Home administration of aerosolized drug therapy (e.g., Pentamidine); administrative services, professional pharmacy services, care coordination, all necessary supplies and equipment (drugs and nursing visits coded separately), per diem

Lay Description
An aerosol is a suspension of solid particles or liquid droplets in a gas. Aerosolized drug therapy is used when rapid absorption and localization effects of the drug are required to produce the appropriate response. They are most commonly used in specific lung diseases that cause breathing difficulties; for example, emphysema, asthma, and COPD. In aerosolized drug therapy, drugs are absorbed through the lungs or bronchial airways through tiny droplets. This code is used to report the administration of aerosolized drug therapy in the home setting and includes the administrative services, professional pharmacy services, care coordination, and all necessary supplies and equipment (e.g. nebulizer) provided on a daily (per diem) basis. The drugs and nursing visits may be reported separately.

S9083-S9088

S9083   Global fee urgent care centers

S9088   Services provided in an urgent care center (list in addition to code for service)

Lay Description

Urgent care centers deliver medical care in a facility outside of a hospital emergency room, and typically, the care is unscheduled and on a walk-in basis. The centers are intended to treat patients who are ill or injured and require immediate care but who do not require the services of a hospital emergency department. Unlike hospital emergency departments, urgent care centers are not open 24 hours a day. These codes are used to report urgent care centers as a global service or as an adjunct code (in addition to the code for the specific service).

S9090

S9090   Vertebral axial decompression, per session

Lay Description

Vertebral axial decompression is a therapy for lower back pain due to herniated lumbar discs or degenerative lumbar disc disease. It uses a computer-driven table to control the disc decompression. For the treatment, a pelvic harness is applied to the patient and the patient lies on the special table and is subjected to a series of cycles as the table is slowly extended and a distraction force is applied via the harness. When the desired tension is reached, it is gradually decreased. This repetitive cycle builds up the patient's tolerance to stronger distraction forces. Each session usually includes 15 cycles lasting about 30 minutes, and 10 to 15 daily treatments are generally administered. Use this code to report each session.

S9097

S9097   Home visit for wound care

Lay Description

This code is used to report a home care visit to care for the patient's wounds, which may include ulcers, burns, pressure sores, open surgical sites, fistulas, tube sites, and tumor erosion sites.

S9098

S9098   Home visit, phototherapy services (e.g., Bili-lite), including equipment rental, nursing services, blood draw, supplies, and other services, per diem

Lay Description

Phototherapy services are prescribed to treat skin disorders, including babies with high bilirubin count. Use this code to report home visits for phototherapy services on a daily (per diem) basis. The code includes all equipment rentals, nursing services, blood draw, supplies and other services.

S9110

S9110   Telemonitoring of patient in their home, including all necessary equipment; computer system, connections, and software; maintenance; patient education and support; per month

Lay Description

Telehealth is the delivery of health-related services via telecommunications equipment, including email, video conferencing, and the transmission of medical images or medical data. The telecommunications most often involve a primary care practitioner with a patient at a remote site and a consulting medical specialist at an urban or referral facility. The originating site is the location of the patient at the time the service is being furnished via a telecommunications system. A fee that is set annually is paid to the originating site. This code represents the telemonitoring of a patient in the home and includes all of the necessary equipment required, including maintenance, patient education and support, and all computer system connections and software. It is billed on a monthly basis.

S9117

S9117   Back school, per visit

Lay Description

Back school may involve one or more instructive sessions where the patient is instructed in anatomy of the spine, the best sleeping positions, and proper body mechanics for standing, lifting, sitting, and doing household chores.

S9122

S9122   Home health aide or certified nurse assistant, providing care in the home; per hour

Lay Description

Home health aides and certified nurse assistants provide routine health care in the patient's home. Their services may include dressing changes, applying topical medications, feeding the patient, monitoring vital signs, and monitoring and reporting changes in heath status. They may also provide help with the patient's personal care, including bathing and dressing and help with toileting.

S9123-S9124

S9123   Nursing care, in the home; by registered nurse, per hour (use for general nursing care only, not to be used when CPT codes 99500-99602 can be used)

S9124   Nursing care, in the home; by licensed practical nurse, per hour

Lay Description

These codes are used to report various home care services provided by a registered nurse (RN) or licensed practical nurse (LPN) on an hourly basis.

Examples of duties usually done by skilled nurses include tube feeding, injections, cardiac and respiratory care, and medication management.

S9125

S9125   Respite care, in the home, per diem

Lay Description
Respite care is the provision of short-term temporary care to a person with a chronic illness or disability. The term "respite care" usually refers to relief provided to a primary caregiver. Use this code to report respite care in the home setting on a daily (per diem) basis.

S9126

S9126   Hospice care, in the home, per diem

Lay Description
Hospice care services are designed to address the physical, mental, emotional, and spiritual needs of terminally ill patients and their families. Hospice care is a palliative service that is provided when a cure is not possible. Services focus on keeping the patient comfortable by relieving pain and other symptoms and supporting the family during the terminal phase of the patient's illness. Hospice services also include bereavement counseling following the patient's death. Hospice care is typically delivered by an interdisciplinary health care team of physicians, nurses, social workers, counselors, home health aides, clergy, therapists, and trained volunteers.

S9127-S9131

S9127   Social work visit, in the home, per diem
S9128   Speech therapy, in the home, per diem
S9129   Occupational therapy, in the home, per diem
S9131   Physical therapy; in the home, per diem

Lay Description
These codes are used to report various services provided by different types of qualified professionals in a home health setting on a per diem basis. Home health includes not only traditional private home settings, but also assisted living quarters, group homes, custodial care facilities, or similar type settings that constitute the patient's place of residence.

S9140-S9141

S9140   Diabetic management program, follow-up visit to non-MD provider
S9141   Diabetic management program, follow-up visit to MD provider

Lay Description
A diabetes management program typically includes an overview of diabetes, as well as instruction in stress management, exercise, meal planning, glucose monitoring, medications, and advice about complications. These codes are used to report a diabetes management program follow-up visit to an MD or a non-MD provider.

S9145

S9145   Insulin pump initiation, instruction in initial use of pump (pump not included)

Lay Description
Insulin pumps are used to deliver rapid-acting insulin continuously throughout the day through a catheter that is placed under the skin. The pump replaces the need for periodic injections of insulin. Prior to using the pump, the patient needs to be instructed in correct use, which includes the basal rate (continuous rate that keeps the glucose level in range overnight and between meals), bolus doses (additional insulin that is given to cover the amount of carbohydrates consumed during a meal), and supplemental doses that may be required to treat high blood sugar. The patient also requires instruction on care of the pump while showering, sleeping, and exercising, and what to do if the pump needs to be removed.

S9150

S9150   Evaluation by ocularist

Lay Description
An ocular prosthesis or artificial eye is a prosthetic unit that is designed to maintain the facial shape and to match the remaining eye as closely as possible for patients who have lost an eye as a result of illness or trauma. An ocularist is an individual who is licensed to design, fabricate, and fit the prosthesis. Use this code to report the evaluation done by an ocularist.

S9152

S9152   Speech therapy, re-evaluation

Lay Description
A speech therapy re-evaluation may be done periodically when the clinician notes a significant improvement or decline or a change that was not anticipated when the plan of care was established. Some state and payer guidelines may require re-evaluations at specific times, but the clinician usually determines when a re-evaluation is indicated. A re-evaluation may not be as extensive as the original evaluation since it is focused on the current treatment. A routine, continuous assessment of the patient's progress is inherent in the treatment and should not be considered a re-evaluation. The re-evaluation is focused on the patient's progress toward the established goals and may include the clinician's judgment on continued care, goal modification, and whether to continue or to terminate the treatment. Typically, the documentation should support the need for further measurements and tests by identifying a significant change in the patient's condition, new clinical findings, or a failure to respond to therapy.

S9208-S9209

S9208 Home management of preterm labor, including administrative services, professional pharmacy services, care coordination, and all necessary supplies or equipment (drugs and nursing visits coded separately), per diem (do not use this code with any home infusion per diem code)

S9209 Home management of preterm premature rupture of membranes (PPROM), including administrative services, professional pharmacy services, care coordination, and all necessary supplies or equipment (drugs and nursing visits coded separately), per diem (do not use this code with any home infusion per diem code)

Lay Description

Preterm labor is regular contractions of the uterus that are accompanied by progressive changes in the cervix prior to 37 weeks of gestation. Preterm premature rupture of the membranes (PPROM) is when the membranes rupture before the onset of uterine contractions and prior to 37 weeks gestation. As an alternative to hospital admission, a woman may opt for home management of her preterm labor or PPROM. In addition to bed rest, medications may be given and a uterine monitor may be used. Tocolytic therapy is the use of drugs to inhibit contractions of the uterus. Acute tocolysis is done to reduce or stop contractions of the uterus and to stop or slow down cervical changes during preterm labor. Maintenance tocolysis is done after acute tocolysis to prevent a recurrence of preterm labor after it has been stopped. Antibiotics may be given for PPROM to prevent infection. The home uterine monitor helps to detect preterm labor. The external device is worn in a belt on the abdomen of a pregnant woman twice a day for one to two hours and records contractions that may be too faint for the patient to recognize. The resulting data is transmitted via telephone modem link to nurses who analyze the data and provide assessment and counseling services to the patient on a daily basis. The uterine monitor consists of a guard ring tocodynamometer that is worn as an abdominal belt, a data transmitter, and a data recorder. Use these codes to report all services involved in home management of preterm labor and PPROM on a daily (per diem) basis. Drugs and nursing visits are to be coded separately. Do not use these codes with any home infusion code.

S9211-S9214

S9211 Home management of gestational hypertension, includes administrative services, professional pharmacy services, care coordination and all necessary supplies and equipment (drugs and nursing visits coded separately); per diem (do not use this code with any home infusion per diem code)

S9212 Home management of postpartum hypertension, includes administrative services, professional pharmacy services, care coordination, and all necessary supplies and equipment (drugs and nursing visits coded separately), per diem (do not use this code with any home infusion per diem code)

S9213 Home management of preeclampsia, includes administrative services, professional pharmacy services, care coordination, and all necessary supplies and equipment (drugs and nursing services coded separately); per diem (do not use this code with any home infusion per diem code)

S9214 Home management of gestational diabetes, includes administrative services, professional pharmacy services, care coordination, and all necessary supplies and equipment (drugs and nursing visits coded separately); per diem (do not use this code with any home infusion per diem code)

Lay Description

Gestational hypertension is the development of high blood pressure in the pregnant woman (usually greater than 140/90) after 20 weeks gestation. Postpartum hypertension is the development of high blood pressure after the completion of labor. Postpartum hypertension may occur in the period just after delivery. Preeclampsia is high blood pressure; swelling of the hands, feet, and face; and excess protein in the urine of a pregnant woman after 20 weeks gestation. If untreated, preeclampsia can lead to serious complications for the mother and the baby. Gestational diabetes is glucose intolerance with first recognition or onset during pregnancy. Use these codes to report the home management of any of the conditions listed above on a daily (per diem) basis. Drugs and nursing visits should be coded separately. Do not report these codes with any home infusion per diem code.

S9325-S9328

S9325 Home infusion therapy, pain management infusion; administrative services, professional pharmacy services, care coordination, and all necessary supplies and equipment, (drugs and nursing visits coded separately), per diem (do not use this code with S9326, S9327 or S9328)

S9326 Home infusion therapy, continuous (24 hours or more) pain management infusion; administrative services, professional pharmacy services, care coordination and all necessary supplies and equipment (drugs and nursing visits coded separately), per diem

S9327 Home infusion therapy, intermittent (less than 24 hours) pain management infusion; administrative services, professional pharmacy services, care coordination, and all necessary supplies and equipment (drugs and nursing visits coded separately), per diem

S9328 Home infusion therapy, implanted pump pain management infusion; administrative services, professional pharmacy services, care coordination, and all necessary supplies and equipment (drugs and nursing visits coded separately), per diem

Lay Description
Home infusion therapy is the intravenous (IV) administration of medication or fluids to patients in their own home. It is done as an alternative to receiving IV therapy in a hospital setting. Nurses and other specially trained individuals provide the insertion and management services of the IV and IV equipment, such as the IV pump. These codes are used to report home infusions for the management of pain on a daily (per diem) basis as an infusion, continuous infusion of 24 hours or more, as an intermittent infusion less than 24 hours, or via an implanted pump. Drugs and nursing visits should be coded separately.

S9329-S9331

S9329 Home infusion therapy, chemotherapy infusion; administrative services, professional pharmacy services, care coordination, and all necessary supplies and equipment (drugs and nursing visits coded separately), per diem (do not use this code with S9330 or S9331)

S9330 Home infusion therapy, continuous (24 hours or more) chemotherapy infusion; administrative services, professional pharmacy services, care coordination, and all necessary supplies and equipment (drugs and nursing visits coded separately), per diem

S9331 Home infusion therapy, intermittent (less than 24 hours) chemotherapy infusion; administrative services, professional pharmacy services, care coordination, and all necessary supplies and equipment (drugs and nursing visits coded separately), per diem

Lay Description
Home infusion therapy is the intravenous (IV) administration of medication or fluids to patients in their own home. It is done as an alternative to receiving IV therapy in a hospital setting. Nurses and other specially trained individuals provide the insertion and management services of the IV and IV equipment, such as the IV pump. These codes are used to report home infusions for the administration of chemotherapy on a daily (per diem) basis as an infusion, continuous infusion of 24 hours or more, or as an intermittent infusion less than 24 hours. Drugs and nursing visits should be coded separately.

S9335

S9335 Home therapy, hemodialysis; administrative services, professional pharmacy services, care coordination, and all necessary supplies and equipment (drugs and nursing services coded separately), per diem

Lay Description
Hemodialysis is done to clear waste and extra fluid from the patient's blood by using a special dialyzer. Two needles are placed into the patient's access site: one into an artery and the other into a vein. They are connected to plastic tubing. This tubing carries the blood to the dialysis machine, which cleanses the blood of excess waste and fluids and returns the clean blood back to the body. The dialysis machine pumps the blood through the dialysis system and controls the temperature, pressure, fluid removal, and treatment time. This code is used to report the administration of hemodialysis. Drugs and nursing visits should be coded separately.

S9336

S9336 Home infusion therapy, continuous anticoagulant infusion therapy (e.g., Heparin), administrative services, professional pharmacy services, care coordination and all necessary supplies and equipment (drugs and nursing visits coded separately), per diem

Lay Description
Heparin is an anticoagulant indicated for the treatment and prevention of blood clots, including pulmonary embolism and deep vein thrombosis. It is also used to ensure patency of indwelling intravenous catheters. Heparin inhibits reactions that lead to the clotting of blood and the formation of fibrin clots. It works by acting as an accelerant in forming antithrombin III-thrombin complex, which deactivates

thrombin. This prevents the conversion of fibrinogen to fibrin. Heparin sodium is derived from bovine or porcine pulmonary or intestinal tissue and standardized for anticoagulant activity. This code is used to report home infusions for the continuous administration of anticoagulant therapy on a daily (per diem) basis. Drugs and nursing visits should be coded separately.

S9338

S9338   Home infusion therapy, immunotherapy, administrative services, professional pharmacy services, care coordination, and all necessary supplies and equipment (drugs and nursing visits coded separately), per diem

Lay Description
Immunotherapy, also known as biological therapy or biotherapy, uses certain characteristics of the immune system to fight diseases, such as cancer, by stimulating the patient's own immune system or by giving the patient immune system components, such as manufactured immune system proteins. This code is used to report home infusions for the administration of immunotherapy on a daily (per diem) basis. Drugs and nursing visits should be coded separately.

S9339

S9339   Home therapy; peritoneal dialysis, administrative services, professional pharmacy services, care coordination and all necessary supplies and equipment (drugs and nursing visits coded separately), per diem

Lay Description
For end stage renal disease (ESRD) patients, peritoneal dialysis is the most common form of home dialysis treatment. A catheter is placed in the peritoneal cavity of the patient. The catheter remains permanently in the peritoneum. During the treatment, dialysate is drained from the peritoneal cavity and is replaced with fresh dialysate, which is allowed to remain in the peritoneum for several hours. At that time, this solution is drained through the catheter and a new bag of dialysate is put into the peritoneum. The peritoneal dialysis may be continuous (CAPD), which involves two to five daily manual treatments. Automated peritoneal dialysis is done with the use of a cycler machine. This machine is programmed to perform three to five fluid exchanges while the patient sleeps. This code is used to report home peritoneal dialysis on a daily (per diem) basis as an infusion, continuous infusion of 24 hours or more, or as an intermittent infusion less than 24 hours. Drugs and nursing visits should be coded separately.

S9340-S9343

S9340   Home therapy; enteral nutrition; administrative services, professional pharmacy services, care coordination, and all necessary supplies and equipment (enteral formula and nursing visits coded separately), per diem

S9341   Home therapy; enteral nutrition via gravity; administrative services, professional pharmacy services, care coordination, and all necessary supplies and equipment (enteral formula and nursing visits coded separately), per diem

S9342   Home therapy; enteral nutrition via pump; administrative services, professional pharmacy services, care coordination, and all necessary supplies and equipment (enteral formula and nursing visits coded separately), per diem

S9343   Home therapy; enteral nutrition via bolus; administrative services, professional pharmacy services, care coordination, and all necessary supplies and equipment (enteral formula and nursing visits coded separately), per diem

Lay Description
Enteral nutrition provides nourishment directly to the digestive tract via a tube for patients whose nutritional needs cannot be met with a regular diet. Feeding tube options include placing a nasogastric or nasoenteric tube through the patient's nose and into the stomach or percutaneous placement of a gastrostomy or jejunostomy tube into the stomach or small intestine. Gravity enteral feedings are poured into the feeding bag and the bag is hung on a pole. The tube from the bag is attached to the feeding tube. Enteral feedings done with a pump are done by connecting the tubes to an electric pump and programming the desired rate. A bolus feeding is achieved by attaching a syringe to the feeding tube and pouring formula into the syringe. It is allowed to flow into the tube by gravity. These codes are used to report home enteral nutrition therapy on a daily (per diem) basis. Drugs and nursing visits should be coded separately.

S9345-S9363, S9370

S9345   Home infusion therapy, antihemophilic agent infusion therapy (e.g., factor VIII); administrative services, professional pharmacy services, care coordination, and all necessary supplies and equipment (drugs and nursing visits coded separately), per diem

S9346 Home infusion therapy, alpha-1-proteinase inhibitor (e.g., Prolastin); administrative services, professional pharmacy services, care coordination, and all necessary supplies and equipment (drugs and nursing visits coded separately), per diem

S9347 Home infusion therapy, uninterrupted, long-term, controlled rate intravenous or subcutaneous infusion therapy (e.g., epoprostenol); administrative services, professional pharmacy services, care coordination, and all necessary supplies and equipment (drugs and nursing visits coded separately), per diem

S9348 Home infusion therapy, sympathomimetic/inotropic agent infusion therapy (e.g., Dobutamine); administrative services, professional pharmacy services, care coordination, all necessary supplies and equipment (drugs and nursing visits coded separately), per diem

S9349 Home infusion therapy, tocolytic infusion therapy; administrative services, professional pharmacy services, care coordination, and all necessary supplies and equipment (drugs and nursing visits coded separately), per diem

S9351 Home infusion therapy, continuous or intermittent antiemetic infusion therapy; administrative services, professional pharmacy services, care coordination, and all necessary supplies and equipment (drugs and visits coded separately), per diem

S9353 Home infusion therapy, continuous insulin infusion therapy; administrative services, professional pharmacy services, care coordination, and all necessary supplies and equipment (drugs and nursing visits coded separately), per diem

S9355 Home infusion therapy, chelation therapy; administrative services, professional pharmacy services, care coordination, and all necessary supplies and equipment (drugs and nursing visits coded separately), per diem

S9357 Home infusion therapy, enzyme replacement intravenous therapy; (e.g., Imiglucerase); administrative services, professional pharmacy services, care coordination, and all necessary supplies and equipment (drugs and nursing visits coded separately), per diem

S9359 Home infusion therapy, antitumor necrosis factor intravenous therapy; (e.g., Infliximab); administrative services, professional pharmacy services, care coordination, and all necessary supplies and equipment (drugs and nursing visits coded separately), per diem

S9361 Home infusion therapy, diuretic intravenous therapy; administrative services, professional pharmacy services, care coordination, and all necessary supplies and equipment (drugs and nursing visits coded separately), per diem

S9363 Home infusion therapy, antispasmotic therapy; administrative services, professional pharmacy services, care coordination, and all necessary supplies and equipment (drugs and nursing visits coded separately), per diem

S9370 Home therapy, intermittent antiemetic injection therapy; administrative services, professional pharmacy services, care coordination, and all necessary supplies and equipment (drugs and nursing visits coded separately), per diem

Lay Description
This group of codes is used to report daily or intermittent infusion therapy services and supplies, other than drugs and nursing visits. Medication is infused through a vein or the subcutaneous tissue.

S9364-S9368

S9364 Home infusion therapy, total parenteral nutrition (TPN); administrative services, professional pharmacy services, care coordination, and all necessary supplies and equipment including standard TPN formula (lipids, specialty amino acid formulas, drugs other than in standard formula and nursing visits coded separately), per diem (do not use with home infusion codes S9365-S9368 using daily volume scales)

S9365 Home infusion therapy, total parenteral nutrition (TPN); 1 liter per day, administrative services, professional pharmacy services, care coordination, and all necessary supplies and equipment including standard TPN formula (lipids, specialty amino acid formulas, drugs other than in standard formula and nursing visits coded separately), per diem

S9366 Home infusion therapy, total parenteral nutrition (TPN); more than 1 liter but no more than 2 liters per day, administrative services, professional pharmacy services, care coordination, and all necessary supplies and equipment including standard TPN formula (lipids, specialty amino acid formulas, drugs other than in standard formula and nursing visits coded separately), per diem

S9367 Home infusion therapy, total parenteral nutrition (TPN); more than 2 liters but no more than 3 liters per day, administrative services, professional pharmacy services, care coordination, and all necessary supplies and equipment including standard TPN formula (lipids, specialty amino acid formulas, drugs other than in standard formula and nursing visits coded separately), per diem

S9368 Home infusion therapy, total parenteral nutrition (TPN); more than 3 liters per day, administrative services, professional pharmacy services, care coordination, and all necessary supplies and equipment including standard TPN formula (lipids, specialty amino acid formulas, drugs other than in standard formula and nursing visits coded separately), per diem

Lay Description

This group of codes is used to report daily parenteral services and supplies, other than nursing visits, associated with total parenteral nutrition (TPN). Parenteral nutrition is administered to the patient through a vein. Since the alimentary tract of a patient with severe pathology does not function adequately for ingesting food normally, nutrients to sustain life must be administered by other methods. Parenteral nutrition solutions are based on the composition of ingredients or nutrients in each product. Scalable TPN ingredients are those that may differ based on lab work or that are ordered based on a concentration basis rather than on the total daily TPN volume.

S9372

S9372 Home therapy; intermittent anticoagulant injection therapy (e.g., Heparin); administrative services, professional pharmacy services, care coordination, and all necessary supplies and equipment (drugs and nursing visits coded separately), per diem (do not use this code for flushing of infusion devices with Heparin to maintain patency)

Lay Description

Heparin is an anticoagulant indicated for the treatment and prevention of blood clots, including pulmonary embolism and deep vein thrombosis. It is also used to ensure patency of indwelling intravenous catheters. Heparin inhibits reactions that lead to the clotting of blood and the formation of fibrin clots. It works by acting as an accelerant in forming antithrombin III-thrombin complex, which deactivates thrombin. This prevents the conversion of fibrinogen to fibrin. Heparin sodium is derived from bovine or porcine pulmonary or intestinal tissue and standardized for anticoagulant activity. This code is used to report home infusions for the intermittent anticoagulant therapy on a daily (per diem) basis. Drugs and nursing visits should be coded separately.

S9373-S9377

S9373 Home infusion therapy, hydration therapy; administrative services, professional pharmacy services, care coordination, and all necessary supplies and equipment (drugs and nursing visits coded separately), per diem (do not use with hydration therapy codes S9374-S9377 using daily volume scales)

S9374 Home infusion therapy, hydration therapy; 1 liter per day, administrative services, professional pharmacy services, care coordination, and all necessary supplies and equipment (drugs and nursing visits coded separately), per diem

S9375 Home infusion therapy, hydration therapy; more than 1 liter but no more than 2 liters per day, administrative services, professional pharmacy services, care coordination, and all necessary supplies and equipment (drugs and nursing visits coded separately), per diem

S9376 Home infusion therapy, hydration therapy; more than 2 liters but no more than 3 liters per day, administrative services, professional pharmacy services, care coordination, and all necessary supplies and equipment (drugs and nursing visits coded separately), per diem

S9377 Home infusion therapy, hydration therapy; more than 3 liters per day, administrative services, professional pharmacy services, care coordination, and all necessary supplies (drugs and nursing visits coded separately), per diem

Lay Description

This group of codes is used to report daily hydration infusion and supplies, other than drugs and nursing visits. Fluids are administered to the patient through a vein. Hydration is used to treat dehydration and electrolyte imbalance. Scalable hydration ingredients are those that may differ based on lab work or that are ordered based on a concentration basis rather than on the total daily volume.

S9379

S9379 Home infusion therapy, infusion therapy, not otherwise classified; administrative services, professional pharmacy services, care coordination, and all necessary supplies and equipment (drugs and nursing visits coded separately), per diem

Lay Description
Infusion therapy is the administration of fluids through a needle or catheter. The infusion is usually intravenous, but may also refer to intracavity, intramuscular, or epidural routes of administration. Home infusion therapy is the administration of the infusion in the patient's home. This code is used to report home infusion therapy that is not otherwise described by other more specific HCPCS Level II codes. The code encompasses administrative services, professional pharmacy services, care coordination, and all necessary supplies and equipment except for drugs and nursing visits.

S9381

S9381 Delivery or service to high risk areas requiring escort or extra protection, per visit

Lay Description
This code is used to report an added charge per visit when an item or service must be delivered in a high crime area. These areas require an escort or extra protection.

S9401

S9401 Anticoagulation clinic, inclusive of all services except laboratory tests, per session

Lay Description
An anticoagulation clinic is an organized outpatient service that monitors and manages the medications used to prevent blood clots. Anticoagulants must be maintained at a level that does not cause too much clotting or too little clotting. There is usually a pharmacist present. The patient's clotting time is determined using an internalized normalized ratio or INR. Medications are then increased or decreased to reach the target INR.

S9430

S9430 Pharmacy compounding and dispensing services

Lay Description
This code is used to report pharmacy fees for the compounding (or mixing) of drug and drug components and the dispensing of the drug.

S9433-S9435

S9433 Medical food nutritionally complete, administered orally, providing 100% of nutritional intake
S9434 Modified solid food supplements for inborn errors of metabolism
S9435 Medical foods for inborn errors of metabolism

Lay Description
Medical foods or food supplements are food stuffs designed and formulated to provide appropriate nutrition to patients who have food allergies or specific problems with digestion or absorption. Inborn errors of metabolism are genetic diseases that cause the incomplete breakdown of various substances or the accumulation of toxic substances that interfere with normal cellular function.

S9436-S9437

S9436 Childbirth preparation/Lamaze classes, nonphysician provider, per session
S9437 Childbirth refresher classes, nonphysician provider, per session

Lay Description
Lamaze is a type of childbirth preparation course. Childbirth preparation courses seek to prepare the woman for coping with pain, progressing through labor, and facilitating delivery of the baby. Women are taught techniques to tolerate pain and to assist the body in a natural childbirth. Techniques include movement, massage, breathing, and exercise. Refresher classes are reviews of the childbirth preparation courses for those women who have previously attended a course.

S9438

S9438 Cesarean birth classes, nonphysician provider, per session

Lay Description
Cesarean birth classes are birth preparation classes designed to explain to women the process of labor, reasons for the cesarian section, the procedure itself, and what to expect after the delivery.

S9439

S9439 VBAC (vaginal birth after cesarean) classes, nonphysician provider, per session

Lay Description
Vaginal birth after cesarean (VBAC) classes are birth preparation classes designed to explain to women the process of labor, the procedure itself, what to expect after the delivery, and any complications that may occur due to the prior cesarean section.

S9441

S9441 Asthma education, nonphysician provider, per session

Lay Description

Asthma education may involve one or more instructive sessions where the patient is taught the anatomy of the lungs, lifestyle changes, triggers, attack prevention, and treatment including the use of medication and medication delivery devices. It may also include self-management and self-monitoring tools to help identify the patient's needs and help them maintain quality of life.

S9442

S9442 Birthing classes, nonphysician provider, per session

Lay Description

Birthing classes seek to prepare the woman for all kinds of issues surrounding childbirth, including breathing, coping with pain, progressing through labor, and vaginal or cesarean delivery of the baby. Women are prepared for the changes that pregnancy brings and the care of a newborn.

S9443

S9443 Lactation classes, nonphysician provider, per session

Lay Description

Lactation classes focus on preparation for breastfeeding, cues from the baby, latching on, length of time to feed, nursing bras, breast pumps, and excess breast milk. Trained counselors are usually available to assist mothers who are encountering difficulties.

S9444

S9444 Parenting classes, nonphysician provider, per session

Lay Description

Parenting classes are lessons and training in the art of parenting. Effective parenting skills include communication skills, stress management, empathy, anger and conflict resolution, boundary and limit setting, rewards and discipline, teamwork, and parenting styles. Parenting classes may be taken for personal growth, but are most often undertaken due to court orders.

S9445-S9446

S9445 Patient education, not otherwise classified, nonphysician provider, individual, per session

S9446 Patient education, not otherwise classified, nonphysician provider, group, per session

Lay Description

Patient education represents patient teaching or training that is not described by other HCPCS Level II codes. Group sessions consist of two or more people, while individual sessions are one-on-one.

S9447

S9447 Infant safety (including CPR) classes, nonphysician provider, per session

Lay Description

Infant safety classes train parents and other caregivers on how to provide safe environments for a newborn and infant. Subjects include car seats, cribs and sleep arrangements, poison prevention, and environmental safety. This code includes cardiopulmonary resuscitation.

S9449

S9449 Weight management classes, nonphysician provider, per session

Lay Description

Weight management classes are training and education related to nutrition, physical activity, stress management, and lifestyle and how they relate to health. They are geared to teaching the patient to reach and maintain an ideal weight.

S9451

S9451 Exercise classes, nonphysician provider, per session

Lay Description

Exercise classes are formal programs of bodily activities that maintain physical fitness and overall health. They are usually performed in a group. Instructors may have formal training. There are generally three types of exercise: flexibility, such as stretching; aerobic, such as cycling, tennis, and swimming; and anaerobic, such as weight lifting. Exercise classes can address all three types or only one.

S9452, S9470

S9452 Nutrition classes, nonphysician provider, per session

S9470 Nutritional counseling, dietitian visit

Lay Description

Nutrition is the provision of the appropriate amount of food, water, vitamins, minerals, and related items that allow an organism to function in a safe and healthy manner. Nutrition classes provide organized instruction in the food and foodstuffs necessary for life. Dietitians are health professionals who specialize in nutrition and meal planning and preparation. Classes are usually group activities that discuss generalities. Counseling involves the dietitian and is usually individualized to a single patient.

S9453

S9453 Smoking cessation classes, nonphysician provider, per session

Lay Description
Smoking cessation classes are organized sessions that provide instruction, assistance, and guidance in the discontinuance of smoking. Smoking usually refers to tobacco smoking, but may also apply to other substances. Smoking cessation can be achieved with or without the assistance of health care professionals and with or without the use of medications. Groups of people who are trying to quit smoking can also provide support to each other.

S9454

S9454 Stress management classes, nonphysician provider, per session

Lay Description
Stress management classes are organized education and training on the techniques and methods of controlling levels of stress, particularly chronic stress, to improve life functioning. Medication can be used to decrease feelings of anxiety and stress. Among the other techniques available are yoga, exercise, meditation, deep breathing, progressive relaxation, time management, planning and decision making, and pet therapy.

S9455-S9465

S9455 Diabetic management program, group session

S9460 Diabetic management program, nurse visit

S9465 Diabetic management program, dietitian visit

Lay Description
A diabetes management program is used to teach a patient how to control and monitor blood glucose levels. The program includes techniques to deal with the emotional and physical problems associated with the disease. It also provides education regarding exercise, nutrition, medication, and monitoring.

S9470

S9470 Nutritional counseling, dietitian visit

Lay Description
Please refer to code S9452 for the description.

S9472

S9472 Cardiac rehabilitation program, nonphysician provider, per diem

Lay Description
A cardiac rehabilitation program is a rehabilitation program for patients who have experienced one or more of the following:

- An acute myocardial infarction within the preceding 12 months

- Coronary artery bypass surgery
- Current stable angina pectoris
- Heart valve repair or replacement
- Percutaneous transluminal coronary angioplasty or coronary stenting
- A heart or heart-lung transplant

Cardiac rehabilitation programs usually include the following components:

- Physician-prescribed exercise each day that items and services are furnished
- Cardiac risk factor modification
- Psychosocial assessment
- Outcomes assessment
- An individualized treatment plan detailing how components are used for each patient

This code represents cardiac rehabilitation services provided by a nonphysician provider.

S9473

S9473 Pulmonary rehabilitation program, nonphysician provider, per diem

Lay Description
Pulmonary rehabilitation (PR) is a program to help improve the quality of life for people with chronic breathing problems. PR may include psychological counseling, breathing strategies, exercise training, ways to conserve energy, and education on the patient's lung disease, including how to manage it. This code includes monitoring services and exercise. Pulmonary rehabilitation items and services are usually prescribed for patients who are diagnosed with moderate to severe COPD, when referred by the physician who is treating the chronic respiratory disease. Report this code when pulmonary rehabilitation services are provided by a nonphysician provider.

S9474

S9474 Enterostomal therapy by a registered nurse certified in enterostomal therapy, per diem

Lay Description
Enterostomal therapy is the care of a stoma, which is a surgically created passageway from the internal body cavity to the outside. A registered nurse certified in enterostomal therapy receives specialized training in the ostomy planning and aftercare. The nurse may work with the patient and surgeons to determine the optimal stoma site, provide surgical aftercare, change the appliance, provide stoma and skin care, and instruct the patient or caregiver on these topics. Enterostomal therapy nurses usually also have specialized training in wound care and incontinence care.

S9475

S9475　Ambulatory setting substance abuse treatment or detoxification services, per diem

Lay Description
Ambulatory setting substance abuse treatment or detoxification services are medically supervised mental and behavioral health services provided in an outpatient environment. Patients arrive at points during the day and return home or to another setting at night. This treatment is aimed at patients with substance abuse problems.

S9476

S9476　Vestibular rehabilitation program, nonphysician provider, per diem

Lay Description
A vestibular rehabilitation program is an organized outpatient program that seeks to train patients with chronic or acute vestibular (inner ear) disorders to deal with or alleviate primary and secondary symptoms. The vestibular rehabilitation therapy is usually exercise based, but may include medications that suppress vestibular functions. Exercises may include the coordination of eye and head movements, balance and walking ability, and fitness and endurance with the goals of decreasing dizziness and visual symptoms, improved balance and ambulation, and increased activity levels. An assessment and therapy plan is usually performed by specially trained physical or occupational therapists.

S9480

S9480　Intensive outpatient psychiatric services, per diem

Lay Description
Intensive outpatient psychiatric services are mental and behavioral health treatments provided in an outpatient setting. Generally, they are at least three hours per day for two or more days per week. The services may address substance abuse disorders, mental or behavioral health issues, or both, which are dual diagnosis programs. These programs are usually used as a step down from acute inpatient care, residential care, or a partial hospitalization program. They may also be viewed as a step up from regular outpatient services.

S9482

S9482　Family stabilization services, per 15 minutes

Lay Description
Family stabilization services are programs, activities, and services that provide participants and their families with employment, family dynamics, economic stability, and reduced barriers. The goal is to keep a family together and united as a cohesive, safe, and productive support system and unit. Many programs operate 24 hours a day, seven days a week.

Family stabilization services involve as many disciplines as required and coordinate services among all professionals and paraprofessionals.

S9484-S9485

S9484　Crisis intervention mental health services, per hour
S9485　Crisis intervention mental health services, per diem

Lay Description
Crisis intervention mental health services are emergency mental and behavioral health care intended to assist in a crisis situation. Crisis situations may be defined as a person's perception or experience of an event or situation that exceeds the person's current resources or coping mechanisms. Crisis intervention seeks to stabilize the person's mental state and prevent immediate harm to the person or others in contact with that person.

S9490

S9490　Home infusion therapy, corticosteroid infusion; administrative services, professional pharmacy services, care coordination, and all necessary supplies and equipment (drugs and nursing visits coded separately), per diem

Lay Description
This code is used to report daily infusion therapy services and supplies of corticosteroids, other than drugs and nursing visits. Medication is infused through a vein.

S9494-S9504

S9494　Home infusion therapy, antibiotic, antiviral, or antifungal therapy; administrative services, professional pharmacy services, care coordination, and all necessary supplies and equipment (drugs and nursing visits coded separately), per diem (do not use this code with home infusion codes for hourly dosing schedules S9497-S9504)
S9497　Home infusion therapy, antibiotic, antiviral, or antifungal therapy; once every 3 hours; administrative services, professional pharmacy services, care coordination, and all necessary supplies and equipment (drugs and nursing visits coded separately), per diem
S9500　Home infusion therapy, antibiotic, antiviral, or antifungal therapy; once every 24 hours; administrative services, professional pharmacy services, care coordination, and all necessary supplies and equipment (drugs and nursing visits coded separately), per diem

S9501 Home infusion therapy, antibiotic, antiviral, or antifungal therapy; once every 12 hours; administrative services, professional pharmacy services, care coordination, and all necessary supplies and equipment (drugs and nursing visits coded separately), per diem

S9502 Home infusion therapy, antibiotic, antiviral, or antifungal therapy; once every 8 hours, administrative services, professional pharmacy services, care coordination, and all necessary supplies and equipment (drugs and nursing visits coded separately), per diem

S9503 Home infusion therapy, antibiotic, antiviral, or antifungal; once every 6 hours; administrative services, professional pharmacy services, care coordination, and all necessary supplies and equipment (drugs and nursing visits coded separately), per diem

S9504 Home infusion therapy, antibiotic, antiviral, or antifungal; once every 4 hours; administrative services, professional pharmacy services, care coordination, and all necessary supplies and equipment (drugs and nursing visits coded separately), per diem

Lay Description
This group of codes is used to report antibiotic, antiviral, or antifungal medication infusion services and supplies, other than drugs and nursing visits. Medication is infused into a vein. The code reported is based on how often the medication is given.

S9529

S9529 Routine venipuncture for collection of specimen(s), single homebound, nursing home, or skilled nursing facility patient

Lay Description
Routine venipuncture needle is the insertion of a needle into a vein to withdraw a specimen of blood for laboratory testing. This code is used to report this service when performed on a single homebound, nursing home, or skilled nursing facility patient.

S9537

S9537 Home therapy; hematopoietic hormone injection therapy (e.g., erythropoietin, G-CSF, GM-CSF); administrative services, professional pharmacy services, care coordination, and all necessary supplies and equipment (drugs and nursing visits coded separately), per diem

Lay Description
Hematopoietic hormones, such as EPO, G-CSF, or GM-CSF, stimulate the production of various types of blood cells. The blood cells usually need replenishment due to exogenous factors, such as

chemotherapy, radiation therapy, or invasive infections. This code includes all services, except for drugs and nursing visits, provided in the patient's home.

S9538

S9538 Home transfusion of blood product(s); administrative services, professional pharmacy services, care coordination and all necessary supplies and equipment (blood products, drugs, and nursing visits coded separately), per diem

Lay Description
A transfusion of blood products is the intravenous infusion of whole blood or blood components into the patient's circulatory system. Blood transfusions are used to replace blood lost during surgery or due to a serious injury, or when the body cannot appropriately create blood due to illness. This code includes all services, except for the blood products, drugs, and nursing visits, provided in the patient's home.

S9542-S9562

S9542 Home injectable therapy, not otherwise classified, including administrative services, professional pharmacy services, care coordination, and all necessary supplies and equipment (drugs and nursing visits coded separately), per diem

S9558 Home injectable therapy; growth hormone, including administrative services, professional pharmacy services, care coordination, and all necessary supplies and equipment (drugs and nursing visits coded separately), per diem

S9559 Home injectable therapy, interferon, including administrative services, professional pharmacy services, care coordination, and all necessary supplies and equipment (drugs and nursing visits coded separately), per diem

S9560 Home injectable therapy; hormonal therapy (e.g., leuprolide, goserelin), including administrative services, professional pharmacy services, care coordination, and all necessary supplies and equipment (drugs and nursing visits coded separately), per diem

S9562 Home injectable therapy, palivizumab, including administrative services, professional pharmacy services, care coordination, and all necessary supplies and equipment (drugs and nursing visits coded separately), per diem

Lay Description
This group of codes is used to report daily injection therapy services and supplies, other than drugs and nursing visits. Medication is injected intravenously or subcutaneously.

S9590

S9590 Home therapy, irrigation therapy (e.g., sterile irrigation of an organ or anatomical cavity); including administrative services, professional pharmacy services, care coordination, and all necessary supplies and equipment (drugs and nursing visits coded separately), per diem

Lay Description

Irrigation therapy is the steady flow of a solution, usually sterile, across or into a wound, organ, or body cavity. It is intended to wash away cellular debris and surface pathogens and, in doing so, promote healing. This code includes all services, except for drugs and nursing visits, provided in the patient's home.

S9810

S9810 Home therapy; professional pharmacy services for provision of infusion, specialty drug administration, and/or disease state management, not otherwise classified, per hour (do not use this code with any per diem code)

Lay Description

This code represents professional pharmacy services for provision of infusion, specialty drug administration, and/or disease state management in home therapy. This code should only be reported when other HCPCS Level II codes do not adequately describe the type of home therapy.

S9900

S9900 Services by a Journal-listed Christian Science practitioner for the purpose of healing, per diem

Lay Description

A Christian Science practitioner is an individual who follows the practice of healing through prayer according to the teachings of Christian Science. This is usually a specifically focused prayer affirming the Christian Scientist beliefs. Any Christian Scientist who has taken an intensive two-week course may be called a practitioner. Full-time practitioners usually have been practicing for several years and must be members of the mother church (the global organization headquartered in Boston). To be journal-listed, the practitioner must be a full-time practitioner and must present evidence of three cases of the healing of non-family members.

S9960-S9961

S9960 Ambulance service, conventional air services, nonemergency transport, one way (fixed wing)

S9961 Ambulance service, conventional air service, nonemergency transport, one way (rotary wing)

Lay Description

Fixed wing (FW) ambulance (airplane) conventional air service is the transportation by a fixed wing aircraft that is certified by the Federal Aviation Administration (FAA) as a fixed wing air ambulance along with the provision of a nonemergency transport, one way, medically. Rotary wing (RW) ambulance (helicopter) conventional air service is the transportation by helicopter that is certified by the Federal Aviation Administration (FAA) as a rotary wing ambulance, including the provision of nonemergency transport, one way.

S9970

S9970 Health club membership, annual

Lay Description

Health club membership is an additional preventive medicine benefit offered by various payers. This code represents the annual fees for a health club, also known as a fitness club or gym. The club or gym is a location that houses exercise equipment, may offer exercise classes, and other educational opportunities.

S9975

S9975 Transplant related lodging, meals and transportation, per diem

Lay Description

This code is used to report the costs of lodging, meals, and transportation for transplant-related companions or care-givers. This code may also be used to report expenses incurred by a living donor.

S9976-S9977

S9976 Lodging, per diem, not otherwise classified

S9977 Meals, per diem, not otherwise specified

Lay Description

These codes are used to report other lodging and meal expenses that are not adequately described by more specific HCPCS Level II codes. These expenses may be reimbursable depending on the circumstances and on payer policy definitions.

S9981-S9982

S9981 Medical records copying fee, administrative

S9982 Medical records copying fee, per page

Lay Description

These codes are used to report charges for reproducing medical or health record pages, electronically or on paper.

S9986

S9986 Not medically necessary service (patient is aware that service not medically necessary)

Lay Description
This code is used when the provider does not believe the item or treatment is medically necessary, which then leads to the question of whether the payer will cover the service. The reporting of this code also indicates that the patient is aware that the service is not medically necessary.

S9988, S9990-S9991

S9988 Services provided as part of a Phase I clinical trial

S9990 Services provided as part of a Phase II clinical trial

S9991 Services provided as part of a Phase III clinical trial

Lay Description
Clinical trials are procedures performed in biomedical or health research development that allow different components to be tested in controlled environments in predefined protocols. A phase one trial is a general screening for safety in a small group of people. Phase one trials seek to determine a safe dose range and to identify any side effects. Phase two trials use a larger group of people to establish effectiveness and safety. Phase three is the final phase of a trial and uses a large group of people to confirm effectiveness, monitor side effects, compare the new treatment to commonly used treatments, and to collect further safety issues.

S9989

S9989 Services provided outside of the United States of America (list in addition to code(s) for services(s))

Lay Description
This code is used to report that the service identified by another HCPCS Level II code was performed outside of the United States.

S9992-S9996

S9992 Transportation costs to and from trial location and local transportation costs (e.g., fares for taxicab or bus) for clinical trial participant and one caregiver/companion

S9994 Lodging costs (e.g., hotel charges) for clinical trial participant and one caregiver/companion

S9996 Meals for clinical trial participant and one caregiver/companion

Lay Description
Transportation, lodging, and meals are not generally reimbursed for participants and caregivers. These codes are used to report these costs when payers do reimburse the expenses.

S9999

S9999 Sales tax

Lay Description
This code is used to report sales tax charged for medical goods and services in some localities.

T

T1000

T1000 Private duty/independent nursing service(s), licensed, up to 15 minutes

Lay Description
Private-duty or independent nursing services involve individuals who provide nursing care on a one-on-one basis to individual patients. This code applies to services provided by licensed individuals, registered nurse, or licensed vocational/practical nurse.

T1001

T1001 Nursing assessment/evaluation

Lay Description
A nursing assessment or evaluation is the gathering and recording of a patient's physiological, psychological, sociological, and sometimes spiritual status. Data are gathered from a nursing point of view, such as information about the need for assistance in daily activities.

T1002-T1004

T1002 RN services, up to 15 minutes

T1003 LPN/LVN services, up to 15 minutes

T1004 Services of a qualified nursing aide, up to 15 minutes

Lay Description
Services provided by each practitioner are recorded in 15-minute increments.

T1005

T1005 Respite care services, up to 15 minutes

Lay Description
Respite care is the provision of short-term temporary care to a person with a chronic illness or disability. The term "respite care" usually refers to relief provided to a primary caregiver.

T1006

T1006 Alcohol and/or substance abuse services, family/couple counseling

Lay Description
This code represents family or couples counseling in relation to alcohol and/or substance abuse services.

T1007

T1007   Alcohol and/or substance abuse services, treatment plan development and/or modification

Lay Description
This code represents the development of a treatment plan and/or its modification, in relation to alcohol and/or substance abuse services.

T1009

T1009   Child sitting services for children of the individual receiving alcohol and/or substance abuse services

Lay Description
This code represents charges for child-sitting services for children of the individual receiving alcohol and/or substance abuse services.

T1010

T1010   Meals for individuals receiving alcohol and/or substance abuse services (when meals not included in the program)

Lay Description
This code represents charges for meals for individuals receiving alcohol and/or substance abuse services. It is used only when meals are not included in the program.

T1012

T1012   Alcohol and/or substance abuse services, skills development

Lay Description
This code represents skills development, which can be work-related, life skills, coping skills, or similar types of skills that are needed to successfully attain a goal in relation to alcohol and/or substance abuse services.

T1013

T1013   Sign language or oral interpretive services, per 15 minutes

Lay Description
This code represents the use of an interpreter for sign language or oral interpretive communication services.

T1014

T1014   Telehealth transmission, per minute, professional services bill separately

Lay Description
Telehealth is the delivery of health-related services via telecommunications equipment. The term encompasses technology that includes email, video conferencing, and the transmission of medical images or medical data. The telecommunications most often involve a primary care practitioner with a patient at a remote site and a consulting medical specialist at an urban or referral facility. An originating site is the location of the patient at the time the service is being furnished via a telecommunications system. A fee that is set annually is paid to the originating site. This code represents the transmission charge for the originating site. A separate payment is made for the professional fee(s) of the physician or practitioner.

T1015

T1015   Clinic visit/encounter, all-inclusive

Lay Description
An all-inclusive fee for a clinic visit or encounter is a predetermined fee that includes all services related to the visit or encounter. These services include facility charges, physician and professional charges, ancillary services, supplies, and drugs.

T1016-T1017

T1016   Case management, each 15 minutes
T1017   Targeted case management, each 15 minutes

Lay Description
Case management is an effort to improve care and to contain costs by having one party manage or coordinate all care delivered to a patient that usually has certain complex illnesses or injuries, including mental and behavioral health issues. Case management may include, but is not limited to, the evaluation of a condition, the development and implementation of a plan of care, the coordination of medical resources, and the appropriate communication to all parties. Targeted case management is targeted to a specific population subgroup.

T1018

T1018   School-based individualized education program (IEP) services, bundled

Lay Description
A school-based individualized education program (IEP) is mandated by the Individuals with Disabilities Act. An IEP is designed to meet the specific educational needs of a child who may have a disability as defined by federal regulations. The IEP is intended to help the child reach educational goals. The child's needs are identified in an evaluation process. Specific instructions are provided to teachers and related providers so that there is a clear understanding of the disability and its effect on the learning process.

T1019-T1020

T1019   Personal care services, per 15 minutes, not for an inpatient or resident of a hospital, nursing facility, ICF/MR or IMD, part of the individualized plan of treatment (code may not be used to identify services provided by home health aide or certified nurse assistant)

T1020 **Personal care services, per diem, not for an inpatient or resident of a hospital, nursing facility, ICF/MR or IMD, part of the individualized plan of treatment (code may not be used to identify services provided by home health aide or certified nurse assistant)**

Lay Description
Personal care services are paraprofessional aide services not directly linked to medical or skilled nursing care. Such services may include activities of daily living such bathing, shopping, and dressing as part of an individualized plan of treatment. This code is not intended for use when a patient has been institutionized in a hospital, nursing facility, or intermediate care facility or is receiving formal home health services.

T1021

T1021 **Home health aide or certified nurse assistant, per visit**

Lay Description
This code identifies a per visit charge for the services provided by a home health aide or certified nurse assistant.

T1022

T1022 **Contracted home health agency services, all services provided under contract, per day**

Lay Description
This code represents the daily rate for all services provided under a contract for home health agency services.

T1023

T1023 **Screening to determine the appropriateness of consideration of an individual for participation in a specified program, project or treatment protocol, per encounter**

Lay Description
This code represents an encounter for the screening used to determine if an individual should participate in a specified program, project, or treatment protocol.

T1024

T1024 **Evaluation and treatment by an integrated, specialty team contracted to provide coordinated care to multiple or severely handicapped children, per encounter**

Lay Description
Multiple disabilities encompass a combination of various challenges and special needs that may include speech, learning, visual, hearing, brain injury, mental retardation, and physical mobility. There may also be sensory loss, behavioral problems, or social issues. The characteristics and severity of these disabilities vary. Severe multiple disabilities include cerebral palsy, severe autism, and brain injuries. An integrated specialty team consisting of practitioners from appropriate practices evaluates the individual with the multiple handicaps and determines which services would be necessary to provide care for the individual.

T1025-T1026

T1025 **Intensive, extended multidisciplinary services provided in a clinic setting to children with complex medical, physical, mental and psychosocial impairments, per diem**

T1026 **Intensive, extended multidisciplinary services provided in a clinic setting to children with complex medical, physical, medical and psychosocial impairments, per hour**

Lay Description
Multiple disabilities encompass a combination of various challenges and special needs that may include speech, learning, visual, hearing, brain injury, mental retardation, and physical mobility. There may also be sensory loss, behavioral problems, or social issues. The characteristics and severity of these disabilities vary. Severe multiple disabilities include cerebral palsy, severe autism, and brain injuries. A multidisciplinary team provides services in a clinic setting to children with complex medical, physical, medical, and psychosocial impairments.

T1027

T1027 **Family training and counseling for child development, per 15 minutes**

Lay Description
Family training and counseling for child development is specialized training and education provided to a family to assist with the child's needs and development.

T1028

T1028 **Assessment of home, physical and family environment, to determine suitability to meet patient's medical needs**

Lay Description
This code represents a visit to and evaluation of an individual's home, physical, and family environment to determine if it is suitable for the patient's medical needs.

T1029

T1029 Comprehensive environmental lead investigation, not including laboratory analysis, per dwelling

Lay Description
This code represents a comprehensive investigation of the lead that may exist in an individual's environment. Lead in the environment may be ingested or inhaled by a child, leading to moderate to severe poisoning that adversely affects the physical and mental health of the individual.

T1030-T1031

T1030 Nursing care, in the home, by registered nurse, per diem

T1031 Nursing care, in the home, by licensed practical nurse, per diem

Lay Description
These codes represent nursing care provided by licensed practitioners in the individual's home.

T1502-T1503

T1502 Administration of oral, intramuscular and/or subcutaneous medication by health care agency/professional, per visit

T1503 Administration of medication, other than oral and/or injectable, by a health care agency/professional, per visit

Lay Description
These codes represent the charge for a health care agency or professional to administer oral, intramuscular, subcutaneous, or other forms of medication.

T1505

T1505 Electronic medication compliance management device, includes all components and accessories, not otherwise classified

Lay Description
An electronic medication compliance management device is a computerized medication dispenser that can dispense individual doses of different medications for up to one month. The device is programmed by the patient's health care provider and delivers the prescribed dose at the prescribed time.

T1999

T1999 Miscellaneous therapeutic items and supplies, retail purchases, not otherwise classified; identify product in "remarks"

Lay Description
This code represents the retail purchase of miscellaneous therapeutic items and supplies that are not otherwise classified in HCPCS codes.

T2001-T2005

T2001 Nonemergency transportation; patient attendant/escort

T2002 Nonemergency transportation; per diem

T2003 Nonemergency transportation; encounter/trip

T2004 Nonemergency transport; commercial carrier, multipass

T2005 Nonemergency transportation; stretcher van

Lay Description
Nonemergency transportation is the delivery or movement of a person in a nonemergency situation to a medical appointment or destination. It generally denotes the use of an emergency transport vehicle, such as an ambulance.

T2007

T2007 Transportation waiting time, air ambulance and nonemergency vehicle, one-half (1/2) hour increments

Lay Description
This code represents the idle or unloaded waiting time that a transport, air ambulance, or nonemergency vehicle spends waiting for a particular patient.

T2010-T2011

T2010 Preadmission screening and resident review (PASRR) level I identification screening, per screen

T2011 Preadmission screening and resident review (PASRR) level II evaluation, per evaluation

Lay Description
Preadmission screening and resident review (PASRR) is a protection for patients with serious mental illness or mental retardation. PASRR is intended to prevent patients from being inappropriately admitted to nursing facilities that cannot provide the specialized care they require. Federal law requires all patients, regardless of payer source, be given a level I identification screening to identify mental illnesses or mental retardation. Level I screens are generally forms completed by hospital discharge planners, community health nurses, or other practitioners defined by state law. Patients who do or may have a mental illness or mental retardation are then referred for a level II evaluation. The level II evaluation is provided to all patients identified in level I and any resident who has experienced a significant change in condition. This level II evaluation is the resident review that is conducted according to federal delineated criteria. Once it is determined that a patient has a mental illness or mental retardation, it must be determined what specialized services are needed and whether the nursing home can provide those services. Types of specialized services and their definition may vary by state.

T2012-T2021

T2012 Habilitation, educational; waiver, per diem

T2013 Habilitation, educational, waiver; per hour

T2014 Habilitation, prevocational, waiver; per diem

T2015 Habilitation, prevocational, waiver; per hour

T2016 Habilitation, residential, waiver; per diem

T2017 Habilitation, residential, waiver; 15 minutes

T2018 Habilitation, supported employment, waiver; per diem

T2019 Habilitation, supported employment, waiver; per 15 minutes

T2020 Day habilitation, waiver; per diem

T2021 Day habilitation, waiver; per 15 minutes

Lay Description
Habilitation is the act of making an individual capable of fitting into and/or functioning in society. The codes indicated here generally refer to people who have disabilities that initially prevent them from functioning independently in society. Habilitation provides the assistance that these people need to attain their goals, wants, and/or needs. Paraprofessionals and professionals usually provide support, training, and any required therapy. Day habilitation may be a full day of directed services or may be an alternate day where recreational activities are the main body of the day.

T2022-T2023

T2022 Case management, per month

T2023 Targeted case management; per month

Lay Description
Case management is an effort to improve care and to contain costs by having one party manage or coordinate all care delivered to patients who have certain complex illnesses or injuries, including mental and behavioral health issues. Case management may include, but is not limited to, the evaluation of a condition, the development and implementation of a plan of care, the coordination of medical resources, and the appropriate communication to all parties. Targeted case management targets a specific population subgroup.

T2024-T2025

T2024 Service assessment/plan of care development, waiver

T2025 Waiver services; not otherwise specified (NOS)

Lay Description
Medicaid may choose to wave certain requirements in conjunction with specialized programs. In these cases, waivers usually refer to permission from the federal government to waive or change certain requirements.

T2026-T2027

T2026 Specialized childcare, waiver; per diem

T2027 Specialized childcare, waiver; per 15 minutes

Lay Description
Specialized childcare usually refers to childcare provided to an individual who has special physical or developmental needs. It may also refer to childcare needed during nonstandard hours, such as overnight, or care for a mildly ill child who cannot attend school or regular daycare. Most states require providers of specialized childcare to be certified, licensed, or otherwise deemed qualified to care for the child. The waiver refers to permission from the federal government to state Medicaid plans to finance services that are not in compliance with federal regulations.

T2028-T2029

T2028 Specialized supply, not otherwise specified, waiver

T2029 Specialized medical equipment, not otherwise specified, waiver

Lay Description
These codes represent specialized supplies or durable medical equipment that is not otherwise identified by other HCPCS Level II codes. The waiver refers to permission from the federal government to state Medicaid plans to finance services that are not in compliance with federal regulations.

T2030-T2031

T2030 Assisted living, waiver; per month

T2031 Assisted living; waiver, per diem

Lay Description
An assisted living facility provides independent living arrangements with varying degrees of medical care and personal and support services. Most are designed to provide assistance with the activities of daily living, such as bathing and dressing. A community dining room or meal service may be available. Minor medical monitoring and assistance may be offered, depending upon state regulations. The waiver refers to permission from the federal government to state Medicaid plans to finance services that are not in compliance with federal regulations.

T2032-T2033

T2032 Residential care, not otherwise specified (NOS), waiver; per month

T2033 Residential care, not otherwise specified (NOS), waiver; per diem

Lay Description
Residential care is long-term care provided in a setting other than the patient's home. This code is used to report residential care that is not adequately described by other HCPCS Level II codes. Varying degrees of independent living, medical care, and

personal and support services may be offered, depending upon state regulations. The waiver refers to permission from the federal government to state Medicaid plans to finance services that are not in compliance with federal regulations.

T2034

T2034   Crisis intervention, waiver; per diem

Lay Description

Crisis intervention is emergency psychological or psychiatric care intended to assist and stabilize individuals who are in an immediate crisis situation. A crisis may refer to any situation where the individual perceives a sudden loss of his/her ability to problem-solve and cope. The waiver refers to permission from the federal government to state Medicaid plans to finance services that are not in compliance with federal regulations.

T2035

T2035   Utility services to support medical equipment and assistive technology/devices, waiver

Lay Description

This code is used to report charges for utility services, such as water and electricity, needed to support medical equipment and assistive technology devices. The waiver refers to permission from the federal government to state Medicaid plans to finance services that are not in compliance with federal regulations.

T2036-T2037

T2036   Therapeutic camping, overnight, waiver; each session

T2037   Therapeutic camping, day, waiver; each session

Lay Description

Therapeutic camping is used to teach life and coping skills in an outdoor wilderness environment. Therapeutic camping may be directed to individuals with mental health, behavioral health, or medical health needs. The waiver refers to permission from the federal government to state Medicaid plans to finance services that are not in compliance with federal regulations.

T2038

T2038   Community transition, waiver; per service

Lay Description

Community transition is the facilitation of the movement of an individual from an institutional environment to community living. The waiver refers to permission from the federal government to state Medicaid plans to finance services that are not in compliance with federal regulations.

T2039

T2039   Vehicle modifications, waiver; per service

Lay Description

This code is used to report charges for a vehicle modification necessary for an individual's functioning. The waiver refers to permission from the federal government to state Medicaid plans to finance services that are not in compliance with federal regulations.

T2040-T2041

T2040   Financial management, self-directed, waiver; per 15 minutes

T2041   Supports brokerage, self-directed, waiver; per 15 minutes

Lay Description

Individuals with serious mental health or substance abuse issues that are actively in recovery are expected to prove self-directed care that includes managing finances, paying bills, and similar financial matters. A financial manager or intermediary supervises and supports these functions. A supports broker assists in defining needs, finding the necessary services, and monitoring the service performance. The waiver refers to permission from the federal government to state Medicaid plans to finance services that are not in compliance with federal regulations.

T2042-T2046

T2042   Hospice routine home care; per diem

T2043   Hospice continuous home care; per hour

T2044   Hospice inpatient respite care; per diem

T2045   Hospice general inpatient care; per diem

T2046   Hospice long-term care, room and board only; per diem

Lay Description

Hospice services are provided to patients who are terminally ill with a medical prognosis of less than six months to live. Routine home care includes hospice services provided in the patient's home for a total of eight hours or less. Continuous home care is provided only during a crisis in which the patient requires continuous nursing care to palliate or manage acute medical symptoms. Respite care is short-term inpatient care provided to relieve the family member or other caretaker. General inpatient care is care in an acute care general hospital for pain control and symptom management. Long-term care is hospice care provided to a patient in a long-term care facility.

T2048

T2048 Behavioral health; long-term care residential (nonacute care in a residential treatment program where stay is typically longer than 30 days), with room and board, per diem

Lay Description
This code is used to report a per diem charge for long-term residential behavioral health care. It is to be used for nonacute care in a residential treatment program where stay is typically longer than 30 days.

T2049

T2049 Nonemergency transportation; stretcher van, mileage; per mile

Lay Description
This code is used to report nonemergency transport of a stretcher patient who is not being medically monitored or treated. Patients most likely transported by stretcher are those individuals who cannot stand or sit independently.

T2101

T2101 Human breast milk processing, storage and distribution only

Lay Description
Human breast milk is the liquid produced by the mammary glands for the nourishment of a human infant. Human breast milk is considered the ideal food for newborns. When a mother cannot produce sufficient quantities of breast milk, the physician may prescribe milk donated by nursing mothers who are not biologically related to the child. This milk is maintained in human milk banks. The banks do not charge for the milk itself, but do charge for the collection, processing, and distribution of the milk.

T4521-T4528

T4521 Adult sized disposable incontinence product, brief/diaper, small, each

T4522 Adult sized disposable incontinence product, brief/diaper, medium, each

T4523 Adult sized disposable incontinence product, brief/diaper, large, each

T4524 Adult sized disposable incontinence product, brief/diaper, extra large, each

T4525 Adult sized disposable incontinence product, protective underwear/pull-on, small size, each

T4526 Adult sized disposable incontinence product, protective underwear/pull-on, medium size, each

T4527 Adult sized disposable incontinence product, protective underwear/pull-on, large size, each

T4528 Adult sized disposable incontinence product, protective underwear/pull-on, extra large size, each

Lay Description
Incontinence garments allow the individual to defecate or urinate somewhat discreetly. The garment is intended to absorb and contain the urine and feces. These garments may be disposable or reusable. It may be a flat diaper or a brief. Disposable garments include those commonly found at supermarkets. Flat reusable cloth diapers are generally rectangular with the same thickness throughout. Fit is accomplished by folding. Reusable briefs come in many varieties and may vary from slightly contoured to fully fitted briefs. There are also fully fitted briefs made of patented materials that are designed to be used with internal pads. Disposable briefs and diapers are intended to be worn once. Adult pull-ons are diapers that can be pulled on like normal undergarments. Protective underwear is intended to further contain any feces or urine and protect outer clothing or bedding.

T4529-T4537

T4529 Pediatric sized disposable incontinence product, brief/diaper, small/medium size, each

T4530 Pediatric sized disposable incontinence product, brief/diaper, large size, each

T4531 Pediatric sized disposable incontinence product, protective underwear/pull-on, small/medium size, each

T4532 Pediatric sized disposable incontinence product, protective underwear/pull-on, large size, each

T4533 Youth sized disposable incontinence product, brief/diaper, each

T4534 Youth sized disposable incontinence product, protective underwear/pull-on, each

T4535 Disposable liner/shield/guard/pad/undergarment, for incontinence, each

T4536 Incontinence product, protective underwear/pull-on, reusable, any size, each

T4537 Incontinence product, protective underpad, reusable, bed size, each

Lay Description
Incontinence garments allow the individual to defecate or urinate somewhat discreetly. The garment is intended to absorb and contain the urine and feces. These garments may be disposable or reusable and may be a flat diaper or a brief. Disposable garments include those commonly found at supermarkets. Flat reusable cloth diapers are generally rectangular with the same thickness throughout. Fit is accomplished by folding. Reusable briefs come in many varieties and may vary from slightly contoured to fully fitted briefs. There are also fully fitted briefs made of patented materials that are designed to be used with internal pads. Some products include an individual disposable liner, shield, guard, pad, or undergarment. Disposable briefs and diapers are intended to be worn once. Underpads and chair pads are intended to provide reusable individual protection.

T4538

T4538 Diaper service, reusable diaper, each diaper

Lay Description
A reusable diaper is a piece of cloth that is intended to absorb and contain the urine and feces. This code represents diapers provided by and maintained by a diaper delivery service.

T4539

T4539 Incontinence product, diaper/brief, reusable, any size, each

Lay Description
This code reports individual disposable pull-on underwear and diapers used for leakage protection and incontinence. These items are used by patients with the inability to voluntarily control bladder or bowel functions or who are unable to use toilet facilities.

T4540-T4544

T4540 Incontinence product, protective underpad, reusable, chair size, each

T4541 Incontinence product, disposable underpad, large, each

T4542 Incontinence product, disposable underpad, small size, each

T4543 Adult sized disposable incontinence product, protective brief/diaper, above extra large, each

T4544 Adult sized disposable incontinence product, protective underwear/pull-on, above extra large, each

Lay Description
Incontinence garments, which absorb and contain the urine and feces, allow the individual to defecate or urinate somewhat discreetly. These garments may be disposable or reusable and may be flat diapers or briefs. Disposable garments include those commonly found at supermarkets. Flat reusable cloth diapers are generally rectangular with the same thickness throughout. The diapers are fitted by folding. Reusable briefs come in many varieties and may vary from slightly contoured to fully fitted briefs. There are also fully fitted briefs made of patented materials that are designed to be used with internal pads. Some products include an individual disposable liner, shield, guard, pad, or undergarment Disposable briefs and diapers are intended to be worn once. Underpads and chair pads are intended to provide reusable individual protection.

T5001

T5001 Positioning seat for persons with special orthopedic needs

Lay Description
Adjustable positioning seat cushions provide skin protection and positioning for individuals with paralysis, deformities, scoliosis, poor muscle control, or other conditions. Positioning seat cushions can aid in manipulation or control of objects, can assist in the performance of specific activities, and can provide added balance and support. Adjustable cushions can be adapted to conform to the individual's special orthopedic needs.

T5999

T5999 Supply, not otherwise specified

Lay Description
This code is used to report supplies that are not otherwise represented by other HCPCS Level II codes.

V

V2020-V2025

V2020 Frames, purchases
V2025 Deluxe frame

Lay Description
Frames are rigid or semi-rigid devices that bear lenses that are held in front of the eyes for vision correction or eye protection. Frames are made from many different materials in many different colors and shapes. The definition of deluxe is generally left to the manufacturer or the insurer.

V2100-V2102

V2100 Sphere, single vision, plano to plus or minus 4.00, per lens

V2101 Sphere, single vision, plus or minus 4.12 to plus or minus 7.00d, per lens

V2102 Sphere, single vision, plus or minus 7.12 to plus or minus 20.00d, per lens

Lay Description
A single vision lens provides one viewing surface in the lens that is concave on the back surface. This concave shape follows the shape of the eye and allows the back of the lens to stay at the same distance when the eye moves. It is used to treat refractive errors that cause the patient to have trouble seeing near or far distances. The sphere is the strength of the long or short sightedness and its value is in diopters. A plus sign (+) in front of the sphere reading indicates the amount of correction for near sight or reading whereas the minus sign (-) indicates the power of correction for far distance correction. If there is not a correction one way or another, it will be listed as plano, 0.00, or P.

V2103-V2114

V2103 Spherocylinder, single vision, plano to plus or minus 4.00d sphere, 0.12 to 2.00d cylinder, per lens

V2104 Spherocylinder, single vision, plano to plus or minus 4.00d sphere, 2.12 to 4.00d cylinder, per lens

V2105 Spherocylinder, single vision, plano to plus or minus 4.00d sphere, 4.25 to 6.00d cylinder, per lens

V2106 Spherocylinder, single vision, plano to plus or minus 4.00d sphere, over 6.00d cylinder, per lens

V2107 Spherocylinder, single vision, plus or minus 4.25 to plus or minus 7.00 sphere, 0.12 to 2.00d cylinder, per lens

V2108 Spherocylinder, single vision, plus or minus 4.25d to plus or minus 7.00d sphere, 2.12 to 4.00d cylinder, per lens

V2109 Spherocylinder, single vision, plus or minus 4.25 to plus or minus 7.00d sphere, 4.25 to 6.00d cylinder, per lens

V2110 Spherocylinder, single vision, plus or minus 4.25 to 7.00d sphere, over 6.00d cylinder, per lens

V2111 Spherocylinder, single vision, plus or minus 7.25 to plus or minus 12.00d sphere, 0.25 to 2.25d cylinder, per lens

V2112 Spherocylinder, single vision, plus or minus 7.25 to plus or minus 12.00d sphere, 2.25d to 4.00d cylinder, per lens

V2113 Spherocylinder, single vision, plus or minus 7.25 to plus or minus 12.00d sphere, 4.25 to 6.00d cylinder, per lens

V2114 Spherocylinder, single vision, sphere over plus or minus 12.00d, per lens

Lay Description
A single vision lens provides one viewing surface in the lens that is concave on the back surface. This concave shape follows the shape of the eye and allows the back of the lens to stay at the same distance when the eye moves. Spherocylinder single vision eyeglass lenses address the correction of one focal power such as nearsightedness or farsightedness, and astigmatism. The sphere is the strength of the long or short sightedness and its value is in diopters. A plus sign (+) in front of the sphere reading indicates the amount of correction for near sight or reading whereas the minus sign (-) indicates the power of correction for far distance correction. If there is not a correction one way or another, it will be listed as plano, 0.00, or P. The cylinder, also measured in + or -, is the measurement for astigmatism.

V2107-V2110

V2107 Spherocylinder, single vision, plus or minus 4.25 to plus or minus 7.00 sphere, 0.12 to 2.00d cylinder, per lens

V2108 Spherocylinder, single vision, plus or minus 4.25d to plus or minus 7.00d sphere, 2.12 to 4.00d cylinder, per lens

V2109 Spherocylinder, single vision, plus or minus 4.25 to plus or minus 7.00d sphere, 4.25 to 6.00d cylinder, per lens

V2110 Spherocylinder, single vision, plus or minus 4.25 to 7.00d sphere, over 6.00d cylinder, per lens

Lay Description
Spherocylinder single-vision eyeglass lenses correct one focal power such as nearsightedness or farsightedness, and astigmatism. Lenses are made from glass or plastic to the specific level of correction required to improve vision. These codes report plus or minus 7.00d sphere and the specific level of astigmatism per lens.

V2111-V2113

V2111 Spherocylinder, single vision, plus or minus 7.25 to plus or minus 12.00d sphere, 0.25 to 2.25d cylinder, per lens

V2112 Spherocylinder, single vision, plus or minus 7.25 to plus or minus 12.00d sphere, 2.25d to 4.00d cylinder, per lens

V2113 Spherocylinder, single vision, plus or minus 7.25 to plus or minus 12.00d sphere, 4.25 to 6.00d cylinder, per lens

Lay Description
Spherocylinder single-vision eyeglass lenses correct one focal power such as nearsightedness or farsightedness, and astigmatism. Lenses are made from glass or plastic to the specific level of correction required to improve vision. These codes report plus or minus 7.25d to plus or minus 12.00d sphere and the specific level of astigmatism per lens.

V2114

V2114 Spherocylinder, single vision, sphere over plus or minus 12.00d, per lens

Lay Description

Spherocylinder single-vision eyeglass lenses correct one focal power such as nearsightedness or farsightedness, and astigmatism. Lenses are made from glass or plastic to the specific level of correction required to improve vision. This code reports plus or minus 12.00d.

V2115

V2115 Lenticular (myodisc), per lens, single vision

Lay Description

Lenticular lenses are designed for very strong prescriptions generally requiring plus or minus 10.00d or higher. The specified prescription power is found in the center of the lens, and the edges are ground down to reduce the weight and thickness of the lens. A myodisc (myopic disk) is a lens with a steep concave curvature that is on the posterior surface of the carrier lens used with low-vision patients that have extreme myopia.

V2118

V2118 Aniseikonic lens, single vision

Lay Description

Aniseikonic lenses are for correction when patients report unequal visual images. This commonly occurs with a cataract, corneal surgical corrections, radial keratotomy, photoreactive keratectomy, laser surgeries, and scleral buckling. The football-shaped lenses have several aspects for correction, including base curve and lens thickness, refractive index, and the difference of magnification between lenses.

V2121

V2121 Lenticular lens, per lens, single

Lay Description

Lenticular lenses are designed for very strong prescriptions generally requiring plus or minus 10.00d or higher. The specified prescription power is found in the center of the lens, and the edges are ground down to reduce the weight and thickness of the lens.

V2199

V2199 Not otherwise classified, single vision lens

Lay Description

A single-vision lens is a piece of glass or plastic shaped to direct light onto the retina so as to produce a clear visual image. Single-vision lenses address either myopia (near-sightedness) or hyperopia (far-sightedness). This code represents a single-vision lens not otherwise classified or described by other HCPCS codes.

V2200-V2202

V2200 Sphere, bifocal, plano to plus or minus 4.00d, per lens

V2201 Sphere, bifocal, plus or minus 4.12 to plus or minus 7.00d, per lens

V2202 Sphere, bifocal, plus or minus 7.12 to plus or minus 20.00d, per lens

Lay Description

Bifocal vision eyeglass lenses address the correction of two focal powers for distance and work such as reading that requires a close-up focus. Lenses are made from glass or plastic to the specific level of correction required to improve vision. The lens provides two viewing surfaces in the lens, which is concave on the back surface. This concave shape follows the shape of the eye and allows the back of the lens to stay at the same distance when the eye moves. The sphere is the strength of the long- or short-sightedness and its value is in diopters. A plus sign (+) in front of the sphere reading indicates the amount of correction for near sight or reading whereas the minus sign (-) indicates the power of correction for far distance correction. No correction one way or another is listed as plano, 0.00, or P.

V2203-V2214

V2203 Spherocylinder, bifocal, plano to plus or minus 4.00d sphere, 0.12 to 2.00d cylinder, per lens

V2204 Spherocylinder, bifocal, plano to plus or minus 4.00d sphere, 2.12 to 4.00d cylinder, per lens

V2205 Spherocylinder, bifocal, plano to plus or minus 4.00d sphere, 4.25 to 6.00d cylinder, per lens

V2206 Spherocylinder, bifocal, plano to plus or minus 4.00d sphere, over 6.00d cylinder, per lens

V2207 Spherocylinder, bifocal, plus or minus 4.25 to plus or minus 7.00d sphere, 0.12 to 2.00d cylinder, per lens

V2208 Spherocylinder, bifocal, plus or minus 4.25 to plus or minus 7.00d sphere, 2.12 to 4.00d cylinder, per lens

V2209 Spherocylinder, bifocal, plus or minus 4.25 to plus or minus 7.00d sphere, 4.25 to 6.00d cylinder, per lens

V2210 Spherocylinder, bifocal, plus or minus 4.25 to plus or minus 7.00d sphere, over 6.00d cylinder, per lens

V2211 Spherocylinder, bifocal, plus or minus 7.25 to plus or minus 12.00d sphere, 0.25 to 2.25d cylinder, per lens

V2212 Spherocylinder, bifocal, plus or minus 7.25 to plus or minus 12.00d sphere, 2.25 to 4.00d cylinder, per lens

V2213 Spherocylinder, bifocal, plus or minus 7.25 to plus or minus 12.00d sphere, 4.25 to 6.00d cylinder, per lens

V2214 Spherocylinder, bifocal, sphere over plus or minus 12.00d, per lens

Lay Description
Bifocal vision eyeglass lenses address the correction of two focal powers for distance and work such as reading that requires a close up focus. Lenses are made from glass or plastic to the specific level of correction required to improve vision. The lens provides two viewing surfaces in the lens that is concave on the back surface. This concave shape follows the shape of the eye and allows the back of the lens to stay at the same distance when the eye moves. The sphere is the strength of the long or short sightedness and its value is in diopters. A plus sign (+) in front of the sphere reading indicates the amount of correction for near sight or reading whereas the minus sign (-) indicates the power of correction for far distance correction. If there is not a correction one way or another, it will be listed as plano, 0.00, or P. The cylinder, also measured in + or -, is the measurement for astigmatism.

V2215

V2215 Lenticular (myodisc), per lens, bifocal

Lay Description
Lenticular lenses are designed for very strong prescriptions generally requiring plus or minus 10.00d or higher. The specified prescription power is found in the center of the lens, and the edges are ground down to reduce the weight and thickness of the lens. A myodisc (myopic disk) is a lens with a steep concave curvature that is on the posterior surface of the carrier lens used with low-vision patients that have extreme myopia.

V2218

V2218 Aniseikonic, per lens, bifocal

Lay Description
Aniseikonic lenses are for correction when patients report unequal visual images. This commonly occurs with a cataract, corneal surgical corrections, radial keratotomy, photoreactive keratectomy, laser surgeries, and scleral buckling. The football-shaped lenses have several aspects for vision correction, including base curve and lens thickness, refractive index, and the difference of magnification between lenses. Bifocal lenses have two visibly identifiable zones of vision divided by a segment line of variable width. Bifocal lenses offer two fixed fields of focus (near/distant) for patients with higher levels of presbyopia.

V2219-V2220

V2219 Bifocal seg width over 28mm
V2220 Bifocal add over 3.25d

Lay Description
Bifocals are corrective lenses with distinct optical regions, each with different corrective features usually treating two different visual problems, e.g., myopia

and astigmatism. Most bifocals are created by molding a reading segment into a specific shape, size, and optical power. The most common reading segment is the D-segment that is 28 mm wide.

V2221

V2221 Lenticular lens, per lens, bifocal

Lay Description
Lenticular lenses are designed for very strong prescriptions generally requiring plus or minus 10.00d or higher. The specified prescription power is found in the center of the lens, and the edges are ground down to reduce the weight and thickness of the lens.

V2299

V2299 Specialty bifocal (by report)

Lay Description
Bifocals are corrective lenses with distinct optical regions, each with different corrective features usually treating two different visual problems, e.g., myopia and astigmatism. This code should be reported when the lens is a specialty lens not described by other HCPCS codes. A report usually accompanies the code so as to explain the special qualities or conditions.

V2300-V2302

V2300 Sphere, trifocal, plano to plus or minus 4.00d, per lens
V2301 Sphere, trifocal, plus or minus 4.12 to plus or minus 7.00d per lens
V2302 Sphere, trifocal, plus or minus 7.12 to plus or minus 20.00, per lens

Lay Description
Trifocal lenses have three visibly identifiable zones of vision divided by two segment lines of variable widths. Trifocal lenses offer three fixed fields of focus (near/intermediate/distant) for patients with higher levels of presbyopia. The lens provides three viewing surfaces in the lens, which is concave on the back surface. This concave shape follows the shape of the eye and allows the back of the lens to stay at the same distance when the eye moves. It is used to treat refractive errors that cause the patient to have trouble seeing near or far distances. The sphere is the strength of the long- or short-sightedness, and its value is in diopters. A plus sign (+) in front of the sphere reading indicates the amount of correction for near sight or reading, whereas the minus sign (-) indicates the power of correction for far distance correction. No correction one way or another is listed as plano, 0.00, or P.

V2303-V2314

V2303 Spherocylinder, trifocal, plano to plus or minus 4.00d sphere, 0.12 to 2.00d cylinder, per lens

V2304 Spherocylinder, trifocal, plano to plus or minus 4.00d sphere, 2.25 to 4.00d cylinder, per lens

V2305 Spherocylinder, trifocal, plano to plus or minus 4.00d sphere, 4.25 to 6.00 cylinder, per lens

V2306 Spherocylinder, trifocal, plano to plus or minus 4.00d sphere, over 6.00d cylinder, per lens

V2307 Spherocylinder, trifocal, plus or minus 4.25 to plus or minus 7.00d sphere, 0.12 to 2.00d cylinder, per lens

V2308 Spherocylinder, trifocal, plus or minus 4.25 to plus or minus 7.00d sphere, 2.12 to 4.00d cylinder, per lens

V2309 Spherocylinder, trifocal, plus or minus 4.25 to plus or minus 7.00d sphere, 4.25 to 6.00d cylinder, per lens

V2310 Spherocylinder, trifocal, plus or minus 4.25 to plus or minus 7.00d sphere, over 6.00d cylinder, per lens

V2311 Spherocylinder, trifocal, plus or minus 7.25 to plus or minus 12.00d sphere, 0.25 to 2.25d cylinder, per lens

V2312 Spherocylinder, trifocal, plus or minus 7.25 to plus or minus 12.00d sphere, 2.25 to 4.00d cylinder, per lens

V2313 Spherocylinder, trifocal, plus or minus 7.25 to plus or minus 12.00d sphere, 4.25 to 6.00d cylinder, per lens

V2314 Spherocylinder, trifocal, sphere over plus or minus 12.00d, per lens

Lay Description

Spherocylinder trifocal vision eyeglass lenses address the correction of focal power such as nearsightedness or farsightedness, and/or astigmatism. Trifocal lenses have three visibly identifiable zones of vision divided by two segment lines of variable widths. Trifocal lenses offer three fixed fields of focus (near/intermediate/distant) for patients with higher levels of presbyopia. Lenses are made from glass or plastic to the specific level of correction required to improve vision. The lens provides three viewing surfaces in the lens, which is concave on the back surface. This concave shape follows the shape of the eye and allows the back of the lens to stay at the same distance when the eye moves. The sphere is the strength of the long- or short-sightedness, and its value is in diopters. A plus sign (+) in front of the sphere reading indicates the amount of correction for near sight or reading, whereas the minus sign (-) indicates the power of correction for far distance correction. No correction one way or another is listed as plano, 0.00, or P. The cylinder, also measured in + or -, is the measurement for astigmatism.

V2315

V2315 Lenticular, (myodisc), per lens, trifocal

Lay Description

Lenticular lenses are designed for very strong prescriptions generally requiring plus or minus 10.00d and higher. The specified prescription power is found in the center of the lens, and the edges are ground down to reduce the weight and thickness of the lens. Trifocal lenses have three visibly identifiable zones of vision divided by two segment lines of variable widths. Trifocal lenses offer three fixed fields of focus (near/intermediate/distant) for patients with higher levels of presbyopia.

V2318

V2318 Aniseikonic lens, trifocal

Lay Description

Aniseikonic lenses are for correction when patients report unequal visual images. This commonly occurs with a cataract, corneal surgical corrections, radial keratotomy, photoreactive keratectomy, laser surgeries, and scleral buckling. The football-shaped lenses have several aspects for vision correction, including base curve and lens thickness, refractive index, and the difference of magnification between lenses. Trifocal lenses have three visibly identifiable zones of vision divided by two segment lines of variable widths. Trifocal lenses offer three fixed fields of focus (near/intermediate/distant) for patients with higher levels of presbyopia.

V2319-V2320

V2319 Trifocal seg width over 28 mm

V2320 Trifocal add over 3.25d

Lay Description

Trifocals are corrective lenses with three distinct optical regions, each with different corrective features usually treating two different visual problems, e.g., myopia and astigmatism. Most trifocals are created by molding a reading segment into a specific shape, size, and optical power. The most common reading segment is the D-segment that is 28 mm wide.

V2321

V2321 Lenticular lens, per lens, trifocal

Lay Description

Lenticular lenses are designed for very strong prescriptions generally requiring plus or minus 10.00d or higher. The specified prescription power is found in the center of the lens, and the edges are ground down to reduce the weight and thickness of the lens.

V2399

V2399 Specialty trifocal (by report)

Lay Description

Trifocals are a corrective lens with three distinct optical regions, each with different corrective features usually treating two different visual problems (e.g., myopia and an astigmatism), with the middle region being a neutral or transition piece. Report this code when the lens is a specialty lens not described by other HCPCS Level II codes. A report usually accompanies the code so as to explain the special qualities or conditions.

V2410

V2410　Variable asphericity lens, single vision, full field, glass or plastic, per lens

Lay Description
Aspheric single-vision lenses address the correction of one focal power such as nearsightedness or farsightedness. They are also a higher quality premium lens, used for patients with slight astigmatism and at the early stages of development of presbyopia. Lenses are made from glass or plastic to the specific level of correction required to improve vision. Report this code for a full field, variable asphericity, single-vision lens.

V2430

V2430　Variable asphericity lens, bifocal, full field, glass or plastic, per lens

Lay Description
Aspherical bifocal vision lenses address the correction of two focal powers for distance and work, such as reading, which requires a close-up focus. They are also a higher quality premium lens used for patients with a slight astigmatism and at the early stages of development of presbyopia. Lenses are made from glass or plastic to the specific level of correction required to improve vision. Report this code for a full field, variable asphericity, bifocal lens.

V2499

V2499　Variable sphericity lens, other type

Lay Description
Light passing through a spherical lens is not all directed at a focal point. This imperfection is known as the lens sphericity. It is the degree of deviation from a sphere. The sphericity of a lens is intended to correct the misfocus of the eye. Spherical lenses are usually used for the main vision correction. The lens acts equally in all meridians.

V2500

V2500　Contact lens, PMMA, spherical, per lens

Lay Description
Polymethyl methacrylate (PMMA) spherical contact lenses are rigid lenses worn directly on the cornea to correct vision and have a spherical anterior (convex) surface and spherical posterior optical zone that approximates the curvature of the sclera. Spherical contact lenses have the same corrective power at each part of the lens, which allows the eye to focus and have clear vision. This code is reported per lens.

V2501

V2501　Contact lens, PMMA, toric or prism ballast, per lens

Lay Description
Polymethyl methacrylate (PMMA) toric or prism ballast contact lenses are rigid lenses worn directly on the cornea to correct vision and have a special curvature designed to correct astigmatism. Astigmatism is a visual defect in which the cornea is not perfectly round. Toric lenses are used when conventional soft or rigid lenses do not correct the defect. This code is reported per lens.

V2502

V2502　Contact lens PMMA, bifocal, per lens

Lay Description
Polymethyl methacrylate (PMMA) bifocal contact lenses are rigid lenses worn directly on the cornea to correct vision. Bifocal contact lenses address the correction of two focal powers for distance and work, such as reading, which requires a close up focus. This code is reported per lens.

V2503

V2503　Contact lens, PMMA, color vision deficiency, per lens

Lay Description
Polymethyl methacrylate (PMMA) contact lenses are rigid lenses worn directly on the cornea to correct vision. Color vision deficiency (a.k.a., color blindness) is a defect in the perception of color. This is usually the inability to distinguish between two or more colors such as red and green. This code represents a specially tinted contact lens that helps the person distinguish between the color for which he or she is deficient.

V2510

V2510　Contact lens, gas permeable, spherical, per lens

Lay Description
A spherical gas permeable contact lens is generally a rigid lens worn directly on the cornea to correct vision and has a spherical anterior (convex) surface and spherical posterior optical zone that approximates the curvature of the sclera. Spherical contact lenses have the same corrective power at each part of the lens, which allows the eye to focus and have clear vision. This lens also allows for oxygen exchange. It consists of materials, such as cellulose acetate butyrate, polyacrylate-silicone, or silicone elastomers, that typically do not attract water.

V2511

V2511　Contact lens, gas permeable, toric, prism ballast, per lens

Lay Description
A gas permeable toric contact lens is generally a rigid lens worn directly on the cornea to correct vision and

has a special curvature designed to correct for astigmatism (a visual defect in which the cornea is not perfectly round). This lens also allows for oxygen exchange. It consists of materials, such as cellulose acetate butyrate, polyacrylate-silicone, or silicone elastomers, that typically do not attract water and are used when conventional soft or rigid lenses do not correct the defect.

V2512

V2512   Contact lens, gas permeable, bifocal, per lens

Lay Description
A gas permeable bifocal contact lens is generally a rigid lens worn directly on the cornea to correct vision and address the correction of two focal powers for distance and work, such as reading, which requires a close-up focus. This lens also allows for oxygen exchange. It consists of materials, such as cellulose acetate butyrate, polyacrylate-silicone, or silicone elastomers, that typically do not attract water.

V2513

V2513   Contact lens, gas permeable, extended wear, per lens

Lay Description
A gas permeable extended wear contact lens is generally a rigid lens intended to be worn directly on the cornea to correct vision and may be worn for an extended period of time (does not have to be taken out of the eye on a daily basis). This lens also allows for oxygen exchange. It consists of materials, such as cellulose acetate butyrate, polyacrylate-silicone, or silicone elastomers, that typically do not attract water.

V2520

V2520   Contact lens, hydrophilic, spherical, per lens

Lay Description
A spherical hydrophilic (soft) contact lens is worn directly on the cornea to correct vision and has a spherical anterior (convex) surface and spherical posterior optical zone that approximates the curvature of the sclera. Spherical contact lenses have the same corrective power at each part of the lens, which allows the eye to focus and have clear vision. This lens consists of a variety of polymer materials that absorb or attract a certain amount of water and is used when conventional soft or rigid lenses do not correct the defect.

V2521

V2521   Contact lens, hydrophilic, toric, or prism ballast, per lens

Lay Description
A hydrophilic toric contact lens is worn directly on the cornea to correct vision and has a special curvature designed to correct for astigmatism (a visual defect in which the cornea is not perfectly round). This lens

consists of a variety of polymer materials that absorb or attract a certain amount of water and is used when conventional soft or rigid lenses do not correct the defect.

V2522

V2522   Contact lens, hydrophilic, bifocal, per lens

Lay Description
A hydrophilic bifocal contact lens is worn directly on the cornea to correct vision and address the correction of two focal powers for distance and work, such as reading, which requires a close up focus. This lens consists of a variety of polymer materials that absorb or attract a certain amount of water, making it more comfortable for the wearer.

V2523

V2523   Contact lens, hydrophilic, extended wear, per lens

Lay Description
A hydrophilic extended wear contact lens is worn directly on the cornea to correct vision and may be worn for an extended period of time (does not have to be taken out of the eye on a daily basis). This lens consists of a variety of polymer materials that absorb or attract a certain amount of water.

V2530-V2531

V2530   Contact lens, scleral, gas impermeable, per lens (for contact lens modification, see 92325)

V2531   Contact lens, scleral, gas permeable, per lens (for contact lens modification, see 92325)

Lay Description
A scleral contact lens is generally a rigid lens worn directly on the sclera that fits underneath the top and bottom eyelids. These lenses are used for patients who have problems wearing conventional lenses, patients with high refractive errors, or for patients with ocular surface disease. It consists of materials, such as cellulose acetate butyrate, polyacrylate-silicone, or silicone elastomers, that typically do not attract water and allow for oxygen exchange.

V2599

V2599   Contact lens, other type

Lay Description
A contact lens is a device that is worn on the cornea to correct vision problems by helping to refocus light onto the retina. This code represents a contact lens that is not detailed in one of the other HCPCS Level II codes.

V2600

V2600 Hand held low vision aids and other nonspectacle mounted aids

Lay Description
A low vision aid or magnifier is a type of magnifying lens used by patients who have impaired vision. This magnifier is handheld or may be used with another piece of equipment, but is not mounted onto glasses.

V2610

V2610 Single lens spectacle mounted low vision aids

Lay Description
A low vision aid or magnifier is a type of magnifying lens used by patients who have impaired vision. This magnifying aid is used on a single lens and mounted onto glasses.

V2615

V2615 Telescopic and other compound lens system, including distance vision telescopic, near vision telescopes and compound microscopic lens system

Lay Description
Telescopic and other compound lens systems, including distance vision telescopic, near vision telescopes, and compound microscopic lens systems, are devices and systems used to improve the vision of a person with low vision. Low vision is defined as reduced vision that is not corrected by spectacles or contact lens. Low vision can vary from moderate (20/70) to near total blindness (more than 20/1,000). Telescopic lens are usually limited by the diameter of the objective lens and the magnification.

V2623

V2623 Prosthetic eye, plastic, custom

Lay Description
An ocular prosthesis is a device that fits over an orbital implant and under the eyelids that produces the appearance of a normal human eye. It is created for a patient with absence or shrinkage of an eye due to a birth defect, trauma, or surgical removal. Eye prostheses assist in maintaining the internal orbital eye structures by filling in the void created by the missing natural eye. A byproduct of the prosthesis allows for a cosmetic enhancement by allowing the patient to appear to have two eyes. A prosthetic eye may be made out of glass, acrylic, silicone, hydroxyapatite, ceramic, or polyethylene.

V2624-V2626

V2624 Polishing/resurfacing of ocular prosthesis
V2625 Enlargement of ocular prosthesis
V2626 Reduction of ocular prosthesis

Lay Description
An ocular prosthesis is a device that fits over an orbital implant and under the eyelids that produces the

appearance of a normal human eye. It is created for a patient with absence or shrinkage of an eye due to a birth defect, trauma, or surgical removal. Eye prostheses assist in maintaining the internal orbital eye structures by filling in the void created by the missing natural eye. A byproduct of the prosthesis allows for a cosmetic enhancement by allowing the patient to appear to have two eyes. A prosthetic eye may be made out of glass, acrylic, silicone, hydroxyapatite, ceramic, or polyethylene. These codes represent work performed on the ocular prosthesis.

V2627

V2627 Scleral cover shell

Lay Description
A scleral cover shell is a device made out of glass or plastic and placed over the cornea and sclera of a damaged eye to give the eye a more natural appearance. It is intended to be worn for a short period of time for cosmetic or reconstructive reasons. It is typically not implanted in the eye.

V2628

V2628 Fabrication and fitting of ocular conformer

Lay Description
An ocular conformer is a temporary eye prosthesis inserted at the completion of the eye surgery and worn for four to eight weeks until a permanent prosthesis is available. This code represents the fabrication and fitting of the ocular conformer.

V2629

V2629 Prosthetic eye, other type

Lay Description
An ocular prosthesis is a device that fits over an orbital implant and under the eyelids that produces the appearance of a normal human eye. It is created for a patient with absence or shrinkage of an eye due to a birth defect, trauma, or surgical removal. Eye prostheses assist in maintaining the internal orbital eye structures by filling in the void created by the missing natural eye. A byproduct of the prosthesis allows for a cosmetic enhancement by allowing the patient to appear to have two eyes. A prosthetic eye may be made out of glass, acrylic, silicone, hydroxyapatite, ceramic, or polyethylene. This code represents a prosthetic eye that is not described by other HCPCS Level II codes.

V2630-V2632

V2630 Anterior chamber intraocular lens
V2631 Iris supported intraocular lens
V2632 Posterior chamber intraocular lens

Lay Description
An intraocular lens (IOL) is an implanted lens used as a replacement for a clouded lens removed in cataract surgery or as a correction for a refraction problem.

When inserted to correct refractive errors, the natural lens is usually not removed. Most IOLs are plastic and contain side struts to hold the lens in place. The anterior chamber is the portion of the eye between the cornea and the iris and is filled with aqueous humor. The iris, along with the choroid and ciliary body, is the midportion of the eye. The posterior chamber is the area between the iris and the rear eye walls. The posterior chamber is filled with the vitreous body. Anterior chamber IOLs can negatively impact the endothelial lining creating corneal complications. IOLs supported by the iris are attached by the struts to the midperipheral iris area. It is believed that iris supported IOLs do not impact the corneal endothelium as much as other types. Posterior chamber IOLs are placed in front of, but do not contact, the natural crystalline lens. Posterior chamber IOLs can cause cataract and pigment dispersion.

V2700

V2700   Balance lens, per lens

Lay Description
Corrective lenses of high powers can become very heavy and thick. A balance lens is similar to another corrective lens (single vision or lined bifocal) that is sized and shaped to appear similar to the other corrective lens. Depending on the patient and the lens, balance lenses may also be used to provide a similar weight as the corrective lens.

V2702

V2702   Deluxe lens feature

Lay Description
This code represents a deluxe lens feature that is not adequately described by other HCPCS Level II codes.

V2710

V2710   Slab off prism, glass or plastic, per lens

Lay Description
A slab off prism is a special lens, with the prismatic effect in the lower half of the lens, used to balance a patient's near vision. Patients whose left and right eyes have a significant difference in power could benefit from the use of a slab-off prism. Two lenses with significant power differences produce different prismatic effects as the eyes move from the distance part of the lens to the reading zone. The prism imbalance can be measured when in the reading zone. A compensating prism can then be incorporated into one of the lenses.

V2715

V2715   Prism, per lens

Lay Description
In optometry, a prism is one device used to correct vision problems. Shifting a corrective lens off the axis can make images appear to be displaced in the same way that a prism displaces images. Prisms are used to correct double vision and positive and negative accommodation problems.

V2718

V2718   Press-on lens, Fresnel prism, per lens

Lay Description
A press-on lens, Fresnel prism, is a prism used to correct vision problems and expand the visual field. Shifting a corrective lens off the axis can make images appear to be displaced in the same way that a prism displaces images. Prisms are used to bend the light so that it produces a clear image to the viewer. Fresnel replaced a large heavy prism lens with small segments. His work was originally developed for lighthouses, but it was adapted for optometry. Press-on lenses are thin flexible pieces of vinyl applied to the back of a corrective lens.

V2730

V2730   Special base curve, glass or plastic, per lens

Lay Description
The base curve in optometry is the measure of the general shape of the lens. On a spectacle lens, it is the flatter curvature of the front surface and on a contact lens, it is the curvature of the back surface. The base curve is the radius of the sphere of the back of the lens that the prescription describes. This code represents a lens that has a special base curve.

V2744

V2744   Tint, photochromatic, per lens

Lay Description
Photochromatic tinted lenses are those in which the degree of tint changes in response to changes in ambient light. Report this code for photochromatic tint per lens.

V2745

V2745   Addition to lens; tint, any color, solid, gradient or equal, excludes photochromatic, any lens material, per lens

Lay Description
Tinted lenses are made by putting coatings on the lens material to reduce the amount of light entering the eye. Report this code for the addition of tint to a lens, any color, solid, gradient or equal, excluding photochromatic.

V2750

V2750   Antireflective coating, per lens

Lay Description
Antireflective coating reduces glare on the surface of a lens and also reduces the reflected glare of headlights to improve nighttime driving. Report this code for antireflective coating, per lens.

V2755
V2755 U-V lens, per lens

Lay Description
UV lenses protect eyes from the potentially harmful ultraviolet rays generated from the sun or other light sources by blocking them from penetrating the lens material and reaching the eye. Report this code per lens.

V2756
V2756 Eye glass case

Lay Description
This code is used to report an eyeglass case. Eyeglass cases hold and protect glasses when they are not being worn.

V2760
V2760 Scratch resistant coating, per lens

Lay Description
Scratch resistant coating is a protective coating applied directly to the lens that reduces the potential for normal scratching or scraping of the lens material, reducing potential lens distortion. Report this code per lens.

V2761
V2761 Mirror coating, any type, solid, gradient or equal, any lens material, per lens

Lay Description
A mirror coating is a highly reflective coating of any color that prevents anyone looking at the lens from seeing anything other than the color of the mirrored lens. Mirror coatings are mainly cosmetic. The person wearing the lens perceives no difference in vision. The coatings are usually applied to sunglasses, but may be applied to any corrective lens. The density of the coating varies with solid mirrors reflecting back more light than other variations. This code represents mirror coating, any gradient or solid, any type, any lens material, per lens.

V2762
V2762 Polarization, any lens material, per lens

Lay Description
Light reflected from a flat surface such as a road or smooth water usually travels in a more horizontal pattern than normal light. Light that travels in one direction more than another is said to be polarized. The polarized light creates a glare that does not allow clear images. Polarized lenses have laminated surfaces that allow only vertically-polarized light to enter, eliminating the glare created by the horizontally-polarized light. The lenses do not prevent glare when the wearer tilts his or her head past 45 degrees. Polarized lenses also reduce the amount of light entering the eye and cannot be used with regular corrective eyeglasses.

V2770
V2770 Occluder lens, per lens

Lay Description
An occluder lens typically is a soft lens that can be worn for up to seven days (extended wear) and is blackened out, blocking vision in the eye wearing it. This type of prosthetic lens in used for treating patients, generally children, with amblyopia, or "lazy eye." The occluder lens forces the development of the amblyopic eye by blocking out all vision in the other eye. This type of lens may also be used in aphakic infants, where patch therapy has failed. This code is reported per lens.

V2780
V2780 Oversize lens, per lens

Lay Description
Oversize lenses are eyeglass lenses that are physically larger than normal lenses. Oversize lenses are sometimes used to create sunglasses that can slip over regular corrective glasses. Most of the time oversize lenses are requested for cosmetic purposes.

V2781
V2781 Progressive lens, per lens

Lay Description
No-line multifocal lenses that provide the needed correction for multiple focal lengths, but do not have a visible seam or line in the lenses are called progressive lenses. Report this code per progressive lens.

V2782-V2783
V2782 Lens, index 1.54 to 1.65 plastic or 1.60 to 1.79 glass, excludes polycarbonate, per lens

V2783 Lens, index greater than or equal to 1.66 plastic or greater than or equal to 1.80 glass, excludes polycarbonate, per lens

Lay Description
The light bending ability of eyeglass lenses is determined by the index of refraction of the lens material. The refractive index is the ratio of the speed of light as it travels through air to the speed of light as it passes through the lenses material. The speed of light is reduced by the amount of its refraction. Lenses that bend light more efficiently have a higher index of refraction than those that bend light less efficiently. Lenses with higher index are thinner and lighter than those lenses of the same power that are made with materials of a lower index. Conventional plastic lenses have a refractive index of approximately 1.50 and glass has an index of 1.52. Any lens material with indexes higher than these are considered high index. High index plastic usually has an index of 1.53 to 1.74. A plastic lens with an index of 1.70 or higher is at least 50 percent thinner than a conventional lens.

V2784

V2784 Lens, polycarbonate or equal, any index, per lens

Lay Description
Polycarbonate is a thin, light material used to create lenses. It has a high impact resistance, which along with its light weight, makes it preferable over other resins. Polycarbonate has a refractive index of 1.59. This lens material blocks both UVA and UVB rays.

V2785

V2785 Processing, preserving and transporting corneal tissue

Lay Description
The cornea is the transparent lens in the front of the eye that covers the iris, the pupil, and the anterior chamber. When the cornea is damaged or diseased it can be replaced, in whole or in part, by a donated cornea from a cadaver. This code is used to report the cost of processing, preserving, and transporting the corneal tissue.

V2786

V2786 Specialty occupational multifocal lens, per lens

Lay Description
Multifocal lenses are corrective lenses that contain one or more lens powers. Bifocals have two powers, trifocals have three, and progressive lenses have many that gradually change from the top of the lens to the bottom. Occupational multifocal lenses are designed for performing a particular job or hobby and are not intended for general use. For example, there are multifocal lenses designed for car mechanics, as well as golfers. Report this code for specialty occupational multifocal lenses, per lens.

V2787-V2788

V2787 Astigmatism correcting function of intraocular lens

V2788 Presbyopia correcting function of intraocular lens

Lay Description
An intraocular lens (IOL) is an implanted lens used as a replacement for a clouded lens removed in cataract surgery or as a correction for a refraction problem. When inserted to correct refractive errors, the natural lens is usually not removed. Most IOLs are plastic and contain side struts to hold the lens in place. Most traditional IOLs are monofocal, providing vision at only one distance—near, intermediate, or far. Patients will most likely have to have corrective lenses for other distances. Toric lenses are used to correct astigmatisms. Presbyopia is a condition where the eye progressively loses the ability to focus on near objects. It is usually part of the aging process. Both the astigmatism and the presbyopia correcting functions

of an intraocular lens are not usually covered by insurance as they are considered premium additions.

V2790

V2790 Amniotic membrane for surgical reconstruction, per procedure

Lay Description
Severe ocular surface diseases, such as Stevens-Johnson syndrome or ocular cicatricial pemphigoid, and injuries damage the corneal epithelial limbus cells. This damage allows the cornea to be enveloped with conjunctival tissue causing scarring and vascularization. A graft is necessary to surgically reconstruct these damaged eyes. An autograft from the patient's undamaged eye may be used or an allograft from the donor's eye may be used. Healthy limbus cells may also be cultivated on an amniotic membrane and transplanted into a severely damaged eye. The membrane provides support and is a carrier for the cultivated cells.

V2797-V2799

V2797 Vision supply, accessory and/or service component of another HCPCS vision code

V2799 Vision item or service, miscellaneous

Lay Description
Report V2797 when the vision supply, accessory, and/or service provided is a component of another HCPCS Level II vision code. This is not to be used to unbundle and report each component separately, but should be used when it is necessary to replace and report only one component of a complex HCPCS Level II code. Report V2799 when the vision service provided is not adequately described by other HCPCS Level II codes.

V5008

V5008 Hearing screening

Lay Description
A hearing screening is a unilateral or bilateral test consisting of the patient's case history, a visual inspection of the ear, pure tone screening within a range of 1000-4000 Hz, speech audiometry, and a self-assessed judgment of hearing difficulty. The screening is conducted by a certified audiologist, speech-language pathologist, or other personnel under the supervision of an audiologist.

V5010-V5020

V5010 Assessment for hearing aid

V5011 Fitting/orientation/checking of hearing aid

V5014 Repair/modification of a hearing aid

V5020 Conformity evaluation

Lay Description
During an assessment for a hearing aid, an audiologist reviews the results of the initial hearing screening with the patient, discusses the type and degree of

hearing loss including the configuration of the loss (whether unilateral or bilateral), the options available based on the information gathered, and costs. The audiologist also obtains audiometric measurements and an impression of the ear canal. The hearing aid is fitted during an orientation in which the audiologist explains how to operate the hearing aid. At this fitting, internal controls of the hearing aid are set or programmed. The patient is scheduled for a conformity evaluation to confirm that the hearing aid is meeting the needs of the patient.

V5030-V5040

V5030   Hearing aid, monaural, body worn, air conduction
V5040   Hearing aid, monaural, body worn, bone conduction

Lay Description
A body worn monaural (one ear) air conduction hearing aid is specifically designed with bigger controls for patients who have less dexterity and have a problem with feedback. It consists of a small box that is clipped to clothing or slips inside a pocket. This connects to a lead to an earphone and attaches to the ear-mould. The bone conduction hearing aid is designed for patients who have an abnormality of the ear canal. Due to drainage, a narrow canal, or no canal at all, the patient is precluded from using an air conduction device. The bone conductor is held onto the mastoid bone by an implanted screw or by using a headband. It works by transmitting vibrations through the skull to the inner ear.

V5050-V5060

V5050   Hearing aid, monaural, in the ear
V5060   Hearing aid, monaural, behind the ear

Lay Description
There are two types of in the ear (ITE) monaural hearing aids available. The full shell aid is for mild to severe hearing loss and is the largest and least expensive available. It covers the entire ear opening and is the most versatile of all the hearing aids. The half-shell/conch aid is for mild to moderately severe hearing loss and is the most popular model. Smaller than the full shell, it covers only the bowl portion of the ear. The behind the ear (BTE) model is connected to the ear by an ear-mold and is used mostly by patients with severe hearing loss, although it can be used for any and all forms of hearing loss. This type is more durable and less flexible than the ITE model.

V5070

V5070   Glasses, air conduction

Lay Description
An air conduction hearing system amplifies sound and directs it into the auditory canal with a thin tube. The device is small and discrete and is worn on the eyeglass frame. The use of a thin tube to direct the amplified sound allows natural ambient sound to also

reach the ear. The eyeglass frame usually holds corrective lenses.

V5080

V5080   Glasses, bone conduction

Lay Description
A bone conduction hearing system transmits sound through mechanical vibrations to the inner ear. The device is small and discrete and is worn on the eyeglass frame. The eyeglass frame usually holds corrective lenses.

V5090

V5090   Dispensing fee, unspecified hearing aid

Lay Description
This code reports the dispensing fee charged by the supplier for the dispensing of a hearing aid that is unspecified or not described by other HCPCS Level II codes.

V5095

V5095   Semi-implantable middle ear hearing prosthesis

Lay Description
A semi-implantable middle ear hearing prosthesis is an alternative to an external acoustic hearing aid for patients with moderate to severe sensorineural hearing loss. The device consists of three components: a magnetic component, a receiver, and a sound processor. The magnetic component is implanted onto the ossicles of the middle ear. The sound processor receives and amplifies sound vibrations and transforms sound pressure into electrical signals, which are transmitted to the receiver. The receiver changes the electrical signals into electromagnetic energy and creates an alternating electromagnetic field with the magnetic component. In turn this electromagnetic field creates varying forces on the implant that cause the bones of the middle ear to vibrate, similar to normal hearing.

V5100-V5110

V5100   Hearing aid, bilateral, body worn
V5110   Dispensing fee, bilateral

Lay Description
A hearing aid is a device that amplifies, modulates, or conducts sound. There are a number of types and sizes with different components. A body worn hearing aid consists of an ear piece connected by a cord to a case containing a microphone, amplifier, battery, and controls that are worn in a pocket or on a belt. The device is usually the size of a deck of cards.

V5120-V5160

V5120   Binaural, body
V5130   Binaural, in the ear
V5140   Binaural, behind the ear
V5150   Binaural, glasses
V5160   Dispensing fee, binaural

Lay Description
Binaural hearing aids are for both ears and are used concurrently to treat bilateral hearing loss. Advantages of wearing two hearing aids include a better understanding of speech and a better ability to localize speech. Hearing aids worn on the body are usually placed in a pocket or on a belt. Binaural hearing aids may also be worn in the ear, behind the ear, or may be incorporated into eyeglass frames.

V5170-V5200

V5170   Hearing aid, CROS, in the ear
V5180   Hearing aid, CROS, behind the ear
V5190   Hearing aid, CROS, glasses
V5200   Dispensing fee, CROS

Lay Description
Contralateral routing of sound (CROS) hearing aids are used for people with one deaf ear and one ear with normal or near normal hearing. The device placed in the deaf ear is a microphone and transmitter. The microphone picks up sound and transmits to the hearing ear. The transmission can be accomplished through a cord joining both hearing aids or may be wireless. The device placed in the normal ear consists of a receiver and an amplifier. Amplified sound from the deaf ear is directed into the ear canal. Most CROS ear molds are of an open design to allow natural sound into the normal ear.

V5210-V5240

V5210   Hearing aid, BICROS, in the ear
V5220   Hearing aid, BICROS, behind the ear
V5230   Hearing aid, BICROS, glasses
V5240   Dispensing fee, BICROS

Lay Description
BICROS is similar to a CROS hearing aid, but is used for people with one deaf ear and one ear that is hard of hearing. The device placed in the deaf ear is a microphone and transmitter. The microphone picks up sound and transmits it to the hearing ear. The transmission can be accomplished through a cord joining both hearing aids or may be wireless. The device placed in the hearing ear consists of a receiver and an amplifier coupled with a regular hearing aid. Signals from both ears are combined and directed into the hearing ear. BICROS ear molds are normally tightly fitted into the ear so as to prevent feedback.

V5241

V5241   Dispensing fee, monaural hearing aid, any type

Lay Description
Monaural hearing aids direct amplified sound to only one ear through a single signal path. Suppliers report this code for the dispensing fee of a monaural hearing aid, any type.

V5242-V5243, V5248-V5249

V5242   Hearing aid, analog, monaural, CIC (completely in the ear canal)
V5243   Hearing aid, analog, monaural, ITC (in the canal)
V5248   Hearing aid, analog, binaural, CIC
V5249   Hearing aid, analog, binaural, ITC

Lay Description
Sound is basically a fluctuation of air pressure and a sound wave is a series of continuous variations in time and amplitude on air pressure. When the fluctuations strike the eardrum, the vibrations are transmitted to the inner ear and ultimately the brain and are perceived as sound. When the fluctuations strike a microphone, they induce corresponding fluctuations or vibrations in the voltage or current of the microphone. These fluctuations or vibrations in the voltage or current are analogs of the sound. Analog hearing aids have a volume control that is adjusted by the patient. They are battery operated and work by converting sound waves to an electronic signal. When the volume is adjusted, all of the sounds are uniformly adjusted.

V5244-V5247, V5250-V5253

V5244   Hearing aid, digitally programmable analog, monaural, CIC
V5245   Hearing aid, digitally programmable, analog, monaural, ITC
V5246   Hearing aid, digitally programmable analog, monaural, ITE (in the ear)
V5247   Hearing aid, digitally programmable analog, monaural, BTE (behind the ear)
V5250   Hearing aid, digitally programmable analog, binaural, CIC
V5251   Hearing aid, digitally programmable analog, binaural, ITC
V5252   Hearing aid, digitally programmable, binaural, ITE
V5253   Hearing aid, digitally programmable, binaural, BTE

Lay Description
Digitally programmable analog hearing aids are battery operated and work by making sound waves larger and breaking them into distinct units. This digital signal is free from distortion and treats soft sounds differently than loud sounds, thus allowing for more clarity of sound, rather than only allowing more volume. The sound waves are converted from an

electronic signal and then passed through an A/D converter. These codes all represent digitally programmable analog monaural hearing aids.

V5248-V5249

V5248 Hearing aid, analog, binaural, CIC
V5249 Hearing aid, analog, binaural, ITC

Lay Description
Please refer to codes V5242-V5243 for the description, coding, and billing information.

V5254-V5261

V5254 Hearing aid, digital, monaural, CIC
V5255 Hearing aid, digital, monaural, ITC
V5256 Hearing aid, digital, monaural, ITE
V5257 Hearing aid, digital, monaural, BTE
V5258 Hearing aid, digital, binaural, CIC
V5259 Hearing aid, digital, binaural, ITC
V5260 Hearing aid, digital, binaural, ITE
V5261 Hearing aid, digital, binaural, BTE

Lay Description
Sound is basically a fluctuation of air pressure and a sound wave is a series of continuous variations in time and amplitude on air pressure. When the fluctuations strike the eardrum, the vibrations are transmitted to the inner ear and ultimately the brain and are perceived as sound. When the fluctuations strike a microphone, they induce corresponding fluctuations or vibrations in the voltage or current of the microphone. These fluctuations or vibrations in the voltage or current are analogs of the sound. Digital hearing aids convert the analog sound into a sequence of numbers that can be translated back into the analog sound. In its digital state, sound can be augmented to cancel feedback, reduce noise, and enhance speech. Digital hearing aids all contain a digital signal processing unit that translates the analog signals into and out of a digital format.

V5262-V5263

V5262 Hearing aid, disposable, any type, monaural
V5263 Hearing aid, disposable, any type, binaural

Lay Description
Disposable hearing aids are made of a soft material that is intended to last the user approximately 40 days. A disposable hearing aid has a mushroom-shaped tip that fits in the ear canal and can be fitted to most adults.

V5264-V5265

V5264 Ear mold/insert, not disposable, any type
V5265 Ear mold/insert, disposable, any type

Lay Description
An earmold is a device composed of plastic or another soft material that is inserted into the ear for sound conduction, ear protection, or sound reduction. Ear molds are shaped to fit precisely into an individual ear. They can be full, which completely fills the ear canal, providing sound reduction, and protection; or partial, which allows in other sound. Ear molds may contain a BTE hearing aid, components of other types of hearing aids, such as a receiver or processor, or may simply be used to protect the ear by blocking loud noises.

V5266

V5266 Battery for use in hearing device

Lay Description
Hearing devices require select batteries to provide power to the listening device. Batteries are available in different brands, sizes, and quantity packs depending on the requirements of the device. This code reports a battery for use in a hearing device.

V5267

V5267 Hearing aid or assistive listening device/supplies/accessories, not otherwise specified

Lay Description
Report this code for hearing aid supplies or accessories that are not adequately described by other HCPCS Level II codes.

V5268

V5268 Assistive listening device, telephone amplifier, any type

Lay Description
Telephone assistive listening devices are used to amplify sound for the hearing impaired. Some of the telephone assistive listening devices available are portable phones, in-line amplifiers, ring signalers, and super phone ringers. This code is reported for any type of telephone amplifier assistive listening device for the telephone.

V5269

V5269 Assistive listening device, alerting, any type

Lay Description
There are two types of alerting assistive listening devices: visual and vibration. The visual alert includes a flashing light, or strobe light, to assist the hearing impaired user in becoming aware of an event such as ringing smoke alarms, doorbells, baby monitors, or alarm clocks. Some patients find that vibrating devices such as pillow shakers or wrist shakers are more effective. This code is used for an alerting assistive listening device of either type.

V5270-V5271

V5270 Assistive listening device, television amplifier, any type

V5271 Assistive listening device, television caption decoder

Lay Description
An assistive listening device used with a television amplifies the audio signal from the television and is generally transmitted through infrared to a headset. Closed captioning decoders are also available for older models of televisions in which a decoder is not built into the system.

V5272

V5272 Assistive listening device, TDD

Lay Description
A TDD is a telecommunication device for the deaf. These include text telephones and teletype machines. These assistive listening devices allow a person with hearing impairment to use the telephone. The device is connected to a small keyboard that allows the user to type the message to be sent. If both the caller and receiver have TDDs, a printed message is read on a screen. However, if the receiver does not have a TDD, the messages are relayed through an operator.

V5273

V5273 Assistive listening device, for use with cochlear implant

Lay Description
An assistive listening device for use with a cochlear implant is designed to amplify the voice in a setting such as a classroom or boardroom directly to the person with the implant without amplifying background noise. These systems include an infrared system with a jack.

V5274

V5274 Assistive listening device, not otherwise specified

Lay Description
Assistive listening devices improve hearing in a specific situation for people with hearing loss. The device emphasizes the one signal that the person is interested in hearing more clearly. This code represents assistive listening devices that are not adequately described by other HCPCS Level II codes.

V5275

V5275 Ear impression, each

Lay Description
Impressions are made of the ear to obtain a hearing device specifically for the individual. The ear canal is visualized through an otoscope to check for wax build up, anomalies, and to check the tympanic membrane. A plug made of soft cotton is inserted just beyond the canal to provide a "wall" for the mold and to ease the removal of debris. The impression material is mixed according to the manufacturer's specifications and loaded into a syringe. The tip of the syringe is placed in the canal and then emptied to fill the ear canal, the pinna, concha, and helix. After the material has set for the time indicated, the impression and cotton wall are removed. The audiologist visualizes the canal with the otoscope to be certain all debris has been removed. Use this code for each impression.

V5281-V5290

V5281 Assistive listening device, personal FM/DM system, monaural (1 receiver, transmitter, microphone), any type

V5282 Assistive listening device, personal FM/DM system, binaural (2 receivers, transmitter, microphone), any type

V5283 Assistive listening device, personal FM/DM neck, loop induction receiver

V5284 Assistive listening device, personal FM/DM, ear level receiver

V5285 Assistive listening device, personal FM/DM, direct audio input receiver

V5286 Assistive listening device, personal blue tooth FM/DM receiver

V5287 Assistive listening device, personal FM/DM receiver, not otherwise specified

V5288 Assistive listening device, personal FM/DM transmitter assistive listening device

V5289 Assistive listening device, personal FM/DM adapter/boot coupling device for receiver, any type

V5290 Assistive listening device, transmitter microphone, any type

Lay Description
This group of codes is used to report frequency modulated/digitally modulated (FM/DM) auditory devices that are used along with hearing aids or independently to help improve hearing. It improves the signal to noise ratio, which helps the patient hear better in an environment with poor acoustics or background noise and helps reduce distances. They are also useful for certain types of hearing deficiencies or disorders, such as auditory processing, attention deficit, and/or autism. With the use of FM/DM technologies, the sound signal is directed from a transmitting device (FM/DM transmitter) through a frequency or digitally modulated signal to a receiving device (FM/DM receiver) that is attached to a hearing device. Some FM/DM technologies are dedicated units, meaning they do not attach to amplification. These self-contained units can be used by people who don't use a hearing aid but suffer from other auditory processing problems. The FM/DM system usually includes a transmitter and a receiving device.

V5298-V5299

V5298   Hearing aid, not otherwise classified

V5299   Hearing service, miscellaneous

Lay Description

These codes represent hearing aids that are not adequately described by other HCPCS Level II codes and a miscellaneous hearing service that is not adequately described by other HCPCS Level II codes.

V5336

V5336   Repair/modification of augmentative communicative system or device (excludes adaptive hearing aid)

Lay Description

An augmentative communicative system or device (excludes adaptive hearing aid) is a method of communication used by people with impairments or restrictions on the production or comprehension of spoken or written language. These systems may generate speech or may consist of a board with pictures to which the person points.

V5362

V5362   Speech screening

Lay Description

Speech screening is a simple test to determine if a person has difficulties with speech that would require further assessment and examination. Generally, a speech screening tests repetitive oral movements of articulation, laryngeal functions of voice, and velopharyngeal function of resonance. Speech that is limited, not easily understood, or that is too loud, too soft, or sounds unusual may signal a speech problem. Screening should be performed in the person's primary language. Language screenings are often done with speech screenings.

V5363

V5363   Language screening

Lay Description

Language screening is a simple test to determine if a person has difficulties with language that would require further assessment and examination. Generally a language screening tests for the understanding and usage of words. Difficulty in understanding instructions, following directions, and/or communicating with other people may signal a language problem. Screening should be performed in the person's primary language. Language screenings are often done with speech screenings.

V5364

V5364   Dysphagia screening

Lay Description

Dysphagia screenings test the difficulty a patient has with the swallowing reflex. There are three phases that are observed: the oral phase, pharyngeal phase, and esophageal phase. The patient is given a small amount of water that is swallowed while the practitioner feels for the swallow above and below the larynx. The patient is observed for delayed swallow, cough on swallowing, drooling, and dysphonia.

NOTES